MORAL PROBLEMS
IN MEDICINE
second edition

Edited, with introductions, by

SAMUEL GOROVITZ, Senior Editor
Department of Philosophy
University of Maryland, College Park

RUTH MACKLIN, Senior Editor
Department of Community Health
Albert Einstein College of Medicine

ANDREW L. JAMETON
Institute for Health Policy Studies
University of California, San Francisco

JOHN M. O'CONNOR
American Philosophical Association
and Department of Philosophy
University of Delaware

SUSAN SHERWIN
Department of Philosophy
Dalhousie University

based on a first edition edited by Samuel Gorovitz, Andrew L. Jameton, Ruth Macklin, John M. O'Connor, Eugene V. Perrin, Beverly Page St. Clair, and Susan Sherwin.

PRENTICE-HALL, INC., Englewood Cliffs, New Jersey 07632

Library of Congress Cataloging in Publication Data

Main entry under title:
   Moral problems in medicine.

   Includes bibliographical references and index.
   1. Medical ethics—Addresses, essays, lectures.
I. Gorovitz, Samuel. [DNLM: 1. Ethics, Medical—
Collected works.   2. Philosophy, Medical—Collected
works.   W 50 M822]
R724.M82 1983   174'.2   82-23133
ISBN 0-13-600742-2

Editorial / production supervision by F. Hubert
Cover design by Wanda Lubelska
Manufacturing buyer: Harry P. Baisley

Printed in the United States of America

10 9 8 7 6 5 4 3 2 1

ISBN 0-13-600742-2

PRENTICE-HALL INTERNATIONAL, INC., *London*
PRENTICE-HALL OF AUSTRALIA PTY. LIMITED, *Sydney*
EDITORA PRENTICE-HALL DO BRASIL, LTDA., *Rio de Janeiro*
PRENTICE-HALL CANADA INC., *Toronto*
PRENTICE-HALL OF INDIA PRIVATE LIMITED, *New Delhi*
PRENTICE-HALL OF JAPAN, INC., *Tokyo*
PRENTICE-HALL OF SOUTHEAST ASIA PTE. LTD., *Singapore*
WHITEHALL BOOKS LIMITED, *Wellington, New Zealand*

Contents

Chapter 4. BIRTH AND DEATH, 270

Chapter 5. HEALTH POLICY, 490

Preface

In 1974, after three years of work, the editorial group that prepared the first edition of this anthology had completed its task. It fell to me to secure a publisher. For six months, I was rebuffed by one publisher after another, including several with whom I had previously worked. Always, the reason was the same: There is no known market for a book of this sort. Prentice-Hall was among those who declined the manuscript. We began to despair of seeing the book in print.

The Prentice-Hall editor chanced to visit my office some months later. He professed genuine interest in my reasons for excoriating the publishing business. I fulminated at him for an hour. A few weeks later, he overcame the conservatism that besets the publishing industry, and Prentice-Hall reversed its decision, took a gamble, and published the first edition.

Within a year, the text had been adopted in over a hundred schools. With a market assured, other publishers rushed to enter the field. In every year since the publication of our first edition, at least one competitor has appeared, and the consideration of the ethical aspects of medical care and health policy has become a standard offering at most universities.

We have welcomed the rapid development of this field and have admired the texts that have provided various advantages over our early effort. Indeed, because there is now such a rich variety of materials available in this area, we were most reluctant to undertake revisions of our own collection. For a time, we were content to use more recent works ourselves. But the field changes fast in many ways, and there was much valuable new material that had not yet been collected into any readily accessible form. We therefore agreed to revise this book to incorporate what we see as the best of the recent work that fits within the basic conception of the anthology as we first framed it. Thus, this second edition is a book of the same kind as the first. It retains an emphasis on issues that arise in the treatment of acute illness, and thus underrepresents the importance of ethical issues in routine primary care. And it includes little historical material, and thus might engender the mistaken impression that concern with ethical matters in medicine is a purely contemporary phenomenon. Yet it is quite a different book in that only about one third of its content appeared in the original edition. Some readers will prefer other approaches, and there will be many choices available to them. Others will favor our approach but will quarrel with some of our decisions about selections and will therefore want to add cases or other supplemental readings to suit their own needs.

The most difficult aspect of preparing this revision was deciding to exclude a great many works that are of high quality and direct bearing on our subject matter. In many cases, the decision to exclude was based on considerations extrinsic to the work itself. For example, we have tried to limit our dependence on the *Hastings Center Report* and *The New England Journal of Medicine,* in which an unusually high proportion of appropriate writings first appeared. In places, we have shifted the emphasis of our selections, for example, by reducing the amount of primary source material in philosophical ethics and increasing the amount of material written from the perspective of religious studies. We have eliminated the pedagogical postscript; we believe it now to be superfluous. We have eliminated the reprinting of oaths and codes because they are now quite readily available elsewhere, and we had to make compromises lest the book be even larger than it is. Also, we have deleted inessential footnotes and renumbered accordingly. Where the best article for our purposes had been anthologized elsewhere, we typically chose nonetheless to include it here. These books are all of the same family, and it is no surprise that they should all bear a family resemblance.

We are grateful to many people for assistance in this project. At Prentice-Hall, Alice Dworkin, Frank Hubert, Ray O'Connell, and Bud Therien have been particularly help-ful. Our work was guided by very valuable ad-vice from Larry McCullough, Stephen Wear, and Bart Gruzalski. And many others, includ-ing several users of the first edition, wrote in-dividual suggestions to us, offered examples of their work, or simply urged us on. They are too numerous to cite, but we are in their debt and

regret that we must inevitably have dis-appointed them in the various decisions we have made.

Finally, we are grateful to our students, who have taught us much over the years about how to approach our subject. We hope this latest effort will serve them well for a time.

Samuel Gorovitz

PREFACE FROM THE FIRST EDITION

This book is designed primarily to provide readings for a consideration of the moral issues in medicine from a philosophical point of view. The included material should be of value both to students training for the health-care professions and to those studying the human-ities. Further, we hope that the book will be of interest to individuals of whatever professional or academic affiliation who are concerned with the evaluative aspects of the decisions forced upon us by modern medicine.

The notion of preparing such a book arose during the second year of the Moral Problems in Medicine Project at Case Western Reserve University. This was a joint undertaking of the Philosophy Department and the School of Medicine. Under the auspices of that project, a seminar concerning moral problems in medi-cine had been developed for undergraduate, graduate, and professional school students. Two aspects of our experience combined to prompt this undertaking.

First, we found it difficult to develop the curriculum. We were continually taxed to find a mixture of philosophical and medical materials that would enable us to pursue the chosen topics advantageously, and the hetero-geneous composition of the class intensified the problem. We resisted the philosopher's in-clination to start from a particular case and venture on a one-way journey to principles, justifications, and meta-ethics. Similarly, we resisted the medical student's proclivity to dwell on the particulars of a case without con-sidering questions of generalization, consis-tency, or conflict of values. In the end, we agreed that our purposes would require both philosophical and medical materials, and a substantial amount of pedagogical caution

and determination as well. To our distress, no suitable materials were readily available. Before attempting to weave the fabric, we had to find the threads one by one.

Second, we gradually came to view our pedagogical efforts as successful. We had sought to promote an increased awareness of the moral dimensions of decision-making in medical contexts and of the importance of the conceptual uncertainties that underlie some of the conventions and practices in health-related areas. While not attempting to take substantive positions on the moral problems at issue, we had sought to increase the com-petence with which students recognized, integrated, and reconciled the various con-siderations relevant to making such decisions. The response from students, and the quality of work that they produced, solidified our belief that we were learning how to achieve such objectives.

We believe that the philosophical perspec-tive is an essential ingredient in the multi-disciplinary approach that is required by moral problems in medicine. This perspective is a distinctive one, demonstrably different from those offered by law, sociology, theology, anthropology, and the rest. For it to interact optimally with the others, it must develop along with them. This book does not itself represent such development; rather, we hope the book will help catalyze the kind of activity that will constitute such development.

There are two basic alternatives in structur-ing a philosophical course in medical ethics. One is to divide the course according to medically conceived topics such as organ transplantation, genetic engineering, eutha-nasia, etc. Such an approach is wholly viable, but we have preferred not to adopt it here. Rather, we have organized the book primarily on the basis of more philosophically inspired categories. Thus, our headings invoke such notions as paternalism, truth, social justice, etc.

No issue discussed here is treated in a complete or thorough way. Further, we do not pretend to have included every important topic or point of view. Instead, we have sought simply to provide sufficient self-contained material of good quality to sustain intensive, well-informed discussion of issues of fundamental importance. Severe limitations of space constrained us to omit further treatment of the issues covered, and to leave out entirely many important topics we would have liked to cover—including, for example, such topics as psychosurgery and behavior control, definitions of health and the medical model, population and birth control, malpractice and iatrogenic injury, issues in pharmacology, and the federal regulatory role in health care research.

A number of the articles included herein contained extensive footnotes and bibliographical references when first published. We have deleted many of these notes in order to make possible the inclusion of several more articles. For those who might wish to use this volume in the classroom, we have appended a pedagogical postscript, including a list of bibliographies.

Several articles appear here for the first time. These include the essays by Bellin, Hare, Metzler, Parfit, and Perrin et al. We are grateful to these authors for making their work available to us. We are particularly indebted to Willard Gaylin, who has done much to bring about public awareness of the moral issues in medicine, for supplying us with the foreword.

We are, of course, grateful to the many authors and publishers who provided permission for the inclusion of works in this book.

We have been aided in various ways in the preparation of this manuscript by Professor Herbert Long, John Merritt, Pat Merritt, Donna Moss, and Gary Schwartz. Our students over the last three years have inspired us and influenced us, and we are grateful to them for that. Rachelle Hollander has played a particularly helpful role in final editorial preparation of the manuscript and in her able handling of the complex and sometimes frustrating process of arranging for all necessary permissions.

Although no grant was made specifically to support the preparation of this manuscript, the book would not have been possible without the activities undertaken in the Moral Problems in Medicine project at Case Western Reserve, supported by the National Endowment for the Humanities under Grant EH-6028-72-111 and by the Exxon Education Foundation, and the Moral Problems in Medicine Institute sponsored by the Council for Philosophical Studies in the Summer of 1974 with the support of the Rockefeller Brothers Fund. Each of these three foundations, by its material support of our participation in directly related projects, has fair claim to view this volume as a partial consequence of that support. Finally, we are grateful to our colleagues at Prentice-Hall for the confidence they expressed in undertaking to publish the volume, for the good advice they have provided along the way, and for the spirit of congeniality with which they have dealt with us—including those inevitable battles about length.

Samuel Gorovitz

Foreword

We tend to become most interested in ethical issues when we are unsure of the direction in which we are heading. Philosophy thrives on self-doubt and self-doubt is a point every sensitive person will reach somewhere along that road from aspiration to fulfillment. When we are young and only aspiring we do not need doubts; we will shape our fantasies in perfect harmony. It is only after we begin to achieve our ends—when we realize that achievement and fulfillment are not necessarily congruent—that we must redefine our goals, guided by our doubts.

Perhaps I am merely saying that success leads to power, and power brings responsibility, and responsibility to a decent human being inevitably leads to anxiety. The urgent interest in medical ethics at this time is a symptom of the success of medicine.

It was not always this way. I look back somewhat enviously at the scientist of the late nineteenth century when medicine was, indeed, all promise and aspiration—when it seemed that science was on the threshold of achieving all the solutions to man's needs.

This attitude persevered well into the present century, symbolized to me by a particular memory. When I first came to college, I was impressed by an unusual archeological detail: a small Victorian building of great charm, albeit somewhat run-down and decrepit, was almost completely surrounded by a functional, massive, ugly-modern building—red brick, as I remember it. The Victorian building, I was later to find out, was the divinity school, and the red brick building was the department of biology. It was a symbol of the state of things then. Biology was about to swallow up theology.

But "swallowing up" is not necessarily destroying. The psychoanalytic concept of introjection describes how that which we devour to destory, with poetic irony, may become a part of us. To absorb something, to take it into you, may also mean that you have unwillingly undertaken its burdens. I think that *has* happened. The scientist, particularly after Hiroshima, has often been the conscience of the nation—what little conscience there has been.

I used to start my lectures in medical ethics to medical students by telling them how funny the subject was twenty years ago when I was in medical school. I could remember only a couple of examples, both of them in retrospect seeming appalling. One had to do with the crisis that might occur if, on the way to the golf course on Sunday morning, you stumbled over a child bleeding to death—the question being whether you were under any obligation to hold up your foursome by stopping to stem the flow of blood. You will be relieved to know that, at least in Ohio twenty years ago, you were under no such obligation.

The other set of problems had to deal with promotion and advertising—the size of the sign you were allowed to have in your window, etc. I remember specifically in Ohio we were not allowed to list our specialties after our names in the Yellow Pages, which fact was told to us with an air of great moral superiority, because certain states permitted such "advertising."

In retrospect, I realize that both of those issues derived from serious ethical conflicts. They arise from the ambiguities of being a man who is at the same time a healer-comforter and a man of commerce. They represent some of the conflict in the individual who has to balance those two roles.

Now, after twenty years, I am in a medical school, this time as a teacher, and the same confusions persist even in understanding the definition and nature of ethics. Two examples may illustrate. At a recent discussion, a group of ward administrators insisted that medical ethics were not neglected at all, at least not on their wards; that they indeed "spent more time on ethical issues than they did on medical issues." I thought this amazing; this was, after all, a general medical ward, and not the chaplain's office. When they explained, however, it became apparent that they were alluding to sociological issues—e.g., the mechanical problems of placing people in nursing homes, clearing the wards of "chronics," etc., and not to ethical dilemmas. This delineated their concept of the ethical issues.

The other example involves a distinguished senior physician attending on a medical ward. He felt that on the whole, ethical questions were indeed, generally neglected—but not on his ward. Here there was no problem. His statement was: "Just as I feel that I have the ultimate responsibility for making all medical decisions, I feel that I must bear the ultimate responsibility for making all ethical decisions." It was said in good faith, and it was not for me to point out to him that there is a fine line between "assumption of responsibility" and arrogation of power. He is, indisputably, an expert on medical decisions, but he is not an expert on ethical decisions. I am not sure whether there are experts in these decisions. The question is: *Should* he be the final arbiter of these decisions any more than the medical student, the nurse, the cleaning lady, or any *one* individual besides himself?

Clearly there persists a confusion about the nature of the problem that is necessary to explore. One has to know the questions before one seeks the answers. To that end I would like to refer briefly to some traditional areas of ethical dilemmas, which will be discussed in greater detail in this book, hoping to indicate how the success of medicine has added urgency to the old problems, has recast them, or has created new problems.

One of the traditional concerns of medical ethics is research on human subjects. Professor Henry Beecher has pioneered in this area. Early work rightly focused on exposing clearly unethical research; it was muckraking in the best sense. There is still, unfortunately, a place for muckraking today.

Beyond this, the rapid development of technology, permitting procedures once never contemplated, is now raising ethical problems of a more complex nature—and confusing some previously settled areas. For example, there has traditionally been a clear separation between standards of "experimental" and "therapeutic" procedure. Consider the recent discussions concerning surgery for revascularization of the heart. This is a difficult procedure used generally in patients crippled with severe angina—with the hope that it also might defer future infarctions. When originally done, it carried a high mortality rate. I needn't tell you that it had a 100 percent morbidity rate, since that is the nature of surgery. It was seen by all as an experimental procedure. However, certain surgical teams have perfected the techniques to a point where the mortality rate in this group is now less than 10 percent. With such dramatic improvements the process is now considered a standard therapeutic option. Compare now how different our attitude would be if we were discussing a drug therapy. If I suggested to you that I had a drug that would relieve the symptoms of angina, with some promise, but no evidence, that it might deter future infarction, would you be reassured by the fact that it caused 100 percent morbidity and 10 percent mortality? Would I even be permitted to market the drug? The operative procedure is not considered experimental because our whole bias toward surgery is different from what it is toward drugs, and for very obvious reasons.

Before the modern era a control mechanism over surgery analogous to drugs would have been unnecessary and foolish. Surgery was a therapy of last resort—often more dreaded than the disease to which it was directed. If the pain and shock of the operation didn't kill you, the post-operative sepsis was likely to. The terror of the patient was sufficient control over the procedure. Now with the advent of sophisticated anesthesia, antisepsis, and antibiotics, serious surgical intervention (e.g., prefrontal lobotomy) can be a routine procedure.

In almost every area considered in this book, it is our success that confounds us. Examine a few. At one time there was no medical need for the physician to consider the *concept* of death. This was because the *fact* of death was generally congruent with the cessation of personhood. We are so built that when we lose those functions which make us human beings by even the crudest definitions, we generally die. With the advent of new techniques in medicine that congruence has been destroyed. So it is now quite possible to sustain life, or to sustain living matter, or to sustain a person beyond the point of previous contemplation. When this happens we are forced to consider the distinctions between human life, living matter, and persons. And so now, we find medical people facing the problems of defining personhood. These philosophical problems have equal urgency in the medical dilemmas at the beginnings of life.

But the recognition of the complexity of problems in these areas becomes most apparent when most specific. At the Columbia Law School as part of curricular development in teaching bioethics, a course was created in which law students, medical students, and seminarians were joined together. They were divided into small research groups of "lawyers," "physicians," and philosopher-theologians. They were charged to design legislation for specific problems of the biological revolution, or to present a convincing rationale as to why their subject should be excluded from the legislative area.

It has been extremely fascinating to see the impact of the medical mind, the legal mind, and the theological mind on one another; to see the differences but also to see the accommodation and growth over a semester. They were instructed to be as futuristic or as present-day oriented as they wished — and the proposals were often startling when cast with the specificity that legislation requires. For example, a contract was written for the hiring of a surrogate mother (i.e., planting a fertilized egg of one couple in the uterus of another woman to bear for nine months). The Surrogate Mother contract is in the service of an honorable old medical tradition, facilitating the desire of parents to have their own "natural" (genetic) child. But when the details are spelled out in the language of contracts the results are unnerving. The surrogate mother should have "rights of first refusal" in case the natural parents decide that they wish to abort. The surrogate mother must fulfill obligatory dietary commitments and interdictions during the gestation period. It is difficult for this to avoid sounding funny, yet renting womb space can be conceived as a respectable alternative, probably preferable to an artificial placenta, for solving the not uncommon problem of a woman who has had her uterus removed, has

perfectly functioning ovaries, produces ova, and wants a "natural" child.

There were other issues considered that were much more of the present. There already exist incorporated, profit-making sperm banks. Artificial insemination with donor sperm is an accepted institution of medicine. Some very simple questions arise. Wouldn't a sperm bank with massive selection and computerized data represent a superior method of donor selection to the current technique of collaring a convenient medical student or intern who needs the money and finds the donation of sperm a more amiable procedure than the donation of blood? What then of criteria and controls? Should there be a free choice of the nature of the donor, and who should make the choice? In the past we have implicitly assumed our task as an imitation of the natural process, and we have attempted to replicate as closely as possible the natural inheritance. The obstetrician does little scientific screening. The traditional donor is, therefore, a poorish (needs the money) medical student (available) healthy and intelligent enough to have survived until, if not through, graduate education, who looks something like the father who is to raise the child (satisfy paternal wants, maintain deception, quiet gossipy speculation).

Appalling as it may seem, this represents the traditional and typical at the current time. One would think that common sense might indicate simple correctives. Why a student? A 60-year-old grandfather who has proved to be a successful sire would seem more logical. Certain late developing diseases with hereditary tendencies could be eliminated (for example, diabetes, arteriosclerotic conditions, etc.). This then introduces some aspects of positive engineering. We are moving from the "having a child" problem to the "having a special child" problem. Should such genetic variables as sex, size, IQ or race be options? Or should they be left to chance? The student legislators mandated matching two variables to the natural parental traits, IQ and size — IQ under the assumption that a child with a high IQ might be disadvantaged with parents of low IQ and size presumably to protect a small mother from a giant fetus. The question of race selection, beyond psychological and sociological consideration, raises problems of constitutional law.

Genetic engineering raises the kind of speculations and choices that boggle the mind and titillate the imagination. But even the less dramatic area of genetic counseling raises distressing dilemmas. Genetic counselors are now adopting the posture that psychiatrists once assumed. They presume to present the facts, eschewing value judgment. Genetic counselors, at this point in time, are geneticists first and counselors second, if at all. The sophisticated psychiatric counselor has abandoned the delusion of objectivity. He is aware that all counseling involves the conscious and unconscious intrusions of the values of the advisor. Because I have yet to meet a value-free psychiatrist, I am skeptical of the genetic counselor's comfort in "only presenting the facts."

The control of behavior is another major area to which this volume devotes substantial attention. Obviously there is a difference now that we have the capacity for mechanical and electronic control of behavior. Also, the specialization of drugs so that they now control specific modalities rather than just ups and downs adds a new dimension to mood modification. We must now ask what, if anything, is the essential ethical difference between injection of a drug, the implantation of a electrode, or the use of normal sensory inputs. The Behavior Control Research Group of the Institute of Society, Ethics and the Life Sciences has been considering this, and my comfortable and comforting biases have already been badly shaken. I started with the usual healthy revulsion against surgically messing with the brain. My emotional aversions gradually were attacked until the only remaining objection I could cling to was the recognition of the irreversibility of surgical destruction. But to a psychiatrist, certain sensory inputs, particularly if initiated early in life, carry the fixity of organic change. If there is a difference between implanting an electrode and implanting an idea, it will require more elegant intellectual attention than it has as yet received.

Finally, the question of transplants and artificial organs really does represent a new field and new conditions under which to consider traditional moral problems. The drama of the new helps illuminate vital old problems which had been relegated to back closets of medical consideration. The problem of priorities is just such an issue, which lay neglected until the transplants highlighted the less glamorous, but urgent areas. It returns us to the example that I offered from my medical school days, and raises the whole question of the marketplace mentality of medicine. There is something distasteful about the concept of selling human life. We have sold chance; we know that. We sell high risk. We will pay someone to work in a submarine. We will pay someone to build a bridge with the sure knowledge that the building of it will take a certain number of lives. But we have not yet arrived at the point where we have allowed the selling of seats in a lifeboat of a sinking ship. Or have we? When we see the posters of the American Hemophilia Society — an authentic, legitimate medical group — presenting the pictures of two young boys, and announcing that one will live a normal life because his father can afford $22,000 a year for treatment and the other one is not going to live because his father cannot afford this, I wonder. I also wonder about the sensitivity of people who would advertise the fact. If it were indeed a fact of necessity that one had no choice but to distribute a life-saving commodity by auction, I might have to live with it, but I wouldn't want to advertise it.

There are, again, no easy answers to the establishment of medical priorities. One seductive solution is to suggest the elimination of them by utilizing chance alone in the form of lotteries. This was suggested by that group of medical, theological, and law students in the experimental course at Columbia Law School. The students felt scarce resources — body parts, for example — ought to be allocated, once medical determinants were the same, by fishbowl lottery with no moral or sociological evaluations. Then, however, they were given the specific case of parents with a six-months' premature baby and their own 6-year-old daughter, and a limited facility needed for survival by both, and asked whether they would want those two names thrown into a fishbowl. The example served to unsettle the majority and to illustrate the difficulty of assuming that chance guarantees equity.

Returning to the question of medical priorities, let us take another undramatic example. Research has always been the most hallowed area of medicine—so much so that a contempt for the general practitioner was commonplace in medical schools. Because the researchers for the most part were running the medical schools, references to the LMD (local medical doctor) carried the tone and implications associated with mention of the village idiot. Nowadays, we are beginning to raise questions, even here, about our priorities. We question whether research in certain life-sustaining areas is justified when that same amount of money might be applied to the distribution of the fruits of research that has already been done. And so we have a conflict. For the first time, to my knowledge, research, which has in general (as distinguished from specific pieces of research) always been treated with the greatest respect, is now being attacked as an elitist phenomenon and, as such, as immoral or unethical.

This, too, is but one part of the larger problem of a redefinition of the physician's role, the physician-patient relationship, the social role of medicine, and, most important, the ethical and political implications of the concept of health.

I would now like to show how such problems evolve, and to indicate some of the social complications of certain "medical" developments. In doing so, it will be necessary to consider three closely related areas. One is the definition of normal; the second is the power of the medical model; and the third is the expansion of individual treatment into social engineering. These are all drawn from the field of psychiatry, but I think they have a validity for the kind of ethical questions that arise in other areas of medicine—they deal, after all, with fundamental problems: freedom and coercion, individual and society, rights versus privileges, definitions of good, etc.

The definition of normalcy has caused particular mischief in the area of mental health, where it is compounded by incorporation into the medical-therapeutic model.

Psychoanalysis liberated whole areas of behavior from the domain of religion and morality, and redefined them in medical terms. A piece of behavior, like a blood-pressure reading or respiratory rate, could now be seen as sick or healthy, neither more nor less. The implication of this was not immediately apparent. To some, this was seen as purely a semantic shift. What was sinful sixty years ago became immoral thirty years ago, and today is merely called sick or immature. To some this was a minor change. We had only changed the name of the game. Health had simply become a new morality. But this is a dangerous underestimation, because in changing the name we changed much more. The changing of the frame of reference to a medical or scientific one had a profound impact on controlling individual action.

The unparalleled power that we place in the hands of the medical man stems directly from the existential fear of death that we all share. The preserver of life has often been exempted from normal limits of behavior. This is true whether he is called a priest or physician, and there have been times when both have literally gotten away with murder. Democratic society prides itself on its toleration of differences in values. However, there are certain areas where one approaches absolutism. Health and sickness is such a polarity. No person aspires to sickness (at least no "healthy" person). We are frightened of sickness because it is the prelude to death. That is why we listen to our lawyer's "advice" but we follow a doctor's "orders." By defining behavior as either healthy or sick the psychiatrist has a profound effect in directing the course of behavior while, with an unbelievable conceit, claiming a neutral stand in the field of morals.

Let me restate what I believe has happened. If a piece of behavior is defined as immoral by a religious authority, the individual still feels free to accept or reject that definition, particularly in our society, which endows religious or moral leaders with little authority or punitive power. It is often easier to change one's religion than to abandon a condemned but desired activity. If, however, you define the very same piece of behavior as "abnormal" or sick, and if the individual can be convinced of your expertise in matters of health, he will often be forced by fear to abandon that activity. He will in addition not feel forced. He will wish to do that which you wish. The universal terror of illness, operating under the imprimatur of the medical establishment, makes coercion in the traditional sense unnecessary. This is a potent force in behavior control which has not been nearly sufficiently analyzed, evaluated, or supervised.

What I am saying is that by changing the frame of reference, we have created a potentially explosive and sociologically significant change. We live in a culture that has always, at least theoretically, respected diversity in moral and religious areas. But we live in a culture in which medicine has always been seen as having certain rights to coercion. In other words, we have resisted coercing people on grounds of their moral right or religious right in recent times, but we have *not* in terms of medical rights. By redefining morality and values into medical terms, we are expanding the mechanism for controlling human behavior. By redefining a piece of behavior as abnormal, rather than immoral, you are subjecting it to the coercive aspects of law. But even without that, you will have the coercive aspects of anxiety in operation.

Even when an organized attempt to avoid the intrusion of values is made, it can never be successful. Psychoanalysis has for years operated with the conceit of a value-free system. Yet time and time again the imposition of values has been demonstrated.

Some unique aspects of the power of the medical model became apparent during meetings of the Behavior Control Research Group evaluating psychosurgery and psychotropic drugs as means of modifying behavior. Much of the discussion of the first conference was on control of violence related to temporal lobe epilepsy. It was interesting to observe the consistency of response in a mixed disciplinary group when confronted by the technologies of those neurosurgeons who went into the brain with scalpels, probes, and electrodes. The general conclusion and feeling of the group seemed to be that if a man is susceptible to rages that have nothing to do with electroencephalographic changes, you have absolutely no right to go in and disturb his brain — even if you can get rid of his rages. However, if there *is* a temporal lobe focus and you can establish that there is a relationship between the focus and the rage, then you *do* have a right to go in and remove the anterior part of the temporal lobe.

This is an interesting concept. I wonder why we are happier and more satisfied with that medical model. I submit that what we are treating anyway is not the focus or EEG change, but the behavior. After surgery, the patient will have, if we are speaking anatomically rather than functionally, a more damaged brain. He may even have greater functional loss — but of a personal rather than interpersonal significance.

Imagine for a moment an EEG change correlated with increased intelligence, creativity, or sensitivity. We are not going to encourage operation on the "abnormality." No, what we want to change is a piece of behavior that we have decided is undesirable. But we all feel uncomfortable in doing it just as a direct matter of behavior control. If we can link it to epilepsy, if we can link it to the epileptic model, even if the only signs of epilepsy are the electroencephalographic changes (and the rages), we feel more secure. There is an illogicality here. If the rages are destructive, if the only way to control them is by surgery, and if we feel that it is legitimate to help a man to facilitate his life by operating on his brain, why not go ahead and do it? We traditionally destroy healthy tissue surgically to enhance life adjustment. Yet few present at the Institute's discussion were prepared to do it when social behavior was involved, unless they had the comfort of the medical model — although the distinction logically pursued may be elusive, arbitrary, capricious, or even nonexistent.

We are happier in the justification of changing behavior when we can utilize a medical model. There are illogicalities, and inequities, here — but the alternatives, as yet not adequately explored, may be even more troublesome. This leads inevitably into the discussion of social engineering and how one may be projected into this area — even when reluctant and resistant. In the nineteenth century, psychiatry and physical medicine were fairly parallel in their views of human pathology. They both saw disease as something imposed on the person from the outside, an invasion, if you will. And they both saw pathology in terms of organ deterioration. If you recall the fact that in the late nineteenth century the majority of patients admitted to psychiatric hospitals were suffering from tertiary syphilis, they weren't too far wrong. The disease then was something external, gross, and bizarre occupying and reducing the individual. The treatment for it became obvious—repel the invader. And you need not worry about definitions of normalcy. The pathological condition was so eccentric that merely removing the eccentricity was presumed to reinstate implicitly the state of normalcy. If someone comes to a doctor with a turnip growing out of his ear, he knows he has to remove the thing, and knows that what remains after the operation is a normal individual, turnipless ears being an implicit part of our definition of normalcy.

Then came the revolution in psychodynamics introduced by Freud. We began to see that people didn't have to be all crazy but only partially so. Healthy, nice, decent people like psychiatrists and judges could be normal in the traditional sense yet have isolated pieces of behavior that were aberrant—phobias, compulsions, etc. The next stage beyond this was the defining of character neuroses. That meant that nothing need necessarily be "crazy" to warrant a classification as abnormal. One could be defined as neurotic on the basis of a constricted character structure. If the personality didn't add up to a productive, happy, or self-fulfilled individual this could be seen as a form of mental illness.

Finally, psychiatry began to conceive of illness in terms of significant behavioral omissions. We decided that there are certain pieces of behavior that *ought* to be present, that *should* be present, that were *normal* to be there. Their absence, therefore, was taken as a sign of neuroses. Now when you begin to raise "ought" questions, of course, you are on that fine borderline between medicine and ethics. This progression into values received added impetus, because simultaneously there was a different model evolving in medicine in general. The therapeutic goal was being replaced by a prophylactic one. When you deal with disease, regardless of how rampant an epidemic, you are dealing with 15, 20, 30 percent of the population. When you're dealing with preventive medicine, you're dealing with 100 percent of the population.

The results of those progressions were inevitable. As psychiatry reduced the criteria for mental illness, it expanded the number of the mentally ill. By requiring less and less to define mental illness, you place larger and larger percentages of the population into the category of the mentally ill. When you then introduce a prophylactic model, you give the privilege of social control of the total population to the physician. This is then added to the considerable powers society has already granted him: the moral imprimatur of the healer, and the coercive privileges of law.

It is now easy to see how we have traveled unwittingly from the safe role of comforter to the sick to the uneasy position of political advocate and social engineer. Yet here we are. The issues are fused and cannot be avoided. Nor should they be. Even if the power of decision is shared, the physician will always be an inevitable and important co-participant. It is an authentic part of his role, and he must be trained for it. He is a value-maker, ethicist, social force, and political influence in the lives of his patient and beyond. He is, whether he wishes to be or not. There is no such thing as a value-free medicine, nor has there ever been. To accept this as a fact of professional life is not arrogance but honesty, and the first step toward that redefinition of the physician's role that is necessitated by the coming of age of medicine. It is our success that demands a new sensitivity, a new humility, and a new training.

Willard Gaylin

INTRODUCTION

THE TRADITIONAL TAXONOMY

Our objective in this book is critically to examine the moral dimensions of decision-making in medical contexts and in contexts involving the biological sciences. By "medical contexts" we refer to the full spectrum of activities pertaining to the provision of health care. These include specific clinical interactions between a physician or other health care provider and patient, and social policy decisions about the allocation of resources as between preventive and curative medicine, therapeutic medicine and medical research, and between health-related expenditures and other kinds of social programs. We also include such conceptual issues as clarification of the concept of health and identification of what kinds of physiological, psychological, or sociological states justify medical intervention. By "the biological sciences" we refer to scientific inquiries into organic and biochemical processes—including both the results of such inquiries and the protocols by which such inquiries are advanced.

The moral problems in medicine have received a great deal of attention in recent years. That attention, however, has not included any systematic attempt to address those problems from the point of view of contemporary analytic philosophy. The problems themselves have been characterized in a taxonomy that is primarily medical and biological in conception, but we shall argue here for the value of a philosophically inspired taxonomy of problems as a valuable new perspective in terms of which familiar problems can be more fruitfully addressed.

We begin by reviewing the traditional way of describing the moral problems in medicine. We cannot here provide any exhaustive account of those problems, but a sense of the subject as it is typically conceived can be conveyed by the brief citation of several general areas, along with a specific illustrative problem within each area. These citations are neither exhaustive nor mutually exclusive.

The Allocation of Limited Resources. At every level, from the individual practitioner to the federal government, needs outstrip resources, and the resulting conflicts about priorities are laden with evaluative questions. Illustration: Given limited governmental capacity to finance health-related endeavors, how much of the available resources should be allocated to improving future health care through basic research, and how much to improving the quality of present health care through support for rural clinics, new medical schools, etc?

The Regulation of Health Care. Medical practice has been largely regulated by the medical profession, but there is a growing sense that it is too important for that. Yet the proper locus and limits of external regulation can only be determined in light of a viewpoint about social and political organization, and the nature of the conflict between social needs and individual rights. Illustration: Under what conditions and for what reasons should mass screening for heritable diseases or severe birth defects via amniocentesis (examination of fetal cells drawn from the amniotic fluid) or other means be required or encouraged as a matter of public policy?

The Use of Human Subjects in Experimentation. Although this issue has received wide attention within the scientific community, with certain codes of conduct having gained acceptance, there are still questions that are vigorously disputed. Illustration: What, precisely, is the nature of informed consent to participation as a subject in an experiment on the part of persons who are disadvantaged with respect to making autonomous decisions—e.g., infants, the mentally retarded, or those who are involuntarily confined?

The Scope of Medical Prerogative. It has been largely conceded that medical decisions should be made by medical professionals, but it is a matter of some dispute what constitutes a medical decision. Illustration: Are these strictly medical questions, and if not, what sort are they—whether a diabetic should be treated with insulin, whether a kidney patient should receive renal dialysis, whether a woman should have an abortion, whether a homosexual or drug user is sick, whether a new drug or surgical procedure is suitable for general use.

Constraint of Research Objectives. Here the issues go beyond the mores of using human subjects to the question of the fundamental purposes and possible effects of research. Illustration: Should experimentation that may lead to the raising of experimental subjects in vitro, via nuclear implantation from human genetic material, be permitted or regulated?

Responsibility for Dependent Persons. Many people deviate from what may be considered normal in the functional capacity of a human being, the reasons for such diminished capacity including retardation, congenital deformity, blindness, severe illness, injury, advanced age, and the like. Medical practice is closely involved in the plight of such persons. But it is not clear what the nature and locus of responsibility are for those who, for whatever reason, are unable to function independently. Illustration: If social policy or law prohibits infanticide in cases of radical deformity or readily demonstrable severe retardation, is there also a communal responsibility to provide resources and facilities for the care of such individuals? Are the problems, principles, and responsibilities different in cases of severe senility or other geriatric infirmity?

Death and Dying. New criteria of death are being shaped, used as guidelines, and affirmed in the courts. But questions remain concerning policy toward the terminally ill. Illustration: What principles should govern decisions concerning euthanasia, withdrawal of costly or scarce life-support systems, determination of narcotic dosages, aggressiveness of treatment of life-threatening infections, and the like, in the terminally ill patient; and what is the relevance, if any, of the patient's age, economic status, or choice?

Commitments of the Medical Profession. The physician's classical commitment to prolong life and relieve suffering places him in conflict situations where adherence to one value requires violation of the other. This is merely a special case of the conflicts inherent in the physician's multiple commitments to his patient, his profession, his own monetary or other career-related interests, the medical profession generally, his community, and his own value structure. Illustration: A physician treating a neighbor's 22-year-old-son on an emergency basis for an injury discovers a large quantity of illegal narcotics in the son's possession. What should the physician's response be to the patient, the neighbor, and the police? Does it matter whether or not the physician is personally an advocate of strict law enforcement with respect to narcotics?

The Physician–patient Relationship. Physicians have a uniquely privileged and powerful position with regard to their patients, and the nature of the actual and optimal relationship between physician and patient is thus a highly charged question for both. Illustration: When a physician discovers an infant to have a heritable disease, and upon testing the ostensible parents discovers that neither is the carrier, what should he tell to whom, and why?

Control of Behavior. The increasing prominence of psychopharmaceutical techniques of behavior control, psychosurgery, behavior modification by aversive conditioning, and the conjectured prospects for intervention via electrode implantation, have all received a good deal of public attention as issues raising moral dilemmas. Confronted by the power of such techniques, one can hardly help but ask what sorts of behavior may justifiably be controlled, by whom, in what ways, for what purposes, in accordance with what values. But less obvious issues also need to be brought to the surface. Illustration: The "medical model" has been debated at length with regard to its appropriateness for conceptualization in mental health or behavior problem areas. But as Willard Gaylin has pointed out, in some ways the medical model itself, with its classification of people by experts into categories of normal or deviant functioning, is an ominously powerful force in general. Given the influence that medical judgments have on attitudes and behavior—what Gaylin calls the physician's special "rights to coercion"—should the concepts of normality that underlie medical practices and public health policy be subjected to greater critical scrutiny from outside the medical profession? Just what are those concepts of normality—how do they limit or in-

fluence therapeutic intervention? Are there credible alternatives to them—and if so, how ought differing models of normality be evaluated?

THE PHILOSOPHICAL TAXONOMY

In an earlier era, the phrase "medical ethics" was frequently taken to refer to a variety of issues concerning the conventions of medical practice. This tradition is reflected even today in the views of the Judicial Council of the American Medical Association, which, in its statement on the principles of medical ethics, addresses attention to such questions as whether physicians may advertise, collect referral commissions, lecture to groups of chiropractors, etc., as well as to questions of social responsibility, confidentiality, and the like, in the interest of rendering "service to humanity with full respect for the dignity of man."

More recently, medical ethics has come to be taken as referring to problems of the sort exemplified in the illustrations above, characterized in terms that are essentially medical or biological. Thus, the focus has shifted to problems of abortion, birth defects, confidentiality in the physician-patient relationship, dying, euthanasia, financing of health care, genetic counseling, human subjects in experimentation, involuntary confinement, etc. This taxonomy persists as the most prominent interpretation of the moral problems in medicine. It is legitimate and useful; the problems thus described are real and important. However, I wish to argue for the concomitant importance of a different taxonomy.

Inquiry into many of the medical contexts that generate moral dilemmas reveals certain common threads of philosophical puzzlement. For example, questions about the right to suicide, about the right of an individual who has committed no crime to be free from involuntary confinement, about a religious group's right to refuse blood transfusions, and about whether the adolescent patient should have access to medical treatment in confidence from parents (who perhaps directly or indirectly cover its costs), all involve issues of personal autonomy and the justifiability of paternalistic intervention. Similarly, questions about responsibility to sustain the lives of seriously deformed newborn infants, like questions about responsibility to sustain the lives of severely deteriorated, terminally ill victims of injury, illness, or advanced age, raise questions about the value of life and the relevance of considerations of quality of life to the assessment of value of life. *Only a consistent point of view about personal autonomy, the justifiability of paternalistic intervention, and the considerations that are relevant to determining the value of life in general or a given life in particular, can allow one to develop a consistent perspective on the various different moral problems in medicine that are reflected in a medically inspired taxonomy.*

There is thus a taxonomy of topics, fundamentally philosophical in conception, that must be addressed as a part of the process of dealing with the moral problems in medicine characterized medically or biologically. These philosophical topics are not new. What is perhaps new is the extent to which clarity about them is demanded for the resolution of pressing problems that arise elsewhere. Typical of such topics are the following:

Autonomy. To what extent is it morally required to allow individuals to act in pursuit of their own aspirations? Does an individual with self-destructive aspirations thereby lose the right to autonomy generally enjoyed by others? Should freedom to act include freedom to follow a foolish or tragic (e.g., suicidal) course of events, or is it justifiable to override another's autonomy paternalistically, as well as for reasons of social benefit? Does respect for a patient's autonomy require honesty on the part of the physician, even when deception seems medically prudent?

Coercion. When is an act voluntary? What conditions must be met for an experimental subject to have volunteered? Do federal programs related to public health or population planning become coercive if they are based on the provision of powerful incentives? Under what conditions is coercion justified in medical contexts?

Normality. Does it make any sense to try to characterize health or illness in terms of a notion of normality? What are the criteria for

distinguishing between desirable and undesirable deviations from physiological or psychological normality for health-related purposes, assuming that the notion of normality is useful?

Naturalness. Can the familiar case be sustained that it is sometimes right to prolong life using natural means but wrong to sustain it by artificial means? Is the distinction between artificial and natural means an intelligible one? Is ''exotic'' life-saving therapy any less natural than routine abdominal surgery or the use of antibiotics?

Rights. Much of the talk about ethical issues in medicine invokes the notion of rights. Is there a right of a fetus to be born, of a patient to have access to his medical record, of a sick person to receive medical treatment, or of a physician to practice where he pleases? Insofar as claims about rights and the resolution of conflicts of rights are obscure, so too are the arguments that involve such claims.

Dependency. Is there a sense in which some individuals can be identified as dependent persons in medically relevant ways? Is anyone genuinely independent? If the notion of dependency is a medically legitimate one, what consequence does a person's being dependent have for the justifiability of paternalistic intervention in his life?

Justice. Is it unjust to distribute health care as a free market commodity, or to consider the social utility of patients in distributing scarce medical resources? Should disputes about damages for medically caused injury be handled by the judicial system or by a special system? Are there unique features of medical situations that raise idiosyncratic problems of justice, or do general considerations of justice apply unaltered in medical contexts?

Needs and Wants. Even granting that one's health-related needs should be met, how are needs to be distinguished from wants that would justify a lesser claim on the benefits of social organization? Insofar as it makes sense to speak of a right to health care, is there a distinction between the need for antibiotic intervention to combat a life threatening infection on the one hand and the desire for cosmetic surgery to alleviate the evidence of aging on the other?

Responsibility. If there can be said to be a right to health care—in the sense that the body politic must make treatment available to individuals suffering from specific diseases the treatments for which are known—is this right to be limited in any way by considerations of personal responsibility? For example, under a system of federally financed free medical care, should the individual whose chronic smoking results in respiratory disease or who is seriously injured because he refused to wear a helmet when riding his motorcycle, be entitled to treatment at public expense, when his imprudent behavior took place in the face of warnings in virtue of which his illness or injury can be viewed to some extent as voluntary?

Personhood. Under what conditions is it appropriate to consider an organism to be a person? What is the relationship between this issue and questions of abortion, the use of fetal tissue in research, and the withdrawal of life support systems from an irreversibly comatose patient?

One could go on at length. The point is merely to show that many familiar philosophical topics are centrally important to the illumination of moral problems in medicine —and, more importantly, that each such philosophical topic cuts across a variety of such problems. Thus, a philosophical inquiry into medical ethics might well focus, say, on the notion of *paternalism,* and investigate the variety of medical and scientific contexts in which that issue arises; likewise for each of the other entries in the philosophical taxonomy. One of the virtues of such an approach is that it enables the philosopher to concentrate on new problems in a way that is familiar and in the use of which he has substantial expertise. An additional virtue of this approach is that it helps those outside philosophy to see connections among medical and scientific problems that are not so easily seen otherwise, and it thereby exhibits more plainly the importance of philosophical inquiry to the resolution of problems of broad social interest.

OLD PROBLEMS AND NEW PROBLEMS

The question of whether death is always and everywhere an evil, whether one has a right willingly to embrace it, and whether life has value independently of the experiences for which it is a precondition, are ancient questions. So too are a number of questions pertaining to the responsibilities of the physician in regard to his patient. Other problems, which seem to arise out of new developments in biomedical research, are largely old problems given new force by recent developments. But there are genuinely new problems as well.

Among the old problems given new force by recent developments are many of those arising in clinical medicine. For example, it is not a new puzzlement to wonder about the appropriate societal constraints on parental reactions to newborn infants who are undesirable by virtue of having certain unanticipated and repugnant characteristics. What is new is the power of the medical profession to save malformed infants who would have died under earlier circumstances. Similarly, what gives deliberations about euthanasia a new urgency is our increased capacity to sustain life beyond reasonable hope of recovery. How one ought to die, and the extent to which one ought to be able to influence or determine the manner and mode of one's death, are old questions. What is new is the power of medical technology to intervene in what were previously dramas that played out largely in their own way.

Our new abilities to gain information also intensify old conflicts. For example, that we can learn via amniocentesis that a fetus is defective sharpens the debate about abortion. We can now identify certain individuals as defective (sometimes grievously) before birth, and hence can circumvent the question of infanticide by advocating early abortion in such instances. Debate about the justifiability of abortion is not new; what is new is our power to perform safe abortions, and the quality of the information that we can bring to bear in some instances in stating the case for abortion.

The genuinely new problems arising from technical developments can be divided into those that arise from developments in health-care technology and those that stem from developments of other sorts. Among the most important developments in health care technology that generate new moral problems are these:

The ability to separate sexual and reproductive activity.

New techniques for obtaining and handling information, including (1) specific testing procedures such as amniocentesis, (2) an understanding of statistical phenomena such as are considered in epidemiology, and (3) the powers of information-handling provided by computerization.

Increased understanding of both the physiological and psychological dimensions of a person—each as a complex set of interrelated systems that can to some extent be separated and acted on independently—e.g., as respiration can be sustained despite renal failure.

The development of psychopharmaceuticals and other technological methods of influencing or controlling behavior.

The ability to conduct research or intervene therapeutically in a way that involves manipulation of human development.

Among the technical developments not directly related to health care, but with substantial impact on questions of health, are the developments in food technology, including the widespread use of chemical food additives, and industrialization, with its attendant pollution of the environment with substances directly related to the pathogenesis of a large variety of diseases.

Each of these areas of technical progress generates or intensifies a cluster of ethically troubling issues. It is hard to overestimate the extent to which our social customs and moral traditions reflect the belief that sexual and reproductive behavior, though distinguishable, are not separable. Now, relatively suddenly, they are quite separable as a result of technical developments. The ramifications of this fact for family structure, educational policy, child-rearing, population planning, and even such a fundamental issue as the right to reproduce, are hardly fathomable at this point. One ramifica-

tion, however, seems clear: questions must now be answered that previously were not even raised.

Our understanding of epidemiology raises some fundamental questions about the competing claims of curative and preventive medicine. Is it justifiable as social policy, for example, that we have allocated $600 million in quest of cures for malignant diseases, and only $30 million to exploration of the carcinogenic effects of environmental pollutants, when there seems to be increasing evidence that a large percentage of malignant disease arises from the presence in the environment of substances that could be regulated? To be sure, curing disease is more dramatic than preventing it, and hence has more appeal both politically and medically. Still, it is not implausible that reflection on the relationship between social responsibility and health would produce arguments in favor of shifting resources dramatically from curative to preventive medicine.

In older, simpler times, an individual was thought to be either alive or dead—the occasional problem being to determine which. Now that we realize that physiological systems deteriorate at different rates and in different ways, we are forced to recognize that, in some of the more difficult cases, whether we have an instance of death or not depends on decisions that we make about which systems have a fundamental importance to our conception of life. Thus, the respiring, digesting, irreversibly comatose quasi-person devoid of neocortical activity challenges us, not to discover whether death or life is present, but to decide which physiological systems are to count in what ways in our deliberations about how to behave in regard to the person or corpse at issue. It is because we understand so much better than we used to what is happening physiologically, and have so much more ability to influence it, that the definition of death is now problematic.

There is no serious question that some use of chemotherapy for psychological purposes is laudable. For example, lithium compounds can transform the lives of certain manic-depressive patients, enabling even some who had required institutionalization to lead happy, productive, stable lives. There seems little basis for dispute about the justifiability of this sort of pharmacological intervention. But the use of drugs such as ritalin as a means of controlling the behavior of inattentive and disruptive school children who lack any identifiable organic deficiency seems a highly suspect use of chemicals to control behavior. Perhaps, after all, it is the school setting that is in need of therapy. But by what principles do we condemn the latter use of drugs while lauding the former?

The horror that some express at the prospects of genetic experimentation results in part from an unwarranted extrapolation from what is presently possible, or even plausible for the foreseeable future, to a fictionalized vision of malevolent geneticists manufacturing humans and quasi-humans in inhumane ways for inhumane purposes. But some genetic research, particularly that involving recombinatory use of genetic material, raises troubling questions now. Thus, the temporary self-imposed moratorium of 1974–75 on such research, and the stringent new guidelines suggested by the research community itself for conducting such experiments safely, reflect the fact that geneticists are now able to create new forms of life with characteristics that are not fully predictable and which, while they fall far short of the fictional mass production of human beings, nevertheless could have substantial impact on the well-being of human beings. And it is explicit in the programs of some of those engaged in such research that a possible future benefit of the work is direct intervention in the genetic development of individual human beings.

Scientific inquiry is a social enterprise supported and conducted at the pleasure of the public whom it ultimately serves. Yet, like medicine, it is practised by a professional elite whose judgments are based on considerations that are essentially obscure in many ways to the public at large. Thus we find, in grappling with questions pertaining to public regulation and public accountability in regard to scientific research, that we must confront traditional questions concerning the proper scope of democratic processes and the prudence of establishing and supporting social institutions that invest power in elite groups charged to act in the interest of a comparatively benighted public.

Two additional points bear mention. First, in the medical context, issues of distributive justice and scarcity are particularly apposite. Medical science is in its infancy. Its successes, largely in the area of infectious diseases and surgical techniques, are impressive. Still, next to nothing is known about the pathogenesis of malignancies, circulatory or cardiac ailments, arthritis, degenerative neurological diseases, and many other conditions. The best and most advanced of medical care, as more and more is learned about the etiology and cure of disease, will for the foreseeable future be in scarce supply. Further, medicine in its entirety will be in competition with other socially valued enterprises for resources that are limited. It will be necessary to address these problems in terms of an unending need to allocate limited resources in the face of competing claims.

Finally, it is clear that there is an inherent conflict between epistemological and ethical aspects of experimentation. For certain kinds of experiments, to inform the subject of the nature of the experiment is to destroy the validity of the experiment at the same time. For examples, if we wish to screen newborn infants for the notorious XYY syndrome, as the first step in a longitudinal study aimed at determining whether or not such individuals are predisposed to antisocial behavior, we cannot inform the parents about the nature of our study without introducing a potentially distorting influence on the relationship between the parents and the children that might itself alter each child's propensity to engage in antisocial behavior. Yet it has been argued that no study of a child is morally permissible without the informed consent of the adults who have responsibility for the child's well-being. Other forms of experimentation that would likely contribute to the general welfare are simply morally repugnant because of their violation of individual rights. For example, we might learn a great deal about language acquisition, with a view toward improving the linguistic ability of underprivileged children, by raising a few children in total isolation from linguistic input for various periods of time—say, two or three years—before immersing them in verbal environments. There should be no question about the scientific utility of such an undertaking, nor should there be any question about its moral unacceptability.

PHILOSOPHY AND MEDICINE

These problems have a special urgency that distinguishes them from many of the issues that philosophers traditionally address. Decisions in clinical medicine do not await philosophical reflection. Nor do government agencies, in establishing regulations that can facilitate or cripple medical research, come to terms as a first step with conflicts between competing ethical theories. Nor do the courts, in ordering life-sustaining treatment of a neonatal monster, come first to some clear general view about the relationship between the value of an individual life and the characteristics of the person whose life it is. Yet these decisions do get made against a backdrop of assumptions and confusions about essentially philosophical topics. For philosophers to address themselves explicitly to those topics as they arise in medical contexts is in no way to abandon the essential character of their philosophical commitments. It is, on the contrary, to do philosophy in a particularly rewarding way, by bringing the strengths of philosophical analysis to bear on problems that engage the immediate interest of physicians, lawyers, policy-makers, legislators, patients, and all the rest of the public in its grand diversity. And for physicians and other health-care professionals to adopt the philosophical perspective is in no way to abandon their commitments to providing care. Rather, it is to broaden the context of sensitivity and understanding within which they provide it—and is thus ultimately to reflect a resolve to provide it in a more humane and enlightened way.

That science exists in the final analysis at the pleasure and for the benefit of society generally is a point to which philosophers generally accede readily. What is perhaps less often noted by them is that philosophy, too, is a social enterprise supported in the final analysis by the public to whose interest it ultimately accrues. It is entirely opportune that philosophers in increasing numbers are addressing their attention to issues with which large portions of the nonphilosophical public can readily identify. When rigorous philosophical work illuminates problems of interest to the public, it is far easier to make the case that the philosophical community, like the scientific, merits public support and respect because it, too, is prepared to respond constructively to pressing social concerns—both because of the essential philosophical interest of those concerns and out of its own sense of social responsibility.

This volume has been prepared in the conviction that both better philosophy and better health care can result from philosophical reflection on medical problems. The chapters that follow have been designed to facilitate such reflection on selected moral problems in medicine. Many moral issues are untreated here that might with equal appropriateness have been included, and even the full range of moral problems in medicine constitutes only a part of the philosophy of medicine. Epistemological issues, such as questions of evidence and predictability, and questions of conceptual clarification, for example, are also important parts of the philosophy of medicine. But the moral problems seem to have a way of commanding center stage, and it is time the philosopher's light was aimed more directly at them.

Samuel Gorovitz

Chapter 1

MORAL PHILOSOPHY

INTRODUCTION

THE NATURE OF ETHICAL THEORY

Of all the areas of inquiry philosophers have engaged in over the centuries, none has been intended as more practical than ethics. Although always putting forward an ideal of some sort, moral philosophers have nonetheless believed that their efforts are addressed to issues in the real world. It is understandable, then, that contemporary philosophers are among those at the forefront of current work in the ''applied'' field of bioethics. Sometimes drawing on traditional theories and writings in the history of philosophy, at other times developing new conceptual approaches to pressing issues in the biomedical domain, philosophers view their practically directed ef-

Portions of this introduction were previously published in an article entitled ''Experimenting on Human Subjects: Philosophical Perspectives,'' by Ruth Macklin and Susan Sherwin. The article appeared in the *Case Western Reserve Law Review*, vol. 25, no. 3 (Spring 1975).

forts as a legitimate extension of the more theoretical aspects of philosophical inquiry.

Ethical theories typically offer moral principles for how we ought to treat people or what sorts of actions are morally permissible. It is not sufficient for an ethical theory merely to assert such principles; it also must offer a justification for them. Moral philosophy is not casuistry, the study of individual cases in an attempt to give specific solutions to problematic ethical dilemmas. Instead, philosophical ethics seeks to offer general moral principles and a thorough justification for their adoption and application in a wide variety of situations in which people might find themselves. The advantage of having a theory, as philosophers have argued at length, is that it enables individual judgments to be systematic and well grounded instead of ad hoc or issued according to whim. To the defender of the latter practices, we can only give the same sort of reply we give to the skeptic who asks, ''Why be rational?'' Skeptics who question the need for or value of ethical theories on the grounds that a systematic or rational approach to individual moral problems is unnecessary or undesirable will probably not be convinced by good reasons of any sort. Their skepticism extends beyond that pertaining to the role of theories in applied ethics. If we include in the notion of "ethical theory" small-scale theories of paternalism, autonomy, and privacy, among others, in addition to the more traditional, comprehensive ethical theories, it is hard to see how moral decision making can take place without those theoretical underpinnings that serve to justify steps at any stage in an argument. The burden of proof lies with the skeptic to show how moral reasoning or ethical judgments can take place in a systematic or rational way in the absence of some background theory.

NORMATIVE ETHICS AND METAETHICS

Concerns of moral philosophers can very roughly be divided into two sorts—normative ethical and metaethical concerns. Normative ethics deals with developing a set of moral principles that tell us what acts or practices are right or wrong, good or bad, obligatory, permissible, or forbidden. This branch of ethics also provides reasons for accepting these principles. Although this may seem to exhaust the important role of moral philosophy, it does not. For in attempting to answer such normative questions as "What actions are right?" or "What things are morally good?" we must have some understanding of what it means to say that something is right or morally good, and of what morality, moral principles, and justification in ethics *are*. These questions in metaethics are about ethics, but they are not sociological questions about what values certain groups accept, nor are they psychological questions that ask why individuals come to hold the moral beliefs or acquire the values they in fact have. Rather, metaethical questions are conceptual questions whose answers help us to understand what we mean when we search for specific principles, and indeed what would count as answers to our normative questions. Studies in metaethics sometimes analyze the nature of moral languages and moral reasoning, such as what is

meant by "good" or "right" and how ethical imperatives function in discourse. Other metaethical inquiries examine the key features and presuppositions of particular normative theories, contemporary ones as well as those in the history of philosophy.

One major area of metaethical inquiry concerns the question whether there are any moral principles that hold for all people at all times. One view maintains that there are absolute values of some kind, despite the facts of cultural diversity in ethical beliefs and practices. The opposing position, known as *ethical relativism,* asserts that no universal moral principles can be held valid for all persons in all circumstances at all times, that moral rightness and wrongness are relative to the particular culture or historical niche in which they happen to be operating. Thus, what is right in the South Sea Islands may not be right in South Carolina, and what was morally required in ancient Sparta may be ethically ruled out today in Switzerland. It is important to see that this brand of ethical relativism denies the very possibility of cross-cultural standards of morality, and therefore, of cross-cultural ethical judgments. In this view, all moral values derive solely from the time or place in which they are practiced, so it is not contradictory to say that slavery was right in the South before the Civil War but wrong throughout the United States today. Ethical relativism is thus a doctrine about the status of moral values and the justification of moral judgments. The selection by Walter T. Stace presents an extensive discussion of the pros and cons of the issue, coming down on the side of ethical absolutism.

Another important concern of philosophers, especially those interested in medical ethics, is the relationship between morality and the law. This is a complex issue, yet one that can be simplified by focusing on a series of basic questions: Are law and morality coextensive; that is, is everything the law requires also morally obligatory? And conversely, is everything that is moral also legally permitted or required? Is disobedience to law itself an immoral act, or are there at least some occasions when to break the law is to pursue a higher moral goal, as in acts of civil disobedience aimed at achieving racial equality or other forms of social justice?

It is easy to produce examples to show that law and morality are not coextensive, since many actions are properly considered immoral but are not and should not be legally forbidden, such as lying in order to gain some personal advantage or breaking a promise to a child because it is inconvenient to keep it. The same is true for the moral status of many laws, such as ones that require alternate side of the street parking or those that prescribe detailed provisions for drawing up a will or a contract. An example that illustrates the many facets of this question is the ongoing debate and recent history concerning the moral and legal status of abortion.

A somewhat different question about law and ethics concerns the use of a legal model for characterizing and understanding morality. Some concepts in ethics, such as the notion of virtue, have no legal analogue; and an ethics of love, such as Christian theology preaches, or of altruism, according to secular morality, are far from the proper domain of law. John Ladd, in ''Legalism and Medical Ethics,'' addresses what he calls ''an ethics of giving and receiving,'' focusing on the differences between an ethics primarily concerned with rights and one primarily concerned with responsibilities seen as deriving from interpersonal relationships.

There are two main sorts of normative ethical theories in the Western philosophical tradition. The first is the *deontological* or *formalist* theory, which holds that the rightness or wrongness of an action is to be determined by examining the sort of action in question, or perhaps the motive with which the action is done. Common to this type of theory is the view that the rightness or wrongness of an action should not depend on its consequences. That is, it is the ''form'' or type of action, the way in which it was done, or the reason behind the doing that are relevant to determining moral rightness or wrongness—not what results the action had. Deontological theories focus on moral duties, along with the related concept of rights.

The other main sort of normative theory is called *teleological* or *consequentialist*. According to this theory, the rightness or wrongness of an action is determined by its actual or expected results. As is true of any other type of normative theory, a consequentialist theory can be used as a tool in moral decision making (before the fact) or as a method of evaluating actions already performed. For the first purpose, determining whether an action is morally right requires us to assess the probable consequences of a proposed action, compared with the probable consequences of other available actions, to see if the action in question would produce a greater balance of good over evil than any other action. To evaluate completed actions, we need to look at the actual consequences and try to determine whether they are better than those of some other action that might have been performed instead.

Still, it is not enough for a consequentialist theory to hold that good or bad results of actions are the relevant factors for judging moral rightness or wrongness. Such theories must also specify a standard for evaluating the goodness or badness of results, and different consequentialist accounts have offered various candidates, among them pleasure, higher states of human happiness or well-being, and an unanalyzable, intuitively known property of goodness. Arguments in favor of any particular criterion for what should be considered *good* consequences of actions constitute part of still another branch of value theory: inquiry into intrinsic goodness. These theoretical relationships can be described in the better-known terminology of *means* and *ends*. Morally right actions are those that serve as a means for achieving a good end—an end that is intrinsically worthwhile, or good in itself. According to this mode of description, the ends are the only thing that can serve to justify the means. Much depends, therefore, on what sorts of ends are deemed good, or intrinsically worthwhile.

In short, deontological theories hold that we can determine the rightness of an action independently of determining its consequences, which is precisely what teleological theories deny. This debate over what are the morally relevant features of actions—the features that make them right or wrong—is a metaethical debate, yet it frequently takes place in the context of a normative theory of ethics. Thus, although normative questions and metaethical questions can be characterized and identified as separate concerns, both are typically embedded in a full-scale ethical theory.

A further word about moral philosophy is in order. Unlike specific ethical codes of behavior or even ethical prescriptions or commandments that derive from religious sources, philosophical ethical theories generally avoid dogmatic principles or rigid, exceptionless commands. One purpose of a sound philosophical ethics is to mediate between an unjustified dogmatism, on the one hand, and an unwarranted moral skepticism, on the other. Hence, philosophical ethics places a premium on the giving of reasons, both in support of the moral principles themselves and against the competing claims of dogmatic ethics and moral skepticism. Moreover, the fundamental moral principles of the most prominent ethical theories can serve as a basis for addressing quite a number of specific issues that arise in biomedical treatment and research.

Yet in spite of the efforts some moral philosophers have made to construct systematic, coherent, comprehensive theories of ethics based on one or more fundamental principles, other writers have been critical of that approach. A major criticism has come from the existentialist school of philosophy, stressing the importance of individuals taking responsibility for their actions. The notion of taking responsibility for one's decisions and actions is the key concept in morality, since according to the existentialist view, a moral agent cannot simply take refuge in an appeal to principles. Based on an underlying premise of freedom of the will, existentialism holds that every agent necessarily chooses how to act in a particular circumstance. Having freely chosen a course of action, the individual becomes responsible, regardless of the role a moral principle might have played in that decision. Existentialists thus stress the role of freedom and responsibility in their view of morality and see little need for formal systems of ethics.

John Dewey argues for a somewhat similar position in the selection from his book, *Theory of the Moral Life*. In his criticism of "customary morality," which blindly accepts moral rules and traditions handed down from one generation to the next, Dewey contends that reflective morality arises out of conflict, out of perplexity

about what to do. To resolve that conflict, a person must weigh competing ends, rights, or responsibilities and arrive at a principled solution based on rational reflection. Dewey does not argue against the value of ethical principles; rather he holds that in the practice of reflective morality, people arrive at suitable ethical principles to guide and justify their actions.

Another approach deserves mention, especially because it gained prominence early in the development of the field now known as bioethics. That approach is *situation ethics,* best known through the writings of its chief proponent, the theologian Joseph Fletcher. Reacting against dogmatic forms of morality, especially those derived from orthodox religious teachings, Fletcher argues that each situation is different and that recognizing the uniqueness of every situation demands that moral agents abandon a rigid adherence to doctrinaire rules and inflexible principles. What is required is to seek a "loving and humane solution" in every situation that poses an ethical dilemma. Fletcher's view has its roots in a Christian ethics of love, and so it is not an altogether nonreligious position. It does, however, seek a methodology for ethical decision making that does not rely on moral rules or universal principles.

Although situation ethics has the virtue of being nondogmatic in its approach to ethical dilemmas, it fails to give clear guidance to the individual perplexed about the morally right thing to do. To tell the pediatrician in a quandary about how aggressively to treat a defective newborn to "choose the loving and humane solution" is simply to restate the problem the physician confronts in other terms. The physician wonders precisely which is the more loving and humane solution: to prolong artificially the infant's less than satisfactory life or to "let nature take its course." The more that situation ethics acknowledges the need to call on some principle or other to guide decision making, the more it resembles traditional ethical theories. Fletcher's writings reveal a distinctly consequentialist bias and might thus be thought of as one variant of utilitarianism, a theory described in the next section.

This discussion of the nature and types of ethical theory has been somewhat abstract, in an attempt to describe the general characteristics of moral philosophy. We turn next to two leading examples of normative ethical theories, one consequentialist and one formalist.

TWO LEADING ETHICAL THEORIES: UTILITARIANISM AND KANT'S THEORY

By way of approaching these illustrative theories, let us first pose a prior question, one that inquires into the nature of persons as entities deserving moral concern. What are the centrally important characteristics of human beings that are relevant to how they ought morally to be treated? The first human characteristic relevant to this concern is that of sentience. Human beings, like other higher forms of animal life, are sentient creatures: that is, they are capable of feeling pleasure and pain under a wide range of predictable circumstances. What is more, people pursue pleasure and seek to avoid pain. Some philosophers and psychologists have gone so far as to claim that pursuit of pleasure and avoidance of pain are the sole factors motivating human behavior. We need not go this far, however, in order to acknowledge the importance of pain and pleasure as determinants of human action. It is this basic fact of sentience, conjoined with the teleological (goal-directed) principle that people seek pleasurable ends and avoid actions with painful or unpleasant consequences, that has led to the widespread acceptance of one prominent ethical theory, utilitarianism.

One of the leading utilitarians, the nineteenth-century English philosopher John Stuart Mill, argued that pleasure is the sole thing that is good as an end. Since each person takes his own pleasure or happiness to be his ultimate aim or goal, toward which all particular activities are a means, Mill claimed that the value that should be maximized in the community as a whole is the greatest happiness of all. For the most part, Mill followed his utilitarian predecessor, Jeremy Bentham, in adopting the "Greatest Happiness Principle" as the fundamental moral principle of his ethical theory. As Mill himself stated, under the principle of utility, "actions are right in pro-

portion as they tend to promote happiness; wrong as they tend to produce the reverse of happiness. By happiness is intended pleasure and the absence of pain; by unhappiness, pain and the privation of pleasure."[1] In order to prevent any misunderstanding of this influential theory, a bit more needs to be said by way of explication and interpretation.

First, it should be emphasized that Mill explicitly disavows the interpretation of his theory as a "gross form" of hedonism. Although he clearly identifies happiness and pleasure, as shown in the quoted statement of the utilitarian principle, Mill nevertheless argues for a qualitative distinction among pleasures in addition to the usual distinction in terms of quantity or amount—the view held by Bentham and others. Mill writes,

> It is quite compatible with the principle of utility to recognize the fact that some kinds of pleasure are more desirable and more valuable than others. It would be absurd that, while in estimating all other things quality is considered as well as quantity, the estimation of pleasure should be supposed to depend on quantity alone.[2]

Thus, although Mill does identify happiness with pleasure, he argues against the mistake of confounding "the two very different ideas of happiness and content." These so-called "higher pleasures" include the pleasures of the intellect, of the feelings and imagination, and of the moral sentiments—all of which are to be accorded a higher value as pleasure than those of "mere sensation."

A second, related point should also be stressed in explicating Mill's view. Utilitarianism might be criticized as being a crass majority-rule doctrine, in which a preference on the part of 51 percent of the population for any action or state of affairs whatsoever renders it morally acceptable. This criticism misinterprets the intent of the utilitarian moral position. Throughout his essay, and especially in the lengthy final chapter entitled "On the Connection Between Justice and Utility," Mill expresses concern for minority rights and, indeed, the basic rights of persons. The claimed weakness of the utilitarian position lies in Mill's response to an objector who asks why society ought to defend a person in the possession of his rights; Mill replies, "I can give him no other reason than general utility."[3] Although nonutilitarians such as Immanuel Kant and John Rawls have found Mill's answer unsatisfactory, a careful reading of Mill's writings reveals a pervasive humane and humanitarian thread woven throughout. A serious problem remains, however, in that the principle of utility alone—as a fundamental moral principle—does not seem able to account for a variety of ethical duties and precepts of justice without the additional corollaries and interpretive remarks offered by Mill and other defenders of utilitarianism.

In summary, it is worth emphasizing again that utilitarians claim that their ethical theory is derivable from certain indisputable facts about human beings: sentience and the tendency of persons to seek pleasure or happiness and avoid pain or unhappiness. It is clear that the utilitarian principle often accurately describes how people actually make judgments about the rightness and wrongness of actions. This ethical principle is frequently the operative criterion that guides many decisions in specific cases of medical treatment and experimentation on humans. In particular, it seems that utility is the underlying moral principle in the notion of the "risk–benefit" equation, an application in the area of research using human subjects.

We now turn to the second basic characteristic of human beings, with which another prominent ethical theory is closely associated. This attribute is rationality, and one major ethical theory that arises largely out of this human characteristic is the doctrine of the eighteenth-century German philosopher Immanuel Kant. Closely linked with the concept of rationality is that of personal autonomy, to which ethical values are attached. Kant's ethical system begins by presupposing rationality and autonomy as fundamental characteristics of persons. He then constructs a moral theory applicable to all rational beings, who possess what he describes as an autonomous, self-legislating will. The inherent autonomy of each person, which is produced by his rationality, requires that each person be treated as a creature having dignity and, therefore, as worthy of respect. To repeat, in Kant's view,

rationality and autonomy are the essential humanity-conferring properties, and they give rise to the moral principle that persons should be accorded dignity and treated with respect.

Kant used the term *rationality* to apply to an attribute of the human species rather than to an attribute of individual persons. As a result, the Kantian framework does not give us a criterion for distinguishing between rational individuals and irrational or nonrational individuals. Instead, it treats the human species (or any other "higher" beings) as having the capacity to reason and form concepts and, hence, as possessing the attribute of rationality. What is required at this point is a brief account of the way in which the concept of rationality and that of autonomy are linked in Kant's theory. We may then see how the human characteristic of rationality gives rise to some fundamental ethical values and moral principles.

Kant's notion of morality is that "its law must be valid, not merely for men, but for all *rational creatures generally,* not merely under certain contingent conditions or with exceptions, but with *absolute necessity.* . . ."[4] This passage makes explicit Kant's concept of morality as one that is applicable to all rational beings rather than one whose application is designed specifically for humans; it also exhibits the tone of his moral philosophy, which has led many to object that it is an implausibly rigid ethical system, since its law commands "with absolute necessity." On the basis of this notion of the nature and scope of morality, Kant formulates his account of the derivation of the commands of ethics:

> Since moral laws ought to hold good for every rational creature, we must derive them from the general concept of a rational being. . . .
>
> Everything in nature works according to laws. Rational beings alone have the faculty of acting according *to the conception* of laws, that is according to principles, *i.e.* have a *will.* Since the deduction of actions from principles requires *reason,* the will is nothing but practical reason.[5]

Kant terms the fundamental moral principle or law of morality *the categorical imperative,* since the moral law commands absolutely (categorically) rather than conditionally (hypothetically).

In the archaic language in which Kant himself expresses it, the categorical imperative states: ''Act only on that maxim whereby thou canst at the same time will that it should become a universal law.''[6] Kant argues that all imperatives of duty can be deduced from this one fundamental principle, since persons can always formulate a maxim for each act they consider performing and then test the maxim for conformity to the fundamental principle, or categorical imperative. If the maxim passes the test, that is, if it can consistently be willed by the agent as a universal law, applicable to all rational creatures, then the contemplated action is morally permissible or morally right. We should emphasize here that this is a purely formal requirement for Kant, a necessary condition for an imperative to count as a moral law. The test Kant postulates is generally referred to, in an alternative formulation, as the requirement of generalization, or universalizability, in ethics. The core idea in all these views is that a moral law is one that holds for all persons similar in relevant respects in all like circumstances. Thus, what is right for one would be right for all similar persons in similar circumstances. Moreover, for a maxim to pass the test of the categorical imperative, it is not a matter of whether or not the agent can will the maxim to be a universal law as a matter of *psychological* fact. For Kant, a formalist, it is a question of *logical* consistency: Maxims that cannot be willed to be universal laws, as prescribed by the categorical imperative, fail either because they lead to a logical contradiction or because such a will would contradict itself. A good will formulates and acts only on those maxims that prescribe our duties; morally right acts are those done for the sake of duty. So, for example, if a person contemplated breaking a promise when it was inconvenient for him to keep it, he would have to formulate a maxim of the following form: It is morally permissible to break promises when it is inconvenient to keep them. This maxim cannot (consistently) be universalized, since if we allowed the possibility that people could break their promises whenever they chose, the very concept of a *promise* would no longer have meaning. An ingredient in the meaning of that concept is the idea that a promise is binding on one who engages in the act. The binding feature of promising is contradicted by a maxim that

enables people to break their promises at will, so such a maxim fails to meet the test of the categorical imperative.

There is but one categorical imperative according to Kant, and yet he offers what he terms a second formulation of this fundamental principle: ''So act as to treat humanity, whether in thine own person or in that of any other, in every case as an end withal, never as means only.''[7] It is not our concern here to debate whether or not this statement is another formulation of the same principle or a new principle based on additional assumptions; we leave that debate to Kantian scholars. The second formulation succeeds in capturing a common moral sentiment: We ought to treat our fellow human beings as ends in themselves and not as mere means or instruments for our own purposes, even to serve so-called ''noble'' aims. It is this second formulation of Kant's categorical imperative that seems especially appropriate as a moral principle applicable in cases of biomedical research on human subjects, for we can always assess proposed actions that use human subjects against the principle that persons should be treated as ends, never as mere means. Kant claims that ''the foundation of this principle is: *rational nature exists as an end in itself.*''[8]

Finally, Kant offers what he considers the third formulation of the categorical imperative, from which the notion of autonomy emerges. The ''third practical principle of the will, which is the ultimate condition of its harmony with the universal practical reason [is] the idea *of the will of every rational being as a universally legislative will.*''[9] This capacity of every human will to be a universally legislating will is what constitutes the principle of autonomy of the will, which according to Kant is claimed to be ''the basis of the dignity of human and of every rational nature.''[10] We can see, then, how the fundamental characteristic of rationality and the derivative concept of autonomy form the foundation for those values most central to our humane moral beliefs. From Kant's moral philosophy we obtain the important value concept of the intrinsic worth or dignity of human beings. In arguing for the central importance of duty in a conception of morality, Kant sums up these interrelationships as follows:

The practical necessity of acting on this principle, i.e. duty, does not rest at all on feelings, impulses, or inclinations, but solely on the relation of rational beings to one another, a relation in which the will of a rational being must always be regarded as *legislative*, since it otherwise could not be conceived as *an end in itself*. Reason then refers every maxim of the will, regarding it as legislating universally, to every other will and also to every action towards oneself; and this not on account of any other practical motive or any future advantage, but from the idea of the *dignity* of a rational being, obeying no law but that which he himself also gives.[11]

The ethical theories of Kant and Mill each propose a basic general principle, according to which any moral agent can test contemplated actions to ascertain their moral rightness or wrongness. In Kant's system, the central moral notion is that of duty, and the intrinsic human values are autonomy and dignity, both derived from the essential human attribute of rationality. Mill bases his theory on the empirically ascertained attribute of sentience in persons, along with the observable goal-directed behavior of human beings in their pursuit of pleasure or happiness and avoidance of pain and suffering. Both basic conceptions of morality found in Kant and Mill seem to be required for a full account of our common moral sentiments and beliefs. In addition, they both provide a general principle under which we can subsume particular actions or subordinate moral rules in order to test their moral acceptability or validity. We need not consider ourselves hedonists in order to accept the utilitarian principle, nor need we adhere, in general, to a duty-oriented conception of ethics in order to acknowledge the importance of the categorical imperative (in any of the formulations Kant suggests).

THE NATURE AND PRACTICE OF APPLIED ETHICS

Despite the care and thought philosophers have invested in formulating systematic theories of ethics, a number of difficulties plague efforts to apply these theories in practical contexts. Although these difficulties should not lead us to conclude that applied ethics is a bogus enterprise or that theories are useless in practice, it is important to recognize the barriers to their easy or straightforward application.

Three main barriers exist: (1) different ethical theories are in competition with one another; (2) ethical theories require interpretation; (3) applied ethics involves much more than the application of ethical principles to individual cases. In the selection entitled "Ethical Engineers Need Not Apply: The State of Applied Ethics Today," Arthur Caplan addresses these and related issues. Some further observations may help to clarify the difficulty of resolving moral problems by a direct appeal to ethical theory.

PROBLEMS IN APPLYING ETHICAL THEORIES: COMPETING ETHICAL PRINCIPLES

The first barrier to easy application is evident in situations where there is an ethical problem or dilemma to be resolved and doctors, nurses, family members, or others disagree about what action to perform. In many (but surely not all) such cases, the dilemma exists precisely because two different ethical principles underlie the competing judgments about what to do. If a dilemma can be traced to tension between two incompatible theories, or competing principles central to those theories, then of course the dilemma cannot be resolved by applying an ethical theory. The problem lies not in the difficulty of application, but alas, in the unsettled metaethical problems of competing theories and disagreements about which principle to accept when two or more are in conflict.

Some of the more common dilemmas confronting health care practitioners illustrate this tension between competing ethical principles or theories. An elderly woman refuses to consent to a proposed surgical amputation of her foot; a surgeon seeks to override her refusal and operate anyway, in the belief that failure to do so will result in the patient's death. The woman's "right to decide," which rests on the principle of autonomy, comes into conflict with a principle of beneficence—"do good whenever possible"—a principle the surgeon might invoke to justify paternalistic behavior. Or a doctor may wish to conceal from a patient the diagnosis of cancer, based on the duty to help the patient maintain hope or on the principle that a physician must refrain from doing harm. A competing duty or moral principle is that which requires people to tell the truth (at least when asked directly), even when the information is distinctly unpleasant.

Another biomedical context in which competing ethical theories yield different answers to the question, ''What is morally permissible?'' is that of human experimentation. Consider this issue in light of the two normative approaches previously discussed: Kant's theory and utilitarian moral theory. Kant could surely approve of experiments in which an intended or hoped-for outcome is some benefit to the subjects themselves. If an experiment is conducted both as a therapeutic attempt and to help others or to further knowledge, it can be acceptable by this standard. Even if the subjects do not themselves need this treatment but merely have an interest in the success of the research for some other reason (for example, if the research is investigating an illness from which a relative suffers or the subjects have a scientific curiosity about the matter or, simply, are acting altruistically), the experiment would still be acceptable.

Nonetheless, Kant might find even these experiments unjustifiable if they could result in a reduction of an individual's ability to function as an independent, autonomous, rational agent. (It is always risky to speculate on what a writer from an earlier time would think about current issues.) But since rationality and autonomy are the most important human characteristics for Kant, they form the basis of his moral framework. Any act that might reduce these capacities would violate an important standard of human dignity and would be inconsistent with the third formulation of the categorical imperative. By this standard, all forms of novel exploratory experimentation on ways of effective behavioral change in humans would be suspect, be they behavior modification techniques, psychosurgery, or new chemical or electrical stimuli to the brain. The notorious syphilis experiment at the Tuskegee Institute, in which unwitting subjects suffering from syphilis were left untreated for more than thirty years, was immoral according to Kant's criterion because it was known that many subjects would become mad in the stage of tertiary syphilis, and it is morally wrong to bring about or promote irrationality.

Kant also argues that being alive must be a fundamental value for everyone. Most people naturally choose life over death. For those who do not, Kant offers arguments to show that everyone who is able to choose has an obligation not to terminate his or her own life. It follows that others must respect this universally binding human end and that any experiment involving the death (or even a serious likelihood of death) of its subjects is wrong. Hence, even if the subjects are willing to risk their lives for the sake of the experiment, they are mistaken, for they ought to value their lives above most other considerations. It is wrong for anyone to violate this fundamental end. The only likely exception to the presumption against experiments involving death would be those cases in which death is imminent without the experiment or where life is otherwise seriously threatened, say, by a high probability of contracting some fatal disease. Even Kant might allow for the possibility of heroic self-sacrifice, however, and then it would be right for subjects to agree to the risk of death in the cause of science.

The utilitarian answer to the question of what experiments are morally justifiable is much easier to formulate, though surely no easier to apply. The utilitarian principle requires us to act in the way that produces the greatest general balance of happiness over unhappiness. In order to determine whether an experiment is justified, a utilitarian must calculate the "expected utility," that is, the good or happiness or welfare likely to come of it. The calculation proceeds by estimating the amount of happiness and multiplying that amount by the probability of its coming about as a result of this experiment, thereby obtaining a measure of the benefit at stake. The utilitarian must then weigh that benefit against the anticipated risk, determined by multiplying the amount of harm by the probablity of its occurrence. The measure is complex, for it must include all the possible good and bad effects of the experiment—including feelings engendered in the general population, feelings of satisfaction or guilt on the part of participants, and consequences of actions taken as a direct result of the experiment. However complex the utilitarian calculation may be, something very much like it appears to be the underlying moral principle in the notion of the risk–benefit equation, as mentioned earlier in discussing Mill's theory.

Utilitarianism permits a wide range of experiments that Kantians would never consider. For instance, utilitarians would probably approve an experiment expected to provide a cure for cancer, even though it was expected to cause its early subjects to develop untreatable cancer; Kantians would surely object. Utilitarians as well as Kantians would object to the Tuskegee syphilis experiments, but on different grounds: Whereas Kantians would object to the loss of the subjects' autonomy as a result of illness and possible insanity, utilitarians would object because the experiments did little good. If the experiments had been better designed and were likely to succeed in producing some significant, useful knowledge leading to beneficial results for humanity, utilitarians might be willing to approve, despite the resulting illness and insanity generated by the tests.

Still, utilitarians do not operate with a simple risk–benefit table that approves any experiment whatsoever where benefit measures higher. They are obliged to choose the option with the best ratio of benefit to risk, and so they have a strong responsibility to minimize risks. It is important to investigate alternative courses of action that might further improve the ratio, even if the benefit already outweighs the risk. In practice, this requirement would prevent Mill and most utilitarians from engaging in many experiments that are threatening to life or that interfere with the basic rights of persons. If a great risk is present, utilitarians would generally assume that the experimenter should wait before performing this particular test and seek a safer means of obtaining the result. However, if no safe alternative can be devised and if the expected benefit clearly outweighs the risk, in terms of happiness or well-being and pain or suffering, utilitarians are obliged to permit experiments that Kantians would unconditionally oppose.

CONCEPTUAL PROBLEMS, FACTUAL UNCERTAINTIES, AND METHODOLOGICAL BARRIERS

Even if all parties to a decision agree on which ethical theory is the correct one to apply, the empirical and methodological difficulties are still formidable, as shown by the foregoing discussion of Kant and Mill. We need only list several stock objections to a relatively straightforward theory such as utilitarianism to be reminded of further difficulties. There is uncertainty in being able to predict outcomes with any reasonable degree of accuracy. There is the range of problems surrounding measurement: whether individual utilities are additive, and if not, how to assign precise values to them; whether it is necessary to compare the utilities of different persons, and if so, how to go about doing so. There are epistemological problems in assigning values to possible outcomes and in whether individual preferences can simply be inferred from people's behavior. Debates persist over whether or not pleasures and pains are commensurable and whether different types of pleasures and pains can or ought to be weighted differently. Some of these difficulties are functions of the state of development of the social sciences. They reflect the fact that the sciences of psychology and sociology (if they are sciences at all) are in their infancy, both as regards the state of theory and also its application in the spheres of prediction and control. If the major difficulties of application can be traced to the state of the art in the social sciences, it is a mistake to focus blame on ethical theories themselves. That is, what stands in the way of being able to apply ethical theory in this range of cases are shortcomings in social science theory and practice.

However, some of the difficulties just noted (for instance, the conceptual and epistemological problems raised by utilitarianism) do not stem from the primitive state of social science but from the elements of philosophical theories themselves. To that extent, the shortcomings lie not so much in efforts to apply the theory but in failure to work out the details of the theory in the first place. A theory that is impossible or exceedingly difficult to apply in practice is flawed in theory as well. Although the heart of a moral theory is the fundamental moral principle or principles it embodies, the theory itself consists of much more than its normative content. There is at least as much controversy among philosophers over the foundations of ethics, over the theory of knowledge that lies behind an acceptance of one or another ethical theory, and over the meanings of basic ethical terms as there is over the selection of the principles themselves.

In applied contexts, sometimes the issues are resolved by getting the participants or disputants to agree on what are the morally relevant considerations. Sometimes the issues are resolved by pointing out that the problem lies not in failure to assent to the same ethical principle but rather in disagreement over the empirical facts or probable outcomes of alternative courses of action. An important aspect of applying ethical theories, then, is attending to the meaning of their central concepts, to the methodology they require, and to the facts that must be gathered before moral principles can be used effectively.

The reflections on morality in this chapter are all examples of metaethical essays. John Dewey analyzes the nature of reflective morality, and Walter Stace probes the controversy between moral absolutists and ethical relativists. John Ladd's reflections are presented within the context of medical ethics, and K. Danner Clouser distinguishes the field of medical ethics from other disciplines with which it might be confused. Arthur Caplan addresses the application of ethical theory, a topic that occupies a large part of the discussion in this introduction and that has occasioned almost as much debate as some of the questions of normative ethics philosophers deal with. Although none of these selections contains the last word on any of the subjects discussed, all of them should help the reader grapple with the moral problems in medicine on which the remainder of this book focuses.

Ruth Macklin

Notes

1. J.S. Mill, *Utilitarianism* (Indianapolis: Bobbs-Merrill, 1957), p. 10.

2. *Ibid.*, p. 12.

3. *Ibid.*, p. 66.

4. Immanuel Kant, *Fundamental Principles of the Metaphysics of Morals,* selection reprinted in Paul Taylor, ed., *Problems of Moral Philosophy,* 2nd ed. (Belmont and Encino, Cal.: Dickenson, 1972), p. 222.

5. *Ibid.*, pp. 223–24.

6. *Ibid.*, p. 229.

7. *Ibid.*, pp. 234–35.

8. *Ibid.*, p. 234.

9. *Ibid.*, p. 236.

10. *Ibid.*, p. 239.

11. *Ibid.*, p. 238.

REFLECTIONS ON MORALITY

From *Theory of the Moral Life*

John Dewey

The intellectual distinction between customary and reflective morality is clearly marked. The former places the standard and rules of conduct in ancestral habit; the latter appeals to conscience, reason, or to some principle which includes thought. The distinction is as important as it is definite, for it shifts the center of gravity in morality. Nevertheless the distinction is relative rather than absolute. Some degree of reflective thought must have entered occasionally into systems which in the main were founded on social wont and use, while in contemporary morals, even when the need of critical judgment is most recognized, there is an immense amount of conduct that is merely accommodated to social usage. In what follows we shall, accordingly, emphasize the difference in *principle* between customary and reflective morals rather than try to describe different historic and social epochs. In principle a revolution was wrought when Hebrew prophets and Greek seers asserted that conduct is not truly conduct unless it springs from the heart, from personal desires and affections, or from personal insight and rational choice.

The change was revolutionary not only because it displaced custom from the supreme position, but even more because it entailed the necessity of criticizing existing customs and institutions from a new point of view. Standards which were regarded by the followers of tradition as the basis of duty and responsibility were denounced by prophet and philosopher as the source of moral corruption. These proclaimed the hollowness of outer conformity and insisted upon the cleansing of the heart and the clarifying of the mind as preconditions of any genuinely good conduct.

One great source of the abiding interest which Greek thought has for the western world is that it records so clearly the struggle to make the transition from customary to reflective conduct. In the Platonic dialogues for example Socrates is represented as constantly raising the question of whether morals can be taught. Some other thinker (like Protagoras in the dialogue of that name) is brought in who points out that habituation to existing moral traditions is actually taught. Parents and teachers constantly admonish the young "pointing out that one act is just, another unjust; one honorable and another dishonorable; one holy and another unholy." When a youth emerges from parental tutelage, the State takes up the task, for "the community compels them to learn laws and to live after the pattern of the laws and not according to their own fancies."

In reply, Socrates raises the question of the foundations of such teaching, of its right to be termed a genuine teaching of virtue, and in effect points out the need of a morality which shall be stable and secure because based upon constant and universal principles. Parents and teachers differ in their injunctions and prohibitions; different communities have different laws; the same community changes its habits with time and with transformations of government. How shall we know who among the teachers, whether individuals or States, is right? Is there no basis for morals except this fluctuating one? It is not enough to praise and blame, reward and punish, enjoin and prohibit. The essence of morals, it is implied, is to know the reason for these customary instructions; to ascertain the criterion which insures their being just. And in other dialogues, it is frequently asserted that even if the mass must follow custom and law without insight, those who make laws and fix customs should have sure insight into enduring principles, or else the blind will be leading the blind.

No fundamental difference exists between systematic moral theory . . . and the reflection

Reprinted with the permission of the Center for Dewey Studies, Southern Illinois University at Carbondale.

an individual engages in when he attempts to find general principles which shall direct and justify his conduct. Moral theory begins, in germ, when any one asks "Why should I act thus and not otherwise? Why is this right and that wrong? What right has any one to frown upon this way of acting and impose that other way?" Children make at least a start upon the road of theory when they assert that the injunctions of elders are arbitrary, being simply a matter of superior position. Any adult enters the road when, in the presence of moral perplexity, of doubt as to what it is right or best to do, he attempts to find his way out through reflection which will lead him to some principle he regards as dependable.

Moral theory cannot emerge when there is positive belief as to what is right and what is wrong, for then there is no occasion for reflection. It emerges when men are confronted with situations in which different desires promise opposed goods and in which incompatible courses of action seem to be morally justified. Only such a conflict of good ends and of standards and rules of right and wrong calls forth personal inquiry into the bases of morals. A critical juncture may occur when a person, for example, goes from a protected home life into the stress of competitive business, and finds that moral standards which apply in one do not hold in the other. Unless he merely drifts, accommodating himself to whatever social pressure is uppermost, he will feel the conflict. If he tries to face it in thought, he will search for a reasonable principle by which to decide where the right really lies. In so doing he enters into the domain of moral theory, even if he does so unwittingly.

For what is called moral theory is but a more conscious and systematic raising of the question which occupies the mind of any one who in the face of moral conflict and doubt seeks a way out through reflection. In short, moral theory is but an extension of what is involved in all reflective morality. There are two kinds of moral struggle. One kind, and that the most emphasized in moral writings and lectures, is the conflict which takes place when an individual is tempted to do something which he is convinced is wrong. Such instances are important practically in the life of an individual, but they are not

the occasion of moral theory. The employee of a bank who is tempted to embezzle funds may indeed try to argue himself into finding reasons why it would not be wrong for him to do it. But in such a case, he is not really thinking, but merely permitting his desire to govern his beliefs. There is no sincere doubt in his mind as to what he should do when he seeks to find some justification for what he has made up his mind to do.

Take, on the other hand, the case of a citizen of a nation which has just declared war on another country. He is deeply attached to his own State. He has formed habits of loyalty and of abiding by its laws, and now one of its decrees is that he shall support war. He feels in addition gratitude and affection for the country which has sheltered and nurtured him. But he believes that this war is unjust, or perhaps he has a conviction that all war is a form of murder and hence wrong. One side of his nature, one set of convictions and habits, leads him to acquiesce in war; another deep part of his being protests. He is torn between two duties: he experiences a conflict between the incompatible values presented to him by his habits of citizenship and by his religious beliefs respectively. Up to this time, he has never experienced a struggle between the two; they have coincided and reënforced one another. Now he has to make a choice between competing moral loyalties and convictions. The struggle is not between a good which is clear to him and something else which attracts him but which he knows to be wrong. It is between values each of which is an undoubted good in its place but which now get in each other's way. He is forced to reflect in order to come to a decision. Moral theory is a generalized extension of the kind of thinking in which he now engages.

There are periods in history when a whole community or a group in a community finds itself in the presence of new issues which its old customs do not adequately meet. The habits and beliefs which were formed in the past do not fit into the opportunities and requirements of contemporary life. The age in Greece following the time of Pericles was of this sort; that of the Jews after their captivity; that following the Middle Ages when secular interests on a large scale were introduced into previous religious and ecclesiastic interests; the present is preëminently a period of this sort with the vast social changes which have followed the industrial expansion of the machine age.

Realization that the need for reflective morality and for moral theories grows out of conflict between ends, responsibilities, rights, and duties defines the service which moral theory may render, and also protects the student from false conceptions of its nature. The difference between customary and reflective morality is precisely that definite precepts, rules, definitive injunctions and prohibitions issue from the former, while they cannot proceed from the latter. Confusion ensues when appeal to rational principles is treated as if it were merely a substitute for custom, transferring the authority of moral commands from one source to another. Moral theory can (i) generalize the types of moral conflicts which arise, thus enabling a perplexed and doubtful individual to clarify his own particular problem by placing it in a larger context; it can (ii) state the leading ways in which such problems have been intellectually dealt with by those who have thought upon such matters; it can (iii) render personal reflection more systematic and enlightened, suggesting alternatives that might otherwise be overlooked, and stimulating greater consistency in judgment. But it does not offer a table of commandments in a catechism in which answers are as definite as are the questions which are asked. It can render personal choice more intelligent, but it cannot take the place of personal decision, which must be made in every case of moral perplexity. Such at least is the standpoint of the discussions which follow; the student who expects more from moral theory will be disappointed. The conclusion follows from the very nature of reflective morality; the attempt to set up ready-made conclusions contradicts the very nature of reflective morality. . . .

We have already noted in passing that the present time is one which is in peculiar need of reflective morals and of a working theory of morals. The scientific outlook on the world and on life has undergone and is still undergoing radical change. Methods of industry, of the production, and distribution of goods have been completely transformed. The basic conditions on which men meet and associate, in work and amusement, have been altered. There has been a vast dislocation of older habits and traditions. Travel and migration are as common as they were once unusual. The masses are educated enough to read and a prolific press exists which supplies cheap reading matter. Schooling has ceased to be the privilege of the few and has become the right and even the enforced duty of the many. The stratification of society into classes each fairly homogeneous in itself has been broken into. The area of contacts with persons and populations alien to our bringing up and traditions has enormously extended. A ward of a large city in the United States may have persons of from a score to fifty racial origins. The walls and barriers that once separated nations have become less important because of the railway, steamship, telegraph, telephone, and radio.

Only a few of the more obvious changes in social conditions and interests have been mentioned. Each one of them has created new problems and issues that contain moral values which are uncertain and disputed. Nationalism and internationalism, capital and labor, war and peace, science and religious tradition, competition and coöperation, *laissez faire* and State planning in industry, democracy and dictatorship in government, rural and city life, personal work and control *versus* investment and vicarious riches through stocks and bonds, native born and alien, contact of Jew and Gentile, of white and colored, of Catholic and Protestant, and those of new religions: a multitude of such relationships have brought to the fore new moral problems with which neither old customs nor beliefs are competent to cope. In addition, the rapidity with which social changes occur brings moral unsettlement and tends to destroy many ties which were the chief safeguards of the morals of custom. There was never a time in the history of the world when human relationships and their accompanying rights and duties, opportunities and demands, needed the unremitting and systematic attention of intelligent thought as they do at present.

From *The Concept of Morals*

Walter T. Stace

Any ethical position which denies that there is a single moral standard which is equally applicable to all men at all times may fairly be called a species of ethical relativity. There is not, the relativist asserts, merely one moral law, one code, one standard. There are many moral laws, codes, standards. What morality ordains in one place or age may be quite different from what morality ordains in another place or age. The moral code of Chinamen is quite different from that of Europeans, that of African savages quite different from both. Any morality, therefore, is relative to the age, the place, and the circumstances in which it is found. It is in no sense absolute.

This does not mean merely—as one might at first sight be inclined to suppose—that the very same kind of action which is *thought* right in one country and period may be *thought* wrong in another. This would be a mere platitude, the truth of which everyone would have to admit. Even the absolutist would admit this—would even wish to emphasize it—since he is well aware that different peoples have different sets of moral ideas, and his whole point is that some of these sets of ideas are false. What the relativist means to assert is, not this platitude, but that the very same kind of action which *is* right in one country and period may *be* wrong in another. And this, far from being a platitude, is a very startling assertion.

It is very important to grasp thoroughly the difference between the two ideas. For there is reason to think that many minds tend to find ethical relativity attractive because they fail to keep them clearly apart. It is so very obvious that moral ideas differ from country to country and from age to age. And it is so very easy, if you are mentally lazy, to suppose that to say this means the same as to say that no universal moral standard exists,—or in other words that

it implies ethical relativity. We fail to see that the word "standard" is used in two different senses. It is perfectly true that, in one sense, there are many variable moral standards. We speak of judging a man by the standard of his time. And this implies that different times have different standards. And this, of course, is quite true. But when the word "standard" is used in this sense it means simply the set of moral ideas current during the period in question. It means what people *think* right, whether as a matter of fact it *is* right or not. On the other hand when the absolutist asserts that there exists a single universal moral "standard," he is not using the word in this sense at all. He means by "standard" what *is* right as distinct from what people merely think right. His point is that although what people think right varies in different countries and periods, yet what actually is right is everywhere and always the same. And it follows that when the ethical relativist disputes the position of the absolutist and denies that any universal moral standard exists he too means by "standard" what actually is right. But it is exceedingly easy, if we are not careful, to slip loosely from using the word in the first sense to using it in the second sense; and to suppose that the variability of moral beliefs is the same thing as the variability of what really is moral. And unless we keep the two senses of the word "standard" distinct, we are likely to think the creed of ethical relativity much more plausible than it actually is.

The genuine relativist, then, does not merely mean that Chinamen may think right what Frenchmen think wrong. He means that what *is* wrong for the Frenchman may *be* right for the Chinaman. And if one enquires how, in those circumstances, one is to know what actually is right in China or in France, the answer comes quite glibly. What is right in China is the same as what people think right in China; and what is right in France is the same as what people think right in France. So that, if you want to know what is moral in any particular country or age all you have to do is to ascertain what are the moral ideas current in that age or country. Those ideas are, *for that age or country,* right. Thus what is morally right is identified with what is thought to be morally right, and the distinction which we made above between these two is simply denied. . . .

To sum up. The ethical relativist consistently denies, it would seem, whatever the ethical absolutist asserts. For the absolutist there is a single universal moral standard. For the relativist there is no such standard. There are only local, ephemeral, and variable standards. For the absolutist there are two senses of the word "standard." Standards in the sense of sets of current moral ideas are relative and changeable. But the standard in the sense of what is actually morally right is absolute and unchanging. For the relativist no such distinction can be made. There is only one meaning of the word standard, namely, that which refers to local and variable sets of moral ideas. Or if it is insisted that the word must be allowed two meanings, then the relativist will say that there is at any rate no actual example of a standard in the absolute sense, and that the word as thus used is an empty name to which nothing in reality corresponds; so that the distinction between the two meanings becomes empty and useless. Finally—though this is merely saying the same thing in another way—the absolutist makes a distinction between what actually is right and what is thought right. The relativist rejects this distinction and identifies what is moral with what is thought moral by certain human beings or groups of human beings. . . .

I shall now proceed to consider, first, the main arguments which can be urged in favour of ethical relativity; and secondly, the arguments which can be urged against it. . . .

There are, I think, [two] main arguments in favour of ethical relativity. The first is that which relies upon the actual varieties of moral "standards" found in the world. It was easy enough to believe in a single absolute morality in older times when there was no anthropology, when all humanity was divided clearly into two groups, Christian peoples and the "heathen." Christian peoples knew and possessed the one true morality. The rest were savages whose moral ideas could be ignored. But all this is

changed. Greater knowledge has brought greater tolerance. We can no longer exalt our morality as alone true, while dismissing all other moralities as false or inferior. The investigations of anthropologists have shown that there exist side by side in the world a bewildering variety of moral codes. On this topic endless volumes have been written, masses of evidence piled up. Anthropologists have ransacked the Melanesian Islands, the jungles of New Guinea, the steppes of Siberia, the deserts of Australia, the forests of central Africa, and have brought back with them countless examples of weird, extravagant and fantastic "moral" customs with which to confound us. We learn that all kinds of horrible practices are, in this, that, or the other place, regarded as essential to virtue. We find that there is nothing, or next to nothing, which has always and everywhere been regarded as morally good by all men. Where then is our universal morality? Can we, in face of all this evidence, deny that it is nothing but an empty dream?

This argument, taken by itself, is a very weak one. It relies upon a single set of facts—the variable moral customs of the world. But this variability of moral ideas is admitted by both parties to the dispute, and is capable of ready explanation upon the hypothesis of either party. The relativist says that the facts are to be explained by the non-existence of any absolute moral standard. The absolutist says that they are to be explained by human ignorance of what the absolute moral standard is. And he can truly point out that men have differed widely in their opinions about all manner of topics including the subject matters of the physical sciences—just as much as they differ about morals. And if the various different opinions which men have held about the shape of the earth do not prove that it has no real shape, either do the various opinions which they have held about morality prove that there is no one true morality.

Thus the facts can be explained equally plausibly on either hypothesis. There is nothing in the facts themselves which compels us to prefer the relativistic hypothesis to that of the absolutist. And therefore the argument fails to prove the relativist conclusion. If that conclusion is to be established, it must be by means of other considerations. . . .

The [second] argument in favour of ethical relativity is also a very strong one. And it does not suffer from the disadvantage that it is dependent upon the acceptance of any particular philosophy such as radical empiricism. It makes its appeal to considerations of a quite general character. It consists in alleging that no one has ever been able to discover upon what foundation an absolute morality could rest, or from what source a universally binding moral code could derive its authority.

If, for example, it is an absolute and unalterable moral rule that all men ought to be unselfish, from whence does this *command* issue? For a command it certainly is, phrase it how you please. There is no difference in meaning between the sentence ''You ought to be unselfish'' and the sentence ''Be unselfish.'' Now a command implies a commander. An obligation implies some authority which obliges. Who is this commander, what this authority? Thus the vastly difficult question is raised of *the basis of moral obligation*. Now the argument of the relativist would be that it is impossible to find any basis for a universally binding moral law; but that it is quite easy to discover a basis for morality if moral codes are admitted to be variable, ephemeral, and relative to time, place, and circumstance.

In this book I am assuming that it is no longer possible to solve this difficulty by saying naïvely that the universal moral law is based upon the uniform commands of God to all men. There will be many, no doubt, who will dispute this. But I am not writing for them. I am writing for those who feel the necessity of finding for morality a basis independent of particular religious dogmas. And I shall therefore make no attempt to argue the matter.

The problem which the absolutist has to face, then, is this. The religious basis of the one absolute morality having disappeared, can there be found for it any other, any secular, basis? If not, then it would seem that we cannot any longer believe in absolutism. We shall have to fall back upon belief in a variety of perhaps mutually inconsistent moral codes operating over restricted areas and limited periods. No

one of these will be better, or more true, than any other. Each will be good and true for those living in those areas and periods. We shall have to fall back, in a word, on ethical relativity.

For there is no great difficulty in discovering the foundations of morality, or rather of moralities, if we adopt the relativistic hypothesis. Even if we cannot be quite certain *precisely* what these foundations are—and relativists themselves are not entirely agreed about them—we can at least see in a general way the *sort* of foundations they must have. We can see that the question on this basis is not in principle impossible of answer—although the details may be obscure; while, if we adopt the absolutist hypothesis—so the argument runs—no kind of answer is conceivable at all.

Relativists, speaking generally, offer two different solutions of the problem, either of which, or perhaps some compromise between the two, might be correct. According to some the basis of morality is in ''emotion.'' According to others it is in ''customs.''. . .

These two views are not really incompatible. For customs surely have their roots in men's feelings. And to say that morality is based on customs is in the end the same as to say that it is based on feelings. One view emphasizes the outward behaviour which exhibits itself in customs; the other view emphasizes the inward feelings which give rise to this behaviour. The dispute is a professional one between rival schools of psychology. It does not affect the larger issues with which we are concerned.

But in spite of the strength of the argument thus posed in favour of ethical relativity, it is not impregnable. For it leaves open one loop-hole. It is always possible that some theory, not yet examined, may provide a basis for a universal moral obligation. The argument rests upon the negative proposition that *there is no theory which can provide a basis for a universal morality*. But it is notoriously difficult to prove a negative. How can you prove that there are no green swans? All you can show is that none have been found so far. And then it is always possible that one will be found tomorrow. So it is here. The relativist shows that no theory of the basis of moral obligation has yet been discovered which could validate a universal morality. Perhaps.

But it is just conceivable that one might be discovered in the course of this book.

It is time that we turned our attention from the case in favour of ethical relativity to the case against it. Now the case against it consists, to a very large extent, in urging that, if taken seriously and pressed to its logical conclusion, ethical relativity can only end in destroying the conception of morality altogether, in undermining its practical efficacy, in rendering meaningless many almost universally accepted truths about human affairs, in robbing human beings of any incentive to strive for a better world, in taking the life-blood out of every ideal and every aspiration which has ever ennobled the life of man. . . .

First of all, then, ethical relativity, in asserting that the moral standards of particular social groups are the only standards which exist, renders meaningless all propositions which attempt to compare these standards with one another in respect of their moral worth. And this is a very serious matter indeed. We are accustomed to think that the moral ideas of one nation or social group may be "higher" or "lower" than those of another. We believe, for example, that Christian ethical ideals are nobler than those of the savage races of central Africa. Probably most of us would think that the Chinese moral standards are higher than those of the inhabitants of New Guinea. In short we habitually compare one civilization with another and judge the sets of ethical ideas to be found in them to be some better, some worse. The fact that such judgments are very difficult to make with any justice, and that they are frequently made on very superficial and prejudiced grounds, has no bearing on the question now at issue. The question is whether such judgments have any *meaning*. We habitually assume that they have.

But on the basis of ethical relativity they can have none whatever. For the relativist must hold that there is no *common* standard which can be applied to the various civilizations judged. Any such comparison of moral standards implies the existence of some superior standard which is applicable to both. And the existence of any such standard is precisely what the relativist denies. According to him the Christian standard is applicable only to Christians,

the Chinese standard only to Chinese, the New Guinea standard only to the inhabitants of New Guinea.

What is true of comparisons between the moral standards of different races will also be true of comparisons between those of different ages. It is not unusual to ask such questions as whether the standard of our own day is superior to that which existed among our ancestors five hundred years ago. And when we remember that our ancestors employed slaves, practiced barbaric physical tortures, and burnt people alive, we may be inclined to think that it is. At any rate we assume that the question is one which has meaning and is capable of rational discussion. But if the ethical relativist is right, whatever we assert on this subject must be totally meaningless. For here again there is no common standard which could form the basis of any such judgments.

This in its turn implies that the whole notion of moral *progress* is a sheer delusion. Progress means an advance from lower to higher, from worse to better. But on the basis of ethical relativity it has no meaning to say that the standards of this age are better (or worse) than those of a previous age. For there is no common standard by which both can be measured. Thus it is nonsense to say that the morality of the New Testament is higher than that of the Old. And Jesus Christ, if he imagined that he was introducing into the world a higher ethical standard than existed before his time, was merely deluded.

Thus the ethical relativist must treat all judgments comparing different moralities as either entirely meaningless; or, if this course appears too drastic, he has the alternative of declaring that they have for their meaning-content nothing except the vanity and egotism of those who pass them. We are asked to believe that the highest moral ideals of humanity are not really any better than those of an Australian bushman. But if this is so, why strive for higher ideals? Thus the heart is taken out of all effort, and the meaning out of all human ideals and aspirations. . . .

I come now to a second point. Up to the present I have allowed it to be taken tacitly for granted that, though judgments comparing different races and ages in respect of the worth of their moral codes are impossible for the ethical relativist, yet judgments of comparison between individuals living within the same social group would be quite possible. For individuals living within the same social group would presumably be subject to the same moral code, that of their group, and this would therefore constitute, as between these individuals, a common standard by which they could both be measured. We have not here, as we had in the other case, the difficulty of the absence of any common standard of comparison. It should therefore be possible for the ethical relativist to say quite meaningfully that President Lincoln was a better man than some criminal or moral imbecile of his own time and country, or that Jesus was a better man than Judas Iscariot.

But is even this minimum of moral judgment really possible on relativist grounds? It seems to me that it is not. For when once the whole of humanity is abandoned as the area covered by a single moral standard, what smaller areas are to be adopted as the *loci* of different standards? Where are we to draw the lines of demarcation? We can split up humanity, perhaps,—though the procedure will be very arbitrary—into races, races into nations, nations into tribes, tribes into families, families into individuals. Where are we going to draw the *moral* boundaries? Does the *locus* of a particular moral standard reside in a race, a nation, a tribe, a family, or an individual? Perhaps the blessed phrase "social group" will be dragged in to save the situation. Each such group, we shall be told, has its own moral code which is, for it, right. But what *is* a "group"? Can anyone define it or give its boundaries? . . .

If these arguments are valid, the ethical relativist cannot really maintain that there is anywhere to be found a moral standard binding upon anybody against his will. And he cannot maintain that, even within the social group, there is a common standard as between individuals. And if that is so, then even judgments to the effect that one man is morally better than another become meaningless. All moral valuation thus vanishes. There is nothing to prevent each man from being a rule unto himself. The result will be moral chaos and the collapse of all effective standards. . . .

Legalism and Medical Ethics

John Ladd

This essay is concerned with some general questions about methodology in medical ethics. As such it belongs under what is generally called "metaethics" or the "logic of ethics," that is, the second-level inquiry into moral concepts, rules, and principles and their logical interrelations. I believe that it is important to get straightened out about some of these methodological questions as a propaedeutic to an inquiry into more substantive moral issues. For, although I believe that metaethics cannot be separated from substantive (or normative)

Reprinted with permission from the author and *The Journal of Medicine & Philosophy,* vol. 4, no. 1, 1979, pp. 70–80.

ethics, I also believe that one cannot pursue the latter in any depth without considering metaethical issues. To paraphrase Kant's famous dictum, "Metaethics without normative ethics is empty, but normative ethics without metaethics is blind."[1]

I want to focus on certain aspects of the kinds of moral problem encountered in medical ethics that raise interesting methodological questions for philosophers. In particular, I shall be concerned with methodological questions created by the concreteness and particularity of moral problems in the medical context, which make it difficult to relate them to the kind of abstract theories that have been generally advanced by philosophers—for example, theories like utilitarianism, Kantianism, intuitionism, natural law and natural rights theories, Rawlsianism, etc. John Stuart Mill called attention to this metaethical problem when he pointed out that the principle of utility is by itself too general and abstract to answer the question, What ought to be done here and now? In order to answer this question, we need, in addition to the principle of utility, secondary principles (namely, practices, rules, concepts, moral notions) to mediate between the abstract super-principle and concrete cases of action or decision making.

"Without such middle principles," Mill wrote, "an universal principle, either in science or in morals, serves for little but a thesaurus of commonplaces for the discussion of questions, instead of a means of deciding them" (Mill 1965, p. 178).[2]

The task for medical ethics, then, is to find appropriate and legitimate secondary principles and categories for dealing with its special problems. In their quest for secondary principles and categories, writers on medical ethics have generally turned to the law. For law, by its very nature, is designed to deal with particular cases, and legal categories, rules, and concepts are much easier to apply directly to concrete situations than are formal and abstract super-principles like the principle of utility or the categorical imperative. Also, because of its flexibility, law appears well adapted to resolve the new kinds of moral problems that arise in the medical context.

Legal answers are readily available for many of these problems, and so it is easy to understand why most problems of medical ethics are discussed in terms of the law. Controversies concerning such diverse matters as euthanasia, paternalism, experimentation, informed consent, organ transplantation, etc., are almost always couched in the language of the law and are treated as ethico-legal issues rather than as either moral or legal issues. As a consequence, it is almost always unclear what the point of issue is in such controversies—for example, Is euthanasia a legal or a moral issue?

Still, the uncritical mingling of legal and moral questions, as well as the indiscriminate use of legal rules and concepts for solving moral problems must be viewed with concern, for they completely distort our perception of the problems and force unacceptable answers on us. I shall refer to this fusion of law and ethics as "legalism."

GENERAL REMARKS ON LEGALISM

By "legalism," I shall mean: "the ethical attitude that holds moral conduct to be a matter of rule following, and moral relationships to consist of duties and rights determined by rules."[3]

The term "legalism" will be used extremely broadly in this article to stand for an attitude or a general approach rather than a specific doctrine. The main thrust of legalism, however, is the legalization of morality and the moralization of law, which generally imply the assimilation of moral and legal issues, of moral reasoning and legal reasoning, and, in general, of moral problems and legal problems. The specific aspect of legalism that I shall focus on is the use of the model of law as a model for the formulation, analysis, and solution of ethical issues.

Although I have misgivings about legalism, I do not wish to disparage the law—as such. What I want to emphasize here is that the function of law, of legal argumentation, and of legal concepts (e.g., rights) is different from the function of ethics, ethical argumentation, and ethical concepts. In Wittgensteinian terms, they are two different language games. The assimilation of functions entirely ignores such things as the use of the law as a socially acceptable and effective means of coping with conflicts of interest and of enforcing socially desirable rules and policies. To put it bluntly, we go to lawyers when we are in trouble and not when we need general advice on how to resolve our personal and social problems. Law usually arises out of conflicts—for example, of interests—and is a social mechanism for resolving conflicts. Ethics, on the other hand, arises out of and is concerned with much wider and deeper perplexities about life and our relations with each other. It follows that different modes of argumentation and different organizing concepts will be relevant and appropriate for ethics from those relevant and appropriate for the law. I shall argue, in as much detail as possible, that the failure to bear in mind the essentially different functions of the two kinds of discourse creates a great deal of confusion, particularly for medical ethics, and for bad ethics and bad jurisprudence.

THE UTILITY OF LEGALISM

We may begin by observing that legalism is not something new, for legalistic ethics or moralistic jurisprudence of the kind I have in mind goes back in Anglo-American society at least as far as Blackstone (1973), who thought that the Common Law was, or ought to be, the embodiment of morality.

There are many reasons for the wide appeal of legalism in popular American ethical thinking and in medical ethics in particular. To begin with, it represents our own peculiar brand of rugged individualism and, as such, has deep roots in American history. Alexis de Tocqueville (1959, vol. 1, p. 290) remarked on the importance of lawyers in American public life and suggested that the language of the law was the "vulgar tongue" of American politics. In a pluralistic society such as ours, a melting pot of diverse religions and ideologies, the language of the law serves as a kind of *lingua franca* for discussions of social and political questions and provides a set of commonly agreed upon ground rules for the settling of conflicts and disagreements, as well as commonly accepted premises for use in public debates.

One practical advantage of law and of the concept of rights in particular is that, insofar as they establish rules of conduct, they serve to define our relationships with strangers as well as with people whom we know. In the medical context, this fact about law and rights is especially important practically, for we may find ourselves in a hospital bed in a strange place, with strange company, and confronted by a strange physician and staff. The strangeness of the situation makes the concept of rights, both legal and moral, a very useful tool for defining our relationships to those with whom we have to deal.

Yet another useful function of law and of the concept of rights is that they serve to define our relationships to impersonal beings like formal organizations—for example, hospitals.[4] This is important because, sooner or later, almost all of the issues relating to such things as euthanasia, the doctor-patient relationship, confidentiality and record keeping, the initiation or termination of treatment, the operations of intensive care units, etc., are tangled up with questions about the rules and regulations of organizations like hospitals or of the medical profession—for example, questions concerning which administrative rules and regulations ought to be adopted, changed, revoked, overridden, ignored, etc.

In sum, legalism serves many useful functions in providing standards for evaluating, criticizing, and ordering social and legal rules through the use of, say, the concept of rights. In particular, as a theory of rights, legalism can be used to protect our interests and concerns against the encroachments, not only of government, but also of formal organizations and professional associations. The Lockean theory of natural rights and other theories of rights were, after all, originally conceived as weapons against the pretensions of absolutist governments. It would seem quite appropriate, therefore, to use the same concepts against more modern versions of tyranny.

Before we decide that legalism provides the only or the most acceptable approach to moral problems in medical ethics, however, we ought to take a second look at the moral bases of legalism and examine some of its implications and limitations. In order to do this, I shall concentrate on the notion of rights, which is a typical legalistic category and one that is very generally used as a bridge concept between law and ethics in discussions of medical ethics.

THE RIGHTS MODEL[5]

Whether we are talking about actual or possible legal rights, human rights, or natural rights, there are certain specific logical properties attached to rights that distinguish them from other moral (and legal) categories. Since the logical properties of rights have been extensively treated in the literature and I have discussed them in some detail elsewhere, I shall examine only three of these properties here: (1) the peremptory nature of rights, (2) the particular kind of interpersonal relationship implied in the appeal to rights, and (3) the ethical importance of distinguishing between the possession and the exercise of a right (see Ladd 1979). If any of these three conditions is omitted or modified when rights are being claimed, the appeal to rights loses its stringency.

The first property of rights is their peremptoriness. That is, unlike other moral considerations, such as appeals for help, rights are the sort of thing that may be demanded peremptorily; to secure them, it is usually permissible to use coercion, either in the form of legal action or in the form of self-help. In general, when a person's rights are involved, many sorts of action are authorized that would otherwise be impermissible. Thus, the right of self-defense, either legal or moral, is used to excuse the killing of another person.

A second important logical property of rights is that they represent a relationship between two persons (or parties): the right-holder and the right-owner.[6] To have a right is to have a right against someone (or against anyone or everyone). The natural and normal situation in which a person asserts a right is when the person against whom he asserts it threatens, neglects, or otherwise appears unwilling to accede to his requests, needs, or demands. There is a sense, therefore, in which the assertion of a right is reactive, that is, it represents a response to another person's actual, probable, or possible negative behavior. In other words, the concept of rights is most characteristically used in an adversary context.

Finally, it is particularly important to note the difference between possessing a right and exercising it. Flathman (1976, pp. 71 ff.) suggests that one can possess a right only if one can choose not to exercise it. In this regard, rights reflect the concept of a person as self-directed or self-governed. Strictly speaking, this condition requires that the right-holder be a competent adult capable of self-directed choice. The idea of a proxy who exercises a person's right is, therefore, an anomaly, or at least it has no moral standing; it might still, of course, serve a useful legal purpose.

Assuming that these three properties are essential to any meaningful assertion of rights, we can see why it is sometimes quite inappropriate ethically to base medical decisions on the notion of rights alone.[7] For medical advice or patients' requests need not be peremptory—that is, put in the form of demands backed by force—and the doctor-patient relationship need not be an adversary relationship. (That is not to say, of course, that it may not turn into an adversary relationship.)

Furthermore, most moral problems that arise in connection with medical decision making simply bypass questions about rights, because none of the parties involved feel it necessary to appeal to their rights—that is, to exercise them. For example, although a patient may have the right to refuse treatment or a doctor may have the right to refuse to treat, it is difficult, if not impossible, for them to discuss rationally with each other what treatment should be undertaken if either of them chooses to exercise his right.[8]

Finally, requests for help from family and friends are not and perhaps ought not to be based on who has a right against whom. For if a request is based on a right, it will more than likely destroy the relationship altogether, because it implies the absence of trust. That is why the appeal to rights is sometimes inappropriate, improper, and immoral, and standing on one's rights is a last-ditch stand, to be taken only after communication has broken down or when there is no communication to begin with.[9]

ANOTHER MODEL: MORAL RELATIONSHIPS AND DUTIES

The disadvantages of the rights model as a conceptual tool for analyzing moral problems in the medical context suggest that we should investigate other possible models. For there must be some other kinds of relationships besides rights relationships, and other sorts of moral categories besides entitlements, that will give us a better understanding of the moral problems that we are concerned about. What we need is a moral principle to cover such things as caring, providing for another person's needs, helping others, etc. More generally, we need an ethics of giving and receiving, that is, an ethics that gives us a moral principle concerning the rightness of giving and receiving that is not based simply on rights or entitlements.

The ethics that I propose bases giving and receiving on certain kinds of interpersonal relationship.[10] The principle may be formulated schematically as follows: A ought to do X for B because A is related to B (ArB) and B needs X (BnX). For example, a mother ought to feed her baby because it is her baby and the baby needs to be fed. The underlying principle of giving and receiving involved here is nicely expressed in the old socialist slogan: from each according to his abilities, to each according to his needs.[11] The mother has the ability, the baby has the need. In the doctor-patient relationship, the doctor has the ability (e.g., the know-how) and the patient has the need.

RESPONSIBILITIES

The moral duties that stem from interpersonal relationships can be brought together under the more general concept of responsibility. By "responsibility," I mean a concern that a person ought to have for another person's welfare by virtue of a special relationship that obtains between him and the other person. Under "welfare" should be included such things as a person's security, health, education, and moral integrity. The formula given in the preceding section may be revised to cover the responsibility relationship: A is responsible for B's welfare (i.e., B's health, education, etc.) because ArB.[12] In this sense of responsibility, parents are responsible for the welfare of their children; friends are responsible for each other's welfare; doctors and nurses are responsible for the welfare of their patients, and so on. Furthermore, being responsible is a kind of virtue, and being irresponsible is a kind of vice; for it is impossible to be a good parent, a good friend, a good doctor, or a good nurse without taking one's responsibilities for the other seriously, that is, acting responsibly toward him, being responsible.

It is obvious, therefore, that fulfilling one's responsibility for a person's welfare differs in important respects from fulfilling a person's rights. To do what a right-holder demands may be inconsistent with one's responsibility to him; for giving someone what he has a right to may in fact not be good for him at all—indeed, it may be quite harmful.[13] By the same token, when a person exercises what is clearly one of his rights he may cause harm to others for whom he is responsible or, for that matter, to himself. For these reasons, therefore, it should be clear that responsibilities belong to a different moral category from the categories of rights-obligations.

A COMPARISON OF THE TWO MODELS

There are at least four important ways in which an ethics of relationships and responsibilities is unlike legalism.[14]

First, the kinds of consideration that are relevant to moral decisions based on moral responsibility are quite different from those that are relevant to decisions based on moral rights. In deciding questions of responsibilities, a much wider range of factors must be taken into account than in deciding questions of rights; a responsible decision may require consideration of such different things as risks and benefits, other relationships, concerns, needs, and abilities of persons affected by and affecting the decision. In addition, in order to make responsible decisions it is usually necessary to "weigh" a number of factors against each other; the final decision often requires what we generally call "judgment." Moral philosophers customarily say that such decisions are the outcome of deliberation, reflection, consultation, and discussion.[15]

Decisions based on rights, on the other hand, are quite different. They do not permit taking into account most of the considerations mentioned, and they do not involve the same kind of weighing, deliberation, judgment, etc., that is called for in cases of responsibility. Indeed, one of the special and distinctive logical properties of a right is that normally, in determining whether to comply with it, one is not permitted to consider any factors other than those directly relating to the status of the right itself and one's ability to do what it requires.[16]

Second, unlike situations where the issue is simply one of rights, attitudes are an essential ingredient of action in an ethics of responsibility; for it is impossible to conceive of moral responsibility apart from an attitude of concern, of caring, and of being solicitous and considerate, etc. Such attitudes are part of the concept of a responsible action. Indeed, even to describe what kind of action is required by a responsibility of a certain sort it often suffices to refer to one of these attitudes. As far as rights are concerned, on the other hand, one's attitudes (and motives) are immaterial; the only thing that counts is that one perform the kind of action required by the right.

Third, in a relationship of responsibility there is a certain kind of antecedent inequality between the parties as far as their needs and abilities are concerned; one person needs to be helped while the other has the ability to help. The rights relationship, on the other hand, is based on the assumption of a certain kind of antecedent equality between the two parties, as is supposed to exist between those entering into a contractual agreement; of course, in actuality, this presumed equality is more often than not fictional. Nevertheless, the notion of "freedom of contract," a basic concept in the ethic of rights, would make no sense if one party were able to impose its will on the other party because of some sort of inequality between them. Thus, where equality in the sense of independence is required by rights relationships, it is of the very essence of responsibility relations that, in some way or other, one person be dependent on the other person. In that sense, the person in question is not a free operator.

The bearing of these conceptual differences between rights and responsibilities on the medical care situation is obvious, for in critically important ways the patient is likely to be in an initial state of dependence and inequality vis-à-vis the doctor; to speak of rights—for example, contractual rights—in such cases is an absurdity. Often, a patient is in no position to assert or exercise a right that he already possesses. Given the prior acceptance of an ethics of rights, the helpfulness of the patient is usually used to justify the assumption of the right to make decisions on the part of the doctor. What I am suggesting is that the unreflective acceptance of an ethics of rights in preference, say, to an ethics of responsibility inevitably leads to moral confusion and irresponsibility of this kind, for the simple reason that the ethics of rights rests on the twin assumptions, often inconsistent, that someone must have the right and that, in the ultimate analysis, rights relationships can only obtain between equals.

On the other hand, the ethics of responsibility implies another sort of equality that is not as obviously a part of an ethics of rights, namely, the equal worth and dignity of individuals, those who are helpless and infirm as well as those who are able and powerful. For an ethics of responsibility requires that all persons involved in the relationship treat each other with equal consideration. Equal consideration here means that help should be matched to needs, rather than to interests, demands, or merit.[17] It also means that the persons involved in the relationship must treat each other with mutual respect and understanding.[18] In other words, persons morally responsibile for others should treat them as ends and not as mere means—all the way through, as it were, and all the time, rather than just partially and occasionally, as is usually the case when morality is reduced, for example, to contractual relations. One way in which the difference between these two conceptions of equality could be put is to say that in an ethics of rights equality is a *terminus a quo,* whereas in an ethics of responsibility it is a *terminus ad quem.*

Finally, responsibility relationships are dynamic—that is, they change and develop through time as the needs and abilities of the persons develop and their conditions change. One important way in which such relationships develop is through open discussion, consultation, argumentation, and persuasion. Where there is disparity in, say, knowledge or maturity, the responsibility project may become educational, in the best sense. The doctor-patient relationship is itself, in many ways, often an educational relationship involving teaching as much as treating; sometimes, indeed, the teaching may be mutual.[19] A good doctor explains to the patient the nature of his disease, the options as far as treatment is concerned, risks, benefits, prognoses, etc. One of his aims is, or ought to be, to educate and thereby to help the patient to accommodate himself to his disease in various sorts of ways. That accommodation is a dynamic process and inevitably brings about changes in the patient himself, if not in the doctor. The outcome aimed at may be thought of as a kind of equality, the equalization of an initial inequality.

An ethics of rights, on the other hand, is static and not subject to the kind of changes and development that characterize the ethics of responsibility. For rights are preexistent and predetermined before the decision process even begins. Thus, the ethics of rights, as such, leaves no room for the kind of mutual education and mutual accommodation that may be necessary to change the situation for the benefit, say, of the patient.[20]

In this article, I have tried to point out some of the difficulties in using the concept of rights indiscriminately as a tool of analysis in medical ethics. I have suggested, as an alternative, the model of relationships and responsibilities, which sometimes gives us a more subtle and human way of dealing with moral problems in the medical context. In conclusion, I want to emphasize once again that the language of ethics is a rich language; it contains a wealth of concepts, principles, and arguments that are available for our use. Therefore, not only ought we to eschew the quest of a slot-mathine ethics or jurisprudence, but we ought also to explore other tools of analysis besides those currently in vogue.

Notes

1. This view of the relationship between metaethics and normative ethics is set forth in Ladd (1973). This article was published in Polish; a typewritten copy of the original English version is available from the author.

2. The same consideration applies to other super-principles such as the categorical imperative, the common good, conforming to nature, etc.

3. I have borrowed this definition from Shklar (1964, p. 1). See also Scheingold (1974).

4. As I have argued elsewhere, formal organizations are not moral beings and cannot, and should not, be perceived as moral persons having moral obligations, moral rights, and moral responsibilities (see Ladd 1970).

5. For a more detailed discussion of the model of rights along the lines suggested here, see Flathman (1976).

6. When considered as a practice, other parties may be involved, as it were, to support or enforce the rights (see Flathman 1976).

7. Strictly speaking, this statement applies only to what I call "proprietary rights," the kind that hold between individuals. It does not apply to what I elsewhere call "ideal rights," "welfare rights" (McCloskey 1965), or "manifesto rights" (Feinberg 1970). The latter set objectives of social policy and legislation and are not directly relevant to the doctor-patient relationship (see Ladd 1979).

8. I do not wish to suggest that a patient's rights are not sometimes entirely ignored by physicians and hospital staffs when medical decisions are made. But I simply want to point out that honesty and honorableness are not requirements that are based on rights; common decency and respect for the patient are moral desiderata quite apart from any rights he may possess.

9. ". . . and when men are friends they have no need of justice" (Aristotle 1155a25).

10. I do not mean relationships of a casual or transient sort, but the kind of relationship that Aristotle called "friendship," which includes family, companions, colleagues, and perhaps even doctors and patients!

11. I have been unable to ascertain the precise source of this slogan, which was already current in French socialist literature before 1848. It is generally attributed to Louis Blanc.

12. For further details about this concept of responsibility, see Ladd (1975).

13. The moral dilemma that this inconsistency between needs and rights presents is familiar to doctors.

14. An ethics of responsibility cannot be applied directly on the impersonal, institutional level simply because responsibility, as conceived here, involves a relationship between persons, whereas formal organizations (e.g., hospitals) are not persons in the sense required (see n. 4).

15. See Aristotle on deliberation (book 3, chap. 3); see also Dewey (1922, pp. 189–209).

16. I call this logical property of rights their "opacity" (see Ladd 1979).

17. This kind of equality was called proportional equality by the French socialists who invented the slogan already mentioned.

18. "... it is of the essence of proper respect that we encourage others to be co-agents, and accept and welcome them as such, each of us, to engage in this enterprise only in ways that are consistent with this attitude" (MacLagan 1960, p. 294).

19. This is one of the main points made in Cassell (1976).

20. The reader should not conclude that I am advocating paternalism, unless it is assumed that education, counseling, and persuasion are by definition "paternalistic."

References

ARISTOTLE. *Nicomachean Ethics.*

BLACKSTONE, WILLIAM. *The Sovereignty of Law,* Edited by Gareth Jones. Toronto: University of Toronto Press, 1973.

CASSELL, ERIC. *The Art of Healing.* Philadelphia: J. B. Lippincott Co., 1976.

DAVIS, JOHN W.; HOFFMASTER, C. B.; and SHORTEN, S., eds., *Biomedical Ethics.* New York: Humana Press, 1978.

DEWEY, JOHN. *Human Nature and Conduct.* New York: Henry Holt & Co., 1922.

FEINBERG, JOEL. "The Nature and Value of Rights." *Journal of Value Inquiry* 4, no. 4 (Winter 1970): 243–57. Reprinted in *Moral Problems in Medicine,* 1st ed., edited by Samuel Gorovitz, Andrew Jameton, Ruth Macklin, John M. O'Connor, Eugene V. Perrin, Beverely Page St. Clair, and Susan Sherwin. Englewood Cliffs, N.J.: Prentice-Hall, Inc., 1976.

FLATHMAN, RICHARD. *The Practice of Rights.* Cambridge: Cambridge University Press, 1976.

LADD, JOHN. "Morality and the Ideal of Rationality in Formal Organizations." *Monist* 54, no. 4 (October 1970): 488–516.

LADD, JOHN. "The Interdependence of Ethical Analysis and Ethics." *ETYKA* 2 (1973): 139–58.

LADD, JOHN. "The Ethics of Participation" In *Participation in Politics,* edited by J. Roland Pennock and John Chapman. New York: Atherton-Lieber, 1975.

LADD, JOHN. "The Definition of Death and the Right to Die." In *Ethical Issues Relating to Life and Death,* New York: Oxford University Press, 1979.

McCLOSKEY, H. J. "Rights." *Philosophical Quarterly* 15 (1965): 115–27.

MacLAGAN, W. G. "Respect for Persons as a Moral Principle. II." *Philosophy* 35, no. 135 (October 1960): 289–305.

MILL, JOHN STUART. "Dr. Whewell on Moral Philosophy." In *Mill's Ethical Writings,* edited by J. B. Schneewind. New York: Macmillan Co., 1965.

SCHEINGOLD, STUART A. *The Politics of Rights.* New Haven, Conn.: Yale University Press, 1974.

SHKLAR, JUDITH. *Legalism.* Cambridge, Mass.: Harvard University Press, 1964.

TOCQUEVILLE, ALEXIS DE. *Democracy in America.* New York: Vintage, 1959.

Some Things Medical Ethics Is Not

K. Danner Clouser

Medical ethics has suddenly moved to center stage. It is vigorously discussed in many quarters; medical schools are in various stages of developing teaching programs dealing with these issues.

Reprinted by permission of the author and the American Medical Association from *JAMA,* vol. 223, no. 7, pp. 787–789. Copyright 1973, American Medical Association.

At this point in its spiraling development, it may be helpful to consider the nature of medical ethics, if only in an effort to stem conceptual sprawl. Conceptual confusion results when ethics tries to be all things to all people. It must trim down to fighting weight, refusing to encompass in its definition all that has been thrust upon it. An explication of "freedom" that included everything anyone has ever meant by the word would be meaningless by virtue of sheer generality, excluding little if anything. So too with "ethics."

My plan is to discuss some things medical ethics is not. A sheer list itemizing what is not ethics would be dictatorial and uninformative. Instead, I will guess at why some disciplines are sometimes thought appropriate housing for medical ethics, and then I will say why that view is mistaken. I will begin with the more obvious distinctions, gathering momentum for the more subtle.

One footnote about this negative approach is in order. Aside from the practical help it may afford those launching programs, there is a systematic point to be made. Determining what is not medical ethics is an important intermediary step in forging a definition of medical ethics. Leaping immediately from intuitive notion to rigid definition cuts off, by definition, consideration of borderline possibilities. The negative intermediate step is a means of reflectively zeroing in on an elusive concept, without strangling the incipient insights and fruitful observations that accrue to the open questioning search for a definition.

Of course, exclusions ought not be arbitrary; they must be justified in the usual systematic way: appeals to key concepts, to consistency, to conceptual economy, and the like. However, the goals of this article are better served by surface descriptions unencumbered by these weightier justifications.

OBVIOUS DISTINCTIONS

At this level, perhaps all we need is a list read with the ring of authority. Medical ethics is not sociology, medical ethics is not history of medicine, medical ethics is not anthropology, nor literature, nor family and community medicine. Actually, medical ethics is seldom considered synonymous with these disciplines, but these disciplines are not infrequently considered the natural home of medical ethics, or at least the executors of its estate. It is instructive to consider why responsibility for ethical deliberations might come to be located (conceptually or actually) within these disciplines. There are several possibilities.

Influence of Science. There is a tendency to lump into one melting pot all that is not "hard" science. To the "hard" scientist all nonscience looks alike—mushy. It seems a place of rampant opinion where one such is as good as any other. If this easy categorization is simply for convenience, it is perhaps tolerable. But it is, in fact, simple-minded and terribly misleading. It ignores those pivotal areas of "hard" science that are really mushy and those critical areas of "soft" disciplines that are really hard. And to be aware of these aspects within one's own discipline is maturing.

Identification with Humanitarianism. Another underlying motivation for identifying ethics with these various camps is the "human" element they all seem to share. On the surface, literature, medical sociology, anthropology, and family and community medicine seem to have a concern with humans as whole beings that other medical sciences do not have. Whether or not this is true is not now to the point. What is to the point is "localized humanitarianism." This is the tendency of disciplines focusing on the whole human and his culture to be saddled with pushing a particular point of view—namely, humanitarianism. In effect these disciplines are forced into being the repository for all responsibility and effort on behalf of kindness, compassion, and general human concern. This does grave injustice both to these disciplines and to human compassion. It strips the disciplines of their true calling and it compartmentalizes human compassion, making it the responsibility of the few rather than the responsibility of everyone.

Linking to Literature. A subtle mistake involved in the uniting of ethics and literature may be the underlying assumption that the study of ethics should motivate one to be ethical. Everyone is aware that literature, drama, and poetry are persuasive and that they can incite to action. And if one assumes the study of ethics should convince students to be ethical, literature and ethics are apt to be coupled, if not identified.

But the validity of an ethical system cannot stand or fall on its capacity to inspire moral behavior—any more than the correctness of a medical therapy depends on its capacity to inspire a patient to follow it. Rather, the student of ethics is developing a skill in working his way through muddled ethical issues and in finding the right action amidst a morass of complicated details.

Whether or not he chooses to do the morally right action is influenced far more by the example of his medical mentor than by anything he could learn in an ethics class. And rightly so. Otherwise ethics might become a series of sermons and exhortations rather than a discipline analyzing actions, principles, and justifications as rigorously and objectively as the subject matter permits.

Related to this confusion is the tendency to regard medical ethics as synonymous with reform movements. Reform may be noble and necessary, but nevertheless it should not be confused with the study of medical ethics. Reform seldom calls for subtle clinical analysis. There is no need for intricate determinations and balancing of competing rights and social effects. What is wrong is clear and obvious, and action is called for to correct it.

In short, there are clear advantages for disciplinary integrity and objectivity in keeping action groups and academic disciplines separate. It is comparable to the separation of the judicial and legislative branches of the government.

Relating to Sociology or Anthropology.
Finally, there is a subtle and mistaken belief causing and in turn strengthened by the relation of ethics with sociology and anthropology. This is the belief that ethics at its best is descriptive, that we can at most discover what things are valued by various peoples at various times and places, but that there exists no way of criticizing and analyzing these values, nor of arguing for what is morally right in current situations. This is avoided by allowing ethics to be its own discipline.

MORE DIFFICULT DISTINCTIONS

The following disciplines are more apt to be confused with ethics. I continue to present simply a sketch of how each differs from ethics. I am making suggestions and giving descriptions more than constructing arguments. If anything of value emerges, it will be as before—by the back door, that is, in saying why medical ethics should *not* be confused with these disciplines.

Law.
The relationship of law and morality has had many volumes dedicated to it. Here, as elsewhere, I simply want to give the layman an intuitive feel for the difference.

Morality is surely external to law: laws are sometimes criticized and even overturned because they are immoral or unjust; frequently laws deal with issues that simply are not moral concerns; and there are matters of morality that cannot be backed by the law because of inconvenience or impossibility of enforcement.

Yet there is overlap, as in instances where immoral behavior is proscribed by law, and becomes punishable (eg, killing, disabling, and breaking promises of a contractual sort). This, of couse, is not all remarkable when we realize that law and morals have much the same purpose: (very roughly) a set of rules we could all agree to that would lead us to live together harmoniously, allowing each of us to achieve his aims and desires insofar as this is compatible with everyone realizing his aims and desires.

The student of medical ethics has a great deal to learn from law in terms of finely-drawn distinctions and helpful concepts. The two are, nevertheless, to be emphatically distinguished. That the law says something about death or fetuses or human experimentation is not the end of the matter. Our quest is for the moral point of view as a critique of current laws and a guide to future ones.

Religion.
As with all the other possible look-alikes, the risk is not that religion and ethics might be thought completely identical. It is rather that they are frequently grouped together under the mistaken belief that they are conceptually entwined. It has often been contended that ethics is impossible without religion. I think this view incorrect, though I will not argue it here.

There are three important points to make in distinguishing religion and ethics:

1. Ethics must have universal appeal. We seek at least a basic set of rules that all rational

men would agree to as moral rules and could urge everyone to follow. Religion is acceptable only to a much smaller subset of this group; we are not required by reason to accept its metaphysical bases, and it would be unjust to insist on such acceptances. Rules and principles based on special knowledge or special commitments can lead only to secret societies, whereas ethics' whole point is to be binding on all, and hence must be understandable and justifiable to everyone.

2. Usually, religion's ethics are more stringent than general ethics. That is, they not only do not go against general ethics, but they require general acts of supererogation—acts above and beyond what could reasonably be *required* of all men. As such, religious ethics can count only on the voluntary commitment of a small remnant of men, whereas general ethics, being a minimal ethic (ie, having only obligations anyone could fulfill) can count on being acceptable to all rational men.

3. Religion is very likely the motivation for many men to be moral. It may well provide impetus, inspiration, or reward for a man's morality. This is probably one reason religion and ethics are popularly lumped together. Though motivation to be moral is extremely important, I think it is not a part of the discipline of ethics, at least not such that an ethical theory would be refuted if it failed to induce moral behavior. Ethics per se should be more like principles of justice and less like political platforms. Ethics can use a sidekick like religion, but he must remain his own man for the sake of objectivity and rigor.

Counseling. Counseling is apt to be regarded the home of medical ethics for a number of reasons: the personal approach, the concern for the total human, its own frequent identification with religion and thereby with ethics. Here I will comment on only two, namely, the elements of ministering and compassion. This is what many take ethics to be all about. I will briefly say why I disagree.

1. Comforting the bereaved, guiding the troubled, and ministering to the dying are noble endeavors. But studying ethics would not equip one for this, nor would counseling skills make one more proficient at ethics. Comforting, counseling, and ministering may well manifest ethical concern; such activity would constitute acts of supererogation for some and performance of duty for others. (For example, it is an obvious duty for counselors, and perhaps for all medical personnel.) So counseling skills are not ethical skills, yet like any other skills, counseling can be used ethically, that is, to fulfill one's moral obligations and commitments.

2. Compassion, closely linked with counseling and ministering, should also be distinguished from ethics as such. It has nothing to do with the study of ethics (though it might motivate one to study ethics) and it is not even a moral obligation. Insofar as compassion is a subjective state or feeling, it could not be required by ethics. But insofar as it is expressed in "compassionate behavior," such behavior may be someone's duty and hence a moral obligation (since doing one's duty is a moral obligation).

Of course, compassion may be personally very important in helping one to fulfill both ethical obligations and ethical commitments, or simply in being well-liked. It is just that ethics obligates us to certain actions (or more accurately, to refraining from certain actions) and not to a feeling or frame of mind in which the obligations should be fulfilled.

Psychiatry. Psychiatry is much like counseling, and might be taken as intimately related to ethics for the same reasons. But I single it out in order to make a special and important point. This concerns life styles or "philosophies of life." At least some approaches in psychiatry and psycho-analysis might be seen as attempts to help the patient mold a new life style or restructure his life plan. In part, it may be this connection with "the good life" that has led people to connect ethics and psychiatry. Again, a distinction is crucial: this time between "the good life" or a "philosophy of life" and morality. Morality *proscribes* many actions (eg, killing, breaking promises, causing pain) but it should not be expected to *prescribe* a way of life. Many styles of life are compatible with living in accord with the basic moral obligations; and many styles of life are compatible with fulfilling one's own moral commitments. Two salient points argue against making a philosophy of life a moral obligation:

1.   All men could never reach agreement on a particular way of life; they could never agree on what goods life should achieve. But we could reach agreement on what men should not do to other men, and hence reach universal agreement on what actions should be forbidden. As long as a philosophy of life is in accord with those proscribed actions, ethics per se can have nothing more to say about it. (Though advice on the effectiveness and satisfaction of any such guide to life will surely flow from many other quarters!)

2.   There is danger in regarding life styles as a matter of morality. It is a common practice, both dangerous and fallacious. It perpetuates moral relativity in that anyone can proclaim his life style as "his" morality and consider it a "moral obligation" to fulfill his life style and plan. His life plan might in fact be highly immoral (doing those things that would be proscribed by universal agreement). And few things are more frightening than immoral actions self-righteously supported with the rhetoric of morality.

CONCLUSIONS

Though I have had to say it in terms of what ethics is not, I have in effect been stressing three basic points: (1) That ethics is a discipline in and of itself, with its own conceptual framework, its own methods, strategies, and purposes. (2) That in studying ethics one ideally develops sensitivity to moral issues and skill in determining the morally right course of action. (The discipline itself will not provide the motivation to live by it anymore than the study of political science will motivate one to become a politician.) (3) Basic moral rules must be universal and will generally proscribe rather than prescribe.

Thus we end at the real starting point. The foregoing has only been ground-clearing, preparing the site for the construction of a definition and description of medical ethics. But that edifice must await another occasion.

From "Ethical Engineers Need Not Apply: The State of Applied Ethics Today"

Arthur L. Caplan

WHAT IS "APPLIED" ABOUT APPLIED ETHICS?

One of the most interesting issues to emerge from the sudden appearance of medical ethics in the past decade is the model of application that underlies much of its work. Medical ethics is often thought to be in the vanguard of research in applied ethics; thus, it is particular-

Reprinted by permission from *Science, Technology, and Human Values*, 6, No. 33, Fall 1980, pp. 24–32.

ly important in assessing the products of research in medical ethics to have a clear picture of the "applied" component of such research. Moreover, any effort to draw implications concerning the validity of applied research for other fields in the humanities and social sciences must itself come to grips with the question of what are the best ways to apply the insights of these fields to science policy.

One commonly espoused belief is that medical ethics is *not* the development and application of any special ethical theories or principles to uniquely govern medicine. Leading contributors to the literature unanimously agree that, whatever else medical ethics may be, it is not the creation of a new ethic or set of normative principles; rather, it involves the application of existing theories, principles, and generalizations from the field of ethics to issues in the domain of medicine. A few citations from some of the standard-bearers of medical ethics should suffice to explain the current model of application. Ronald Munson, in *Intervention and Reflection: Basic Issues in Medical Ethics,* notes that

> medical ethics is specifically concerned with moral principles and decisions in the context of medical practice, policy and research. Moral difficulties connected with medicine are so complex and important that they require special attention. Medical ethics gives them this attention, but it remains a part of the discipline of ethics.[1]

K. Danner Clouser in his article on "bioethics" in the *Encyclopedia of Bioethics* begins with a disclaimer to the effect that,

> Medical ethics is a special kind of ethics only insofar as it relates to a particular realm of facts and concerns and not because it embodies or appeals to some special moral principles or methodology. ... It consists of the same moral principles and rules we would appeal to, and argue for, in ordinary circumstances. It is just that in medical ethics these familiar moral rules are being applied to situations peculiar to the medical world. We have only to scratch the surface of medical ethics and we break through to the issues of "standard" ethics as we have always known them.[2]

Similarly, Tom Beauchamp, in the introduction to ethical theory in his anthology, *Bioethics,* notes that, in doing applied normative ethics

> ... ethicists attempt to explicate and defend positions on critical moral problems such as civil disobedience, abortion, and sexual discrimination. ... The term "applied" is used because more general ethical principles are applied in an attempt to resolve these moral problems.[3]

The sense of application that emerges from these definitions is quite straightforward. Applied ethics is distinguished as a field of inquiry by the distinctive nature of the issues it addresses. Dilemmas, cases, and problematic practical issues are the glue that holds medical ethics together. The object of inquiry in medical ethics, or any branch of applied ethics, is to use existing theories of ethics to solve moral problems in a particular profession or type of activity.[4]

THE APPLIED/THEORETICAL DISTINCTION IN THE SCIENCES

This model of medical ethics—a version of conceptual engineering—meets many of the needs mentioned earlier in describing the causal circumstances surrounding the genesis of this field. If medical ethics is understood as the attempt to bridge the theoretical and the practical between medicine and ethical theories, it holds out the prospect of providing "expert" solutions to the many headaches and dilemmas posed by advances in the biomedical sciences. It also remains firmly embedded within the field of ethics proper. For, while many philosophers might find it difficult to tolerate medical ethics if it threatened to develop as an alternative to existing conceptions of ethical theory, they regard it as perfectly palatable when seen as the mechanical application of available theories to the nitty-gritty of medical practice.

However, real problems confront this view of applied ethics, both for those now working in areas like medical ethics and for those in other fields who might turn to applied ethics as a model for dealing with normative issues in science generally. The relationship thought to obtain between applied ethics and ethical theory obviously parallels the relationship often thought to obtain between science and technology or between pure and applied science. The practitioners of applied ethics see the theoretical aspects of ethics as confined to the pure or basic side of ethics. Practitioners of applied ethics depict themselves as moral "engineers" who take theoretical insights from the basic researchers and apply them to the resolution of concrete moral dilemmas. However, there are a number of reasons for being suspicious of the adequacy of the view that applied ethics derives its applied characteristics as a variant of engineering.

It is far from clear that the distinction between pure and applied, or theory and application, can be taken very far even within the sciences.[5] In many areas of applied or technological science, theoretical or purely conceptual issues dominate. Ecology, for example, has always been viewed as one of the most applied biological sciences. Yet the individuals in ecology concerned with resource management, pest control, water pollution, and species preservation are currently embroiled in some of the hottest theoretical disputes in all of biology. Disputes about group selection, predator-prey dynamics, optimal foraging and the evolution of castes and sex now swirl through the literature of ecology in a steady (and dizzying) procession.[6] Similar tales of boundary fuzziness between theory and application can be told for many other areas within the social and the natural sciences.[7]

Not only are those who invoke this engineering metaphor inaccurately describing the relationships that obtain between theory and application in the sciences, they are also overlooking some important attributes of the "applied" sciences. Theoretical concerns *per se* do not always serve to distinguish basic from applied work in science. Nor do those concerned with technology or application always aim at a concrete problem or dilemma to orient their research. Indeed, it is often the case in so-called applied science that finding solutions to problems is of less interest than investigating the assumptions or circumstances giving rise to problems in the first place. And problem solving should not be confused with policy making. As those who have engaged in the latter activity know all too well, the goals and constraints of research aimed at aiding public policies may have little if anything to do with applied research. One need only consider recent disputes about IQ testing, busing for school desegregation, or the efficacy of incarceration as a deterrent to crime to see how different policy prescriptions are from applied or technological research in fields such as behavioral genetics or criminology.[8]

PROBLEMS FOR THE ETHICAL ENGINEERING VIEW

The notion that normative issues in science or medicine can be handled as simple engineering problems is an unfortunate one. This view of applied ethics has done much to distort the work of those in various areas of applied ethics. It has also done much to disappoint those in the professions and in government when hoped-for moral resolutions to sticky ethical problems fail to emerge from pages and pages (or hours and hours) of moral analysis.

Applied ethics is not of necessity an atheoretical enterprise. In many areas within medicine problems arise for which existing moral theories have no answers. Questions about the moral standing of the comatose, the senile, or the retarded may require recourse to the concepts of moral philosophy, but no single moral theory has, or claims to provide, a definitive answer for the proper treatment and care that ought to be given to individuals in these categories.

In many problem areas, no *single* moral theory can lay claim to the mantle of truth. For example, it is not easy to select a principle of justice for resolving cases of triage or allocation in medicine. Devotees of desert, social worth, utility, merit, and need will inevitably conflict as a direct result of their eagerness to apply particular moral rules.

Most importantly, as is the case in many applied sciences, applied ethics as a field sits astride a fascinating theoretical issue internal to the very enterprise. There are many ways currently in vogue for constructing theories in ethics. Some moral philosophers, such as John Rawls,[9] start with abstract idealizations of society and build out to the real world of moral phenomena. Others, such as Robert Nozick,[10] begin with certain theories of human nature and economic rationality and attempt to construct moral systems consistent with these views. But these are not the only starting points for moral theorizing. One might want to start with a rich base of moral phenomena and, inductively, construct a moral theory that captures the richness and complexity of moral life. Medicine is a fruitful place to seek just this sort of data. Thus, medical ethics or other areas of applied ethics research force (or should force) attention to the issue of what is the best research program to follow to construct a moral theory. Far from being *a*theoretical, medical ethics and its related enterprises in applied ethics compel attention to deep philosophical questions about optimal research strategies in ethical theorizing. Only a strict adherence to the engineering model of applied ethics forecloses attention to this very real theoretical issue in the context of applied ethics.[11]

This point has weight beyond the boundaries of medical ethics. For a similar issue confronts anyone attempting to engage in policy research or normative inquiry in the sciences. Should policy work be guided by existing insights, concepts, and generalizations with all their attendant theoretical baggage, or does the philosopher or historian of science have to start from empirical scratch.[11]

Not only does the engineering model of applied ethics give a false impression of the theoretical richness involved in such work, but it often holds out promises that cannot be fulfilled. Dilettantes are not well-tolerated in medicine. Nor is expertise, even in moral matters, greatly absent. It is simply naïve to think that a well-trained philosopher can step boldly into the emergency room or neonatal unit and immediately dissolve moral conundrums by dint of expertise in moral theory. Sometimes not enough facts are available for finding fast solutions. Sometimes the philosopher does not have the foggiest idea of exactly what problem should be the grist for the mill of moral theory. And it is often presumptuous to think that health professionals of moderate intelligence would fail through years and years of practice to discern solutions to moral quandaries capable of quick and easy resolution. It is simply ludicrous to think that all that has stood between medicine and moral insight is the application of a few key principles wielded by some moral virtuoso.

The persistence of certain moral dilemmas in medicine should discourage any thought that quick and easy solutions are forthcoming. Conceptual confusion and miscommunication can, of course, often be cited as the sole causes for

disagreement about moral issues, but achieving conceptual clarification is not the same as finding a solution to a moral dilemma. The difference becomes quickly apparent to anyone who has taken on the assignment of constructing a code of ethics, a patient bill of rights, an intensive care unit admissions policy, or guidelines for a national health insurance scheme. Answers to these policy problems can be found; rarely are they fashioned solely out of the cloth of extant theory in ethics.

Another problem confronts the engineering model of applied ethics which has broader implications for those undertaking policy research. The engineering model presumes that those involved in the analysis and solution of a moral problem or quandary always recognize that the nature and description of the problem or quandary is not in dispute.[12] In other words, the task of describing the problem to be addressed is left to those seeking a solution from the applied ethicist. In reality, however, it is often uncertain exactly what normative issue the applied ethicist is being called upon to grapple with. . . .

WHAT SHOULD APPLIED ETHICS BE?

The main thrust of this essay has been to critique what I have termed the "engineering" view of applied ethics as an inadequate conception of what is involved in applied normative inquiry. But critiques, to be truly useful, must be supplemented with some suggestions of what else might be involved in this activity. It is easy enough to poke fun at a simplistic model of ethical engineering. What other tasks exist for the person interested in applied normative research beyond technical engineering?

A number of interesting theoretical issues are raised in the course of attempting to do applied ethics. The applied context is one in which preconceived ideas about the formulation of strategies and the adequacy of given data bases for theory in ethics can easily be examined. Applied contexts also present useful opportunities for examination of the scope and adequacy of existing moral theories. The feasibility of various moral views is at least as interesting as the implications of these views for solving moral quandaries. Theoreticians are always in danger of oversimplifying, overidealizing, or underestimating the complexity of human behavior. The opportunity to use applied contexts to refashion and reshape normative views is at least as enticing as the opportunity to reshape normative views of scientific methodology through case studies in the history and sociology of science.[13]

Applied ethicists are also in a good position to highlight tacit values that may be operating in a given professional, personal, or institutional context. A knowledge of ethics is helpful in attempting descriptive or comparative research in normative matters. Indeed, without the availability of a rich taxonomy of descriptive values, the possible pragmatic contributions of applied ethics are seriously compromised.[14]

Numerous epistemological issues arise in applied contexts as well. The validity of claims to privileged knowledge or expertise are best pondered in real-world settings. The need for conceptual clarification and explication is particularly strong in social contexts that remain highly isolated and insular from general social values and norms.

Even the nature of problem solving itself poses important theoretical issues for those doing applied work. Are there special modes of reasoning that must be used to divine answers to real and unavoidable moral quandaries? Are particular forms of practical reasoning or casuistic logic required in certain applied settings?[15] Given the relatively low esteem in which positivist models of explanation are held by many humanists, how vulnerable is the engineering model of application—solution by subsumption under general principles—to the many criticisms leveled against nomological explanation via deduction as a model of scientific explanation?[16] And, is it the case that the model of theory structure inherent in the engineering view of ethics—where ethical theories are seen as hierarchical pyramids of deductively linked generalizations—will stand up under close scrutiny?[17]

Humanists and social scientists interested in science and technology know all too well how intractable these kinds of issues are. Moreover, the pressures and demands of the real world do not provide an optimal environment for supporting the kinds of inquiry necessary to examine these issues with great depth or rigor. The fact remains that, despite the very real demands placed on those who undertake normative policy work in terms of time and in terms of demands for answers, these kinds of questions must be addressed. Minimally, those called upon to suppy policy answers must have some idea of the risks and costs associated with technical fixes even if they are normative ones.

MORALS FOR NORMATIVE POLICY RESEARCH

The experience of those working in applied fields of ethics such as medical ethics should not be ignored either by those already engaged in policy research or by those tempted at the prospect. Every discipline feels it has something to offer in the way of expertise to those making policy and when the opportunity arises it is hard to resist the temptation to make pronouncements as an expert. There are, however, many models other than that of expert technician. Theoretician, diagnostician, educator, coach, conceptual policeman, and skeptic are all supplemental or alternative roles to that of technician.

Normative policy inquiry demands a firsthand knowledge of the values, organization, and practices of the groups or communities under investigation. It is one thing to convince scientists and society to take normative issues concerning science seriously. It is quite another *to be taken seriously* in formulating answers to policy issues. Finally, historians, philosophers, and sociologists of science must be aware of all the moral and political dangers inherent in being taken seriously when they are analyzing issues in science with strong moral dimensions. The strait between the Scylla of co-optation and the Charybdis of carping is narrow. The voyage demands constant critical attention to both the nature of the models underlying the research and the complexity of the enterprise.

Notes

1. Ronald Munson, ed., *Intervention and Reflection: Basic Issues in Medical Ethics* (Belmont, CA: Wadsworth, 1979), p. 2.

2. K. Danner Clouser, "Bioethics," in W. Reich, ed., *The Encyclopedia of Bioethics* (New York: The Free Press, 1978), vol. I, p. 115.

3. Tom L. Beauchamp and LeRoy Walters, eds., *Contemporary Issues in Bioethics* (Belmont, CA: Dickenson, 1978), p. 3.

4. This view of medical ethics as a form of moral engineering is reflected in the organization of most anthologies and texts on the subject. Most begin with presentations of key ethical theories before moving on to presentations of problem cases or dilemmatic situations. A neophyte to the field quickly learns the proper way of approaching moral issues in applied ethics is theory first, then the analysis of cases. See Sissela Bok, "The Tools of Bioethics," in *Ethics in Medicine,* Stanley Reiser, William Curran, Arthur Dyck, eds. (Cambridge, MA: MIT Press, 1977), pp. 737–41.

5. Joseph Agassi, "Between Science and Technology," 47 *Philosophy of Science* (1980): 82–99.

6. For example, see M.E. Gilpin, *Group Selection in Predator-Prey Communities* (Princeton, NJ: Princeton University Press, 1975): Paul Colinvaux, *Why Big Fierce Animals Are Rare* (Princeton, NJ: Princeton University Press, 1978); and E.R. Pianka, *Evolutionary Ecology* (New York: Harper & Row, 1974).

7. The *locus classicus* for the analysis of the theory application distinction in the social sciences is Alvin Gouldner's "Theoretical Requirements of the Applied Social Sciences," 17 *American Sociological Review* (1957): 92–102.

8. Many criticisms of policy advocacy masquerading as basic research can be found in the selections included in Hilary Rose and Steven Rose, eds., *Ideology of/in the Natural Sciences* (Cambridge, MA: Schenkman, 1979).

9. John Rawls, *A Theory of Justice* (Cambridge, MA: Harvard University Press, 1971).

10. Robert Nozick, *Anarchy, State and Utopia* (New York: Basic Books, 1974).

11. Some interesting ruminations on these issues are to be found in Dorothy Nelkin's introduction to her anthology, *Controversy: Politics of Technical Decisions* (Beverly Hills, CA: Sage, 1979), pp. 18–21; and in the essays by Sanford A. Lakoff, "Science Policy Studies: The Policy Perspective" and M.J. Mulkay, "Sociology of the Scientific Research Community," in I. Spiegel-Rosing and D. de Solla Price, eds., *Science, Technology and Society,* (Beverly Hills, CA: Sage, 1977).

12. See Robert Veatch, *Case Studies in Medical Ethics* (Cambridge, MA: Harvard University Press, 1977); and Tom L. Beauchamp and J. F. Childress, *Principles of Biomedical Ethics* (New York: Oxford University Press, 1979). Neither book devotes significant attention to the issue of case description or individuation.

13. R. M. Burian, "More Than a Marriage of Convenience: On the Inextricability of History and Philosophy of Science," 44 *Philosophy of Science* (1977): 1–42.

14. See C.L. Bosk, *Forgive and Remember* (Chicago, IL: University of Chicago Press, 1979), for an example of careful systematics in a medical setting.

15. This claim is made in A.R. Jonsen, "Can an Ethicist Be a Consultant?" in V. Abernethy, ed., *Frontiers in Medical Ethics* (Cambridge, MA: Ballinger, 1980), pp. 157–72.

16. See the introduction to Fred Suppe's *The Structure of Scientific Theories,* 2nd ed. (Urbana, IL: University of Illinois Press, 1977), for a useful summary of these criticisms.

17. See A.L. Caplan, "Testability, Disreputability and the Structure of the Modern Synthetic Theory of Evolution," 13 *Erkenntnis* (1978): 261–78, for a critique of this model of theory structure. Also see E. McMullin, "The Criterion of Fertility and the Unit for Appraisal in Science," 39 *Boston Studies in the Philosophy of Science* (1976): 395–432.

Chapter 2

PROVIDER AND PATIENT

INTRODUCTION

This chapter deals with the moral problems that pervade the relationship between providers of health care and patients, and also the relationship among various groups of health care providers. Philosophers are generally agreed that the need for a system of ethics arises to a significant degree out of the existence of conflict. Discord may arise among persons in their wants, desires, or interests; at other times a conflict is best described in terms of a clash of moral principles. These principles are among those that lie at the heart of our social institutions and practices, as well as those that reflect our commonly held moral beliefs. If the need for having an ethical system does, indeed, occur as a result of conflicts among persons or principles, then a satisfactory ethical theory must attempt to examine these various conflicts and propose methods that offer some hope of resolving them.

Some conflicts emerge as a result of different perspectives that different persons have, whether those perspectives represent permanent features of their situation or temporary disparities in points of view. For example, the status of being a patient is one that confers certain properties on anyone who occupies that status. One such property is that of dependency. Especially in the case of the hospitalized patient, the individual freedom and decision-making autonomy that are normally present and give rise to fundamental rights in our society are diminished, if not altogether abolished. In addition to the sorts of conflict that arise because of differing points of view, others may emerge as a result of differing *roles* or positions that persons occupy. Problems of both types are examined in the chapter sections entitled "The Physician–Patient Relationship" and "The Nurse."

One of the major issues that generates conflicts between persons with different perspectives or different roles is the tension between autonomy and paternalism. Our moral sentiments and beliefs in the field of medical ethics reflect the overall value scheme or ethical system that we hold. One of the major background assumptions of this scheme or system is the fact that our culture values highly the autonomy of persons—their independence and self-reliance, their ability to do things for themselves. Freedom from authoritarian rule and dislike of totalitarian practices serve to characterize not only our political democratic ideals but also, in large measure, our social institutions, including the family; one can readily observe the antiauthoritarianism and antipaternalistic bias that pervades American values.

While this may be an assumption of our overall cultural system of ethics, situations arise in medical practice that lead some people to believe that one type of interference with the autonomous actions of others is justified. These are acts done for the health-related benefit or welfare of those who suffer the interference. Since one of the major goals (indeed, some say the principal goal) of a health care system is to benefit individual patients, it is argued sometimes that it is perfectly appropriate, if not morally obligatory, for those administering health care to take actions that benefit patients, even if these actions interfere with or neglect the patient's autonomy. This issue is dealt with in the section entitled ''Autonomy and Paternalism.'' This section contains both essays that deal with the relation between the concepts of autonomy and paternalism and essays that discuss the morally appropriate stance to take with respect to concrete issues in medical practice.

In the selection from *On Liberty*, Mill states that we never have a right to interfere with another person merely in order to benefit that person. Mill justifies that view on utilitarian grounds, but the same position sometimes rests on the belief that individuals have dignity and therefore deserve the respect that is expressed in honoring their decisions in matters that concern only themselves. The remainder of the essays in this section deals with applying the concepts of autonomy and paternalism to the realm of medical decision making.

Buchanan expresses the view that many physicians believe a paternalistic model is appropriate for characterizing the relationship between physicians and patients. He goes on to describe the model and then offers challenges to it. The excerpts from judicial opinions by Wright and Underwood provide examples of attempts to recognize patients' rights to make their own decisions in cases where human life is at stake.

One way to deal with an apparent conflict, such as the one between autonomy and paternalism, is to attempt to show that the conflict is not as acute as many believe. The selection by Miller does this by distinguishing four senses of autonomy and presenting arguments intended to establish the claim that the apparent conflict between autonomy and the appropriate exercise of medical judgment is not as sharp as it seems to be. Another way to deal with an apparent conflict between values is to suggest that in some situations the best way to achieve a value is to act in a way that appears to be intended to achieve the opposite value. An example of this is presented by Cassell, who claims that the function of medicine is to preserve autonomy. In saying this, however, he does not mean to say that a practitioner ought never to act against the patient's expressed wishes. Rather, he argues that in some cases, though certainly not all, the patient's illness interferes with the patient's autonomy, and thus, to treat the illness against the patient's wishes can be justified on the grounds that curing the illness will restore the patient to wholeness and make the patient capable of exercising autonomy.

In the final selection in this section, Veatch attempts to clarify various models that might characterize the physician-patient relationship. Of particular interest regarding autonomy and paternalism are what he calls the Priestly Model and the Contractual Model. Because of its broad perspective, Veatch's paper provides a good link to the issue of the relationship between the physician and the patient.

Let us turn now to a more detailed look at the specific types of moral problems in the physician-patient relationship. Although being a patient is, for most people, a relatively temporary state, it is nonetheless significant in the emotional investment and anxiety produced, largely as a result of fear, uncertainty, and the pervasive threat to bodily integrity. One of the salient features of the patient's life in an era of impressive medical technology and advanced therapeutic procedures is the so-called ''dehumanization'' a person may suffer. A closely related aspect is the occurrence of diminished autonomy and freedom of choice, which can be observed as well in other institutionalized populations (for example, prisoners, the elderly, and the mentally retarded). Taken together, these two facets of patient life may be seen as constituting a threat to fundamental human rights. A related problem is physicians' frequent failure to view things from the patient's perspective.

Moreover, conflicts can arise within the physician's role itself. There are several different ways in which this role can be construed, and the issue is further complicated by the several aims or goals embodied in this role. The physician has a special set of duties and obligations, in addition to the usual sorts of duties that all persons possess by virtue of their membership in human society. Within the physician's role, conflicts may occur between two or more of the acknowledged goals of medical practice—for example, the aim of alleviating the pain and suffering of the sick versus that of contributing new knowledge to medical science. This particular conflict may occur in cases in which new drugs or modes of treatment are contemplated; it is often hard to draw a clear-cut line between "pure" therapy and treatment when an element of innovation is present. In practice the existence of conflicts of interest (the patient's, society's, the medical profession's), as well as the sometimes divergent goals of medicine, may cause moral dilemmas, and there is no universal ethical prescription that can provide a solution.

Yet there are principles of varying degrees of strength that might be adopted by a physician, such as the view propounded in the selection by Hans Jonas. "In the course of treatment," writes Jonas, "the physician is obligated to the patient and to no one else. He is not the agent of society, nor of the interests of medical science, the patient's family, the patient's co-sufferers, or future sufferers from the same disease. The patient alone counts when he is under the physician's care." This principle sets up a clear order of priorities among the subgoals embodied in the physician's role; however, not everyone would agree to it. Even where agreement is secured, problematic cases may still arise that require reflective moral judgments.

The selections in the section subtitled "The Physician-Patient Relationship" begin with an essay by May, who attempts to meet the need for an adequate characterization of that relationship by distinguishing codes, contracts, and covenants. May suggests that seeing the physician as having made a covenant may lead to an ethically adequate way of conceiving the physician's role. In order to indicate the fact that the physician's role is complex and contains several ethical dimensions, Jonsen develops various interpretations of the often cited maxim of physicians, "Do no harm."

The papers by Freud and Kasper feature discussions of the psychological problems posed by the attitudes of physicians and patients toward each other. These attitudes are sometimes expressions of unconsciously felt needs that relate to a person's sense of worth or dignity. The medical context can both threaten people and, especially in the case of physicians, help to fulfill them. The essay by Jonas makes suggestions for dealing with serious ethical questions facing physicians who fail to appreciate their own fallibility or the complexity of the moral issues they face.

The papers by Calland and Groves put more emphasis on patients. Calland, himself a physician, recounts his experiences as a patient and his feelings and thoughts concerning those experiences. He makes some recommendations about vitally needed reforms in patient treatment, especially with respect to specialists' failure to work together to meet the patient's needs. Groves focusses on four classes of patients most physicians dread. He believes that, in coming to grips with the fact that patients of these sorts do exist and with the feelings that attempting to treat these patients can produce, physicians may be able to be more effective in dealing with them.

In the final section of the chapter, entitled "The Nurse," the complex moral problems faced by nurses are examined. Many of these problems arise from the fact that nurses often feel they are in a position of subservience to physicians. All of the selections in this section deal with various aspects of this situation.

Jameton discusses the hard choices faced by nurses when they work under the supervision of those who are incompetent or who abuse patients. Rather than give rules that nurses might follow in dealing with such problems, Jameton presents considerations that are relevant to deciding whether or not to take personal risks to avoid participating in activities that harm patients.

The problem posed by the fact that physicians are seen to have authority over nurses is addressed by Ladd. He suggests that, since physicians and nurses do not have sufficient agreement about goals and methods to make an authoritarian system function effectively, we should work toward more democratic pro-cedures involving consultation and collaboration.

In presenting an analysis of the nurse's role in the present-day health-care structure, Harding argues that nursing is in effect an industrialized form of "women's work" and that the most powerful forces shaping today's health-care system are not sufficiently supportive either of the nurse's goals of caring and curing or of efforts to give health-care workers, such as nurses, greater control over their working conditions.

John O'Connor

AUTONOMY AND PATERNALISM

From *On Liberty*

John Stuart Mill

The object of this essay is to assert one very simple principle, as entitled to govern absolutely the dealing of society with the individual in the way of compulsion and control, whether the means used be physical force in the form of legal penalties or the moral coercion of public opinion. That principle is that the sole end for which mankind are warranted, individually or collectively, in interfering with the liberty of action of any of their number is self-protection. That the only purpose for which power can be rightfully exercised over any member of a civilized community, against his will, is to prevent harm to others. His own good, either physical or moral, is not a sufficient warrant. He cannot rightfully be compelled to do or forbear because it will be better for him to do so, because it will make him happier, because, in the opinions of others, to do so would be wise or even right. These are good reasons for remonstrating with him, or

From John Stuart Mill, *On Liberty*, edited by Currin V. Shields, Copyright © 1956, by The Liberal Arts Press, Inc. Reprinted by permission of The Bobbs-Merrill Company, Inc.

reasoning with him, or persuading him, or entreating him, but not for compelling him or visiting him with any evil in case he do otherwise. To justify that, the conduct from which it is desired to deter him must be calculated to produce evil to someone else. The only part of the conduct of anyone for which he is amenable to society is that which concerns others. In the part which merely concerns himself, his independence is, of right, absolute. Over himself, over his own body and mind, the individual is sovereign.

It is, perhaps, hardly necessary to say that this doctrine is meant to apply only to human beings in the maturity of their faculties. We are not speaking of children or of young persons below the age which the law may fix as that of manhood or womanhood. Those who are still in a state to require being taken care of by others must be protected against their own actions as well as against external injury. For the same reason we may leave out of consideration those backward states of society in which the race itself may be considered as in its nonage.

The early difficulties in the way of spontaneous progress are so great that there is seldom any choice of means for overcoming them; and a ruler full of the spirit of improvement is warranted in the use of any expedients that will attain an end perhaps otherwise unattainable. Despotism is a legitimate mode of government in dealing with barbarians, provided the end be their improvement and the means justified by actually effecting that end. Liberty, as a principle, has no application to any state of things anterior to the time when mankind have become capable of being improved by free and equal discussion. Until then, there is nothing for them but implicit obedience to an Akbar or a Charlemagne, if they are so fortunate as to find one. But as soon as mankind have attained the capacity of being guided to their own improvement by conviction or persuasion (a period long since reached in all nations with whom we need here concern ourselves), compulsion, either in the direct form or in that of pains and penalties for noncompliance, is no longer admissible as a means to their own good, and justifiable only for the security of others.

It is proper to state that I forego any advantage which could be derived to my argument from the idea of abstract right as a thing independent of utility. I regard utility as the ultimate appeal on all ethical questions; but it must be utility in the largest sense, grounded on the permanent interests of man as a progressive being. Those interests, I contend, authorize the subjection of individual spontaneity to external control only in respect to those actions of each which concern the interest of other people. If anyone does an act hurtful to others, there is a *prima facie* case for punishing him by law or, where legal penalties are not safely applicable, by general disapprobation. There are also many positive acts for the benefit of others which he may rightfully be compelled to perform, such as to give evidence in a court of justice, to bear his fair share in the common defense or in any other joint work necessary to the interest of the society of which he enjoys the protection, and to perform certain acts of individual beneficence, such as saving a fellow creature's life or interposing to protect the defenseless against ill usage—things which whenever it is obviously a man's duty to do he may rightfully be made

responsible to society for not doing. A person may cause evil to others not only by his actions but by his inaction, and in either case he is justly accountable to them for the injury. The latter case, it is true, requires a much more cautious exercise of compulsion than the former. To make anyone answerable for doing evil to others is the rule; to make him answerable for not preventing evil is, comparatively speaking, the exception. Yet there are many cases clear enough and grave enough to justify that exception. In all things which regard the external relations of the individual, he is *de jure* amenable to those whose interests are concerned, and, if need be, to society as their protector. There are often good reasons for not holding him to the responsibility; but these reasons must arise from the special expediencies of the case: either because it is a kind of case in which he is on the whole likely to act better when left to his own discretion than when controlled in any way in which society have it in their power to control him; or because the attempt to exercise control would produce other evils, greater than those which it would prevent. When such reasons as these preclude the enforcement of responsibility, the conscience of the agent himself should step into the vacant judgment seat and protect those interests of others which have no external protection; judging himself all the more rigidly, because the case does not admit of his being made accountable to the judgment of his fellow creatures.

But there is a sphere of action in which society, as distinguished from the individual, has, if any, only an indirect interest: comprehending all that portion of a person's life and conduct which affects only himself or, if it also affects others, only with their free, voluntary, and undeceived consent and participation. When I say only himself, I mean directly and in the first instance; for whatever affects himself may affect others through himself; and the objection which may be grounded on this contingency will receive consideration in the sequel. This, then, is the appropriate region of human liberty. It comprises, first, the inward domain of consciousness, demanding liberty of conscience in the most comprehensive sense, liberty of thought and feeling, absolute freedom of opinion and sentiment on all subjects, practical or speculative, scientific, moral, or theological. The liberty of expressing and publishing opinions may seem to fall under a different principle, since it belongs to that part of the conduct of an individual which concerns other people, but, being almost of as much importance as the liberty of thought itself and resting in great part on the same reasons, is practically inseparable from it. Secondly, the principle requires liberty of tastes and pursuits, of framing the plan of our life to suit our own character, of doing as we like, subject to such consequences as may follow, without impediment from our fellow creatures, so long as what we do does not harm them, even though they should think our conduct foolish, perverse, or wrong. Thirdly, from this liberty of each individual follows the liberty, within the same limits, of combination among individuals; freedom to unite for any purpose not involving harm to others: the persons combining being supposed to be of full age and not forced or deceived.

No society in which these liberties are not, on the whole, respected is free, whatever may be its form of government; and none is completely free in which they do not exist absolute and unqualified. The only freedom which deserves the name is that of pursuing our own good in our own way, so long as we do not attempt to deprive others of theirs or impede their efforts to obtain it. Each is the proper guardian of his own health, whether bodily *or* mental and spiritual. Mankind are greater gainers by suffering each other to live as seems good to themselves than by compelling each to live as seems good to the rest.

Medical Paternalism

Allen Buchanan

I

There is evidence to show that among physicians in this country the medical paternalist model is a dominant way of conceiving the physician-patient relationship. I contend that the practice of withholding the truth from the patient or his family, a particular form of medical paternalism, is not adequately supported by the arguments advanced to justify it. Beyond the issue of telling patients the truth is the distinction between "ordinary" and "extraordinary" therapeutic measures, a distinction which, I argue, both expresses and helps to perpetuate the dominance of the medical paternalist model.

There are two main types of arguments against paternalism. First are the arguments that rely upon a theory of moral rights rooted in a conception of personal autonomy. These ar-

From *Philosophy & Public Affairs*, Vol. 7, no. 4 (Summer 1978). Copyright © 1978 by Princeton University Press. Reprinted by permission of Princeton University Press and the author.

guments are more theoretically interesting and perhaps in the end they are the strongest arguments against paternalism. Second are the arguments that meet the paternalist on his own ground and then attempt to cut it from beneath him by showing that his arguments are defective. I shall concentrate on the second type of antipaternalist argument because I wish my arguments to have some practical effect, and I believe that this goal can best be achieved if they are directed against paternalist justifications which are actually employed by the practitioners of medical paternalism. Further, the arguments I advance require a minimum of theoretical baggage. The strength of a rights-based attack on paternalism depends ultimately upon whether a rational foundation for the relevant theory of rights can be produced. It would be unfortunate if successful attacks on medical paternalism had to await the development and defense of a full-blown theory of moral rights. By articulating the inadequacy of the justifications which the paternalist himself advances, however, one need rely only upon the moral views to which the paternalist himself subscribes. My goal, then, is to present effective criticisms of medical paternalist practices which rely upon a minimal base of moral agreement between the paternalist and his critic.

II

Paternalism is usually characterized as interference with a person's liberty of action, where the alleged justification of the interference is that it is for the good of the person whose liberty of action is thus restricted.[1] To focus exclusively on interference with liberty of *action* however, is to construe paternalism too narrowly. If a government lies to the public or withholds information from it, and if the alleged justification of its policy is that it benefits the public itself, the policy may properly be called paternalistic.

On the one hand, there may be a direct connection between such a policy and actual interference with the citizen's freedom to act. In order to withhold information from the public, agents of the government may physically interfere with the freedom of the press to gather, print, or distribute the news. Or government officials may misinform the public in order to restrict its freedom to perform specific acts. The police, for example, may erect signs bearing the words ''Detour: Maintenance Work Ahead'' to route unsuspecting motorists around the wreckage of a truck carrying nerve gas. On the other hand, the connection between withholding of information and actual interference with freedom of action may be indirect at best. To interfere with the public's freedom of information the government need not actually interfere with anyone's freedom to act—it may simply not divulge certain information. Withholding information may preclude an *informed* decision, and it may interfere with attempts to reach an informed decision, without thereby interfering with a person's freedom to decide and to act on his decision. Even if I am deprived of information which I must have if I am to make an informed decision, I may still be free to decide and to act.

Granted the complexity of the relations between information and action, it seems plausible to expand the usual characterization of paternalism as follows: paternalism is interference with a person's freedom of action or freedom of information, or the deliberate dissemination of misinformation, where the alleged justification of interfering or misinforming is that it is for the good of the person who is interfered with or misinformed. The notion of freedom of information is, of course, unsatisfyingly vague, but the political examples sketched above along with the medical examples to follow will make it clearer. We can now turn to a brief consideration of evidence for the claim that medical paternalism is a widespread phenomenon in our society.

III

The evidence for medical paternalism is both direct and indirect. The direct evidence consists of the findings of surveys which systematically report physicians' practices concerning truth-telling and decision-making and of articles and discussions in which physicians and others acknowledge or defend paternalistic medical practices. The indirect evidence is more subtle. One source of indirect evidence for the pervasiveness of medical paternalist attitudes is the language we use to describe physician-patient interactions. Let us now consider some of the direct evidence.

Though there are many ways of classifying cases of medical paternalism, two distinctions are especially important. We can distinguish between the cases in which the patient is legally competent and those in which the patient is legally incompetent; and between those cases in which the intended beneficiary of paternalism is the patient himself and those in which the intended beneficiary is the patient's guardian or one or more members of the patient's family. The first distinction classifies cases according to the *legal status of the patient,* the second according to the *object of paternalism.*

A striking revelation of medical paternalism in dealings with legally competent adults is found in Donald Oken's essay, ''What to Tell Cancer Patients: A Study of Medical Attitudes.''[2] The chief conclusion of this study of internists, surgeons, and generalists is that ''. . . there is a strong and general tendency to withhold'' from the patient the information that he has cancer. Almost 90 percent of the total group surveyed reported that their usual policy is not to tell the patient that he has cancer. Oken also notes that ''no one reported a policy of informing every patient.'' Further, Oken reports that some physicians falsified diagnoses.

> Some physicians avoid even the slightest suggestion of neoplasia and quite specifically substitute another diagnosis. Almost everyone reported resorting to such falsification on at least a few occasions, most notably when the patient was in a far-advanced stage of illness at the time he was seen.[3]

The physicians' justifications for withholding or falsifying diagnostic information were uniformly paternalistic. They assumed that if they told the patient he had cancer they would be depriving him of all hope and that the loss of hope would result in suicidal depression or at least in a serious worsening of the patient's condition.

A recent malpractice case illustrates paternalistic withholding of information of a different sort. As in the Oken study, the object of paternalism was the patient and the patient was a legally competent adult. A bilateral thyroidectomy resulted in permanent paralysis of the patient's vocal cords. The patient's formerly healthy voice became frail and weak. The damage suit was based on the contention that by failing to tell the patient of the known risks to her voice, the physician had violated his duty to obtain informed consent for the operation. The physician's testimony is clearly paternalistic.

> In court the physician was asked ''You didn't inform her of any dangers or risks involved? Is that right?'' Over his attorney's objections, the physician responded, ''Not specifically. . . . I feel that were I to point out all the complications—or even half the complications—many people would refuse to have anything done, and therefore would be much worse off.''[4]

There is also considerable evidence of medical paternalism in the treatment of legally incompetent individuals through the withholding of information from the patients or their guardians or both.[5]

The law maintains that it is the parents who are primarily responsible for decisions concerning the welfare of their minor children.[6] Nonetheless, physicians sometimes assume primary or even total responsibility for the most awesome and morally perplexing decisions affecting the welfare of the child.

The inescapable need to make such decisions arises daily in neonate intensive care units. The most dramatic decisions are whether to initiate or not initiate, or to continue or discontinue life-sustaining therapy. Three broad types of cases are frequently discussed in recent literature. First, there are infants who are in an asphyxiated condition at birth and can be resuscitated but may suffer irreversible brain-damage if they survive. Second, there are infants with Down's syndrome (mongolism) who have potentially fatal but surgically correctable congenital cardiovascular or gastrointestinal defects. Third, there are infants with spina bifida, a congenital condition in which there is an opening in the spine and which may be complicated by paralysis and hydrocephaly. New surgical techniques make it possible to close the spine and drain the fluid from the brain, but a large percentage of the infants thus treated suffer varying degrees of permanent brain-damage and paralysis.

A. Shaw notes that some physicians undertake the responsibility for making decisions about life and death for defective newborns in order to relieve parents of the trauma and guilt of making a decision. He cites the following comment as an example of this position.

> At the end it is usually the doctor who has to decide the issue. It is . . . cruel to ask the parents whether they want their child to live or die. . . .[7]

We have already seen that the information which physicians withhold may be of at least two different sorts. In the cases studied by Oken, physicians withhold the diagnosis of cancer from their patients. In the thyroidectomy malpractice case the physician did not withhold the diagnosis but did withhold information about known risks of an operation. The growing literature on life or death decisions for defective neonates reveals more complex paternalistic practices. Some physicians routinely exclude parents from significant participation in decision-making either by not informing the parents that certain choices can or must be made, or by describing the child's condition and the therapeutic options in such a skeletal way as to preclude genuinely informed consent.

A case cited by Shaw is a clear example of a physician withholding from parents the information that there was a choice to be made.

> Baby A was referred to me at 22 hours of age with a diagnosis of esophageal atresia and tracheo-esophageal fistula. The infant, the firstborn of a professional couple in their early thirties had obvious signs of mongolism, about which they were fully informed by the referring physician. After explaining the nature of the surgery to the distraught father, I offered him the operative consent. His pen hesitated briefly above the form and then as he signed, he muttered, "I have no choice, do I?" He didn't seem to expect an answer and I gave him none. The esophageal anomaly was corrected in routine fashion, and the infant was discharged to a state institution for the retarded without ever being seen again by either parent.[8]

The following description of practices in a neonate intensive care unit at Yale illustrates how parents may be excluded because of inadequate information about the child's condition or the character of various therapeutic options.

> Parents routinely signed permits for operation though rarely had they seen their children's defects or had the nature of various management plans and their respective prognoses clearly explained to them. Some physicians believed that parents were too upset to understand the nature of the problems and the options for care. Since they believed informed consent had no meaning in these circumstances, they either ignored the parents or simply told them that the child needed an operation on the back as the first step in correcting several defects. As a result, parents often felt completely left out while the activities of care proceeded at a brisk pace.[9]

Not every case in which a physician circumvents or overrides parental decision-making is a case of paternalism toward the parents. In ignoring the parents' primary legal respon-

sibility for the child, the physician may not be attempting to shield the parents from the burdens of responsibility—he may simply be attempting to protect what he perceives to be the interests of the child.

These examples are presented, not as conclusive evidence for the claim that paternalist practices of the sorts discussed above are widespread, but as illustrations of the practical relevance of the justifications for medical paternalism, which I shall now articulate and criticize.

IV

In spite of the apparent pervasiveness of paternalistic practices in medicine, no systematic justification of them is available for scrutiny. Nonetheless, there appear to be at least three main arguments which advocates of paternalism could and sometimes do advance in justification of withholding information or misinforming the patient or his family. Since withholding information seems to be more commonly practiced and advocated than outright falsification, I shall consider the three arguments only as justifications of the former rather than the latter. Each of these arguments is sufficiently general to apply to each of the types of cases distinguished above. For convenience we can label these three arguments (A) the Prevention of Harm Argument, (B) the Contractual Version of the Prevention of Harm Argument, and (C) the Argument from the Inability to Understand.

The Prevention of Harm Argument is disarmingly simple. It may be outlined as follows.

> 1. The physician's duty—to which he is bound by the Oath of Hippocrates—is to prevent or at least to minimize harm to his patient
>
> 2. Giving the patient information X will do great harm to him.
>
> 3. (Therefore) It is permissible for the physician to withhold information X from the patient.

Several things should be noted about this argument. First of all, the conclusion is much weaker than one would expect, granted the first premise. The first premise states that it is the physician's *duty* to prevent or minimize harm to the patient, not just that it is *permissible* for him to do so. However, since the weaker conclusion—that withholding information is permissible—seems more intuitively plausible than the stronger one, I shall concentrate on it.

Second, the argument as it stands is invalid. From the claims that (1) the physician's duty (or right) is to prevent or minimize harm and that (2) giving information X will do the patient great harm, it does not follow that (3) it is permissible for the physician to withhold information X from the patient. At least one other premise is needed: (2') giving information X will do greater harm to the patient on balance than withholding the information will.

The addition of (2') is no quibble. Once (2') is made explicit we begin to see the tremendous weight which this paternalist argument places on the physician's powers of judgment. He must not only determine that giving the information will do harm or even that it will do great harm. He must also make a complex comparative judgment. He must judge that withholding the information will result in less harm on balance than divulging it. Yet neither the physicians interviewed by Oken nor those discussed by Shaw even mention this comparative judgment in their justifications of withholding information. They simply state that telling the truth will result in great harm to the patient or his family. No mention was made of the need to compare this expected harm with harm which might result from withholding the information, and no recognition of the difficulties involved in such a comparison was reported.

Consider two of the cases described above: a terminal cancer case and the thyroidectomy case. In order to justify withholding the diagnosis of terminal cancer from the patient the physician must not only determine that informing the patient would do great harm but that the harm would be greater on balance than whatever harm may result from withholding information. Since the notion of "great harm" here is vague unless a context for comparison is supplied, we can concentrate on the physician's evidence for the judgment that the harm of informing is greater on balance than the harm of withholding. Oken's study showed that the evidential basis for such comparative judgments was remarkably slender.

> It was the exception when a physician could report known examples of the unfavorable consequences of an approach which differed from his own. It was more common to get reports of instances in which different approaches had turned out satisfactorily. Most of the instances in which unhappy results were reported to follow a differing policy turned out to be vague accounts from which no reliable inference could be drawn.

Oken then goes on to focus on the nature of the anticipated harm.

> It has been repeatedly asserted that disclosure is followed by fear and despondency which may progress into overt depressive illness or culminate in suicide. This was the opinion of the physicians in the present study. Quite representative was the surgeon who stated, "I would be afraid to tell and have the patient in a room with a window." When it comes to actually documenting the prevalence of such ontoward reactions, it becomes difficult to find reliable evidence. Instances of depression and profound upsets came quickly to mind when the subject was raised, but no one could report more than a case or two, or a handful at most. . . . The same doctors could remember many instances in which the patient was told and seemed to do well.[10]

It is not simply that these judgments of harm are made on the basis of extremely scanty evidence. The problem goes much deeper than that. To say simply that physicians base such judgments on extremely weak evidence is to overlook three important facts. First, the judgment that telling the truth would result in suicidal depression is an unqualified *psychiatric* generalization. So even if there were adequate evidence for this generalization or, more plausibly, for some highly qualified version of it, it is implausible to maintain that ordinary physicians are in a position to recognize and assess the evidence properly in a given case. Second, it is doubtful that psychiatric specialists are in possession of any such reliable generalization, even in qualified form. Third, the paternalist physician is simply assuming that suicide is not a rational choice for the terminally ill patient.

If we attempt to apply the Prevention of Harm Argument to cases in which the patient's family or guardian is the object of paternalism, other difficulties become apparent. Consider cases of withholding information from the parents of a neonate with Down's syndrome or spina bifida. The most obvious difficulty is that premise (1) states only that the physician has a duty (or a right) to prevent or minimize harm to the patient, not to his family. If this argument is to serve as a justification of paternalism toward the infant patient's family, the advocate of paternalism must advance and support one or the other of two quite controversial premises. He must either add premise (1′) or replace premise (1) with premise (1″):

> (1′)   If X is a guardian or parent of a patient Y and Y is the patient of physician Z, then X is thereby a patient of physician Z as well.
>
> (1″)   It is the duty of the physician to prevent or minimize harm to his patient and to the guardian or family of his patient.

Since both the law and common sense maintain that one does not become a patient simply by being related to a patient, it seems that the best strategy for the medical paternalist is to rely on (1″) rather than on (1′).

Reliance on (1″), however, only weakens the case for medical paternalism toward parents of defective neonates. For now the medical paternalist must show that he has adequate evidence for psychiatric predictions the complexity of which taxes the imagination. He must first determine all the relevant effects of telling the truth, not just on the parents themselves, but on siblings as well, since whatever anguish or guilt the parents will allegedly feel may have significant effects on their other children. Next he must ascertain the ways in which these siblings—both as individuals and as a peer group—will respond to the predicted anguish and guilt of their parents. Then the physician must determine how the siblings will respond to each other. Next he must consider the possible responses of the parents to the responses of the children. And, of course, once he has accomplished all of this, the physician must look at the other side of the question. He must con-sider the possible harmful effects of withholding information from patients or of preventing them from taking an active part in decision-making. The conscientious paternalist must consider not only the burdens which the exercise of responsibility will allegedly place upon the parents, and indirectly upon their children, but also the burdens of guilt, self-doubt, and shame which may result from the parents' recognition that they have abdicated their responsibility.

In predicting whether telling the truth or withholding information will cause the least harm for the family as a whole, the physician must first make intrapersonal comparisons of harm and benefit for each member of the family, if the information is divulged. Then he must somehow coalesce these various intrapersonal net harm judgments into an estimate of the total net harm which divulging the information will do to the family as a whole. Then he must make similar intrapersonal and interpersonal net harm judgments about the results of not telling the truth. Finally he must compare these totals and determine which course of action will minimize harm to the family as a whole.

Though the problems of achieving defensible predictions of harm as a basis for paternalism are clearest in the case of defective neonates, they are in no way peculiar to those cases. Consider the case of a person with terminal cancer. To eliminate the complication of interpersonal net harm comparisons, let us suppose that this person has no relatives and is himself legally competent. Suppose that the physician withholds information of the diagnosis because he believes that knowledge of the truth would be more harmful than withholding the truth. I have already indicated that even if we view this judgment of comparative harm as a purely clinical judgment—more specifically a clinical psychiatric judgment—it is difficult to see how the physician could be in a position to make it. But it is crucial to note that the notions of harm and benefit appropriate to these deliberations are not exclusively clinical notions, whether psychiatric or otherwise. In taking it upon himself to determine what will be most beneficial or least harmful to this patient the physician is not simply making ill-founded medical judgments which someday might be confirmed by psychiatric research. He is making *moral* evaluations of the most basic and problematic kind.

The physician must determine whether it will be better for the patient to live his remaining days in the knowledge that his days are few or to live in ignorance of his fate. But again, this is a gross simplification: it assumes that the physician's attempt to deceive the patient will be successful. E. Kübler-Ross claims that in many, if not most, cases the terminally ill patient will guess or learn his fate whether the physician withholds the diagnosis from him or not.[11] Possible harm resulting from the patient's loss of confidence in the physician or from a state of uncertainty over his prospects must be taken into account.

Let us set aside this important complication and try to appreciate what sorts of factors would have to be taken into account in a well-founded judgment that the remainder of a person's life would be better for that person if he did not know that he had a terminal illness than if he did.

Such a judgment would have to be founded on a profound knowledge of the most intimate details of the patient's life history, his characteristic ways of coping with personal crises, his personal and vocational commitments and aspirations, his feelings of obligation toward others, and his attitude toward the completeness or incompleteness of his experience. In a society in which the personal physician was an intimate friend who shared the experience of families under his care, it would be somewhat more plausible to claim that the physician might possess such knowledge. Under the present conditions of highly impersonal specialist medical practice it is quite a different matter.

Yet even if the physician could claim such intimate personal knowledge, this would not suffice. For he must not only predict, but also *evaluate*. On the basis of an intimate knowledge of the patient as a person, he must determine which outcome would be *best* for that person. It is crucial to emphasize that the question which the physician must pose and answer is whether ignorance or knowledge will make possible a life that is better *for the patient himself.* The physician must be careful not to confuse this question with the question of whether ignorance or knowledge would make for a better life for the physician if the physician were terminally ill. Nor must he confuse it with the question of whether the patient's life would be a *better life*—a life more valuable to others or to society—if it ended in ignorance rather than in truth. The question, rather, is whether it would be better *for the patient himself* to know or not to know his fate.

To judge that a certain ending of a life would be best for the person whose life it is, is to view that life as a unified process of development and to conclude that that ending is a fitting completion for that process. To view a human life as a unified process of development, however, is to view it selectively. Certain events or patterns of conduct are singled out as especially significant or valuable. To ascertain the best completion of a person's life for that person, then, is to make the most fundamental judgments about the value of that person's activities, aspirations, and experiences.

It might be replied that we do make such value judgments when we decide to end the physiologic life of a permanently comatose individual. In such cases we do make value judgments, but they are not judgments of this sort. On the contrary, we believe that since this individual's experience has ended, his life-process is already completed.

When the decision to withhold information of impending death is understood for what it is, it is difficult to see how anyone could presume to make it. My conjecture is that physicians are tempted to make these decisions in part because of a failure to reflect upon the disparity between two quite different kinds of judgments about what will harm or benefit the patient. Judgments of the first sort fall within the physician's competence as a highly trained medical expert. There is nothing in the physician's training which qualifes him to make judgments of the second sort—to evaluate another human being's life as a whole. Further, once the complexity of these judgments is appreciated and once their evaluative character is understood, it is implausible to hold that the physician is in a better position to make them than the patient or his family. The failure to ask what sorts of harm/benefit judgments may properly be made by the physician in his capacity as a physician is a fundamenal feature of medical paternalism.

There is a more sophisticated version of the attempt to justify withholding of information in order to minimize harm to the patient or his family. This is the Contract Version of the Prevention of Harm Argument. The idea is that the physician-patient relationship is contractual and that the terms of this contract are such that the patient authorizes the physician to minimize harm to the patient (or his family) by whatever means he, the physician, deems necessary. Thus if the physician believes that the best way to minimize harm to the patient is to withhold information from him, he may do so without thereby wronging the patient. To wrong the patient the physician would either have to do something he was not authorized to do or fail to do something it was his duty to do and which was in his power to do. But in withholding information from the patient he is doing just what he is authorized to do. So he does the patient no wrong.

First of all, it should be noted that this version is vulnerable to the same objections just raised against the non-contractual Argument from the Prevention of Harm. The most serious of these is that in the cases of paternalism under discussion it is very doubtful that the physician will or even could possess the psychiatric and moral knowledge required for a well-founded judgment about what will be least harmful to the patient. In addition, the Contract Version is vulnerable to other objections. Consider the claim that the patient-physician relationship is a contract in which the patient authorizes the physician to prevent or minimize harm by whatever means the physician deems necessary, including the withholding of information. This claim could be interpreted in either of two ways: as a descriptive generalization about the way physicians and patients actually understand their relationship or as a normative claim about the way the physician-patient relationship should be viewed or may be viewed.

As a descriptive generalization it is certainly implausible—there are many people who do not believe they have authorized their physician to withhold the truth from them, and the legal doctrine of informed consent supports their view. Let us suppose for a moment that some people do view their relationship to their physician as including such an authorization and that there is nothing morally wrong with such a contract so long as both parties entered into it voluntarily and in full knowledge of the terms of the agreement.

Surely the fact that some people are willing to authorize physicians to withhold information from them would not justify the physician in acting toward other patients as if they had done so. The physician can only justify withholding information from a particular patient if this sort of contract was entered into freely and in full knowledge *by this* patient.

What, then, is the physician to do? Surely he cannot simply assume that all of his patients have authorized him to withhold the truth if he deems it necessary. Yet if in each case he inquires as to whether the patient wishes to make such an authorization, he will defeat the purpose of the authorization by undermining the patient's trust.

There is, however, a more serious difficulty. Even the more extreme advocates of medical paternalism must agree that there are some limits on the contractual relationship between physician and patient. Hence the obligations of each party are conditional upon the other party's observing the limits of the contract. The law, the medical profession, and the general public generally recognize that there are such limits. For example, the patient may refuse to undergo a certain treatment, he may seek a second opinion, or he may terminate the relationship altogether. Moreover, it is acknowledged that to decide to do any of these things the patient may—indeed perhaps must—rely on his own judgment. If he is conscientious he will make such decisions on consideration of whether the physician is doing a reasonable job of rendering the services for which he was hired.

There are general constraints on how those services may be rendered. If the treatment is unreasonably slow, if the physician's technique is patently sloppy, or if he employs legally questionable methods, the patient may rightly conclude that the physician has not lived up to the implicit terms of the agreement and terminate the relationship. There are also more special constraints on the contract stemming from the special nature of the problem which led the patient to seek the physician's services in the first place. If you go to a physician for treatment of a skin condition, but he ignores that problem and sets about trying to convince you to have cosmetic nose surgery, you may rightly terminate the relationship. These general and special constraints are limits on the agreement from the patient's point of view.

Now once it is admitted that there are any such terms—that the contract does have some limits and that the patient has the right to terminate the relationship if these limits are not observed by the physician—it must also be admitted that the patient must be in a position to discover *whether* those limits are being observed. But if the patient were to authorize the physician to withhold information, he might deprive himself of information which is relevant to determining whether the physician has observed the limits of the agreement.

I am not concerned to argue that authorizing a physician to withhold information is logically incompatible with the contract being conditional. My point, rather, is that to make such an authorization would show either that (a) one did not view the contract as being conditional or that (b) one did not take seriously the possibility that the conditions of the contract might be violated or that (c) one simply did not care whether the conditions were violated. Since it is unreasonable to expect a patient to make an unconditional contract or to ignore the possibility that conditions of the contract will be violated, and since one typically does care whether these conditions are observed, it is unreasonable to authorize the physician to withhold information when he sees fit. The Contract Version of the Argument from the Prevention of Harm, then, does not appear to be much of an improvement over its simpler predecessor.

There is one paternalist argument in favor of withholding of information which remains to be considered. This may be called the Argument from the Inability to Understand. The main premise is that the physician is justified in withholding information when the patient or his family is unable to understand the information. This argument is often used to justify paternalistic policies toward parents of defective infants in neonate intensive care units. The idea is that either their lack of intelligence or their excited emotional condition prevents parents from giving informed consent because they are incapable of being adequately informed. In such cases, it is said, "the doctrine of informed consent does not apply."[12]

This argument is also vulnerable to several objections. First, it too relies upon dubious and extremely broad psychological generalizations —in this case psychological generalizations about the cognitive powers of parents of defective neonates.

Second, and more importantly, it ignores the crucial question of the character of the institutional context in which parents find themselves. To the extent that paternalist attitudes shape medical institutions, this bleak estimate of the parental capacity for comprehension and rational decision tends to be a self-fulfilling prophecy. In an institution in which parents routinely sign operation permits without even having seen their newborn infants and without having the nature of the therapeutic options clearly explained to them, parents may indeed be incapable of understanding the little that they are told.

Third, it is a mistake to maintain that the legal duty to seek informed consent applies only where the physician can succeed in adequately informing parents. The doctor does not and cannot have a duty to make sure that all the information he conveys is understood by those to whom he conveys it. His duty is to make a reasonable effort to be understood.[13]

Fourth, it is important to ask exactly why it is so important not to tell parents information which they allegedly will not understand. If the reason is that a parental decision based on inadequate understanding will be a decision that is harmful to the *infant,* then the Argument from the Inability to Understand is not an argument for paternalism toward *parents.* So if this argument is to provide a justification for withholding information from parents for *their* benefit then the claim must be that their failure to understand will somehow be harmful to *them.* But why should this be so? If the idea is that the parents will not only fail to understand but become distressed because they realize that they do not understand, then the Argument from the Inability to Understand turns out not to be a new argument at all. Instead, it is just a restatement of the Argument from the Prevention of Harm examined above—and is vulnerable to the same objections. I conclude that none of the three justifications examined provide adequate support for the paternalist practices under consideration. If adequate justification is to be found, the advocate of medical paternalism must marshal more powerful arguments.

V

So far I have examined several specific medical paternalist practices and criticized some general arguments offered in their behalf. Medical paternalism, however, goes much deeper than the specific practices themselves. For this reason I have spoken of "the medical paternalist model," emphasizing that what is at issue is a paradigm, a way of conceiving the physician-patient relationship. Indirect evidence for the pervasiveness of this model is to be found in the very words we used to describe physicians, patients, and their interactions. Simply by way of illustration, I will now examine one widely used distinction which expresses and helps perpetuate the paternalist model: the distinction between "ordinary" and "extraordinary" therapeutic measures.

Many physicians, theologians, ethicists, and judges have relied on this distinction since Pius XII employed it in an address on "The Prolongation of Life" in 1958. In reply to questions concerning conditions under which physicians may discontinue or refrain from initiating the use of artificial respiration devices, Pius first noted that physicians are duty-bound "to take the necessary treatment for the preservation of life and health." He then distinguished between "ordinary" and "extraordinary" means.

> But normally one is held to use only ordinary means—according to circumstances of persons, places, times, and culture—means that do not involve any grave burden for oneself or another.[14]

Though he is not entirely explicit about this, Pius assumes that it is the right of the physician to determine what will count as "ordinary" or "extraordinary" means in any particular case.

In the context of the issue of when a highly trained specialist is to employ sophisticated life-support equipment, it is natural to assume that the distinction between "ordinary" and "extraordinary" means is a distinction between higher and lower degrees of technological sophistication. The Pope's unargued assumption that the medical specialist is to determine what counts as "ordinary" or "extraordinary" reinforces a technological interpretation of the distinction. After all, if the distinction is a technological one, then it is natural to assume that it is the physician who should determine its application since it is he who possesses the requisite technical expertise. In my discussions with physicians, nurses, and hospital administrators I have observed that they tend to treat the distinction as a technological one and then to argue that since it is a technological distinction the physician is the one who should determine in any particular case whether a procedure would involve "ordinary" or "extraordinary" means.[15]

Notice, however, that even though Pius introduced the distinction in the context of the proper use of sophisticated technical devices and even though he assumed that it was to be applied by those who possess the technical skills to use such equipment, it is quite clear that the distinction he explicitly introduced is not itself a technological distinction. Recall that he defines "ordinary" means as those which "do not involve any grave burden for oneself or another." "Extraordinary" means, then, would be those which do involve a grave burden for oneself or for another.

If what counts as "extraordinary" measures depended only upon what would constitute a "grave burden" to the patient himself, it might be easier to preserve the illusion that the decision is an exercise of medical expertise. But once the evaluation of burdens is extended to the patient's family it becomes obvious that the judgment that a certain therapy would be "extraordinary" is not a technological or even a clinical, but rather a *moral* decision. And it is a moral decision regardless of whether the evaluation is made from the perspective of the patient's own values and preferences or from that of the physician.

Even if one is to evaluate only the burdens for the patient himself, however, it is implausible to maintain that the application of the distinction is an exercise of technological or clinical judgment. For as soon as we ask what would result in "grave burdens" for the patient, we are immediately confronted with the task of making moral distinctions and moral evaluations concerning the quality of the patient's life and his interests as a person.

When pressed for an explanation of how physicians actually apply the distinction between "ordinary" and "extraordinary" therapeutic measures, the director of a neonate intensive care unit explained to me that what counts as "ordinary" or "extraordinary" differs in "different contexts." Surgical correction of a congenital gastrointestinal blockage in the case of an otherwise normal infant would be considered an "ordinary" measure. But the same operation on an infant with Down's syndrome would be considered extraordinary.

I am not concerned here to criticize the moral decision to refrain from aggressive surgical treatment of infants with Down's syndrome. My purpose in citing this example is simply to point out that this decision *is* a moral decision and that the use of the distinction between "ordinary" and "extraordinary" measures does nothing to help one make the decision. The use of the distinction does accomplish something though: it obscures the fact that the decision *is* a moral decision. Even worse, it is likely to lead one to mistake a very controversial moral decision for a "value-free" technological or clinical decision. More importantly, to even suggest that a complex moral judgment is a clinical or technological judgment is to prejudice the issue of *who* has the right to decide whether life-sustaining measures are to be initiated or continued. Once controversial moral decisions are misperceived as clinical* or technological decisions it becomes much easier for the medical paternalist to use the three arguments examined above to justify the withholding of information. For once it is conceded that his medical expertise gives the physician the right to make certain decisions, he can

then argue that he may withhold information where this is necessary for the effective exercise of this right. By disguising complex moral judgments as medical judgments, then, the "ordinary/extraordinary" distinction reinforces medical paternalism.

VI

In this paper I have attempted to articulate and challenge some basic features of the medical paternalist model of the physician-patient relationship. I have also given an indication of the powerful influence this model exerts on medical practice and on ways of talking and thinking about medical treatment.

There are now signs that medical paternalism is beginning to be challenged from within the medical profession itself.[16] This, I believe, is all to the good. So far, however, challenges have been fragmentary and unsystematic. If they are to be theoretically and practically fruitful they must be grounded in a systematic understanding of what medical paternalism is and in a critical examination of justifications for medical paternalist practices. The present paper is an attempt to begin the task of such a systematic critique.

Notes

1. See, for example, G. Dworkin's paper "Paternalism," in S. Gorovitz et al., *Moral Problems in Medicine,* 1st ed., (Englewood Cliffs, NJ; Prentice-Hall, 1976), p. 18.
2. In *Moral Problems in Medicine,* 1st ed., p. 112. Oken's study was first published in 1967.
3. Oken, p. 113.
4. *Malpractice Digest* (St. Paul, MN: The St. Paul Property and Liability Insurance Company, July-August 1977), p. 6.
5. It is interesting to note that acccording to both the usual and the expanded characterization of paternalism stated above, only a person who has certain physical and mental capacities can be an object of paternalism, since it is only when these capacities are present that it is correct to speak of interfering with that individual's freedom of action, misinforming him, or withholding information from him.

6. For a helpful summary, see J. A. Robertson and N. Fost, "Passive Euthanasia of Defective Newborn Infants: Legal Considerations," *The Journal of Pediatrics* 88, no. 5 (1976): 883–889.

7. Shaw, "Dilemmas of 'Informed Consent' in Children," *The New England Journal of Medicine* 289, no. 17 (1973): 886. Reprinted in this volume.

8. Shaw, p. 885.

9. R. Duff and A. Campbell, "Moral and Ethical Dilemmas in the Special-Care Nursery," *The New England Journal of Medicine* 289, no. 17 (1973): p. 893. Reprinted in this volume.

10. Oken, "What to Tell Cancer Patients," pp. 112, 113.

11. Kübler-Ross, excerpts from *Death and Dying,*

quoted in *Moral Problems in Medicine,* 1st ed., p. 122.

12. Duff and Campbell, "Moral and Ethical Dilemmas," p. 893.

13. I would like to thank John Dolan for clarifying this point.

14. Pius XII, "The Prolongation of Life," in Reiser et al., *Ethics in Medicine,* (Cambridge, MA: MIT Press, 1977), pp. 501–504.

15. These discussions occurred in the course of my work as a member of the committee which drafted ethical guidelines for Children's Hospital of Minneapolis.

16. See, for example, A. Waldman, "Medical Ethics and the Hopelessly Ill Child," *The Journal of Pediatrics* 88, no. 5 (1976): 890–892.

From "Application of President and Directors of Georgetown College"

J. Skelly Wright

Mrs. Jones was brought to the hospital by her husband for emergency care, having lost two thirds of her body's blood supply from a ruptured ulcer. She had no personal physician, and relied solely on the hospital staff. She was a total hospital responsibility. It appeared that the patient, age 25, mother of a seven-month-old child, and her husband were both Jehovah's Witnesses, the teachings of which sect, according to their interpretation, prohibited the injection of blood into the body. When death without blood became imminent, the hospital sought the advice of counsel, who applied to the District Court in the name of the hospital for permission to administer blood. Judge Tamm of the District Court denied the application, and counsel immediately applied to me, as a member of the Court of Appeals, for an appropriate writ.

Excerpted from the decision 331 F.2d 1000. (D.C. Cir.), certiorari denied, 377 U.S. 978 (1964). Reprinted as it appeared in *Experimentation with Human Beings,* ed. J. Katz (N.Y: Russell Sage Foundation, 1972), pp. 551–52.

I called the hospital by telephone and spoke with Dr. Westura, Chief Medical Resident, who confirmed the representations made by counsel. I thereupon proceeded with counsel to the hospital, where I spoke to Mr. Jones, the husband of the patient. He advised me that, on religious grounds, he would not approve a blood transfusion for his wife. He said, however, that if the court ordered the transfusion, the responsibility was not his. I advised Mr. Jones to obtain counsel immediately. He thereupon went to the telephone and returned in 10 or 15 minutes to advise that he had taken the matter up with his church and that he had decided that he did not want counsel.

I asked permission of Mr. Jones to see his wife. This he readily granted. Prior to going into the patient's room, I again conferred with Dr. Westura and several other doctors assigned to the case. All confirmed that the patient would die without blood and that there was a better than 50 per cent chance of saving her life with it. Unanimously they strongly recommended it. I then went inside the patient's room. Her appearance confirmed the urgency which had been represented to me. I tried to communicate with her, advising her again as to what the doctors had said. The only audible reply I could hear was ''Against my will.'' It was obvious that the woman was not in a mental condition to make a decision. I was reluctant to press her because of the seriousness of her condition and because I felt that to suggest repeatedly the imminence of death without blood might place a strain on her religious convictions. I asked her whether she would oppose the blood transfusion if the court allowed it. She indicated, as best I could make out, that it would not then be her responsibility. . . .

[I] signed the order allowing the hospital to administer such transfusions as the doctors should detemine were necessary to save her life. . . .

Before proceeding with this inquiry, it may be useful to state what this case does not involve. This case does not involve a person who, for religious or other reasons, has refused to seek medical attention. It does not involve a disputed medical judgment or a dangerous or crippling operation. Nor does it involve the delicate question of saving the newborn in preference to the mother. Mrs. Jones sought medical attention and placed on the hospital the legal responsibility for her proper care. In its dilemma, not of its own making, the hospital sought judicial direction. . . .

If self-homicide is a crime, there is no exception to the law's command for those who believe the crime to be divinely ordained. The Mormon cases in the Supreme Court establish that there is no religious exception to criminal laws, and state *obiter* the very example that a religiously inspired suicide attempt would be within the law's authority to prevent. . . . But whether attempted suicide is a crime is in doubt in some jurisdictions, including the District of Columbia.

The Gordian knot of this suicide question may be cut by the simple fact that Mrs. Jones did not want to die. Her voluntary presence in the hospital as a patient seeking medical help testified to this. Death, to Mrs. Jones, was not a

religiously commanded goal, but an unwanted side effect of a religious scruple. . . . Nor are we faced with the question of whether the state should intervene to reweigh the relative values of life and death, after the individual has weighed them for himself and found life wanting. Mrs. Jones wanted to live.

A third set of considerations involved the position of the doctors and the hospital. Mrs. Jones was their responsibility to treat. The hospital doctors had the choice of administering the proper treatment or letting Mrs. Jones die in the hospital bed, thus exposing themselves, and the hospital, to the risk of civil and criminal liability in either case. It is not certain that Mrs. Jones had any authority to put the hospital and its doctors to this impossible choice. The normal principle that an adult patient directs her doctors is based on notions of commercial contract which may have less relevance to life-or-death emergencies. It is not clear just where a patient would derive her authority to command her doctor to treat her under limitations which would produce death. The patient's counsel suggests that this authority is part of constitutionally protected liberty. But neither the principle that life and liberty are inalienable rights, nor the principle of liberty of religion, provides an easy answer to the question whether the state can prevent martyrdom. Moreover, Mrs. Jones had no wish to be a martyr. And her religion merely prevented her consent to a transfusion. If the law undertook the responsibility of authorizing the transfusion without her consent, no problem would be raised with respect to her religious practice. Thus, the effect of the order was to preserve for Mrs. Jones the life she wanted without sacrifice of her religious beliefs.

The final, and compelling, reason for granting the emergency writ was that a life hung in the balance. There was no time for research and reflection. Death could have mooted the cause in a matter of minutes, if action were not taken to preserve the *status quo*. To refuse to act, only to find later that the law required action, was a risk I was unwilling to accept. I determined to act on the side of life.

From *In re Brooks Estate*

Robert C. Underwood

On and sometime before May 7, 1964, Bernice Brooks was in the McNeal General Hospital, Chicago, suffering from a peptic ulcer. She was being attended by Dr. Gilbert Demange, and had informed him repeatedly during a two-year period prior thereto that her religious and medical convictions precluded her from receiving blood transfusions. Mrs. Brooks, her husband and two adult children are all members of the religious sect commonly known as Jehovah's Witnesses. Among the religious beliefs adhered to by members of this group is the principle that blood transfusions are a violation of the law of God, and that transgressors will be punished by God. . . .

Mrs. Brooks and her husband had signed a document releasing Dr. Demange and the hospital from all civil liability that might result from the failure to administer blood transfusions to Mrs. Brooks. The patient was assured that there would thereafter be no further effort to persuade her to accept blood.

Notwithstanding these assurances, however, Dr. Demange, together with several assistant State's attorneys, and the attorney for the public guardian of Cook County, Illinois, appeared before the probate division of the circuit court with a petition by the public guardian requesting appointment of that officer as conservator of the person of Bernice Brooks and further requesting an order authorizing such conservator to consent to the administration of whole blood to the patient. . . . Thereafter, the conservator of the person was appointed, consented to the administration of a blood transfusion, it was accomplished and apparently successfully so, although appellants now argue that much distress resulted from transfusions due to a "circulatory overload.". . .

Appellees argue that society has an overriding interest in protecting the lives of its

Excerpted from the decision 32 Ill.2d 361, 205 N.E.2d 435 (1965). Reprinted as it appeared in *Experimentation with Human Beings*, ed. J. Katz (N.Y.: Russell Sage Foundation, 1972), pp. 559–60.

citizens which justifies the action here taken. . . .

We believe Jefferson's fundamental concept that civil officers may intervene only when religious "principles break out into overt acts against peace and good order" has consistently prevailed. . . .

. . . It seems to be clearly established that the First Amendment of the United States Constitution, as extended to the individual States by the Fourteenth Amendment to that constitution, protects the absolute right of every individual to freedom in his religious belief and the exercise thereof, subject only to the qualification that the exercise thereof may properly be limited by governmental action where such exercise endangers, clearly and presently, the public health, welfare or morals. Those cases which have sustained governmental action as against the challenge that it violated the religious guarantees of the First Amendment have found the proscribed practice to be immediately deleterious to some phase of public welfare, health or morality. The decisions which have held the conduct complained of immune from proscription involve no such public injury and no danger thereof.

Applying the constitutional guarantees and the interpretations thereof heretofore enunciated to the facts before us we find a competent adult who has steadfastly maintained her belief that acceptance of a blood transfusion is a violation of the law of God. Knowing full well the hazards involved, she has firmly opposed acceptance of such transfusions, notifying the doctor and hospital of her convictions and desires, and executing documents releasing both the doctor and the hospital from any civil liability which might be thought to result from a failure on the part of either to administer such transfusions. No minor children are involved. No overt or affirmative act of appellants offers any clear and present danger to society—we have only a governmental agency compelling conduct offensive to appellant's religious principles. Even though we may consider appellant's beliefs unwise, foolish or ridiculous, in the absence of an overriding danger to society we may not permit interference therewith in the form of a conservatorship established in the waning hours of her life for the sole purpose of compelling her to accept medical treatment forbidden by her religious principles and previously refused by her with full knowledge of the probable consequences. In the final analysis, what has happened here involves a judicial attempt to decide what course of action is best for a particular individual, notwithstanding that individual's contrary views based upon religious convictions. Such action cannot be constitutionally countenanced. . . .

While the action of the circuit court herein was unquestionably well-meaning, and justified in the absence of decisions to the contrary, we have no recourse but to hold that it has interfered with basic constitutional rights.

Accordingly, the orders of the probate division of the circuit court of Cook County are reversed.

Autonomy and the Refusal of Lifesaving Treatment

Bruce L. Miller

Contemporary, normative ethics—both theoretical and applied—has reacted against utilitarianism because of its tendency to regard the individual as little more than a recipient of good and evil. To avoid the pernicious effect of this notion, many philosophers have insisted that the concept of a person as an autonomous agent must have a central and independent role in ethical theory.[1] From this position there is firm ground to resist coercion and its less forceful, but more pervasive, cousins: manipulation and undue influence. It also provides a warrant for treating a person's own choices, plans, and conception of self as generally dominant over what another believes to be in that person's best interest.

In biomedical ethics, the concept of a person as an autonomous agent places an obligation on physicians and other health professionals to respect the values of patients and not to let their own values influence decisions about treatment. The conflict of patient values and physician values becomes most troublesome when a patient refuses treatment needed to sustain life and a physician believes that the patient should

Reprinted with permission from the author and *The Hastings Center Report*, August 1981. © Institute of Society, Ethics and the Life Sciences, 360 Broadway, Hastings-on-Hudson, N.Y. 10706.

be treated. The conflict can be resolved by taking a firm line on autonomy: any autonomous decision of a patient must be respected. On the other hand, the physician's obligation to preserve life can be placed above the patient's right to autonomy and refusals of treatment can then be overridden when they conflict with "medical judgment."[2] The notion of medical judgment used here is not clear, and it may only be a gloss for "what doctor thinks best." Neither extreme position is tenable; both are insensitive to the complexities of such cases, and the second removes the right to autonomy altogether. But, the conflict between autonomy and medical judgment is not as sharp as it seems.

FOUR CASES

Consider the following cases.

Case 1. A doctor, sixty-eight years of age, had been retired for five years after severe myocardial infarction. He was admitted to a hospital after a barium meal had shown a large and advanced carcinoma of the stomach. Ten days after palliative gastrectomy was performed, the patient collapsed with a massive pulmonary embolism and an emergency embolectomy was done on the ward. When the patient recovered, he asked that if he had a further cardiovascular collapse no steps should be taken to prolong his life, for the pain of his cancer was more than he would needlessly bear. He wrote a note to this effect in his case records and the hospital staff knew of his feelings.[3]

Case 2.   A forty-three-year-old man was admitted to the hospital with injuries and internal bleeding caused when a tree fell on him. He needed whole blood for a transfusion but refused to give the necessary consent. His wife also refused. Both were Jehovah's Witnesses, holding religious beliefs that forbid the infusion of whole blood. The hospital lawyer brought a petition to the home of a judge. The patient's wife, brother, and grandfather were present to express his strong convictions. The grandfather said that the patient "wants to live very much . . . He wants to live in the Bible's promised new world where life will never end. A few hours here would nowhere compare to everlasting life." The judge was concerned with the patient's capacity to make such a decision in light of his serious condition. She recognized the possibility that the use of drugs might have impaired his judgment. The hospital lawyer replied that the patient was receiving fluid intravenously but no drugs that could impair his judgment. He was conscious, knew what the doctor was saying, was aware of the consequences of his decision, and had with full understanding executed a statement refusing the recommended transfusion and releasing the hospital from liability. The judge went to the patient's bedside. She asked him whether he believed that he would be deprived of the opportunity for "everlasting life" if transfusion were ordered by the court. His response was, "Yes. In other words, it is between me and Jehovah; not the courts. . . . I'm willing to take my chances. My faith is that strong. . . . I wish to live, but not with blood transfusions. Now get that straight." The patient had two young children. There was a family business and money to provide for the children, and a large family willing to care for them.[4]

Case 3.   A thirty-eight-year-old man with mild upper respiratory infection suddenly developed severe headache, stiff neck, and high fever. He went to an emergency room for help.

The diagnosis was pneumococcal meningitis, a bacterial meningitis almost always fatal if not treated. If treatment is delayed, permanent neurological damage is likely. A physician told the patient that urgent treatment was needed to save his life and forestall brain damage. The patient refused to consent to treatment saying that he wanted to be allowed to die.[5]

Case 4.   A fifty-two-year-old married man was admitted to a medical intensive care unit (MICU) after a suicide attempt. He had retired two years earlier because of progressive physical disability related to multiple sclerosis (MS) during the fifteen years before admission. He had successfully adapted to his physical limitations, remaining actively involved in family matters with his wife and two teenage sons. However, during the three months before admission, he had become morose and withdrawn. On the evening of admission, while alone, he had ingested an unknown quantity of diazepam. When his family returned six hours later, they found the patient semiconscious. He had left a suicide note. On admission to the MICU, physician examination showed several neurologic deficits, but no more severe than in recent examinations. The patient was alert and fully conversant. He expressed to the house officers his strong belief in a patient's right to die with dignity. He stressed the "meaningless" aspects of his life related to his loss of function, insisting that he did not want vigorous medical intervention should serious complications develop. This position appeared logically coherent to the MICU staff. However, a consultation with members of the psychiatric liaison service was requested. During the initial consultation the patient showed that the onset of his withdrawal and depression coincided with a diagnosis of inoperable cancer in his mother-in-law, who lived in another city. His wife had spent more and more time satisfying her mother's needs. In fact, on the night of his suicide attempt, the patient's wife and two sons had left him alone for the first time to visit his mother-in-law.[6]

In the first two cases, the most compelling intuition is to respect the refusal of treatment. The patients are competent, exercising their right of autonomy to refuse treatments they believed not in their interest. The patient in Case 1 believed further resuscitation was needless, for it would only briefly prolong a life of great suffering. His concern was for life on earth. The patient in Case 2 believed the transfusions would deprive him of salvation. His concern for life hereafter made whatever life on earth he could get from the transfusions insignificant. In Case 2 the Superior Court and Court of Appeals recognized the patient's right to refuse transfusion and none was given. Though the patient's chances were thought very slim, he recovered and was discharged from the hospital. In Case 1, two weeks after the embolectomy the patient suffered acute myocardial infarction; his heart was restarted five times in one night. He recovered to linger for three weeks in a coma. On the day his heart stopped, plans were being made to put him on a respirator. The Jehovah's Witness was fortunate, retaining his life on earth without risking the loss of life everlasting. The physician was not so lucky; his right to an autonomous decision concerning the manner of his own death fell victim to the technological imperative—"If you *can* do it, you *should* do it."

Cases 3 and 4, however, incline to the view that patient autonomy may be overridden by medical judgment. In Case 3 there is no apparent reason to justify the death of this otherwise healthy victim of meningitis. His medical condition is not hopeless, as was the condition of the doctor in Case 1, nor does he have a religious objection to treatment like the Jehovah's Witness in Case 2. Our intuition is to treat him against his will. In Case 4 the patient's disability may give us pause; it does prevent a full life, yet he had managed until his mother-in-law became ill and the family began attending to her needs. We might expect that family discussion of the problem could lead to a resolution that would restore the patient's desire to live.

At first glance the position that although there is a right to autonomy from which patients can refuse lifesaving treatment, the right is not absolute and sometimes medical judgment can override it is a tenable one; for there is nothing surprising about a right that is not absolute.[7] However, acknowledging the limits of rights does not mean that rights can be over-

ridden when their exercise conflicts with others' judgments. If medical judgment can override the right to refusal of treatment, then all four patients should have been treated against their will, for in each case a physician believed that the patient should be treated. If this is implausible, given our intuitions on Cases 1 and 2, then we have to say that autonomy is supreme and the refusals of lifesaving treatment should have been respected in all four cases.

One way around this impasse is to develop a list of conditions that must be taken into account to determine whether a refusal of treatment should be respected,[8] for example, age of the patient, life expectancy with and without treatment, the level of incapacity with and without treatment, the degree of pain and suffering, the effect of the time and circumstances of death on family and friends, the views of the family on whether the patient should be treated, the views of the physician and other medical staff, and the costs of treatment. This is a plausible approach; with it the refusal of treatment for meningitis can be justifiably overridden and the refusal of treatment for the doctor suffering from cancer justifiably respected. The meningitis patient is young and will recover without residual defect to lead a full life; the cancer patient will die soon in any case, is suffering greatly, and even though resuscitated is not likely to survive with a capacity for conscious awareness.

The problem with this approach is twofold. First, the list of characteristics is so vague, and hence subject to alternative interpretations, that the right to autonomy, and with it the right to refuse lifesaving treatment, can again be overruled. In practice it might turn out that refusals of treatment would be respected only if there were few negative consequences and everyone agreed with the decision. Second, this view shifts the focus from the patient's refusal to the patient's condition. Appealing to a list of diagnostic and prognostic features and to the consequences for others of treatment versus nontreatment makes the decision one *about* the patient rather than one *by* the patient. The patient's refusal becomes simply one of many factors to weigh in arriving at a decision. But the thrust of placing the patient's right to autonomy in the forefront of medical ethics is to counteract just that tendency to secure those decisions *for* patients that are appropriately theirs. An approach that preserves this priority must be developed.

FOUR SENSES OF AUTONOMY

If the concept of autonomy is clarified, we will have a more rigorous understanding of what the right to autonomy is and what it means to respect that right, thus illuminating the problems regarding refusals of lifesaving treatment. At the first level of analysis it is enough to say that autonomy is self-determination, that the right to autonomy is the right to make one's own choices, and that respect for autonomy is the obligation not to interfere with the choice of another and to treat another as a being capable of choosing. This is helpful, but the concept has more than one meaning. There are at least four senses of the concept as it is used in medical ethics: autonomy as free action, autonomy as authenticity, autonomy as effective deliberation, and autonomy as moral reflection.[9]

Autonomy as Free Action. Autonomy as free action means an action that is voluntary and intentional. An action is voluntary if it is not the result of coercion, duress, or undue influence. An action is intentional if it is the conscious object of the actor. To submit oneself, or refuse to submit oneself, to medical treatment is an action. If a patient wishes to be treated and submits to treatment, that action is intentional. If a patient wishes not to be treated and refuses treatment, that too is an intentional action. A treatment may be a free action by the physician and yet the patient's action is not free. If the meningitis victim is restrained and medication administered against his wishes, the patient has not voluntarily submitted to treatment. If the patient agrees to pain relief medication, but is given an antibiotic without his knowledge, the patient voluntarily submitted to treatment, but it was not a free action because he did not intend to receive an antibiotic. The doctrine of consent, as it was before the law gave us the doctrine of *informed* consent, required that permission be obtained from a patient and that the patient be told what treatment would be given; this maintains the right to autonomy as free ac-

tion. Permission to treat makes the treatment voluntary and knowledge of what treatment will be given makes it intentional.

Autonomy as Authenticity. Autonomy as authenticity means that an action is consistent with the person's attitudes, values, dispositions, and life plans. Roughly, the person is acting in character. Our inchoate notion of authenticity is revealed in comments like, "He's not himself today" or "She's not the Jane Smith I know." For an action to be labeled "inauthentic" it has to be unusual or unexpected, relatively important in itself or its consequences, and have no apparent or proffered explanation. An action is unusual for a given actor if it is different from what the actor almost always (or always) does in the circumstances, as in, "He always flies to Chicago, but this time he took the train." If an action is not of the sort that a person either usually does or does not do, for example, something more like getting married than drinking coffee, it can still be a surprise to those who know the person. "What! George got married?"

A person's dispositions, values, and plans can be known, and particular actions can then be seen as not in conformity with them. If the action is not of serious import, concern about its authenticity is inappropriate. To ask of a person who customarily drinks beer, "Are you *sure* you want to drink wine?" is to make much of very little. If an explanation for the unusual or unexpected behavior is apparent, or given by the actor, that usually cuts off concern. If no explanation appears on the face of things or if one is given that is unconvincing, then it is appropriate to wonder if the action is really one that the person wants to take. Often we will look for disturbances in the person's life that might account for the inauthenticity.

It will not always be possible to label an action authentic or inauthentic, even where much is known about a person's attitudes, values, and life plans. On the other hand, a given disposition may not be sufficiently specific to judge that it would motivate a particular action. A generous person need not contribute to every cause to merit that attribute. If a person's financial generosity is known to extend to a wide range of liberal political causes, not making a contribution to a given liberal candidate for political office may be inauthentic. On the other hand, most people have dispositions that conflict in some situations; an interest in and commitment to scientific research will conflict with fear of invasive procedures when such an individual considers being a subject in medical research. Many questions about this sense of autonomy cannot be explored here, for example, whether there can be authentic conversions in a persons' values and life plans.

Autonomy as Effective Deliberation. Autonomy as effective deliberation means action taken where a person believed that he or she was in a situation calling for a decision, was aware of the alternatives and the consequences of the alternatives, evaluated both, and chose an action based on that evaluation. Effective deliberation is of course a matter of degree; one can be more or less aware and take more or less care in making decisions. Effective deliberation is distinct from authenticity and free action. A person's action can be voluntary and intentional and not result from effective deliberation, as when one acts impulsively. Further, a person who has a rigid pattern of life acts authentically when he or she does the things we have all come to expect, but without effective deliberation. In medicine, there is no effective deliberation if a patient believes that the physician makes all the decisions. The doctrine of *informed* consent, which requires that the patient be informed of the risks and benefits of the proposed treatment and its alternatives, protects the right to autonomy when autonomy is conceived as effective deliberation.

Gerald Dworkin has shown that an effective deliberation must be more than an apparently coherent thought process.[10] A person who does not wear automobile seat belts may not know that wearing seat belts significantly reduces the chances of death and serious injury. Deliberation without this knowledge can be logically coherent and lead to a decision not to wear seat belts. Alternatively, a person may know the dangers of not wearing seat belts, but maintain that the inconvenience of wearing them outweighs the reduced risk of serious injury or death. Both deliberations are noneffective: the first because it proceeds on ignorance of a crucial piece of information; the second because it assigns a nonrational weighting to alternatives.

It is not always possible to separate the factual and evaluative errors in a noneffective deliberation. A patient may refuse treatment because of its pain and inconvenience, for example, kidney dialysis, and choose to run the risk of serious illness and death. To say that such a patient has the relevant knowledge, if all alternatives and their likely consequences have been explained, but made a nonrational assignment of priorities, is much too simple. A more accurate characterization may be that the patient fails to appreciate certain aspects of the alternatives. The patient may be cognitively aware of the pain and inconvenience of the treatment, but because he or she has not experienced them, may believe that they will be worse than they really are. If the patient has begun dialysis, assessment of the pain and inconvenience may not take into account the possibilities of adapting to them or reducing them by adjustments in the treatment.

In order to avoid conflating effective deliberation with reaching a decision acceptable to the physician, the following must be kept in mind: first, the knowledge a patient needs to decide whether to accept or refuse treatment is not equivalent to a physician's knowledge of alternative treatments and their consequences; second, what makes a weighting nonrational is not that it is different from the physician's weighting, but either that the weighting is inconsistent with other values that the patient holds or that there is good evidence that the patient will not persist in the weighting; third, lack of appreciation of aspects of the alternatives is most likely when the patient has not fully experienced them. In some situations there will be overlap between determinations of authenticity and effective deliberation. This does not undercut the distinctions between the senses of autonomy; rather it shows the complexity of the concept.

Autonomy as Moral Reflection. Autonomy as moral reflection means acceptance of the moral values one acts on.[11] The values can be those one was dealt in the socialization process, or they can differ in small or large measure.

In any case, one has reflected on these values and now accepts them as one's own. This sense of autonomy is deepest and most demanding when it is conceived as reflection on one's complete sets of values, attitudes, and life plans. It requires rigorous self-analysis, awareness of alternative set of values, commitment to a method for assessing them, and an ability to put them in place. Occasional, or piecemeal moral reflection is less demanding and more common. It can be brought about by a particular moral problem and only requires reflection on the values and plans relevant to the problem. Autonomy as moral reflection is distinguished from effective deliberation, for one can do the latter without questioning the values on which one bases the choice in a deliberation. Reflection on one's values may be occasioned by deliberation on a particular problem, so in some cases it may be difficult to sort out reflection on one's values and plans from deliberation using one's values and plans. Moral reflection can be related to authenticity by regarding the former as determining what sort of person one will be and in comparison to which one's actions can be judged as authentic or inauthentic.

RESOLVING APPARENT CONFLICTS

The distinction of four senses of autonomy can be used to resolve the apparent conflict between autonomy and medical judgment that the four cases generate. The action of the Jehovah's Witness in Case 2 is autonomous in at least three of the senses. It was a free action because it was voluntary and intentional. The patient was not being coerced and knew what he was doing. It was an authentic action because it was demanded by a strongly held religious belief. A Jehovah's Witness who accepted transfusion under the circumstances would be regarded as one who lacked the strength of commitment to resist earthly temptations; this would not be cause for blame, for it is understandable and, if you are not a Jehovah's Witness, commendable. The action was the result of effective deliberation because the patient knew he had a choice, was aware of the alternatives and their

consequences, evaluated them on his values, and made a choice. The situation was so clear and his belief so strong that the deliberation probably did not take much time and thought; effective deliberation is long and painstaking only when the matter for decision is perceived to be difficult. Whether the patient engaged in moral reflection is difficult to determine. The case is not sufficiently detailed to know whether the patient ever carefully reflected on his religious beliefs. One can have strong beliefs without ever having thought carefully about them. Further, since no position has been taken on just what the standards for adequate moral reflection are, it is not possible to make a determination even if all the facts were there. Whether one can, or should, choose a life plan or a religious belief by reasoned inquiry (effective deliberation at the most general level) is a matter of controversy in philosophy and theology.

In Case 1, the physician with cancer, the refusal of treatment was a free action, authentic, and the result of effective deliberation. The decision to treat the patient after he had refused resuscitation in the event of cardiovascular collapse was clearly a violation of his autonomy. He did not voluntarily submit to treatment; he was treated against his will even though no force or threat of force had to be used. He did not intend to submit to treatment, his conscious desire was not to be treated. The authenticity of the refusal of treatment is less a matter of identifying a particular strong belief and showing that the action is in accord with it, than it is a matter of the patient announcing that further resuscitation would incur needless suffering. Because this patient is a physician who has seen such suffering and is now undergoing it, it is more likely that the assertion is coming from the patient's values, and not as something that is not an authentic expression of himself. The refusal also appears to be the result of effective deliberation: the patient knew the alternatives and their consequences, his assessment and weighting of them cannot be regarded as nonrational or a lack of appreciation. Again we do not know whether and how this patient has reflected on the fundamental values that determine his judgment, but to require that he subject them to some sort of reflection before his wishes have to be respected would be to set the standards of autonomy too high.

In Case 4, the man with MS who attempted suicide, the action of the patient is a free action, that is, voluntary and intentional, and it is the result of effective deliberation, but it is not authentic. This was the outcome of the case:

> The patient had too much pride to complain to his wife about his feelings of abandonment. He was able to recognize that his suicide attempt and his insistence on death with dignity were attempts to draw the family's attention to his needs. Discussion with all four family members led to improved communication and acknowledgment of the patient's special emotional needs. After these conversations, the patient explicitly retracted both his suicidal threats and his demand that no supportive medical efforts be undertaken.[12]

It is tempting to say that the actions of the patient, the suicide attempt and the refusal of treatment, were not free actions because they were neither voluntary nor intentional. Even though the patient was not coerced directly by another, he was pressured into the actions by his condition and the circumstances of his mother-in-law's terminal illness. Further, it was not an intentional action because he did not *really* want to die; he wanted attention and support. This position is not defensible. First, the claim that the actions were not voluntary rests on the fact that the pressure of circumstances as a motivating factor can be as strong as the direct threat of another person. Indeed, it is easy to imagine cases where it would be stronger. It is important to preserve a clear and distinct concept of voluntariness, and treat similar but distinguishable situations under a different rubric.

Second, the claim that his action was not intentional, that is, not his conscious object, is wrong for two reasons. It fails to distinguish the action of taking the overdose of diazepam from his saying that he wanted no treatment and that he wanted to die with dignity. It was his conscious desire to take the diazepam and to refuse treatment; whether it was his conscious desire to die with dignity is a separate matter. Its answer requires adducing considerations that belong to the notion of autonomy as authenticity. The belief that the patient did not want to

die depends on knowing that he had gotten on very well for many years, that his change of view was coincident to the illness of his mother-in-law and the family's attention to her, that a desire to die is not consistent with the values revealed by the past several years of the patient's life, and that there is no apparent or proffered explanation of a change in values but instead an explanation of the alleged desire for death with dignity as a way of asserting his demands on his family. His suicide attempt, the taking of diazepam, and refusal of treatment were free actions, but they were not authentic.

The claim that the patient's taking of diazepam was the result of effective deliberation is more difficult to defend. The hospital staff regarded the explanation as logically coherent, but the appearance of logical coherence is not sufficient for effective deliberation. If the patient lacked relevant knowledge, made a nonrational assignment of weights to alternatives or failed to appreciate one of the alternatives or its consequences, then the decision to take an overdose and request that lifesaving measures not be started would not be the result of effective deliberation. The case description lacks the detail required to reach a definite conclusion on all of these. The most difficult is whether the patient overestimated the difficulty of continuing his life as a victim of MS; it is hard to imagine that he lacked knowledge, and even though we might regard his weighting of death versus continued life in his condition as mistaken, the severity of his condition and the difficulty of coping with it do not readily support a claim that it is not a rational weighting. Further, he is the person with MS and he is the one who has suffered it for fifteen years; for another person to believe that the patient fails to appreciate the severity of his condition seems on its face to discount the most relevant experience. On the other hand, his appreciation at the time of the attempted suicide might be said to have been altered by the perceived threat to his care and comfort. More information is required to decide this; even if his action is ultimately regarded as the result of effective deliberation, it is still not authentic. One might even say that the lack of authenticity influences the effectiveness of the deliberation. More strongly, if an action is not authentic, whether it is the result of effective deliberation becomes somewhat irrelevant; it is rather like asking whether a person effectively decided a matter based on values or plans that were not his own. As in the other cases, we have no clear evidence that the patient ever engaged in moral reflection, or if he did that the values and life plans he reflected about had direct bearing on the issues presented by his attempted suicide. It does seem that a person who has had to manage his life with a seriously debilitating illness must have given some thought to what is important to him and what sort of life plan is suited to him.

In the case of the patient in the emergency room with meningitis, his refusal of treatment is autonomous in the sense of free action. But is it authentic and the result of effective deliberation? This is difficult to determine unless someone in the emergency room knew the patient well or is able to get to know the patient well. Presumably no one knows him and there is not enough time to get to know him; if treatment is delayed there is risk of brain damage and death. Assuming that the patient has the capacity for autonomy in all four senses, treating him would be contrary to his autonomy in the sense of free action; whether it would be a violation of his autonomy in the senses of authenticity, effective deliberation, and moral reflection cannot be determined. Treating him would make possible his further deliberation on whether he wished to live. On balance, it is more respectful of autonomy, given all four senses, to treat him against his will. On the other hand, it might be argued that meningitis has made the patient incompetent. Though the patient has voluntarily and intentionally refused treatment, his disease has removed his capacity to act authentically or to effectively deliberate. If this is so, then the patient's refusal is not an autonomous action, and the obligation to respect the autonomy of patients would not be abridged by treating the patient against his wishes.

A BRIDGE BETWEEN PATERNALISM AND AUTONOMY

This discussion shows that there is no single sense of autonomy and that whether to respect a refusal of treatment requires a determination of what sense of autonomy is satisfied by a patient's refusal. It also shows that there need not be a sharp conflict between autonomy and medical judgment. Jackson and Youngner argue that preoccupation with patient autonomy and the right to die with dignity pose a "threat to sound decision making and the total (medical, social and ethical) basis for the 'optional' decision."[13] Sound decision making need not run counter to patient autonomy; it can involve a judgment that the patient's refusal of treatment is not autonomous in the appropriate sense. What sense of autonomy is required to respect a particular refusal of treatment is a complex question.

If a refusal of lifesaving treatment is not a free action, that is, is coerced or not intentional, then there can be no obligation to respect an autonomous refusal. It is important to note that if the action is not a free action then it makes no sense to assert or deny that the action was autonomous in any of the other senses. A coerced action cannot be one that was chosen in accord with the person's character and life plan, nor one that was chosen after effective deliberation, nor one that was chosen in accord with moral standards that the person has reflected upon. The point is the same if the action is not intentional. When a refusal of treatment is not autonomous in the sense of free action, the physician is obliged to see that the coercion is removed or that the person understands what he or she is doing. Is it possible that coercion cannot be removed or that the action cannot be made intentional? This could be the case with an incompetent patient, not externally coerced, but subject to an internal compulsion, or who lacked the capacity to understand his or her situation. For incompetent patients the question of honoring refusals of treatment does not arise; it is replaced by the issue of who should make decisions for incompetent patients, an issue beyond the scope of this article.

If a refusal of treatment is a free action but there is reason to believe that it is not authentic or not the result of effective deliberation, then the physician is obliged to assist the patient to effectively deliberate and reach an authentic decision. This is what happened in Case 4. It is not required that everyone bring about, make possible, or encourage another to act authentically and/or as a result of effective deliberation. Whether such an obligation exists depends on at least two factors: the nature of the relationship between the two persons and how serious or significant the action is for the actor and others. Compare the relationships of strangers, mere acquaintances, and buyer and seller on the one hand, with those of close friends, spouses, parent and child, physician and patient, or lawyer and client. To borrow, and somewhat extend, a legal term, the latter are fiduciary relationships; a close friend, parent, spouse, physician, or lawyer cannot treat the other person in the relationship at arms' length, but has an obligation to protect and advance the interests of the other. For example, we have no obligation to advise a mere acquaintance against making an extravagant and unnecessary purchase, though it is an option we have so long as we do not go so far as to interfere in someone else's business. The situation is different for a good friend, a close relative, or an attorney who is retained to give financial advice.

The other factor, the seriousness of the action, is relevant to medical and nonmedical contexts. If, inspired by the lure of a "macho" image, my brother impulsively decides to buy yet another expensive automobile, how I respond will depend on how it will affect him and his dependents. If a patient refuses a treatment that is elective in the sense that it might benefit him if done but will not have adverse consequences if not done, a physician can accept such a refusal even though it is believed not to be the result of effective deliberation. On the other hand, if the refusal of treatment has serious consequences for the patient, the physician has the obligation to at least attempt to get the patient to make a decision that is authentic and the result of effective deliberation. For the patient with meningitis who refuses treatment (Case 3) the consequences of the refusal are indeed serious, but there is no opportunity to determine whether the decision is authentic and the result of effective deliberation and, if not, to encourage and make possible an authentic and effectively deliberated decision.

A crucial issue is whether a refusal of lifesaving treatment that is autonomous in all four senses can be justifiably overridden by medical judgment. It will help here to compare the Jehovah's Witness case with a somewhat fanciful expansion of the meningitis case. The former's refusal is autonomous in three of the four senses and could be judged autonomous in the sense of moral reflection if we knew more about the patient's acceptance of his faith and had a clear idea of the criteria for moral reflection. Though the beliefs of Jehovah's Witnesses are not widely shared, and many regard as absurd the belief that accepting a blood transfusion is prohibited by biblical injunction, their faith has a fair degree of social acceptance. Witnesses are not regarded as lunatics. This is an important factor in the recognition of their right to refuse transfusion. Suppose that the meningitis victim had a personal set of beliefs that forbid the use of drugs, that after years of reflection he came to the view that it was wrong to corrupt the purity of the body with foreign substances. Suppose that he acts on this belief consistently in his diet and medical care, that he has carefully thought about the fact that refusal in this circumstance may well lead to death, but he is willing to run that risk because his belief is strong. This case is parallel to the Jehovah's Witness case; the principal difference is that there is no large, organized group of individuals who share the belief and have promulgated and maintained it over time. One reaction is to regard the patient as mentally incompetent, with the central evidence being the patient's solitary stance on a belief that requires an easily avoided death. An alternative approach is to not regard the patient as incompetent, but to see treatment as justified paternalism. Finally, the position could be that a refusal of lifesaving treatment that is fully autonomous, that is, in all four senses, must be respected even though the belief on which it is founded is eccentric and not socially accepted. Which approach to take would require an analysis of incompetence, a definition of paternalism, and an examination of when it is justified.[14] Defining paternalism as an interference with autonomy in one or more of the four senses might be an illuminating approach.

The conflict between the right of the patient to autonomy and the physician's medical judgment can be bridged if the concept of autonomy is given a more thorough analysis than it is

usually accorded in discussions of the problem
of refusal of lifesaving treatment. In some cases
where medical judgment appears to override
autonomy, the four senses of autonomy have
not been taken into account.

Notes

1. Alan Donagan, *The Theory of Morality* (Chicago:
   The University of Chicago Press, 1977); Ronald
   Dworkin, *Taking Rights Seriously* (Cambridge:
   Harvard University Press, 1977); John Rawls,
   A Theory of Justice (Cambridge: Harvard Univer-
   sity Press, 1971).
2. David L. Jackson and Stuart Youngner, "Pa-
   tient Autonomy and 'Death with Dignity,'"
   The New England Journal of Medicine 301 (1979),
   404.
3. This case is drawn from W. St. C. Symmers,
   Sr., "Not Allowed to Die," *British Medical Journal* 1 (1968), 442; it is reprinted in Tom L.
   Beauchamp and James F. Childress, *Principles of
   Biomedical Ethics* (New York: Oxford University
   Press, 1979), p. 263.
4. This case is drawn from *In Re Osborne,* 294 A.2d
   372 (1972).
5. This case is drawn from Eric J. Cassell, "The
   Function of Medicine," *Hastings Center Report* 6
   (1976), 16.
6. This case is drawn from Jackson and Youngner,
   p. 406.
7. *Ibid.,* p. 408.
8. Mark Siegler, "Critical Illness: The Limits of
   Autonomy" *Hastings Center Report* 8(1977),
   12-15.
9. Beauchamp and Childress, pp. 56-62; Donagan, p. 35; Gerald Dworkin, "Autonomy and
   Behavior Control," *Hastings Center Report*
   6(1976), 23; and "Moral Autonomy" in H.
   Tristram Engelhardt and Daniel Callahan,
   Morals, Science and Society, (Hastings Center,
   1978), p. 156; Harry G. Frankfurt, "Freedom
   of the Will and the Concept of a Person," *The
   Journal of Philosophy* 68(1971), 5; Bernard Gert
   and Timothy J. Duggan, "Free Will as the
   Ability to Will" *Nous* 13 (1979), 197; Charles
   Taylor, "Responsibility for Self" in Amelie
   Rorty, ed. *The Identities of Persons* (Berkeley:
   University of California Press, 1976).
10. Gerald Dworkin, "Paternalism" in Richard A.
    Wasserstrom, ed. *Morality and the Law* (Belmont:
    Wadsworth Publishing Co., 1971).
11. This brief account draws on Dworkin, "Moral
    Autonomy," and Taylor.
12. Jackson and Youngner.
13. *Ibid.,* p. 405.
14. Dworkin, "Paternalism"; Bernard Gert and
    Charles M. Culver, "Paternalistic Behavior,"
    Philosophy and Public Affairs 6(1976), 45; and
    "The Justification of Paternalism," in Wade L.
    Robison and Michael S. Pritchard, eds. *Medical
    Responsibility: Paternalism, Informed Consent, and
    Euthanasia* (Clifton, N.J.: Humana Press,
    1979), pp. 1-14.

From "What Is the Function of Medicine?"[1]

Eric J. Cassell

Thought about the care of dying patients has changed over the past several decades. The question raised initially concerned physicians' obligations towards the dying. As the technical power of medical practice increased, thought was given as to whether "ordinary" or "extraordinary" means must be used to keep the terminally ill alive. In more recent times, the emphasis has shifted from the obligations of physicians, to the patient as a possessor of rights. A glance at bibliographies of bioethics will show the same increasing preoccupation with the rights of the sick in all areas of medical care. Whether one sees the topic of the dying patient from the point of view of physicians' obligations or patients' rights, it is clearly concerned with the doctor–patient relationship. I am going to examine the issue of the patient's right to be allowed to die to see what it can tell us about the doctor-patient relationship and equally what it can reveal about the intimately related question—what is the function of medicine?

It is reasonable to start by seeing what universe of patients we are talking about. It seems to me that we are talking about three classes of patients. First are those patients whose disease is completely curable but if untreated will probably be fatal. The serious infectious diseases such as the bacterial meningitides or septicemias come to mind as examples. But also included would be surgical emergencies such as hemorrhage, shock, head injuries or perforated ulcers.

A second group of patients are those whose disease is *not* curable but who will, with continued treatment, live in functional health for a variable but meaningful time. In this class are patients with heart failure, certain malignan-

cies such as Hodgkins' disease, patients with end-stage renal disease who require regular dialysis with the artificial kidney, and persons with certain chronic anemias who need repeated transfusions. This class of patients is expanding as more cancers become responsive to chemotherapy and other diseases are controlled by newer therapy. The key characteristic of these patients is not simply that they live longer but that they require continuing treatment to remain alive.

The final group are the terminally ill. Their disease is not curable, and treatment offers nothing beyond the prolongation of their dying.

Although it is the contributions of technology and physicians to the sufferings of this latter group, paradoxically, that initially raised the issues I am examining, the question of the patient's right to be allowed to die was gradually extended to the former two groups in both theory and practice.

An example from each of the first two groups should help unpack the issues:

A thirty-eight year old man who had a mild upper respiratory infection suddenly developed severe headache, stiff neck, and a high fever. He went to a local emergency room for help. Brief examination confirmed the physician's suspicion that the man had meningitis. Based on the story of the illness and the age of the patient, the most likely diagnosis was pneumococcal meningitis. This kind of bacterial meningitis is almost uniformly fatal if not treated, and if simple antibiotic treatment is delayed, although cure will result, permanent neurological damage is likely. The doctor told the patient the problem and how important urgent treatment was to save his life and forestall brain damage. The patient refused consent for treatment saying that he wanted to be allowed to die.

Does such a patient have a right to be allowed to die? On the face of it the answer must be yes. That is because the patient cannot be legally treated without his consent. But I would guess that it would be a rare hospital where such a patient would not be treated against his will. The physicians would ask for a psychiatric consultation to declare the patient incompetent and then start therapy. Since penicillin works equally well against the bacteria whether the patient wants to die or not, he would recover.

Why is my expectation (and sincere hope) that such a patient would be treated despite his declared wish to be allowed to die? When a patient enters the hospital (or doctor's office) for help, he enters into a relationship with the treating physicians—and by extension the hospital itself. While the nature of that relationship is still obscure, we know that when the physician enters the relationship he acquires a responsibility for the patient that *cannot* be morally relieved merely by the patient's refusal to consent for treatment. But more simply, the physician could not stand aside and allow the patient to die from a disease otherwise easily treated without feeling that he, the doctor, was responsible for the death. Much is said of the patient's rights in the doctor-patient relationship, but the patient also has obligations. In giving himself into the responsibility of another, he is obligated not to injure the other morally or legally by making it impossible for the physician to act on the responsibility. In coming into the emergency room for help (he could have *not come* at all) he caused the physician and the hospital to become responsible for him without beforehand limiting the nature and degree of their responsibility. Although not meaningful in this case, such antecedent limits might allow the physician to refuse to enter the relationship.

In the situation I have described, by refusing treatment, the patient is effectively committing suicide. As opposed to going out a high window, here he is enlisting the aid of others in his suicide. On the other hand, if he is not committing suicide, his motives are not clear. Therefore, if he resists treatment, the doctors might reasonably believe that the patient does not know what he is doing. The element of time appears to play a part. But time for what? A different but similar situation may make clear what function time serves and what is lacking in this case of the man with meningitis.

A Jehovah's Witness, injured in an accident, comes to the hospital bleeding profusely. Blood transfusions are necessary to save the patient's life before surgery can be done to stop the bleeding. The Jehovah's Witness refuses transfusions. While there will probably be much agonizing over the decision, or even recourse to the courts, the patient's right to refuse treatment (even though death will follow) may be—indeed has been, acknowledged. The situations are similar. The condition is curable, but without treatment death results. What is very different is that the patient's motive is well known to us and has been expressed by a durable agent, his church, over time. Further, the patient's decision is consistent with a set of beliefs well known to us, whatever we may think about them.

In addition to highlighting the element of time in allowing the reason for the decision to be expressed over time, time to be durable and time to be known to us, the case makes another important point. The Jehovah's Witness did not ask to be allowed to die, he asked to be permitted to refuse treatment. That the decision may result in his death is not relevant. It is not death that is chosen, it is treatment (and its effects—religious in this instance) that is being refused. We do not say that the soldier on a hazardous mission chose death, we say that he was courageous. On reflection, I think that you will see that most, if not all, instances chosen to highlight the discussion of patients' rights to die in medical care are instances of the right to refuse the *consequences* of treatment of which death may be only one, and the least important at that.

From the first group of patients, those whose disease is curable but who will die without treatment, I must conclude from my experience of how medicine is practiced in the United States that the patient's right to be allowed to die will not be honored and that the thing truly being requested is the right to refuse treatment. Further, at least one reason the request will not be granted is that insufficient time is present to assess the patient's motives if they are not otherwise clear.

I believe the issues will be clarified by considering the second class of patients, those whose disease is not curable but for whom continued treatment will provide functional life over a long period. As I noted earlier, this class of patients is daily enlarged by medical advances, as chronic diseases from cancer to emphysema are more successfully treated. Instead of the man with bacterial meningitis, let us pose the case of a patient with sickle cell anemia requiring repeated transfusions, or a patient with chronic renal failure who needs dialysis with an artificial kidney several times weekly. If such a patient were to refuse treatment could the same course be followed as with the man in the emergency room? It seems unlikely. It has been the case that a patient who refused further artificial kidney dialysis was declared incompetent on the basis of the fact that his refusal constituted suicide. But what happened then? Did the doctors in that kidney unit tie him down on the dialysis couch time after time and week after week? If it was a patient with anemia who required continued transfusions, would the doctors force the transfusions on the patient? Again and again and again? That seems counterintuitive. But if it is not reasonable, why not?

. . . There are several crucial differences between situations like this and those represented by the man with meningitis. In this instance when the patient refuses treatment and asks to be allowed to die, can we claim that he does not know what he is doing? Obviously not. Patients with chronic diseases requiring long-term therapy are usually very knowledgeable. They have had plenty of time to learn about the disease, its treatment, and the consequences of both disease and treatment. Such patients learn from books, from physicians and nurses, and perhaps most importantly from other patients. Not only is the information available, but, the patient has time to test his beliefs against time and the arguments of others. Certainly at the point of refusing further therapy the patient will be exposed to considerable argument and discussion that can test his reasons and reasoning. The process is two-sided. As the patient has had time to acquire knowledge and test his beliefs, his doctors have had time to know the patient. During the weeks, months, or years that they

have been treating him, the staff has an opportunity to know whether the patient's refusal of treatment and desire to die is consonant with all the other things they know of him.

When the man with meningitis refuses treatment and asks to be allowed to die, it does not appear to me to be a truly autonomous act. However, when dialysand refuses further dialysis, his action appears to me to be much more the exercise of his autonomy. To clarify my reasoning it is necessary to look more closely at the concept of autonomy as it applies to medical care. As these last decades have seen the emphasis shift, in the critical and theoretical examination of medicine, from the doctor's obligations to the patient's rights, there has been increasing discussion of the importance of the patient's autonomy. Autonomy appears to be the basis for the demand for informed consent. Patients' autonomy is also, it seems to me, the basis of the move to demystify medicine and make the patient a partner in his or her care. As a society we have come to place increasing value on autonomy. Indeed we often mark ourselves in part by our autonomy. But what is autonomy?

Gerald Dworkin argues[2] that autonomy requires both *authenticity* and *independence*. Authenticity is the true selfness of a person. The degree to which their beliefs, ideas or actions are truly *their* ideas, beliefs or actions despite whatever source they may have had. Someone is authentic to the degree that they are uniquely themselves.

Independence, it appears to me, is above all freedom of choice. Freedom of choice requires three things: first, knowledge about the area where choice is to be made. One cannot be considered to be making a free choice if he does not know what the choices are. Knowledge alone is not sufficient. To have freedom of choice one must also be able to reason, to think clearly, otherwise the knowledge is of little use. Finally, one must have the ability to act on one's choice, otherwise freedom of choice is meaningless.

When philosophers and lawyers (and many others) talk about rights they often speak as though the body does not exist. When they discuss the rights of patients they act as if a sick person is simply a well person with an illness appended. Like putting on a knapsack, the illness is added but nothing else changes. That is simply a wrong view of the sick. The sick are different than the well[3] to a degree dependent on the person, the disease, and the circumstances in which they are sick and/or are treated.

Let us see what autonomy means to a sick person, or conversely what does illness do to autonomy. Let me start with authenticity. Is an ugly Paul Newman authentic? Am I my authentic self as I writhe in pain? Am I my authentic self when I am foul-smelling from vomitus or feces, lying in the mess of my illness? It is common to hear patients say that they do not want visitors ''to see me like this.'' In the first days after a mastectomy, it seems reasonable when the patient questions her authenticity—after all, body-image helps make up our authentic self. And, finally, is that my authentic father lying there, hooked up to tubes and wires, weak and powerless? It is clear that illness can impair authenticity.

But if illness has an effect on authenticity, what does it do to independence? If freedom of choice requires knowledge, then the sick do not have the same freedom of choice as the well. Knowledge, for the sick person, is incomplete and (for the very sick) never can be complete even if the patient is a physician. For even the best understood disease there are large gaps in understanding. Causes may be obscure and outcomes vary in probability. But the sick person cannot deal in percentages when what is wanted is certainty. For the doctor caring for the patient, these gaps are of less importance and uncertainty is his constant companion. Besides, as Jerimiah Berondess has pointed out, it is vastly easier for a physician to know what to do than to know what is the matter.

. . . In the simplest terms, it is difficult to be clear headed in pain or suffering. I have said previously that the very sick may have impairment in the ability to reason abstractly even when their mental function is seemingly intact.[4] Thus not only is knowledge incomplete for the ill, but the capacity to operate on the knowledge is disturbed. The final element necessary for meaningful free choice is the ability to act. Illness so obviously interferes with the ability to act as to require almost no comment. It should be pointed out, however, that a pa-

tient does not have to be bedridden to be unable to act, the fear of action born of uncertainty may be just as disabling.

It is reasonable to conclude that illness interferes with autonomy to a degree dependent on the nature and severity of the illness, the person involved, and the setting. The sick person is deprived of wholeness by the loss of complete independence and by the loss of complete authenticity. What helps restore wholeness? It should first be pointed out that autonomy is a relational term. Autonomy is exercised in relation to others; it is encouraged or defeated by the action of others as well as by the actor. For this reason wholeness can be restored to the sick (in the terms of autonomy) in part by family and friends. However, there are limits to the capacity of family or friends in returning autonomy to the sick, particularly in acute illness. This is true of both terms of autonomy, authenticity and independence. This is because the well, even the most loving well, are forced to turn aside from the ugliness, foulness, pain and suffering of sickness. Merely the smell of illness and its mess is difficult to surmount for most people. They are unable to see the sick person in the bed completely apart from the illness and when sickness itself does not turn them aside, the setting will. Visitors in intensive care areas commonly cannot decide where to look and often end up staring more at the monitors and the equipment than at the patient. That person on the bed is simply not the authentic loved one, friend, or relative. These things are especially true during acute illness although when sickness lasts longer the family may successfully overcome their distaste. But further the family is also injured by damaged authenticity of the beloved sick person. As the sick person is not whole, neither are they. Similarly family and friends cannot usually restore independence to the sick person. They, too, do not have the knowledge of the illness and although they can supply the ability to reason, their thinking is also clouded by emotion—by fear, concern, and doubt. Finally, while the family and friends can (and usually do) provide some surrogate ability to act for the sick person, they, like he, cannot act against the most important thief of autonomy, the illness.

There is one relationship from which

wholeness can be returned to the patient and that is the relationship with the doctor. The doctor-patient relationship can be the source from which both authenticity and independence can be returned to the patient. The degree of restoration will depend on both patient and doctor and is subject to the limits imposed by the disease. *I am also well aware that by his actions or lack of them, the physician can further destroy rather than repair the patient's autonomy. But here I am not speaking of what harm can be done but what good can be done. In the same manner, when I speak of the use of a good and potent drug, I would not focus on its misuse even though it may often be misused, nor concentrate primarily on its side effects, but speak rather of how it can and should be employed.*

The physician, in his relationship with the patient, can help restore authenticity. The mess of illness does not repel him and through training he is protected from defensiveness at the pain of others. For these reasons, he can see the person amidst and within the illness. He can see a parent where there is a father or a craftsman, attorney or mother, all aside from the sickness surrounding them. If he has known the patient for a long time he knows the person has a history or he can construct that history from conversation. He has he ability to talk of the future if he chooses (as in all of this) to use that ability. He helps restore authenticity by teaching the sick person how to reassert himself above his disability, by teaching how to be whole when the body is not whole.

The physician can also help return independence to the patient. He has the knowledge of the disease and the circumstances that the patient and family lack and he can search out the knowledge of the person that is necessary to make his medical knowledge meaningful to the patient. He can supply the ability to reason and help bridge the gaps in the patient's ability to reason. Finally, he can provide surrogate ability to act, against the illness if nowhere else. In so doing, the patient can be shown how to act in his own behalf and by that means reach a measure of control over his circumstances.

I must stop now and ask the central question raised by the issue of the patient's right to be allowed to die or right to refuse the consequences of treatment. Is the function of medicine to preserve biological life or is the function of medicine to preserve the person as he defines himself?

I believe that the function of medicine is to preserve autonomy and that preservation of life is neither primary nor secondary but rather subservient to the primary goal. This issue is confused by several factors. First, it is obvious that the best way to preserve autonomy is to cure the patient of the disease that impairs autonomy and return him to his normal life. In normal life, doctors and medical care are irrelevant. The second thing that confuses the issue is that the threats to life and well-being, and therefore autonomy, have been organized into a system of knowledge and a mode of thought called medical science which centers around concepts of disease. Doctors are trained to concentrate on disease and the system of thought, often forgetting the origins of the system in the human condition. That body of medical science and the derivative technology has acquired an existence now independent of its original function—understanding the sicknesses which rob persons of their independence and authenticity. The issue is further confused because in the last few centuries of the history of medicine, the underlying focus of medicine has been the preservation of the body and biological life. But until the last two generations it did not matter what the philosophy was, the tools of medical practice were so poor that medical care (although perhaps not surgery) had to function through the agency of the patient. The patient did or did not follow the regimen or work with the physician. The major tool of medicine was the doctor-patient relationship itself. Where that is the case, to preserve the relationship, to keep it functioning, requires the active participation of the patient. Where the patient's function is necessary, so is some measure of his autonomy represented. And it does not matter here whether the patient's autonomy was expressed primarily by the patient or, primarily by the physician, so long as the actions and outcome were authentic to the patient, or at least perceived by the patient as authentic to himself. That may be difficult to conceive in this era of ''I can do it myself'' but is, I believe, supportable from the perspective of previous eras. But, in this time of technological effectiveness, life at all costs seems to be a slogan and becomes a reality in the face of which autonomy is easily destroyed. This last thirty or forty years of medical history should not be allowed to eclipse the goals of the previous two thousand years. For me, and I believe, for most of the history of medicine, the function of medicine is the preservation of autonomy.

Let us return to the cases. The patient with pneumococcal meningitis is treated against his will (correctly, I think) because the physicians have not had time to know whether his desire to avoid treatment is authentic while they do know it to be suicidal. Further, the only consequences of treatment that can be perceived are a return to health. It appears reasonable to me that *where doubt exists* doctors should always err on the side of preserving life. While there may not always be hope where there is life, there are usually more options. Indeed, in this instance, after he is well again the patient can, if he wishes, commit suicide.

The patient with end stage renal disease presents a different problem. We allow him to refuse treatment and, thus, die because in his knowledge of the disease and its treatment and in our knowledge of him acquired during his treatment, we know his actions to be authentic.

Further, allowing him to act on his desire preserves his independence. Here it is clear that the patient is not choosing death but rather avoiding the consequences of treatment which to the patient means a life the living of which is unsupportable. The issue is sharpened in the case of the terminally ill. If biological life is medicine's goal then the patient should be kept alive as long as possible. If the preservation of autonomy is the goal of medicine then one must do everything possible to maintain the integrity of the person in the face of death.

To medicine, as to mankind, death should not matter, life matters.

Notes

1. With the assistance of Nancy McKenzie. This work was supported in part by grants from the Henry Blum Research Fund and the Robert Wood Johnson Foundation.
2. Gerald Dworkin. "Autonomy and Behavior Control," *Hastings Center Report,* 6 (February 1976), 23–28.
3. Eric J. Cassell. *The Healer's Art.* New York: Lippincott, 1976, 47–83.
4. Eric J. Cassell. *The Healer's Art,* p. 38.

Models for Ethical Medicine in a Revolutionary Age

Robert M. Veatch

Most of the ethical problems in the practice of medicine come up in cases where the medical condition or desired procedure itself presents no moral problem. Most day-to-day patient contacts are just not cases which are ethically exotic. For the woman who spends five hours in the clinic waiting room with two screaming

Reprinted with permission from the author and *The Hastings Center Report,* vol. 2, no. 3, June 1972, pp. 5–7. © Institute of Society, Ethics and the Life Sciences, 360 Broadway, Hastings-on-Hudson, N.Y. 10706.

children waiting to be seen for the flu, the flu is not a special moral problem; her wait is. When medical students practice drawing bloods from clinic patients in the cardiac care unit—when teaching material is treated as material—the moral problem is not really related to the patient's heart in the way it might be in a more exotic heart transplant. Many more blood samples are drawn, however, than hearts transplanted. It is only by moving beyond the specific issues to more basic underlying ethical themes that the real ethical problems in medicine can be dealt with.

Most fundamental of the underlying themes of the new medical ethics is that health care must be a human right, no longer a privilege limited to those who can afford it. It has not always been that way, and, of course, is not anything near that in practice today. But the norm, the moral claim, is becoming increasingly recognized. Both of the twin revolutions have made their contribution to this change. Until this century health care could be treated as a luxury, no matter how offensive this might be now. The amount of real healing that went on was minimal anyway. But now, with the biological revolution, health care really is essential to "life, liberty, and the pursuit of happiness." And health care is a right for everyone because of the social revolution which is really a revolution in our conception of justice. If the obscure phrase "all men are created equal" means anything in the medical context where biologically it is clear that they are not equal, it means that they are equal in the legitimacy of their moral claim. They must be treated equally in what is essential to their humanity: dignity, freedom, individuality. The sign in front of the prestigious, modern hospital, "Methadone patients use side door" is morally offensive even if it means nothing more than that the Methadone Unit is located near that door. It is strikingly similar to "Coloreds to the back of the bus." With this affirmation of the right to health care, what are the models of professional-lay relationships which permit this and other basic ethical themes to be conveyed?

1. THE ENGINEERING MODEL

One of the impacts of the biological revolution is to make the physician scientific. All too often he behaves like an applied scientist. The rhetoric of the scientific tradition in the modern world is that the scientist must be "pure." He must be factual, divorcing himself from all considerations of value. It has taken atomic bombs and Nazi medical research to let us see the foolishness and danger of such a stance. In the first place the scientist, and certainly the applied scientist, just cannot logically be value-free. Choices must be made daily—in research design, in significance levels of statistical tests, and in perception of the "significant" observations from an infinite perceptual field, and each of these choices requires a frame of values on which it is based. Even more so in an applied science like medicine choices based upon what is "significant," what is "valuable," must be made constantly. The physician who thinks he can just present all the facts and let the patient make the choices is fooling himself even if it is morally sound and responsible to do this at all the critical points where decisive choices are to be made. Furthermore, even if the physician logically could eliminate all ethical and other value considerations from his decision-making and even if he could in practice conform to the impossible value-free ideal, it would be morally outrageous for him to do so. It would make him an engineer, a plumber making repairs, connecting tubes and flushing out clogged systems, with no questions asked. Even though I strongly favor abortion reform, I am deeply troubled by a physician who really believes abortion is murder *in the full sense* if he agrees to either perform one or refer to another physician. Hopefully no physician would do so when confronted with a request for technical advice about murdering a postnatal human.

2. THE PRIESTLY MODEL

In proper moral revulsion to the model which makes the physician into a plumber for whom his own ethical judgments are completely excluded, some move to the opposite extreme, making the physician a new priest. Establishment sociologist of medicine Robert N. Wilson describes the physician-patient relationship as religious. "The doctor's office or the hospital room, for example," he says, "have somewhat the aura of a sanctuary;" ". . . the patient must view his doctor in a manner far removed from the prosaic and the mundane."

The priestly model leads to what I call the "As-a syndrome." The symptoms are verbal, but the disease is moral. The chief diagnostic sign is the phrase "speaking-as a. . . ." In counseling a pregnant woman who has taken Thalidomide, a physician says, "The odds are against a normal baby and "speaking-as-a-physician that is a risk you shouldn't take." One must ask what it is about medical training that lets this be said "as-a-physician" rather than as a friend or as a moral man or as a priest. The problem is one of generalization of expertise: transferring of expertise in the technical aspects of a subject to expertise in moral advice.

The main ethical principle which summarizes this priestly tradition is "Benefit and do no harm to the patient." Now attacking the principle of doing no harm to the patient is a bit like attacking fatherhood. (Motherhood has not dominated the profession in the Western tradition.) But Fatherhood has long been an alternative symbol for the priestly model, "Father" has traditionally been a personalistic metaphor for God and for the priest. Likewise, the classical medical sociology literature (the same literature using the religious images) always uses the parent-child image as an analogy for the physician-patient relationship. It is this paternalism in the realm of values which is represented in the moral slogan "benefit and do no harm to the patient." It takes the locus of decision-making away from the patient and places it in the hands of the professional. In doing so it destroys or at least minimizes the other moral themes essential to a more balanced ethical system. While a professional group may affirm this principle as adequate for a professional ethic, it is clear that society, more generally, has a much broader set of ethical norms. If the professional group is affirming one norm while society affirms another for the same circumstances, then the physician is placed in the uncomfortable position of having to decide whether his loyalty is to the norms of his professional group or to those of the broader society. What would this larger set of norms include?

a. Producing Good and Not Harm.

Outside of the narrowest Kantian tradition, no one excludes the moral duty of producing good and avoiding harm entirely. Let this be said from the start. Some separate producing good and avoiding evil into two different principles placing greater moral weight on the latter, but this is also true within the tradition of professional medical ethics. The real difference is that in a

set of ethical norms used more universally in the broader society producing good and avoiding harm is set in a much broader context and becomes just one of a much larger set of moral obligations.

b. Protecting Individual Freedom.

Personal freedom is a fundamental value in society. It is essential to being truly human. Individual freedom for both physician and patient must be protected even if it looks like some harm is going to be done in the process. This is why legally competent patients are permitted by society to refuse blood transfusions or other types of medical care even when to the vast majority of us the price seems to be one of great harm. Authority about what constitutes harm and what constitutes good (as opposed to procedures required to obtain a particular predetermined good or harm) cannot be vested in any one particular group of individuals. To do so would be to make the error of generalizing expertise.

c. Preserving Individual Dignity.

Equality of moral significance of all persons means that each is given fundamental dignity. Individual freedom of choice and control over one's own life and body contributes to that dignity. We might say that this more universal, societal ethic of freedom and dignity is one which moves beyond B. F. Skinner.

Many of the steps in the hospitalization, care, and maintenance of the patient, particularly seriously ill patients are currently an assault on that dignity. The emaciated, senile man connected to life by IV tubes, tracheotomy, and colostomy has difficulty retaining his sense of dignity. Small wonder that many prefer to return to their own homes to die. It is there on their own turf that they have a sense of power and dignity.

d. Truth-telling and Promise-keeping.

As traditional as they sound, the ethical obligations of truth-telling and promise-keeping have retained their place in ethics because they are seen as essential to the quality of human relationships. It is disturbing to see these fundamental elements of human interaction compromised, minimized, and even eliminated supposedly in order to keep from harming the patient. This is a much broader problem than the issue of what to tell the terminal carcinoma patient or the patient for whom there has been an unanticipated discovery of an XYY chromosome pattern when doing an amniocentesis for mongolism. It arises when the young boy getting his measles shot is told "Now this won't hurt a bit" and when a medical student is introduced on the hospital floor as "Doctor." And these all may be defended as ways of keeping from harming the patient. It is clear that in each case, also, especially if one takes into account the long range threat to trust and confidence, that in the long run these violations of truth-telling and promise-keeping may do more harm than good. Both the young boy getting the shot and the medical student are being taught what to expect from the medical profession in the future. But even if that were not the case, each is an assault on patient dignity and freedom and humanity. Such actions may be justifiable sometimes, but the case must be awfully strong.

e. Maintaining and Restoring Justice. Another way in which the ethical norms of the broader society move beyond concern for helping and not harming the patient is by insisting on a fair distribution of health services. What we have been calling the social revolution, as prefigurative as it may be, has heightened our concern for equality in the distribution of basic health services. If health care is a right then it is a right for all. It is not enough to produce individual cases of good health or even the best aggregate health statistics. Even if the United States had the best health statistics in the world (which it does not have), if this were attained at the expense of inferior health care for certain groups within the society it would be ethically unacceptable.

At this point in history with our current record of discriminatory delivery of health services there is a special concern for restoring justice. Justice must also be compensatory. The health of those who have been discriminated against must be maintained and restored as a special priority.

3. THE COLLEGIAL MODEL

With the engineering model the physician becomes a plumber without any moral integrity. With the priestly model his moral authority so dominates the patient that the patient's freedom and dignity are extinguished. In the effort to develop a more proper balance which would permit the other fundamental values and obligations to be preserved, some have suggested that the physician and the patient should see themselves as colleagues pursuing the common goal of eliminating the illness and preserving the health of the patient. The physician is the patient's "pal." It is in the collegial model that the themes of trust and confidence play the most crucial role. When two individuals or groups are truly committed to common goals then trust and confidence are justified and the collegial model is appropriate. It is a very pleasant, harmonious way to interact with one's fellow human beings. There is an equality of dignity and respect, an equality of value contributions, lacking in the earlier models.

But social realism makes us ask the embarrassing question. Is there, in fact, any real basis for the assumption of mutual loyalty and goals, of common interest which would permit the unregulated community of colleagues model to apply to the physician-patient relationship?

There is some proleptic sign of a community of real common interests in some elements of the radical health movement and free clinics, but for the most part we have to admit that ethnic, class, economic, and value differences make the assumption of common interest which is necessary for the collegial model to function are a mere pipedream. What is needed is a more provisional model which permits equality in the realm of moral significance between patient and physician without making the utopian assumption of collegiality.

4. THE CONTRACTUAL MODEL

The model of social relationship which fits these conditions is that of the contract or covenant. The notion of contract should not be loaded with legalistic implications, but taken in its more symbolic form as in the traditional religious or marriage "contract" or "covenant." Here two individuals or groups are interacting in a way where there are obligations and expected benefits for both parties. The obligations and benefits are limited in scope, though, even if they are expressed in somewhat vague terms. The basic norms of freedom, dignity, truth-telling, promise-keeping, and justice are essential to a contractual relationship. The premise is trust and confidence even though it is recognized that there is not a full mutuality of interests. Social sanctions institutionalize and stand behind the relationship, in case there is a violation of the contract, but for the most part the assumption is that there will be a faithful fulfillment of the obligations.

Only in the contractual model can there be a true sharing of ethical authority and responsibility. This avoids the moral abdication on the part of the physician in the engineering model and the moral abdication on the part of the patient in the priestly model. It also avoids the uncontrolled and false sense of equality in the collegial model. With the contractual relationship there is a sharing in which the physician recognizes that the patient must maintain freedom of control over his own life and destiny when significant choices are to be made. Should the physician not be able to live with his conscience under those terms the contract is not made or is broken. This means that there will have to be relatively greater open discussion of the moral premises hiding in medical decisions before and as they are made.

With the contractual model there is a sharing in which the patient has legitimate gounds for trusting that once the basic value framework for medical decision-making is established on the basis of the patient's own values, the myriads of minute medical decisions which must be made day in and day out in the care of the patient will be made by the physician within that frame of reference.

In the contractual model, then, there is a real sharing of decision-making in a way that there is realistic assurance that both patient and physician will retain their moral integrity. In this contractual context patient control of decision-making in the individual level is assured without the necessity of insisting that the patient participate in every trivial decision. On the social level community control of health care is made possible in the same way. The lay community is given and should be given the status of contractor. The locus of decision-making is thus in the lay community, but the day-to-day medical decisions can, with trust and confidence, rest with the medical community. If trust and confidence are broken the contract is broken.

Medical ethics in the midst of the biological and social revolutions is dealing with a great number of new and difficult ethical cases: in vitro fertilization, psychosurgery, happiness pills, brain death, and the military use of medical technology. But the real day-to-day ethical crises may not be nearly so exotic. Whether the issue is in an exotic context or one which is nothing more complicated medically than a routine physical exam, the ethos of ethical responsibility established by the appropriate selection of a model for the moral relationship between the professional and the lay communities will be decisive. This is the real framework for medical ethics in a revolutionary age.

THE PHYSICIAN–PATIENT RELATIONSHIP

Code and Covenant or Philanthropy and Contract?

William F. May

When it first broke in the news the Summer of 1975, the case of the Marcus twins (gynecologists at a teaching hospital in New York City) posed in vivid circumstances several difficult and illuminating problems in professional ethics; problems which worry both laymen and doctors. The usual analysis of such problems, which appeals to the language of Philanthropy and Contract, boggles at the Marcus case. The categories of Code and Covenant (which are related to Philanthropy and Contract as *genera* to *species*) offer at least the beginnings of solutions to the professional ethical problems embodied in the case.

The Marcus brothers were physicians who, although technically expert (they wrote one of the best current textbooks on gynecology) and professionally and sympathetically involved, allowed themselves to become addicted to barbiturates, to miss appointments, and to offer consultation, diagnosis, and treatment while under the observable influence of drugs. They retained skill and expertise enough, however, to refrain from killing any of their patients. Their colleagues and the institutions in which they worked were slow to blow the whistle on them.

The Marcus case poses ethical problems for the professional. At what point is a doctor who prescribes drugs for himself misusing his technical expertise? At what point does a professional's duty to laymen override his duties to his fellow professionals? At what point does professional courtesy become professional whitewash? Is there a duty to a profession, as distinct from a duty to those individuals who

Reprinted by permission from the author and *The Hastings Center Report*, vol. 5, no. 6, Dec. 1975, pp. 29–38. © Institute of Society, Ethics and the Life Sciences, 360 Broadway, Hastings-on-Hudson, N.Y. 10706.

practice the profession and those who benefit from its practice? These problems tend to concern the layman more than the experts in moral philosophy. Professional moralists tend to apply their analytical skills to issues they find intellectually interesting. They tend to solve moral puzzles rather than outline the foundations for professional character. They have produced in recent years elegant work on abortion, euthanasia, organ transplants, scarce medical resources and other subjects tantalizing at a theoretical level. The layman meanwhile is concerned with more prosaic questions. He wonders whether the doctor's real loyalty is to the patient or to the guild. Are medical societies, hospitals, and other health agencies ready and willing to weed out incompetent or unscrupulous practitioners? Will the profession find ways of challenging those doctors who order unwarranted surgery, charge fees that always press against the ceiling, play Ping Pong with referrals, process patients through their office with the speed of salts, or commit the sick to the hospital with indecorous haste?

Such blatantly unethical behavior (perhaps its self-evident wrongness explains why the professional moralist seldom attends to it) stirs the layman's anger. The profession seems to belong to an elite, utterly beyond the reach of his criticism. Certainly the physician is beyond serious challenge from the nurse and the social worker. His professional hegemony is well-nigh total over other health professionals. As long as doctors are in scarce supply and badly distributed, they are also beyond the reach of consumer criticism—except through the melodramatic, spotty, random, and sometimes, in its own right, unjust resort to the malpractice suit. For the same reason to date, they have not been seriously limited—except for the demands of paperwork—by outside agencies—the government, Blue Shield, and insurance companies. Under current conditions, the maintenance of professional standards of conduct depends largely on the doctor's own internal sense of professional obligation and on the willingness of the profession to enforce standards of conduct on its members.

This essay on the basis of professional ethics will therefore divide into two questions; why, despite the existence of medical codes and enforcement procedures, is the medical profession reluctant to engage in serious self-criticism? How are the concepts of code and covenant useful in interpreting professional duties and in establishing their obligatory power?

When the *New York Times* first carried its story on the Marcus brothers, it seemed a potentially scandalous reminder that the profession is loath to accept responsibility for professional discipline. The death of the gynecologists exposed both the ineffectualness of the well-intentioned New York Medical Society and the possible lack of zeal of the teaching hospital in protecting patients from two derelict professionals.

As it turned out, the case was not quite so pure an instance of *noblesse néglige* as it first appeared. The New York Hospital did write a letter terminating the services of the gynecologists. (Unfortunately for the reputation of the hospital and the profession, the termination date set in the letter preceded their death only by seventeen days, and, at a stage so far along the road of addiction that the body weight of these six footers at death was 115 and 100 pounds each.) Officials also made the point that the work of professionals is always monitored by colleagues in the hospital but they conceded that such controls would not apply to the Marcus brothers' private practice. In this as in other cases of solo practice, the patient—certainly the unsophisticated patient—is unprotected by the profession from its incompetent or unscrupulous members.

Whatever the final disposition of the Marcus brothers' case, a fundamental problem remains—and grows—that deserves the attention of moralists; that is, the tension in medical ethics between obligations to patients and obligations to one's fellow professionals. The tendency in the profession is to take the latter duties more seriously than the former. Professional ethics has traditionally had two social vectors: one concerned with behavior toward patients or clients; the other, with conduct toward one's colleagues. When concern for colleagues prevails, professional ethics reduces itself to courtesy within a guild. Certain arguable responsibilities to patients (such as informing them about incompetent treatment) are not simply eclipsed, they are professionally denied, that is, they are viewed as a breach of the discretionary bonds that pertain within the guild. Thus an inversion occurs. A report on incompetent or unethical behavior to patients becomes a breach in "professional ethics," that is, a breach in courtesy.

There are many reasons both material and ideological for the reluctance of doctors to engage in professional self-criticism and regulation. First, like any professional group, doctors find themselves in a complex, interlocking network of relations with fellow professionals: they extend favors, incur debts; exchange referrals; intertwine personal histories. The bond with fellow professionals grows, while ties with patients seem transient. Further, any society organized around certain ends tends to generate a sense of community among professional staff members serving those ends. This experience of collegiality becomes an end in its own right and subtly takes precedence over the needs of the population served. Hence criticism gets muted.

Second, professional self-regulation may be even more difficult to achieve in medicine because self-criticism seems somewhat more natural to lawyers and academicians whose work goes on in an adversarial or, at least, a disputatious setting. The doctor, however, has a special role in relation to his patients, quasi-priestly-parental, which seems more severely subverted by criticism. Trust is a very important ingredient in the relationship; criticism seems outside the boundaries of professional behavior.

Third, the doctor's authority, while great, is precarious. The analogy often drawn between the authority of the modern doctor and the traditional power of the parent and priest obscures an important difference between them in the security of their status. The modern doctor's position, while exalted, is inherently less stable. Apotheosized by many of his patients, he is resented bitterly if his hand slips publicly but once. The reason for this instability lies in differing sources to authority. Parents and priests in traditional society derived their authority from sacred powers perceived to be creative, nurturant, and beneficent. Given this positive derivation of power, human defect in the authority figure could be tolerated. The power of good would prevail despite human lapse. The modern doctor's authority, however, is reflexively derived from a grim negativity; that is, from the fear of death. This self-same power of death that exalts him and makes him the most highly paid, the most authoritative, professional in the modern world threatens to bring him low if through his own negligence, unscrupulousness or incompetence, he endangers the life of his patient. Thus while the modern physician enjoys much more prestige and authority than the contemporary teacher or lawyer, his position as a professional is, in one sense, more precarious than theirs. Resentment against him is potentially much greater. Professional self-criticism in academic life or in the law seems like child's play compared with medicine. The slothful teacher deprives me merely of the truth; the negligent lawyer forfeits my money, or at worst, my freedom; but the incompetent doctor endangers my life. The stakes seem much higher in the case of medicine. The profession is tempted to draw its wagons around in a circle when any of its members are challenged.

Fourth, Americans of all walks of life have a morally healthy suspicion of officiousness. They are loath to press charges against their neighbors or colleagues. They are peculiarly sensitive to the injustice and hypocrisy of those who are zealous about the sliver in their neighbor's eye while unmindful of the beam in their own. Better, then, to comply with moral standards in one's own professional conduct, but, beyond that, to live and let live. It is difficult, after all, to tell the difference between an honest mistake and culpable negligence. Who can know enough about a particular medical case to second-guess the physician in charge? Is it not better to keep one's mouth shut? Must a person be his colleague's keeper?

This revulsion against officiousness deserves sympathy, but it fails to respect fully the special moral situation of the professional. Professionals are those who, on the basis of their special knowledge and competence, claim final right to pass judgment in professional matters on colleagues or would-be colleagues. The state honors and supports this right when it establishes licensing procedures under the control of professionals and backs up these procedures by prosecuting imposters and pretenders. In effect, the state sanctions a monopoly (a limitation on the supply of professionals) from which, to be sure, patients profit, but also from which the professional profits—handsomely, financially. If the professional were in fact, a freelance entrepreneur (as the myth would have it) without the protection of the monopoly, he would not fare nearly so well.

Professional accountability therefore cannot be restricted to the question of one's own personal competence; it includes also the question of the competence of the guild. The right to pass judgment on colleagues carries with it the duty so to judge; otherwise doctors profit from a monopoly established by the state without enforcing those standards the need for which alone justified the monopoly. The license to practice is based on the prior license to license. If the license to practice carries with it the duty to practice well, the license to license carries with it the duty to judge and monitor well.

Ethical standards sag and falter when they are no longer accepted as universally binding. The usual test of whether an individual holds an ethical principle to be universally valid is whether he concedes its application not only to others but to himself. No one can make of himself an exception. The famous confrontation between King David and Nathan the prophet was devoted to that point. The king who makes judgments and enforces laws shall live by the law himself.

Today, however, in professional ethics, the test of moral seriousness may depend not simply upon personal compliance with ethical principles, but upon the courage to hold others accountable. Otherwise, the doctor's oath to his patients has yielded to the somewhat tarnished majesty of the guild.

A fifth and final cause for reserve in pressing for disciplinary action is neither exclusively modern nor American. It is prepared for in principle as far back as the Hippocratic Oath. The ancient oath made an important distinction between two sets of obligations: those that pertain to the doctor's treatment of his patients and those he accepts toward his teacher and his teacher's progeny. Obligations to one's fellow professionals flow from an original indebtedness of the student to his teacher; consequently, they acquire a gravity that makes them take precedence over obligations to patients.

To explore this distinction in obligations, we will need to press back into alternative ways of conceptualizing professional ethics and corresponding perceptions of its binding power. For this reason, in the second section of this essay, we will examine certain root terms for interpreting professional obligation, specifically the concepts of code, covenant, philanthropy, and contract. This investigation will take us beyond the somewhat narrower issue of professional discipline with which we began, but it remains a topic to which, in closing, we will need to return.

The Hippocratic Oath is a useful place to begin not only because of its prominence in medicine, but because it forces reflection on the distinction between code and covenant. The oath itself includes three elements: first, codal duties to patients; second, covenantal obligations to colleagues; and, third, the setting of both within the context of an oath to the gods, specifically, the gods of healing.

The duties of a physician toward his patients, as elaborated in the oath, include a series of absolute prohibitions (against performing surgery, assisting patients in attempts at suicide or abortion, breaches in confidentiality, and acts of injustice or mischief toward the patient and his household, including sexual misconduct); more positively, the physician must act always for the benefit of the sick (the chief illustration of which is to apply dietetic measures according to the physicians best judgment and

ability), and, more generally, to keep them from harm and injustice.

The second set of obligations, directed to the physician's teacher, his teacher's children and his own, require him to accept full filial responsibilities for his adopted father's personal and financial welfare, and to transmit without fee his art and knowledge to the teacher's progeny, his own, and to other pupils, but only those others who take the oath according to medical law.

In his monograph on the Hippocratic Oath, Ludwig Edelstein characterizes those obligations that a physician undertakes toward his patients as an ethical code and those assumed toward the professional guild and its perpetuation as a covenant. Just why this difference in terminology is appropriate, Edelstein does not say. In my judgment, the chief reason for resorting to the word covenant in describing the second set of obligations is the fact of indebtedness. The doctor may have duties to his patients, but he owes something to his teacher. He is the beneficiary of goods and services received to which his filial services are responsive. This is one of the hallmarks of covenant. Both the Hammurabi Code and the Mosaic Law detail those statutes that will give shape to a civilization; in this respect, they are alike. But the biblical covenant differs in that it places the moral duties of the people within the all-important context of a divine act of deliverance: ''I am the Lord thy God who brought thee out of the land of Egypt, the house of bondage.'' Thus the promises which the people of Israel make at Mt. Sinai to obey the statutes of God are responsive to goods already received. Analogously, in the Hippocratic Oath, the physician undertakes obligations to his teacher and his progeny out of gratitude for services already rendered. It will be one of the contentions of this essay that the development of the practice of modern medicine for understandable reasons, has tended to reinforce this particular and ancient distinction between code as the ruling ideal in relations to patients, but not with altogether favorable consequences for the moral health of the profession.

The Hippocratic Oath, of course, includes a third element: the vow or religious oath proper, directed to the gods. ''I swear by Apollo, the physician, and Aesculapius and health and all-heal and all the Gods and Godesses that, according to my ability and judgment, I will keep this oath and stipulation.'' A religous reference appears again in the statement of duties to patients: ''In purity and holiness I will guard my life and art''; and the promise-maker finally petitions: ''If I fulfill this oath and do not violate it, may it be granted to me to enjoy life and art . . . ; if I transgress it and swear falsely, may the opposite of all this be my lot.''

This religious oath, in the literal sense, makes a ''professional'' out of the man who takes it. He professes or testifies thereby to the power of healing of which his duties to patients and his obligations to his teacher are a specification. Swearing by Apollo and Aesculapius is at the ontological root of his life. He professes those powers by which his own state of being is altered. Henceforth he is a professional, a professor of healing.

It is an intriguing, but not quite resolvable, question as to whether this oath is an ingredient of a covenant or simply a part of the full meaning of a code. In some respects, it is like a covenant. The physician makes a promise which has a reference to the gods from whom the profession of healing is utlimately derived. This religious promise becomes then the basis for that secondary promise or covenant which the physician makes to care for his teacher and for those duties which he undertakes toward his patients. His promise by the gods gives gravity and shape to the whole. Yet in two important respects the oath itself differs from a biblical covenant: it offers no prefatory statement about the actions of the divine to which the human promise is responsive; and, second, its form is such as to deemphasize the responsive nature of the physician's action, for he swears *by* the gods instead of promises *to* the gods to undertake his professional duties.

Similarly, the question can be raised as to whether this religious vow should be interpreted as part of the full meaning of a code, but, to argue this case, the concept of code needs to be expanded to include more than it means currently in the medical profession.

The word ''code'' in current professional

ethics usually has two meanings—depending on the way in which professional duties are mediated. It can refer alternatively to those *unwritten* and habitual modes of behavior that are transmitted chiefly in a clinical setting from generation to generation of physicians or to those *written* codes, beginning with the Hippocratic Oath and concluding with the various AMA codes that have had wide currency in this country. Technical proficiency is the prized ideal in the informal codes of behavior passed on from doctor to doctor; the ideal of philanthropy (that is, the notion of gratuitous service to humankind) looms larger in the more official, engraved tablets of the profession.

Code, however, covers a third form of activity—above and beyond habitual modes of behavior and collections of written statutes—it refers also to special languages, coded messages, and solemn oaths within special groups. It is this third aspect of code which may be most ethically illuminating; for it implies a special initiation, a profession of allegiance, the possession of a key, and a mutual understanding available only to those who have undergone an alteration in their being which privileges them to use the codebook, the vocabulary, and the technical proficiency.

This third dimension of code prompted us to suggest that the religious vow in the Hippocratic Oath might be interpreted in codal as well as convenantal terms. The professional not only enters into a relationship with a patient, colleague, or a guild, but also makes a *profession* in and through which his being is altered. He recognizes that his subsequent life for good or ill is derived from this profession. Whenever the medical guild fails to recognize this third aspect of code, it reduces itself to the ideal of technical proficiency alone or it tries to elevate itself to the compensatory and ultimately pretentious concept of philanthropy.

THE CURRENT CODAL IDEAL OF TECHNICAL PROFICIENCY

Both the ideal of technical proficiency and the skills that go with it are transmitted largely in a clinical setting. A code operating in this milieu shapes human behavior in a fashion somewhat similar to habits and rules. A habit, as Peter Winch has pointed out,[1] is a matter of doing the same thing on the same kind of occasion in the same way. A moral rule is distinct from a habit in that the agent in this instance *understands what is meant* by doing the same thing on the same kind of occasion in the same way. Both habits and rules are categorical, universal, and to this degree ahistorical; they do not receive their authority from particular events by which they are authorized or legitimated. They remain operative categorically on all similar occasions. *Never* assist patients in attempts to suicide or abortion or never break a confidence except under certain specified circumstances.

A code is usually categorical and universal in the aforementioned sense but not in the sense that it is binding on any and all groups. Hammurabi's code is obligatory only for particular peoples. Moreover, inner circles within certain societies—whether professional or social groups—develop their special codes of behavior. We think of code words or special codes of behavior among friends, workers in the same company, or professionals within a guild. These codes offer directives not only for the content of action, but also for its form. In its concern with appropriate form, a code, partly understood, moves in the direction of the aesthetic. It becomes less concerned with what is done or why it is done than with how it is done; so reduced, a code becomes preoccupied with matters of style and decorum. Thus medical codes include directives not only on the content of therapeutic action, but also on the fitting style for professional behavior including such matters as dress, discretion in the household, fitting behavior in the hospital, and prohibitions on self-advertisement.

Insofar as a code becomes more exclusively concerned with style, image, and decorum, it runs the danger of detaching itself from its ontological root. Style functions to protect the stylist from the assaults of life (and death) and to preserve him also from any alterations in his own being. This tendency to move ethics in the direction of aesthetics, rather than ontology, is conveniently illustrated in the work of the modern novelist who is most associated with the aesthetic ideal of a code—Ernest Hemingway.

The ritual killing of a bull in the short stories and novels of Hemingway offers a paradigm for the professional; the bullfighter symbolizes an ethic in which stylish performance becomes everything.

> . . . the bull charged and Villalta charged and just for a moment they became one. Villalta became one with the bull and then it was over. (*In Our Time*, Hemingway).

For the Hemingway hero, there is no question of permanent commitments to particular persons, causes, or places. Robert Jordan of *For Whom the Bell Tolls* does not even remember the "cause," "power," or "profession" for which he came to Spain to fight. Once he is absorbed in the ordeal of war, the test of a man is not a cause to which he is committed but his conduct from moment to moment. Life is a matter of eating, drinking, loving, hunting, and dying well; Jordan can no longer "profess" a cause or sustain a long-term commitment; just like Catherine in *A Farewell to Arms,* he must die. Hemingway writes about lovers, briefly joined, but rarely about marriage or the family. Just for a moment, lovers become one and then it is over.

The bullfighter, the wartime lover, the doctor—all alike—must live by a code that eschews involvement; for each there comes a time when the thing is over; matters are terminated by death. At best, one can hope to escape from the pain of time; thus the aesthetic aspires to the timeless. Men must learn to live beautifully, stylishly, fittingly. Discipline is all, according to the aesthetic code. There is a right and a wrong way to do things. And the wrong way usually results from a deficiency in technique or from an excessive preoccupation with one's ego. The bad bullfighter either lacks technique or he lets his ego—through fear or vanity—get in the way of his performance. The conditions of beauty are technical proficiency and a style wholly purified of disruptive preoccupation with oneself. Literally, however, when the critical moment is consummated, it is over, it cannot shape the future. Partners must fall away; only the code remains.

For several reasons, the medical profession has been attracted to the aesthetic ideal of code for its interpretation of its ethics. First, such a code requires one to subordinate the ego to the more technical question of how a thing is done and done well. At its best, the discipline of a code cultivates the aesthetic. It encourages a proficiency that is quietly eloquent. It conjoins the good with the beautiful. Since the technical demands of medicine have become so great, the standards of the guild are largely transmitted by apprenticeship to those whose preeminent skills define the real meaning of the profession. All the rest is a question of disciplining the ego to the point that nervousness, fatigue, faint-heartedness, and temptations to self-display (including gross efforts at self-advertisement) have been smoothed away.

A code is additionally attractive in that it does not, in and of itself, encourage personal involvement with the patient; and it helps free the physician of the destructive consequences of that personal involvement. Compassion, in the strictest sense of the term, "suffering with," has its disadvantages in the professional relationship. It will not do to pretend that one is the second person of the Trinity, prepared with every patient to make the sympathetic descent into his suffering, pain, particular form of crucifixion, and hell. It is enough to offer whatever help one can through finely honed services. It is imporant to remain emotionally free so as to be able to withdraw the self when those services are no longer pertinent, when as Hemingway says, "it is over." Such is the attraction of the codal ideal of technical proficiency.

THE IDEAL OF A COVENANT

A covenant, as opposed to a code, has its roots in specific historical events. Like a code, it may give inclusive shape to behavior, but it always has reference to a specific historical exchange between partners leading to a promissory event. Edelstein was quite right in distinguishing code from covenant in the Hippocratic Oath. Rules governing behavior toward patients have a different right to them from that fealty which a physician owes to his teacher. Loyalty to one's instructor is founded in a specific historical event—that original transaction in which the student received his

knowledge and art. He receives, in effect, a specific gift from his teacher which deserves his life-long loyalty, a gift that he perpetuates in his own right and turn as he offers his art without fee to his teacher's children and his own progeny. Covenant ethics is responsive in character.

In its ancient and most influential form, a covenant usually included the following elements: first, an original experience of gift between the soon-to-be convenanted partners; and, second, a covenant promise based on this original or anticipated exchange of gifts, labors, or services. However, these temporal and contractual elements of a covenant were but two aspects of a tripartite concept: a covenant included not only an involvement with a partner in time, and a responsive contract, but the notion of a change of being; a covenanted people is a people changed utterly by the covenant. This third aspect of covenant is, like the third aspect of the concept code, ontological in nature. The aesthetic code attempts to remove style from time; a contract has a limited duration in time, but a covenant imposes a change on all moments. A mechanic can act under a contract, and then, when not fixing the piston, act without regard to the contract, but a covenanted people is covenanted while eating, sleeping, working, praying, stealing, cheating, healing, or blundering. Paul remarks, in effect, "When you eat, eat to the glory of God, and when you fast, fast to the glory of God, and when you marry, marry to the glory of God, and when you abstain, abstain to the glory of God."[2] When the professional is initiated, he is covenanted, and the physician is a healer when he is healing, and when he is sleeping, when he is practicing, and when he is malpracticing.

A covenant changes the shape of the whole life of the covenanted. It changes the totality of the subsequent life of the covenanted in two ways: first, it contains very specific contractual obligations; the law of Moses, and the Talmudic code based on this law changed the life of the covenanted, by specifying not only the way in which God was to be worshipped, but in their methods of stewing kids; a physician contracts not only to do no harm, but specifically to educate free of charge other professionals' kids. However, the covenant changes are not restricted to the codified and specified changes. It alters the covenanted pervasively in his being; at the beginning of the oath, the physician seals himself, and his whole life, to the gods through his profession. This second change is ontological.

The scriptures of ancient Israel are littered with such covenants between men and controlled throughout by that singular covenant which embraces all others. The covenant between God and Isreal includes the aforementioned elements: (1) a gift (the deliverance of the people from Egypt); (2) an exchange of promises (at Mt. Sinai); and (3) the shaping of all subsequent life by the promissory event. God "marks the forehead" of the Jews forever, as they respond by accepting an inclusive set of ritual and moral commandments by which they will live. These commands are both specific enough to make the future duties of Israel concrete (e.g., the dietary laws), yet summary enough (e.g., love the Lord thy God with all thy heart . . .) so as to require a fidelity that exceeds any specification.[3]

For some of the reasons already mentioned, the bond of covenant, in the classical period, tended to define and bind together medical colleagues to one another, but it did not figure large in interpreting the relations between the doctor and his patients. The doctor receives his professional life from his teacher; this gift establishes a bond between them and prompts him to assume certain life-long duties not only toward the teacher (and his financial welfare), but toward his children. This symbolic bond with one's teacher acknowledged in the Hippocratic Oath is strengthened in modern professional life by all those exchanges between colleagues to which reference was made in the opening section of this essay—referrals, favors, personal confidences, and collaborative work on cases. Thus loyalty to colleagues is a responsive act for gifts already, and to be, received.

Duties to patients are not similarly interpreted in the medical codes as a responsive act for gifts or services received. This is the essential feature of covenant conspicuously missing in the interpretation of professional duties to patients from the Hippocratic Oath to the modern codes of the AMA. Compensatorily,

the profession has tended to elaborate the codal ideal of philanthropy.

PHILANTHROPY VERSUS COVENANTAL INDEBTEDNESS

The medical profession includes in its written codes an ideal that Hemingway never shared and that seldom looms large in the ethic of any self-selected inner group—the ideal of philanthropy. The medical profession proclaims its dedication to the service of mankind. This ideal is implicitly at work in the Hippocratic Oath and the culture out of which it emerged;[4] it continues in the Code of Medical Ethics originally adopted by the American Medical Association at its national convention in 1847 and it is elaborated in contemporary statements of that code.

This ideal of service, in my judgment, succumbs to what might be called the conceit of philanthropy when it is assumed that the professional's commitment to his fellow man is a gratuitous, rather than a responsive or reciprocal, act flowing from his altered state of being. Statements of medical ethics that obscure the doctor's prior indebtedness to the community are tainted with the odor of condescension. The point is obvious if one contrasts the way in which the code of 1847 interprets the obligations of patients and the public to the physician, as opposed to the obligations of the physician to the patient and the public. On this particular question, I see no fundamental change from 1847 to 1957.

Clearly the duties of the patient are founded on what he has received from the doctor:

The members of the medical profession, upon whom is enjoined the performance of so many important and arduous duties, toward the community, and who are required to make so many sacrifices of comfort, ease, and health, for the welfare of those who avail themselves of their services, certainly have a right to expect and require that their patients should entertain a just sense of the duties which they owe to their medical attendants. (Art. II, Sect. I, "Obligations of Patients to Their Physicians," Code of Medical Ethics, American Medical Association, May 1847; Chicago: A.M.A. Press, 1897.)

In like manner, the section on the Obligations of the Public to Physicians (Art. II, Sect. 1) emphasizes those many gifts and services which the public has received from the medical profession and which are the basis for its indebtedness to the profession.

> The benefits accruing to the public, directly and indirectly, from the active and unwearied beneficiaries of the profession, are so numerous and important that physicians are justly entitled to the utmost consideration and respect from the community.

But turning to the preamble for the physician's duties to the patient and the public, we find no corresponding section in the code of 1847 (or 1957) which founds the doctor's obligations on those gifts and services which he has received from the community. Thus we are presented with the picture of a relatively self-sufficient monad, who, out of the nobility and generosity of his disposition and the gratuitously accepted conscience of his profession, has taken upon himself the noble life of service. The false posture in all this blurts out in one of the opening sections of the 1847 code. Physicians "should study, also, in their deportment so as to unite tenderness with firmness, and condescension with authority, so as to inspire the minds of their patients with gratitude, respect and confidence."

I do not intend to demean the specific content of those duties which the codes set forth in their statement of the duties of physicians to their patients, but I am critical of the setting or context in which they are placed. Significantly the code refers to the *Duties* of Physicians to their Patients but to the *Obligations* of Patients to their Physicians. The shift from "Duties" to "Obligations" may seem slight, but, in fact, I believe it is a revealing adjustment in language. The AMA thought of the patient and public as *indebted* to the profession for its services but the profession has accepted its *duties* to the patient and public out of noble conscience rather than a reciprocal sense of indebtedness.

Put another way, the medical profession imitates God not so much because it exercises power of life and death over others, but because it does not really think itself beholden, even partially, to anyone for those duties to patients which it lays upon itself. Like God, the profession draws its life from itself alone. Its action is wholly gratuitous.

Now, in fact, the physician is in very considerable debt to the community. The first of these debts is already adumbrated in the original Hippocratic Oath. He is obliged to someone or some group for his education. In ancient times, this led to a special sense of covenant obligation to one's teacher. Under the conditions of modern medical education, this indebtedness is both substantial (far exceeding the social investment in the training of any other professional) and widely distributed (including not only one's teachers but those public monies on the basis of which the medical school, the teaching hospital, and research into disease, are funded).

In view of the fact that many more qualified candidates apply for medical school than can be admitted and many more doctors are needed than the schools can train, the doctor-to-be has a second order of indebtedness for privileges that have almost arbitrarily fallen his way. While the 1847 code refers to the "privileges" of being a doctor it does not specify the social origins of those privileges. Third, and not surprisingly, the codes do not make reference to that extraordinary social largesse that befalls the physician, in payment for services, in a society where need abounds and available personnel is limited. Further, the codes do not concede the indebtedness of the physician to those patients who have offered themselves as subjects for experimentation or as teaching material (either in teaching hospitals or in the early years of practice). Early practice includes, after all, the element of increased risk for patients who lay their bodies on the line as the doctor "practices" on them. The pun in the word but reflects the inevitable social price of training. This indebtedness to the patient was most recently and eloquently acknowledged by Judah Folkman, M.D., of Harvard Medical School in a Class Day Address.

> In the long run, it is better if we come to terms with the uncertainty of medical practice. Once we recognise that all our efforts to relieve suffering might on occasion cause suffering, we are in a position to learn from our mistakes and appreciate the debt we owe our patients for our

education. It is a debt which we must repay—it is like tithing.

I doubt that the debt we accumulate can be repaid our patients by trying to reduce the practice of medicine to a forty-hour week or by dissolving the quality of our residency program just because certain groups of residents in the country have refused, through legal tactics, to be on duty more than every fourth or fifth night or any nights at all.

And, it can't be repaid by refusing to see Medicaid patients when the state can't afford to pay for them temporarily.

But we can repay the debt in many ways. We can attend postgraduate courses and seminars, be available to patients at all hours, teach, take recertification examinations; maybe in the future even volunteer for national service; or, most difficult of all, carry out investigation or research."[5]

The physician finally is indebted to his patients not only for a start in his career. He remains unceasingly in their debt in its full course. This continuing reciprocity of need is somewhat obscured for we think of the mature professional as powerful and authoritative rather than needy. He seems to be a self-sufficient virtuoso whose life is derived from his competence while others appear before him in their neediness, exposing their illness, their crimes, or their ignorance, for which the professional, as doctor, lawyer, or teacher, offers remedy.

In fact, however, a reciprocity of giving and receiving is at work in the professional relationship that needs to be acknowledged. In the profession of teaching, for example, the student needs the teacher to assist him in learning, but so also the professor needs his students. They provide him with regular occasion and forum in which to work out what he has to say and to rediscover his subject afresh through the discipline of sharing it with others. Likewise, the doctor needs his patients. No one can watch a physician nervously approach retirement without realizing how much he has needed his patients to be himself.

A convenantal ethics helps acknowledge this full context of need and indebtedness in which professional duties are undertaken and discharged. It also relieves the professional of the temptation and pressure to pretend that he is a demigod exempt from human exigency.

CONTRACT OR COVENANT

While criticizing the ideal of philanthropy, I have emphasized the elements of exchange, agreement, and reciprocity that mark the professional relationship. This leaves us with the question as to whether the element of the gratuitous should be suppressed altogether in professional ethics. Does the physician merely respond to the social investment in his training, the fees paid for his services, and the terms of an agreement drawn up between himself and his patients, or does some element of the gratuitous remain?

To put this question another way: is covenant simply another name for a contract in which two parties calculate their own best interests and agree upon some joint project in which both derive roughly equivalent benefits for goods contributed by each? If so, this essay would appear to move in the direction of those who would interpret the doctor-patient relationship as a legal agreement and who want, on the whole, to see medical ethics draw closer to medical law.

The notion of the physician as contractor has certain obvious attractions. First, it represents a deliberate break with more authoritarian models (such as priest or parent) for interpreting the role. At the heart of a contract is informed consent rather than blind trust; a contractual understanding of the therapeutic relationship encourages full respect for the dignity of the patient, who has not, because of illness, forfeited his sovereignity as a human being. The notion of a contract includes an exchange of information on the basis of which an agreement is reached and a subsequent exchange of goods (money for services); it also allows for a specification of rights, duties, conditions, and qualifications limiting the agreement. The net effect is to establish some symmetry and mutuality in the relationship between the doctor and patient.

Second, a contract provides for the legal enforcement of its terms—on both parties—and thus offers both parties some protection and recourse under the law for making the other accountable for the agreement.

Finally, a contract does not rely on the pose of philanthropy, the condescension of charity.

It presupposes that people are primarily governed by self-interest. When two people enter into a contract, they do so because each sees it to his own advantage. This is true not only of private contracts but also of that primordial social contract in and through which the state came into being. So argued the theorists of the eighteenth century. The state was not established by some heroic act of sacrifice on the part of the gods or men. Rather men entered into the social contract because each found it to his individual advantage. It is better to surrender some liberty and property to the state than to suffer the evils that would beset men apart from its protection. Subsequent enthusiasts about the social instrument of contracts,[6] have tended to measure human progress by the degree to which a society is based on contracts rather than status. In the ancient world, the Romans made the most striking advances in extending the areas in which contract rather than custom determined commerce between people. In the modern world, the bourgeoisie extended the instrumentality of contracts farthest into the sphere of economics; the free churches, into the arena of religion. Some educationists today have extended the device into the classroom (as students are encouraged to contract units of work for levels of grade); more recently some women's liberationists would extend it into marriage and still others would prefer to see it define the professional relationship. The movement, on the whole, has the intention of laicizing authority, legalizing relationships, activating self-interest, and encouraging collaboration.

In my judgment, some of these aims of the contractualists are desirable, but it would be unfortunate if professional ethics were reduced to a commercial contract. First, the notion of contract suppresses the element of gift in human relationships. Earlier I verged on denying the importance of this ingredient in professional relations, when I criticized the medical profession for its conceit of philanthropy, for its self-interpretation as the great giver. In fact, this earlier criticism was not an objection to the notion of gift but to the moral pretension of a profession whenever it pretends to be the exclusive giver. Factually, the professional is also the beneficiary of gifts received. It is unbecom-

ing to adopt the pose of spontaneous generosity when the profession has received so much from the community and from patients, past and present.

But the contractualist approach to professional behavior falls into the opposite error of minimalism. It reduces everything to tit for tat. Do no more for your patients than what the contract calls for. Perform specified services for certain fees and no more. The commercial contract is fitting instrument in the purchase of an appliance, a house, or certain services that can be specified fully in advance of delivery. The existence of a legally enforceable agreement in professional transactions may also be useful to protect the patient or client against the physician or lawyer whose services fall below a minimal standard. But it would be wrong to reduce professional obligation to the specifics of a contract alone.

Professional services in the so-called helping professions are directed to subjects whose needs are in the nature of the case rather unpredictable. The professional deals with the sickness, ills, crimes, needs, and tragedies of humankind. These needs cannot be exhaustively specified in advance for each patient or client. The professions therefore must be ready to cope with the contingent, the unexpected. Calls upon services may be required that exceed those anticipated in a contract or for which compensation may be available in a given case. These services moreover are more likely to be effective in achieving the desired therapeutic result if they are delivered in the context of a fiduciary relationship that the patient or client can really trust.

Contract and covenant, materially considered, seem like first cousins; they both include an exchange and an agreement between parties. But, in spirit, contract and covenant are quite different. Contracts are external; covenants are internal to the parties involved. Contracts are signed to be expediently discharged. Covenants have a gratuitous, growing edge to them that spring from ontological change and are directed to the upbuilding of relationships.

There is a donative element in the upbuilding of covenant—whether it is the covenant of marriage, friendship, or professional relationsip. Tit for tat characterizes a commercial transaction, but it does not exhaustively define the vitality of that relationship in which one must serve and draw upon the deeper reserves of another.

This donative element is important not only in the doctor's care of the patient but in other aspects of health care. In a fascinating study of *The Gift Relationship,* the late economist, Richard M. Titmuss, compares the British system of obtaining blood by donations with the American partial reliance on the commercial purchase and sale of blood. The British system obtains more and better blood, without the exploitation of the indigent, which the American system has condoned and which our courts have encouraged when they refused to exempt non-profit blood banks from the antitrust laws. By court definition, blood exchange becomes a commercial transaction in the United States. Titmuss expanded his theme from human blood to social policy by offering a sober criticism of the increased commercialism of American medicine and society at large. Recent court decisions have tended to shift more and more of what had previously been considered as services into the category of commodity transactions with negative consequences he believes for the health of health delivery systems.[7] Hans Jonas has had to reckon with the importance of voluntary sacrifice to the social order in a somewhat comparable essay on "Human Experimentation." Others have done so on the subject of organ transplants.

The kind of minimalism that a contractualist understanding of the professional relationship encourages produces a professional too grudging, too calculating, too lacking in spontaneity, too quickly exhausted to go the second mile with his patients along the road of their distress.

Contract medicine encourages not only minimalism, it also provokes a peculiar kind of maximalism, the name for which is "defensive medicine." Especially under the pressure of malpractice suits, doctors are tempted to order too many examinations and procedures for self-protection. Paradoxically, contractualism simultaneously tempts the doctor to do too little and too much for the patient—too little in that one extends oneself only to the limits of what is specified in the contract, yet, at the same time, too much in that one orders procedures useful in protecting oneself as the contractor even though not fully indicated by the condition of the patient. The link between these apparently contradictory strategies of too little and too much is the emphasis in contractual decisions on self-interest.

Three concluding objections to contractualism can be stated summarily. Parties to a contract are better able to protect their self-interest to the degree that they are informed about the goods bought and sold. Insofar as contract medicine encourages increased knowledge on the part of the patient, well and good. Nevertheless the physician's knowledge so exceeds that of his patient that the patient's knowledgeability alone is not a satisfactory constraint on the physician's behavior. One must at least, in part, depend upon some internal fiduciary checks which the professional (and his guild) accept.

Another self-regulating mechanism in the traditional contractual relationship is the consumer's freedom to shop and choose among various vendors of services. Certainly this freedom of choice needs to be expanded for the patient by an increase in the number of physicians and paramedical personnel. However, the crisis circumstances under which medical services are often needed and delivered does not always provide the consumer with the kind of leisure or calm required for discretionary judgment. Thus normal marketplace controls cannot be relied upon fully to protect the consumer in dealings with the physician.

For a final reason, medical ethics should not be reduced to the contractual relationship alone. Normally conceived, ethics establishes certain rights and duties that transcend the particulars of a given agreement. The justice of any specific contract may then be measured by these standards. If, however, such rights and duties adhere only to the contract, then a patient might legitimately be persuaded to waive his rights. The contract would solely determine what is required and permissible. An ethical principle should not be waivable (except to give way to a higher ethical principle). Professional ethics should not be so defined as to permit a physician to persuade a patient to waive rights that transcend the particulars of their agreement.

The Donative mode seems to provide for a more satisfactory analysis than the philanthropic or the contractual, but it shares their flaws. Analysis based on Donative elements suggests that the professional fulfills his contract, lives up to his specified technical code, and then, gratuitously, throws in something extra to sweeten the pot. All of these tools of analysis allow the analyst to evade the uncomfortable and demanding ontological implications of Initiatory Code, Covenant as Chosen, and Profession as transformation. The ontological changes implied in Secret Code, Covenanted People, and Profession of a mystery are complete changes in substance which affect the total life of the professional. A carpenter who contracts to build a chair, when he eats an ice cream cone, does not eat it as a carpenter, nor, when he gets his union card, does he imply that his initiation has changed him utterly, relating him, before everything else, to the mystery of chair making or shellac. A profession of a mystery, in theological terms changes one from damned to saved; in professional terms, from a man who studies medicine, to a man who at all times embodies healing. Malpractice, then, is rather like the sin against the Holy Ghost, uncomfortable for those sinned against, but utterly negating the identity of the sinner. A professional eats to heal, drives to heal, reads to heal, comforts to heal, rebukes to heal, and rests to heal. The transformation is radical, and total. The Hippocratic Oath, under this ontological aspect, can be summrized: *aut medicus aut nihil;* from this moment, I am a healer or I am (literally) nothing. He takes his identity from that which he professes, and that which he professes, to which he is covenanted, whose code he will embody, transcends him and transcends his colleagues.

TRANSCENDENCE AND COVENANT

Two characteristics of covenantal ethics have been developed in the course of contrasting it with the ideal of philanthropy and the legal instrument of contracts. As opposed to the ideal of philanthropy that pretends to wholly gratuitous altruism, covenantal ethics places the service of the professional within the full context of goods, gifts, and services received; thus covenantal ethics is responsive. As opposed to the instrument of contract that presupposes agreement reached on the basis of self-interest, covenantal ethics may require one to be available to the covenant partner above and beyond the measure of self-interest; thus covenantal ethics has an element of the gratuitous in it.

We have to reckon now with the potential conflict between these characteristics. Have we developed our notion of covenant too reactively to alternatives without paying attention to the inner consistency of the concept itself? On the one hand, we had cause for suspecting those idealists who founded professional duties on a philanthropic impulse, without so much as acknowledging the sacrifice of others by which their own lives have been nourished. Then we have reasons for drawing back from those legal realists and positivists who would circumscribe professional life entirely within the calculus of commodities bought and sold. But now, brought face to face, these characteristics conflict. Response to debt and gratuitous service seem opposed principles of action.

Perhaps our difficulty results from the fact that we have abstracted the concept of covenant from its original context within the transcendent. The indebtedness of a human being that make his life—however sacrificial—inescapably responsive cannot be fully appreciated by totaling up the varying sacrifices and investments made by others in his favor. Such sacrifices are there; and it is lacking in honesty not to acknowledge them. But the sense that one is inexhaustably the object of gift presupposes a more transcendent source of donative activity than the sum of gifts received from others. For the biblical tradition this transcendent was the secret root of every gift between human beings, of which the human order of giving and receiving could only be a sign. Thus the Jewish scriptures enjoin the covenanted people: when you harvest your crops, do not pick your fields too clean. Leave something for the sojourner for you were once sojourners in Egypt. Farmers obedient to this injunction were responsive, but not simply mathematically responsive to gifts received from the Egyptians or from strangers now drifting through their own land. At the same time, their actions could not be construed as wholly gratuitous. Their ethic of service to the needy flowed from Israel's original and continuing state of neediness and indebtedness before God. Thus action which, at a human level, appears gratuitous, in that it is not provoked by a specific gratuity from another human being, at its deepest level, is but gift answering to gift. This responsivity is theologically expressed in the New Testament as follows: "In this is love, not that we loved God, but that He loved us . . . if God so loved us, we also ought to love one another." (I John 4:10–11) In some such way, covenant ethics shies back from the idealist assumption that professional action is and ought to be wholly gratuitous and from the contractualist assumption that it be carefully governed by quotidian self-interest in every exchange.

A transcendent reference may also be important in laying out not only the proper context in which human service takes place but also the specific standards by which it is measured. Earlier we noted some dangers in reducing rights and duties to the terms of a particular contract. We observed the need for a transcendent norm by which contracts are measured (and limited). By the same token, rights and duties cannot be wholly derived from the particulars of a given covenant. What limits ought to be placed on the demands of an excessively dependent patient? At what point does the keeping of one covenant do an injustice to obligations entailed in others? These are questions that warn against a covenantal ethics that sentimentalizes any and all involvements, without reference to a transcendent by which they are both justified and measured.

FURTHER REFLECTIONS ON COVENANT

So far we have discussed those features of a covenant that affect the doctor's conduct toward his patient. The concept of covenant has further consequences for the patient's understanding of his role as patient, for the accountability of health institutions, for the placement of institutional priorities within other national commitments, and, finally, for such collateral problems as truth-telling.

Every model for the doctor-patient relationship establishes not only a certain image of the doctor, but also a specific concept of the patient. The image of the doctor as priest or parent encourages dependency in the patient. The image of the doctor as skillful technician encourages the patient to think of himself as passive host to a disease. The doctor and his technical procedures are the only serious agent in the relationship. The image of the doctor as covenanter or contractor bids the patient to become a more active participant both in the prevention and the healing of disease. He must bring a will-to-live and a will-to-health to the partnership.

Differing views of disease are involved in these differing patterns of relationship to the doctor. Disease today is usually interpreted by the layman as an extraordinary state, discrete and episodic, disjunctive from the ordinary condition of health. Illness is a special time when the doctor is in charge and the layman renounces authority over his life. This view, while psychologically understandable, ignores the build-up, during apparent periods of health, of those pathological conditions that invite the dramatic breakdown when the doctor "takes over."

The cardiovascular accident is a case in point. Horacio Fabrega[8] has urged an interpretation of disease and health that respects more fully the processive rather than the episodic character of both disease and health. This interpretation, I assume, would encourage the doctor to monitor more continuously health and disease than ordinarily occurs today, to share with the patient more fully the information so obtained, and to engage the layperson in a more active collaboration with the doctor in health maintenance.

The concept of covenant has two further advantages for defining the professional relationship, not enjoyed by models such as parent, friend, or technician. First, covenant is not so restrictively personal a term as parent or friend. It reminds the professional community that it is not good enough for the individual doctor to be a good friend or parent to the patient, it is important also that whole institutions—the hospital, the clinic, the professional group—keep covenant with those who seek their assistance and sanctuary. Thus the concept permits a certain broadening of accountability beyond personal agency.

At the same time, however, the notion of the covenant also permits one to set professional responsibility for this one human good (health) within social limits. The professional covenant concerning health should be situated within a larger set of covenant obligations that both the doctor and patient have to other institutions and priorities within the society at large. The traditional models for the doctor-patient relationship (parent, friend) tend to establish an exclusivity of relationship that obscures these larger responsibilities. At a time when health needs command $120 billion out of the national budget, one must think about the place that the obligation to the limited human good of health has amongst a whole range of social and personal goods for which men are compacted together as a society.

Although a covenantal ethic has implications for other collateral problems in biomedical ethics, I will restrict myself simply to one final issue that has not been viewed from the perspective of covenant: the question of truth-telling.

Key ingredients in the notion of covenant are promise and fidelity to promise. The philosopher, J. I. Austin drew the distinction, now famous, between two kinds of speech: descriptive and performative utterances. In ordinary declarative or descriptive sentences, one describes a given item within the world. (It is raining. The tumor is malignant. The crisis is past.) In performative utterances, one does not merely describe a world; in effect, one alters the world by introducing an ingredient that would not be there apart from the utterance. Promises are such performative utterances. (I, John, take Thee, Mary. We will defend your country in case of attack. I will not abandon you.) To make or to go back on a promise is a very solemn matter precisely because a promise is world-altering.

In the field of medical ethics, the question of truth-telling has tended to be disposed of entirely as a question of descriptive speech. Should the doctor, as technician, tell the patient he has a malignancy or not? If not, may he lie or must he merely withhold the truth?

The distinction between descriptive and performative speech expands the question of the truth-telling in professional life. The doctor, after all, not only tells descriptive truths, he also makes or implies promises. (I will see you next Tuesday. Despite the fact that I cannot cure you, I will not abandon you.) In brief, the moral question for the doctor is not simply a question of telling truths, but of being true to his promises. Conversely, the total situation for the patient includes not only the disease he's got, but also whether others desert him or stand by him in his extremity. The fidelity of others will not eliminate the disease, but it affects mightily the human context in which the disease runs its course. What the doctor has to offer his patient is not simply proficiency but fidelity.

Perhaps more patients could accept the descriptive truth if they experienced the performative truth. Perhaps also they would be more inclined to believe in the doctor's performative utterances if they were not handed false diagnoses or false promises. That is why a cautiously wise medieval physician once advised his colleagues: "Promise only fidelity!"

THE PROBLEM OF DISCIPLINE REVISITED

The conclusion of this essay is not that covenantal ethics should be preferred to the exclusion of some of those values best symbolized by code and contract. If we return to the problem of discipline with which we began, we can see that both alternatives have resources for professional self-criticism.

Those who live by a code of technical proficiency have a standard on the basis of which to discipline their peers. The Hemingway novel, especially *The Sun Also Rises,* is quite clear about this. Those who live by a code know how to ostracize deficient peers. Indeed, any "ingroup," professional or otherwise, can be quite ruthless about sorting out those who are "quality" and those who do not have the "goods."

Medicine is no exception. Ostracism, in the form of discreetly refusing to refer patients to a doctor whose competence is suspected, is probably the commonest and most effective form of discipline in the profession today.

Defendents of an ethic based on code might argue further that deficiencies in enforcement today result largely from too strongly developed a sense of covenantal obligations to colleagues and too weakly developed a sense of code. From this perspective, then, covenant is the source of the problem in the profession rather than the basis for its amendment. Covenantal obligation to colleagues inhibits the enforcement of code.

A code alone, however, will not in and of itself solve the problem of professional discipline. It provides only a basis for excluding from one's own inner circles an incompetent physician. But, as Eliot Freidson has pointed out in *Professional Dominance,* under the present system, the incompetent professional, when he is excluded from a given hospital, group practice, or informal circle of referrals, simply moves his practice and finds another circle of people of equal incompetence in which he can function. It will take a much stronger, more active and internal sense of covenant obligation to patients on the part of the profession to enforce standards within the guild beyond local informal patterns of ostracism. In a mobile society with a scarcity of doctors, local ostracism simply hands on problem physicians to other patients elsewhere. It does not address them.

Code patterns of discipline not only fall short of adequate protection for the patient, they also fail to be collegially responsible to the troubled physician. To ostracize may be the lazy way of handling a colleague when it fails altogether to make a first attempt at remedy and to address the physician himself in his difficulty.

At the same time, it would be unfortunate if the indispensable interest and pride of the medical profession in technical proficiency were allowed to lapse out of an expressed preference for a professional ethic based on covenant. Covenant fidelity to the patient remains unrealized if it does not include proficiency. A rather sentimental existentialism unfortunately assumes that it suffices morally for

human beings to be "present" to one another. But in crisis, the ill person needs not simply presence but skill, not just personal concern but highly disciplined services targeted on specific needs. Code behavior, handed down from doctor to doctor, is largely concerned with the transmission of technical skills. Covenant ethics, then, must include rather than exclude the interests of the codes.

Neither does this essay conclude with a preference for covenant to the total exclusion of the interests of enforceable contract. While the reduction of medical ethics to contract alone incurs the danger of minimalism, patients ought to have recourse against those physicians who fail to meet minimal standards. They ought not to be dependent entirely upon disciplinary measures undertaken within the profession. There ought to be appeal to the law in cases of malpractice and for breach of contract explicit or implied.

On the other hand, a legal appeal cannot be sustained in the case of an injustice without assistance and testimony from physicians who take their obligations to patients and their profession seriously. If, in such cases, fellow physicians simply herd around and protect their colleague like a wounded elephant, the patient with just cause is not likely to get far. Thus the instrument of contract and other avenues of legal redress can be sustained only by physicians who have a sense of obligation to the patient and the profession. Needless to say, it would be better for all concerned if professional discipline and continuing education were so vigorously pursued within the profession as to cut down drastically on the number of cases that needed to reach the courts.

The author inclines to accept covenant as the most inclusive and satisfying model for framing questions of professional obligation. Covenant fidelity includes the code duty to become technically proficient; it includes the obligation to meet the minimal terms of contract, but it also requires much more. Moreover, this surplus of obligation may be to the final advantage not only of patients but also of colleagues. The Marcus case, or, if not that one, others like it, suggest a failure in covenant responsibilities not only to patients but to troubled colleagues.

Notes

1. *The Idea of a Social Science and its Relation to Philosophy* (New York: Humanities Press, 1958).
2. A paraphrase of Rom. 4:5–8 and I Cor. 10:31.
3. The most striking contemporary restatement of an ethic based on covenant is offered by Hemingway's great competitor and contemporary as a novelist—William Faulkner. See especially "Delta Autumn" and "The Bear" and *Intruder in the Dust.*
4. See P. Lain-Entralgo, *Doctor and Patient* (New York: McGraw-Hill, 1969), for his analysis of the classical fusion of *techne* with *philanthropia,* skill in the art of healing combined with a love of mankind defines the good physician.
5. *New York Times,* Op. Ed. Page, June 6, 1975.
6. Sir Henry Sumner Maine, *Ancient Law* (London: Oxford University Press, 1931).
7. Titmuss does not acknowledge that physicians in the United States have helped prepare for this commercialization of medicine by their substantial fees for services (as opposed to salaried professors in the teaching field or salaried health professionals in other countries).
8. Horacio Fabrega, Jr., "Concepts of Disease: Logical Features and Social Implications," *Perspectives in Biology and Medicine,* Vol. 15, No. 4, Summer 1972.

Do No Harm

Albert R. Jonsen

The maxim "do no harm" is often identified as a primary principle of the ethics of the medical profession. A book on malpractice begins "what is needed . . . is a return to basics, to the first principle of medicine, *primum non nocere;* therein lies the answer to the malpractice crisis."[1] Henry Beecher wrote, "if doctors were certain of the benefit of penicillin, for example, yet did not use it, their decision could be construed as running counter to the basic rule of the physician, *primum non nocere.*"[2] A medicolegal expert, writing on "brain death," refers to "the leading axioms of . . . medical ethics, which include . . . *primum non nocere.*"[3] A notable 19th Century text on medical ethics, Simon's *Deontologie Medicale* (1845) insists, "No physician should ever forget the unbending moral precept: do no harm."[4]

Most physicians who quote the venerable text know little of its origin and are unaware of the range of possible meanings it might have in

From *Annals of Internal Medicine,* vol. 88, no. 6, June 1978. Reprinted by permission of the author and the American College of Physicians.

arguing a case in medical ethics. Usually, the maxim is abruptly cited, as if its import is quite obvious. For example, several physicians offer it as a manifest refutation of what they consider unethical informed consent requirements: "Are we needlessly frightening our patients [by the informed consent process] and contributing to the morbidity and mortality of our procedures . . . *primum non nocere.*"[5]

After some remarks about the origin of the maxim and the form in which it is quoted, this paper will suggest four ways in which it might be used in a discussion of medical ethics. These four uses are "ideal types," that is, they are constructed out of occasional allusions to the maxim, which only hint at some fuller argument that might be put together in order to make some ethical point about medical practice. This method of constructing four ideal types of usage is made necessary by the rather surprising dearth of extended arguments based on the maxim. Despite its frequent citation, neither physicians nor philosophers seem to have pressed it very far as a principle of ethical analysis or argument. One such effort, however, has come to my attention and, in the conclusion of this article, I will propose it as an example of the complexity hidden in this apparently obvious phrase.

THE ORIGIN AND FORM
OF THE MAXIM

Those who cite *primum non nocere* often attribute it to the Hippocratic Oath. It is not part of the Oath, although the Oath does contain a similar expression: "I will use treatment to help the sick according to my ability and judgment, but I will never use it to injure or wrong them."[6] The actual phrase "do no harm" appears in another work of the Hippocratic literature, *The Epidemics.* This work, which has been called "the most remarkable product of Greek science,"[7] is a collection of clinical observations made by Greek physicians as they went on their "epidemia," or rounds to various cities and islands. The entire work is devoted to descriptions of signs and symptoms, with occasional remarks about therapeutics. However, in Chapter Eleven of Book I, four peculiar sentences break abruptly into the scientific text. They have a moralistic tone, with something of a copybook naivete.

> Declare the past, diagnose the present, fortell the future; practice these acts. As to diseases, make a habit of two things—to help, or at least to do no harm. The art has three factors, the disease, the patient, the physician. The physician is servant of the art. The patient must cooperate with the physician in combatting the disease.[8]

In the midst of this brief excursus into medical philosophy appears the aphorism that has won fame as the primary principle of medical ethics. Like the entire passage, it is left unexplained and neither its purpose nor its application is made clear by the text. Its succinctness and directness, however, have endeared it to generations of physicians who recognize in it the ideal and the peril of their labors.

The Latin words *primum non nocere* are translated "above all, [or first of all] do no harm." There is no justification in the Greek

text for the "above all." The Greek text is quite stark: "to practice about diseases, two things: to help or not to harm." The origin of the word "primum" is obscure. None of the major modern commentators on the Hippocratic literature mentions it. Professor Oswei Temkin, in a personal communication to the author, states, "I do not know the origin of *primum non nocere,* though I am sure it has its roots in the Hippocratic passage. As with other old medical dicta, it is very difficult, if not impossible to trace the exact origin." In my own search for the source of "primum," I noted that Galen, the great commentator on Hippocrates, rephrases the maxim and, in rephrasing it, does insert the Latin expression, "imprimis," that is, above all. However, he adds it not to the "harm" phrase but to the "help" one: The physician must aim *above all* at helping the sick; if he cannot, he should not harm them.[9]

The two words, "at least," often associated with the maxim, pose another exegetical oddity. The standard English translation by W. H. S. Jones reads, "to help or, at least do no harm."[10] The classic French version by E. Littré translates, "avoir dans les maladies, deux choses en vue; être utile ou du moins ne pas nuire."[11] Again, the Greek text does not allow for these additional words and, again, I can find no trace of their origin. Its presence in the maxim, although not literal, has seemed to many natural and congenial, as if expressing a resigned acknowledgment of the impotence of medicine; you will probably not do much good, but *at least* don't make things worse! This reflection brings us directly to the interpretation and use of this first principle of medical ethics.

THE FIRST USE:
MEDICINE AS A MORAL
ENTERPRISE

Medical skills, in particular the administration of drugs and use of surgery, are designed to effect a change for the better in a physical state or process that distresses, debilitates, or may destroy the life of a person. These same skills can, however, be turned to other purposes: they can create such defective states in a healthy person for purposes of venality, revenge, or torture. They can be directed to benefit, but out of motives of personal profit or aggrandizement rather than the good of the patient. When it is said that the first duty of the physician is to do no harm, it may be intended to assert that practitioners of medicine have the obligation to consider their art as a moral enterprise.

"Medicine as a moral enterprise" might imply that medical skills are, somehow, intrinsically and of themselves, meant to be used for human benefit. "Do no harm" is a warning against their abuse. Although it would be difficult to demonstrate the intrinsically beneficial nature of the medical enterprise, this idea does appear throughout Eastern and Western medicine in the continued insistence that a physician must never refuse to treat a person in need. The inscription on the Asklepieon at the Acropolis reads, "[the physician] should be like a god; savior equally of slaves, of paupers, of rich men, of princes, to all a brother, because we are all brothers."[12] The Hindu Oath states, "You shall assist brahmins, venerable persons, poor people, women, widows and orphans and anyone you meet on your rounds, as if they were your relatives."[13] The Chinese code of Sun Ssumiao (7th Century A.D.) affirms, "aristocrat or commoner, poor or rich, aged or young, beautiful or ugly, friend or enemy, native or foreigner, educated or uneducated, all are to be treated equally."[14]

Indeed, the medical art itself is considered sacred in many traditions, for it is said to come directly from the hand of God and is intended to heal the creatures of God. The prayer of Maimonides ends, "Almighty God, thou has chosen me in thy mercy to watch over the life and death of thy creatures. I now apply myself to my profession. Support me in this great task so that it may benefit mankind."[15] A long tradition, then, supports the view that the physicians are not morally free to dispose of their skills entirely as they see fit, but are bound by the origin, nature, and purpose of their art to use them only for human benefit.

Medicine as a moral enterprise may also mean that, even if the medical skills are indifferent in themselves, they so affect areas of unmistakable human good and evil, such as health and illness, that their use should be guided solely by those needs of others. The physician should be so strongly motivated to secure the good of his or her patient that all other motives will be banished or subordinated. "Do no harm," in this sense, is an injunction to take to heart the motive of acting only for the benefit of the sufferer.

Whether one attends to the nature of the enterprise or to the motives of its practitioners, one cannot fail to notice the ethical importance of "caring." To possess medical skills *is to be able to care for the sick.* As the origin of the English word "care" reveals, caring means being "troubled by another's trouble." The agreement to care, even in a most formal sense, is itself a moral act, for it initiates a series of activities explicitly designed to affect another person as a response to that person's manifest need. Here, as in innumerable other human interactions, the possibility of responsible or irresponsible acts, of praiseworthy or reprehensible behavior, of selfless or selfish motives, in short, of moral action, arises. It is here that "do no harm" in its meaning "do no mischief" applies most fittingly. To assume some power over another so that the other will benefit is to assume care.

In this first usage, then, "do no harm" is an injunction that admonishes medical practitioners that they enter a moral enterprise and exhorts them to have motivations that will focus their skills on the well-being of their patients. The ethical roots of this use are as deep as any ethical roots can go. The maxim, meant in this sense, is equivalent to the first principle or axiom of all morality. As Aquinas wrote, "This is the first precept of the natural law, good is to be done and promoted and evil is to be avoided."[16] John Locke stated the first principle of the natural law as "all being equal and independent, no one ought to harm another in his life, health, liberty or possessions."[17] In this first use, then, the maxim stands for a self-evident first principle of moral discourse. It serves to affirm the moral nature of medical practice as a whole and to enjoin practitioners to hold motives agreeable to that nature.

Stated at a level of such generality, the maxim provides little concrete direction. It would seem only to exclude malicious uses of medical skills. However, common moral opinion would find such acts reprehensible. No principle peculiar to medical ethics seems needed to condemn them. A physician who excises a kidney not because it is diseased, but because it is the kidney of his enemy, is an evil person who only coincidentally has surgical skills. Similarly, a physician who tortures is a moral reprobate who only *per accidens* has a license to practice medicine. In this first usage, then, something most important about medicine in general is announced, but nothing very illuminating about any particular moral problems is provided.

THE SECOND USE:
DUE CARE

The second principle of the Principles of Medical Ethics of the American Medical Association requires physicians ''to strive continuously to improve their medical knowledge and skill . . .'' Medicine is a practice based on a fusion of several sciences, joined to clinical experience. Use of that science and experience in clinical judgment requires accurate information, clear reasoning, sensitive observation, and, occasionally, manual dexterity. Each of these is attained and improved through exercise and through critical reappraisal by oneself and others. They are reappraised in view of certain standards. Attending to these standards and applying them to particular patients is ''due care.'' Benefit should result from applying due care; harm may result from failing to do so. In this use, the maxim could refer both to medical practices in general, calling for their continued improvement by research, and to the skills of particular practitioners, demanding continued study and upgrading.

The admonition to take due care follows reasonably from the maxim in its first use. If medicine is a moral enterprise, under the imperative of benefiting the patient, the specific acts of medicine, diagnosis and therapy, should meet standards which will assure, with some certainty, the beneficial outcome. Just as the maxim in its first use stated the ethical basis of undertaking care, so in this use, it urges the one

who has undertaken care to *take care*. It enjoins careful assessment, careful procedures, careful evaluation, careful follow-up. For example, it is an act of carelessness for a physician to fail to perform a thorough rectal examination on a patient presenting with rectal bleeding. A casual diagnosis of hemorrhoids may mask the presence of rectal cancer. It is a careless act to treat bronchitis with the antibiotic chloramphenicol which, while very effective, can have fatal complications and is properly indicated only in serious infections, such as typhoid fever. It is careless to ignore, as happened in a leading malpractice case, persistent foul odor from a leg cast which, to the careful practitioner, would suggest the inception of gangrene.

This second use is where questions of morality become issues of legality, for claims of malpractice frequently assert failure to take due care in accord with accepted standards of practice. Several questions arise: Has a physician been negligent? What are accepted standards? What is the boundary between negligence and the fallibility intrinsic to medical knowledge and reasoning? However, there are more objective questions about the very nature of medical knowledge. Contemporary biomedical science makes possible elaborate description of diseases but, because of the plethora of information, may retard identification of the particular illness in a particular patient. Contemporary therapies can have significant theoretical and practical effects in general but may be very difficult to assess in particular patients. The concept of due care, then, not only enjoins carefulness in the practitioner but also reexamination of the methodology of clinical reasoning.

The first use of the maxim has an absolute tone: It declares the morality of medical practice and permits no exceptions. The second use, on the other hand, admits of degrees of carefulness, from the long process of diagnosis and treatment of neoplasms to the rushed repair of serious trauma. One cannot argue about whether a physician should do harm in the sense of the first use of the maxim: It is obvious that to do so would be unethical. However, in the second sense, there can be interminable arguments about *how much care* the ethical physician must take.

THE THIRD USE:
RISK–BENEFIT RATIO

Any assessment of medical procedures that is carried out in order to establish standards of due care reveals that the outcome of most procedures is only predictable with relative certainty. Some procedures promise an almost certain benefit, which may not, however, come about in a particular application. Other procedures that will certainly benefit entail certain or probable concomitant harm. It has become possible, because of epidemiologic and statistical methods, to determine in quantitative terms some of these possibilities. Thus, the experience of open heart surgery for replacement of multiple valves shows mortality risks of 5% to 20%; use of the anaesthetic halothane carries a risk of causing hepatic dysfunction estimated to be in the range of 1 in 5000 cases. Clinical trials are constantly being designed and carried out to ascertain efficacy and safety of operations and drugs.

Due care requires that these statistics be collected. The careful practitioner will be aware of them as he attempts to match therapy to disease, although one's own experience, one's clinical intuitions, and one's understanding of the nature of statistics should breed caution in their use. "Medical statistics," writes "Pappworth, "are like bikinis, concealing what is vital while revealing much that is interesting."[18] Still, the practitioner can use them to steer clear of dangerous or inefficacious treatment. However, any particular patient is a statistic of one. Each patient will respond uniquely; there may be allergic or idiosyncratic reactions. Here, the practitioner, approaching the individual patient, must base a risk-benefit assessment not only on statistics, but also on a focused and full knowledge of the person and the illness. That knowledge will never comprehend the uniqueness of the person but can, by refined experience and sophisticated clinical methodology, draw closer and closer to that uniqueness.

This statistical and clinical risk-benefit equation is not only an element in the diagnostic and therapeutic judgments of the practitioner; it is also an element in the decision of the patient to accept treatment. Physicians may know, statistically and clinically, how much risk of failure or of harm a procedure entails. But patients alone can know how much risk they wish to run and how much they desire the possible benefits. All persons have a "risk budget," as Charles Fried has observed. They calculate in rough ways, out of their experience, emotions, and energy, the extent of security and danger they will accept in their lives.[19]

The *Oxford English Dictionary* defines risk as "exposure to mischance or peril." Although the risk itself is an actuality, as a set of circumstances constituting the exposure, the harm is a possibility. Decisions taken about risks are decisions to place oneself in an exposed position, to dispense with certain securities and protections. When persons do so, they are more uncertain about the consequent situation than they would otherwise be, but only in relation to a certain plan of life. There is, of course, a radical uncertainty about every next situation, given the contingency of existence. But the risks taken within life plans have to do with voluntary steps into more exposed, less protected states of affairs.

In this usage, "do no harm," refers, on the one hand, to the physician's educated assessment of risks. It commands that those procedures be selected that carry the best chance for success with the lowest risk of harm. In this sense, Dr. L. J. Henderson rephrased the maxim as "try to do as little harm as possible."[20] On the other hand, it refers to the patient's own assessment of how those risks and chances fit a lifestyle, with its own personal goals, strengths, and weaknesses. Here the maxim seems to be assimilated into a familiar form of ethical discourse sometimes called "utilitarian." The objective statement of the equation is translated into a personal "felicific calculus" and choices are made in terms of how the calculation would reveal ways to maximize the goods and minimize the evils of a person's experienced life in its present and future.

In this usage, the word "harm" must be given much more content than in the two previous usages. Although a discussion of harm might begin with an enumeration of possible physical detriments, as is usual in discussions of medical procedures, the scope of meaning quickly expands to wider realms of human experience. Thus, at a first level of meaning, harm might signify an intrusion by physical means upon the physical integrity of oneself or another, leaving an effect of some duration. The intrusion may come from a voluntary or involuntary agent or from an inanimate object or power. One can be harmed by man or beast, by lead weight or lightning, by scalpel or scopolamine. The intrusion comes about because no effort is made, or no effort succeeds, in warding it off. Its effect is more than transient, as a hurt can be, but remains debilitating for a time or permanently. It reduces one's ability to defend oneself, leaving a wounded integrity.

Without distortion, this primitive notion can be expanded from the physical to the psychologic realm, even though psychologic integrity is a more vague concept. Perhaps it can be defined as the ability to respond appropriately and effectively to intellectual and emotional challenges, such as loss or danger. Here the agents of harm move beyond the physical to the psychologic. They include threats, lies, ridicule, shame.

Finally, physical and psychologic integrity imply social integrity, the ability to maintain oneself as a whole person by initiating action and responding to others. This integrity can be harmed by cutting off human contacts, by distorting communication, by rendering ineffectual all efforts at self preservation. At the heart of harming and being harmed is the notion of the ability to respond to challenge. A harmful act is one that cannot be warded off, and its harmful effect is a decreased ability to defend oneself, physically, psychologically, or socially. Response, measured and timely, is the sign of integrity.

"Harming," then, may describe any action or event that results in prolonged diminished ability to respond to physical, psychologic, or social challenge. In this usage, then, the risk to physical integrity is assumed into the wider scope of risks to the personal integrity of patients. Patients alone are capable of assessing the boundaries of this personal integrity, because it is coterminous with their selfhood. However, it is not uncommon that the patient is incapable of making or expressing an assessment. When this happens, someone must make a surrogate assessment. In such cases, the surrogate, who may or may not be the physician, must attempt to be "in place of the other." The complexities of this question cannot be discussed here. It should only be noted that if the surrogate is a physician, his duty to do no harm extends not only to controlling the risk of physical harm, but also to adopting the "felicific calculus" of the patient, attempting to imagine in some general way the entire range of possible insults to personal integrity of his patient.

THE FOURTH USE: THE BENEFIT–DETRIMENT EQUATION

Many medical procedures not only carry risk of harm, but necessarily bring about some detriment at the same time as they effect a benefit. Any amputation will, in one and the same act, remove a diseased part in order to save life and always leaves the patient with a physical and, sometimes, a psychologic deficit. Administration of powerful alkylating agents, such as nitrogen mustards, for treatment of lymphomas, produces almost invariably unpleasant and sometimes serious side-effects. Drawing blood for careful monitoring of a tiny premature baby's blood gases significantly reduces the baby's blood volume. Some of these necessarily associated detriments can be remedied; some must be borne.

In situations such as these, the maxim might be rephrased as, "do no harm unless that harm is necessarily associated with a compensating benefit." A certain benefit must be balanced against a certain detriment. Here again, as in the previous risk-benefit usage, a felicific calculus can be employed. How does one sum the benefits and the detriments in terms of a desired life plan? Here also, the physician should know, from science and experience, the ratio, and use it to eliminate disproportionate approaches and inform the patient about the effects of that therapeutic plan that seems most reasonable. Here again, the patient alone is in a position to make the calculation. One person chooses to live even as a quadriplegic; another prefers the limited life on dialysis to the risks of transplantation; a third rejects chemotherapy, which he considers too unpleasant even though it may prolong life.

There are, however, certain problems of benefit-detriment that do not fit easily into the felicific calculus. These are problems in which the benefit accrues to one party and the detriment to another. Four current problems in medical ethics are of this type: abortion, allocation of scarce biomedical resources, nontherapeutic experimentation on subjects incapable of consent, and sterilization of carriers of deleterious genes. In such cases, certain evils are visited upon some in order that others might benefit. Classic utilitarian reasoning, although vaunting its solution to such problems, has generally been considered at its weakest in coming to grips with the distribution of benefits and burdens to different parties.

Another manner of moral reasoning, traditionally called the Principle of Double Effect was designed to deal with problems of this sort. Although much criticized in recent years, from within and without the camp of Roman Catholic moral theologians, who were its creators, it seems at least to ask the right question: Under what circumstances can one be said to act morally when one of the multiple effects of that action is an evil? The death of a fetus, the danger to a nonconsenting subject, refusal of dialysis, the imposed sterility of a dysgenic male are all evils. Is their occurrence or permission justified by some good, presumably "greater," for some other or others?

In its most traditional form, the double-effect argument depends on the distinction between directly intended and indirectly intended (or merely permitted) effects. The object of the direct intention must be a good in itself or, at least, be morally indifferent. An act good in itself could cause a foreseen, but unintended evil result, but no good result, no matter how great, could justify an act vitiated by an intrinsically evil object. Recent attempts by Catholic theologians to untangle this ethical intricacy have turned on the notion of "proportionate reason," which is not merely a "serious reason" but rather an explanation of how the evil effect is an inextricable by-product of a good that one is obliged to perform.[21] Outside

the theologians' camp, philosopher Philippa Foot argues that it is the concept of positive and negative duties, rather than the intended and the foreseen effects, that determines the justifiability of an evil effect.[22]

We will not enter the debate about the strengths and weaknesses of double-effect reasoning. We simply note that, in arguments about the morality of multiple effects, participants often believe that some of these are undesirable and, perhaps, immoral. They also believe that something other than "greater good of another or of the greater number" must be proposed to justify the commission or permission of an evil effect. They seek for "serious" or "overriding" reasons. The abortion debate, in some of its forms, is the classic example. Abortion is a medical act that has two associated consequences: the mother's well-being and the death of the fetus. Many make an ethical case for abortion by admitting that the fetal death is undesirable and perhaps immoral, but then cite one or several reasons that they consider "to override" or "to justify" that effect. Freedom to control one's own body is considered by some to be such a reason; others refuse to allow this to outrank the right to life of the fetus.

In this use, then, "do no harm" is an imperative that calls for double-effect reasoning in order to reach a conclusion about the morality of an action. It calls for the proposal of serious or proportionate reasons for allowing some detriment that is necessarily concomitant with a desired benefit.

A PARADOXICAL USE

Recently, several authors have invoked the principle "do no harm" to justify involuntary euthanasia. Philosopher-physician H. Tristram Engelhardt writes:

> In the field of medicine, the need is to recognize an ethical category, a concept of wrongful continuance of existence, . . . [which] presupposes that life can be of a negative value such that the medical maxim *primum non nocere* would not require sustaining life.[23]

The proposal is, at first sight, paradoxical. Does not one harm another by allowing him to die? Can sustaining life be properly called harming?

A review of the several uses of the maxim may put Dr. Engelhardt's proposal in perspective. If "do no harm" is intended to bear the meaning of the first usage, always having the motive to care for the other, termination of painful or a seriously debilitated existence might be considered a "caring act." However, this appears to beg the question: Can deprivation of life, of any quality, be a good for the one deprived? The second usage, due care, at first sight, seems irrelevant for it is primarily procedural. However, it may be highly relevant. Due care consists of assessing medical actions in relation to certain goals. It might be argued that sustaining life of low quality is not a goal of medical actions because medicine is concerned only with restoration of health in some functional sense. Medical actions that cannot achieve this are improper and may be ethically discontinued. The physician judges this action to be beyond his or her responsibility. The third usage, risk-benefit equation, bears only on the question, often moot, about whether continued care might possibly bring about restoration. The fourth use, benefit-detriment equation, is most often invoked. If seen as felicific calculus, it is flawed by being always a surrogate judgment and also by the logical peculiarities inherent in the suggestion that someone would be "better off dead." It seems that both benefit and detriment must be experienced in order to be evaluated.

Finally, if the fourth use is seen as a good reasons argument, the good reasons must be scrutinized in terms of some broader ethical theory that gives the criteria whereby a reason is measured as good. For example, Father Richard McCormick proposes such criteria based upon a theological foundation:

> In all of these instances—instances where the life could be saved—the discussion is couched in terms of the means necessary to preserve life. But often enough it is the kind of, the quality of life thus saved (painful, poverty-stricken and deprived, away from home and friends, oppressive) that established the means as extraordinary. *That* type of life would be an excessive hardship for the individual. It would distort and jeopardize his

grasp on the overall meaning of life. Why? Because, it can be argued, human relationships—which are the very possibility of growth in love of God and neighbor—would be so threatened, strained, or submerged that they would no longer function as the heart and meaning of the individual's life as they should. Something other than the "higher more important good" would occupy first place. Life, the condition of other values and achievements, would usurp the place of these and become itself the ultimate value. When that happens, the value of human life has been distorted out of context.[24]

It seems reasonable to invoke the "do no harm" maxim as a justification for termination of life.[24] The logic of this justification, however, must move through usage two and four, "due care" and "good reasons." The substance of the argument is difficult to make because standards of due care for the dying and the irretrievably comatose are very insufficiently developed by physicians and because theories of good reason for action are very skimpily designed by philosophers. Physicians who do not understand the "end of medicine" and philosophers who do not appreciate the "end of man" are unlikely to succeed in providing the substance of that argument.[26,27]

CONCLUSION

Several generalizations may be drawn about the "do no harm" argument. First, the ancient maxim serves in a variety of ways, each of which represents a somewhat different mode of ethical discourse. We have noted at least four that can be designated as an absolute principle, a counsel of prudence, a calculation of acceptability, a rule of double effect. When the maxim appears, its role as one or another of these should be recognized and the argument analyzed accordingly. Secondly, the maxim as absolute principle and counsel of prudence is directed at the physician as moral agent, urging that he or she have certain motives, intentions, and ways of judging. As calculus of acceptability and as rule of double effect, it is directed primarily at the patient and only indirectly at the physician, for it is the recipient of care who must accept risks and find reasons proportionate. Only occasionally will the physician have to exercise surrogate judgment about these. The "do no harm" maxim, in the third and fourth uses, affirms that physician ethics must be centered on respect for the autonomy of patients. The benefit to others commanded by the absolute principle that initiates the moral enterprise of medicine is seen to be the benefit of fostering the independence of patients. Harming touches not only the body but also the person in his or her personality and community.

In conclusion, it may appear that dwelling on the negative apodosis of the maxim, "do no harm," rather than upon the positive protasis, "be of benefit," creates the impression of a minimalist morality. This may be. But, if we recall the version of the maxim, "at least do no harm," we may see it not so much as a morality of lower limits, but as an admonition to humility. When good persons possess great powers and wield them on behalf of others, they sometimes fail to recognize the harm done as they ply their beneficent craft. The medical profession has such power and its practitioners usually intend to use it well. They must become sensitive to its shadow side. A character in a recent novel states the case for humility well: "I was less morally ambitious than you . . . I didn't aspire to do good: that seemed too difficult. I only wanted not to do harm."[28] Only wanting not to do harm, we may conclude, is difficult enough!

Notes

1. Kramer C: *The Negligent Doctor.* New York, Crown Publishing, 1968, p. 17
2. Beecher H: *Research and the Individual.* Boston, Little-Brown, 1970, p. 94
3. Van Till HAH: Diagnosis of death in comatose patients under resuscitation treatment: A critical review of the Harvard Report. *Am J Law Med* 2:1-40, 1976
4. Simon M: *Deontologie Medicale.* Paris, J. B. Bailliere, 1845, p. 269
5. Kaplan SR, Greenwald RA, Rogers AI: Neglected aspects of informed consent. *N Engl J Med* 296:1127, 1977
6. Jones WHS: *Hippocrates I.* Cambridge, Harvard University Press, 1923, p. 165
7. *See* Reference 6, p. 141
8. *See* Reference 6, p. 165, Cf. Jonsen A: Do no harm, in *Philosophical Medical Ethics: Its Nature and Significance,* edited by Spicker SF, Engelhardt HT Jr. *Philosophy and Medicine Series, vol. 3.* Dordrecht, Holland, D. Reidel Publishing Co., 1977, pp. 27-41
9. Galen: *Commentarium I in Hippocratis libri I Epidemiorum,* c. 50. Leipzig, C. Cnoblochius, 1828, vol. 17A, p. 148
10. *See* Reference 6, p. 165
11. Littré E. *Ouevres Complès d'Hippocrate,* vol. II. Paris, J.B. Bailliere, 1839–1869, p. 635
12. Etziony MB: *The Physicians Creed.* Springfield, Charles C Thomas Publishing, 1973, p. 21.
13. *See* Reference 12, p. 15
14. *See* Reference 12, p. 20
15. *See* Reference 12, p. 30
16. Aquinas: *Basic Writings,* edited by Pegis A. New York, Random House, 1945, II, 773 (I-II, 94, 2)
17. Locke J: *Two Treatises of Government,* edited by Cook T. New York, Hafner Publishing, 1947, p. 73
18. Pappworth MH: *Primer of Medicine.* New York, Appleton-Century-Crofts, 1971, p. 41
19. Fried C: *Anatomy of Values.* Cambridge, Harvard University Press, 1971, p. 177
20. Henderson LJ: The physician and the patient as a social system. *N Engl J Med* 212:819–823, 1937
21. Knauer P: The hermaneutic principle of double effect. *Natural Law Forum* 12:132–162, 1962
22. Foot P: The problem of abortion and the doctrine of double effect. *Oxford Rev* 5:5–15, 1967
23. Engelhardt HT: Aiding the death of young children, in *Beneficent Euthanasia,* edited by Kohl M. Buffalo, Prometheus Books, 1975, p. 187
24. McCormick R: To live or let die. *JAMA* 229:173–175, 1974
25. Jonsen A. Garland M: *The Ethics of Newborn Intensive Care.* Berkeley, Institute for Governmental Studies, 1976
26. Gustafson, J: *The Contribution of Theology to Medical Ethics.* Milwaukee, Marquette University Press, 1975
27. Kass L: Regarding the end of medicine and the pursuit of health. *Public Interest* 40:11–42, 1970
28. Lurie A: *The War Between the Taits.* New York, Random House, 1975, p. 271

From "The Doctor-Patient Relationship"

Anna Freud

. . . Even if the doctor contributes a good deal to [the doctor-patient relationship] I think it is only fair to say that the patient contributes more. . . . Your patients will be ill and therefore they need a doctor. They will have bodily pains; they expect you to cure them. . . . One would expect that this is a straight-forward relationship, that the doctor . . . enters the patient's life as a new person with new qualities, that the patient reacts to him as such, that the patient values his knowledge, appreciates his attitude, and chooses him like one chooses other professional people in life. . . . But curiously enough the relationship between . . . patient and doctor does not remain the same. Elements enter it which cannot be explained by the present reality at all. We are surprised by it, we have to search for the origin. For example . . . many patients over-evaluate their doctors. . . . Their doctor is the best in the world. Their dentist is the best. Enormous expectations are raised—he will help, he will cure, he will fulfill all expectations. This gives you a warm glow of satisfaction. It's nice to be thought such a remarkable person until, a week later, the scene changes. You are no good at all—such an ignorant person has never existed. You don't fulfill the expectations. You have promised something and you can't carry it out. The patient is deeply disappointed in you, and you become dejected. Am I really as bad as that? . . . Until, when this same sequence has repeated itself a number of times, you become alerted to it and you realize this is not you at all. You are neither as good, nor as bad, neither as efficient nor as inefficient as the patient sees you. He evidently has turned you into somebody else. And this belief is strengthened by further discoveries, namely that the patient doesn't only expect you to fulfill

the contract to be cured by you, but that he expects you to like him or, if it is in analysis, even to love him, to be interested in him, to prefer him to other patients. He comes to you with details of his life, which have really nothing to do with the doctor-patient relationship on a reality basis, and you realize that now you have ceased to be what you set out to be—the person to cure this particular individual; you have become an important person in his life, somebody who is loved, hated, on whom demands are made, from whom the patient wants interest, intimacy, preference, and suddenly you feel this must be somebody quite definite from the patient's past. He treats you as if you were his parent. He obeys you as if you had authority over him, or he fights against you as if he were a rebellious child. And suddenly you find that instead of having a sensible patient before you, you have become what we call an object of his transference, namely the whole load of feeling left over from earlier years—unfulfilled, disappointed—has been unloaded onto you. You are in the center of his interest, and he expects you to play the role that you are given.

What can you do with this most disturbing doctor-patient relationship? . . .

I think that all doctors use the transferred positive relationships from the patients for their own advantage. The patient is in a state of submission, admiration, obedient to the doctor. All the better. So long as this whole trend is positive, you can use it for your own ends; you will find that your prescriptions work better, your commands are obeyed, and at least the psychological side of the patient's illness—and we know there is mostly a psychological side—will be influenced favorably. Doctors have done that always. They have done it without knowing it. It's only when this attitude becomes negative that you are in trouble. . . .

To understand what is going on can be of enormous help in your profession. It will save you a lot of annoyance. It will make you very careful how to act or how to make use of the patient's personal relationship. It will do something to your self-esteem when you know that this changing picture of yourself is not your fault. It will help you to stand firm and, as in so many other walks of life, understanding the difficulties of the situation will ease them. It will ease it especially with regard to one particular point. The patient uses the doctor . . . not only to replace people of a lost past, he also uses him to represent in the outside world parts of his own person. For instance, a patient may be quite aware of the fact that either his eating habits or his drinking habits, or any other habits are injurious to his health, but he doesn't feel that he has the strength inside to combat the injurious habits. Then he will give you the role, to represent that part of himself which should control the eating and drinking. Many women who want to lose weight look for a doctor who gives them a diet, where they could diet themselves by eating less. But that is very difficult. It is easier to have the figure of the forbidding agency outside, and then either to obey or to revolt. The same is true about drinking. The same is true about people with heart trouble who cannot bring themselves to be really careful of their bodies. It's easier to have the forbidding agency outside, which in itself does not yet guarantee obedience. . . .

But even that isn't the whole story yet. I have another point to make for you. [You will discover] how badly adult and sensible people take care of their own bodies. After all, our body, our health is one of our most valuable possessions, if not the most valuable one altogether. Wouldn't you expect all your patients to take the greatest care of their bodies, never to do anything that is injurious to their health, carefully to avoid infections, damage, dangers and, if they are ill, to take the right measures immediately. Wouldn't that be eminently sensible behavior? But there are very few adults, reasonable as they may be otherwise, who show such sensible behavior. This lack of good sense in health matters will make your future work extremely difficult. It will make it all the more difficult because you will feel, "I just can't understand it. After all it's his

body. Why doesn't he take better care of it? Why does he expect me to do it instead of doing it himself?" You wouldn't be at all astonished about that point, if you had the opportunity to watch the human being's relationship to his body from the very beginning. . . .

If you have the chance to observe children in their second year of life, you will make the surprising discovery that they treat their bodies as if they were not their own. Their bodies belong to their mothers which is only natural since it is not so very long ago—in the intrauterine stage—that the infant's body was actually part of the mother's. Neither in his first nor in his second year can the infant do anything for the care of his body. There is, in the beginning, even no barrier to self-injury and the baby would draw blood from his face if the mother did not see to the cutting of his nails. What we call the pain barrier is established gradually during the first year and the child's aggression deflected with it from his own body to the world outside.

We even think that the infant begins to love and respect his own body to the degree it is loved and respected by the mother, i.e., for the mother's sake. As regards the toddler, we certainly feel that he needs more than our guardian angel to keep alive in spite of the attractions of heights, stairs, water, fire, scissors, knives, and whatever other dangerous objects he may meet. He has, at this time of life, no appreciation of danger and he will inevitably injure himself unless he is protected. Pediatricians, child analysts and other workers in the field have learned to judge the quality of mothering available to a young child by the numbers of accidents in which he has been involved.

The child's intelligence has to mature before he learns to appreciate that fire burns and water drowns, that not everything is edible, etc. What he learns last of all is submission to the rules of hygiene and obedience in medical matters. At school age even, and right up to adolescence, many children act as if it were their privilege to do the most harmful and dangerous things to their bodies, while it is the parent's duty and privilege to protect them. [You] know how difficult it is to keep a child in bed with a fever, with an infection, that the dietary rules are felt by the child as a deep offense, a deprivation, a sign of not being liked. Even the ill child would eat what is bad for him, or the child would, for its own reasons, not eat even if he were starving himself. . . .

But what about you and the doctor-patient relationship? I only tell you these stories so that you can understand where all the irrational attitudes of your adult patients towards their health and towards their bodies come from. It is true you deal with adults, but every adult who is ill, who has fever, who is in pain, or who expects an operation, returns to childhood in some way. He feels small and helpless, and due to the ease with which he transfers feelings of the past onto you, you become the parent, you own his body. It is now your duty to look after him, and it is his privilege to be naughty about it: he feels well protected by you because he feels that somehow you will see to it that he doesn't do the wrong thing. You may get angry about it, but you will not be angry, if you remember that this adult before you is in reality a child, once more the child who has entrusted his body for safekeeping to an adult.

This brings us to the end point and perhaps to one of the most difficult tasks of the doctor in the doctor-patient relationship. The patient, as you see from the various points I made, will do his best to push you into the place of parental authority, and he will make use of you as parental authority to the utmost. You must understand that. On the other hand, you must not be tempted to treat him as a child. You must be tolerant towards him as you would be towards a child and as respectful as you would be towards a fellow adult, because he has only gone back to childhood so far as he's ill. He also has another part of his personality which has remained intact, and that part of him will resent it deeply, if you make too much use of your authority.

From "The Doctor and Death"

August M. Kasper

The physician's training stresses "scientific objectivity," and physicians are often fond of mistaking themselves for scientists. There are some very useful similarities between science and medicine, but whereas a scientist is interested in death, a doctor is against it. It is indeed possible to be a physician and a scientist, but it is a rare combination in practice. The physician qua physician is committed to a credo which is far different from that of the scientist, even if we insist that such tenets as knowability, order, and inductive method are articles of faith. Medical practitioners have the wistful audacity, thank God, to blindly insist that pain is bad and life is to be preserved. This patent value judgment is the basis of medicine, and

Excerpted with permission of author and publisher from *The Meaning of Death*, edited by H. Feifel (N.Y.: McGraw-Hill, 1959). Copyright © 1959 by McGraw-Hill Inc.

only coincidentally has it anything to do with knowledge of observable reality. Some doctors wish to be scientists in order to gain mastery over life by treating people as interesting things. It is this orientation which permits a doctor to speak of a "good" case of leukemia; that is, the case in question corresponds closely to the standard description of a certain disease entity, so that the adjective "good" is correctly, if disturbingly, used. This oddly inhuman perspective makes it possible for the doctor to observe, codify, diagnose, and treat, free from interfering preoccupations with horrors of disease and fear of death. The layman, hearing the doctor so speak and act, often gets the idea that the physician is cold and is treating the patient as a "thing," but the layman doesn't recognize that all such talk and activity is premised on the idea that life should be maintained and pain avoided. I cannot be sure whether it is a good thing or not, but the doctor will often conceal his own fear of pain and death behind his prerogative to be "objective" or "scientific.". . .

There is the frustration of the young doctor's orientation toward the hopelessly ill, toward those whom he knows can respond only with gratitude, and often not even that. These are the people in dreary wards and cheerless rooms. They lie quietly, dreaming perhaps, but looking for all the world like the doctor's "first patient." They need to have certain things done: indolent ulcers must be cleaned, draining wounds dressed, fetid mouths tended, fecal impactions removed, and very often, because no other way will do, they must be sustained by fluids dripped into failing, clogging veins. And this last tenderness gives a name to the whole tour of mercy: "watering the vegetables." The dying are thus not neglected, but they are very rarely approached with hope or even interest, because, I suppose, they simply will not feed the doctor's narcissism by responding and getting well. Their care is demanding, frustrating, and far from helpful to the medical magician's self-esteem.

Later, in the hospital years, one again sees clearly the formal, if unwritten, code: doctors should never become personally "involved" while working at their profession. This is sometimes carried to the extreme I witnessed while an intern. A very competent and kindly surgeon was performing an operation on a nine-year-old boy which could only extend the youngster's life a few weeks longer at the most. During surgery, the doctor remarked that it was a shame that this boy would not live to marry and have sons of his own. The interns, residents, and nurses who heard this remark later speculated about why it had been made. The consensus seemed to be that it was, at least, in bad taste and might even be explained by assuming that the surgeon had been drinking before surgery. They were wrong, I believe; but this very excellent doctor did often drink heavily *after* the day's work. He seemed to have reached the necessary truth, but like the fabled neurotic, he was unhappy about it.

. . . the doctor continues his maternal identification and vicarious dependency by caring for others. This ordinarily works very well because he helps people, and they are grateful and "like" him. But everyone knows how fickle is the affection of the "helped" person, how his dependency is felt as a weakness in which he has submitted to the helper, the physician; the doctor fears and the patient broods on the turning of the tables. The doctor works hard to keep the relationship from changing; traditionally, this omnipotent help is not even contaminated (made realistic) by talk of money for services rendered—as if both parties preferred the God-supplicant arrangement. Besides this, or as part of it, the doctor often is pretty unpleasant about people who don't understand how wonderful he is; on this point, one might consult nurses, curious patients, and Armed Forces personnel who had to command doctors. All this then to indicate that the doctor keeps his power, his patients' love, and his invulnerability by fending off death and illness. And when the magic doesn't work, the doctor who still believes the myth is in serious danger of disillusionment and disgrace. Such a doctor has often treated his patients so highhandedly that the latter will actually sense the situation and find some small comfort in the spiteful revenge of dying. We talk about positive and negative transference, but most doctors accept the first as their normal, just due, and any other reaction as recalcitrance or ingratitude. A convenient notion, an enviable viewpoint, but the doctor who subscribes to it simply cannot face the anger and rejection of the hurt and disappointed patient. Most doctors would rather not ever have to, but it is necessary at times—if only for the reason given by Hippocrates: "And by seeing and announcing beforehand those who will live and those who will die, he will thus escape censure." If we could, without censure, maintain our reputation for omnipotence, I wonder how often we would admit our inadequate skills.

If a doctor's death is dismayingly incredible to the dreamer in everyone, it is even more poignantly noted when a medical man hears of a psychiatrist's suicide, a surgeon's pancreatic cancer, or an internist's coronary occlusion. Here even the initiated are awed by the surrender of the specalist to his intimately familiar foe. Specialization would seem to offer some fascinating opportunities for more specific resolution of the search that leads men into the "noble art." I am not in a position to compare one specialty with another in this regard, but I would like to say a word about my own. Psychiatrists, often thought to be so far from organic disease, pain and death, hear a lot about how these things affect people. But if a surgeon hides behind his mask, a psychiatrist has an even more effective shield. I do not mean the couch, which is good in its way, but rather that wonderful step in intellectualization whereby we alter the quality of reality through nomenclature. This allows us to treat a man's fear of death as we would a fear of things in the dark. In practice, this is a good idea, i.e., it works because phobias are irrational fears. But where there isn't anything in the dark, there is death, and the man who doesn't recognize death is unlikely to preserve his life effectively. So it happens that the psychiatrist can deny death as he denies the apparent source of any other phobia, and some seem to take advantage of this possibility, although Freud wrote, "If you would endure life, be prepared for death." An even more elaborate formulation is often interpreted as meaning that we die because we "wish" it or are physically impelled toward it. Again this may be, but I imagine we would die whether or not it were so. It is the over-simplification and misunderstanding of such concepts that make the playwright and novelist depict us as unctious, smug possessors of secrets that would give man complete freedom from anxiety, guilt, and death. It seems to me however, that psychiatrists are less likely to give this impression now than previously, perhaps because we are understood better and understand more.

Almost all doctors are reluctant to make and reveal serious diagnoses. While touched by pain and saddened by each patient's death, they often contrive to show their feelings in devious and distorted ways. I recently saw a woman in consultation who gave a perceptive picture of the two types of doctors she had encountered during some twenty years of being treated for pulmonary tuberculosis. Doctors had assumed a God-like stature in her mind because her life literally depended on their judgment and treatment. Because of this she was unable to express any resentment directly to them. She said that at one extreme was the doctor who was solicitous, overly kind, protective, but afraid of her illness and its possible consequences. He seemed uncomfortable in touching her and took elaborate, sometimes extreme, precautions against becoming infected by her. He was so concerned and fearful that on many occasions he behaved too conservatively in his treatment and was reluctant to do anything that inconvenienced or hurt her. At the other pole, there was the doctor who was rough, brusque, and practically manhandled her. She liked being so treated to some extent because at least it made her feel respected as a person of some strength. However, this type of man told her very little about her progress, minimized her symptoms, and laughed at her complaints. Once when a chest X ray was made, he only told her that if anything was wrong, he would call her. He then let her worry for several weeks until she finally called him—only to be told that the chest plate was negative, and what the devil did she expect him to do: call every patient who had a negative X ray? The patient said she felt most doctors were probably inclined toward one or the other extreme, and that they were able to be pleasant, warm, and personable only as long as there was nothing seriously wrong with the patient, that is, so far as their own specialty was concerned. It is painfully evident to this woman that technical excellence cannot substitute for personal courage and warmth in the doctor's task to help his patient. She would be happy if she could deceive herself about her doctor, but her sensitivity to his feelings prevents it.

It is often unfortunately true that the seriously or hopelessly ill patient senses the doctor's emotions clearly. The doctor's disillusionment, depending on his maturity, will show as sympathy, anger, disgust, indifference, interest, disappointment, or embarrassment. Though not exhaustive, this list suggests the many ways a patient may perceive how his doom affects his physician. The hardest to bear is indifference because it is so defensive, so weak, that the patient cannot believe that which such a man tells him. I have sometimes seen attitudes closer to anger rouse a man from guilt and dread and keep him emotionally with his family until the real death. Those feelings at the opposite pole—true grief, sympathy—are most supportive for the dying one, not only because he feels loved, but because he then sees that the living need his help. He feels called upon to soothe the physician's hurt, to comfort those who will mourn, to assure men of their dignity. Such a man will live his life to the end, as well and as productively as he ever was able.

And the doctor will help to this end if he can know his own fear and weakness and hope. Realizing the human condition, he will not be too disturbed by his failure and disillusionment. He can function as comforter and, while not promising life, can offer hope.

From "Philosophical Reflections on Experimenting with Human Subjects"

Hans Jonas

EXPERIMENTATION ON PATIENTS

So far we have been speaking on the tacit assumption that the subjects of experimentation are recruited from among the healthy. To the question "Who is conscriptable?" the spontaneous answer is: Least and last of all the sick—the most available source as they are under treatment and observation anyway. That the afflicted should not be called upon to bear additional burden and risk, that they are society's special trust and the physician's particular trust—these are elementary responses of our moral sense. Yet the very destination of medical research, the conquest of disease, requires at the crucial stage trial and verification on precisely the sufferers from the disease, and their total exemption would defeat the purpose itself. In acknowledging this inescapable necessity, we enter the most sensitive area of the whole complex, the one most keenly felt and most searchingly discussed by the practitioners themselves. This issue touches the heart of the doctor-patient relation, putting its most solemn obligations to the test. Some of the oldest verities of this area should be recalled.

Reprinted with deletions by permission of author and *Daedalus,* Journal of the American Academy of Arts and Sciences, Boston, Massachusetts. Spring 1969, *Ethical Aspects of Experimentation with Human Subjects.*

THE FUNDAMENTAL PRIVILEGE OF THE SICK

In the course of treatment, the physician is obligated to the patient and to no one else. He is not the agent of society, nor of the interests of medical science, the patient's family, the patient's co-sufferers, or future sufferers from the same disease. The patient alone counts when he is under the physician's care. By the simple law of bilateral contract (analogous, for example, to the relation of lawyer to client and its "conflict of interest" rule), he is bound not to let any other interest interfere with that of the patient in being cured. But manifestly more sublime norms than contractual ones are involved. We may speak of a sacred trust; strictly by its terms, the doctor is, as it were, alone with his patient and God.

There is one normal exception to this—that is, to the doctor's not being the agent of society vis-à-vis the patient, but the trustee of his interests alone—the quarantining of the contagious sick. This is plainly not for the patient's interest, but for that of others threatened by him. (In vaccination, we have a combination of both: protection of the individual and others.) But preventing the patient from causing harm to others is not the same as exploiting him for the advantage of others. And there is, of course, the abnormal exception of collective catastrophe, the analogue to a state of war. The physician who desperately battles a raging epidemic is under a unique dispensation that suspends in a nonspecifiable way some of the strictures of normal practice, including possibly those against experimental liberties with his patients. No rules can be devised for the waiving of rules in extremities. And as with the famous shipwreck examples of ethical theory, the less said about it the better. But what is allowable there and may later be passed over in forgiving silence cannot serve as a precedent. We are concerned with nonextreme, nonemergency conditions where the voice of principle can be heard and claims can be adjudicated free from duress. We have conceded that there are such claims, and that if there is to be medical advance at all, not even the superlative privilege of the suffering and the sick can be kept wholly intact from the intrusion of its needs. About this least palatable, most disquieting part of our subject, I have to offer only groping, inconclusive remarks.

THE PRINCIPLE OF "IDENTIFICATION" APPLIED TO PATIENTS

On the whole, the same principles* would seem to hold here as are found to hold with "normal subjects": motivation, identification, understanding on the part of the subject. But it is clear that these conditions are peculiarly difficult to satisfy with regard to a patient. His physical state, psychic preoccupation, dependent relation to the doctor, the submissive attitude induced by treatment—everything connected with his condition and situation makes the sick person inherently less of a sovereign person than the healthy one. Spontaneity of self-

---

*Early in this essay, Jonas argues that morally permissible use of human beings in medical experimentation requires that they be those persons with a maximum of identification, understanding, and spontaneity—the most highly motivated, the most highly educated, and the least "captive" members of the community. *Ed.*

offering has almost to be ruled out; consent is marred by lower resistance or captive circumstance, and so on. In fact, all the factors that make the patient, as a category, particularly accessible and welcome for experimentation at the same time compromise the quality of the responding affirmation that must morally redeem the making use of them. This, in addition to the primacy of the physician's duty, puts a heightened onus on the physician-researcher to limit his undue power to the most important and defensible research objectives and, of course, to keep persuasion at a minimum.

Still, with all the disabilities noted, there is scope among patients for observing the rule of the "descending order of permissibility" that we have laid down for normal subjects, in vexing inversion of the utility order of quantitative abundance and qualitative "expendability." By the principle of this order, those patients who most identify with and are cognizant of the cause of research—members of the medical profession (who after all are sometimes patients themselves)—come first; the highly motivated and educated, also least dependent, among the lay patients come next; and so on down the line. An added consideration here is seriousness of condition, which again operates in inverse proportion. Here the profession must fight the tempting sophistry that the hopeless case is expendable (because in prospect already expended) and therefore especially usable; and generally the attitude that the poorer the chances of the patient the more justifiable his recruitment for experimentation (other than for his own benefit). The opposite is true.

NONDISCLOSURE AS A BORDERLINE CASE

Then there is the case where ignorance of the subject, sometimes even of the experimenter, is of the essence of the experiment (the "double blind" control group-placebo syndrome). It is said to be a necessary element of the scientific process. Whatever may be said about its ethics in regard to normal subjects, especially volunteers, it is an outright betrayal of trust in regard to the patient who believes that he is receiving treatment. Only supreme importance of the objective can exonerate it, without making it less of a transgression. The patient is definitely wronged even when not harmed. And ethics apart, the practice of such deception holds the danger of undermining the faith in the *bona fides* of treatment, the beneficial intent of the physician—the very basis of the doctor-patient relationship. In every respect, it follows that concealed experiment on patients—that is, experiment under the guise of treatment—should be the rarest exception, at best, if it cannot be wholly avoided.

This has still the merit of a borderline problem. This is not true of the other case of necessary ignorance of the subject—that of the unconscious patient. Drafting him for nontherapeutic experiments is simply and unqualifiedly impermissible; progress or not, he must never be used, on the inflexible principle that utter helplessness demands utter protection.

When preparing this paper, I filled pages with a casuistics of this harrowing field, but then scratched out most of it, realizing my dilettante status. The shadings are endless, and only the physician-researcher can discern them properly as the cases arise. Into his lap the decision is thrown. The philosophical rule, once it has admitted into itself the idea of a sliding scale, cannot really specify its own application. It can only impress on the practitioner a general maxim or attitude for the exercise of his judgment and conscience in the concrete occasions of his work. In our case, I am afraid, it means making life more difficult for him.

It will also be noted that, somewhat at variance with the emphasis in the literature, I have not dwelt on the element of ''risk'' and very little on that of ''consent.'' Discussion of the first is beyond the layman's competence; the emphasis on the second has been lessened because of its equivocal character. It is a truism to say that one should strive to minimize the risk and to maximize the consent. The more demanding concept of ''identification,'' which I have used, includes ''consent'' in its maximal or authentic form, and the assumption of risk is its privilege.

NO EXPERIMENTS ON PATIENTS UNRELATED TO THEIR OWN DISEASE

Although my ponderings have, on the whole, yielded points of view rather than define prescriptions, premises rather than conclusions, they have led me to a few unequivocal yeses and noes. The first is the emphatic rule that patients should be experimented upon, if at all, *only* with reference to *their* disease. Never should there be added to the gratuitousness of the experiment as such the gratuitousness of service to an unrelated cause. This follows simply from what we have found to be the *only* excuse for infracting the special exemption of the sick at all—namely, that the scientific war on disease cannot accomplish its goal without drawing the sufferers from disease into the investigative process. If under this excuse they become subjects of experiment, they do so *because,* and only because, of *their* disease.

This is the fundamental and self-sufficient consideration. That the patient cannot possibly benefit from the unrelated experiment therapeutically, which he might from experiment related to his condition, is also true, but lies beyond the problem area of pure experiment. Anyway, I am discussing nontherapeutic experimentation only, where *ex hypothesi* the patient does not benefit. Experiment as part of therapy—that is, directed toward helping the subject himself—is a different matter altogether and raises its own problems, but hardly philosophical ones. As long as a doctor can say, even if only in his own thought: ''There is no known cure for your condition (or: You have responded to none); but there is promise in a new treatment still under investigation, not quite tested yet as to effectiveness and safety; you will be taking a chance, but all things considered, I judge it in your best interest to let me try it on you''—as long as he can speak thus, he speaks as the patient's physician and may err, but does not transform the patient into a subject of experimentation. Introduction of an untried therapy into the treatment where the tried ones have failed is not ''experimentation on the patient.''

Generally, there is something ''experimental'' (because tentative) about every individual treatment, beginning with the diagnosis itself; and he would be a poor doctor who would not learn from every case for the benefit of future cases, and a poor member of the profession who would not make any new insights gained from his treatments available to the profession at large. Thus, knowledge may be advanced in the treatment of any patient, and the interest of the medical art and all sufferers from the same affliction as well as the patient may be served if something happens to be learned from his case. But this gain to knowledge and future therapy is incidental to the *bona fide* service to the present patient. He has the right to expect that the doctor does nothing to him just in order to learn.

In that case, the doctor's imaginary speech would run, for instance, like this: "There is nothing more I can do for you. But you can do something for me. Speaking no longer as your physician but on behalf of medical science, we could learn a great deal about future cases of this kind if you would permit me to perform certain experiments on you. It is understood that you yourself would not benefit from any knowledge we might gain; but future patients would." This statement would express the purely experimental situation, assumedly here with the subject's concurrence and with all cards on the table. In Alexander Bickel's words: "It is a different situation when the doctor is no longer trying to make [the patient] well, but is trying to find out how to make others well in the future."

But even in the second case of the non-therapeutic experiment where the patient does not benefit, the patient's own disease is enlisted in the cause of fighting that disease, even if only in others. It is yet another thing to say or think: "Since you are here—in the hospital with its facilities—under our care and observation, away from your job (or, perhaps, doomed), we wish to profit from your being available for some other research of great interest we are presently engaged in." From the standpoint of merely medical ethics, which has only to consider risk, consent, and the worth of the objective, there may be no cardinal difference between this case and the last one. I hope that my medical audience will not think I am making too fine a point when I say that from the standpoint of the subject and his dignity there is a cardinal difference that crosses the line between the permissible and the impermissible, and this by the same principle of "identification" I have been invoking all along. Whatever the rights and wrongs of any experimentation on any patient—in the one case, at least that residue of identification is left him that it is his own affliction by which he can contribute to the conquest of that affliction, his own kind of suffering which he helps to alleviate in others; and so in a sense it is his own cause. It is totally indefensible to rob the unfortunate of this intimacy with the purpose and make his misfortune a convenience for the furtherance of alien concerns. The observance of this rule is essential, I think, to attenuate at least the wrong that nontherapeutic experimenting on patients commits in any case.

Iatrogenic Problems in End-Stage Renal Failure

Chad H. Calland, M.D.

The problem of a patient with end-stage renal failure can be viewed as a set of simple alternatives. He can undergo long-term chronic hemodialysis, he can have a successful kidney transplantation, or he can die. Since the third alternative is usually considered unacceptable to all concerned, every effort is made by the physician to achieve one of the first two alternatives. At this point a simple problem becomes extremely complex.

The problem is complex for a host of reasons, but I intend to focus upon the division that exists between the nephrologist and the transplant surgeon, and the moral and ethical problems in the physician-patient relation that develop as a consequence. Both specialists work desperately to solve the problem of end-stage renal failure. Each honestly believes that he has "the true answer"—if only it could be perfected. Unfortunately, it is the patient who suffers because of these differing but equally legitimate endeavors and opinions.

METHODS OF OBSERVATION

I was a victim of chronic membranous nephritis, which culminated in end-stage renal failure, dialysis in hospitals, dialysis at home and five renal transplantations. Interested readers may find the case report fairly well documented in the lay press.[1,2] Since I have experienced nearly every conceivable complication of both methods of therapy, I feel uniquely qualified to comment upon these treatments and their problems.

Aside from my personal involvement, I have had the opportunity to know and to share the experiences of patients undergoing both hemodialysis and transplantation in the three centers where I have been treated. Time on dialysis and time in the post-operative period grows long, and the opportunity is excellent for close,

Reprinted by permission of The New England Journal of Medicine, vol. 283, no. 7, Aug. 17, 1979. pp. 334–336.

meaningful interplay among patients in similar straits. I enjoyed the added advantage that the patients did not regard me as a doctor. I was simply another patient who happened to be a doctor, and they felt free to share their problems with me. My observations are not scientific, and are not presented as such. However, I can comment upon the experiences of 40 to 50 patients and some of their families; the pattern is so strikingly similar that it is clinically meaningful to me and worthy of report.

OBSERVATIONS

Patients on Chronic Dialysis

The pattern of response of these patients is striking to me because it differs so greatly from that described in the literature. Patients I have read about seem to be wrapped up in coping with mechanisms which are not useful, such as psychotic, neurotic or behavior disorders, or the organic brain syndrome that accompanies uremia.[3]

On the other hand, patients I have known on dialysis seem to be concerned about very real problems. To be held to an 800-ml total intake of fluids per day is most difficult. Restrictions on consumption of sodium and potassium make any kind of meal unpalatable. Restraints on travel even further constrain an already regimented, complicated and compromised life style.

A young woman wonders whether anyone will ever marry her, or whether she should even consider marriage. A young husband wonders whether he can, or even should, sire children and, if he does, who will support them. Older, more established patients on dialysis wonder if the struggle to live is worth the effort and money that must be put forth for the rest of their lives. Patients with growing children wonder whether these children's lives would be more damaged by continuing hemodialysis or by "accidental" unplugging of the shunt, so that at least their family's future would be more financially secure.

Many of these conflicts are considered by most psychiatrists to be evidence of depressive or paranoid ideation. I cannot emphasize strongly enough that, in this group of patients, these fears are well founded and are based in reality. It is real, for example, that some employers will not lend money for necessary equipment, nor give time off for treatment. It is real that friends and neighbors, even when positively helpful, regard the dialysis patient as a marginal person—here today, gone tomorrow. It is real that the patient's own tenuous grasp on the future is reflected constantly in his own professional and financial dealings (promotions are delayed, and arrangements for mortgages and insurances are difficult, if not impossible).

Patients on dialysis are accustomed to being told by the doctor, "You are doing fine"—usually after the latest measurements of electrolytes and creatinine. The patient then thinks to himself, "If I'm doing fine, why do I feel so rotten?" After undergoing correction of several days' accumulation of metabolites in a few hours, who could feel well with the resultant cerebral edema?[4-6] Who, with a hematocrit of 17 per cent, feels well enough to function when he cannot climb his own stairway because of dyspnea?

After a number of such visits to the doctor, the patient begins to think that perhaps his very real symptoms of fatigue, dyspnea, muscle weakness and so forth are products of a deranged mind, so that he begins to conceal them because he is ashamed. Eventually, the time comes when the patient complains of nothing, and the doctor is thus wholly unaware of these symptoms, just as he is unaware of the other (marital, financial and social) difficulties that the patient is experiencing.

Patients on hemodialysis know these facts better than the physician does, because the patient alone experiences them—often in isolation. Is it any wonder that the patient feels less valuable than any healthy person and doubts the worth of his struggle?[7,8] Is it necessary to postulate psychiatric disorders to understand the self-evident?

Is dialysis "the true answer" for all patients?

Patients with Transplants

On the other hand, after successful transplants, patients have even greater difficulties to cope with because, almost without exception, they have undergone the problems of hemodialysis. They can now view life from a different perspective, free from machines, tubes, dialysates, supplies, dietary, fluid and travel restrictions, anemia, the mess of cleaning up after a run, and all the shunt or fistula problems that plague the patient on hemodialysis. Nonetheless, patients with transplants continue to share the anxieties of their friends who remain on hemodialysis, and, in addition, they carry the constant burdens of fear of rejection and of the primary complications of immunosuppressive therapy: Cushingoid faces, infections, cancer, diabetes, capillary fragility, osteoporosis, glaucoma, cataracts and acne.

They may also face worse mental depression. Despite a successful graft, their employment, marital, insurance, mortgage and financial situations have not improved because not enough data have yet been gathered about life expectancy after successful transplantation. The longest known survival is 15 years, and this fact does not satisfy anyone, let alone insurance underwriters.

Cosmetic problems crop up. An 18-year-old guitarist stops taking steroids because "they puff up my face" and make him unattractive on the bandstand. As a result, he loses his kidney, refuses hemodialysis and dies. A dedicated young nurse finds her complexion and facial appearance so unpleasant that she finds it necessary to "go underground," and she becomes a member of a "hippie" set. A young couple find the uncertainty of the future so unbearable that they separate, and the recipient commits suicide. In an older man with no rejection problems whatsoever meningoencephalitis (a result of immunosuppressive therapy?) develops, and he loses his executive position after 10 weeks off the job. A long-term recipient with good graft function acquires *Pneumocystis carinii* infection after the fourth transplant and dies from alveolar-capillary block. A young man dies after his fourth transplant from lymphosarcoma (caused by immunosuppression?).

Is transplantation "the true answer" for all patients?

THE PROBLEM

The problem devolves into the simple fact that the nephrologist and the transplant surgeon, within two different disciplines and ideologies, do not speak freely with one another to find "the true answer" for any individual patient. These specialists should be working and co-operating together as friends and colleagues for the benefit of each patient, but instead they work at odds, to the detriment of all their patients. And neither specialist informs or consults fully with the patient and his family about their needs and desires. The doctor is thus at a disadvantage of his own making—the terrible disadvantage of having knowledge of his patients' feelings about illness and treatment concealed from him.

If the nephrologist could only know what goes on within his patients' lives, which he cannot, he would pay more attention to the quality of life and less attention to the quantity of life and to the disparities of the blood-brain barrier.[9] Why do so many dialysis patients "hang around" transplant clinics? Why do so few patients with successful transplants return to their primary doctors? Why, therefore, does the nephrologist believe that there are so few with successful transplants who view life in a different way, and enjoy what they find? Why is the transplant surgeon so overburdened with patients who are no longer within his province? The unpleasant answer is that the nephrologist has devoted his attention to his patients' biochemical findings rather than to his patients.

The transplant surgeon has minimized the morbidity and mortality of graft rejection and of immunosuppressive therapy. His endeavors are supported by his accumulated data on graft survival and patient survival; when reporting his statistics, he does not mention his patients' fractures, infections, bleeding and other problems. Younger patients are often willing to risk these side effects to achieve a greater freedom in life style. Frequently, older patients are not willing to accept these risks when they have done well on dialysis and have, perhaps, only a few years left to live.

But how often is the patient (and his family) given a truly informed choice?

DISCUSSION

It is the fragmentation of medical care and understandable lack of information that the nephrologist and the transplant surgeon have to work with that create a schism between these two physicians. The schism may be all well and good from the academic point of view, but, in the end, it is the patient who suffers. These two men should work as a team, not as competitors. It is sad that they think they have to justify what they do by their scientific training. Is it necessary to cite length of survival after either mode of treament? Is it necessary to state how many dollars are saved by this or that? To many patients, the point that is most important is the quality of life, whether by hemodialysis or by transplantation. These are some data that cannot be quantified in years, dollars, kilograms or any other numbers, but are gathered in the often intangible experiences of life.

Dialysis and transplantation should be complementary forms of therapy, and I believe strongly that the patient should have a doctor who is interested in the art of medicine—namely, the care of the patient, so that he may return to a more nearly "normal" life, whatever that means to him, not what it means to the doctor.

The primary reasons, I hope, that we became physicians were to love and help our fellow man. But the polemic that exists among physicians "doing their own thing" does not help anyone.

A lay person criticizing physicians for their divisiveness would be called "sour grapes." But I have seen both sides of the fence, and I want to make proper commentary before more patients suffer.

Notes

1. Hano A: Incredible ordeal of Chad Calland, M. D. Redbook 137: 94, September, 1971

2. Five kidneys and two years of hell. San Francisco Chronicle 107: 9, January 11, 1971
3. Menninger KA: Paranoid psychosis with uremia. J Nerv Ment Dis 60:26–34, 1924
4. Scheitlin W, Hunziker A: Die Beeinflussung des Liquorchemismus durch Hämodialyse beim urämischen Patienten. Schweiz Med Wochenschr 92:673–676, 1962
5. Kennedy AC, Linton AL, Eaton JC: Urea levels in cerebrospinal fluid after haemodialysis, Lancet 1:410–411, 1962
6. Cowie J, Lambie AT, Robson JS: The influence of extracorporeal dialysis on the acid-base composition of blood and cerebrospinal fluid. Clin Sci 23:397–404, 1962
7. Tsaltas TT: Psychiatric aspects of dialysis. Vinculum 3 (3):3–4, 1970 (Published by Cobe Laboratories, Inc. Denver, Colorado)
8. Schreiner GE: Mental and personality changes in the uremic syndrome. Med Ann DC 28:316–323: 362, 1959
9. Moschcowitz E: Essays on the biology of disease: Uremia. J Mt Sinai Hosp NY 15:38–48, 1948

Taking Care of the Hateful Patient

James E. Groves

Admitted or not, the fact remains that a few patients kindle aversion, fear, despair or even downright malice in their doctors. Emotional reactions to patients cannot simply be wished away, nor is it good medicine to pretend that they do not exist. Doctors cannot avoid occasional negative feelings toward the "obnoxious patient,"[1] the whining "self-pitier"[2] or the help rejecting "crock."[3] Like that of Faust, the doctor's ideal is to "know all, love all, heal all, "[4] but when this ideal of the perfect physician collides with the quotidian realities of caring for sick and troubled patients, a number of processes may ensue: there may be "helplessness in the helper"[5]; there may be unconscious punishment of the patient[2]; there may be self-punishment by the doctor[4]; and there may be inappropriate confrontation of the patient[6]; and there may be a desperate attempt to avoid or to extrude the patient from the care-giving system.[7,8]

A 51-year-old attorney specializing in medical negligence was enraged when his many complaints were ultimately diagnosed as multiple sclerosis. Known for his flashy wardrobe and courtroom pyrotechnics, he roamed from doctor to doctor, refusing to understand the nature of his illness and threatening to sue the previous "bastard" who had tried to help him. He was like Job (xiii:4), who raged, "ye are forgers of lies, ye are all physicians of no value." He adamantly refused treatment and demanded more and more tests and consultations. Eventually, his doctors did not return his calls for appointments and were frightened and depressed about him. How long this situation might have continued is not known, because at this point—to the relief of all concerned—he was stopped by an exacerbation of his demyelinating process that required hospitalization in a chronic-care facility.

This vignette illustrates a "hateful patient"— one whom most physicians would dread to treat. The present communication addresses "countertransference" feelings toward the patient, except for two situations that are thoroughly treated elsewhere: feelings toward the obviously suicidal patient[4]; and idiosyncratic bias reactions confined to a particular doctor with certain kinds of patients.[2,9] The latter group of reactions is determined by specific psychologic processes (usually unconscious) in one doctor; in such a case, the remedy of transferring the patient may well be appropriate, since the idiosyncracies of one physician are not highly likely to be those of another. Here,

Reprinted by permission of the author and *The New England Journal of Medicine*, vol. 298, no. 16, April 20, 1978, pp. 883–887.

discussion will center on patients for whom most physicians would harbor negative feelings and for whom transfer is not usually helpful to the patient.

HATE IN THE LITERATURE OF MEDICINE

The medical student and the doctor find little help in the literature. Even Osler fails in this regard. Nowhere in his *Principles and Practice of Medicine*[10] does he allude to personal feelings that the difficult patient may stir up; his other writings[11,12] are sermons, more inspirational than practical. Modern textbooks of medicine have a few pages on the doctor-patient relationship,[13,14] but their most negative appellation for a patient is "exasperating,"[15] and they generally suggest that the physician disown negative feelings in favor of integrity, truth, humor and compassion. Psychiatry too, with certain notable exceptions,[2,3,9] has failed to help the rest of medicine with the feelings that patients stir up; even when feelings are addressed directly,[16] the advice tendered is most likely to be, transfer to a colleague who can stand the patient. This gap is particularly odd because psychiatry has been fascinated with the negative side of the doctor-patient relationship since the turn of the century.

"Countertransference" is the word that Freud coined to mean emotional reactions to a patient that are determined by the psychoanalyst's own unconscious conflict. Later on, "countertransference" assumed for some a broader meaning of unconscious and conscious unbidden and unwanted hostile and sexual feelings toward the patient—feelings that were seen to impede the treatment and to reflect poorly on the analyst. Although Freud himself was rather candid about his own countertransference reactions, his scientific attitude about it was often difficult for his early followers to emulate.

In 1949 the prestigious *International Journal of Psycho-Analysis* published a paper written by a pediatrician and psychoanalyst named D. W. Winnicott and entitled "Hate in the Countertransference."[17] In it he acknowledged outright hatred for some patients in certain circumstances. This hatred—and even the murderous wishes associated with it—he compared with the occasional inevitable dislike of the normal mother for her demanding infant. He noted that the apparent innocence of nursery rhymes and lullabys betrays such hatred mixed with maternal love ("Down will come baby/Cradle and all"). The publication of "Hate in the Countertransference" was a benchmark in the study of such feelings; subsequently, papers about countertransference were less defensive. Such feelings have gradually come to be regarded not only as a painful visitation but also as a necessary clue guiding the psychiatrist's conceptualization and technic. Likewise, the study of countertransference phenomena can guide other physicians, especially in the management of four classes of patients: dependent *clingers;* entitled *demanders;* manipulative *help-rejecters;* and self-destructive *deniers.* At times, a single patient may epitomize more than one of these classes. The following portraits are stereotypes.

DEPENDENT CLINGERS

Clingers escalate from mild and appropriate requests for reassurance to repeated, perfervid, incarcerating cries for explanation, affection, analgesics, sedatives and all forms of attention imaginable. They are naïve about their effect on the physician, and they are overt in their neediness. They may have no discernible medical illness, or they may have severe, chronic or life-threatening disorders; but whatever their medical problems, what is common to them as a group is their self-perception of bottomless need and their perception of the physician as inexhaustible. Such dependency may eventually lead to a sense of weary aversion toward the patient. When the doctor's stamina is exhausted, a referral for psychiatric examination may be adamantly put forth in frustrated tones that the patient (correctly) interprets as rejection. Psychiatric referrals made in this context are destined to fail utterly.

A 23-year-old "exotic dancer" of no little beauty consulted a resident in medicine because of fatigue. This male resident was eventually able to make the diagnosis of lupus. He took care in explaining the mild nature of her particular course. She responded intelligently with questions pertinent to prognosis and eventually asked him whether he would follow her, long-term, for this chronic illness. Flattered and touched, he vowed to do so. Later that day she telephoned briefly to thank him.

During the next week she visited with a question about her medication. In the following week she called twice, once professing great fear that she would die and another time to thank him again. As weeks passed, her calls and visits became more frequent, and her thanks dwindled to nothing. He began to dread her calls.

By the end of two months she was calling him daily, in the office and at home. What had begun as a minuet ultimately became a fandango. He changed programs; she soon was involved in a similar situation with another resident in the same clinic.

Early signs of the clinger are the patient's genuine gratitude, but to an extreme degree, and the doctor's feelings of power and specialness to the patient, an emotion not unlike puppy love. Later on, the doctor and the patient have different feelings toward each other. The doctor becomes the inexhaustible mother; the patient becomes the unplanned, unwanted, unlovable child. Early identification of this situation is helpful, but its corrective may be applied—if done skillfully—at any point short of a complete blowup. The clinger must be told as early in the relationship as possible, and as tactfully and firmly as possible, that the physician has not only human limits to knowledge and skill but also limitations to time and stamina. Written follow-up appointments are placed in the patient's hand, the doctor says, "so long," and never, "good-bye," and the patient is firmly reminded not to call except during office hours or in an emergency. This approach is not cruelty or rejection. It is in the best interest of patient care to protect the patient from promises that cannot be kept and from illusions that are bound to shatter.

ENTITLED DEMANDNESS

Demanders resemble clingers in the profundity of their neediness, but they differ in that—rather than flattery and unconscious seduc-

tion—they use intimidation, devaluation and guilt-induction to place the doctor in the role of the inexhaustible supply depot. They appear less naïve about their effect on the physician than clingers and buttress their hold on the doctor by threatening punishment. The patient may try to control the physician by withholding payment or threatening litigation. The patient is unaware of the deep dependency that underlies these attacks on the doctor. The physician, in turn, does not recognize that the hostility is born of terror of abandonment. Moreover, such patients often exude a repulsive sense of innate deservedness as if they were far superior to the physician. This attitude is to shield them from awareness that the physician seems to have power over life and death. Obviously, this sense of innate and magical entitlement to everything that is wanted is depressing (and therefore often enraging) to the busy physician, who may have had to surrender many dreams of omnipotence and omniscience over the years of training. The physician becomes fearful about reputation, enraged that the patient is not cooperative and grateful and—eventually—secretly ashamed, as if the patient's devaluating demands were realistic. But this very "entitlement," repulsive as it may be, is resorted to by the patient in an effort to preserve the integrity of the self in a world that seems hostile or during an illness that seems terrifying. "Entitlement" serves for some persons the functions that faith and hope serve in better adjusted ones. The usual impulse toward entitlement is a wish to point out suddenly and devastatingly that the patient has earned little, medically or in larger society, and deserves little. But this course would be an assault on the very psychologic foundations that support such a patient. Entitlement is such a patient's religion and should not be blasphemed.

Because the lawyer with multiple sclerosis in the first vignette was entitled, he was vulnerable to counterattack. But because he had so much actual power to harm his caregivers, counterattack did not in fact occur. Because his terror and entitlement were concealed beneath the trappings of real achievement, neither was his bombast recognized for what it was—a pathetic sham. Thus it was not addressed in service of the patient's best interest. The physician should never gainsay the patient's entitlement. The most helpful therapeutic strategy with the entitled demander is to support the entitlement but to rechannel it in the direction of the indicated regimen. His doctor might have said,

> I know you're mad about this and mad at the other doctors. You have reason to be mad. You have an illness that makes some people give up, and you're fighting it. But you're fighting your doctors too. You say you're entitled to repeated tests, damages for suffering and all that. And you are entitled—entitled to the very best medical care we can give you. But we can't give you the good treatment you deserve unless you help. You deserve a chance to control this disease; you deserve all the allies you can get. You'll get the help you deserve if you'll stop misdirecting your anger to the very people who are trying to help you get what you deserve—good medical care.

Such an approach acknowledges the patient's entitlement—not to have unreasonable demands met or to bully others but to what is realistically good care. The physician must be aware of the litigiousness of such patients and may to a certain extent practice "defensive medicine," but need not be bullied or actually defensive. The doctor also should beware of getting entangled in complicated logical (or illogical) debates with the patient. Rather, there should be tireless repetition of the theme of acceptance that the patient deserves first-rate medical care.

MANIPULATIVE HELP-REJECTERS

Help-rejecters, or "crocks,"[3] are familiar to every practicing physician. Like clingers and demanders, they appear to have a quenchless need for emotional supplies. Unlike clingers, they are not seductive and grateful; unlike demanders they are not overtly hostile. They actually seem the opposite of entitled; they appear to feel that no regimen will help. Appearing almost smugly satisfied, they return again and again to the office or clinic to report that, once again, the regime did not work. Their pessimism and tenacious nay-saying appear to increase in direct proportion to the physician's efforts and enthusiasm. When one of their

symptoms is relieved, another mysteriously appears in its place. Apparently, what is sought is not relief of symptoms. What is sought is an undivorcible marriage with an inexhaustible caregiver. Such patients seem to use their symptoms as an admission ticket to a relationship that cannot be sundered so long as symptoms exist. Thus, they are often accused of "masochism" and are said to be reaping unjustified "secondary gain." Such patients frequently deny being depressed and typically refuse referral to a psychiatrist. Lipsitt[3] records the case of one such patient who had 10 operations in 12 years, multiple visits to a dozen clinics and a chart that was four volumes long. "Only once was the term depression mentioned in . . . her record and that appeared in . . . 1956," some 13 years after she had begun her hegira. Another patient whom he studied had 829 visits to 26 clinics in 36 years; she "said of herself, 'I have a *bisel* of *tsuri*'" (a smidgen of trouble).

These behaviors elicit first in the physician anxiety that a treatable illness has been overlooked, next irritation with the patient and, finally, depression and self-doubt in the doctor. But the depression originally is not in the doctor—it is usually in the patient. Although it is important to suspect depression in the help-rejecter, it is hazardous to imply that he or she is too dependent or immature to get better or that unconscious manipulation is going on. Such an approach simply precipitates a new round of doctor-shopping. Rather, it may be helpful to "share" the pessimism—to say that the treatment may not be entirely curative. Even if it is, regular follow-up visits (hence, at intervals determined by the doctor) are put forth as necessary for the maintenance of any modest gains. In this way, the patient's fear of losing the doctor may be partly allayed, and the patient may be able to follow the treatment plan without fear of engineering his or her own abandonment. .

Pathologic dependency presents in one of its extremes as *manipulativeness*—an intense, covert, contradictory, self-defeating attempt to get needs met. It is the behavioral manifestation of a need by the patient to get close to but at the same time to maintain safe distance from sources of emotional support. (Occasional patients feel so empty that, paradoxically, to get needs met threatens them with engulfment; they are so famished that closeness may actually make them feel merged with someone else and therefore not really alive.) Such patients seem to have a deathly fear of that which they most crave[8]:

> A young woman in her twenties was hospitalized for control of brittle diabetes mellitus. Cachectic and hateful, she appeared to drive people away. She had a long history of psychiatric hospitalizations, multiple suicide attempts, abysmal relationships and an implacable resistance to cooperating in the management of her illness. Yet she clung to hospitalization. On the day before discharge she simultaneously infected her intravenous lines with feces and spiked a high temperature and threatened to sign out against medical advice. Raging and septic, she had to be physically restrained from leaving prematurely.

The remedy here is not to interpret the pathologic "solution" to the "need/fear dilemma," which is unconsciously being acted out by the patient. Such an action would be useless and harmful. Rather, limits on unrealistic expectations, limits on demanding hostility and—most of all—repeated appeals to entitlement are again invoked. The doctor, by a consistent, firm manner, conveys that the patient will not be allowed to become so close as to be engulfed nor so distant as to starve. Gentle, simple reasoning with this patient is better than complicated explanations.

To refer help-rejecters for psychiatric evaluation is never easy. If a psychiatric illness is thought to be present, one tactic for helping the patient accept psychiatric consultation is to schedule another appointment with the patient for a time after the consultation is to occur. In this way, the doctor can convey that the consultation is an adjunct to medical treatment, not abandonment.

SELF-DESTRUCTIVE DENIERS

Self-destructive deniers display unconsciously self-murderous behaviors, such as the continued drinking of a patient with esophageal varices and hepatic failure. This type of denial must be distinguished from other forms of denial, such as the "forgetting" of a brawny cardiac patient told not to shovel snow—a type of denial that evokes anxiety in the physician. Grossly self-destructive denial, on the other hand, stirs up malice. To make this distinction, it is important first to recognize that some patients—called "major deniers"[18]—deny without any self-destructive intent. They prize their independence and deny infirmity and chafe bitterly under the restrictions that a medical regimen imposes. But their denial is probably adaptive because they appear to survive longer than nondeniers.[18] The doctor working with a "major denier" should work cheerfully with the denial. Appeals to the patient's sense of sturdiness are harnessed to the necessary regimen. "Major deniers" tend to be likable and hard-working patients who respond to person-to-person medical advice delivered with a light touch and focused on maintenance of good health. Doomsaying, authoritarian approaches typically fail because the patient easily denies bad news.

The self-destructive denier is an entirely different story. Such patients are not independent and using the defense of denial in an attempt to survive. Rather, they are at base profoundly dependent and have given up hope of ever having needs met. Such patients seem to glory in their own destruction. They appear to find their main pleasure in furiously defeating the physician's attempts to preserve their lives. They may represent a chronic form of suicidal behavior; often they let themselves die.

> A 45-year-old alcoholic man was familiarly called "Old George" by members of the emergency-ward staff. They had seen him a hundred times over six years for visits ranging from acute gastrointestinal bleeds to a subdural hematoma (after a fall that he barely survived). It became a standing joke that the more carefully Old George was tended and the more thoroughly he was worked up, the more furiously he drank. He was released from his hospitalization for the subdural hematoma on Monday, stitched up for multiple lacerations on Tuesday, allowed to "sleep it off" in the back hall on Wednesday, casted for a fractured arm on Thursday and admitted with wildly bleeding esophageal varices on Friday. The staff worked frantically through the night, pumping in

whole blood as fast as it would go, but at 4 A.M. the intern pronounced Old George dead, the junior resident muttered, "thank God," under his breath, and the senior resident said, "amen," quite audibly.

What the physician can do to help self-destructive deniers is quite limited. The starting point for the care of such a patient is to recognize without shame or self-blame that they provoke in their caregivers the fervent wish that they would die and "get it over with." Many physicians, recognizing in themselves such a wish, recoil—by temperament and by training. When the doctor encounters the expertly self-destructive patient, he or she is caught between the ideal of rescuing the patient on the one hand and the unwanted wish for the patient to die on the other. Depending on how mature the physician is about such hateful feelings, malice toward the patient will be either conscious and associated with little guilt or self-reproach[4] or hidden and a cause of feelings of dread, self-blame, gratuitously heroic rescue efforts or a flat, bland, given-up and hopeless attitude. The optimal care of the chronically self-murderous patient entails a psychiatric consultation for the patient to ascertain whether treatable depression exists. If the patient refuses such a consultation (and most do) the primary physician may have to fight the impulse to abandon the patient. It is crucial to recognize the limitations that such patients pose for even the most ideal caregivers and to work with diligence and compassion to preserve the denier as long as possible, just as one does with any other patient with a terminal illness.

DISCUSSION

The "hateful patient," then, is the patient who—by a variety of behaviors related to profound dependency—stimulates a series of negative feelings in most doctors. Dependent *clingers* evoke aversion. Entitled *demanders* evoke fear and then counterattack upon entitlement. Manipulative *help-rejecters* evoke guilt and feelings of inadequacy. Self-destructive *deniers* (unlike "major deniers," who generally stir up

affection mingled with anxiety) evoke all these negative feelings, as well as malice and, at times, the secret wish that the patient will "die and get it over with."

Day in and day out, however, the physician routinely helps most patients establish better contact with reality, better adaptation to painful illnesses and better relations with families, friends and other caregivers. What is it about the patient "everybody hates" that compromises these workaday skills? It is probably the additional burden of having to deny or disown the intense, hateful feelings kindled by the dependent, entitled, manipulative or self-destructive patient. What the behaviors of such patients teach over time is that it is not how one feels about them that is most important in their care. It is how one behaves toward them: the doctor who begins to feel aversion toward the patient should begin to think of setting limits on dependency. The doctor who begins to feel the impulse to counterattack should begin to think of rechanneling entitlement into expectations of realistically good medical care. The doctor who begins to feel depressed with the patient's smug help-rejecting should begin to think of "sharing pessimism" so that the patient's losing the symptom is not equated with losing the doctor. And the doctor who begins to wish that the patient would die should begin to grasp the possibility that the patient wishes to die.

Negative feelings about medical and surgical patients constitute important clinical data about the patient's psychology. When the patient creates in the doctor feelings that are disowned or denied, errors in diagnosis and treatment are more likely to occur. Disavowal of hateful feelings requires less effort than bearing them. But such disavowal wastes clinical data that may be helpful in treating the "hateful patient."

Notes

1. Martin PA: The obnoxious patient, Tactics and Techniques in Psychoanalytic Therapy. Vol 2. Countertransference. Edited by PL Giovacchini, New York, Jason Aronson, 1975, pp 196–204

2. Hackett TP: Which patients turn you off? It's worth analyzing. Med Econ 46(15):94–99, 1969

3. Lipsitt DR: Medical and psychological characteristics of "crocks." Int J Psychiatry Med 1:15–25, 1970

4. Maltsberger JT, Buie DH: Countertransference hate in the treatment of suicidal patients. Arch Gen Psychiatry 30:625–633, 1974

5. Adler G: Helplessness in the helpers. Br J Med Psychol 45:315–326, 1972

6. Adler G, Buie DH: The misuses of confrontation with borderline patients. Int J Psychoanal Psychother 1:109–120, 1972

7. Groves JE: Management of the borderline patient on a medical or surgical ward: the psychiatric consultant's role. Int J Psychiatry Med 6:337–348, 1975

8. Idem: Violence and sociopathy in the general hospital: psychotic and borderline patients on medical and surgical wards, The MGH Handbook of Liaison Psychiatry. Edited by TP Hackett, NH Cassem. St. Louis, CV Mosby (in press)

9. Bibring GL: Psychiatry and medical practice in a general hospital. N Engl J Med 254:366–372, 1956

10. Osler W: Principles and Practice of Medicine. Twelfth edition. Edited by T. McCrae, New York, Appleton-Century, 1935

11. Idem: Aequanimitas. Third edition. New York, Blakiston, 1943

12. Idem: Selected Writings: 12 July 1849 to 29 December 1919. London, Oxford University Press, 1951

13. Cecil-Loeb Textbook of Medicine. Edited by PB Beeson, W. McDermott. Philadelphia, WB Saunders, 1975

14. Harrison's Principles of Internal Medicine. Eighth edition. Edited by GW Thorn, RD Adams, E Braunwald, et al. New York, McGraw-Hill, 1977

15. Harrison's Principles of Internal Medicine[14], p 1955

16. Kolb LC: The psychoneuroses, Cecil-Loeb Textbook of Medicine. Eleventh edition. Edited by PB Beeson, W McDermott, Philadelphia, WB Saunders, 1963, pp 1709–1727

17. Winnicott DW: Hate in the counter-transference. Int J Psychoanal 30:69–74, 1949

18. Hackett TP, Cassem NH: Psychological reactions to life-threatening illness, Psychological Aspects of Stress. Edited by H Abram. Springfield, Illinois, CC Thomas, 1970, pp 29–43

THE NURSE

Making Hard Choices

Andrew L. Jameton

What should nurses do when they find they are working with someone who is incompetent or abusive to patients? This topic will be developed in connection with two philosophical issues underlying moral problems that nurses face. The first issue is that of *complicity*. What is a nurse's personal responsibility for the wrongoings of other personnel? Second is the issue of *sacrifice*. What is the nurse's responsibility as a professional to sacrifice personal interests or to take risks on behalf of patients? Are nurses obligated to be saints, heroes, or heroines?

A. MORAL DISTRESS IN THE HOSPITAL

Hospitals present a chiaroscuro of beneficial and harmful practices. From one point of view to labor in the hospital is to labor in the pits. Like Eugene O'Neill's Hairy Ape, the coal stoker at the ship's furnaces below deck, nurses, respiratory therapists, and residents stoke the furnaces of suffering under an unceasing fluorescent glare, along clattering halls coated not in soot but painted pale green, white, or pink. Attendings, like wealthy passengers on the catwalk above, stop briefly to marvel at the spectacle and depart to the dining room. From another point of view this picture is outrageously distorted. Health care is noble and beautiful. The health care team heals the sick and succors the dying. Intimate contact with human suffering elevates us. Medical techniques, although not perfected, are glowing marvels compared to the dark remedies of the past. Health care professionals express the most powerful tradition of humane ideals of any occupation.

Since urgent good and gruesome evil cohabit in the hospitals, nurses work in ambiguity and contradiction. Since they do both good and bad to patients, nurses ask themselves whether the enterprise as a whole justifies continuing cooperation with the things that are in their judgment reprehensible. That someone else generally makes the decision to undertake a risky procedure does not relieve the feeling of complicity in wrong, since nurses are "hands on" in many procedures.

Nurses feel guilt and real moral distress when they perform procedures that they feel are morally wrong but can find no way to avoid. Common instances causing this distress are:

1. A nurse is assigned to perform a painful test on a child when the child is dying, and it seems to the nurse that the test is irrelevant to the child's welfare.

2. A nurse in the adult intensive care unit is assigned to care for a patient who the nurse believes is dead. A machine pumps the chest and the heart beats, but the brain is dead.

3. In the newborn intensive care unit, a nurse cares for a severely damaged infant that she feels in her heart cannot survive. She punctures its heel each day to take blood tests.

4. The nurse is tending a patient who is about to have surgery and has signed the consent forms for it. Yet the nurse suspects from the patient's conversation that the patient has no comprehension of the seriousness of the choice.

5. A surgeon fails to wash his hands before examining a patient in the ICU and ignores the nurse's reminder.[1]

These cases are more than failures to realize an ideal; they involve actions the nurses judge to be morally wrong. Nurses can thus be very critical of the hospitals in which they work. "I wonder if we should even work here. It seems like an immoral place to work," said one Coronary Care Unit nurse just before she quit her job. Frances J. Storlie reports similar remarks. "Politics, or catering to the doctors—that's what counts around here.   There is an overriding feeling of doing McDonald's nursing."[2] But nurses work at hospitals and contribute to the setting. Are staff nurses to blame for what is going on? Is this painful sense of guilt that nurses feel legitimate?

The American Nurses' Association "Code for Nurses" gives a straightforward, partial answer to this question. The code states unequivocally

Point 3: The nurse acts to safeguard the client and the public when health care and safety are affected by incompetent, unethical, or illegal practice of any person. (1976)[3]

It is unprofessional, therefore, to cooperate in acts that, in the nurse's judgment, unethically impose risks on patients. But this is merely the beginning of the inquiry. Does failure to meet this duty require one to feel guilty? What can one do when a situation like this comes up? Do nurses really have any choice about these things? To examine these questions, consider a common but difficult case: What can and should nurses do about incompetent medical practitioners?

B.   DEALING WITH MEDICAL INCOMPETENCE

There is an old joke that beds are dangerous because so many people die in them. From that point of view hospital beds are particularly dangerous. In 1964 a study showed that 20 percent of patients on the wards of a teaching hospital suffered iatrogenic harm.[4] *Iatrogenic* illness is that caused by medical, nursing, or other health care interventions. In a more recent study reported in 1981 the combined medical, nursing, and other health care error rate was 36 percent. Nine percent of these errors were life-threatening, and 2 percent of these killed patients (or .7 percent of all patients admitted). This is a *conservative* estimate; if there was any doubt about the medical source of an untoward event, it was not counted. The authors attributed the 150 percent increase in errors since 1964 to increasingly complex medical technology.[5] A recent study of surgical errors with adverse outcomes found fewer errors but worse consequences. It found a 1 percent error rate, an overall mortality rate of 55 percent, average excess hospitals costs of $40,000 per client, and an average 40 days excess hospitalization.[6]

These studies do not show that patients should stay out of the hospital; patients might have been even worse off if they had stayed at home. Instead, the studies show that coping with errors is part of everyday hospital work.

What should nurses do when they detect mistakes in their own work, that of other nurses, physicians, or other hospital workers? To consider the issue, let us look at an extreme case, not simply the excusable mistakes of a competent clinician, but the chronic mistakes of an incompetent one. The following incident took place in the late 1970s in a medium-sized private teaching hospital.

> Dr. Hyde performed four surgeries at Mt. Citadel Hospital during a four-month period. All four were for slowly growing cancers in debilitated elderly patients. All four patients died slow, painful deaths in the Intensive Care Unit. There was a consensus among the ICU nurses and residents that Dr. Hyde performed the surgeries for marginal indications, that he performed them badly, and that he atrociously mismanaged their follow-up care in the unit. Said Nurse Robin, "He wrote orders that were just ridiculous."

How did the ICU staff nurses deal with this problem?

> The ICU nurses did their best to see that each of Dr. Hyde's patients got the best care possible under the circumstances. They carried out the residents' instructions as quickly as possible and

delayed fulfilling Dr. Hyde's less competent changes in their orders.

They did not complain through hospital channels. In their opinion, the head nurse and the medical director were weak and would not help. The residents concurred in this judgment and so complained through very indirect channels. Staff were not yet sure whose side the new Director of Nursing was on. Moreover, seeing her would require going over the head nurse.

The nurses hesitated to use any "outside" channels, not because they feared losing their jobs, but they did fear a possible libel suit. When they looked at the case records, they could not find any obvious defects in them; however, the patients were in bad shape.

They did not discuss their concerns with Dr. Hyde because they hated him. Everybody hated him. Besides, they were sure that he knew he was incompetent, and his air of theatrical insincerity discouraged frank discussion.

The nurses did not discuss it with any of the families. Only Mr. Apple had family actively involved in his care. His sister suspected that Dr. Hyde was not managing the case well. The nurses stood by when she asked Dr. Hyde how Mr. Apple was doing. "He's doing fine," said Dr. Hyde.

Later, the sister asked Nurse Robin privately, "Why is he still in a coma?" "What could I say?" commented Ms. Robin months later, "The patient has rotted for a month. It is too late to say, 'Somebody blew it,' I am just a nurse. All I know is that his patients don't do well. At this point, confidence in the doctor was about all the health care we had to offer."

The nursing staff hoped that Mr. Apple's sister would ask if a second opinion was needed. When they induced her to ask this, the nurses said, "YES!" The sister consulted the Director of Surgery at the hospital, an excellent surgeon whom the nurses regarded as beyond reproach. But he whitewashed the case in his report to the sister and in his notes in the record. No problems were mentioned concerning the indications for surgery, the surgery itself, or the post-surgical management. Ms. Robin said, "I felt physically ill."

The staff nurses engaged in a number of rituals to ease their tension. When Dr. Hyde's four patients filled half the ICU beds and Mr. Apple's sister came to visit, the staff lined up all four patients in exactly the same position with their respirator hoses in exactly parallel alignment.

They labelled that part of the ICU "The Dr. Hyde Memorial Isolation Room." When the last patient died, Ms. Robin cowled herself in a sheet like a nun "to escort Mr. Apple to his Heavenly Rest."

Before Dr. Hyde got to a fifth patient, a quiet, informal agreement was reached between him and the Chief of Surgery. He was not to perform any surgeries at Mt. Citadel without first consulting closely with the Chief, and all surgery had to be performed with another surgeon.

A month after Mr. Apple died, Ms. Robin ran into his sister on the street. She asked again what the nurses thought of Dr. Hyde. Ms. Robin still could not bring herself to say anything critical. That she never talked openly with his sister remains for her one of the most painful and doubtful issues about her own actions. Ms. Robin asks, "What do you do when you know what you have no right to know?"[7]

Cases like these are extremely painful and complex. There are three questions that we should ask about this particular case. First, what was Ms. Robin's obligation to say something to the patient or do something about the problem? Second, what courses of actions were available to her? And third, did she really have a choice?

There are many things she considered and should have considered in ascertaining her obligations. Some of the most immediate questions are:

Was She Sure the Doctor Was Incompetent? Absolute certainty that there is a problem is not required. In health care one always has to work under conditions of uncertainty. The unit may have been in the grip of coincidence and mass hysteria. But since Dr. Hyde's orders appeared "ridiculous" to everyone, surely there was adequate evidence to raise the issue.

Was This an Issue of Protecting the Patient? The ANA Code is clear that protection is owed to the patient, but in this case the primary harm had already been done. It was too late to interfere with the surgery. Yet, during his stay in the ICU, further harm to Mr. Apple might have been prevented by discussing the issue with his sister. After he was dead, or nearly dead, protecting him was no longer the issue; instead, the issue became one of protecting future patients.

The duty to protect patients could call for some unusual actions. For example, if Ms. Robin saw that a *fifth* patient were scheduled for the same kind of surgery with Dr. Hyde, would she have a duty to speak to that patient?

Would the Patient or the Family Lose Faith in Health Care? We don't know what would have happened. Perhaps the sister would have lost faith in the nurse for challenging her confidence in the doctor, but in this case her confidence already seemed weak. Moreover, health care should not be an article of faith. Good results are sometimes obtained by admitting errors to patients. Such admissions help clients better understand what is happening to them when unexpected side-effects occur. In addition patients may appreciate the trust shown them through frankness.

Does the Patient Want to Know? If the patient asks, then there is good reason to think the patient wants to know. In this case Mr. Apple's sister, who can be regarded as a legitimate proxy for the patient, asked. If the patient does not ask, matters are less clear. Some hold that the patient's views should prevail, and so we should not challenge patients who choose incompetent clinicians. They know more about their needs than we do as observers; they may be getting things from their doctors that we do not recognize.

This position will not do, however. It is part of the practice of a profession to make judgments about its practitioners. Dr. Hyde may have had a convincing bedside manner, but the patient was also entitled to a professional judgment of Dr. Hyde's overall competence as a surgeon. Assessing basic competencies of practitioners is not like trying to judge acupuncturists or faith healers who claim a different *kind* of competence. Ms. Robin is a nurse; Dr. Hyde is a physician. Although they are not members of the same profession, their professions overlap, and so she was in a position to make judgments about his competence.

Would Disclosure Expose Ms. Robin to Personal Risks? Every health professional who thinks of whistle-blowing rightly worries about retaliation. She could be seen as a troublemaker and lose the confidence and cooperation of other nurses and physicians. Moreover, patients are natural hostages for retaliation. A physician may react to a request for a second opinion by dropping the patient or creating difficulties with a subsequent patient. Nurses who blow the whistle are sometimes fired—never for blowing the whistle, but for some unrelated infraction of the rules. Would this have happened in this case? We just don't know.

Are There Any Conflicting Obligations? Hospital workers owe loyalty to other workers. But, in this case, Ms. Robin *hated* Dr. Hyde. If she owed him any loyalty, it was of the most abstract kind based merely on his occupation. She had a much stronger relationship with Mr. Apple's sister, and perhaps even with the comatose Mr. Apple. Discussing the matter with the client's sister would also have helped to break down the "professional/patient barrier," which is frequently an obstacle to nurse/patient relations.

Were Her Motives Pure? It would not do for health professionals to go about blaming each other for the problems of health care. Was she displacing onto Dr. Hyde her justified hostility toward physicians as a group and her own guilt over the inadequacies of Mt. Citadel Intensive Care? Or, in deciding not to disclose, was she avoiding trouble and protecting herself? These are the things one learns only through time and by looking at other choices: Does one admit one's *own* errors? Is one complaining about everything?

There is the beginning here of a case for disclosure: Mr. Apple's sister asked for information; Ms. Robin had information of which she was pretty sure; protection of the patient was at issue. Countervailing considerations were present, but they were not as strong in this case as in many others.[8] In spite of their feeling that they could have done more, Ms. Robin and other nurses did help to prevent further harm. They brought the case, admittedly indirectly, to the attention of the Chief of Surgery. Although he was unwilling to act for the record, he restricted Dr. Hyde's activities. Instead of making a summary judgment on the case, we should consider some of the general philosophical questions raised by it.

C. COOPERATION IN WRONGDOING

Hospital staff nurses rarely undertake what they regard as questionable procedures by themselves on their own initiative or as team leaders. They usually find themselves involved in bad practice through cooperation with others. The preceding case was just one extreme example. General principles to keep in mind in setting limits on cooperation are:

1. *What is the seriousness of the harm involved?* The more serious the danger posed to this patient or to future patients, the stronger the call to action. The practitioner causing the harm may be competent, incompetent, well-meaning, or uncaring, but these considerations are not as relevant as the amount of harm.

2. *Does this happen often?* The more chronic the problem in one's institution, the more reason to address it. As an instance of a class of cases or as an indication of some more general problem, a case gains importance as a focus of noncooperation. Steps taken against a general problem may prevent further harm of that kind. Noncooperation, whether it succeeds in this case or not, gains a symbolic value where the case is an instance of a more general problem. Noncooperation in a particular case can make a vivid statement about more general issues.

3. *Are there ways to prevent the harm or future occurrences of it?* Refusing to participate in the care of a patient or speaking to the head nurse or supervisor may prevent an incident or lead to changes in the future. Even if there is no recourse, some acts are so wrong that one should not cooperate in them, whatever the consequences.

4. *What is the nurse's role in causing the harm?* One's responsibility grows as one becomes more closely involved in causing the harm. A nurse is responsible for administering a harmful medication even though the act is done at the instruction of a physician. Although this is a fine point, the nurse who cares for a patient after a questionable surgery is in a morally safer position than a nurse who prepares the patient for surgery.[9]

5. *What is the nurse's attitude with regard to the harm?* A nurse who wholeheartedly supports a ques-

tionable procedure is more actively responsible for it than a nurse who acts reluctantly.[10]

In brief, nurses generally are *accountable* for harmful practices in which they are involved even though they do not initiate it themselves. As the profession becomes more autonomous, the responsibility of nurses for health practices increases. Thus, if health care continues to have problems, nurses will become responsible for them, not merely as accomplices, but as principal agents.

D. HOW TO PROCEED WITH COMPLAINTS

What should one do about one's own mistakes or those of others? What should one do first? The ANA "Code for Nurses" is specific about what steps to take.

First,

> . . . concern should be expressed to the person carrying out the questionable practice and attention called to the possible detrimental effects upon the client's welfare.

The next step, if needed, is to consult "the responsible administrative person."

Then,

> If indicated, the practice should then be reported to the appropriate authority within the institution, agency, or larger system.

The Code states that such an authority or mechanism for reporting to an authority should have

> . . . an established mechanism for the reporting and handling of incompetent, unethical, or illegal practice within the employment setting so that such reporting can go through official channels and be done without fear of reprisal.

The Code also says that

> Local units of the professional association should be prepared to provide assistance . . .

Finally, if a problem persists,

The problem should be reported to other appropriate authorities such as the practice committees of the appropriate professional organizations or the legally constituted bodies concerned with licensing of specific categories of health workers or professional practitioners.[11]

One of the problems is that there are so *many* ways one can proceed. And there are more ways than the ANA mentions. One can speak to the client or the client's family. One can go to the courts or newspapers. Or one could go to one's union.

Virtually all hospitals have established a mechanism for filing *incident reports*. Nurses are expected to file these reports on every untoward incident—a bad drug reaction, a fall or spill, a drunken practitioner. Hospitals like to have these as a documentary basis if any legal actions occur and for discussing changes in procedures. These reports have defects, however. Most incident reports are simply filed. The report is not an instrument useful to nurses in discussing their mistakes.[12] Instead, it is an instrument of administration.

Coping with bad *medical* practice can be an extremely delicate matter. Not only are nurses relatively powerless in relationship to physicians in these matters, but physicians regard the problem of bad medical practice as one of extreme delicacy. Most procedures are complex and mined with legal pitfalls.[13]

In California the Board of Medical Quality Assurance oversees licensure and discipline of physicians. It has a procedure by which *anyone* can make a complaint simply by filing a form. The board will always respond with an investigation. The Civil Code

> . . . provides nearly absolute immunity for persons who communicate ". . . information . . . to any hospital, hospital medical staff, professional society, medical or dental school, professional licensing board or division, committee or panel of such licensing board, peer review committee, or underwriting committee . . . when such communication is intended to aid in the evaluation of the qualifications, fitness, character, or insurability of a practitioner of the healing arts and does not represent as true any matter not reasonably believed to be true."[14]

In spite of these many options, and in spite of written assurances of protection, many nurses view whistle-blowing as a hazardous and ineffective venture.

> "I don't know why I bother to fill this out," she complained. "I've worked in this unit for more than seven years, and in that time I've filed exactly three reports about medical practice. Nothing is ever done. . . . You document what you observed, and you darn well better have proof. You know it doesn't matter when a doctor is complaining about a nurse. No one asks for proof of what he says, but if I complain about a physician's practice, I'm just not taken seriously. . . . Nothing is ever done."[15]

Are nurses right in this judgment? In spite of these problems, 80 percent of respondents to an *R.N.* survey reported that they have been able to take effective action in response to medical errors.[16] If procedures were used more widely and actively, would the air clear and action be taken? The only way to find out is to use these mechanisms and to create new ones.

E.   CONSCIENTIOUS OBJECTION

The forms of recourse previously mentioned follow established channels. Another form of recourse is simply to refuse to cooperate with a procedure even if ordered to do it. Refusals to cooperate in employment situations resemble *conscientious objection* or *civil disobedience* when one's noncooperation violates the employer's policies or the conditions of employment, and when one's protest is based on issues of conscience.

Civil disobedience in order to make a public point about a moral issue has been prominent in the birth control movement. Emma Goldman, Van Kleek Allison, Margaret Sanger, and Ethel Byrne all violated laws in the early part of the century in order to marshal support for the legalization of contraception. While she was in jail, Margaret Sanger tried to distribute birth control information among other prisoners.[17]

The issue of conscientious objection has arisen recently in connection with abortion.

Although abortions are legal, some nurses object to them strongly on grounds of conscience. Nurses who object should not be required to cooperate with them, not because they might provide bad care, but because they should not be required to cooperate in actions they regard as wrong. Thelma Schorr, for example, argues

> There are many nurses who see an abortion as an unconscionable act, and certainly they should never be placed in the position of having to nurse patients who have chosen to have their pregnancies terminated. Just as a patient's freedom to choose must be respected, so must a nurse's. But it is also that nurse's responsibility to protect both the patient's freedom and her own by refusing to work in a situation which she finds morally offensive.[18]

Institutions should make arrangements to make conscientious noncooperation possible. For example, the International Labour Conference recommends

> Nursing personnel should be able to claim exemption from performing specific duties, without being penalized, where performances would conflict with their religious, moral, or ethical convictions and where they inform their supervisor in good time of their objection so as to allow the necessary alternative arrangements to be made to ensure that essential nursing care of patients is not affected.[19]

Analogously, bad nursing and medical practice can also be seen as issues of conscience—if not of private conscience, then at least of professional conscience. It is not at all unusual for nurses to refuse to carry out questionable orders by physicians. Physicians often carry out the orders themselves without much conflict. For instance, the nurse may say, "I won't give an injection for this much morphine; you'll have to do it yourself." The physician says, "All right. I'll do it." Or a nurse may refuse to work on a unit until a mishandled case is resolved. This may galvanize the nurses and physicians who remain into holding the meetings needed to get the problem resolved promptly.

If one felt strongly about an issue, one could go further. A nurse could say, "Anyone who comes near this patient does so at their peril,'' and physically prevent procedures from being done. In 1974, the Feminist Women's Health Center in Los Angeles stole the equipment from a substandard abortion clinic in order to prevent its operation.[20] In another case aides at a nursing home sued their employers because supervisors were ordering aides to engage in abusive procedures, such as disciplining patients with cold showers.

Nurses and physicians have found highly varied ways in which to cope with conflicts between their standards of practice and the rules under which their work is conducted. For example, it is still the law in California that newborn babies' eyes be washed with silver nitrate as a prophylactic against gonorrhea. In the judgment of many clinicians this is unnecessary in many cases. When parents refuse to consent to the procedure, newborn units vary in their reactions. The personnel in one unit insists on performing the procedure because it is required by law. If they have to, they sign and file the consent forms themselves. In another unit, they simply forget about it. In another, they do it and don't tell the parents. In another, they document doing the procedure and don't do it. In still another, they make up a very light wash of silver nitrate and wash it out very quickly. This variety of reactions indicates the depth and difficulty of finding ways to proceed when one is morally distressed and facing institutional constraints.

F. IS THERE REALLY A CHOICE?

Many of the institutional practices that we regret appear to us as contraints—like natural laws that limit our actions. There are many things we just can't do. For example, we can't make a hospital committee listen when it won't. In some conceivable sense of ''can,'' perhaps one *can* make it listen, but to do so would require nearly impossible quantities of energy and involve great personal risks or violations of principles one holds dear. Indeed, there are really two very different kinds of limits on our ability to choose. There are limits of physical and psychological possibility, and limits of conventions and ethics.

An important viewpoint on human possibility is that of Jean Paul Sartre.[21] He believed that we are completely free to choose, no matter what circumstances we are in. He emphasized that what ethics says one can and cannot do does not exhaust the possibilities that are open. Ethics, for example, says that we should not force a committee to listen to us by waving a gun at its members, but we still ''can.''

Sartre believed that most of us find this freedom awesome and frightening. It makes us responsible for everything that goes on around us. So we try to escape this freedom. We pretend to ourselves that we are forced to do things when we are not. When a nurse, for example, tells a patient, ''You must do this because the doctor ordered it,'' both the nurse and patient pretend that they must act because of the doctor's order, but in fact either one could make another choice.

In this way, we use ethics to escape from freedom. A nurse who asks a bioethicist, ''What should I do?'' may be told that ethics does not provide a definite answer. Instead of rejoicing that ethics leaves room for choice, the nurse regrets that no rule or principle forces a definite course of action. Although Sartre saw this regret as natural, he offered no comfort for it. He believed that there is no significant morality except that of honest choice and personal responsibility.

This is one of the deeper meanings of *accountability*. Nurses who work in hospitals are accountable for their choices there because they choose to work there and make choices in that setting when they could be making other choices. Many nurses leave nursing precisely because they morally reject hospital working conditions. Burnout can be a moral statement. Since the good that nurses do in hospitals must also be credited to their account, it is a legitimate choice to stay in the hospital, to accomplish as much as one can there, and to struggle for changes. What Sartre wants to emphasize is that such courses of action represent free *choices,* not necessities. In remaining in the hospital setting, nurses thereby become responsible for complicity in wrongs done there.

Another point of view emphasizes the limits on individuals set by ethical claims of institutions. Immanuel Kant gives expression to this position.

> Many affairs which are conducted in the interest of the community require a certain mechanism through which some members of the community must passively conduct themselves with artificial unanimity, so that the government may direct them to public ends, or at least prevent them from destroying those ends.[22]

The government is not the only institution that demands "artificial unanimity." Any large, complex enterprise requires the smooth cooperation of many persons to accomplish its ends, and hospitals are no exception. If the hospital were to become the site of daily discussions of the aims, goals, and morality of health care, there would be little time left for work. It is difficult for us to reconcile our conception of ourselves as autonomous agents with our understanding that the hospital can accomplish its goals only through major cooperative effort.

A very basic choice is forced on those who work in hospitals by the existence of prevalent and systematic problems in health care. If one fails to resist exploitation, incompetence, and corrupt practices, one becomes responsible for them. If one resists them, one enters into conflict with conventional conceptions of behavior for employees and thereby risks reprisals. One has to choose between complicity and self-sacrifice, or enter the uncomfortable middle of ground of irony. Ethics does not give a clear answer as to which path one must choose. Instead, one is free to move in the direction of the kind of world one personally desires to create.

G. RISKS AND PERSONAL SACRIFICES

Should nurses take risks or sacrifice personal interests for the sake of patient care?

In any society some sacrifice of one's interests is demanded of all. Paying taxes, engaging in politics, and avoiding harm to others involve getting less than one could otherwise, but they are necessary contributions to the common good. If we did not generally make such contributions, we would all be worse off.

Sacrifices thought of as *charity* or volunteer work are not usually required but are generally praised. Such activities create personal rewards, partly through personal costs.

Health care is traditionally considered a charitable enterprise, and sacrifices for the health of patients are thought to be honorable and ethical. Exposing oneself to disease in order to care for the sick is a traditional health care virtue. Similarly, it is a virtue to risk one's job in order to protect one's patient.

Health professionals generally place the good of the patient first. That means that if nurses' interests on occasion have to be sacrificed for the sake of the patient, then nurses should sacrifice them. But how much one should sacrifice is unclear. One can extend oneself to levels of *sainthood* and *heroism*. Being extremes, such actions are necessarily rare. If heroism and sainthood were required, they would then be conventional and no longer exceptional.[23] They must then be morally *optional*. At the same time, our moral ideals stand ready to praise sainthood and acts of heroism and to make them meaningful.

At the same time, nurses in particular should be wary of the temptations of self-sacrifice. Nurses—like women in general in Western culture—have traditionally been called upon to sacrifice themselves. Under calls to idealism, they have been asked to work long hours for low wages and to show deference to physicians—to bring them chairs and charts, not to benefit patients, but to benefit physicians. Self-abnegation by women nurses conforms to traditional gender discrimination. Self-sacrifice by nurses is thus best directed only toward patients and acts that strengthen nurses as a group. It is perhaps better to think in terms of acts of heroism than of saintliness.[24]

The following considerations are useful in considering whether to take personal risks in order to avoid complicity in harming patients:

1. Personal sacrifice is justified only where there is some possibility that something may be achieved by it. That "something" can be taken quite broadly, such as avoiding complicity in wrongdoing.

2. The greater the risk of harm to the patient or to

future patients, the greater the obligation to make some sacrifice (if needed and efficacious) to reduce the risk.

3. It is more important to think in terms of having a good defense for what one does than it is to think in terms of avoiding risks. It is hard to fault someone who

   a. acts sincerely,

   b. gives clearly articulated reasons that others can understand,

   c. consults with others in making decisions, and

   d. acts publicly and on the record.

4. One should assess personal risk realistically. One should not frighten oneself into paralysis with tales of unlikely and horrendous consequences.

5. It is both prudent and morally acceptable to take steps to protect oneself. For example, in a tightly managed hospital it is helpful not to be vulnerable on other grounds.)

6. What are others doing? If someone thinks something is morally wrong, there are likely to be others who agree. Act collectively whenever possible.

7. Nursing is a profession, not a calling. It does not call for unlimited commitment.

8. Taking risks in order to protect patients is a well-established conventional obligation of the health professions.

H. REVIEWING THE CASE

These brief reflections do not produce, even in retrospect, a definite course of action for Nurse Robin to have pursued in regard to Dr. Hyde. Yet, they help to clarify the moral problems created by the case and underline the considerations relevant to making a decision.

To review the case in terms of the discussion, on one hand, the harm Dr. Hyde was doing was serious and recurrent. But on the other, Ms. Robin was for the most part indirectly involved in it. Her main direct involvement was to carry out Dr. Hyde's instructions for Mr. Apple's postoperative care. It is a standard professional responsibility for nurses to protect patients from harm due to incompetence. Nurse Robin's primary responsibility was to prevent harm to Mr. Apple, who by this time was practically beyond harm, but she also had less well-defined responsibilities to future patients. On one hand the simpler and less dramatic remedies prescribed by the ANA Code looked unpromising. But on the other, nurses are entitled to take more irregular measures where demanded by professional conscience. Other options Ms. Robin might have chosen include circumventing the head nurse and going directly to the new Director of Nursing, refusing to work on the unit until the problem was solved, speaking privately with Mr. Apple's sister, or informing the Medical Director of the unit that she intended to speak with the family unless something were done about Dr. Hyde.

These more forceful steps were shrouded in uncertain impact and personal risk. It is understandable that she did not consider undertaking any of them a light matter. The liability Ms. Robin incurred should be placed in the context of collective responsibility. She did less than she might have in a context where others habitually did less than they could and where institutional lacunae made remedies difficult. The unavailability of simple remedies was the result of collective actions and omissions attributable to the hospital and the health professions.

Speaking to Mr. Apple's sister would have had an uncertain impact on Dr. Hyde's future practice, but clearly there was something to be gained from approaching her. Ms. Robin might have given the family a clearer opportunity to seek legal redress for malpractice, an action which appears justified. The least strong reason for not answering the sister's questions was probably the most powerful cause for withholding information; there is sometimes a deep gulf between professionals and lay persons that resembles the tension between separate cultures. More reasonable considerations for not responding to the sister might include a tacit acceptance of responsibility as an employee of the hospital not to foster suits against it, a reasonable rejection of malpractice as a sound mode of professional discipline, or a general distaste for retribution.

Doubt about what direction to move is best resolved by considering what sort of health care delivery system Ms. Robin would like to see created in the long run. Would she like to see the separation between professionals and patients fostered, or would she like to see patients have more information about and control over their care? Whatever the actual consequences of her action might have been, it could have performed a symbolic function toward this end. If she aspired to a more open health care system, then speaking to Mr. Apple's sister was certainly justified. The only question remaining is whether it would have been heroic to do so or not. The personal risks to which Ms. Robin might have exposed herself with other choices are inestimable since none of these roads were taken, and the question of heroism cannot be resolved. We can only judge that her actual choices were not heroic.

The case is a good example of a class of cases common in the study of ethics in health care. It is sufficiently complex that putting the ethical considerations in order is itself an interesting and thought-provoking task, and coming to a judgment requires appeal to at least three different kinds of considerations.

1. Relatively concrete events in the case play a crucial role in giving direction to final judgments about the case. For example, that Mr. Apple's sister asked more than once for information rules out a host of considerations about the nurse's responsibility to manage information for patients and their families.

2. What might be called "political" considerations—the nurse's long run hopes for the structure of health care delivery—provide specific commitments needed to resolve uncertainty about consequences and philosophical principles.

3. General philosophical considerations help us to identify the ethical issues and to appreciate their generality, but general philosophical questions do not have to be resolved in order to make a decision with regard to the case. For example, the question of balancing self-interest against the interest of others, although relevant to understanding the case, does not have to be answered to make a judgment. Indeed, the more specific responsibilities of professionals for patients provide much clearer direction, and even these falter before the realities of the working world.

Philosophical principles do not so much provide a resolution to problems like these as they help us to appreciate the significance of a resolution. Cases of this kind aid the study of ethics by helping us to understand philosophical principles more concretely and to indicate what issues philosophers should address. The appropriate role of philosophy in such cases is not the *application* of ethical theory, as suggested by the common ascription of the rubric ''applied ethics'' to the study of ethics in health care. Instead, such cases provide important information and direction for the continuing growth and development of philosophical theory.

Notes

1. For recent rates of hand-washing, see Richard K. Albert and Francis Condie, ''Hand-Washing Patterns in Medical Intensive-Care Units,'' *The New England Journal of Medicine* 304 (1981):1465–66. In relationship to patient contacts, nurses wash their hands about twice as much as physicians. But, since nurses have the bulk of contact with patients, most unwashed contacts are with nurses. Respiratory therapists are *tops* at hand-washing.

2. Frances J. Storlie, ''Burnout: The Elaboration of a Concept,'' *American Journal of Nursing* 79 (1979), p. 2108.

3. The AMA code has a similar provision: A physician should deal honestly with patients and colleagues, and strive to expose those physicians deficient in character or competence, or who engage in fraud or deception (AMA, 1980).

4. Elihu M. Schimmel, ''The Hazards of Hospitalization,'' *Annals of Internal Medicine* 60 (1964): 100–110.

5. Knight Steel et al., ''Iatrogenic Illness on a General Medical Service at a University Hospital,'' *The New England Journal of Medicine* 304 (1981):638–42.

6. Nathan P. Couch et al., ''The High Cost of Low-Frequency Events: The Anatomy and Economics of Surgical Mishaps,'' *The New England Journal of Medicine* 304 (1981):634–37.

7. I chose a nurse/doctor problem because such problems are so often discussed by nurses. I am unsure whether the incompetence of other nurses is mentioned less often because it is a simpler or a more difficult problem.

8. This judgment is itself a form of ''second-guessing'' arrived at over several years' con-

templation. I was present during the last weeks of this case. Should I have done more about it? If so, what? Dr. Hyde is still in practice. Should I do something now?

9. In this and the next point, I am reflecting a distinction made by some Catholic ethics texts between *formal* and *material* cooperation. To cooperate in evil *formally* is either to choose or to desire the evil act itself, or to cooperate knowingly in actions that are a means to that evil act. To cooperate *materially* is to be involved not as a means and not to wish for the evil outcome. I *formally* cooperate when I loan my brother my car when he asks me if he can use it to rob a bank. If he comes to me after the robbery and asks me to hide him, and this is the first I have heard it, hiding him would only be *material* cooperation. Formal cooperation is morally more culpable than material cooperation. See for example, Joseph B. McAllister, *Ethics: With Special Application to the Medical and Nursing Professions,* Second Edition (Philadelphia: W. B. Saunders Company, 1955), pp. 97–98.

10. One cannot find permanent refuge in mental reservations (except under the most repressive conditions). Chronic reluctance eventually becomes bad faith and as morally problematic as wholehearted cooperation in evil.

11. All quotes here are from Point 3.2 of the American Nurses' Association "Code for Nurses" (1976).

12. Physicians practice the regular ritual of the morbidity and mortality conference. In this conference physicians confess their errors and discuss them openly and critically. This is a way of improving practice and displaying frankness, humility, and competence. See Charles L. Bosk, "Occupational Rituals in Patient Management," *The New England Journal of Medicine* 303 (1980):71–76. To the best of my knowledge, nurses have no similar protected, regular setting in which to discuss mistakes openly.

13. William E. Mitchell, Jr., "How to Deal with Poor Medical Care," *Journal of the American Medical Association* 236 (1976):2875–77, describes some sound procedures and considerations for dealing with poor medical care. The procedures also reflect the difficulty in getting anything done.

14. California Medical Association and Board of Medical Quality Assurance, "Physician Responsibility . . . A Joint Statement," January, 1980. This pamphlet is quoting from California Civil Code, Section 43.8.

15. Storlie, "Burnout," p. 2110.

16. Linda Stanley, "Dangerous Doctors: What to Do When the M.D. Is Wrong," *R.N.* 42, 3 (March 1979):25.

17. Edward H. Madden and Peter H. Hare, "Civil Disobedience in Health Services," in Warren T. Reich, ed., *Encyclopedia of Bioethics* Vol. IV (New York: The Free Press, 1978), p. 159.

18. Thelma Schorr, "Issues of Conscience," *American Journal of Nursing* 72 (1972):61.

19. International Labour Conference, "Text of the Recommendation Concerning Employment and Conditions of Work and Life of Nursing Personnel, Submitted by the Drafting Committee," *Provisional Record,* Sixty-Third Session, Geneva, 1977, p. 21B/5.

20. Madden and Hare, "Civil Disobedience," p. 160.

21. For a brief account of Sartre's views, see "Existentialism Is Humanism (1946)."

22. Immanual Kant, "What Is Enlightenment," translated by Lewis White Beck, in *Foundations of the Metaphysics of Morals and What Is Enlightenment* (Indianapolis: The Bobbs-Merrill Company, Inc., 1959), p. 87.

23. J. O. Urmson, "Saints and Heroes," in Joel Feinberg, ed., *Moral Concepts* (New York: Oxford University Press, 1970), pp. 60–73.

24. Saintliness has stronger connotations of moral goodness than heroism. A hero or heroine can be noble but not necessarily moral. Heroism can be episodic, but saintliness requires a long track record. Physicians are more often described as heroic than saintly, and we have such concepts as *heroic intervention* and *heroic medicine.* Saintliness has been more closely associated with nursing, especially as a result of nursing's early associations with religious orders.

Some Reflections on Authority and the Nurse

John Ladd

As is evident from the chapters in this volume, there are a number of different problems confronting nurses collectively and individually. In this chapter, I want to focus on some of the moral quandaries faced by nurses that originate in what Touster calls the "complex and compelling system of authority which inhibits independence and transforms that moral character of her work largely into questions of obedience, disobedience, or evasion of authority."[1] I use the term "quandary" advisedly, because I want to stress the connotation of a "subjective perception" of the dilemma.[2] For, although many of the problems connected with authority appear to be moral dilemmas, strictly speaking, they are not really dilemmas at all and should therefore, for logical and ethical reasons, be handled quite differently from dilemmas.[3] If we try to clarify some logical and ethical aspects of the concept of authority, especially as it relates to nursing, we may make some headway in determining where the real issues lie and how to approach them.

First, a few comments are in order concerning what I shall call the *social issues* relating to nursing, namely, all those problems connected with the generally inferior social and economic status assigned to nurses in the medical hierarchy. As Touster and others have pointed out, present-day oppression and exploitation of nurses can, in large measure, be explained historically, for, in the past, nurses generally belonged to the lower social and economic classes and have almost always been women. When viewed sociologically, these facts may explain why in nursing circles today there is so much emphasis on the conception of nursing as a profession; by becoming professionals, nurses will be able to enter the middle class and

From Stuart F. Spicker and Sally Gadow, eds., *Nursing Images and Ideals.* Copyright © 1980 by Stuart F. Spicker. Published by Springer Publishing Company, Inc., New York. Used by Permission.

so achieve social parity with other middle-class professionals, including doctors.[4]

For obvious reasons, these social problems loom large in the consciousness of nurses and of women in general. But there is not much that a philosopher can do about oppression and exploitation, whether it be economic or sexist, except to deplore it. We should not forget, however, that things are changing. Our age is an age of revolutions, not merely political revolutions, but biological, technological, social, and sexual revolutions. The winds of change are upon us and there is no reason to believe that the social, economic, and sexist status of nurses will remain the same as it has been in the past.

These revolutions, like all revolutions, also create many ethical problems that are interesting and that are enormously complex and troublesome: e.g., questions like how much of the old to cast away and how much to retain? What methods can and should be used to secure the necessary changes? What should be the long-range goals as contrasted with the short-range goals? These questions are already incorporated into public debates over such things as reverse-discrimination, fair employment practices, and unionization.

Let us suppose, however, that as a result of revolutions of this type the social issues connected with nursing are resolved, or at least transformed so radically that it will no longer be true that being a nurse means being female, uneducated, and lower class, or that being a doctor means being male, educated, and upper class. Other important ethical problems encountered by nurses would still remain to be resolved, in particular, ethical problems relating to authority and role differentiation. These problems were aired by Plato a long time ago, quite independently of the particular social issues that nurses are concerned with today. We should not forget that Plato was one of the first philosophers to advocate the equality of the sexes and that although he firmly believed in authority and role differentiation, he certainly did not believe in male domination. Authoritarianism is not necessarily sexist or economically exploitative.

AUTHORITY AND POWER

Any discussion of authority—including the authority of doctors, hospital administrators, head nurses, deans, judges, and generals—must begin by distinguishing between power and authority. Authority always carries the connotation of legitimacy, which power does not. Following de Jouvenal, I shall define "power" as the "capacity to make oneself obeyed," that is, the capacity to make others do what one wants them to do against their own desires and preferences and against their will.[5] There is no question that individual physicians and organizations, such as hospitals, wield a great deal of power, or "clout," and that nurses, as well as patients, are often "forced" to do things or to suffer things that they would prefer, often with good reason, not to do or not to suffer. How to respond to power when it is illegitimate, illegal, or immoral raises many interesting ethical questions, but they are of a different sort from questions about how to respond to authority. Here Touster's term "evasion" seems entirely appropriate: if someone sticks a gun in your ribs, either literally or figuratively, evasion is an entirely appropriate response. If, therefore, the alleged authority of physicians and hospital managers is simply a matter of power, then the moral principles governing a nurse's or a patient's proper responses to their orders would not differ essentially from the principles that mandate a person's responses to the orders of one of his captors in, say, a concentration camp: that is, subterfuge, escape, resistance, and sabotage.

But we are not concerned here with power as such—which need not be, and often is not, legitimate—but with authority in the sense that it connotes legitimacy. Although "authority" is sometimes defined as "legitimate power," or, if you wish, as "legal power" or "morally justified power," in order to avoid confusion, it is better to regard power as an adjunct of

authority or a consequence of authority rather than as definitive of it. After all, Plato found no need for power in his republic; the authority of the philosopher-king was founded on reason, not on power. Let us therefore try to analyze the concept of authority without reference to the concept of power.

The best way to understand the concept of authority is to approach it from the point of view of the individual who is subject to it. Authority calls for respect rather than fear. Respect for authority, in turn, implies the right to command rather than the power to coerce. For, in Hart's words, "to command is characteristically to exercise authority over men, not power to inflict harm, and though it may be combined with threats of harm a command is primarily an appeal not to fear but to respect for authority."[6]

Insofar as authority is based on respect rather than on fear, it is something that is accepted voluntarily; the acceptance of authority implies a willingness to comply with the commands of authority on the part of the subject. The authority commands, and the subject obeys, because, for one reason or another, he acknowledges that the authority has the right to command and that he or she, on that account, has the duty to obey. Thus, de Jouvenal says: "To follow authority is a voluntary act. Authority ends where voluntary assent ends."[7]

It is assumed that the subject is willing to comply with the commands of an authority even when the particular acts demanded are contrary to his or her own personal wishes, desires, or interests. In addition, the subject obeys the command not because of its content or because it is rational, but simply because it is commanded by an authority that he or she has accepted.[8] In other words, authority is to be obeyed not because what it commands is reasonable, but because it is reasonable to obey its commands. In this sense, the *ipse dixits* of an authority serve *eo ipso* as binding reasons for a person to do or to refrain from doing something. For this reason, authority is often said to imply the "voluntary surrender of judgment" or the "voluntary abdication of choice" on the part of the subject in the area over which authority rules.[9]

However, it should be observed that, strictly

speaking, assent, i.e. acceptance, is by itself neither sufficient nor necessary to make a person an authority over others; it is possible for people to *think* that they ought to obey a person who actually has no right to command them, just as it is also possible for people to *think* that they need not obey a person who actually does have such a right. If the authority is legitimate, then it is more nearly accurate to say that people subject to it *ought* to accept the authority, that is, ought to assent to its right to command, and so *ought* to obey its commands.

To say that people ought to accept an authority and to obey its commands means that there is a good reason for them to do so. But there is no good reason for people to accept and obey an authority if the authority claimed has no basis; the claim that a person has the right to command others must have a basis or ground. As with rights in general, if the right to command has no basis, then there is no reason for accepting and obeying what is claimed to be an authority. Hence, if the claimant is unable to provide the kind of validation or justification required of authority, the claim to authority falls to the ground; it has no logical or moral force.[10] It follows that the *burden of proof* lies on the claimant to show that the authority claimed is legitimate, rather than on those over whom the authority is claimed; the latter are not obliged to provide their own counterarguments against the claim of authority.[11]

SPURIOUS AUTHORITIES AND THE LIMITS TO AUTHORITY

It is impossible to understand what is at issue in many of the ethical problems relating to authority and nursing, unless we take into consideration that, in many cases, people do not really have the authority that they claim to have. Let us call such persons *spurious authorities* (or "false authorities"). As I have already pointed out, there is no valid reason, much less a moral reason, for accepting a spurious authority; if the authority is spurious, one has no moral obligation to comply with his commands and one should not feel "guilty" about not doing so. Therefore, whether or not to comply with the demands of a spurious authority

does not, strictly speaking, present a moral dilemma, that is, a situation in which one is forced to choose between conflicting duties.[12]

It should also be pointed out that there are always limits to the scope of an authority, not only limits as regards those over whom it has jurisdiction, but also as regards the kind of conduct that it may command. With the possible exception of the Almighty, there is no such thing as an unlimited authority; that is, the right of one person to command is always restricted to one group of people, one sphere of action, in short, to one specific context.[13] Thus, granting that a physician has a certain kind of authority over, say, a nurse or a patient, that authority does not extend over everything conceivable that the nurse or the patient might do or wish to do.[14] If a person tries to command others who do not come under his or her authority, or tries to command them in matters that do not come under that authority, that person is said to "exceed his or her authority." Based on what I have already said, it thus follows that no one has the duty to obey the commands of a person when that person exceeds his or her authority. The limits of an authority are part and parcel of the validation (or justification) of authority, since the limits of one's obligation to obey have the same basis as the obligation to accept and obey.[15]

By now, the intent of my argument should be clear. The duty of a nurse to comply with the orders of a doctor or administrator depends on the nature, source, and limits of that person's authority. If that authority is spurious, or the orders exceed the person's authority, the nurse may be in a quandary. However, there is no moral dilemma. Although it may be prudent to comply with a doctor's or administrator's order because he has power, it is not ethically necessary to justify noncompliance as such. In other words, it is not necessary for a nurse to "think up" a special reason for not complying with an order such as that it is morally wrong: for example, to lie to a patient. Ethically, the correct response to the order to lie to a patient is either that the doctor has no right to tell the nurse what to do—i.e., the doctor has no authority—or that the doctor has no right to tell the nurse to do that particular thing—i.e., he has exceeded his authority. In other words, the nurse is not required to defend her refusal with a counterargument, for example, to the effect that she has a duty to the patient that conflicts with her duty to the doctor. For, in such cases, she has no duty to the doctor at all.[16]

BASES OF AUTHORITY

In investigating the basis of authority in medicine—whether it be the authority of the physician, of the hospital administrator, or of whomever else—over other persons, say, nurses or patients, we must recognize at the very outset that the issues are complicated and that the relationships in question may involve many different kinds of authority. But we should be careful not to allow the complexity of the relationships to conceal the spuriousness of some claims to authority on the part of doctors or other professionals in the health-care system. Once again, it should not be forgotten that the burden of proof always falls on the doctor, hospital administrator, or whoever else makes the authority claim. Ethically, then, it is always proper to respond to an order by asking: Why should I obey you? What is the basis of your authority?[17]

There are, of course, many different bases of authority and, accordingly, many different kinds of authority. In order to determine what grounds there might be for authority in medicine, say, the authority of the doctor over a nurse or over a patient, let us examine some possible answers to the question: Why should we obey A., an authority?

Let us start with the distinction between authorities for *beliefs* and authorities over *conduct.* By the former, which might be called "intellectual" or "cognitive" authority, I mean the kind of authority that is used to establish the truth of some proposition or other. Technically, an argument that uses authority in this way is called "an argument from authority." An argument from authority is based on the general principle that if one has good reason to believe that A. knows p and asserts p, then one has a sufficiently good reason to believe p oneself—on A.'s word, so to speak. It is often highly reasonable to "take the word" of someone who knows something better than we do,

e.g., the word of an expert who has specialized technical knowledge that we do not possess. The authority of the doctor is often this type of intellectual authority, the authority of an expert, whose word we readily take, as to what is ailing us, because it is in our own interest to do so. But it is not self-evident that this kind of authority makes the physician an authority over conduct.

It has often been maintained that a person who has specialized knowledge—i.e., who is an authority in the intellectual sense—automatically has authority over conduct or practical authority—e.g., the right to command. This is the position taken in Plato's *Republic.* The rulers in the Republic have special knowledge on how to rule; therefore, they have the right to rule and others have the duty to obey. Their intellectual qualifications, as experts in ruling, *eo ipso* make them into authorities over conduct, or practical authorities. Doctors are sometimes thought to have authority over conduct for the same sort of reason. However, before the transition from authority in the intellectual sense to authority in the practical sense—i.e., over conduct—can be considered valid, some additional theoretical underpinning is needed. In Plato's case, the transition is justified by reference to his twofold doctrine that knowledge is virtue and that ethical knowledge is a *techné*—i.e., the kind of knowledge possessed by experts. There are, of course, serious philosophical objections to both doctrines.[18] But in any case, it is far from obvious that doctors possess the kind of knowledge and virtue required of rulers in Plato's Republic.

It hardly seems necessary to dwell on the absurdity of the idea that intellectual authority automatically gives a person the right to order people around. There is nothing extraordinary about the fact that we have to rely on others for specialized information of various sorts, and that we have to accept what they say on authority. But, at that, it still is possible for an individual to decide what to do and what not to do, based on the authoritative information that he or she has received from others. It is obvious that in dealing with scientific matters, it is almost always necessary to take the word of expert authorities. But in this regard, medical science is ostensibly no different from, say, physics and engineering. No one who is an authority in one of these fields thereby acquires the authority to make decisions for other people. As I have already suggested, anyone who wishes to base a doctor's right to command on his superior knowledge must be prepared to *show* that doctors know more about (medical?) ethics than others and are more virtuous than their nurses or their patients.[19]

BASES OF AUTHORITY: LEGITIMATION AND VALIDATION

Let us now turn to authority over conduct, i.e., the kind of practical authority that generates the obligation to accept and obey orders on the part of persons subject to it. As I have already remarked, authority in this sense requires the abdication of choice with regard to what a subject does or does not do. The question before us is: by what right does one person require someone else's abdication of choice?

Before trying to answer this question we should note that not all authority has or needs a moral basis. There are many kinds of activities that require authority but that are not moral activities per se. Consequently, we must allow for other types of legitimation and validation besides moral justification.

If we take a broad look at authority, we see a great variety of activities that require authorities of one sort or another: for example, authorities are needed in playing games, e.g., captains of teams and umpires; for running orderly meetings, e.g., chairpersons; for operating businesses, e.g., managers; and so on. Employer-employee relations almost always involve some kind of authority of the employer over the employee.

From these considerations, it follows that some legitimate authorities do not need a moral basis and that consequently not all obligations to accept and obey an authority are moral obligations. For it should be obvious that different bases generate different kinds of obligations on the part of those affected. For example, if the authority has only a legal basis, then it will generate only a legal obligation, unless we assume that every legal obligation is also a moral obligation.[20]

The issues involved here will be easier to discuss if we break down the question about the basis of authority into two separate questions: Why is authority needed, i.e., what makes it legitimate? And, why should an individual accept and comply with a particular authority? Although for the purpose of this chapter we need to keep these questions separate, it will become clear that when we take up the ethical issues relating to authority they tend to become indistinguishable. It will be convenient to refer to the process of establishing the legitimacy of an authority as *legitimation* and the process of establishing the obligation to accept and obey an authority as *validation*.[21] Let us begin with legitimation.

Turning to modes of legitimation, we should note that many authorities acquire their legitimacy on the ground that they fill an essential need. Thus, organizations generally need authorities in order to operate efficiently: the authority coordinates, organizes, and plans, while others are expected to acknowledge this authority and to comply with the orders. Let us call the kind of authority that is adopted for the sake of efficiency *organizational authority*. Formal organizations of all kinds, including health-care bureaucracies and hospitals, involve organizational authority of a special sort, namely, a hierarchy of authorities.

Questions about the legitimacy of particular organizational authorities generally revolve around their so-called rationality, that is, their efficiency and effectiveness in promoting a goal and the worthiness of the goal itself. Assuming that one of the goals of a hospital is to provide treatment facilities, then its managerial structure, i.e., the structure of authority, might be legitimized in terms of its ability to facilitate this goal.

Among goals that may be used to legitimize organizational authority, some may be moral, some may be nonmoral, and some may be downright immoral. Activities such as games may be subsumed under nonmoral types. Organized crime and totalitarian organizations exemplify the immoral type.

For our purposes, only the first two kinds of

organized activities are of interest. Let us assume that the health-care authorities we are concerned with do not fall under the category of organized crime.

Let us now turn to the second question: why should a person accept and comply with the orders of an authority? In particular, why obey the captain, the chairperson, or the boss? Disregarding questions of incentives and disincentives, i.e., rewards and sanctions that proceed from power rather than from authority, we are really concerned here with finding good reasons for accepting and complying with the commands of an authority as such.

In the case of organizational authority, which is our concern here, it is often easy to answer these questions. For example, in games and in meetings, it is reasonable to comply with the commands of the authority because doing so makes the activity in which one is participating more efficient and effective. Here, the motive or ground for accepting the authority in question is the acceptance of the goal, and the recognition that a particular authority structure is a means to that goal. In Kant's words, to will the end is to will the means.

Sometimes, one shares the goal with others, in particular, with the person who is the authority. In that case, we have validation based on participation: sharing the goal. On the other hand, there are cases in which the person subject to an authority does not share the goals that legitimize that authority. When goals diverge, compliance seems to be less voluntary than when they converge. Therefore, divergence requires some kind of extraneous validation. Much of the logic of authority, that is, of validation, hinges on whether there is a convergence or a divergence of goals.

CAN AUTHORITY HAVE A MORAL BASE?

Up to this point we have examined the bases of authority independently of their moral implications. It is obvious that many kinds of activities require the acceptance of an authority where moral considerations are irrelevant, peripheral, or adventitious. But, it is time to turn to

a more direct consideration of the ethical aspects of legitimation and validation, which might be called the moral justification of an authority and of compliance with that authority. So far, the analysis has been in terms of what Kant called a "hypothetical imperative." We must now examine these questions from the point of view of ethics, that is, in terms of the categorical imperative.

Moral justification is distinguished from nonmoral legitimation and validation in that moral requirements take precedence over other sorts of requirements. Morality in general consists of a set of standards and principles that take precedence over other systems of rules and other enterprises, and that can be used to criticize, judge, and evaluate these other systems of rules and enterprises.[23]

We may begin with two simple and obvious kinds of justification that fit a large number of cases in which the acceptance of authority and obedience are morally required—namely, those based on contract, e.g., a contract of employment, and those established by law, e.g., the authority of a police officer, judge, or tax collector.[24]

I shall call the moral justification involved here *extrinsic justification,* because it depends on extrinsic factors, e.g., the making of a contract or a law. Without the contractual or the legislative act that creates the obligation, there would be no obligation and obedience would not be morally binding.

It should be noted that these two types of extrinsic justifications generally presuppose that the individual bound thereby does not share the goals of the authority structure. That is, they involve cases in which goals diverge. Industrial organizations provide good examples, for those subject to the authority of management and the foreman are bound to obey them by virtue of a contract of employment and not because they expect to share in the profits of the organization.

Without wishing to prejudge the issue, we might ask at this point whether the authority of a doctor over a nurse is just one of these two kinds. Is the obligation to obey simply based on contract or on law? Obviously the answer is: sometimes, but not always. A nurse, like any employee, is bound by the terms of a contract and, like other citizens, is bound to observe the law. But there may be other reasons for accepting medical authority. Let us consider what they might be.

Before proceeding, it should be observed that neither contracts nor law can require persons to do anything immoral. There are limits to contracts and limits to law, in theory at least. The nurse's moral integrity and her moral responsibilities to the patient as a person set limits to what may be required by contracts or law. An implied condition, e.g., of a contract, from a moral point of view, is that one not be required to deceive or abandon the helpless.

Apart from legitimation and validation, on the one hand, and extrinsic moral justification on the other hand, can the authority structure in medicine and nursing be morally justified? One answer might be that authority is morally justifiable if it serves a moral purpose, a morally worthy goal. Such might be the utilitarian answer.

The complexities are immediately apparent. What is the goal of medicine or of the health-care system? Is there a single, comprehensive goal of such determinateness that it could be used to justify the right of certain persons, e.g., doctors, to exercise authority over others?

Let us grant that in certain contexts authority is needed and is morally desirable—for example, in the operating room. In an operating room, the authority of the surgeon might be likened to the authority of the conductor of an orchestra: the surgeon is the chief performer and the one who "orchestrates" the proceeding. Let us grant that the aim of the procedure is to save the patient's life, i.e., a morally worthy goal. But here, as with the orchestra, we are dealing with a precisely defined, limited enterprise involving goals that we may assume are shared by all the parties involved, or, perhaps, to be more nearly accurate, we should say that they ought to be shared by all of them.

The fact is, however, that when we examine other contexts and other health-care activities, the goals are not that simply defined. In fact, there is a multiplicity of divergent goals: the doctor may be concerned to cure, the nurse may want to help the patient to adjust, and the patient may be principally worried about how to pay for everything. The divergence of goals among parties in the health-care setting accounts for the fact that there is a great deal of noncompliance and evasion, e.g., in hospitals, since it undermines the rational underpinning of the authority structure insofar as it is founded on voluntary participation.

In closing, I would like to suggest that our society relies too much on authoritarian structures to organize cooperative activities. Authoritarian structures depend for their legitimacy and effectiveness on common agreement about goals and methods. This kind of agreement is not universally found in the present-day health-care situation. It is not found in many other institutions either, e.g., in universities.[25] In the absence of the conditions that are necessary for authority, we ought to look for other ways of working together.

As an alternative, we might try to find more "democratic" procedures, procedures involving mutual counseling, consultation, and collaboration. Mutual accommodation and persuasion should take the place of one person issuing commands to others below. In the long run, such methods are the only ones that can hold up under rational scrutiny in situations in which there is a divergence of goals, concerns, and interests, but where there is still a modicum of goodwill.

Notes

1. This essay was originally presented in response to Professor Saul Touster's "Decision-Making in the Nurse/Physician Relationship: Authority, Obedience and Collaboration," a paper presented at a conference on "Nursing and the Humanities: A Public Dialogue," held at the University of Connecticut Health Center, Farmington, November, 1977.

2. According to the dictionary, quandary refers "to the subjective aspect of a dilemma and emphasizes perplexity and vacillation."

3. By a "moral dilemma" I mean an unavoidable situation in which one is forced to choose between performing one obligation rather than another, or to choose between evils, rights or wrongs, duties, and so on. A good example of a

moral dilemma in this sense is having to choose between saving a person's life and telling a lie. In philosophical jargon, a dilemma represents a clash between prima facie duties. As I have argued elsewhere, there are many other kinds of ethical problems besides those arising from dilemmas. See my "The Task of Ethics," in Warren Reich (ed.), *The Encyclopedia of Bioethics*, New York: Macmillan, 1978, vol. 1, pp. 400–07.

4. See Burton J. Bledstein, *The Culture of Professionalism: The Middle Class and the Development of Higher Education in America*. New York: Norton, 1977. Strictly speaking, nursing lacks some of the essential perquisites of a profession, as Touster points out.

5. See Bertrand de Jouvenal, *Sovereignty* (trans. J. F. Huntington). Chicago: University of Chicago Press, 1957, p. 32. In calling it a capacity, I want to stress the counterfactual aspect of power. Frequently, there is no need for a person with power to exercise that power, e.g., the power that goes with a gun, because the desires and preferences of the parties in fact coincide or they obey out of habit. Such is the case with charismatic power, for example. But power, in the sense of might, usually comes into play in marginal cases, since it is generally not the most effective way of controlling the behavior of others. Obviously, a great deal more needs to be said about power. It should be stressed that here we are concerned with power only in the narrow political and social sense and a sense that makes it possible to differentiate between the power of a doctor or administrator and his authority.

6. H.L.A. Hart, *The Concept of Law*. Oxford: Clarendon Press, 1961, p. 20.

7. de Jouvenal, *Sovereignty*, p. 33.

8. See Hobbes's distinction between counsel and command: "Now counsel is a precept in which the reason of my obeying it, is taken from the thing itself which is advised; but command is a precept, in which the cause of my obedience depends on the will of the commander." *De Cive*, S.P. Lamprecht (ed.), New York: Appleton-Century-Crofts, 1949, p. 155.

9. See Richard B. Friedman, "On the concept of authority in political philosophy," reprinted in Richard E. Flathman, (ed.), *Concepts in Social and Political Philosophy*, New York: Macmillan, 1973, especially pp. 127 ff.

10. It makes no difference whether the claimant claims the authority for someone else or for himself.

11. The point is a logical or ethical one; in the absence of reasons for accepting a person as an authority, his alleged authority reduces to power, brute power, if you will.

12. See note 3, *supra*. Elsewhere, I call this kind of dilemma a "conflict of obligations." See my "Remarks on the conflict of obligations," *Journal of Philosophy*, September 11, 1958.

13. Inasmuch as totally dependent human beings, e.g., infants and idiots, cannot have obligations, the concept of authority has no immediate applicability to them.

14. Perhaps this consideration points to one way of distinguishing between power and authority; power can be unlimited, authority cannot. The power of a kidnapper over a captive often is close to being unlimited.

15. The *locus classicus* for an argument aimed at establishing the limits of authority is John Locke's *A Letter Concerning Toleration*. New York: Liberal Arts Press, Bobbs-Merrill, 1950. Locke argues that legislation regarding religion is impermissible because it is not authorized in the original contract establishing the civil authority.

16. Logically the two possible types of moral argumentation involve the difference between what may be called "refutation" and "confutation." Showing that you have no duty to do *x*, i.e., refuting the claim, must be distinguished logically from showing that you have a duty not to do *x*, i.e., confuting the claim. See my "The issue of relativism," in John Ladd, (ed.), *Ethical Relativism*. Belmont, California: Wadsworth, 1973.

17. I assume that "to obey" is to comply with a *command* in contradistinction to complying with a request, a piece of advice or other kinds of guidance. See Hobbes's distinction quoted above in note 8.

18. For a critique of the concept of ethics as a *techné* see my "Egalitarianism and elitism in ethics," *L'Egalité*, V, Brussels, 1978.

19. Simply *saying* so is not sufficient to make it true.

20. For a critique of this notion, see my "Legal and moral obligation," in J. Roland Pennock and John Chapman, (eds.), *NOMOS XII: Political and Moral Obligation*. New York: Atherton Press, 1970.

21. There is, as far as I know, no standard use for these terms in discussions of authority by philosophers and political theorists.

22. We shall see that this difference may be crucial in the present inquiry, for nurses and doctors often have different goals in mind with regard to a patient, and the patient himself may have a different goal from that of the doctor or that of the nurse.

23. For more on this concept of morality, see my *The*

Structure of a Moral Code, Cambridge, Mass.: Harvard University Press, 1957.

24. Elsewhere I have expressed some reservations about these kinds of obligation, but they are immaterial to the present issue. See my "Legal and moral obligation," in J. Roland Pennock and

John Chapman, (eds.), *NOMOS XII: Political and Moral Obligation.* New York: Atherton Press, 1970.

25. The decline of authority in our society has been called the "eclipse" or the "twilight" of authority.

From "Value-Laden Technologies and the Politics of Nursing"

Sandra Harding

THE ORGANIZATION OF HEALTH CARE

Health care has been organized in a variety of ways, as the history and sociology of medicine reveal. In our society health care is organized around hospitals and vast numbers of hierarchically-organized workers—from research physicians to nurses' aides. Nurses themselves exist at several intermediate levels in this hierarchy. In the following account, the outlines of which are no doubt familiar to many readers, I wish to bring out some peculiar and significant features of nursing which are easy to overlook if one fails to see the function nursing performs within the overall structure of health care. The organization of the labor of nursing is grasped, I shall argue, only if one understands nursing as an industrialized form of traditional women's work. Thus the position of nursing is located in the structure of health care in much the same way as domestic labor is situated in the structure of social life in general. In particular, the service ethic which in part attracts women to nursing is "cooled out" for lower levels of nurses through techniques of industrial management and in part through the substitution of a "professional" ethic for the service ethic. These subversions of the service ethic result in nurses' "natural" social strengths as well as

their training being turned against them and against those they are charged to care for and cure. I turn first to remind you of the particular way the labor of nursing has been organized.

Educated women employed outside the home have tended to cluster in the so-called helping professions. In addition to nursing, the most obvious of these occupations are secretarial work, teaching, social work, psychology, and the paramedical services of occupational, physical, and speech therapy. There are two reasons for this clustering. First of all, women have had few other options for paid employment. Secondly, all of these jobs call upon the social strengths women have developed in their traditional roles in the family—nurturing, caring, doing the "housekeeping" tasks. In the helping professions the social strengths of women are mobilized on behalf not just of the family but of the whole society.[1] The negative side of this segregation of the work force is that until very recently women have been systematically prevented from entering not only any areas of the work force where they might obtain high salaries, but also any areas where their duties would not be consistent with their feminine roles in the family. They have been especially prevented from entering any of the policymaking roles in the economy, in government, in education, and in health care.

It is no accident that the helping professions emerged on a significant scale in the middle of the 19th century. They can be seen as the psychosocial counterpart of the move in material production which relocated economic activity out of the small-scale and personal atmosphere of the individual home and into the large-scale and impersonal setting of the factory. The trend in both material production and in the production of services has been toward breaking down complex production processes into increasingly specialized and repetitive activities. This division of labor and accompanying specialization is necessary if there is to be centralized control of production processes. And centralized control is necessary if just a few people are to extract the maximum profit from the labor of production which is performed mainly by others. The particular recent forms of industrialization of the production of both material goods and psychosocial services have been useful for the accumulation of both political power and wealth by a minority of people. In the case of health care, the hospital has become the hub of the wheel of the production of services, and it is here that the structure and value of nursing are more obvious.

There are two striking features that nursing shares with the other kinds of women's work, including the domestic labor from which it emerged. The first of these is the contradiction between the social value of the work and the public recognition of this value. The second is the way that the service ethic—the ethic of altruism that is in part responsible for attracting women to nursing—is "cooled out" and subverted. It is "cooled out" in different ways for different ranks of nurses. As long as they are not recognized, these "cooling out" devices prevent nurses from organizing to change the conditions of their labor—that is, from organizing to change the technologies under which health-care is delivered. Thus nursing is like other kinds of women's work in that the special strengths of women are turned against both women themselves and against those for whom they are expected to care.

I turn first to the contradiction between the social value of nursing and the public recognition of this value. This contradiction appears once we note the three features which distinguish the labor of health care from other kinds of industrial labor. First of all, the in-

troduction of a new technology—a new way of organizing labor—makes most industries less labor-intensive. Such "substitute technologies" allow the production of more goods with less human labor. However, technological change in health care has required the hiring and training of vast numbers of additional workers to operate the various new machines and instruments. At the same time, the full number of existing staff is required to provide the continuing services. This increase in the health-care work force is due to the "add-on" character of most of the technological changes in health care. These changes do not merely substitute a new way of accomplishing a task for an old way but, instead, accomplish things not possible before.[2] The number of workers needed to provide health care has vastly increased, and the greatest increase has been in the lower-level workers—nurses, technicians, and nurses' aides.

Secondly, the social value of health care is immediately and unquestionably obvious.[3] It is obvious first to the workers themselves. The factory worker may wonder about the value of a new flavor of cat food or about the value of the 19th brand of can opener she is involved in producing, but health is a "product" the value of which is immediately apparent to health-care workers. The social value of health care is also perfectly clear to everyone else in the society: we wonder about the value of the cat food or the can opener, but we never question the value of health. We want it, and the more of it the better. And who provides all of this valuable health care? While only 8 percent of health-care workers are doctors, 50 percent are nurses. The remaining 42 percent is divided among the fields of dentistry, pharmacy, clinical laboratory services, environmental control, secretarial and office services, and various other miscellaneous categories.[4] This, too, is obvious to the nurses themselves, if less so to the rest of society. A nurse in a municipal hospital says with only slight exaggeration: "You could imagine a hospital with no doctors. Everything would get done just the same. But try to imagine a hospital with no nurses. It would be chaos. The patients would all die of neglect."[5]

In the third place, in the "factory" of health care, the hospital, there is extraordinary functional interdependence among workers who have very different rank within the hospital and very different social status in the outside world. This too distinguishes health-care workers from other industrial workers.

> A surgical operation commonly requires the cooperative efforts of a team whose members range in rank from surgeon to aides. The surgeon has had eight or more years of post-college training; he may earn more than $50,000 a year and sit on one of the hospital's key management committees, on the almost all-powerful medical board or even on the board of directors. The aides may have no high school education, earn less than $7000, and lack even the authority to make a simple suggestion. But in the operation itself they are both essential participants, as the aide can easily demonstrate by making a small but fatal mistake.[6]

The nurse's contribution to health care is as crucial as that of any other health-care worker. This contradiction in the nurse's importance and her rank in the hospital hierarchy is mirrored by the contradiction in the doctor's importance and his rank in the hospital hierarchy. Given his *functional* importance, the doctor has a vastly inflated status within the hospital. As the technology of health care becomes increasingly that of an industrial assembly line, the doctor more and more becomes just one among many production workers, one skilled worker among many. He works right alongside the nurses, aides, and technicians and his work is continually observed by these, his inferiors in rank. It is these "inferiors," and usually they alone, who are witnesses to all of his failures— his faulty diagnoses, unnecessary postoperative complications, and the like.[7] But, as an integral part of hospital management, he has the highest rank in the institution.

Nurses are low paid and many of the mundane jobs doctors used to do have been transferred to nurses. The division of labor in health care is spectacular. And narrow job definitions are enforced through hierarchical control within the health system. A nurse writes in the journal *Nursing Outlook:*

> So often I knew the patient better than the physician and had scientifically based reasons for wanting to initiate a certain action—yet I was

prevented from doing so without being given equally valid reasons. The goal seemed to be to keep the institution operating at a smooth pace and to placate the other professional people, rather than to help the patient to meet his needs.[8]

Individual nurses perform an increasingly small portion of the process of producing health care. As with any labor industrialized in this way, it becomes easy for workers to lose sight of the final "product" of such specialized labor. Nurses report again and again the vast gap between what they are capable of and trained to do on the one hand, and what in fact the hierarchy of hospital work allows them to do on the other hand. One nurse says: "We're really like secretaries pushing papers around. All we do is dispense pills to the patients."[9] And a nurse educator with 12 years nursing experience behind her says:

> Let's face it, nursing is a rotten job. You have no control over hours, you rotate shifts, work weekends and holidays. You get moved from floor to floor. Sometimes you're the only one with fifty patients and yet the supervisor comes in and yells at you and you think, what do they expect from me?[10]

In this respect, nursing is organized exactly like the rest of "women's work." Thus the high social value of the huge contribution of nurses to health care is not rewarded in commensurable income, appropriate social status inside or outside the institution, or proportionate control over either the working conditions of nursing or the way in general in which health care is delivered.

The second striking feature nursing shares with other kinds of women's work is the way that the social ethic is "cooled out" and subverted. It is cooled out in different ways for different ranks of nurses, ways appropriate to their social statuses in the larger society—their "absolute" social statuses.

This preservation of absolute social status in the ranked division of labor inside the hospital is characteristic of hospital worker in general. Doctors are 98 percent white, 93 percent male, and predominantly from upper and upper-middle class families. Nurses and technicians are usually lower-middle class and white; 98

percent of nurses and about 70 percent of technicians are women. Aides, cooks, and maids are the lower-class men and women. In the big northern cities these are usually black, Chicano, or Puerto Rican. In New York City's municipal hospitals, for instance, between 80 and 90 percent are nonwhite.[11] The preservation of different absolute statuses within the nursing ranks insures that nurses will find it difficult to identify and to organize around shared goals.

For the practical nurses, nurses' aides, and other health-care workers in the lower ranks of the hospital hierarchy, the hierarchical control of the conditions under which health care is delivered eventually alienates them from the content of their work. As the Ehrenreichs report:

> Conditions (in even the best hospitals), however, are enough to undermine the efforts of even the most dedicated workers—understaffing, inadequate supplies and equipment, obstructive red tape, priorities given to non-patient care functions, etc. In their training or orientation, lower-level workers are warned against taking it all too seriously. "Do not try to achieve perfection in everything, because, admirable as it is, it is an invitation to failure and often is most impracticable," warns one text for practical nurses. (*Personal and Vocational Relationships in Practical Nursing,* Carmen F. Ross, Philadelphia 1969, p. 103). Suggestions and innovations from the ranks are not encouraged, and are usually viewed as "troublemaking." An aide told us, "You go to your supervisor [about a patient care problem]. She doesn't do anything. Eventually, *you* stop caring, too." Again and again we heard the refrain. "After a while you just don't give a damn." You become the adjusted, "industrialized" worker for whom hospital work is just a job.[12]

Through techniques of "industrial management," workers at the lower levels of nursing are forced to accept and adjust to the class divisions preserved within health care, and to deny the service ethic which was in part responsible for attracting them to health care.

One might think that the recent trend toward unionization of hospital workers would alleviate this situation. However, unions do not challenge either the way work is organized or the nature or quality of the "product" workers produce. As in other unions, hospital unions succeed—when they do—simply in getting more pay for jobs no matter how meaningless and dead-end they are. And as in other industries, hospitals pass on to consumers the wage increases won by unions. Thus by failing to challenge the organization of health-care labor or the nature of the health care "produced," unions in fact force the needs of the worker to be in conflict with the needs of the consumer of health care.[13] This can be regarded as the final subversion of the service ethic.

On the other hand, for higher-level health workers such as registered nurses, the ideology of professionalism leads them to deny the class divisions among health-care workers and to divert their service ethic into a professional "ethic."[14] In the professional "ethic" it is not service to the patient—caring and curing—but loyalty to the institution which guides their perception of and ability to deliver health care.

This is not a description of the professional "ethic" that is likely to comfort professionals, because the ideal to which professionals overtly pay allegiance is a very different one. Just a few years ago, as astute a social observer as Paul Goodman thought it uncontroversial to say that "professionals are autonomous individuals beholden to the nature of things and the judgment of their peers, and bound by an explicit or implicit oath to benefit their clients and the community."[15] This ideal has been a powerful social force motivating many who have entered law, medicine, and university life. Has the ideal really functioned to guide professionals in serving the needs of clients and community? A skeptical answer to this question has been emerging from recent examinations of the struggles of the rising middle class in 19th-century America.

The first clue toward understanding how professions in fact function is to note that from a legal point of view a profession is a monopoly: ". . . a profession is an organized occupational group which has been granted a monopoly over the performance of certain functions and a certain degree of autonomy in carrying them out."[16] Among the monopolies the medical profession has been granted are exclusive rights to police medical workers, to set standards for entering the various fields of medical work, to practice surgery, to prescribe drugs, to classify people as fit or unfit for various duties or functions.[17] From a historical perspective, these monopolies on professional services emerged as the middle class sought to entrench its interests institutionally. In one of the recent studies, Burton Bledstein argues that the "cult of professionalism" emerged only with the help of the developing modern university, catering to middle-class students and finding it profitable to promote its role as gatekeeper to the profession. The modern university provides the foundation for the "true professionals" who insist that equality of opportunity and that democratic goals are identical with meritocratic ones. Since "merit will always find its true reward," professionals can confidently identify life with work and career. Since their high social status is taken as a reflection of that invisible hand of fate correctly rewarding merit, they can pride themselves on the way in which they bring both native talent and subsequent training to solve crucial social problems, simultaneously advancing both themselves and the interests of society at large.[18]

When we consider nursing, it becomes apparent that nurses have never even been encouraged to be professionals in Goodman's ideal sense at all. Bound by the rules of institutional hierarchy, they are allowed neither to function as autonomous individuals "beholden to the nature of things," nor, consequently, to act in accordance with what they perceive to be the greatest benefit for their patients and the community. Moreover, in the legal sense, nursing has only the most superficial resemblance to its presumably by definition coequal sibling professions. Like members of all the other "health professions" except for doctors, registered nurses as a group are in fact subordinate to and supervised by the medical profession itself.[19] The ideology of RNs requires that they recognize their "proper place" in the hierarchy of health care. . . .

I have been arguing that we can grasp the technology of contemporary nursing only when we see nursing as an industrialized form of "women's work." Let me summarize the features of nursing which also characterize the

domestic work from which nursing as an occupation emerged and which today's nurses still perform as their second job.

The labor of the modern family is also characterized by hierarchy and by division of labor. The male is official manager, he is the breadwinner and decision-maker. The female is domestic laborer, peforming the repetitive and menial physical labor of family life as well as providing the bulk of the psychological and social services the family requires—the caring and curing of child care and husband-tending, organizing the social life of the family, and so on. Without her labor, he could not spend the time required in training for and performance of his job: his salary actually covers the wages of two workers. For most women of every class, the discrimination and low pay they face in the public labor market make marriage and "family service" look like the most attractive way for them to "earn a living."[20] But the altruistic ethic of service finds perhaps its purest expression in the ideology of women's role in the family—the ideology of the loyal and happy housewife. It makes domestic labor justifiable as a pseudo-career and obscures to outsiders (that is, to husbands and policy-makers) the fact that women's domestic labor is both socially necessary and given virtually no public recognition—not in terms of income, status, or power to determine the conditions of labor.

Furthermore, the ethic of altruism is systematically subverted into an ethic of loyalty to the prevailing structure of the family as an institution and to the husband's interests, right or wrong. This prevents housewives both from identifying and from acting to promote the best interests of their children, of themselves, of the larger community, or, indeed, of their husbands. (I distinguish between men's best interests and their best interests as the dominant culture has defined these. Requiring massive "support forces" at home and dominating others are examples of the latter but not the former.) This subversion of the altruistic ethic into the ethic of loyal wife has been the topic of much recent literature documenting the gruesome details of contemporary domestic life from child-beating, wife-beating, and the high incidence of "mental illness" and depression in married women to the systematic support women provide to the related and inequitable hierarchies of both domestic and political life.[21]

Finally, efforts to "industrialize" domestic labor have been plagued with the same "cooling out" of the service ethic characteristic of the lower echelons of nursing, and for the same reasons. Both privately hired workers, such as maids and house cleaners, and publicly hired workers, such as those in many of the new day-care centers, are paid so little and given so little power over the conditions of their labor that it requires what can only be seen as an almost fanatic dose of altruism for them to continue to identify and serve the real needs of their "clients" or charges. In many cases, they understandably come to regard their industrialized domestic labor as "just a job." The exceptions to this rule are significant. Only community-organized domestic labor—whether in parent-run nurseries or, more broadly, in some of the communal living groups—has succeeded in industrializing domestic labor and yet maintaining the service ethic. In these cases the new ways of organizing labor were selected with an interest in maximizing desirable social relations as defined by the workers.

It seems characteristic of "women's work"—whether at home or in the "helping professions"—that it is technologized not to suit the needs of the women working or of their "charges," but to serve the interests of other powerful groups in society from which women are systematically excluded.

What are these "other groups" whose interests have in fact shaped contemporary health care? Three forces have been dominant since the end of the Second World War. These are the academic medical empires, the health-care financiers, and the health-care profiteers.[22] Their interests are not always identical with the interests of the recipients of health-care, nor with the interests of health-care workers. Sometimes the interests of the decision-makers actually conflict with patients' and nurses' interests.

Research and education are the main interests of the academic medical establishment. The academicians

contributed to the scientific and technological advances in medicine following World War II. However they gained their dominant position in the health-care delivery system not because of the scientific and technical advances, but because they used the prestige from federal research grants to insure plenty of paying patients to fill their beds.[23]

Often the interests of the academic establishment support good health care. Because of basic research, antibiotics were discovered and they contributed greatly to human health. However, there are many cases where the interests of the medical academy conflict with the interests of patients. The overriding desire for experimental results can lead to the use of inadequately tested drugs on patients; hospitals are often organized into many specialty clinics which further the education of medical students and the interests of researchers but which frequently result in confused, discouraged, and sometimes mistreated patients.[24]

The largest of the private financiers of health care is Blue Cross. However, Blue Cross was initially organized by hospitals, and it pays only for health care delivered in hospitals even though the concentration of health care delivered in hospitals does not always maximize benefits to patients. Two sorts of objections may be raised to restricting the delivery of health care to hospitals. In the first place, the concentration of medical resources in hospitals makes these resources less available to patients under some conditions: and, secondly, some kinds of health "problems" (impending death, childbirth, and chronic illness) are accompanied by emotional and physical needs better served at home.[25]

Finally, the third force shaping contemporary health care is the health profiteers. Hospital supply companies and drug companies in particular have reaped huge profits from scientific discoveries, profits paid for by patients; and, furthermore, they have contributed to the concentration of health care in hospitals.[26]

Thus the nature and structure of nursing have in effect been the consequences of the ability of these three groups of policy-makers to translate their interests into practice. The ability of nurses to care and cure is limited by the power of these three forces to determine which of the alternative technologies of health care will be brought into existence.[27] None of these policy-makers has an interest in giving greater control over working conditions to health-care workers, and none has caring and curing as his highest priority.

Notes

1. For accounts of why women cluster in the helping professions and of the history of the emergence of the helping professions, see Margaret Adams, "The Compassion Trap," in *Woman in Sexist Society*, (eds.) V. Gornick and B. Moran, New York: Basic Books, 1971; Susan Reverby, "Health: Women's Work," in *Prognosis Negative: Crisis in the Health Care System*, (ed.) D. Kotelchuck, New York: Random House, 1976; and Eli Zaretsky, *Capitalism, The Family and Personal Life*, New York: Harper and Row, 1976.

2. Barbara Caress, "The Health Workforce: Bigger Pie, Smaller Pieces," *Prognosis Negative: Crisis in the Health Care System*, (ed.) D. Kotelchuck, New York: Random House, 1976, p. 169; Ivan L. Bennett, Jr., "Technology as a Shaping Force," in *Doing Better and Feeling Worse*, (ed.) J. H. Knowles, New York: W. W. Norton, 1977, p. 126.

3. John and Barbara Ehrenreich, "Hospital Workers: A Case Study in the 'New Working Class,'" *Prognosis Negative: Crisis in the Health Care System*, (ed.) D. Kotelchuck, New York: Random House, 1976, p. 186.

4. Caress, p. 168.

5. Ehrenreich, *op. cit.*, p. 188.

6. *Ibid.*, p. 187–188.

7. *Ibid.*, p. 188.

8. Quoted in Reverby, *op. cit.*, p. 176.

9. *Ibid.*, p. 175.

10. *Ibid.*

11. Ehrenreich, *op. cit.*, p. 189.

12. *Ibid.*, p. 191.

13. *Ibid.*, p. 192.

14. *Ibid.*, p. 191.

15. Quoted in Thomas L. Haskell, "Power to the Experts," *The New York Review* XXIV, Oct. 13, 1977, p. 28.

16. Ehrenreich, *op. cit.*, p. 193.

17. *Ibid.*

18. Burton J. Bledstein, *The Culture of Professionalism: The Middle Class and the Development of Higher Education in America*, New York: Norton, 1977. I have critically examined the ideal of a meritocracy in "Equality of Opportunity, Meritocracy, and the Democratic Ethic," *Philosophical Forum*, X(1979).

19. Ehrenreich, *op. cit.*, p. 195.

20. Francine D. Blau, "Women in the Labor Force: An Overview," in *Women: A Feminist Perspective*, (ed.) Jo Freeman, Palo Alto: Mayfield, 1975.

21. Pauline Bart, "Depression in Middle-Aged Women"; in *Woman in Sexist Society*, (eds.) V. Gornick and B. Moran, New York: Basic Books, 1971; Jessie Bernard, "The Paradox of the Happy Marriage," in the same volume; Dair Gillespie, "Who Has the Power? The Marital Struggle," *Journal of Marriage and the Family*, 1971.

22. David Kotelchuck, "The Health-Care Delivery System," in *Prognosis Negative: Crisis in the Health Care System*, (ed.) Kotelchuck, New York: Random House, 1976, p. 2.

23. *Ibid.*

24. *Ibid.*

25. *Ibid.*

26. *Ibid.*

27. A valuable discussion of obstacles to change in health care is Robert R. Alford's *Health Care Politics: Ideological and Interest Group Barriers to Reform*, Chicago: University of Chicago Press, 1975.

Chapter 3

TRUTH
AND INFORMATION

INTRODUCTION

In Chapter Two there was a consideration of the ethical problems that arise out of conflicts in perspectives and conflicts of roles that different persons have. In this chapter we deal with problems arising from two other sorts of conflict that a particular person may face.

First, there are conflicts between two or more moral principles to which a person subscribes but which cannot be simultaneously followed because of special circumstances. Dilemmas of informed consent appear generally to be of this type. Attempts to resolve disputes about these matters almost always appeal to one moral principle or another, and the particular principles involved are often agreed to by the disputants as being fundamental to our moral way of life. The disagreement in such cases rests on a matter of priorities. Which ethical principle ought one to invoke when two or more come into conflict with one another? Disputes of this sort are considered in the sections entitled "Consent" and "Disclosure."

Second, conflict within a person may also

arise because of a person's *conflicting loyalties*— loyalty to two or more persons, institutions, or groups. Most of the conflicting loyalties that fall into this class are explored in the section entitled "Privacy and Confidentiality." Indeed, most situations in which the ethical issues focus on privacy, rights of privileged communication, and confidentiality are of this type.

Examining the issues raised in the section entitled "Consent," we find there are two closely related concerns to which the readings are addressed. One of these is primarily ethical, and the other is concerned with knowledge or belief.

The ethical concern is addressed in the selection by Cardozo, who forcefully states a basic moral position concerning the human being's right to determine what shall be done with his or her own body, and in the paper by Donagan, who traces the way in which the recognition of human beings as deserving of respect has led to an increased sensitivity to the need for obtaining consent from patients and experimental subjects. Donagan sees this as a shift away from utilitarianism toward a deontological view on ethical matters.

With respect to the question of knowledge or belief, it is evident that the notion of "being informed" is none too clear. A great variation exists in both the amount and kind of information that one may possess, and as a result, there are different degrees of being informed. A question that demands some careful reflection is this: How much information and what specific sorts of information ought a person have before his consent can properly be said to be "informed?" This question and a number of closely related ones are debated in the selections by Ingelfinger and Demy, while Preston Burnham responds to the problem satirically in his "consent form for hernia patients." Many physicians claim that patients, or lay persons in general, can never be fully informed in the requisite sense; in order to meet such a requirement, patients would have to know as much as the physician knows about diseases, risks, complications, statistics about similar cases, and perhaps a range of other facts. If being fully informed entails the possession of knowledge of this scope and depth, consent could rarely be given for most routine therapeutic procedures, much less for a variety of experimental procedures employing human subjects. We must, then, reasonably expect to adopt some standard other than "full and complete information" on which to base consent. A problem still remains in determining precisely what this standard should be. Focus should probably lie in the area of ascertaining what information is relevant to a patient's or experimental subject's granting consent, and even though judgments about relevance are also subject to dispute, the problem seems to be more manageable.

Aside from these issues concerning what it is to be informed and how we can tell in any specific case when a person really is informed, there are a number of closely related concerns that have moral implications. One is the question of the ability or competence of persons to give their consent; another issue is the way in which consent is obtained; and still another relates to the occasional need to gain consent from someone other than the patient himself. All these overlap and raise many of the same problems, but each has a somewhat different focus. In thinking about the topic of informed consent, we need to distinguish a variety of specific issues, conceptual as well as ethical. The conceptual ones include an inquiry into the concept of competence, in the sense required for a person to grant his consent for research or treatment. The paper by Roth, Meisel, and Lidz deals with this topic. The authors describe tests of competency to consent to treatment and claim that circumstances play an important role in determining which elements of which tests are emphasized in determining competency to consent. A related question is to what extent a person who is a patient, and thus in a vulnerable and perhaps emotionally insecure state, is capable of remembering information presented in informed consent procedures. This is discussed by Robinson and Merav.

The ethical concerns and those dealing with knowledge and belief are brought together in the selection by Loftus and Fries, the response to that selection, and their reply. Loftus and Fries agree that the principle of informed consent is correct, but they ask if there is not a danger in supplying too much information to prospective subjects in experiments. One of the central issues is whether researchers, in obtaining informed consent, have the right (or, indeed, the obligation) to weigh the possible benefits and harms that arise from disclosing all possibly relevant information to prospective subjects; or is this question of harms and benefits irrelevant since the subject has the right to the information.

A special set of moral problems is singled out for more detailed examination in the section entitled "Disclosure," which contains essays dealing with the provision of information to patients. These moral problems involve some sort of conflict between the precept that one ought to tell the truth and some other prominent ethical directive; here again, two generally held moral principles come into conflict, and both cannot be followed simultaneously. Few, if any, moral philosophers have maintained the ethical principle enjoining truth-telling in an absolutist form—for example, "always, in all kinds of circumstances, tell the truth, the whole truth, and nothing but the truth"; or "never lie, under any circumstances." Immanuel Kant is the philosopher most often cited as a defender of absolutist moral principles prohibiting lying. But Kant's views on this matter lend themselves to varying interpretations, some of which construe his position as more flexible in matters of truth-telling than the standard interpretation allows.

In any case, while there may be few defenders of an absolutist principle prescribing truth-telling, there are still two major areas where disagreement can arise. One concerns the circumstances or conditions that justify departures from truth-telling and how these are to be weighed in a specific case. The other lies in the type of justification offered by two different ethical theories. Duty theorists, those who subscribe to a deontological ethical theory, claim that one of our *prima facie* duties as moral agents is to tell the truth. But, they would add, this duty can be overridden by other, more important duties, such as the duty to preserve life and health whenever possible. Utilitarians, or more generally, consequentialists, might agree both on the general principle that people ought to tell the truth and on just which particular circumstances justify departing from this moral principle. The justification offered by the utilitarian would be quite different from that of the deontologist, however. The utilitarian would say that truth-telling as a general moral practice, and perhaps in particular cases as well, is justified by the predominance of its good consequences over bad ones. Departures from truth-telling are seen as justifiable, at least sometimes, if the benefit accomplished by lying outweighs whatever good could be accrued from adhering to the moral principle of telling the truth. Indeed, two persons, each of whom subscribes to a different moral theory, might agree on everything about a particular case except the moral justification for the action judged to be morally right or morally wrong. These sorts of disagreements are proper subjects of discussion for ethical theorists, but do not usually affect the sorts of problems faced by people who are involved in situations requiring moral decision making.

It seems, not surprisingly, that few practitioners in the health sciences are concerned specifically with the application of abstract moral principles enjoining truth-telling—or anything else—to their daily practices. Instead, they view moral problems as arising directly out of situations they encounter where interests conflict or where people's rights are open to question. Indeed, Hartmann claims that in such situations one must not look to ethical theory for a solution. Rather, one should make a choice according to conscience and then accept the consequences of that choice.

We observed earlier that there is much current concern about patients' rights; there is also a concern for the rights of other groups or classes of persons whose presumed rights have not been previously identified or claimed in medical situations, such as the rights of children, retarded persons, and prisoners used as experimental subjects. One specific right claimed on behalf of patients is their alleged "right to know." Just what it is that patients are supposed to have a right to know varies from case to case, and in some instances it is far from clear. Some obvious candidates for things a patient could be said to have the right to know are: the specific disease or ailment he has; what the prognosis is for him, in particular; general statistics about people who have this disease or condition, sometimes described in terms of the patient's "chances" for living or dying; and others that come readily to mind. There are many physicians who oppose telling a patient very bad news about his condition or his life chances. Of course physicians do not usually couch their views in terms of the morality of lying to patients. Instead, they emphasize the importance of helping the patient maintain hope. Sometimes this is linked directly to the patient's medical condition; other times, it is seen as a separate yet significant aspect of the doctor's relationship with his patient.

Salzman argues in this connection that in psychotherapeutic situations one should distinguish between honesty and truth. He says that the therapist must be honest with the patient, although the question of when to communicate judgments honestly is a matter of technique. He also stresses the fact that to put forward an educated guess as though it were established truth can be as harmful to a patient as simply lying.

We can readily see that the morality of telling the patient the truth must be pitted against other values that are deemed important, such as preservation of the health and well being of fellow human beings. Indeed, if it is true that some patients are likely to be worse off, in any sense, as a result of knowing the severity of their condition or the prognosis, then perhaps these patients ought not be told. The difficulty lies in whether anyone can ascertain just which patients are likely to be harmed and which will benefit from knowing the truth.

Another set of reasons offered by those who advocate withholding information from terminally ill patients revolves around the notion of denial. Physicians frequently claim that the mechanism of denial with respect to our own death operates in most of us and that, furthermore, there are good psychological reasons why this defense exists and ought not be invaded by well-meaning doctors, family members, or others. Some writers on this subject add that the denial mechanism is so strong that even when a patient is told bluntly about his condition, he may not "process" the information correctly and thus may not really be aware of what he has been told. There is, however, another view that the dying know they are dying, even without being told, and that terminally ill persons have guessed "the truth" even when everyone concerned has tried to hide the facts from them.

So it appears that before we can directly confront the moral problem of what to tell seriously ill persons, we must address a number of factual questions. Might telling such patients the truth harm more than benefit them? Is there a general answer to this question, or can the question only be asked of each particular patient? What criteria exist for determining whether or not a patient can "handle" the truth? If there are no easily identifiable criteria, then how do doctors themselves come to know these sorts of psychological facts about their patients? There are also some questions of a more or less factual sort regarding the issue of denial. Does the denial mechanism operate in everyone? How can doctors tell whether or not the mechanism is operative in a particular patient? If they cannot really know, should this inability affect their decision to tell or not to tell patients the truth?

Even apart from the philosophically problematic issues surrounding the notion of rights, the answer to the question of what doctors ought to tell patients is complicated by still other factors. These factors are related to some issues that are dealt with in the section concerning paternalism on the part of physicians. Sometimes a paternalistic argument is based on an appeal to the medical knowledge and therapeutic expertise of doctors; specifically, their medical knowledge and experience are cited as reasons why they know best when, what, and how much to tell patients. Occasionally other sorts of factors are mentioned—for example, the greater likelihood that the physician will be more rational and objective about the patient's condition than the patient himself; hence, whatever sorts of decisions might need to be made are more appropriately made by the doctor than by the patient, who may be highly emotional or under stress. But simply pointing out these factors does not provide a solution to the question of what to tell patients or whether or not to withhold information. In order to rebut the opposing view that patients have "the right to know" all the relevant facts about their own condition, an argument still needs to be offered to show that acts of paternalism are sometimes justified. If, as some people argue, the physician's obligation to prevent harm to patients is the primary moral consideration, then the solution to this problem tends to favor the physician's discretionary judgments. If, on the other hand, ensuring patients' rights and maintaining adult patients' autonomy are the major moral considerations, then the solution seems to be that physicians should tell patients all they want to know. But, here again, there will always be debates about how to determine whether or not a patient "really" wants to know, so some judgments will inevitably have to be made by even the most frank and open physicians. As we shall see in some of the cases presented in this section, a measure of paternalism is sometimes justifiable. But this simply cannot be assumed; it must be demonstrated with cogent reasons.

Many of these difficult issues are discussed in the rest of the readings in this section. Vaisrub wonders if physicians who claim the right to inform patients about impending death are not really presuming to play a role that is inappropriate. Collins argues that there are good reasons to withhold the truth from some patients and that physicians should cultivate the "fine" art of lying. In his essay Weir presents three reasons for believing that truth-telling in medicine is a moral obligation. Among these are his view that patients are autonomous persons and that the physician-patient relationship is built on mutual trust. Appleton gives a utilitarian argument for psychiatrists' telling patients the truth: it will make the therapy more effective.

It is interesting to note, as pointed out by Novack and others, that physicians' attitudes concerning whether or not to tell a patient that he or she has cancer seem to have changed dramatically in recent years in favor of telling. Whether this shift reflects an increased concern with ethical issues or reflects other factors is a topic for additional study. There does seem to be a consensus, however, that if the patient is to be told the truth about a potentially fatal condition, and Novack's study indicates that more physicians say they would tell the truth, the information must, if possible, be presented in a nonthreatening way. The selection from Cope illustrates this.

In an essay related to these themes, Bok stresses the need for trust between patient and physician regarding the use of placebos. She points out that prescribing placebos can undermine patients' confidence and notes that many people do not seem sensitive to this as use of placebos seems innocuous almost by definition. The theme of trust is also addressed by Kempner, who discusses the practice of having surgery performed by residents rather than the surgeon with whom the patient has dealt. Kempner attempts to work out a solution that would enable patients to be told the truth without upsetting the system that is used to train surgeons.

Most people agree that consent for research or treatment must be voluntary, granted by mentally competent, rational, and properly informed agents. All of these concepts require clear analysis and explication so we can develop useful and applicable criteria in practice when informed consent must be obtained. It is especially important to protect those individuals who are incapable of providing fully informed or fully voluntary consent on their own behalf, thus necessitating an inquiry into justifiable and unjustifiable modes of paternalism. In the absence of a careful analysis of these issues, we risk making our practical criteria too weak or too strong, too vague or too ambiguous, and therefore, inappropriate or hard to apply. Philosophical analysis can help us sharpen our thinking, not only for abstract or theoretical purposes but also to aid in developing clear, practical criteria for applying the concept of informed consent, along with other central concepts in medical ethics.

The problems considered in the section entitled "Privacy and Confidentiality" fall into the category of conflicting loyalties, especially in those cases involving confidentiality, privileged communication, and privacy. Should a patient's confidence ever be violated? Is medical confidentiality abused? If so, in what ways? Are there special problems that arise in this area in the case of psychotherapy? For example, if a psychiatric patient tells his therapist that he has suicidal impulses or has made a suicide attempt or is reading books about fast-acting, lethal drugs, where does the therapist's obligation lie? Ought he to maintain his patient's confidentiality and not inform anyone? Or should he alert the patient's family or even, perhaps, others to the possibility that the person might make a suicide attempt? How high should the probability be that this patient could make a successful suicide attempt in order to justify the therapist's violating confidentiality? Can such probabilities even be meaningfully assessed? Some might claim that the principle, "Always maintain confidentiality," is fully acceptable no matter what the consequences. Adherence to such dogmatic principles is rare, however. But most people believe that physicians' primary obligation is to their patients. Another response is that steps taken to preserve a patient's life fulfill this obligation, and therefore, violating confidentiality is justified. This can now be identified as largely a dispute about the facts of a specific case, since the parties to the moral dispute appear to agree on their main ethical principle. One might argue, however, that new value issues enter the dispute when we consider whether or not it is more appropriate to place a higher priority on keeping trust than on preserving life. In this example, it is hard to imagine that anyone would value keeping trust over preserving life, but the matter is not as simple as this description implies. It is not a question here of a direct life-saving act, but rather, a small step in a chain of acts—a step that is based on a subjective judgment of probabilities by one physician. Nevertheless it is questionable whether a closer or more detailed look at a case's facts would provide the sort of evidence that could settle this dispute. An ethical issue like this, in the last analysis, may be reduced to a question of one's ultimate value preferences.

The moral presumption seems to be on the side of breaking doctor-patient confidentiality in cases in which a patient shows evidence of being potentially dangerous to other persons. Here, it might reasonably be argued, the physician has an overriding moral duty to prevent harm to innocent persons, and this obligation supersedes the narrower or weaker obligation to maintain confidentiality. But whether this reason is offered to justify breaking confidence or to support taking coercive measures, the strength of the position rests on the knowledge that a physician or therapist has to make judgments about the likelihood of a patient's committing acts of violence or harm to others. The dilemma must be viewed as a genuine ethical conflict—one that poses two alternative courses of action, each of which has moral reasons that can be urged on its behalf.

The selection by Cass and Curran gives the legal background of the topic of confidentiality. Chayet's article discusses the problem mentioned previously of the psychiatrist's patient who talks of committing a crime and also of the privileged communication between patient and psychiatrist. Chayet argues that only if the psychiatrist is convinced his patient will commit a crime that will result in injury or harm to persons or property does the psychiatrist have the right (indeed, the obligation) to inform the authorities. He also expresses the view that psychiatrists should not be required to testify in court about communication with patients, since in effect the patient would be forced to testify against him or herself. Daley discusses questions, including legal questions, concerning psychiatrists' ability to predict violence. He claims that psychiatrists probably cannot predict violence more accurately than the layperson, but the perception of others that psychiatrists can predict violence may make a difference in the way the law deals with what is called the "duty to warn."

Halleck discusses the problem faced by psychiatrists who work in university clinics when asked for information about students by schools and prospective employers. Gaylin raises questions about the ethical propriety of a medical journal's running an FBI wanted poster that told of a person with a condition that might require treatment by one of the specialists for whom the journal was intended. Gaylin points out that there is a serious ethical issue concerned in this case. Rosner and those who responded to his article discuss the ethical issues involved in a program in which a medical association collaborates with an insurance company in peer review of outpatient psychiatric treatment. In the final selection in this section, Abrams, Buckner and Levin discuss an emergency room case that raises issues concerning confidentiality and the fundamental responsibility of physicians.

John O'Connor

CONSENT

From *Schloendorff v. New York Hospital*

Benjamin N. Cardozo

. . . Every human being of adult years and sound mind has a right to determine what shall be done with his own body; and a surgeon who

From B. N. Cardozo, *Schloendorff v. N.Y. Hospital* 211 N.Y. 127, 129, 105 N.E. 92, 93 (1914) as it appears in *Experimentation with Human Beings,* Jay Katz ed. (New York: Russell Sage Foundation, 1972), p. 526.

performs an operation without his patient's consent commits an assault, for which he is liable in damages. (*Pratt* v. *Davis,* 224 Ill. 300; *Mohr* v. *Williams,* 95 Minn. 261.) This is true except in cases of emergency where the patient is unconscious and where it is necessary to operate before consent can be obtained. . . .

From "Informed Consent in Therapy and Experimentation"

Alan Donagan

INFORMED CONSENT TO THERAPY

It has never been disputed that a necessary condition of the coming into existence of the relation between himself and his patient that is the source of a physician's professional responsibilities is that the patient have sought treatment from him, or that a sufficient condition of that relation's ceasing to exist is that the patient communicate to the physician his decision to terminate it. Except in emergencies, that a prospective patient asks for treatment does not suffice to make him a patient: physicians have always maintained that, as provided in the fifth section of the American Medical Association's *Principles of Medical Ethics,* "A physician may choose whom he will serve" (AMA 1964; from Katz 1972, p. 313). However, it has never been questioned that a patient's consent is necessary to his being a patient, and consequently that

Reprinted with permission from the author and *The Journal of Medicine & Philosophy,* 1977, vol. 2, no. 4, pp 310–327.

withdrawal of that consent terminates his being one.

Once a physician-patient relationship exists, what responsibilities to the patient does the physician incur by virtue of it? The Hippocratic oath, in its various forms,[1] lays down only one comprehensive responsibility, which is formulated as follows in the version reproduced by Katz: "I will follow that system of regimen which, according to my ability and judgment, I consider for the benefit of my patients, and abstain from whatever is deleterious and mischievous" (Katz 1972, p. 311). Taken strictly, this binds the physician, as long as the physician-patient relationship endures, to treat his patients for their benefit, but according to what he, not they, judge that benefit to be, and to what he, not they, judge will most promote it.

When the bulk of his patients have little power, influence, or education, that is how a physician will tend to conduct himself toward them. But it is now a long time since a physician could claim that he ought so to treat his patients without being unintentionally comic.

Consider the following exchange in a case heard as late as 1961 (*Moore* v. *Webb,* 345 S.W. 2d, Mo. 1961). A patient had consulted a surgeon about toothache. He was advised that extractions would be necessary, and he consented to that, but claimed at the same time to have insisted that they should be only partial. After X-ray examination, the surgeon decided that a complete extraction would be beneficial; and, without any further consultation, when the patient presented himself for the operation, extracted all his teeth. The patient sought to recover damages for an operation to which he had not consented. At the trial this passage occurred between surgeon and plaintiff's attorney:

> . . . I think you should strive to do for the patient what is the best thing over a long period of time for the patient. We tried to abide by that.
> Q: Isn't that up to the Patient? A: No, I don't think it should be. If they go to a doctor they should discuss it. He should decide . . .
> Q: Isn't this up to the patient? . . . If I want to keep these teeth can't I do it? A: You don't know whether they are causing you trouble.
> Q: That is up to me, isnt' it? A: Not if you came to see me it wouldn't be. [Katz 1972, p. 649].

That this dialogue seems to belong in the captions of a silent movie shows how out-of-date is the conception of the physician-patient relation it presents. But in what ways is it out of date?

In an influential paper published in 1956, the psychiatrists Thomas Szasz and Marc Hollender distinguished three basic models of the physician-patient relation, more than one of which may be combined in any actual specimen of it. The first, or "activity-passivity" model, they describe as "the oldest conceptual model," and characterize it as "based on the effect of one person on another in such a way and in such circumstances that the person acted upon is unable to contribute actively, or is considered inanimate." According to it, a patient resembles a helpless infant, and a physician an active parent. The second, or "guidance-cooperation" model, they describe as underlying much of medical practice, and characterize it as one in which both patient and

physician are active, but in which "the patient is expected to 'look up to' and to 'obey' his doctor" and is "neither to question nor to argue or disagree with the orders he receives." The prototype of this model is the relation between "the parent and his (adolescent) child." The third, or "mutual participation" model, is characterized as "predicated on the postulate that equality among human beings is desirable," and as an "interaction" in which physician and patient "(1) have approximately equal power, (2) [are] mutually interdependent (i.e., need each other), and (3) engage in activities that will be in some ways satisfactory to both." Sometimes relations satisfying this model are "overcompensatory," but sometimes they are medically necessary, as for example in the treatment of most chronic illnesses, where "the patients' own experiences provide valuable and important clues for therapy" and the program of treatment "is principally carried out by the patient" (Szasz and Hollender 1956; from Katz 1972, pp. 229–30).

Although profoundly suggestive, the Szasz-Hollender models partly obscure the change from which the informed consent requirement has grown by confounding two distinct generic physician-patient relations, which I shall call the treatment relation and the choice of course of treatment relation. For our purposes, it is the latter that counts.

The Szasz-Hollender models largely hold for the treatment relation: that is, the therapeutic relation between physician and patient as treatment is actually going on. This relation appears to have three specific kinds: (1) physician active and patient wholly passive, as in surgery under a general anaesthetic; (2) patient active as well as physician, but merely in following the physician's specific instructions; and (3) patient active as well as physician, and deciding many substantive questions of treatment for himself. By contrast, there seem to be only two specific kinds of choice of course of treatment relation: (1) physician chooses the patient's course of treatment until either terminates the physician-patient relation; and (2) physician proposes, patient decides. The Szasz-Hollender triad obscures the fact that each of the two kinds of choice of course of treatment relation is compatible with each of the three kinds of treatment relation. For example, a choice of course of treatment relation in which the physician chooses is perfectly compatible with a treatment relation in which the patient, a diabetic say, decides for himself many therapeutic questions. Likewise, a choice of course of treatment relation in which a patient, having rejected his physician's first recommendation, and, after inquiring about alternatives that are medically acceptable to his physician, chooses another is perfectly compatible with his choosing a course of treatment in which he will be in the most passive of all treatment relations—surgery under a general anaesthetic.

There are, of course, cases in which there is no distinction between course of treatment and treatment, as when a patient agrees to have a flu shot. But there will be a distinction wherever a course of treatment is complex. Advancing a claim to decide on the course of treatment one is to undergo in no way encroaches upon the physician's authority over how that course of treatment is to be carried out.

The express requirement of informed consent to therapy, I suggest, is no more than the formal recognition of a change taking place in the predominant form of physician-patient relation: a change from a "physician decides" kind of choice of course of treatment relation to a "physician proposes, patient decides" kind. And physicians who exhibit the deepest understanding of the physician-patient relation have seen in this change of realization of something present in it all along. Consider the following statement by Otto E. Guttentag: "the *original* and, indeed, the basic justification for our profession [is that] . . . one human being is in distress, in need, crying for help; and another fellow human being is concerned and wants to assist him. The cry for help and the desire to render it precipitate the relationship. Here *both* the healing and the sick persons are subjects, fellow-companions, partners to conquer a common enemy who has overwhelmed one of them. Theirs is a relationship between two 'I's' . . . I have called it 'mutual obligation of equals'" (Guttentag 1953; from Ladimer and Newman 1963, p. 65).

In the majority of the writings known to me in which the requirement of informed consent is accepted (I had almost said "all," but I have made no systematic count), that requirement is grounded upon one or another of three principles, which, although not identical, are nevertheless connected, namely: (1) that in nature as it is known to us, human beings have a dignity and worth that is unique; (2) the Kantian principle that a human being is never to be used merely as a means, but always at the same time as an end; and (3) a principle laid down in the Declaration of Independence, which, as we shall see, is far from merely political, that every human being is endowed with an inalienable right to life, liberty, and the pursuit of happiness. In many of those writings, as in Guttentag's paper, these principles are explicitly or implicitly acknowledged to have been transmitted, in Western societies, largely through the Judaeo-Christian religious tradition, in which it is held that, unlike the innocent beasts, man is "created in the image of God, and tempted by the devil" (Guttentag 1953; from Ladimer and Newman 1963, p. 69). Of course, despite their historical connection, the conception of man expressed in this doctrine is logically separable from any belief in God or the devil.

In an important and justly influential statement on the ethics of consent, Paul Ramsey has shown that the requirement of consent is connected with the fidelity human beings owe one another in their interactions: "The principle of an informed consent [he wrote] is a statement of the fidelity between the man who performs medical procedures and the man on whom they are performed. . . . Fidelity is between man and man in these procedures. Consent expresses or establishes this relationship, and the requirement of consent sustains it" (Ramsey 1970, p. 5). But connecting the requirement of consent with "the faithfulness that is normative for all the . . . moral bonds of life with life" is only the first stage in its justification: Ramsey correctly went on to derive faithfulness itself from the unique dignity of man: "A human being is more than a patient or experimental subject; he is a *personal* subject—every bit as much a man as the physician-experimenter" (Ramsey 1970, p. 5). And that, of course, returns us to the first of the three principles above.

Recognition of every human being as having a unique dignity as human, and as therefore being an end in every relation in which others may morally stand to him, entails that no human being may legitimately be interfered with in pursuing his conception of his happiness in whatever way seems best to him, provided that in doing so he does not himself violate human dignity. A man is not deprived of his right to life, liberty, and the pursuit of happiness by preventing him from taking away the lives and liberty of others, or interfering with their pursuit of happiness, even if that can only be done at the cost of his life or liberty. An inalienable right may be forfeited. Nor does one violate another's human dignity by forcibly preventing him from killing himself, or destroying his own capacity to lead a human life. But no human being has the right to impose on another his view of that other's happiness, or of how that other's happiness may best be promoted. Paul Ramsey has drawn the corollary for medical practice, by adapting a saying of Lincoln: "No man is good enough to cure another without his consent" (Ramsey 1970, p. 7).

For this reason, no physician in the Western moral tradition has ever questioned that for a physician to lay hands on a patient's body (to "touch" him, in legal parlance) in any way to which that patient has not consented is wrong. Common lawyers call that wrong "assault and battery." The legal principle was stated in a celebrated opinion of Chief Judge Cardozo: "Every human being of adult years and sound mind has a right to determine what shall be done with his own body; and a surgeon who performs an operation without his patient's consent, commits an assault, for which he is liable in damages" (*Schloendorff* v. *New York Hospital* 105 N.E. 92; N.Y. 1914). As Marcus L. Plant has put it, in a magisterial article, "It is the patient's prerogative to accept medical treatment or take his chances of living without it" (Plant 1968, p. 650).

Yet although physicians seem never to have disputed this important principle, as the case of *Moore* v. *Webb* discussed above shows, some of them were slow to grasp its implications. By merely consulting a physician, and not discontinuing treatment, a patient does not confer on that physician the right to administer whatever treatment he judges best. Before embarking on any course of treatment, a physician must secure his patient's consent to it; and he cannot secure consent unless he informs his patient, in words that patient can understand, of the nature and character of the course of treatment proposed. The most frequent complaints of patients in civil actions against physicians for battery have not been that treatment was administered without consent, or that their consent was obtained by outright misrepresentation, but rather that they were not informed of important parts of what would be done (e.g., that the patient was informed of what would be done to his prostate, but not that, in order to do it, his spermatic cords would be severed and tied off), or that they were informed in technical or ambiguous language they did not understand (e.g., that the patient was told that a mastectomy would be peformed, but did not understand that mastectomy is the removal of a breast). It is now generally conceded that, if any such complaint is true in fact, the physician has committed a grave wrong. And a physician is simply not competent if he is unable to describe, in words intelligible to his patients, everything that could matter to them as patients about the character of any course of treatment he proposes.

Avoidance of battery, however, is not enough to satisfy the principle of consent. For, in deciding whether or not to consent to a proposed course of treatment, a patient will certainly want to take into account any hazards that may be collateral to administering the proposed treatment. But here a difficulty arises. Nobody questions that good medical practice may require a physician to be reticent in discussing a patient's condition with him, if telling the full truth may disturb the patient needlessly and perhaps jeopardize his recovery. Many physicians conceived this duty of reticence to extend to what they should tell certain patients, especially those liable to be very disturbed by it, of hazards collateral to treatments proposed. And when Plant wrote on the subject, medical and legal opinion were in agreement that what information about collateral hazards a physician is called upon to divulge to a patient is a matter of expert medical judgment (see Plant 1968, p. 656; Mills 1974, p. 307).

A very little reflection will show that, in a

physician-patient relation in which the patient decides upon the course of treatment proposed by the physician, this agreed opinion was muddled. Having conceded that, except in emergencies, it is for a responsible adult patient to decide whether or not he is to receive any proposed course of treatment, it is inconsistent to allow that he may be refused information essential to forming an intelligent judgment on the question. Indeed, for a physician to assume the right to conceal a certain hazard is to make that hazard count for nothing in the patient's deliberations, and so in part to usurp the prerogative to decide. Unless a physician is prepared to maintain that his patient is no longer responsible, and the public is rightly becoming reluctant to accept a physician's word on that, the patient has a right to all the information he needs to make a judgment.

Nor is it for the physician to decide what that information is. It is true, and as far as I know undisputed, that only a medical expert is qualified to judge what benefits are to be hoped for from a proposed treatment, and their probability, and what evils are to be feared, and their probability. Having reached a scientific conclusion on these questions, he will then try to judge what values and disvalues his patient would reasonably assign to the respective probabilities that those hopes and those fears will be realized, and will recommend a course of treatment accordingly. However, the judgment he makes as to what values and disvalues a patient ought to assign to those probabilities is patently not an exercise of his medical expertise. The surgeon general is within his medical province in informing us that cigarette smoking imperils our health; but he would not be if he were to add that we ought to account that peril of more weight than satisfying our craving to smoke. Again, simplifying a set of cases that have been litigated: a physician is within his medical province in advising his patient that while a serious prostate ailment can be cured by a certain treatment with 90 percent probability, there is a 20 percent probability that a collateral result will be infertility or diminished sexual capacity; but it is as a man, and not as a medical expert, that he proceeds to judge that the high probability of the cure hoped for should outweigh the low probability of the collateral harm that is feared.

It is for the patient, not for the physician, to decide such questions, although most patients give a good deal of weight to their physician's advice.

It follows that, as a U.S. Appellate Court ruled in *Canterbury* v. *Spence* (464 F 2d 772, CA DC 1972): "The test for determining whether a particular peril may be divulged is its materiality to the patient's decision: all risks potentially affecting the decision must be unmasked" (quoted in Simonaitis 1973a; 1973b, p. 91). What is material to a patient's decision depends upon what values and disvalues *he* assigns to the respective probabilities of various possible outcomes of a proposed course of treatment, and not on those his physician thinks ought to be assigned to them. For example, different patients will assign very different disvalues to slight chances of death or serious disability, and they have the right to act on those they assign.

As these complexities became apparent, even physicians who advocated the principle of informed consent began to speak of "the fallacy [of] . . . uncritically accepting [informed consent] as an easily attainable goal, whereas it is often beyond our full grasp" (Beecher 1962, p. 145). Those less favorable to the principle derided it as irksome, superfluous, and often gratuitously distressing (e.g., Burnham 1966), and even as calculated to empty surgeons' consulting rooms (Irvin 1963). Both reactions agree that the principle of informed consent cannot be a binding practical principle, but at best is an ideal to be approximated. To the extent that a principle is morally binding, it must be capable of being observed.

But can the principle of informed consent not be so formulated as to be capable of being observed? Is it not a logical development of the perfectly orthodox doctrine of the physician-patient relationship set out by Guttentag?

That an exact and applicable doctrine of informed consent is possible was soon demonstrated by the activities of courts in developing one. And so, in part from investigations of their problems with malpractice suits, physicians began to work out a practicable professional principle. Sober discussions such as those of Mills have largely established that there is "a line of reasonable disclosure . . . that is consistent with good medical practice and that affords reasonable legal safety'' (Mills 1974, p. 307; cf. Meisel 1975, Mills 1975). And this line is morally as well as legally obligatory. The principal difficulty discerned by Beecher in requiring informed consent is that the physician often does not know all the collateral risks incurred in undergoing a certain treatment. Experimenters are necessarily even more in the dark than therapists. Since physicians can only be required to do what they can do, the principle of informed consent cannot be interpreted as requiring them to provide all the information whatever that would be material to a patient's decision, but only all the information at the disposal of a competent practitioner, and any special knowledge they may have acquired themselves. They can also be required to inform their patients that, medicine being an inexact science, there is a small chance in any radical treatment of grave unforeseeable collateral effects, and that there may also be unforeseeable contingencies with harmful results.

In twenty years time it is predictable that cases such as *Canterbury v. Spence* will be perceived as no more than registering a logical development in medical practice arising from a distinction physicians had already drawn between their province as scientific practitioners and their province as medical advisers. It has, after all, been in no small part through the educative efforts of physicians that patients have been learning that they must accept ultimate responsibility for whatever courses of treatment they undergo, and that they cannot blame their physicians when risks they decide to take become realities.

A recently reported "clinicosociologic" conference perhaps allows us a glimpse of the view that will prevail in the future. The case was discussed of an eighty-six-year-old lady, who was able to communicate with her physicians and supply an accurate medical history, but who because of failures of memory had assigned legal responsibility for her affairs to a guardian. She was found to have an asymptomatic abdominal aortic aneurysm. The rupture of such an aneurysm is immediately fatal, if complete, and fatal within hours to days if partial. Often, however, it can be prevented surgically, by elective aneurysm replacement.

The physician, after telephoning a surgeon, decided that the risks of such surgery were too great and recommended against it. His recommendation was discussed with the guardian and accepted, but not with the patient. Six months later the aneurysm partially ruptured, and, in the emergency room, a different surgeon discussed with her what should be done, making clear the risks of surgery, now very much greater. Despite those risks, she chose it. The guardian could not be reached. Thirty hours after surgery she died. Two remarks on the case by Dr. Gerald Perkoff are of great interest. On the initial decision not to operate, he said: "[I]t was a mistake not to have operated earlier when she was well. . . . Had this patient interacted personally with the surgeon at the time of her first visit, it clearly would have been preferable. . . . Either the internist or the surgeon, or both, should have insisted upon a consultation visit" (Cryer and Kissane 1976, p. 918). What matters here is less Perkoff's disagreement with the original physician's recommendation than his insistence that the patient should have been given the opportunity to decide. And on the second, and fatal, decision to operate, he said: "[T]he question I asked myself . . . is "Can a physician do other than treat a patient if the patient is completely informed and desires treatment?" The answer I gave was that there is no other choice but to treat such a patient" (Cryer and Kissane 1976, p. 918).

INFORMED CONSENT TO EXPERIMENTATION

Therapeutic medicine is inescapably experimental: for, since no two patients are medically identical, even in a case in which prognosis after treatment is regarded as unproblematic, every physician ought to be alert should *this* one, after all, turn out to be exceptional. However, even when, with his informed consent, a highly risky treatment is administered to a patient, in therapeutic experimentation the end that determines whether or not that treatment is administered is the patient's good. That, incidentally, it may advance medical science, and so presumably benefit many human beings in the future, is a secondary and nondetermining consideration.

Medical science advanced rapidly in the past century because the haphazard experimentation inseparable from any intelligently administered medical treatment was supplemented by systematic experimentation, more or less well designed. Some of it was abhorrent. For example, valuable results on the transmission of venereal diseases were obtained by methods differing from the abominations punished at Nuremberg only in scale and in that the wretched subjects were procured by deceit rather than by force (Veressayev 1916; Pulvertaft 1952). But such cases were a minority. The great nineteenth-century authority, Claude Bernard, both preached and practiced, as "the principle of medical morality," that one is "never to carry out on a human being an experiment that cannot but be injurious to him in some degree, even if the outcome could be of great interest to science, that is to say, the health of other human beings" (quoted in McCance, 1950; from Ladimer and Newman 1963, p. 72). However, in Walter Reed's classic experimental investigation at Havana in 1900 of how yellow fever is transmitted, and in subsequent experiments by Richard P. Strong in the Philippines on plague and beriberi, it was held permissible to carry out procedures that could be nothing but harmful, provided that the subjects were volunteers. In these experiments there was no question of carrying out any procedure known to be gravely harmful or lethal; but procedures were permitted that could not but have been harmful to some degree, and that could have been gravely harmful or lethal, and sometimes were (see Lasagna 1969, pp. 449–52).

In this paper, it is assumed that a human being is entitled to volunteer the use of his body for at least some risky experiments (see previous section). Hence it will also be assumed that the genuine consent of human subjects to risky experiments for which they are entitled to volunteer is a sufficient condition of the moral permissibility of those experiments. But whether it is also a necessary condition has been questioned, in view of the magnitude of the benefits to mankind at large of the experiments

of Reed, Strong, and others. Is it wrong to sacrifice the health of a few, or even their lives, for the sake of the lives and health of the many, both now and in the future?

At the Nuremberg trials, the defense recognized that if the voluntary consent of the human subjects to an experiment is essential to its legal permissibility, as the tribunal ultimately ruled that it is (*Trials, Nuremberg*, 2:181–82), then the case for the defendants was hopeless. And so it had no choice but to argue that such consent is not legally essential. The argument for this position by Dr. Robert Servatius, on behalf of Dr. Karl Brandt, although primarily legal, is of very great ethical interest (*Trials, Nuremberg*, 2:126–130). Its cardinal points were three. (1) A state may demand a sacrifice from an individual on behalf of the community; and decisions as to what the interests of the community are, what those interests require, and how great a sacrifice may be demanded are all to be made by the state alone. (2) There are no pertinent valid distinctions to be drawn between conscripting somebody for military service, ordering somebody to drop an atomic bomb, and requiring somebody to submit to medical experimentation. (3) In the history of medicine, numerous experiments have been carried out on human beings without their informed consent; and "looking through the medical literature, one cannot escape the growing conviction that the word 'volunteer,' where it appears at all, is used only as a word of protection and camouflage" (*Trials, Nuremberg*, 2:128).

The most embarrassing of Servatius's three points, namely, 3, morally tended to support the prosecution. It is true that numerous experiments have been carried out by physicians on unconsenting human beings, but for most of the present century at least, they have been the shame of medicine. And even if the word "volunteer" in the report of an experiment is for protection and camouflage, that only shows that camouflage was thought necessary—and why should it have been, unless it was acknowledged that to experiment on a human being without his consent is wrong? It should be added that Servatius seems to have been mistaken as to the facts. Although there are strong objections to some of the kinds of volunteers that have been used as subjects in the United States—for example, imprisoned or condemned criminals—there is also good evidence that most of them have genuinely been volunteers (see Katz 1972, pp. 1020–26, 1028–34).

Servatius's first two points, however, are in no way weakened by the failure of his third. Yet they are formulated in terms of a political theory that is anathema to those who uphold classical Western, that is nonstatist, political theories, and the conceptions of the human good that go with them. But it is plain that his first point would be unaffected as an argument against the requirement of consent had he spoken of a genuinely democratic society instead of *a* state, and of the institutions of a genuinely democratic society instead of *the* state. Genuinely democratic societies have been known to compel unwelcome actions in the name of social goods, although not always the same goods as those in the name of which undemocratic societies have acted.

A second adjustment that must be made in order fairly to appraise Servatius's arguments is to separate their appraisal from all the circumstances of the Nuremberg medical case not directly relevant to them. As I read the published volumes, most if not all the accused would justly have been condemned even had the necessity of consent not been affirmed by the tribunal, on the ground that the scientific incompetence of some of the experimental designs, and the nonmedical purposes of others, would have left no choice but to pronounce the experimenters guilty of gratuitous killing, mutilating, and other forms of injury (*Trials, Nuremberg,* 1:73–74; see also Alexander 1949). There is every reason to suppose that, even if the first two points in Servatius's argument were to be accepted, modifying them according to a less obnoxious political theory, the number of sanctioned dangerous experiments would be comparatively few, as would the number of deaths and serious injuries caused by them.

Once they have been sanitized in this way, Servatius's two points are not shocking at all, academically at least: they are straightforward applications of a disputed but academically respectable doctrine, namely, utilitarianism in its generalized form, according to which what is right is defined as what is for the greatest *good* of the greatest number. (Its most familiar specific form is the hedonistic one of Bentham and Mill, in which good is identified with happiness.) Hence it is not surprising that, during the very period in which the organized medical profession was preparing to reaffirm at Helsinki the Nuremberg principle of informed consent, many individual physicians were concluding that that principle need not be observed in responsibly conducted scientific experimentation. What the Nuremberg tribunal really condemned, they appear to have thought, was not experimentation without informed consent, but only atrocious experimentation. Indeed, in 1962, in a passage endorsed by Beecher himself, Walter Modell wrote: "I . . . think that when society confers the degree of physician on a man it instructs him to experiment on his fellow. I think that when a patient goes to a physician for treatment, regardless of whether he consents to it, he is also unconsciously presenting himself for the purpose of experimentation" (Modell 1962, p. 146).

What happens when those who thus unconsciously present themselves for experimentation become conscious of it was demonstrated in the Jewish Chronic Diseases Hospital Case, which began less than two years after Modell wrote. (For documentation, see Katz 1972, pp. 9–65.) That case is particularly important, because the experiment involved was perfectly harmless and was from a scientific point of view admirably conducted. The facts of the case pertinent to the present study are as follows. In the summer of 1963, at the request of an outside cancer research institute, the medical director of the hospital agreed to permit physicians from the institute to inject into twenty-two patients suspensions of cells obtained from cultures of human cancer tissue, in order to determine the mechanism and rate of rejection of the injected material by debilitated but noncancerous subjects. It was asserted by the experimenters that spoken consent was obtained from the subjects, but it was not disputed that the subjects were not told that what was to be injected contained cancer cells. The reason given for this reticence was that, although the experiment was neither harmful nor hazardous, if the dread word "cancer" had been used the subjects would have been misled and unnecessarily distressed. Ultimately, the medical director of the hospital and the principal investigator were found by the Board of Regents of the University of the State of New York (which has jurisdiction over all licensed professions excluding that of law) to be guilty of fraud and deceit in the practice of medicine.

Much sympathy was rightly expressed for the physicians thus censured. For they had acted in good conscience, even if erroneously; and they had done nothing different in kind from what many others had done or advocated. And some sympathizers went further. Had the censured physicians not achieved a significant if modest scientific result, at the cost of no harm to anybody beyond a temporary mild discomfort? Why then should the attorney general for New York, in a memorandum to the Board of Regents, have written as though he was addressing the Nuremberg tribunal (Katz 1972, pp. 44–48)?

The answer emerges from what the defenders of experimentation without informed consent wrote in the years that followed; for it became evident that, if from excusing what was done in the Jewish Chronic Diseases Hospital Case (which they seldom mentioned, although they cannot but have had it in mind) they were to pass on to justifying it, they would have no option but to present a sanitized version of the defense offered by Servatius at Nuremberg.

With exemplary courage, a number of them did so. The most forthright was Walsh McDermott, in some "Opening Comments" that have already outlived the 1967 Colloquium they introduced. He put forward a democratic version of Servatius's first point in these words: "... as a society we enforce the social good over the individual good across a whole spectrum of nonmedical activities every day, and many of these activities ultimately affect the health or the life of an individual.... [W]hen the conflict is head on, when the group interest and the individual interest are basically irreconcilable ... we try to depersonalize the process by spreading responsibility for decision throughout a framework of legal institutions"

(McDermott 1967, p. 39). It should be noticed that McDermott acknowledged that "we" only "try to depersonalize" this process, without noting that those societies that have succeeded are unappealing as models.

He also enriched Servatius's second point with an additional example of a head-on conflict between individual interest and social interest that is resolved according to the latter, namely, "the decision to impose capital punishment" (McDermott 1967, p. 39). But, in declaring that situations in clinical medicine "in which it clearly seems to be in the best interests of society that [certain scientific] information be obtained ... [which] can be obtained only from studies on certain already unlucky individuals" belong to the same "hard core" of cases as situations requiring military conscription or capital punishment, he did not substantially differ from Servatius (McDermott 1967, p. 40).

The same two points recur in papers by Guido Calabresi, Louis L. Jaffe, and Louis Lasagna, which arose out of conferences arranged by the American Academy of Arts and Sciences, and were published in *Daedalus* for Spring 1969. Calabresi, indeed, furnished yet another example of Servatius's second point: "Many activities are permitted, even though *statistically* we know they will lose lives, since it costs too much to engage in these activities more safely, or to abstain from them altogether" (Calabresi 1969, p. 387). All three followed McDermott in concluding that, in the Helsinki Declaration, and in subsequent promulgations by such bodies as the U.S. Food and Drug Administration and the National Institutes of Health, our society either has mistaken the nature of its own morality, as evidenced by the practices it sanctions, or is hypocritical. Its error or hypocrisy ought to be corrected by repudiating the requirement of informed consent. But even when that correction has been made, the problem will remain of how nonvolunteer research subjects are to be obtained. At this point Jaffe assured his readers that his argument was not "the ominous prolegomenon to a program for conscripting human guinea pigs" (Jaffe 1969, p. 407), and those who accept the utilitarian argument would probably do the same. Calabresi, for example, declared that right-minded scholars "ought to be devoting themselves to the development of a workable but not too obvious control system . . . " (Calabresi 1969, p. 405). Jaffe himself looked to developments in the common law. Lasagna appeared to imagine that all would be well if physicians and public alike would only embrace situation ethics.[2] None made any significant advance upon McDermott's ironical conclusion: "Obviously we cannot convene a constitutional convention of the Judaeo-Christian culture and add a few amendments to it. Yet, in a figurative sense, unless we can do something very much like that . . . the problem, at its roots, is unsolvable and we must continue to live with it" (McDermott 1967, p. 41; cf. McDermott 1970).

It is regrettable that these distinguished physicians and lawyers should have assumed that generalized utilitarianism is the only moral position pertinent to examining the cases which, according to their second point, are of the same kind as the "hard core" ones in medical experimentation. It is true by definition that, from the point of view of generalized utilitarianism, the only thing that counts in settling any moral question is what would be for the greatest good of the greatest number. But there are other moral positions, among them the Judaeo-Christian one, according to which a variety of nonutilitarian considerations may count.

Setting aside Servatius's case of dropping an atomic bomb on a city, on the ground that it is dubious whether that is permissible on either utilitarian or Judaeo-Christian grounds, let us consider the cases offered by Servatius, McDermott, and Calabresi. In the Judaeo-Christian moral tradition, it is held permissible for a civil society to attach penal sanctions to its laws, in extreme cases even the sanction of death, without ceasing to treat the persons so punished as ends; for when laws themselves have a moral sanction, to punish those who break them in itself treats them as genuinely responsible for their deeds. Punishment is not inflicted primarily for deterrence or reformation, but as what the criminal deserves. Again, in compelling citizens to serve in a just war on threat of punishment, a civil society only com-

pels them to uphold a good common to them all, and not primarily the good of others. The very concept of a common good has fallen into disrepute partly because it has become confounded with the idea of the good of the many as opposed to that of the few. Even though the Judaeo-Christian tradition applauds a sacrifice by one man for his fellows, it utterly denies the right of his fellows, no matter how many, to compel that sacrifice (see Ramsey 1970, pp. 28, 107–8). Finally, while certain kinds of laxity in safety regulations are morally objectionable, for example, allowing a machine tended by human beings to be used when it is only a question of time when it will blow up, other kinds are not, for example, allowing the use of a machine that would be dangerous in the hands of an unskilled operator. Laxities of the latter kind, even when it is statistically predictable that some injuries will result, and not necessarily to the negligent operator, do not sacrifice the few to the many: they merely allow, without compelling, many to risk being among the few. Hence, from a Judaeo-Christian point of view, securing nonvolunteer subjects for medical research is *not* an action of the same kind as conscripting for military service, imposing capital punishment, or tolerating certain kinds of risky activities: they have nonutilitarian justifications, it does not.

And so we come to the first point. If a piece of medical research would be for the greatest good of the greatest number, then according to generalized utilitarianism, nonvolunteer subjects may be procured for it by one or other of the only two possible methods: lawful compulsion as in the Nuremberg case, or deception as in the Jewish Chronic Diseases Hospital case. Is this justification of those methods acceptable?

The consensus reached by the organized medical profession is that it is not acceptable. And, in a case study such as this, that is the principal thing to be said. Among physicians, "there is essentially no valid argument about the basic principle that informed consent—or whatever may be its legal equivalent in a specialized situation—is a prerequisite for human experimentation" (Edsall 1969, p. 468). They recognize that they have neither legal nor moral authority to compel non-volunteers to be experimental subjects; and the great majority of them would repudiate, as unprofessional, any suggestion that they experiment on conscripts provided by the state. And most of them now agree that it is equally inadmissible to procure experimental subjects by deception, whether by misrepresentation or by withholding information those subjects would consider material.

It is not disputed that observing the requirement of informed consent may delay otherwise desirable scientific progress. But David D. Rutstein's doctrine is now widely accepted that "ethical constraints that prohibit certain human experiments are similar in their effects as are scientific constraints on the design of experiments" (Rutstein 1969, p. 529). To use his example, in research on infectious hepatitis, it is a scientific constraint that no laboratory animal has been found that is susceptible to hepatitis, in which the large quantities of the virus needed for vaccine manufacture can be grown, and it is an ethical constraint that "it is not ethical to use human subjects for the growth of a virus for any purpose" (Rutstein 1969, p. 529).

Hermann L. Blumgart has succinctly formulated the accepted reason why the requirement of informed consent must be satisfied, and it is the familiar Judaeo-Christian one: "To use a person for an experiment without his consent is untenable; the advance of science may be retarded, but more important values are at stake" (Blumgart 1969, p. 256). Preeminent among those values is respecting the autonomy of potential experimental subjects. The decision whether or not they are to participate can only be theirs. Admittedly, invading their autonomy may be good for science and good for most people. But, in Beecher's words, "a particularly pernicious myth is the one that depends on the view that ends justify means. A study is ethical or not at its inception. It does not become ethical merely because it turned up valuable data. Sometimes such a view is rationalized by the investigator as having produced the most good for the most people. This is blatant statism. Whoever gave the investigator the god-like right to choose martyrs?" (Beecher 1966a, pp. 34-35). He might have added that those who fancy they are playing God are nearly always possessed by devils.

RETROSPECT

The history has been outlined of two cases in which the medical profession confronted a conflict between a supposed moral constraint on professional practice and the attainment of two of its supposed ends—the health of each patient, and the health of the community at large. In both, the issue was between conceptions of moral duty, that on the one side being based on unconditional respect for persons as ends, each of those on the other alleging a requirement that a certain producible good be maximized: in the first, an individual good; in the second, a universal or "utilitarian" one. For both of the latter "consequentialist" positions appeal was made to ends that have important places in the practice of medicine. Hence both were perceived at once to have serious claims to acceptance, and were ably defended.

The history of how the conflict between the anticonsequentialist position and its consequentialist rivals was resolved is of the greatest interest to moral philosophy. From the beginning, physicians were forced to consider what is implicit in the traditional—and imperfectly understood—relation between physician and patient on which medical morality ultimately depends, and to investigate whether what on the surface seem plainly to be ultimate ends of medicine—in therapy, the health of the individual patient, and in experimentation, the health of the community at large—can justify weakening the commitment to respect for human beings that was more and more seen to underlie the traditional physician-patient relation. The result, as we have seen, was the reaffirmation of the less obvious position. The doctrine was repudiated that admittedly good consequences can justify attaining them by means in which the respect owed to human beings as such is violated. And in the process, the "common moral knowledge" implicit in the best traditional medical practice was consciously formulated as a general truth. There was a transition from common moral knowledge to knowledge of the kind Kant called "philosophical."

As Kant recognized, any such transition raises further philosophical problems. Having identified the ethical principles that are the foundation of a certain part of our common moral knowledge, we must go on to investigate the nature of those principles and how they are justified—to construct what he called a "metaphysic of morals," that is, a philosophical theory of morality.

And a further problem can be discerned. The moral principle implicit in the traditional conception of the physician-patient relationship rests on the conception of all human beings as autonomous ends in themselves, whose existence is beyond price. But do the theoretical medical sciences regard human beings in that way? Do they not rather lead to the concept of man which William James called "medical materialism"? If so, can these two points of view be reconciled? Or is medicine afflicted with multiple personality? But that is for another study.

Notes

1. The ancient text of the Hippocratic oath, in which, e.g., the physician forswears surgery, differs from later Christian versions of it (see Sigerist 1961, 2:301–4). Ludwig Edelstein (1943) has established that its origin was Pythagorean. The heart of all versions of it, however, is that the physician is to act "in purity and holiness" solely for the benefit of the sick, and never to their harm.
2. That there can be such a thing as "situation ethics" as opposed to "rule ethics" is a gross error, which has a common ancestry with the discredited educational fallacy that there is such a thing as "teaching children" as opposed to "teaching subjects." Any rational system of moral rules has to do with how human beings ought to act in different situations, and, when from a moral point of view situations differ relevantly, it must treat them differently. But this in no way entails that there are not kinds of action that are wrong in all situations, e.g., murder—accurately defined to exclude such justifiable forms of homicide as self-defense. The contention that experimenting on a responsible adult

human being without his consent is wrong in all situations entails neither that all situations should be treated in the same way nor that there are no situations in which it is permissible to experiment on a human being without his consent—e.g., certain kinds of situations, not discussed in this paper, in which responsibility is impaired. While conceding too much to doctrines of situation ethics fashionable at the time, Fletcher (1967) indirectly brings out how little doubt "situational" approaches throw on the requirement of informed consent. See also Ramsey (1970, p. 6n.), and, for a devastating general criticism of situation ethics, his *Deeds and Rules in Christian Ethics* (1967).

References

ALEXANDER, LEO. "Medical Science under Dictatorship." *New England Journal of Medicine*, vol. 241 (1949); excerpts from pp. 39, 43 in Katz (1972), p. 302.

American Medical Association. *Opinions and Reports of the Judicial Council*. Chicago: American Medical Association, 1964. In Katz (1972), pp. 313–14.

BEECHER, HENRY K. "Experimentation in Man." *Journal of the American Medical Association* 169 (1959): 461–78.

BEECHER, HENRY K. "Some Fallacies and Errors in the Application of the Principle of Consent in Human Experimentation." *Clinical Pharmacology and Therapeutics* 3 (1962): 141–45.

BEECHER, HENRY K. "Consent in Clinical Experimentation: Myth and Reality." *Journal of the American Medical Association* 195 (1966): 34–35. (a) Excerpts in Katz (1972), pp. 583, 638.

BEECHER, HENRY K. "Ethics and Clinical Research," *New England Journal of Medicine* 274 (1966): 1354–60. (b) Reprinted in *Biomedical Ethics and the Law*, edited by J. M. Humber and Robert F. Almeder. New York: Plenum Press, 1976. Page references to the latter. Excerpts in Katz (1972), pp. 307–10.

BLUMGART, HERRMAN L. "The Medical Framework for Viewing the Problem of Human Experimentation." *Daedalus* (Spring 1969), pp. 248–74.

BURNHAM, PRESTON J. "Medical Experimentation in Humans." *Science* 152 (1966): 448–50. Excerpts in Katz (1972), pp. 658–59.

CALABRESI, GUIDO. "Reflections on Medical Experimentation in Humans." *Daedalus* (Spring 1969), pp. 387–405. Reprinted in Freund (1970).

CRYER, PHILIP E., and KISSANE, JOHN M., eds.

"Clinicosociologic Conference: Decisions regarding the Provision or Withholding of Therapy." *American Journal of Medicine* 61 (1976): 915–23.

EDELSTEIN, LUDWIG. *The Hippocratic Oath.* Baltimore: Johns Hopkins Press, 1943.

EDSALL, GEOFFREY. "A Positive Approach to the Problem of Human Experimentation." *Daedalus* (Spring 1969), pp. 463–79. Excerpt in Katz (1972), p. 559.

FLETCHER, JOHN. "Human Experimentation: Ethics in the Consent Situation." *Law and Contemporary Problems* 32 (1967): 620–49.

FREUND, PAUL A., ed. *Experimentation with Human Subjects.* New York: George Braziller, Inc., 1970.

GUTTENTAG, OTTO E. "The Problem of Experimentation on Human Beings: The Physician's Point of View." *Science* 117 (1953): 206–10. In Ladimer and Newman (1963), pp. 63–69. Excerpts in Katz (1972), pp. 918–19.

IRVIN, WILLIAM J. "Now, Mrs. Blare, about the Complications . . . ." *Medical Economics* 40 1963): 102–8. Excerpts in Katz (1972), pp. 393–94.

JAFFE, LOUIS L. "Law as a System of Control." *Daedalus* (Spring 1969), pp. 406–26. Reprinted in Freund (1970). Excerpts in Katz (1972), pp. 721–22, 929–30, 1040.

KANT, IMMANUEL. *Grundlegung zur Metaphysik der Sitten.* 2d ed. Riga: J. F. Hartknoch, 1786.

KATZ, JAY. *Experimentation with Human Beings.* New York: Russell Sage Foundation, 1972.

LADIMER, IRVING, and NEWMAN, ROGER W. *Clinical Investigation in Medicine.* Boston: Law-Medicine Research Institute, Boston University, 1963.

LASAGNA, LOUIS L. "Special Subjects in Human Experimentation." *Daedalus* (Spring 1969), pp. 449–62. Reprinted in Freund (1970). Excerpt in Katz (1972), p. 381.

McCANCE, R. A. "The Practice of Experimental Medicine." *Proceedings of the Royal Society of Medicine* 44 (1950): 189–94. In Ladimer and Newman (1963), pp. 48–57.

McDERMOTT, WALSH. "Opening Comments to Colloquium: The Changing Mores of Biomedical Research." *Annals of Internal Medicine* 67, suppl. 7 (1967): 39–42. Excerpts in Katz (1972), pp. 316–18.

McDERMOTT, WALSH. "Comment on [Jaffe]. 'Law as a system of Control.' " In *Experimentation with Human Subjects,* edited by Paul A. Freund. New York: George Braziller, Inc., 1970. Excerpts in Katz (1972), pp. 926–27, 931.

MEISEL, ALAN. "Informed Consent—the Rebuttal." *Journal of the American Medical Association* 234 (1975): 615.

MILLS, DON HARPER. "Whither Informed Consent?" *Journal of the American Medical Association* 229 (1974): 305–10.

MILLS, DON HARPER. "Informed Consent—the Rejoinder." *Journal of the American Medical Association* 234 (1975): 616.

MODELL, WALTER. "Let Each New Patient Be a Complete Experience." *Journal of the American Medical Association* 174 (1960): 1717–19. In Ladimer and Newman (1963), pp. 73–78. Excerpt in Katz (1972), pp. 826–27.

MODELL, WALTER. "Comment [on Beecher 1962]." *Clinical Pharmacology and Therapeutics* 3 (1962): 145–46. Excerpt in Katz (1972), p. 316.

PIUS XII. "Address to the First International Conference on the Histopathology of the Nervous System, September 14, 1952." *Acta Apostolicae Sedis* 44 (1952): 779. Translated in Ladimer and Newman (1963), pp. 276–86.

PLANT, MARCUS L. "An Analysis of 'Informed Consent.' " *Fordham Law Review* 36 (1968): 639–72. Excerpts in Katz (1972), pp. 599–600.

PULVERTAFT, R. J. V. "The Individual and the Group in Modern Medicine." *Lancet,* vol. 2 (1952). Excerpts in Katz (1972), pp. 291, 707, 825.

RAMSEY, PAUL. *Deeds and Rules in Christian Ethics.* New York: Charles Scribner's Sons, 1967.

RAMSEY, PAUL. *The Patient as Person: Explorations in Medical Ethics.* New Haven, Conn.: Yale University Press, 1970.

RUTSTEIN, DAVID D. "The Ethical Design of Human Experiments." *Daedalus* (Spring 1969), pp. 523–41. Excerpts in Katz (1972), pp. 906–7.

SIGERIST, HENRY E. *A History of Medicine.* New York: Oxford University Press, 1961.

SIMONAITIS, JOSEPH E. "More about Informed Consent, Part I," *Journal of the American Medical Association* 224 (1973): 1831–32. (*a*)

SIMONAITIS, JOSEPH E. "More about Informed Consent, Part II." *Journal of the American Medical Association* 225 (1973): 91. (*b*)

SZASZ, THOMAS S., AND HOLLENDER, MARC H. "A Contribution to the Philosophy of Medicine—the Basic Models of the Doctor-Patient Relationship," *Archives of Internal Medicine,* vol. 97 (1956). Excerpts from pp. 585–87 in Katz (1972), pp. 229–30.

Trials of War Criminals at the Nuernberg Military Tribunals under Control Council Law No. 10. Vols.

1-2, "The Medical Case," Neurnberg, October 1946–April 1949. Washington, D.C.: Government Printing Office, n.d. (Cited as *Trials, Nuremberg*.) Excerpts in Katz (1972), pp. 292-306.

VERESSAYEV, VIKENTY. *The Memoirs of a Physician.* Translated by Simeon Linden. New York: Alfred A. Knopf, Inc., 1916. Excerpts in Katz (1972), pp. 284-91.

Tests of Competency to Consent to Treatment

Loren H. Roth, Alan Meisel, and Charles W. Lidz

The concept of competency, like the concept of dangerousness, is social and legal and not merely psychiatric or medical.[1] Law and, at times, psychiatry are concerned with an individual's competency to stand trial, to make a will, and to contract.[2-5] The test of competency varies from one context to another. In general, to be considered competent an individual must be able to comprehend the nature of the particular conduct in question and to understand its quality and its consequences.[3, 6] For example, in *Dusky v. United States* the court held that to be considered competent to stand trial an individual must have "sufficient present ability to consult with his lawyer with a reasonable degree of rational understanding—and . . . a rational as well as a factual understanding of the proceedings against him."[7] A person may be considered competent for some legal purposes and incompetent for others at the same time.[3] An individual is not judged incompetent merely because he or she is mentally ill.[6]

There is a dearth of legal guidance illuminating the concept of competency to consent to medical treatment.[8-11] Nevertheless, competency plays an important role in determining the validity of a patient's decision to undergo or forego treatment. The decision of a person who is incompetent does not validly authorize a physician to perform medical treat-

From *The American Journal of Psychiatry*, vol. 134:4, pp. 279-284, 1977. Copyright 1977, the American Psychiatric Association. Reprinted by permission of the author and the American Psychiatric Association.

ment.[12] Conversely, a physician who withholds treatment from an incompetent patient who refuses treatment may be held liable to that patient if the physician does not take reasonable steps to obtain some other legally valid authorization for treatment.[13]

In psychiatry the entire edifice of involuntary treatment is erected on the supposed incompetency of some people to voluntarily seek and consent to needed treatment.[14] In addition, the acceptability of behavior modification for the patient who is considered dangerous,[15] the resolution of ethical issues in family planning (i.e., sterilization),[16, 17] and the right to refuse psychoactive medications[18]—to cite only a few of the more prominent examples—turn in part on the concept of competency.

As we explain in our companion paper in this issue of the *Journal*,[19] competency is theoretically one of the independent variables that is determinative in part of the legal validity of a patient's consent to or refusal of treatment. There is therefore a need to specify how competency can be determined. Related questions include the following: Who raises the question of competency? When is this question raised? and Who makes the determination? Answers to these questions are beyond the scope of this paper.

The objective of the present inquiry is to make sense of various tests of competency, to analyze their applicability to patients' decisions to accept or refuse psychiatric treatment, and to illustrate the problems of applying these tests by clinical case examples from the consultation service of the Law and Psychiatry Program of Western Psychiatric Institute and Clinic.

In a brief presentation it is impossible to provide any serious linguistic analysis of a number of words that are frequently used in discussions of competency—words such as "responsible,"[20] "rational" or "irrational,"[21,22] "knowing,"[23, 24] "knowingly," (p. 99)[25] "understandingly,"[24] or "capable."[26] These words are often used interchangeably without sufficient explanation or clear behavioral referents. Only the rare scholarly article attempts to explain with precision what is meant by such terms;[11] judicial decisions or statutes generally do not.

In evaluating tests for competency several criteria should be considered. A useful test for competency is one that, first, can be reliably applied; second, is mutually acceptable or at least comprehensible to physicians, lawyers, and judges; and third, is set at a level capable of striking an acceptable balance between preserving individual autonomy and providing needed medical care. Reliability is enhanced to the extent that a competency test depends on manifest and objectively ascertainable patient behavior rather than on inferred and probably unknowable mental status.[6]

TESTS FOR COMPETENCY

Several tests for competency have been proposed in the literature; others are readily inferable from judicial commentary. Although there is some overlap, they basically fall into five categories: 1) evidencing a choice, 2) "reasonable" outcome of choice, 3) choice based on "rational" reasons, 4) ability to understand, and 5) actual understanding.

Evidencing a Choice

This test for competency is set at a very low level and is the most respectful of the autonomy of patient decision making.[10] Under this test the competent patient is one who evidences a preference for or against treatment. This test focuses not on the quality of the patient's decision but on the presence or absence of a decision. This preference may be a yes, a no, or even the desire that the physician make the

decision for the patient. Only the patient who does not evidence a preference either verbally or through his or her behavior is considered incompetent. This test of competency encompasses at a minimum the unconscious patient; in psychiatry it encompasses the mute patient who cannot or will not express an opinion.

Even such arch-defenders of individual autonomy as Szasz have agreed that patients who do not formulate and express a preference as to treatment are incompetent. In answer to a question about the right to intervene against a patient's will, Szasz has stated,

> It is quite obvious, and I make this abundantly clear, that I have no objection to medical intervention vis-à-vis persons who are not protesting, . . . [for example,] somebody who is lying in bed catatonic and the mother wants to get him to the hospital and the ambulance shows up and he just lies there.[27]

The following case example illustrates the use of the test of evidencing a choice:

> *Case 1.* A 41-year-old depressed woman was interviewed in the admission unit. She rarely answered yes or no to direct questions. Admission was proposed; she said and did nothing, but looked apprehensive. When asked about admission, she did not sign herself into the hospital, protest, or walk away. She was guided to the inpatient ward by her husband and her doctor after being given the opportunity to walk the other way.

This test may be what one court had in mind when, with respect to sterilization of residents of state schools, it ruled that even legally incompetent and possibly noncomprehending residents may not be sterilized unless they have formed a genuine desire to undergo the procedure.[28]

The guidelines proposed by the U.S. Department of Health, Education, and Welfare concerning experimentation with institutionalized mentally ill people also point in this direction by requiring even the legally incompetent person's "assent to such participation . . . when . . . he has sufficient mental capacity to understand what is proposed and to express an opinion as to his or her participation"[29], (at

46.504c). Although this low test of competency does not fully assure patient's understanding of the nature of what they consent to or what they refuse, it is behavioral in orientation and therefore more reliable in application; it also guards against excessive paternalism.

"Reasonable" Outcome of Choice

This test of competency entails evaluating the patient's capacity to reach the "reasonable," the "right," or the "responsible" decision.[10, 30] The emphasis in this test is on outcome rather than on the mere fact of decision or how it has been reached. The patient who fails to make a decision that is roughly congruent with the decision that a "reasonable" person in like circumstances would make is viewed as incompetent.

This test is probably used more often than might be admitted by both physicians and courts. Judicial decisions to override the desire of patients with certain religious beliefs not to receive blood transfusions may rest in part on the court's view that the patient's decision is not reasonable.[31] When life is at stake and a court believes that the patient's decision is unreasonable, the court may focus on even the smallest ambiguity in the patient's thinking to cast doubt on the patient's competency so that it may issue an order that will preserve life or health. For example, one judge issued an order to allow amputation of the leg of an elderly moribund man even though the man had clearly told his daughter before his condition deteriorated not to permit an amputation.[32, 33]

Mental health laws that allow for involuntary treatment on the basis of "need for care and treatment."[34] without requiring a formal adjudication of incompetency in effect use an unstated reasonable outcome test in abridging the patient's common-law right not to be treated without giving his or her consent. These laws are premised on the following syllogism: the patient needs treatment; the patient has not obtained treatment on his or her own initiative; therefore, the patient's decision is incorrect, which means that he or she is incompetent, thus justifying the involuntary imposition of treatment.

The benefits and costs of this test are that social goals and individual health are promoted at considerable expense to personal autonomy. The reasonable outcome test is useful in alerting physicians and courts to the fact that the patient's decision-making process may be, but not necessarily is, awry. Ultimately, because the test rests on the congruence between the patient's decision and that of a reasonable person or that of the physician, it is biased in favor of decisions to accept treatment, even when such decisions are made by people who are incapable of weighing the risks and benefits of treatment. In other words, if patients do not decide the "wrong" way, the issue of competency will probably not arise.

Choice Based on "Rational" Reasons

Another test is whether the reasons for the patient's decision are "rational," that is, whether the patient's decision is due to or is a product of mental illness.[10, 22] As in the reasonable outcome test, if the patient decides in favor of treatment the issue of the patient's competency (in this case, whether the decision is the product of mental illness) seldom if ever arises because of the medical profession's bias toward consent to treatment and against refusal of treatment.

In this test the quality of the patient's thinking is what counts. The following case example illustrates the use of the test of rational reasons:

Case 2. A 70-year-old widow who was living alone in a condemned dilapidated house with no heat was brought against her will to the hospital. Her thinking was tangential and fragmented. Although she did not appear to be hallucinating, she seemed delusional. She refused blood tests, saying, "You just want my blood to spread it all over Pittsburgh. No, I'm not giving it." Her choice was respected. Later in the day, however, when her blood pressure was found to be dangerously elevated (250 over 135 in both arms), blood was withdrawn against her will.

The test of rational reasons, although it has clinical appeal and is probably much in clinical use, poses considerable conceptual problems; as a legal test it is probably defective.[10] The problems include the difficulty of distinguishing rational from irrational reasons and drawing inferences of causation between any irrationality believed present and the valence (yes or no) of the patient's decision. Even if the patient's reasons seem irrational, it is not possible to prove that the patient's actual decision making has been the product of such irrationality. The patient's decision might well be the same even if his or her cognitive processes were less impaired. For example, a delusional patient may refuse ECT not because he or she is delusional but because he or she is afraid of it, which is considered a normal reaction. The emphasis on rational reasons can too easily become a global indictment of the competency of mentally disordered individuals, justifying widespread substitute decision making for this group.

The Ability to Understand

This test—the ability of the patient to understand the risks, benefits, and alternatives to treatment (including no treatment)—is probably the most consistent with the law of informed consent.[19] Decision making need not be rational in either process or outcome: unwise choices are permitted. Nevertheless, at a minimum the patient must manifest sufficient ability to understand information about treatment, even if in fact he or she weighs this information differently from the attending physician. What matters in this test is that the patient is able to comprehend the elements that are presumed by law to be a part of treatment decision making. How the patient weighs these elements, values them, or puts them together to reach a decision is not important.

The patient's capacity for understanding may be tested by asking the patient a series of questions concerning risks, benefits, and alternatives to treatment.[35] By providing further information or explanation to the patient, the physician may find deficiencies in understanding to be remediable or not.[36] The following case examples illustrate the use of the test of the ability to understand:

Case 3. A 28-year-old woman who was unresponsive to medication was approached for consent to ECT. She initially appeared to be unaware of the examiner. Following an explanation of ECT, she responded to the request to explain its purposes and why it was being recommended in her case with the statement, "Paul McCartney, nothing to zero." She was shown a consent form for ECT that she signed without reading. Further attempts to educate her were unsuccessful. It was decided not to perform the ECT without seeking court approval.

Case 4. A 44-year-old woman who was diagnosed as having chronic schizophrenia refused amputation of her frostbitten toes. She was nonpsychotic. Although her condition was evaluated psychiatrically as manifesting extreme denial, she understood what was proposed and that there was some risk of infection without surgery. Nevertheless, she declined. She stated, "You want to take my toes off; I want to keep them." Her decision was respected. She agreed to return to the hospital if things got worse. A month later she returned, having suffered an auto-amputation of the toes. There was no infection; she was rebandaged and sent home.

Some of the questions raised by this test of competency are, What is to be done if the patient can understand the risks but not the benefits or vice versa? Alternatively, what if the patient views the risks as the benefits? The following case example illustrates this problem:

Case 5. A 49-year-old woman whose understanding of treatment was otherwise intact, when informed that there was a 1 in 3,000 chance of dying from ECT, replied, "I hope I am the one."

Furthermore, how potentially sophisticated must understanding be in order that the patient be viewed as competent? There are considerable barriers, conscious and unconscious and intellectual and emotional,[37] to understanding proposed treatments. Presumably the potential understanding required is only that which would be manifested by a reasonable person provided a similar amount of information. A few attempts to rank degrees of understanding have been made.[38] However, this matter is highly complex and beyond the scope of the present inquiry. Certainly, at least with respect to nonexperimental treatment, the patient's potential understanding does not have to be perfect or near perfect for him or her to be considered competent, although one court seemed to imply this with respect to experimental psychosurgery.[39] A final problem with this test is that its application depends on unobservable and inferential mental processes rather than on concrete and observable elements of behavior.

Actual Understanding

Rather than focusing on competency as a construct or intervening variable in the decision-making process, the test of actual understanding reduces competency to an epiphenomenon of this process.[19] The competent patient is by definition one who has provided a knowledgeable consent to treatment. Under this test the physician has an obligation to educate the patient and directly ascertain whether he or she has in fact understood. If not, according to this test the patient may not have provided informed consent.[19] Depending on how sophisticated a level of understanding is to be required, this test delineates a potentially high level of competency, one that may be difficult to achieve.

The provisional decision of DHEW to mandate the creation of consent committees to oversee the decisions of experimental subjects,[29] (at 46.506) implicitly adopts this test, as does the California law requiring the review of patient consent to ECT[40]. Controversial as these requirements may be, they require physicians to make reasonable efforts to ascertain that their patients understand what they are told and encourage active patient participation in treatment selection.[41]

The practical and conceptual limitations of this test are similar to those of the ability-to-understand test. What constitutes adequate understanding is vague, and deficient understanding may be attributable in whole or in part to physician behavior as well as to the patient's behavior or character. An advantage that this test has over the ability-to-understand test, assuming the necessary level of understanding can be specified a priori, is its greater reliability. Unlike the ability-to-understand test, in which the patient's comprehension of material of a certain complexity is used as the basis for an assumption of comprehension of other material of equivalent complexity (even if this other material is not actually tested), the actual understanding test makes no such assumption. It tests the very issues central to patient decision making about treatment.

DISCUSSION

It has been our experience that competency is presumed as long as the patient modulates his or her behavior, talks in a comprehensible way, remembers what he or she is told, dresses and acts so as to appear to be in meaningful communication with the environment, and has not been declared legally incompetent. In other words, if patients have their wits about them in a layman's sense[19] it is assumed that they will understand what they are told about treatment, including its risks, benefits, and alternatives. This is the equivalent of saying that the legal presumption is one of competency until found otherwise.[42] The Pandora's box of the question of whether and to what extent the patient is able to understand or has understood which has been disclosed is therefore never opened.

In effect, the test that is actually applied combines elements of all of the tests described above. However, the circumstances in which competency becomes an issue determine which elements of which tests are stressed and which are underplayed. Although in theory competency is an independent variable that determines whether or not the patient's decision to accept or refuse treatment is to be honored, in practice it seems to be dependent on the interplay of two other variables, the risk/benefit ratio of treatment and the valence of the patient's decision, i.e., whether he or she consents to or refuses treatment.

The phrase "risk/benefit ratio of treatment" is used here in a shorthand way to express the fact that people who determine patient competency make this decision partly on the basis of the risks of the particular treatment being considered and the benefits of that treatment. We do not mean to imply that any formal calculation is made or that any given ratio is determinative of competency. The problems of who decides what is a risk and what is a benefit, the relative weights to be attached to risks and benefits, and who bears the risks and to whom the benefits accrue (e.g., the patient, the clinician, society), are beyond the scope of the present inquiry.

Table 1 illustrates the interplay of the valence of the patient's decision and the risk/benefit ratio of treatment. When there is a favorable risk/benefit ratio to the proposed treatment in the opinion of the person determining competency and the patient consents to the treatment, there does not seem to be any reason to stand in the way of administering treatment. To accomplish this, a test employing a low threshold of competency may be applied to find even a marginal patient competent so that his or her decision may be honored (cell A). This is what happens daily when uncomprehending patients are permitted to sign themselves into the hospital. Similarly, when the risk/benefit ratio is favorable and the patient refuses treatment, a test employing a higher threshold of competency may be applied (cell B). Under such a test even a somewhat knowledgeable patient may be found incompetent so that consent may be sought from a substitute decision maker and treatment administered despite the patient's refusal. An example would be the patient withdrawing from alcohol who, although intermittently resistive, is nevertheless administered sedative medication. In both of these cases, in which the risk/benefit ratio is favorable, the bias of physicians, other health professionals, and judges is usually skewed toward providing treatment. Therefore, a test of competency is applied that will permit the treatment to be administered irrespective of the patient's actual or potential understanding.

However, there is a growing reluctance on the part of our society to permit patients to undergo treatments that are extremely risky or for which the benefits are highly speculative. Thus if the risk/benefit ratio is unfavorable or questionable and the patient refuses treatment, a test employing a low threshold of competency may be selected so that the patient will be found competent and his or her refusal honored (cell C). This is what happens in the area of sterilization of mentally retarded people, in which, at least from the perspective of the retarded individual, the risk/benefit ratio is questionable. On the other hand, when the risk/benefit ratio is unfavorable or questionable and the patient consents to treatment, a test using a higher threshold of competency may be applied (cell D), preventing even some fairly knowledgeable patients from undergoing treatment. The judicial opinion in the well-known *Kaimowitz* psychosurgery case delineated a high test of competency to be employed in that experimental setting.[39]

Of course, some grossly impaired patients cannot be determined to be competent under any conceivable test, nor can most normally functioning people be found incompetent merely by selective application of a test of competency. However, within limits and when the patient's competency is not absolutely clearcut, a test of competency that will achieve the desired medical or social end despite the actual condition of the patient may be selected. We do not imply that this is done maliciously either by physicians or by the courts; rather, we believe that it occurs as a consequence of the strong societal bias in favor of treating treatable pa-

TABLE 1   Factors in Selection of Competency Tests

Patient's Decision	Risk/Benefit Ratio of Treatment	
	Favorable	Unfavorable or Questionable
Consent	Low test of competency (cell A)	High test of competency (cell D)
Refusal	High test of competency (cell B)	Low test of competency (cell C)

tients so long as it does not expose them to serious risks.

CONCLUSIONS

The search for a single test of competency is a search for a Holy Grail. Unless it is recognized that there is no magical definition of competency to make decisions about treatment, the search for an acceptable test will never end. "Getting the words just right" is only part of the problem. In practice, judgments of competency go beyond semantics or straightforward applications of legal rules; such judgments reflect social considerations and societal biases as much as they reflect matters of law and medicine.

Notes

1. Shah SA: Dangerousness and civil commitment of the mentally ill: some public policy considerations. Am J Psychiatry 132:501–505, 1975
2. Allen RC, Ferster EZ, Weihofen H: Mental Impairment and Legal Incompetency. Englewood Cliffs, NJ, Prentice-Hall, 1968
3. Hardisty JH: Mental illness: a legal fiction. Washington Law Review, 48:735–762, 1973
4. Alexander GJ, Szasz TS: From contract to status via psychiatry. Santa Clara Lawyer 13:537–559, 1973
5. Group for the Advancement of Psychiatry Committee on Psychiatry and Law: Misuse of Psychiatry in the Criminal Courts: Competency to Stand Trial. Report 89. New York, GAP, 1974
6. Green MD: Judicial tests of mental incompetency. Missouri Law Review 6:141–165, 1941
7. Dusky v United States, 362 US 405 (1960) (per curiam)
8. Informed consent and the dying patient. Yale Law Journal 83:1632–1664, 1974
9. Mental competency of patient to consent to surgical operation or treatment. American Law Reports Annotated, Third Series 25:1439–1443, 1969
10. Friedman PR: Legal regulation of applied behavior analysis in mental institutions and prisons. Arizona Law Review 17:39–104, 1975
11. Shapiro MH: Legislating the control of

behavior control: autonomy and the coercive use of organic therapies. Southern California Law Review 47:237–356, 1974
12. Demers v Gerety, 515 P 2d 645 (NM 1973)
13. Steele v Woods, 327 SW 2d 187, 198 (Mo 1959)
14. Peszke MA: Is dangerousness an issue for physicians in emergency commitment? Am J Psychiatry 132:825–828, 1975
15. Halleck SL: Legal and ethical aspects of behavior control. Am J Psychiatry 131:381–385, 1974
16. Grunebaum H, Abernethy V: Ethical issues in family planning for hospitalized psychiatric patients. Am J Psychiatry 132:236–240, 1975
17. Relf v Weinberger, 372 F Supp 1196 (DC 1974)
18. Michels R: The right to refuse psychoactive drugs: case studies in bioethics. Hastings Center Report 3(3):10–11, 1973
19. Meisel A, Roth LH, Lidz CW: Toward a model of the legal doctrine of informed consent. Am J Psychiatry 134:285–289, 1977
20. A Draft Act Governing Hospitalization of the Mentally Ill, revised. US Public Health Service Publication 51. Washington, DC, US Government Printing Office, 1952, pp. 6, 26, 27
21. In re Yetter, 62 D&C 2d 619, 624 (CP Northampton County, Pa 1973)
22. Stone AA: Mental Health and Law: A System in Transition. US Department of Health, Education, and Welfare Publication 75-176. Rockville, Md. National Institute of Mental Health, 1975, p. 68
23. US Department of Health, Education, and Welfare: Protection of human subjects. Federal Register 39:18914–18920, May 30, 1973
24. Moore v Webb, 345 SW 2d 239, 243 (Mo 1961)
25. Friedman PR: Legal regulation of applied behavior analysis in mental institutions and prisons. Arizona Law Review 17:39–140, 1975
26. New York City Health and Hospital Corp v Stein. 335 NYS 2d 461, 465 (NY 1972)
27. McDonald MC: And things get rough. Psychiatric News. Nov 5, 1975, pp. 13–14
28. Wyatt v Aderholt, 368 F Supp 1383, (MD Ala 1974)
29. US Department of Health, Education, and Welfare: Protection of human subjects: proposed policy. Federal Register 39 30647, 30657, Aug 23, 1974
30. United States v George, 239 F Supp 752 (D Conn 1965)
31. Cantor NL: A patient's decision to decline life-saving medical treatment: bodily integrity versus the preservation of life. Rutgers Law Review 26:228–264, 1973

32. Judge OKs amputation of south sider's leg. Pittsburgh Press, June 4, 1975, p 1

33. Amputate order more human than judicial, Larsen says. Pittsburgh Press, June 8, 1975, p 1

34. Developments in the law—civil commitment of the mentally ill. Harvard Law Review 87: 1190–1406, 1974

35. Miller R, Willner HS: The two-part consent form. N Engl J Med 290:964–966, 1974

36. Ingelfinger FJ: Informed (but uneducated) consent N Engl J Med 287:465–466, 1972

37. Katz J: Experimentation with Human Beings. New York, Russell Sage Foundation, 1972, pp 609–673

38. Olin GB, Olin HS: Informed consent in voluntary mental hospital admissions. Am J Psychiatry 132:938–941, 1975

39. Kaimowitz v Michigan Department of Mental Health, Civil Action 73-19434-AW (Wayne County, Mich, Cir Ct 1973)

40. California enacts rigid shock therapy controls. Psychiatric News, Feb 5, 1975, pp 1, 4–7

41. Szasz RS, Hollender MH: The basic models of the doctor/patient relationship. Arch Intern Med 97:585–592, 1956

42. Lotman v Security Mutual Life Insurance Co. 478 F 2d 868 (Bd Cir 1973)

From "Informed (but Uneducated) Consent"

Franz J. Ingelfinger

The trouble with informed consent is that it is not educated consent. Let us assume that the experimental subject, whether a patient, a volunteer, or otherwise enlisted, is exposed to a completely honest array of factual detail. He is told of the medical uncertainty that exists and that must be resolved by research endeavors, of the time and discomfort involved, and of the tiny percentage risk of some serious consequences of the test procedure. He is also reassured of his rights and given a formal, quasi-legal statement to read. No exculpatory language is used. With his written signature, the subject then caps the transaction, and whether he sees himself as a heroic martyr for the sake of mankind, or as a reluctant guinea pig dragooned for the benefit of science, or whether, perhaps, he is merely bewildered, he obviously has given his "informed consent." Because established routines have been scrupulously observed, the doctor, the lawyer, and the ethicist are content.

But the chances are remote that the subject really understands what he has consented to—in the sense that the responsible medical investigator understands the goals, nature, and hazards of his study. How can the layman comprehend the importance of his perhaps not receiving, as determined by the luck of the draw, the highly touted new treatment that his roommate will get? How can he appreciate the sensation of living for days with a multilumen intestinal tube passing through his mouth and pharynx? How can he interpret the information that an intravascular catheter and radiopaque dye injection have an 0.01 per cent probability of leading to a dangerous thrombosis or cardiac arrhythmia? It is moreover quite unlikely that any patient-subject can see himself accurately within the broad context of the situation, to weigh the inconveniences and hazards that he will have to undergo against the improvements that the research project may bring to the management of his disease in general and to his own case in particular . . . .

Nor can the information given to the experimental subject be in any sense totally complete. It would be impractical and probably unethical for the investigator to present the nearly endless list of all possible contingencies; in fact, he may not himself be aware of every untoward thing that might happen. Extensive detail, moreover, usually enhances the subject's confusion. Epstein and Lasagna showed that comprehension of medical information given to untutored subjects is inversely correlated with the elaborateness of the material presented.[1] The inconsiderate investigator, indeed, conceivably could exploit his authority and knowledge and extract "informed consent" by overwhelming the candidate-subject with information.

Ideally, the subject should give his consent freely, under no duress whatsoever. The facts are that some element of coercion is instrumental in any investigator-subject transaction. Volunteers for experiments will usually be influenced by hopes of obtaining better grades, earlier parole, more substantial egos, or just mundane cash. These pressures, however, are but fractional shadows of those enclosing the patient-subject. Incapacitated and hospitalized because of illness, frightened by strange and impersonal routines, and fearful for his health and perhaps life, he is far from exercising a free power of choice when the person to whom he anchors all his hopes asks, "Say, you wouldn't mind, would you, if you joined some of the other patients on this floor and helped us to carry out some very important research we are doing?" When "informed consent" is obtained, it is not the student, the destitute bum, or the prisoner to whom, by virtue of his condition, the thumb screws of coercion are most relentlessly applied; it is the most used and useful of all experimental subjects, the patient with disease.

When a man or woman agrees to act as an experimental subject, therefore, his or her consent is marked by neither adequate understanding nor total freedom of choice. The conditions of the agreement are a far cry from those visualized as ideal. Jonas would have the subject identify with the investigative endeavor so that he and the researcher would be seeking a common cause: "Ultimately, the appeal for volunteers should seek . . . free and generous endorsement, the appropriation of the research purpose into the person's [i.e., the subject's] own scheme of ends."[2] For Ramsey,

"informed consent" should represent a "covenantal bond between consenting man and consenting man [that] makes them . . . joint adventurers in medical care and progress."[3] Clearly, to achieve motivations and attitudes of this lofty type, an educated and understanding, rather than merely informed, consent is necessary.

Although it is unlikely that the goals of Jonas and of Ramsey will ever be achieved, and that human research subjects will spontaneously volunteer rather than be "conscripted,"[4] efforts to promote educated consent are in order. In view of the current emphasis on involving "the community" in such activities as regional planning, operation of clinics, and assignment of priorities, the general public and its political leaders are showing an increased awareness and understanding of medical affairs. But the orientation of this public interest in medicine is chiefly socioeconomic. Little has been done to give the public a basic understanding of medical research and its requirements not only for the people's money but also for their participation. The public, to be sure, is being subjected to a bombardment of sensation-mongering news stories and books that feature "breakthroughs," or that reveal real or alleged exploitations—horror stories of Nazi-type experimentation on abused human minds and bodies. Muckraking is essential to expose malpractices, but unless accompanied by efforts to promote a broader appreciation of medical research and its methods, it merely compounds the difficulties for both the investigator and the subject when "informed consent" is solicited.

The procedure currently approved in the United States for enlisting human experimental subjects has one great virtue: patient-subjects are put on notice that their management is in part at least an experiment. The deceptions of the past are no longer tolerated. Beyond this accomplishment, however, the process of obtaining "informed consent," with all its regulations and conditions, is no more than an elaborate ritual, a device that, when the subject is uneducated and uncomprehending, confers no more than the semblance of propriety on human experimentation. The subject's only real protection, the public as well as the medical profession must recognize, depends on the conscience and compassion of the investigator and his peers.

Notes

1. Epstein LC, Lasagna L: Obtaining informed consent: form or substance. Arch Intern Med 123:682–688, 1969

2. Jonas H: Philosophical reflections on experimenting with human subjects. Daedalus 98: 219–247, Spring, 1969

3. Ramsey P: The ethics of a cottage industry in an age of community and research medicine. N Engl J Med 284:700–706, 1971

4. Jonas, Philosophical reflections.

From "Informed Opinion on Informed Consent"

Nicholas J. Demy

To the Editor.—As a radiologist who has been sued, I have reflected earnestly on advice to obtain Informed Consent but have decided to "take the risks without informing the patient" and trust to "God, judge, and jury" rather than evade responsibility through a legal gimmick . . . .

President Truman had a sign on his desk to remind him that "the buck stops here." So with the physician. He may not be God, judge, and jury, but he is their surrogate and must speak alone with the patient as Moses did with God on Mt. Sinai. Think what the Ten Commandments would be if a committee or a TEAM had gone up there to discuss the terms.

Alfidi's form and arguments are appropriate for the patient with a serious problem who is referred to the Cleveland Clinic or to some other medical Mecca for a special examination. Such patients have already been primed and know the score, but in a general radiologic practice many of our patients are uninformable and we would never get through the day if we had to obtain their consent to every potentially harmful study. We do not have the resident and nursing staff to act as our angels and interpreters. The practice of medicine is a matter of individual communication and good rapport with the patient . . . .

We still have patients with language problems, the uneducated and the unintelligent, the stolid and the stunned who cannot form an Informed Opinion to give an Informed Consent; we have the belligerent and the panicky who do not listen or comprehend. And then there are the Medicare patients who comprise 35% of general hospital admissions. The bright ones wearily plead to be left alone; protoplasm grows old and awfully tired, and longs for immortality elsewhere; they do not even want the Routine Profile of gall bladder, intravenous pyelogram, barium enema, and gastrointestinal tract, much less the Rule Out angiogram. As for the apathetic rest, many of them were kindly described by Richard Bright as not being able to comprehend because "their brains are so poorly oxygenated." Try talking cold turkey to them. Asking a patient with the Sword of Damocles hanging over his head to sign an Informed Consent may be smart protection but it sounds as gruesome as an Executioner getting a pardon from his victim before the axe descends.

Why instill fear and then argue to allay it? Patients—like lovers—change their minds or their vows.

"Yes," I answered you last night;
   "No," this morning, sir, I say.
Colors seen by candle-light
   Will not look the same by day.

Reprinted with permission of author and publisher from *Journal of the American Medical Association* 217:5, 696–97, August 2, 1971. Copyright 1971, the American Medical Association.

If a complication arises after the procedure, patients can deny, and have denied, that they understood what they were signing or that the Informed Consent included the complication they suffered despite the adjuvant paragraph to cover the unexpected: "It would be impractical and probably misleading . . . to describe in detail all the complications . . . '' The law says you cannot sign away your rights in advance of a procedure and the courts have upheld awards in the face of signed Informed Consents. You may still be sued.

A lawyer will see to that.

Informed Consent: Recall by Patients Tested Postoperatively

George Robinson and Avraham Merav

It is the patient's right to determine whether he will or will not undergo surgical treatment, and it is the responsibility of the surgeon to provide information for the patient so that he can make an intelligent decision based upon comprehension of the intended procedure. Variations in the standards of adequacy of such information and recent changes in laws across our nation make judgments on the details and validity of informed consent very difficult.[1] Several recent legal decisions have transferred evaluation of the adequacy of informed consent from physicians to the jury, and it is now the latter who may decide whether adequate information has been supplied to permit the patient to make a sensible decision with respect to treatment. Certainly, when he is considering whether to undergo a major operation the patient requires information as to the possibility of death or injuries from potential complications. He is also entitled to an expert evaluation of the alternatives to surgical treatment.

The extent to which physicians must inform patients has recently been determined to be that information which is material to the decision-making process. Information regarding complex technological methods, surgical procedures, and prosthetic devices is difficult to transmit to the wide spectrum of patients. Total comprehension by patients, even those with a medical background, may be impossible to achieve, yet the physician is duty bound to inform. By training and experience, the surgeon is accustomed to rendering a prospective analysis of a clinical problem and to evaluating methods alternative to surgery. He should therefore be able to present this material to the patient in a comprehensible form. Documentation of this transmittal of information in the patient's clinical records has been shown to be desirable.

We have made a conscientious effort to obtain fully informed consent from all our patients undergoing cardiac procedures. Since January, 1975, tape recordings have been made of the informed consent conversations; these recordings were made with the knowledge and permission of the patients. In a carefully structured but informal session one or two days prior to operation, the elements of informed consent were systematically covered in considerable detail.

The outline of information included in each interview was as follows:

1. Diagnosis and nature of the illness

2. Proposed operation, surgical techniques to be employed, and prosthetic devices to be used (if applicable)

Reprinted with permission from the authors and The Annals of Thoracic Surgery, vol. 22, no. 3, September 1976, pp. 209–212.

3. Risk of death resulting from the operative procedure

4. Potential complications of operation and prosthetic devices (if applicable)

5. Benefits of the proposed operative procedure

6. Alternative methods of management and their chances for failure or success

7. Acknowledgment by the patient of his understanding of all explanations and answering of questions

We were first alerted to the major loss of recall that occurs following the informed consent interview when 2 patients, both of whom were convalescing normally at ten days and six weeks after their operations, denied any recollection of the preoperative recorded interview. A formal study of recall by postoperative testing was then initiated.

MATERIALS AND METHODS

Between 4 and 6 months following operation, 20 patients were selected for reinterview to determine the capacity of each to recall the details of their informed consent interview. Each of these patients had convalesced uneventfully after a satisfactory postoperative course. Patient selection was otherwise totally random. Ages ranged between 35 and 66 years, with a mean age of 52 years. Nine patients had undergone operation for atherosclerotic heart disease, and 11 patients had been operated upon for acquired valvular heart disease. Recordings were also made at the time of the second interview. All patients had been hospitalized one or more times previously for diagnostic or therapeutic purposes, and none had had their operations performed as emergency procedures.

All informed consent interviews were conducted by one author (G. R.), and all reinterviews were conducted by the second author (A. M.). Before reinterview the original tape recording was replayed, and a chart of the points discussed in each category of informed consent was prepared for rapid reference. At the reinterview each category of the consent procedure was reviewed twice to determine the

patient's ability to recall. *Primary recall* was the response to general questions in each category of consent (1 to 6). Questions asked during the primary recall portion of the reinterview were identical for all patients. An effort was made to avoid suggesting responses. The questions were:

Do you remember having an interview with Dr. Robinson before your operation?

Tell me what you remember of the interview.

What were you told about what was wrong with you—the diagnosis?

What were you told about the operation to be performed?

Were you told of risks or dangers associated with the operation?

Were any of the possible complications associated with the operation discussed? What were they?

Were you told in what way the operation would help you?

Were you told about methods of treatment other than operation?

Following this, the itemized list of topics from the prepared chart was then reviewed with the patient. The patient was asked if each item had been discussed originally and, if affirmative, what the substance of the conversation was. The response of the patient to questions regarding specific items known to have been discussed in the original interview was designated *secondary recall*. Suggestions of correct responses were unavoidable in testing for secondary recall.

Accuracy of primary and secondary recall was then graded 0 to 100% in each of the categories 1 through 6 of the informed consent interview. If there was no recall of a category having been discussed, a score of 0 was given. Partial scores were awarded according to the degree of recall in each category. No deductions were made for denial, fabrication, or errors of attribution.

RESULTS

Findings upon reinterview indicated generally poor retention in all categories of informed con-

Recall of Informed Consent Interview by 20 Patients 4 to 6 Months Postoperatively

Category of Informed Consent Information	% Primary Recall	% Secondary Recall
1. Diagnosis and nature of illness	33	46
2. Proposed operation	26	50
3. Risks of the operative procedure	35	42
4. Potential complications	10	23
5. Benefits of the proposed operation	29	47
6. Alternative methods of management	43	43
Average	29	42

sent information. The Table indicates the average scores achieved by 20 patients reinterviewed in each of the 6 categories. The poorest scores were achieved in the single category of potential complications: there was 10% primary recall and, with the suggestion of appropriate responses, a secondary recall of 23% out of a possible 100% for this category. The average recall in all categories was 29% for primary and 42% for secondary recall. Thus, even with the influence of suggestion and a point-by-point review of every item covered in the original interview, patients could remember only 42% of the items that had been covered in the informed consent interview. The Figure illustrates the scores achieved by percentage groups in each category and demonstrates the improvement in secondary recall. Of the 20 patients tested, 17 scored 50% or less on primary recall and 12 scored 50% or less on secondary recall. The lowest individual score achieved was 3% primary and 3% secondary recall, and the highest score achieved was 57% primary and 87% secondary recall.

Errors made by patients in the repeat interview had qualitative differences. They may be described as failure to recall; positive denial of a truth; fabrication, or the assertion of an untruth or falsehood; and errors of attribution.

Each of the 20 patients failed to recall major parts of the interview. Sixteen of the 20 patients positively denied that certain major items had been discussed at all. Of these 16 patients who made positive denials, 13 denied having been informed on multiple (maximum of eight) significant items of information. After failure

to recall and denial, the next most common error was fabrication, or the assertion of an untruth or falsehood. This was present to a significant degree in 13 of the 20 patients reinterviewed. A common error (and one that is quite understandable) was attribution of information gathered from other sources to the informed consent interview.

Two patients voluntarily complained that the preoperative interviews were very brief, inferring that they were not informative. One of these stated that "all he did was lift up my shirt, put a stethoscope on my heart, and that was it." The recorded portion alone of this informed consent conference was 24 minutes long. The second complaint about brevity of the interview came from a patient whose recording lasted 23 minutes. The unrecorded portions of each consultation visit easily exceeded 10 additional minutes.

Noteworthy was a significant difference in the self-assurance with which patients responded to questions in reinterviews. The quality of responses to questions often indicated some doubt or lack of certainty. Three patients were considered to have a quality of response that indicated near total self-assurance in being correct in the details of recall. The poorest score of all 20 patients reinterviewed was achieved by a patient who responded authoritatively and expressed no doubts regarding his recollections. Two other patients, who scored fifteenth and seventeenth, respectively, also had the same quality of response: they were frequently in error but never in doubt.

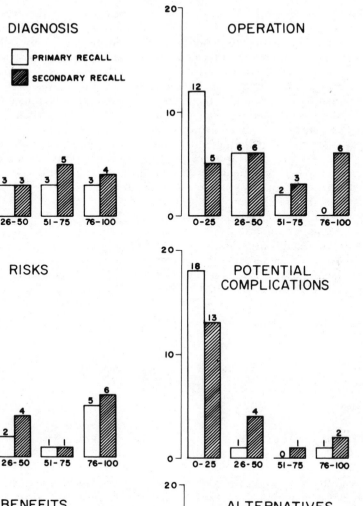

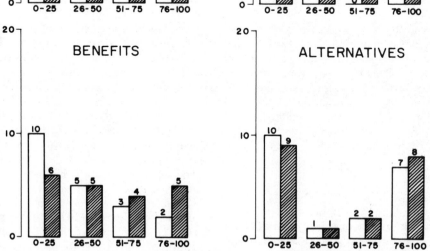

Primary and secondary recall in each category of informed consent. Vertical axis indicates number of patients; horizontal axis indicates scores in percent.

COMMENT

Despite meticulous attention to detail by the surgeon in a carefully conducted informed consent procedure, all of 20 patients tested between 4 and 6 months postoperatively failed to recall accurately what had transpired at their interview. The informed consent had been given in a simple, direct, and uncomplicated manner in the form of a dialog between the patient and the surgeon. There were repeated instances in each conversation in which the patient was asked if he understood the explanations, and questions were answered as they arose. We believe, therefore, that all patients completely understood the information imparted and that they gave a truly informed consent to their operations. Noteworthy is the fact that the patients studied had been educated by their previous experience with their disease; all had chronic heart disease and had been hospitalized many times for diagnostic and therapeutic procedures. This study calls attention to the fact that, while these patients were well informed and comprehended their situations prior to operation, they subsequently forgot most of what they had understood and made other qualitative errors in their attempts to recall the consent interview. We believe it is essential to document in some way the details of informed consent so that it becomes a permanent part of the clinical record, since memory of the event is unreliable.

Note

1. Nick WV: Informed consent—the new decisions. Bull Am Coll Surg 59:12, 1974

From "Medical Experimentation on Humans"

Preston J. Burnham

Having read the News and Comment headed "Human experimentation: New York verdict affirms patient's rights," I believe I understand the situation well enough to attempt to help lay committees develop a series of forms for obtaining patients' infomed consent. I am working now on forms . . . for our standard operations . . . .

CONSENT FORM FOR HERNIA PATIENTS:

I, _____, being about to be subjected to a surgical operation said to be for repair of what my doctor thinks is a hernia (rupture or loss of belly stuff—intestines—out of the belly through a hole in the muscles), do hereby give said doctor permission to cut into me and do duly swear that I am giving my informed consent, based upon the following information:

Operative procedure is as follows: The doctor first cuts through the skin by a four-inch gash in the lower abdomen. He then slashes through the other things—fascia (a tough layer over the muscles) and layers of muscle—until he sees the cord (tube that brings the sperm from testicle to outside) with all its arteries and veins. The doctor then tears the hernia (thin sac of bowels and things) from the cord and ties off the sac with a string. He then pushes the testicle back into the scrotum and sews everything together, trying not to sew up the big arteries and veins that nourish the leg.

Possible complications are as follows:

1. Large artery may be cut and I may bleed to death.

2. Large vein may be cut and I may bleed to death.

3. Tube from testicle may be cut. I will then be sterile on that side.

4. Artery or veins to testicles may be cut—same result.

5. Opening around cord in muscles may be made too tight.

6. Clot may develop in these veins which will loosen when I get out of bed and hit my lungs, killing me.

7. Clot may develop in one or both legs which may cripple me, lead to loss of one or both legs, go to my lungs, or make my veins no good for life.

8. I may develop a horrible infection that may kill me.

9. The hernia may come back again after it has been operated on.

10. I may die from general anesthesia.

11. I may be paralyzed if spinal anesthesia is used.

12. If ether is used, it could explode inside me.

13. I may slip in hospital bathroom.

14. I may be run over going to the hospital.

15. The hospital may burn down.

I understand: the anatomy of the body, the pathology of the development of hernia, the surgical technique that will be used to repair the hernia, the physiology of wound healing, the dietetic chemistry of the foods that I must eat to cause healing, the chemistry of body repair, and the course which my physician will take in treating any of the complications that can occur as a sequel of repairing an otherwise simple hernia.

Patient
Lawyer for Patient
Lawyer for Doctor
Lawyer for Hospital
Lawyer for Anesthesiologist
Mother-in-law
Notary Public

Informed Consent May Be Hazardous to Health

Elizabeth F. Loftus and James F. Fries

Before human subjects are enrolled in experimental studies, a variety of preliminary rituals are now required. These include an explanation of the nature of the experimental procedure and a specific elaboration of possible adverse reactions. The subjects, in turn, can either withdraw from the experiment or give their "informed consent." These rituals are said to increase the subjects' understanding of the procedures but, perhaps more important,

Reprinted by permission from *Science*, vol. 204, p. 6, April 6, 1979. Copyright 1979 by the American Association for the Advancement of Science.

they came into existence because of a strong belief in the fundamental principle that human beings have the right to determine what will be done to their minds and bodies.

Some, on the other hand, consider that the purpose of informed consent is not protection of subjects, but rather protection of investigators and sponsoring institutions from lawsuits based on the charge of subject deception should a misadventure result. But lawsuits arise in any case; subjects simply claim that they did not understand the rituals. It is reasonable, then, to ask whether the putative beneficiary, the subject, might be harmed rather than helped by the current informed consent procedure.

A considerable body of psychological evidence indicates that humans are highly suggestible. Information has been found to change people's attitudes, to change their moods and feelings, and even to make them believe they have experienced events that never in fact occurred. This alone would lead one to suspect that adverse reactions might result from information given during an informed consent discussion.

An examination of the medical evidence demonstrates that there is also a dark side to the placebo effect. Not only can positive therapeutic effects be achieved by suggestion, but negative side effects and complications can similarly result. For example, among subjects who participated in a drug study after the usual informed consent procedure, many of those given an injection of a placebo reported physiologically unlikely symptoms such as dizziness, nausea, vomiting, and even mental depression. One subject given the placebo reported that these effects were so strong that they caused an automobile accident. Many other studies provide similar data indicating that to a variable but often scarifying degree, explicit suggestion of possible adverse effects causes subjects to experience these effects. Recent hypotheses that heart attack may follow coronary spasm indicate physiological mechanisms by which explicit suggestions, and the stress that may be produced by them, might prove fatal. Thus, the possible consequences of suggested symptoms range from minor annoyance to, in extreme cases, death.

If protection of the subject is the reason for obtaining informed consent, the possibility of iatrogenic harm to the subject as a direct result of the consent ritual must be considered. This clear cost must be weighed against the potential benefit of giving some people an increased sense of freedom of choice about the use of their bodies. The current legalistic devices, which are designed in part to limit subject recourse, intensify rather than solve a dilemma.

The features of informed consent procedures that do protect subjects should be retained. Experimental procedures should be reviewed by peers and public representatives. A statement to the subject describing the procedure and the general level of risk is reasonable. But detailed information should be reserved for those who request it. Specific slight risks, particularly those resulting from common procedures, should not be routinely disclosed to all subjects. And when a specific risk is disclosed, it should be discussed in the context of placebo effects in general, why they occur, and how to guard against them. A growing literature indicates that just as knowledge of possible symptoms can cause those symptoms, so can knowledge of placebo effects be used to defend against those effects. A move in this direction may ensure that a subject will not be at greater risk from self-appointed guardians than from the experiment itself.

Letters: "Uninformed Consent"

Some reform may be needed in the procedure for gaining informed consent from "human subjects" asked to participate in an experiment, but the reasons advanced in "Informed consent may be hazardous to health," by Loftus and Fries (Editorial, 6 April, p. 11) obscure the fundamental issues.

Reprinted by permission from *Science*, vol. 205, pp. 644, 646–647, August 17, 1979. Copyright 1979 by the American Association for the Advancement of Science.

The editorial begins with the noncontroversial statement that "before human subjects are enrolled in experimental studies, a variety of preliminary rituals are now required.... These rituals... came into existence because of a strong belief in the fundamental principle that human beings have the right to determine what will be done to their minds and bodies." Still, one wonders at the use of "ritual" in this connection, associated as "ritual" is with the notion of an idle exercise, empty of substantive import. It is true of course that when arresting officers inform arrestees of their rights, the officers tend to recite them like a catechism, but it would hardly be termed a ritual.

Having stated the principle, the authors go on to claim that "A considerable body of psychological evidence indicates that humans are highly suggestible. Information has been found to change people's attitudes, to change their moods and feelings, and even to make them believe they have experienced events that never in fact occurred." From this premise it is astonishingly concluded, "This alone would lead one to suspect that adverse reactions might result from information given during an informed consent discussion." The premise is remarkable for its understatement. It is common knowledge and not the science of psychology which tells us that if someone we trust informs us that our house is on fire and our children are burning, our moods will assuredly change; if someone we trust informs us falsely of such an event, our mood will also change and we may be made to believe something that never in fact occurred. The principle behind the informed consent procedure is not threatened by such facts; the subject has a prima facie right to determine what will be done with his or her mind and body in or out of an experiment, and the opportunity to make that determination is frustrated if information is withheld or deception practiced by the experimenter. How is a subject to decide rationally about participating in an experiment if information is withheld or he or she is being deceived?

We wonder at the relevance of the "dark side to the placebo effect" to the assertion that informed consent may be "harmful." If volunteer subjects are informed that they may or may not be getting a placebo and that placebos sometimes or occasionally have adverse effects, that information is required if they are to exercise their rights. They are entitled to the most complete information in deciding whether to participate or withdraw.

The editorial then proceeds to medical matters in support of the claim that informed consent is potentially harmful. It cites, for example, "hypotheses that heart attack may follow coronary spasm," which hypotheses "indicate

physiological mechanisms by which explicit suggestions, and the stress that may be produced by them, may prove fatal." The authors conclude, "Thus the possible consequences of suggested symptoms range from minor annoyance to, in extreme cases, death." One expects (hopes?) that a subject with heart spasms who might die from being informed about possible further symptoms would not be asked to participate in experiments in which details of the experiment (whether given or withheld) are dangerous to his life and health. For that, after all, is what the editorial was about; the relationship between a *voluntary subject* in an experiment and the experimenter. It was not about the special peculiarities of the client-doctor relationship.

If one of us has a heart spasm we will very likely seek the services of a doctor, but not as an experimental subject. In contracting for those services we can expect that the doctor will do what he can to help reduce suffering and restore health. In consultation with a doctor, a client may even insist that there are some things he or she doesn't want to know, and the doctor may have some hard choices. But even in the doctor-client context the prima facie right to full information on matters which may affect our minds and bodies prevails. Balancing those rights against putative harms in that context is a delicate business which we need not go into since, as noted above, the editorial is about human subjects in scientific experimentation. The two contexts must be kept distinct and explicitly so even where they involve the same doctor and the same subject.

Finally, the most mischievous conceptual confusion is in the penultimate paragraph. It says ". . . the possibility of iatrogenic harm to the subject as a direct result of the consent ritual must be considered. This clear cost must be weighed against the potential benefit of giving some people an increased sense of freedom of choice about the use of their bodies." What is distressing is the failure to make the absolutely crucial distinction between rights and benefits, a distinction which is the cornerstone of our legal and moral system. When a police officer informs a suspect of his rights and how they might be exercised, he is not conferring a benefit. Borrowing the regional usage of the editorial, we find it "scarifying" that some experimenters on human subjects have less comprehension of such matters than the cop on the beat.

Ruth Barcan Marcus
Bruce Kuklick
Sacvan Bercovitch
Center for the Advanced Study in the
Behavioral Sciences, 202 Junipero Serra
Boulevard, Stanford, California 94305

Individuals vested in certain beliefs and unfamiliar with the nuances of a topic sometimes react to the subject of a discussion and not to its substance; this phenomenon is strikingly illustrated by the above letter. The respondents have characterized a statement strongly in favor of human rights as an attack upon such rights. Their response contains colorful but inaccurate rhetoric and a truly novel theory concerning the predictability of heart attack. We welcome the opportunity to recapitulate our arguments.

We strongly uphold the right of individuals to determine for themselves what will be done to their minds and bodies. The basic right to self-determination, however, is threatened by two forces represented in the current "rituals" offered in the name of "informed consent." An informed consent ritual is an attempt to defend the underlying "right"; it is not in itself, either legally or ethically, a "right." It is justified *only* to the extent that it actually promotes self-determination. We very deliberately chose the term "ritual" to distinguish certain practices from the underlying "right" to self-determination. The ethical question with such "rituals" is whether or not they are the best possible ones to ensure that the "right" is protected.

The threats are these. First, institutional lawyers dictate the form of recommended consent forms, so that the forms become releases designed to protect the institution, not information designed to inform the individual. One has only to read a few such forms to note the legal language, the requirement for witnesses, and the obvious intent. We point out this happening, emphasize that it does not even protect the institution, and urge that the practice stop.

Second, those who have been formulating informed consent rituals have not paid sufficient attention to the injury that may be caused by the ritual itself. We point out, and our respondents agree, that harm may result from ill-considered offerings of "information." The harm may take the form of suggested symptoms, induced anxiety, panic-related accidents, or serious physiological reactions. The respondents would argue that all individuals have a right to this information, and that all must receive it. But does a right to harm people exist? The right of free speech has, in American legal and ethical thinking since Holmes, been specifically held to deny the right to cry "fire" in a crowded theatre. Thus, the action of unnecessarily evoking anxiety reactions which can lead to physical harm cannot be a "right"; it is this property of present informed consent rituals that we criticize.

The consent form is inescapably a part of the experimental procedure. If it has potential for harm, the subject must be warned against this possibility just as surely as against the other hazards of an experiment. Current consent form rituals constitute human experimentation, but oddly enough they have not been subjected to as rigorous control as other forms of human experimentation. Who is going to watch the watchdog?

What, then, shall we tell our subject? "Full disclosure" is often naïvely equated with "full knowledge." In point of fact, more comprehension is generally achieved by transmission of smaller amounts of clearly stated information than by prodigious quantities of "fine print." "Full access" is a more reasonable approach, and is the one which we urge. For example, a consent form might in two or three sentences outline the experiment and accurately define the expected level of risk in terms of a universally understood referent. (As dangerous as . . . the drawing of blood, a tonsillectomy, an airplane trip.) The reverse of the form, or a separate booklet, a copy of which the subject would retain, could contain all additional information that might be desired.

Nothing should be withheld from those who wish to know it. Similarly, nothing should be forced down the throats of those who do not wish to know. For those individuals who choose to know all, there are numerous ways in which information about potential adverse side effects can be presented to them. Whatever way is chosen, it is wise to include a discussion of the placebo effect and its potential for adverse reactions, since this may mitigate the adverse effects. This recommendation, of course, is one of offering access to *more* information than is currently the custom.

We closed our editorial by noting that in some instances subjects might be at greater risk from their self-appointed guardians than from the experiment; it was precisely individuals such as our respondents that we had in mind. They would not allow the risks of informed consent to be considered; this, they say, is "mischievous." They reflexly defend actions alleged to be in defense of a fundamental right

without considering whether such actions actually defend or threaten the right of individuals to determine what will be done to their minds or bodies. These obtuse advocates of full information unfailingly argue that "more is better"; they argue for protection of the subject even as their rituals increase that subject's peril. Human beings have a right to access to information that will affect them, but they simultaneously have the right to choose when they have had enough.

James F. Fries
Elizabeth F. Loftus

*Center for Advanced Study
in the Behavioral Sciences*

DISCLOSURE

From "Ethical Duties Towards Others: Truthfulness"

Immanuel Kant

The exchange of our sentiments is the principal factor in social intercourse, and truth must be the guiding principle herein. Without truth social intercourse and conversation become valueless. We can only know what a man thinks if he tells us his thoughts, and when he undertakes to express them he must really do so, or else there can be no society of men. Fellowship is only the second condition of society, and a liar destroys fellowship. Lying makes it impossible to derive any benefit from conversation. Liars are, therefore, held in general contempt. Man is inclined to be reserved and to pretend. Reserve is *dissimulatio* and pretence *simulatio*. Man is reserved in order to conceal faults and shortcomings which he has; he pretends in order to make others attribute to him merits

Reprinted with permission of the publisher from Immanuel Kant, *Lectures on Ethics*, trans. Louis Infield (New York: Harper & Row, 1963), pp. 147–54.

and virtues which he has not. Our proclivity to reserve and concealment is due to the will of Providence that the defects of which we are full should not be too obvious. Many of our propensities and peculiarities are objectionable to others, and if they became patent we should be foolish and hateful in their eyes. Moreover, the parading of these objectionable characteristics would so familiarize men with them that they would themselves acquire them. Therefore we arrange our conduct either to conceal our faults or to appear other than we are. We possess the art of simulation. In consequence, our inner weakness and error is revealed to the eyes of men only as an appearance of well-being, while we ourselves develop the habit of dispositions which are conducive to good conduct. No man in his true senses, therefore, is candid. Were man candid, were the request of Momus[1] to be complied with that Jupiter should place a mirror in each man's heart so that his disposition might be visible to all, man would have to be better constituted and to possess good principles. If all men were good there would be no need for any of us to be reserved; but since they are not, we have to keep the shutters closed. Every house keeps its dust-bin in a place of its own. We do not press our friends to come into our water-closet, although they know that we have one just like themselves. Familiarity in such things is the ruin of good taste. In the same way we make no exhibition of our defects, but try to conceal them. We try to conceal our mistrust by affecting a courteous demeanour and so accustom ourselves to courtesy that at last it becomes a reality and we set a good example by it. If that were not so, if there were none who were better than we, we should become neglectful. Accordingly, the endeavour to appear good ultimately makes us really good. If all men were good, they could be candid, but as things are they cannot be. To be reserved is to be restrained in expressing one's mind. We can, of course, keep absolute silence. This is the readiest and most absolute method of reserve, but it is unsociable, and a silent man is not only unwanted in social circles but is also suspected; every one thinks him deep and disparaging, for if when asked for his opinion he remains silent people think that he must be taking the worst view or he would not be averse from expressing it. Silence, in fact, is always a treacherous ally, and therefore it is not even prudent to be completely reserved. Yet there is such a thing as prudent reserve, which requires not silence but careful deliberation; a man who is wisely reserved weighs his words carefully and speaks his mind about everything excepting only those things in regard to which he deems it wise to be reserved.

We must distinguish between reserve and secretiveness, which is something entirely different. There are matters about which one has no desire to speak and in regard to which reserve is easy. We are, for instance, not naturally tempted to speak about and to betray our own misdemeanours. Every one finds it easy to keep a reserve about some of his private affairs, but there are things about which it requires an effort to be silent. Secrets have a way of coming out, and strength is required to prevent ourselves betraying them. Secrets are

always matters deposited with us by other people and they ought not to be placed at the disposal of third parties. But man has a great liking for conversation, and the telling of secrets adds much to the interest of conversation; a secret told is like a present given; how then are we to keep secrets? Men who are not very talkative as a rule keep secrets well, but good conversationalists, who are at the same time clever, keep them better. The former might be induced to betray something, but the latter's gift of repartee invariably enables them to invent on the spur of the moment something non-committal. . . .

If I announce my intention to tell what is in my mind, ought I knowingly to tell everything, or can I keep anything back? If I indicate that I mean to speak my mind, and instead of doing so make a false declaration, what I say is an untruth, a *falsiloquium*. But there can be *falsiloquium* even when people have no right to assume that we are expressing our thoughts. It is possible to deceive without making any statement whatever. I can make believe, make a demonstration from which others will draw the conclusion I want, though they have no right to expect that my action will express my real mind. In that case I have not lied to them, because I had not undertaken to express my mind. I may, for instance, wish people to think that I am off on a journey, and so I pack my luggage; people draw the conclusion I want them to draw; but others have no right to demand a declaration of my will from me. Thus the famous Law[2] went on building so that people might not guess his intention to abscond. Again, I may make a false statement (*falsiloquium*) when my purpose is to hide from another what is in my mind and when the latter can assume that such in my purpose, his own purpose being to make a wrong use of the truth. Thus, for instance, if my enemy takes me by the throat and asks where I keep my money, I need not tell him the truth, because he will abuse it; and my untruth is not a lie (*mendacium*) because the thief knows full well that I will not, if I can help it, tell him the truth and that he has no right to demand it of me. But let us assume that I really say to the fellow, who is fully aware that he has no right to demand it, because he is a swindler, that I will tell him the truth, and I do not, am I then a liar? He has decieved me and I deceive him in return; to him, as an individual, I have done no injustice and he cannot complain; but I am none the less a liar in that my conduct is an infringement of the rights of humanity. It follows that a *falsiloquium* can be a *mendacium*—a lie—especially when it contravenes the right of an individual. Although I do a man no injustice by lying to him when he has lied to me, yet I act against the right of mankind, since I set myself in opposition to the condition and means through which any human society is possible. If one country breaks the peace this does not justify the other in doing likewise in revenge, for if it did no peace would ever be secure. Even though a statement does not contravene any particular human right it is nevertheless a lie if it is contrary to the general right of mankind. If a man spreads false news, though he does no wrong to anyone in particular, he offends against mankind, because if such a practice were universal man's desire for knowledge would be frustrated. For, apart from speculation, there are only two ways in which I can increase my fund of knowledge, by experience or by what others tell me. My own experience must necessarily be limited, and if what others told me was false, I could not satisfy my craving for knowledge. A lie is thus a *falsiloquium in praejudicium humanitatis*, even though it does not violate any specific *jus quaesitum* of another. In law a *mendacium* is a *falsiloquium in praejudicium alterius*; and so it must be in law; but morally it is a *falsiloquium in praejudicium humanitatis*. Not every untruth is a lie; it is a lie only if I have expressly given the other to understand that I am willing to acquaint him with my thought. Every lie is objectionable and contemptible in that we purposely let people think that we are telling them our thoughts and do not do so. We have broken our pact and violated the right of mankind. But if we were to be at all times punctiliously truthful we might often become victims of the wickedness of others who were ready to abuse our truthfulness. If all men were well-intentioned it would not only be a duty not to lie, but no one would do so because there would be no point in it. But as men are malicious, it cannot be denied that to be punctiliously truthful is often dangerous. This has given rise to the concep-

tion of a white lie, the lie enforced upon us by necessity—a difficult point for moral philosophers. For if necessity is urged as an excuse it might be urged to justify stealing, cheating and killing, and the whole basis of morality goes by the board. Then, again, what is a case of necessity? Everyone will interpret it in his own way, and, as there is then no definite standard to judge by, the application of moral rules becomes uncertain. Consider, for example, the following case. A man who knows that I have money asks me: "Have you any money on you?" If I fail to reply, he will conclude that I have; if I reply in the affirmative he will take it from me; if I reply in the negative, I tell a lie. What am I to do? If force is used to extort a confession from me, if my confession is improperly used against me, and if I cannot save myself by maintaining silence, then my lie is a weapon of defence. The misuse of a declaration extorted by force justifies me in defending myself. For whether it is my money or a confession that is extorted makes no difference. The forcing of a statement from me under conditions which convince me that improper use would be made of it is the only case in which I can be justified in telling a white lie. But if a lie does no harm to anyone and no one's interests are affected by it, is it a lie? Certainly. I undertake to express my mind, and if I do not really do so, though my statement may not be to the prejudice of the particular individual to whom it is made, it is none the less *in praejudicium humanitatis*. Then, again, there are lies which cheat. To cheat is to make a lying promise, while a breach of faith is a true promise which is not kept. A lying promise is an insult to the person to whom it is made, and even if this is not always so, yet there is always something mean about it. If, for instance, I promise to send some one a bottle of wine, and afterwards make a joke of it, I really swindle him. It is true that he has no right to demand the present of me, but in Idea it is already a part of his own property.

. . . But though we are entitled to form opinions about our fellows, we have no right to spy upon them. Everyone has a right to prevent others from watching and scrutinizing his actions. The spy arrogates to himself the right to watch the doings of strangers; no one ought to presume to do such a thing. If I see two people whispering to each other so as not to be heard, my inclination ought to be to get farther away so that no sound may reach my ears. Or if I am left alone in a room and I see a letter lying open on the table, it would be contemptible to try to read it; a right-thinking man would not do so; in fact, in order to avoid suspicion and distrust he will endeavour not to be left alone in a room where money is left lying about, and he will be averse from learning other people's secrets in order to avoid the risk of the suspicion that he has betrayed them; other people's secrets trouble him, for even between the most intimate of friends suspicion might arise. A man who will let his inclination or appetite drive him to deprive his friend of anything, of his fiancée, for instance, is contemptible beyond a doubt. If he can cherish a passion for my sweetheart, he can equally well cherish a passion for my purse. It is very mean to lie in wait and spy upon a friend, or on anyone else, and to elicit information about him from menials by lowering ourselves to the level of our inferiors, who will thereafter not forget to regard themselves as our equals. Whatever militates against frankness lowers the dignity of man.

Notes

1. Momus, the god of mockery and censure, demanded that a little door be made in man's breast, that he might see his secret thoughts.
2. The reference is to John Law (1671–1729) and his Mississippi venture.

From "Truthfulness and Uprightness"

Nicolai Hartmann

VALUATIONAL CONFLICTS BETWEEN TRUTHFULNESS AND THE SO-CALLED "NECESSARY LIE"

Truthfulness as a value, with its specific moral claim, admits of no expection at all. What is called the necessary lie is always an anti-value—at least from the point of view of truthfulness as a value. No end can justify deliberate deception as a means—certainly not in the sense of causing it to cease to be a moral wrong.

Still we are confronted here with a very serious moral problem, which is by no means solved by the simple rejection of each and every lie. There are situations which place before a man the unescapable alternative either of sinning against truthfulness or against some other equally high, or even some higher, value. A

From "Truthfulness and Uprightness" by Nicolai Hartmann, reprinted with permission from *Ethics*, vol. 2, trans. Stanton Coit (New York: Humanities Press; London: George Allen and Unwin Ltd., 1932), pp. 281–85.

physician violates his professional duty, if he tells a patient who is dangerously ill the critical state of his health; the imprisoned soldier who, when questioned by the enemy, allows the truth about his country's tactics to be extorted from him, is guilty of high treason; a friend, who does not try to conceal information given to him in strictest personal confidence, is guilty of breach of confidence. In all such cases the mere virtue of silence is not adequate. Where suspicions are aroused, mere silence may be extremely eloquent. If the physician, the prisoner, the possessor of confidential information will do their duty of warding off a calamity that threatens, they must resort to a lie. But if they do so, they make themselves guilty on the side of truthfulness.

It is a portentous error to believe that such questions may be solved theoretically. Every attempt of the kind leads either to a one-sided and inflexible rigorism concerning one value at the expense of the rest, or to a fruitless casuistry devoid of all significance—not to mention the danger of opportunism. Both rigorism and casuistry are offences against the intention of genuine moral feeling. The examples cited are so chosen that truthfulness always seems to be inferior to the other value which is placed in opposition to it. It is the morally mature and seriously minded person who is here inclined to decide in favour of the other value and to take upon himself the responsibility for the lie. But such situations do not permit of being universalized. They are extreme cases in which the conflict of conscience is heavy enough and in which a different solution is required according to the peculiar ethos of the man. For it is inherent in the essence of such moral conflicts that in them value stands against value and that it is not possible to escape from them without being guilty. Here it is not the values as such in their pure ideality which are in conflict; between the claim of truthfulness as such and the duty of the soldier or friend there exists no antinomy at all. The conflict arises from the structure of the situation. This makes it impossible to satisfy both at the same time. But if from this one should think to make out a universal justification of the necessary lie, one would err, as much as if one were to attempt a universal justification for violating one's duty to one's country or the duty of keeping one's promise.

Nevertheless a man who is in such a situation cannot avoid making a decision. Every attempt to remain neutral only makes the difficulty worse, in that he thereby violates both values; the attempt not to commit oneself is at bottom moral cowardice, a lack of the sense of responsibility and of the willingness to assume it; and often enough is also due to moral immaturity, if not to the fear of others. What a man ought to do, when he is confronted with a serious conflict that is fraught with responsibility, is this: to decide according to his best conscience; that is, according to his own living sense of the relative height of the respective values, and to take upon himself the consequences, external as well as inward, ultimately the guilt involved in the violation of the one value. He ought to carry the guilt and in so doing become stronger, so that he can carry it with pride.

Real moral life is not such that one can stand guiltless in it. And that each person must step by step in life settle conflicts, insoluble theoretically, by his own free sense of values and his own creative energy, should be regarded as a feature of the highest spiritual significance in complete humanity and genuine freedom. Yet one must not make of this a comfortable theory, as the vulgar mind makes of the permissible lie, imagining that one brings upon oneself no guilt in offending against clearly discerned values. It is only unavoidable guilt which can preserve a man from moral decay.

Truth, Honesty, and the Therapeutic Process

Leon Salzman

A basic premise of a therapeutic relationship and an essential part of the contract the patient makes in establishing it is to be honest and

Reprinted with permission of author and publisher from the *American Journal of Psychiatry* 130:11, 1281–82, November 1973. Copyright 1973, the American Psychiatric Association.

truthful. Although the concepts of honesty and truth are rarely mentioned in the psychiatric or psychoanalytic literature, Freud referred to them constantly. He stated:

The psychoanalytic treatment is founded on truthfulness. A great part of its educative effect and its ethical value lies in this very fact . . . .

Since we demand strict truthfulness from our patients, we jeopardize our whole authority if we let ourselves be caught by them in a departure from the truth.[1]

In order for the therapeutic process to be useful to our patients, they must tell us what concerns them, with a minimum of distortion or withholding, to the extent that their emotional capacity and cognitive integrity permit. What is the therapist's part in this arrangement? How much should he tell or withhold from the patient? To communicate our feelings, attitudes, observations, or interpretations to our patients may be essential to the process of therapy, but at times such communication can be destructive. Is this countertransference or simply an essential part of the therapeutic arrangement?

THE DISTINCTION BETWEEN HONESTY AND TRUTH

First, we must clarify our concepts. Honesty is not the same as truth, although the two are related. Webster defines truth as "the state of being the case: fact," while honesty is defined as "fairness and straightforwardness of conduct or adherence to the facts. I would like to suggest that honesty is a dynamic concept that is based on an individual's sincere and objective attempt to appraise a total situation and that is limited by his inability to be totally unbiased. Truth, on the other hand, is a matter of definition and varies according to the framework in which it is established—whether scientifically, as in natural laws, or morally; as determined by man or God. As Oppenheimer has stated, "Truth is so largely defined by how you find it."[2] He meant simply that what is true depends upon how one sets out to determine the truth.

This distinction is crucial in a discussion of the place of truth, honesty, and trust in the therapeutic process. For example, we must recognize that honesty is not exclusively a moral issue, since it is determined by the degree of freedom the person has to explore, express, and determine the truths in his environment. A person's honesty is strongly influenced by the amount of neurotic defenses he has and the degree of distortion he unconsciously imposes

on the environment by such behaviors as denial, projection, or dissociation. The degree of honesty a person expresses is determined by the amount of security and self-esteem he has, which allows him to be more or less honest in seeing a situation as it really is. Dishonesty, whether consciously elaborated or unconsciously demonstrated, is a defensive maneuver designed to support a neurotic system. We distinguish between the deliberate and the unconscious liar only because we still tend to assign moral judgments to those types of distortion.

Is the child lying when he tells you about the fire engine drawn by elephants and led by a maharajah, à la Dr. Seuss, or is he simply using his imagination? Are our patients being dishonest when they deny that they are irritated when we cut short their hours—because they are afraid we will get angry and terminate therapy? Is a patient being dishonest when he unconsciously falsifies a childhood experience by remembering it as having been bitten by a dog rather than as having kicked and hurt the dog?

These examples illustrate some of the vagaries of the concept of honesty and demonstrate why it cannot simply be appraised but must be understood in the context of the experience. Honesty is the potential to see a situation for what it is; it is achieved only when one has a minimal need to defend oneself against anxiety because one has sufficient self-regard. Whether we communicate this honest appraisal of a situation in a truthful statement or withhold it for reasons we believe are justified, our goal in the training of therapists should certainly be to encourage and develop basic honesty in our human contacts. Dishonesty is the inevitable consequence of the neurotic structure and occurs when a person's defenses demand some distortion of reality—by total reversal, slight distortion, exaggeration, minimizing, shading, etc. In therapy, this tendency is generally not categorized as dishonesty but rather is considered a problem of defense. The therapist should refrain from moralizing judgments and recognize that these distortions are a necessary activity in the neurotic state.

This link between neurosis and dishonesty has led many theorists, particularly Horney and Sullivan, to consider neuroses immoral and to classify them as "ethical diseases." Certainly the neurotic is dishonest but, since he is unable to make any choices, his dishonesty is imposed upon him by his neurosis. He does not wish it and would like to rid himself of it. The psychotic individual, whether his psychosis is of an organic or psychological origin, likewise describes events and experiences in a manner that deviates widely from fact. These reports are labeled delusions, hallucinations, faulty perceptions, confabulations, and the like. The issue of honesty or truth is not raised in regard to them, although we occasionally designate malingering as a deliberate attempt to deceive or defraud. In therapy we prefer to talk about defenses rather than honesty, since the problem of honesty is very loaded with ethical and theological judgments.

The matter of honesty leads us to an examination of the concept of truth. There are many interesting definitions of truth. All of them are true, yet none of them is entirely true. And this is precisely the limitation of the concept of truth, unless we believe in an absolute truth. To say that something is absolutely true is immediately to tell a lie, for truth is entirely dependent on our frame of reference, as Einstein plainly demonstrated in his experiments in relativity. Yet if we limit our definition of truth to some relativistic or indeterminate sense, we have chaos. Consequently, civilized societies have agreed on some basic truths as a foundation for morality.

HONESTY AND TRUTH IN THERAPY

In the therapeutic process honesty is an essential for patient and therapist. It is unthinkable that a rational, humanistic, nonauthoritarian healing process can take place without it. Yet it is too often demanded of the patient and not often enough required of the therapist. Many therapies, such as magic, proceed in an atmosphere that could be described as dishonest, but these are not subsumed under the strict category of psychotherapy by mutual exchange, as defined by Freud.

What needs to be clarified is not whether one should be honest, but how to use our honest evaluations in an effective way. This is exclusively a question of technique, or at least it should be. Although we should not knowingly deviate from honest appraisals in our therapeutic work, we must constantly decide how best to utilize these appraisals. The question is not when should we be honest but when should we communicate our honest observations so that they most effectively serve the therapeutic process. In the case of a patient with incipient schizophrenia, there is no question about *whether* we should interpret to him a dream caused by severe anxiety that presages emotional disorganization; it is only a matter of *when* to do it. Likewise, we must decide *when* to inform a patient that we dislike some behavior and find it obnoxious (not should we or should we not).

The therapist's honesty in appraising such situations must be assumed and required without question. *What* we communicate, however, is a different question from whether or not we honestly appraise the total situation. We must not confuse honesty with technique, for without a basic honesty the therapy itself is in jeopardy and the technical problem never arises.

Unfortunately, for many therapists this decision never occurs, for they automatically decide to withhold unpleasant or distressful observations from patients because of their own inability to handle the consequences. In such cases, however, we are not dealing with honesty or truth but with an incompetent or immature therapist who has greater concern for his own welfare than for that of his patient. At times, of course, it may be the overwhelming characterological problems of the patient that put the therapist on the defensive, and one must acknowledge that this can happen to any therapist, however skillful, experienced, or mature.

On the matter of truth I think we can be much clearer. I cannot visualize many situations in which an untruth can be justified in the healing profession. Certainly we can argue endlessly about the dilemma of the patient with incurable cancer, but aside from this, I think we would all agree that in the psychotherapeutic process an untruth is never justified. This must be clearly distinguished from withholding the truth for definable reasons. Our rationalizations may be incorrect, our justifications fallacious, but withholding the truth is quite different from telling a patient a lie. Freud made this clear in his statement quoted above. Certainly it is easy to justify withholding the truth from patients for reasons ostensibly beneficial to them when we are really protecting ourselves. It is easy to blame failures in therapy on our patients when our own skills are at fault. But this is a matter of recognizing our own deficiencies. In my opinion our patients are better able to handle unpleasant material than we ever give them credit for.

Yet here again we must not confuse technique with truth. In the present state of development of psychological theory our interpretations and observations are a long way from being verifiable, and consequently we may not be withholding a *truth* if we refrain from making an interpretation, but only an *opinion*. We can establish some honesty in our appraisal only if we allow ourselves the freedom to examine human experience from a standpoint that is not biased or preconceived. The truthfuless of these observations will be determined somewhere far in the future.

At present we work only with skilled guesses, approximations, and rudimentary scientific observations and we must never fool ourselves about this fact. Frequently we present our educated guesses and approximations to our patients as though they were established truths.

Such misrepresentations are as harmful as lying or withholding, and perhaps more so, since they occur so frequently. We must avoid the temptation to use our status to establish a set of "truths" that may be far removed from any acceptable definition of truth.

The purpose of distinguishing between honesty and truth in therapy is to stress the wisdom of using certain technical interventions in the therapeutic process. Although there is no virtue in a doctrine of absolute truthfulness in the therapeutic process, there seems never to be a justification for deception. But just as honesty is relative to the patient's sense of security, so much we recognize that the therapist is also human, and therefore subject to neurotic difficulties, defending himself with denials, and seeing less than the whole truth. We hope, however, that he has less need for such defenses than the patient does, and consequently we believe we have a right to expect less deception on his part.

Notes

1. Freud S: Introductory lectures, in Complete Psychological Works, standard ed. Translated and edited by Strachey J. London, Hogarth Press, 1963.
2. Oppenheimer JR: The Open Mind. New York, Simon and Schuster, 1955.

Playing Supergod

Samuel Vaisrub

How should we tell a patient with a fatal disease the truth? And having told it, how do we prepare him for dying? These questions are discussed widely in current medical and lay

Reprinted with permission from the *Journal of the American Medical Association* 218:4, 588, October 25, 1971. Copyright 1971, American Medical Association.

publications as well as on televised panels in which physicians share concerns with attorneys, clergymen, and psychiatrists.

These concerns are not new. Until recently, however, the central question was not *how* to tell a patient the truth, but *whether* to tell it. Opinions were divided. Those who favored leveling with the patient marshalled persuasive arguments for so doing. After all, truth is considered to be a moral-religious imperative. To withhold it is sinful, as well as harmful and impractical. Why deprive the patient of a compelling incentive for setting his business affairs in order and making his peace with God?

Less self-righteous, those who oppose informing the patient were often too self-conscious to present their views with convincing forcefulness. Yet, they have a strong case. The truth about imminent death is not a philosophical abstraction to be discussed with cool detachment. It is a statement which may be as lethal to the spirit as its message is to the body. To many patients—even to those who insist on being told the truth—certitude of impending death may prove to be an unbearable burden. The emotional state provoked by the revelation may dim rather than brighten judgment for setting one's house in order or for preparing to face one's Creator.

It may even be argued that foreknowledge of death is contrary to Nature's plan or God's will. No mortal to-date has received a Divine estimate of his remaining days on earth. Nor has Nature provided this kind of information. Unlike fear or pain which often serve a protective purpose, intimation of mortality, apparently, has no survival value in the evolutionary process of natural selection.

Must, then, the physician set himself above Nature and play Supergod?

Should Doctors Tell the Truth?

Joseph Collins

This is not a homily on lying. It is a presentation of one of the most difficult questions that confront the physician. Should doctors tell patients the truth? Were I on the witness stand and obliged to answer the question with "yes" or "no," I should answer in the negative and appeal to the judge for permission to qualify my answer. The substance of this article is what that qualification would be.

Though few are willing to make the test, it is widely held that if the truth were more generally told, it would make for world-welfare and human betterment. We shall probably never know. To tell the whole truth is often to perpetrate a cruelty of which many are incapable. This is particularly true of physicians. Those of them who are not compassionate by nature are made so by experience. They come to realize that they owe their fellow-men justice, and graciousness, and benignity, and it becomes one of the real satisfactions of life to discharge that obligation. To do so successfully

they must frequently withhold the truth from their patients, which is tantamount to telling them a lie. Moreover, the physician soon learns that the art of medicine consists largely in skillfully mixing falsehood and truth in order to provide the patient with an amalgam which will make the metal of life wear and keep men from being poor shrunken things, full of melancholy and indisposition, unpleasing to themselves and to those who love them. I propose therefore to deal with the question from a pragmatic, not a moral standpoint.

"Now you may tell me the truth," is one of the things patients have frequently said to me. Four types of individuals have said it: those who honestly and courageously want to know so that they may make as ready as possible to face the wages of sin while there is still time; those who do not want to know, and who if they were told would be injured by it; those who are wholly incapable of receiving the truth. Finally, those whose health is neither seriously disordered nor threatened. It may seem an exaggeration to say that in forty years of contact with the sick, the patients I have met who are in the first category could be counted on the fingers of one hand. The vast majority who demand the truth really belong in the fourth category, but there are sufficient in the second—with whom my concern chiefly is—to justify considering their case.

One of the astonishing things about patients is that the more serious the disease, the more silent they are about its portents and manifestations. The man who is constantly seeking reassurance that the vague abdominal pains indicative of hyperacidity are not symptoms of cancer often buries family and friends, some of whom have welcomed death as an escape from his burdensome iterations. On the other hand, there is the man whose first warning of serious disease is lumbago who cannot be persuaded to consult a physician until the disease, of which the lumbago is only a symptom, has so far progressed that it is beyond surgery. The seriousness of disease may be said to stand in direct relation to the reticence of its possessor. The more silent the patient, the more serious the disorder.

The patient with a note-book, or the one who is eager to tell his story in great detail, is rarely very ill. They are forever asking. "Am I going to get well?" and though they crave assistance they are often unable to accept it. On the other hand, patients with organic disease are very chary about asking point blank either the nature or the outcome of their ailment. They sense its gravity, and the last thing in the world they wish to know is the truth about it; and to learn it would be the worst thing that could happen to them.

This was borne in upon me early in my professional life. I was summoned one night to assuage the pain of a man who informed me that he had been for some time under treatment for rheumatism—that cloak for so many diagnostic errors. His "rheumatism" was due to a disease of the spinal cord called locomotor ataxia. When he was told that he should submit himself to treatment wholly different from that which he had been receiving, the import of which any intelligent layman would have divined, he asked neither the nature nor the probable outcome of the disease. He did as he was counselled. He is now approaching seventy and, though not active in business, it still engrosses him.

Had he been told that he had a disease which was then universally believed to be progressive, apprehension would have depressed him so heavily that he would not have been able to offer the resistance to its encroachment which has stood him in such good stead. He was told the truth only in part. That is, he was told his "rheumatism" was "different"; that it was dependent upon an organism quite unlike the one that causes ordinary rheumatism; that we have preparations of mercury and arsenic which kill the parasite responsible for this disease, and that if he would submit himself to their use, his life would not be materially shortened, or his efficiency seriously impaired.

Many experiences show that patients do not want the truth about their maladies, and that it is prejudicial to their well-being to know it, but none that I know is more apposite than that of a lawyer, noted for his urbanity and resourcefulness in Court. When he entered my consulting room, he greeted me with a bonhomie that bespoke intimacy, but I had met him only twice—once on the golf links many years before, and once in Court where I was appearing as expert witness, prejudicial to his case.

He apologized for engaging my attention with such a triviality, but he had had pain in one shoulder and arm for the past few months, and though he was perfectly well—and had been assured of it by physicians in Paris, London, and Brooklyn—this pain was annoying and he had made up his mind to get rid of it. That I should not get a wrong slant on his condition, he submitted a number of laboratory reports furnished him by an osteopath to show that secretions and excretions susceptible of chemical examinations were quite normal. His determination seemed to be to prevent me from taking a view of his health which might lead me to counsel his retirement. He was quite sure that anything like a thorough examination was unnecessary but he submitted to it. It revealed intense and extensive disease of the kidneys. The pain in the network of nerves of the left upper-arm was a manifestation of the resulting autointoxication.

I felt it incumbent upon me to tell him that his condition was such that he should make a radical change in his mode of life. I told him if he would stop work, spend the winter in

Honolulu, go on a diet suitable to a child of three years, and give up exercise, he could look forward confidently to a recovery that would permit of a life of usefulness and activity in his profession. He assured me he could not believe that one who felt no worse than he did should have to make such a radical change in his mode of life. He impressed upon me that I should realize he was the kind of person who had to know the truth. His affairs were so diversified and his commitments so important that he *must* know. Completely taken in, I explained to him the relationship between the pain from which he sought relief and the disease, the degeneration that was going on in the excretory mechanisms of his body, how these were struggling to repair themselves, the procedure of recovery and how it could be facilitated. The light of life began to flicker from the fear that my words engendered, and within two months it sputtered and died out. He was the last person in the world to whom the truth should have been told. Had I lied to him, and then intrigued with his family and friends, he might be alive to-day.

The longer I practice medicine the more I am convinced that every physician should cultivate lying as a fine art. But there are many varieties of lying. Some are most prejudicial to the physician's usefulness. Such are: pretending to recognize the disease and understand its nature when one is really ignorant; asserting that one has effected the cure which nature has accomplished, or claiming that one can effect cure of a disease which is universally held to be beyond the power of nature or medical skill; pronouncing disease incurable which one cannot rightfully declare to be beyond cessation or relief.

There are other lies, however, which contribute enormously to the success of the physician's mission of mercy and salvation. There are a great number of instances in support of this but none more convincing than that of a man of fifty who, after twenty-five years of devotion to painting, decided that penury and old age were incompatible for him. Some of his friends had forsaken art for advertising. He followed their lead and in five years he was ready to gather the first ripe fruit of his labor.

When he attempted to do so he was so immobilized by pain and rigidity that he had to forego work. One of those many persons who assume responsibility lightly assured him that if he would put himself in the hands of a certain osteopath he would soon be quite fit. The assurance was without foundation. He then consulted a physician who without examining him proceeded to treat him for what is considered a minor ailment.

Within two months his appearance gave such concern to his family that he was persuaded to go to a hospital, where the disease was quickly detected, and he was at once submitted to surgery. When he had recovered from the operation, learning that I was in the country of his adoption, he asked to see me. He had not been able, he said, to get satisfactory information from the surgeon or the physician; all that he could gather from them was that he would have to have supplementary X-ray or radium treatment. What he desired was to get back to his business which was on the verge of success, and he wanted assurance that he could soon do so.

He got it. And more than that, he got elaborate explanation of what surgical intervention had accomplished, but not a word of what it had failed to accomplish. A year of activity was vouchsafed him, and during that time he put his business in such shape that its eventual sale provided a modest competency for his family. It was not until the last few weeks that he knew the nature of his malady. Months of apprehension had been spared him by the deception, and he had been the better able to do his work, for he was buoyed by the hope that his health was not beyond recovery. Had he been told the truth, black despair would have been thrown over the world in which he moved, and he would have carried on with corresponding ineffectiveness.

The more extensive our field of observation and the more intimate our contact with human activity, the more we realize the finiteness of the human mind. Every follower of Hippocrates will agree that "judgment is difficult and experience fallacious." A disease may have only a fatal ending, but one does not know; one may know that certain diseases, such as general paresis, invariably cause death, but one does not know that tomorrow it may no longer be true. The victim may be reprieved by acciden-

tal or studied discovery or by the intervention of something that still must be called divine grace. . . .

Truthtelling in Medicine

Robert Weir

''To tell or not to tell'' is a moral problem central to physician–patient relationships. How much ''truth'' is necessary—or advisable—in communicating a diagnosis to a patient? When and what should a physician communicate to a patient known to be dying? How much information is necessary for a patient to be ''informed''—and thus give informed consent—prior to going to surgery? What are the defining limits of informed consent for randomized clinical trails which may or may not prove beneficial for a particular patient? What are the advantages and disadvantages of informing patients about the possible use of placebos? How much deception with parents is morally permissible in communicating the prognosis—or cause of death—of a defective neonate?

Because of its centrality in a number of clinical contexts, truthtelling in medicine is one of the recurring themes in the field of biomedical ethics. Two problems exist, however, in the interpretations of truthtelling in the bioethical literature. First, the classic case of truthtelling—the case of the dying patient—dominates the scene to the point that many discussions of truthtelling in medicine rarely get beyond an analysis of conversations with terminal patients. Second, much of the literature on truthtelling in other medical contexts (e.g., those requiring informed consent) tends to be contextually isolated, suggesting that the moral requirements of truthtelling in one clinical situation have no application to other clinical situations.

From *Perspectives in Biology and Medicine*, Autumn 1980, pp. 95–112. Reprinted by permission of the author and the University of Chicago Press. © 1980 by the University of Chicago.

I intend to discuss the issue of truthtelling by focusing on its two dimensions of truth and truthfulness, showing how the requirement of truthtelling applies to two different clinical contexts, and putting forth reasons for regarding truthtelling as a moral obligation applicable to all medical fields. The clinical contexts are those involving dying patients and genetic counselees, the former chosen because it is the traditional ''paradigm case'' of truthtelling and the latter because genetic counseling is representative of a number of medical fields in which physicians regularly confront the issue of truthtelling with patients who are not dying. My purpose will be to demonstrate, using genetic counseling as the comparative context, that the issue of truthtelling in medicine is richer, more complex, and more central to the entire medical enterprise than it seems when limited to the traditional context of dying patients or when analyzed solely in one of the new clinical contexts requiring informed consent. The perspective from which I will be working is an understanding that the pivotal thinkers in Western philosophical and religious traditions have been in general agreement that (in Sissela Bok's words) ''truthful statements are preferable to lies in the absence of special considerations'' [p. 30].[1]

THE PHYSICIAN AS TRUTH-CONTROLLING AUTHORITY

There can be little question that physicians are regarded as authority figures in their relationships with patients, nurses, and virtually everyone else in a hospital setting who has not received a medical degree. The precise reasons for their status as authority figures are varied and include their roles as restorers of health, masters of a technical knowledge, decision makers in crisis situations, combatants against disease and death, dispensers of powerful drugs, and choreographers of a vast array of technological procedures and equipment. In a nutshell, physicians possess a highly specialized knowledge and perform a number of highly specialized tasks which are valued by persons who are dependent on them.

It is the possession of a specialized knowledge which is relevant to the issue of truthtelling in medicine. Dying patients seeking information—and persons seeking genetic counseling—are caught up in a dependency relationship in which a medical expert controls highly significant or risk-laden knowledge which is not generally accessible to nonmedical persons. Certain parts of this knowledge may be sought (and sometimes secured) from nonmedical sources, but in order to secure the most accurate and complete knowledge relevant to their medical conditions, both dying patients and persons seeking genetic counseling are dependent on an authority figure whose training gives him or her special access to the knowledge—or truth—being sought.

This relationship of dependency—and the role of the physician as a truth-controlling authority—is illustrated by an exchange of comments between two highly respected geneticists at a conference sponsored by the Hastings Center. D. J. H. Brock, professor of human genetics at the University of Edinburgh, and Arno Motulsky, professor of medical genetics at the University of Washington, compared notes on the issue of truthtelling in the following manner:

BROCK: Take the example of myotonic dystrophy. A man in his early thirties just contracting the disease comes in for counseling. *In the interest of efficiency,* surely the genetic counselor *should describe in very real terms what is going to happen to him,* what the prognosis is. If he doesn't do it, this man who is minimally affected at the time simply cannot see the need to curtail his reproduction. He can't see that there is any point in

doing this, unless it is spelled out to him in very clear terms what the eventual outcome of the disease is going to be. *And yet this would seem to me to be totally inhumane.*

MOTULSKY: You have an alternative to what you can tell this man. You can tell him, "Your case is rather mild. Many people with the disease have a mild case. However, the disease can be very bad." Then proceed to tell him about severely affected cases.

You don't have to take the props out from under a man. I try to give the patients some hope. *Giving the patient the truth and all the unadorned facts is erring against the ethos of medicine* by which we try to help the patient. Sometimes, withholding of all information is in *the best interest of the patient.* If I think it is better that a man not be told that he has cancer, I will not tell him. As a physician, I have to make this decision myself. It is hard. I can share and discuss with my colleagues, but ultimately it is my decision. *To give the whole truth to every patient is not humane.* [p. 98, emphasis added][2]

As suggested by these comments, physicians often understand themselves to have the right of controlling (or at least managing) the truth, whether the immediate context is a dying patient's room, a counseling room in a genetics clinic, or some other clinical setting. Working out of the perspective of medical paternalism, physicians sometimes think they know more about a patient's needs, interests, and emotional stability than the patient does and withhold potentially damaging information to protect the patient from possibly undergoing an emotional catastrophe. As controllers of vital information, they conclude that the withholding of all (or at least a significant part) of such information is often in "the best interest of the patient."

Because this accepted role is common in the medical profession, there are numerous clinical situations in which a physician may choose to control the truth a patient receives simply by withholding all or part of the relevant information. Two such situations involve dying patients who seek information about their medical conditions and persons genetically at risk who seek scientific and mathematical information about a particular genetic disease. The two geneticists quoted above obviously think there are close parallels between the two situations and appear to agree that in both kinds of situations the "withholding of all information" or at least the withholding of some of the "truth and all the unadorned facts" is a proper part of the physician-patient relationship because such practices are in the patient's best interests.

Is the physician-patient relationship generally understood by both parties to include the right of physicians to control the truth by withholding some or all of the relevant medical information? Are the situations of dying patients and persons genetically at risk sufficiently alike in moral terms that to answer the questions of truthtelling in one situation is also to answer them in the other? What, in fact, does it mean to engage in truthtelling in these clinical situations?

WHAT CONSTITUTES THE TRUTH IN THESE MEDICAL CONTEXTS?

In much of the medical literature which addresses the issue of truthtelling with dying patients, the actual nature of "the truth" is taken to be self-evident. The question, "Should dying patients be told the truth?" is taken to be a question in reference to the correctness or incorrectness (e.g., inaccurate euphemisms) of what a patient may be told about her medical condition. When understood in this manner, the truth rather obviously means logical truth or verbal accuracy—the correspondence of verbal statements to reality. Thus, years ago, when William Kelly and Stanley Friesen[3] did a survey of cancer patients, and when Donald Oken[4] did a survey of physicians who treat cancer patients, portions of the questions regarding truthtelling were left unstated: "Do you want to be told (the medical evidence)?" or "What is your usual policy about telling patients (what the medical data are)?"

Understood in this way—with no reference to the veracity of the speaker—the truth for dying patients means nothing more or less than an accurate representation of the medical facts: an accurate diagnosis (e.g., stage IV cancer of the cervix) followed by an accurate prognosis (it is terminal), backed up with evidence accumulated through biopsies, lab tests, and surgery. Put another way, the truth for dying patients is frequently interpreted to mean a Cronkite-like statement of the medical findings: "And that's the way it is. . . . ."

In a similar manner, the truth for persons genetically at risk is generally understood to mean nothing more or less than an accurate representation of the genetic evidence: an accurate diagnosis (e.g., Duchenne muscular dystrophy), accompanied by an accurate family history, interpretation of the inheritance pattern (X-linked recessive), recurrence risks, prognosis (rapid deterioration, likely terminal during the teenage years), and possibilities of treatment if any exist. Depending upon the particular disease, the truth communicated during a counseling session can often be backed up with clinical evidence: chromosome studies, biochemical tests on blood and urine, skin biopsies, and so forth.

The problem which confronts genetic counselors at this point, however, is that the truth in terms of scientific accuracy is often difficult to determine and, at times, simply impossible to know because of the comparatively elementary state of the science. It was, after all, as recently as 1956 that the normal chromosomal number in humans was determined to be 46 and only in 1959 that a genetic disease (Down's syndrome) was traced to a chromosomal aberration.[5] The extent of scientific knowledge yet to be discovered in human genetics can only be estimated by observing the number of incomplete tables in medical genetics textbooks, or by noting the extraordinary recent gains in genetic knowledge (as reflected in the five editions of Victor McKusick's *Mendelian Inheritance in Man*) and surmising that much more is yet to come.[6]

An additional problem is the complexity of the genetic evidence already known. If, for example, all that a genetic counselor had to do to tell the truth was to identify genetic conditions caused by alleles at a single chromosomal locus and then interpret the etiology of the condition in terms of autosomal dominant, autosomal recessive, or X-linked inheritance patterns, the relation between verbal accuracy and scientific evidence could be drawn fairly easily. When, however, an unusual genetic condition is present and the affected individual's pedigree shows no readily identifiable pattern, a counselor must consider a variety of factors which can affect gene expression: penetrance, expressivity, pleiotrophy, sex-limited traits, variable onset age, polygenic inheritance, and so forth [pp. 73–80].[7] The truth—in terms of accuracy—can in these circumstances be very elusive.

WHAT ABOUT TRUTHFULNESS WITH PATIENTS AND COUNSELEES?

There is another dimension to truthtelling in medicine which we have not yet covered. The first dimension is an objective one: the accuracy of what a patient or counselee is told about the medical facts. The second and morally more important dimension is a subjective one: the intended result of what is said to a patient or counselee. As Bok correctly observes, the moral question "of whether you are lying or not is not *settled* by establishing the truth or falsity of what you say. In order to settle this question, we must know whether you *intend your statement to mislead* [p. 23].[1]

Truth and truthfulness are obviously closely related, and, up to a point, each is indispensable to the other. Fortunately for all of us, the two frequently come together in the written and verbal communications we have with other people. If this were not the case, there would be little possibility for any of us ever to participate in intelligent, trustworthy conversations with other persons. We would be constantly alert lest we be confused by someone who was not reporting factual information correctly, or lest we be misled by someone who was deliberately trying to deceive us.

On those occasions when, in retrospect, we become convinced that meaningful communication has broken down, our reaction usually varies depending upon our assessment of why the communication has broken down. If we find out that the information we were given was wrong, we are likely to have second thoughts about going to that person again for the same kind of information. When we need factual data of the same sort the next time, we will probably consult another person who we hope will be more competent and will be able to

"get the facts straight." If, however, we become convinced that communication has broken down because the person lied to us or in some other manner tried to deceive us, our reaction is likely to be much different and much more intense. The excuse we might make for the person in the first case ("everybody makes mistakes") simply does not fit the person in the second case. Rather than offering excuses for the person or perhaps questioning the person's competence in a certain area of knowledge, we are apt to be resentful, disappointed, and suspicious in any further dealings we have with that individual.

What the truth/truthfulness distinction points to, therefore, is the difference between epistemological certainty and moral choice [pp. 6–31].[1] For a person to be able to "speak the truth" depends upon that person's knowledge of a certain sphere of information and ability to give an accurate representation of that knowledge. In medicine, as in any other field, communication sometimes breaks down for the undeniable reasons of human ignorance and fallibility: a physician may tell a patient something which the physician thinks is correct, whereas in reality the physician has made a mistake and given the wrong diagnosis or prognosis. For a person to be able to "speak truthfully" depends, in contrast, not on that person's knowledge or professional competence in some field, but on the person's moral choice to be honest and straightforward in speech. In medicine, again as in any other field, communication breaks down for the simple reason of moral choice: a physician may give a patient factually correct information and nevertheless intend to mislead the patient through a deceitful use of that information.

Physicians sometimes depart from truthfulness with dying patients by engaging in what Robert Veatch describes as "the big lie": a rationalization of lying by which a physician engages in self-deception as well as deception of a patient [pp. 222–229].[8] Two particular forms of the big lie described by Veatch are deliberate decisions not to be honest with patients. In the "truthful lie" (or, more correctly, the technically true lie), physicians attempt to fulfill the obligation of telling the truth by spewing medical jargon, while at the same time avoiding any communication of the medical evidence which the patient can understand. A physician's words to a patient may be technically true (e.g., "You have a neoplasm with the characteristics of a leimyosarcoma with possible secondary metastatic growth"), but the physician intentionally deceives the patient by using a highly specialized language which few nonmedical persons understand. In "indirect communication," physicians rationalize that "direct, immediate, blunt talk" is harmful to a patient and should be replaced by communication which can be handled by the patient because it is suggestive only. Again, the physician's words to a patient may be technically correct, but the physician is dishonest because he communicates through intentionally ambiguous terminology and evasive responses to questions. When either of these forms of the big lie occurs, physicians are blameworthy not because they give inaccurate information or withhold some of the medical facts, but because they are less than truthful with patients who trust them and expect them to be honest.

The same sort of problems often characterize the communications between genetic counselors and their counselees. In fact, counselors who want to avoid being truthful can find any number of alternatives which are personally and professionally satisfactory. For instance, a counselor who anticipates that the genetic information to be communicated will have a serious impact on an individual's life or marriage may give an accurate diagnosis and then modify the actual prognosis with overly optimistic statements and false assurances. Thus counselors working with members of choreic families do on occasion, after having accurately diagnosed Huntington's disease, engage in false reassurances along the line that "medical science will find a cure" in the next two or three decades or that "lightning never strikes twice in the same place" [p. 4].[9] Or, alternatively, a counselor may correctly identify a general category of genetic disease (chromosomal aberration, inborn error of metabolism, etc.), but decide to deceive counselees regarding which disease in the category is at issue. Thus, in the "unexpected chromosome" case in which a pregnant woman had amniocentesis performed for the purpose

of detecting Trisomy 21, the counselor could have chosen to give the woman a technically true statement (e.g., the amniocentesis "confirmed the presence of an extra chromosome"), yet intentionally deceive her by not telling her that the extra chromosome detected was a Y chromosome (giving the fetus the XYY sex chromosome configuration) rather than the extra twenty-first chromosome, which would be present if the fetus had Trisomy 21 [pp. 137–139].[10] In either of these instances, one of the results of not being honest with counselees is that they may, because they have been misled by the counselor, make decisions about procreation or abortion or some other important matter which they would not have made if the counselor had been truthful with them.

WHAT CONSTITUTES THE PROBLEM OF TRUTHTELLING IN THESE SITUATIONS?

As illustrated by the Kelly-Friesen and Oken studies cited previously, the problem of telling dying patients the truth often hangs on the moral conflict between the patient's right to know the truth and the patient's welfare if the truth cannot be handled. The Kelly-Friesen study indicates that the overwhelming majority of patients with cancer (89 percent), as well as patients without known cancer (82 percent), want to be told that they have an irreversibly terminal condition if that is what the medical evidence indicates. The Oken study, in sharp contrast, shows that 88 percent of the physicians in one major hospital have a personal policy of not telling patients that they have cancer even if that is clearly indicated by the medical evidence. A more recent study of physicians' attitudes in another hospital shows that, while the responding physicians indicate unanimous agreement that cancer patients have "the right to know" and 98 percent of the group report an unspecified policy of telling the patients the truth, the majority of the physicians (91 percent) sometimes do not tell patients the truth because of "personal and emotional factors" (such as possible patient depression or undefined suicidal tendencies).[11] Thus physicians, as controllers of a specialized knowledge, sometimes decide on paternalistic grounds to withhold information which they agree patients have a right to know.

Put in an alternate way, the moral conflict in telling dying patients is between advocates who argue along deontological lines (the physician has a duty to tell the patient the truth) and others who argue along consequentialist lines (to hear the truth might harm the patient). Even though utilitarian arguments are occasionally put forth for telling patients the truth, the utilitarian arguments which surface most often in this debate are similar to Motulsky's statement quoted earlier: "Withholding of all information is in the best interest of the patient." Thus euphemisms, circumlocutions, and lies are sometimes regarded by physicians as justifiable means of achieving the desirable ends of maintaining a patient's hope, preventing the patient from getting depressed, and avoiding the possibility that some patients who cannot cope with medical reality will attempt suicide.

As to the failure to be truthful with dying patients, a physician's personal attitudes toward death and toward dying patients may be colored by a tendency to deny the reality of death and to postpone having to admit that, despite his specialized knowledge and skills, another patient is irretrievably dying. As suggested by the Oken study and backed up by the research of Herman Feifel et al., physicians do have a problem confronting the reality of death and admitting their technical limitations before that inevitable fact [pp. 201–202].[12] The result is that it is psychologically easier for some physicians to be dishonest and deceptive with dying patients than to confront—personally and with the patient—the unpleasant tasks imposed by a policy of honesty.

It is obvious from the Brock-Motulsky comments quoted earlier that the same kind of moral conflict regarding truth and truthfulness exists among medical geneticists. Brock suggests (for the wrong reason) that a genetic counselor is obligated to describe "in very real terms what is going to happen" to the man with myotonic dystrophy. Namely, the condition the man has inherited is a progressive myotonia, accompanied by expressionless facial muscles, cataracts, decreased functional activity of the gonads, frontal baldness (in males), mental deterioration, abnormal heart activity, and death between the ages of 40 and 60 due to congestive heart failure [pp. 126–127].[13]* Motulsky's response is to give a consequentialist argument regarding truth and truthfulness: out of concern for the man's welfare (possible loss of hope), either (a) withhold some of the relevant medical facts from the patient (do not tell him the truth), or (b) give an overly optimistic diagnosis and prognosis (do not be truthful with him).

Other factors add to the problem of truthtelling with counselees. One of these factors is the rapidity with which new genetic information is being accumulated. Hymie Gordon observes that "scarcely a week passes without a new syndrome being delineated, a new diagnostic procedure being proposed or additional statistical insights being provided" [p. 1223].[14] When a field of science is expanding this rapidly, it is difficult for a genetic counselor to keep abreast of new developments. Consequently, a counselor's knowledge (or lack of it) regarding the diagnosis and possible treatment of "new" genetic diseases sometimes imposes a practical limit to the truth which can be told a counselee.

Another factor which contributes to the problem of truthtelling in medical genetics is the extraordinary ease with which risk figures can be manipulated to fit the value system of the counselor. A simple shift in wording—from telling a woman she has a 50 percent chance of having a defective child to telling her she has a 50 percent chance of having a normal child—"colors" the accuracy of the statement. Or, to illustrate the problem further, suppose that a woman has some reason to think she may be a carrier of Niemann-Pick disease and comes to see a genetic counselor. The truth (accuracy of information) and truthfulness (honesty) she receives may well be influenced by a counselor's moral judgments regarding amniocentesis, abortion, the actual effects of this disease in young children, the importance of this woman having children, and the possible transmission of a genetic condition which is characterized by neurological degeneration and death around the age of 5 years. If a

*Editors' Note: Myotonic Dystrophy is not always accompanied by all of the conditions listed.

counselor wishes to deter the woman from having a child, he may emphasize the risk (25 percent) of producing a genetically affected child. If the counselor chooses to be optimistic, he may downplay the risk by indicating that there is a 75 percent chance of producing a normal child. If, in addition, the counselor thinks that amniocentesis is a safe diagnostic procedure and selective abortion a morally justifiable option should Niemann-Pick disease be detected prenatally, he may emphasize that the chance of producing a normal child is drastically improved once amniocentesis and abortion are part of the picture.

Still another factor which complicates the issue of truthtelling in medical genetics—in contrast to truthtelling with dying patients—is the frequent failure of counselees to understand genetic information. As Elisabeth Kübler-Ross[15] and Avery Weisman[16] have demonstrated, dying patients often have predictable psychological reactions when told the truth about their dying. The immediate reaction is denial of the truth, followed in many instances in a rather unsystematic fashion by anger, bargaining, depression, and, sometimes, acceptance of the truth that he has an irreversible medical condition and is dying. Yet a dying patient—when no longer going through denial—does not have to understand the specifics of the case (e.g., the particular form of sarcoma) to know intuitively that the truth communicated by the physician is a prediction of irreversible decline and death. Because there is no known therapy which will alter the medical condition, a dying patient's understanding of the medical facts is irrelevant to the ultimate outcome.

In contrast, a person receiving information that she has or carries a genetic disease needs to have at least a minimal understanding of the etiology of the disease, the severity of the disease, and the probabilities of the disease's recurrence—if that person is to use the truth in making decisions about the future. A counselee undoubtedly undergoes some of the same initial psychological reactions to the truth that a dying patient does, but in order to accept the framework of reality imposed by the truth communicated by the counselor, a counselee must understand the implications that truth has on

her own individual health picture, marriage plans, and possibilities of procreation. And the difficulty many counselees have in understanding genetic information and mathematical risk figures is a significant reason why truthtelling in genetic counseling is a problematic enterprise.

TRUTHTELLING AS A MORAL OBLIGATION IN MEDICINE

We now arrive at the heart of the issue. Numerous variables involved in physician-patient relationships have direct bearing on the issues of truthtelling: the power imbalance between physician and patient, the specialized knowledge possessed by the physician, legal requirements and potential legal liabilities for the physician, occasional uncertainty as to whether a patient wants or can handle troubling information, decisions on the part of the patient which are dependent upon accurate information honestly rendered, the physician's interest in not harming the patient, and so forth.

Given these variables, truthtelling in the physician–patient relationship can be—and is—interpreted in three ways. Telling patients the truth and being truthful with them can be regarded as a legal requirement imposed on the traditional physician-patient relationship by recent court decisions. Telling the truth and being truthful with patients can be considered, as evidenced by the Brock-Motulsky exchange, a contextually limited privilege granted by physicians when they consider it appropriate and withheld when they judge it not in the best interests of a particular patient. Or telling the truth and being truthful with patients can be interpreted as a moral obligation on the part of physicians which must be carried out in all but the most exceptional circumstances.

When truthtelling is interpreted as a legal requirement with little or no additional moral significance, physicians easily become defensive about this unnecessary intrusion of the law into the traditional physician–patient relationship. Brought about by the patients' rights movement, malpractice suits, and laws mandating freedom of information, the requirement of truthtelling represents a legal obstacle course which must be successfully maneuvered by physicians in all branches of medicine.

The practical implications of this view are several, and together they represent a troubling perspective on the practice of medicine—and on the relationship between medicine, law, and ethics.

1. Virtually all of the obstacles in this course have to do with the sort of information giving which will satisfactorily fulfill the requirements of the law and protect physicians from malpractice suits. The result is a minimalist understanding of truthtelling which equates the truth with legally protective documents (e.g., informed consent documents) and disregards any particular responsibility for truthfulness in speech because verbal deception is not likely to bring about legal problems.

2. Because the legal instruments now used in medicine are regarded as primarily serving the purpose of protecting physicians from legal liability, they easily come to represent for some physicians unnecessary paperwork which merely complicates the physician–patient relationship. If a physician chooses to do so, he or she can react to this paperwork burden by making sarcastic comments to patients about the legal forms (''I think these are silly, but our lawyers tell us we have to use them''), thus suggesting to patients that they really need not take the forms seriously because, after all, doctors are ''good guys'' who do not need lawyers telling them how to conduct their business.

3. By equating the truth with legally required forms, and by making derogatory remarks about the forms, some physicians end up practicing defensive medicine: patients are given information about their conditions and about recommended medical procedures because the law requires it, not because patients have a right to the information and may benefit from knowing it. In this defensive approach to medicine, the truth (e.g., information about surgical risks) is reluctantly told out of professional self-interest, and truthfulness with patients can easily suffer through the deceptive use of legal forms.

Illustrative of this defensive approach to truthtelling are the practices of some physicians

with dying patients and with persons who may be genetically at risk. An internist who has a legalistic and self-protective understanding of truthtelling may attempt to forestall future legal problems by informing the relatives of a dying patient that the patient is irretrievably dying, but never get around to telling the patient the truth or being truthful with that particular patient. An obstetrician may give genetic counseling to a woman or couple at risk merely to avoid the possibility of being sued for negligence in a ''wrongful life'' suit, while being very critical of the courts because of the time and effort required to do an accurate family medical history.[17] Or, alternatively, a genetic counselor in a prenatal genetic counseling session may, for similar legalistic and self-protective reasons, make informed consent documents (e.g., for amniocentesis, for a national chromosomal registry) the focal point of the counseling session by giving a detailed reading of the documents, but never inform the counselees that they give up the right to confidentiality when they sign one of the forms.

When truthtelling is interpreted as a contextually limited privilege, it can be granted or withheld at the discretion of any physician in any clinical context. Accurate information and candid communication can be withheld any time the physician in charge of a patient decides the truth and truthfulness are not ''in the patient's best interests''—regardless of the patient's physical, mental, or emotional status. As long as the physician stays within the boundaries of the law, there is no compelling reason to engage in truthtelling with any given patient or to have a consistent policy of truthtelling which carries over from one patient (or clinical context) to another.

As with the legalistic perspective on truthtelling, there are several practical implications of this view.

1. This interpretation clearly subsumes the responsibility of telling the truth and being truthful with patients under the paternalistic model of the medical profession. Even when, as in the study by Dennis Novack and his colleagues, physicians acknowledge that patients have a right to the truth, that ''right'' is ignored when the physician judges that telling a par-

ticular patient the truth would do harm to the patient.[11] In other words, a physician, because of presumed greater wisdom and acknowledged greater power in this context, decides to interfere with the patient's freedom by withholding information and/or intentionally engaging in deception.

2. Physicians who determine that truthtelling would bring harm to a patient are often thereby making psychiatric and moral judgments for which they have no special qualifications. Having the knowledge and skill to make an accurate diagnosis in a particular case in no way gives a physician special qualifications to know that telling this patient the truth will bring about greater harm to the patient than withholding the truth; or that this patient, upon hearing accurate information honestly rendered, will immediately lose all hope and go into suicidal depression; or that this patient's "best interests" are limited to whatever the physician happens to know about the patient through limited contact in a clinical setting.

3. By making truthtelling a context-limited privilege, physicians who function under the paternalistic model frequently set up a list of criteria by which only certain patients qualify for the privilege. The study by Novack and colleagues is again illustrative. When asked about their policy of telling cancer patients (who may or may not have a terminal form of the disease) the truth about their conditions, approximately half of the responding physicians listed the patient's age, the patient's intelligence, the patient's emotional stability, the patient's expressed wish to be told, and the wishes of the patient's relatives as "frequent factors" in determining whether or not to tell patients the truth about their cancer.

4. The decision "to tell or not to tell" in this paternalistic model is thus dependent on isolated factors in a particular clinical context which are frequently nonmedical in nature and, more important, the physician's perception of these factors. Telling the truth and being truthful depend not so much on the status of the law or on acknowledged patient rights as on a physician's belief that a particular patient "qualifies" for the privilege. Therefore, one patient may be given accurate information and honest counsel by a physician, whereas in the next room another patient whose medical condition, psychological status, and personal interests are roughly the same as the first patient's may be denied the truth and given evasive answers by the same physician because, for any number of fleeting variables, the physician believes that this patient does not qualify for the privilege.

It is not necessary at this point to give additional examples of this approach to truthtelling in medicine because of the prominence of the paternalistic model in virtually all medical fields. Suffice it to say that, as we have seen, physicians with dying patients and genetic counselors with counselees sometimes do not engage in truthtelling because they believe that some patients/counselees cannot understand the information and/or will be harmed by the information and its impact on their lives. In either case, the patients and counselees are denied a "privilege" which could be granted them: an accurate diagnosis and a straightforward assessment of what the diagnosis means.

When truthtelling is interpreted as a moral obligation in medicine, it cannot be restricted to the use of legally required documents or the occasional granting of a privilege to patients who qualify. Its status is different from and more extensive than codes of law or moral rules of thumb (e.g., "Tell patients the truth when they qualify for it") which have limited application to physician-patient relationships in differing clinical contexts. Rather, as a moral obligation or duty, it applies generally to all physician-patient relationships involving mentally competent patients—including those relationships in which there is no usage of legal forms and in which there is wide disparity of patient age, intelligence, ability to articulate, emotional stability, socioeconomic status, marital status, and so forth.

The claim need not and should not be made that truthtelling is an absolute duty which obligates all physicians in all clinical contexts always to tell the truth and be truthful with their patients. To do so would be to take away the freedom of physicians as responsible moral agents. Instead, the claim which can and should be made is that truthtelling is a prima facie duty which obligates all physicians in all clinical contexts to tell the truth and be truthful with their patients unless there is a conflicting and stronger duty which takes precedence in a particular clinical context. The ''unless clause'' does not weaken the claim that truthtelling with patients is a moral obligation applicable to all physicians. It merely acknowledges that there could be exceptional circumstances (e.g., a clear, indisputable indication that truthtelling would lead to an attempted suicide by the patient) in which another obligation to a particular patient would override the physician's truthtelling responsibility.

If truthtelling is a moral obligation in medicine, why is this the case? Why should truthtelling in medicine be regarded as a moral obligation rather than merely a legal requirement or physician-controlled privilege? There are, in my judgment, three persuasive reasons.

First, the most common arguments against truthtelling with patients—those coming from the perspective of medical paternalism—do not stand up to examination. Granted that the ancient moral principle of nonmaleficence (''above all, do no harm'') continues as a vital part of morally responsible medical practice, there are serious reasons for questioning the frequency with which it is used as a rationalization for not telling patients the truth and being truthful with them. How, for instance, can a physician after very limited contact with a patient know that truthtelling with that patient would be more harmful than withholding relevant information and being dishonest with the patient? Even when the issue at hand is as vital as a patient's emotional health, or the restoration of the patient's physical health, or the prolongation of the patient's life, how can a physician know that this particular patient—in the absence of relevant medical information and an honest assessment of alternatives—''agrees'' with the decision which has been made in his behalf?

The limitations of this paternalistic model—sometimes referred to as ''benevolent deception''—can rather easily be demonstrated. Suppose that an internist decides to withhold diagnostic information from a dying patient because she believes the truth will be more harmful to the patient than not knowing the diagnosis. In other words, she determines

that it will be better for this patient to live out the remaining days of his life in ignorance and deception than in knowledge and truthfulness—and presumes that the patient would agree with that judgment. To make an accurate judgment along these lines would require intimate knowledge of the patient's life history, the ways in which he copes with personal crises, his feelings of obligation to family and career and friends, the sorts of things he would want to do to ''put his house in order,'' and the hierarchy of values by which he governs his life.[18]

Given the highly specialized and impersonal character of modern medicine, it is exceedingly unlikely that any physician could plausibly claim to have access to such personal information or would feel confident in making other highly invasive decisions in this particular patient's behalf. In fact, it is unlikely that the physician could confidently claim such predictive and evaluative capabilities even if the decision were being made in behalf of one of her close friends.

The same problem exists in genetic counseling. Take, for example, the case of myotonic dystrophy mentioned earlier. A man in his early thirties comes in for genetic counseling and is diagnosed as being in the early stage of a progressively degenerating disease which will increasingly affect his hands, eyes, facial muscles, reproductive organs, and heart function and will cause his death, possibly within 10 years. For a counselor in this situation to withhold relevant information and to deceive the man about his genetic future is to make the predictive and evaluative judgment for the counselee himself that it would be better to live out the remaining years in ignorance than in knowledge. In order to presume accuracy in such a judgment, the counselor would need to know all of the things mentioned above in the case of the dying patient, plus highly personal information about the man's reproductive plans, his feelings of responsibility in running a 50/50 risk of passing on the disease, his long-range personal and professional goals, and other highly valued aspects of his life which are dependent upon normal eyesight and muscle performance. Given the limited contact genetic counselors have with counselees, the possession of this kind of knowledge about any particular counselee would be highly improbable.

Second, truthtelling is a moral obligation in medicine because patients and counselees are autonomous persons. Even though they are in a dependency relationship with a medical authority who possesses specialized knowledge about their bodies, they in no way can be said—short of being defined as prisoners—to have given up their personal autonomy when they entered that medical context. As persons, they have the right to autonomy shared by all persons: namely, the right to choose a life plan and make decisions relative to that life plan. The life plan may be well conceived or poorly thought out, praiseworthy or blameworthy, consistently followed or rarely achieved in fact. The point is that all persons, within certain legal constraints, have a moral right to determine the course of action they intend to follow in their lives, to make specific plans which are likely to bring that desired course of action into reality, and to make independent decisions along life's way which have direct bearing on that chosen course of action.

In order to make the right decisions relative to a chosen life plan, autonomous persons—inside and outside of medical contexts—need to have accurate information and honest advice at crucial points along the way. No person is likely to come close to realizing his or her life plan if critical decisions are made in the absence of important factual data or under deception. The relative achievement of a life plan is even less likely if critical decisions are made by someone else on an individual's behalf, especially if that someone else has only a limited knowledge of the individual based on minimal interpersonal contact.

Given their status as autonomous persons, patients in medical contexts have a legitimate claim to accurate information about their medical conditions and to an honest interpretation of the ramifications of that information by the physician. They do not need nor should they lay claim to "the whole truth": surely patients and counselees need not be told all of the myriad scientific details known by the physician in a specific case. But in order to make correct decisions relative to their chosen life plan, they do have a right to the truth which may be

relevant to that life plan and to the sort of truthfulness which will provide them with an honest assessment of alternatives available to them. With dying patients, that means an accurate diagnosis of the disease and a candid appraisal of the disease's probable trajectory, the possibilities and limitations of available therapy programs, and the advisability of choosing a social context other than the hospital (e.g., home, hospice) for dying. With counselees, it means an accurate diagnosis of the genetic disease the person has or carries (if a diagnosis can be made) and honest judgments regarding the severity of the disease, the inheritance risks, the usual effects of the disease on a family unit, the benefits of available therapies, the "track records" of health care institutions in the area, and so forth. Only when such truth and truthfulness are provided by the physician can patients or counselees make responsible decisions about the future which awaits them.

Third, truthtelling is a moral obligation in medicine because of the fiduciary relationship between physician and patient. As in other professional relationships built on confidence and trust (e.g., lawyer–client, priest–confessor), the physician-patient relationship has a number of unstated expectations at its center: the physician will not inflict unnecessary pain on the patient, the physician will not divulge confidential information about the patient, the patient will follow the physician's medical recommendations, and so on. While any physician who departs significantly from some of these expectations might be legally liable, the expectations are only implicitly contractual in nature, and in many physician-patient relationships the expectations have no basis other than the confidence and trust engendered by the relationship itself.

One of the expectations vital to the physician-patient relationship concerns truth and truthfulness in communication. When physicians ask patients questions about their personal medical history and current physical problems, they expect true and nondeceptive responses and proceed in their task as physicians trusting that the answers they have been given are accurate and trustworthy. Should later lab results or other evidence prove that they have been misled or deceived, the physicians will undoubtedly judge that important time and energy has been wasted and will have serious reservations about continuing to see these particular patients.

In the same way, because a fiduciary relationship is a two-way street, patients also expect the truth and nondeceptive communication from their physicians (should evidence prove this point wrong, physician-patient relationships are worse off than I imagine). By entering into a relationship in which specialized knowledge and vitally important personal information can best be secured when communicated by the physician, patients proceed through periods of anxiety and uncertainty trusting that they are being given accurate information about their conditions and honest responses to their questions. Should a dying patient later find out that she has been the victim of a conspiracy of silence, or a counselee later discover that he has been given misleading statements or false reassurances about a genetic disease, these patients will undoubtedly feel betrayed by persons whom they had trusted. If such feelings of betrayal occur in a significant percentage of patients, the resulting damage to the foundation of trust on which physician-patient relationships are based would be monumental.

One final comment. Sometimes discussions of truthtelling in medicine focus on the manner of communicating with patients, with physicians arguing that it is emotionally harmful for patients to be confronted with ''the brutal truth.'' Having given three reasons for telling patients the truth and being truthful with them, I do not intend to suggest that truthtelling has to be done or should be done in a blunt, brutal, insensitive, or sadistic manner. Obviously, the factors of timing and communication dynamics need to be adapted to the circumstances of particular patients. The point is that patients have a right to the truth and truthfulness—communicated with compassion, understandable language, empathy, and respect.

Notes

1. Bok, S. *Lying: Moral Choice in Public and Private Life*. New York: Pantheon. 1978.
2. Discussion section. In *Ethical Issues in Human Genetics*, edited by B. Hilton, D. Callahan, M. Harris, et. al. New York: Plenum, 1973.
3. Kelly, W. D., and Friesen, S. R. Do cancer patients want to be told: *Surgery* 27:322–326, 1950.
4. Oken, D. What to tell cancer patients. JAMA 175:86–94, 1961.
5. McKusick, V. A. *Human Genetics*, 2d ed. Englewood Cliffs, N.J.: Prentice-Hall, 1969.
6. McKusick, V. A. *Mendelian Inheritance in Man*, 5th ed. Baltimore: The Johns Hopkins Univ. Press, 1978.
7. Thompson, J. S., and Thompson, M. W. *Genetics in Medicine*, 2d ed. Philadelphia: Saunders, 1973.
8. Veatch, R. M. *Death, Dying, and the Biological Revolution*. New Haven, Conn.: Yale Univ. Press, 1976.
9. Pearson, J. S. H. D. *Handbook for Health Professionals*. New York: Committee to Combat Huntington's Disease, n. d.
10. Veatch, R. M. *Case Studies in Medical Ethics*. Cambridge, Mass.: Harvard Univ. Press, 1977.
11. Novack, D. H.; Plumer, R.; Smith, R. L.; et al. Changes in physicians' attitudes toward telling the cancer patient. *JAMA* 241:897–900, 1979.
12. Feifel, H.; Hanson, S.; Jones R.; et al. Physicians consider death. *Proc. Am. Psychol. Assoc. Conv.*, pp. 201–202, 1967.
13. Nora, J. J., and Fraser, F. C. *Medical Genetics: Principles and Practice*. Philadelphia: Lea & Febiger, 1974.
14. Gordon, H. Genetic counseling: considerations for talking to parents and prospective parents. *JAMA* 217:1215–1225, 1971.
15. Kübler-Ross, E. *On Death and Dying*. New York: Macmillan, 1969.
16. Weisman, A. *On Dying and Denying*. New York: Behavioral Publications, 1972.
17. Curran, W. J. Genetic counseling and wrongful life. *Am. J. Public Health* 68:501–502, 1978.
18. Buchanan, A. Medical paternalism. *Philos. Public Affairs* 7:370–390, 1978.

The Importance of Psychiatrists' Telling Patients the Truth

William S. Appleton

A former professor of medicine at a leading university is said to have expelled a third-year student from the wards, the school, and medicine in front of 50 colleagues during grand rounds. The student's offense? He told a patient he had cancer.

As the student, frightened and near tears, was about to go, the professor called him back and said: "Now you have a small idea of what it is like to be told you have cancer."

I have always thought, as did many of the students who repeated it, that this story meant the professor did not believe in telling patients they were going to die. Looking back, it seems equally plausible that he wanted his students to understand the emotional impact of such a pronouncement on the patient.

To summarize current medical opinion on the matter: Tell the patient the truth about whether or not he has a fatal illness if he really wants to know. (There is extensive discussion in the medical and psychiatric literature about how to tell which patients really do want to know, how the patient will react once informed, and how to identify those patients who should be protected from the truth about fatal illnesses.)

THE SPIRIT OF DIAGNOSIS

Psychiatrists have frequently criticized internists and surgeons for indulging in charades that not only do not fool the fatally ill patient but also confuse and disorient him. My colleagues often admonish physicians and surgeons to "communicate," to tell the patient the truth more often.

The irony of the psychiatrist's position in all this becomes overwhelmingly apparent as one

Reprinted with permission of author and publisher from *American Journal of Psychiatry*, 129:6 742–45, December 1972. Copyright 1972, the American Psychiatric Association.

examines the same problem in the field of mental illness. In the teaching hospital in which I work, in the many institutions I have visited, and in the hospitals where I have trained, too often psychiatric patients were told nothing about their illness.

The psychiatrist usually reasons that schizophrenia and depression are not predictable diseases with known causes. Therefore, to tell a patient he or she is so afflicted would have no therapeutic or prognostic meaning. He correctly believes the spirit of diagnosis to be not one of mere labeling but rather one of suggesting causation, therapeutic action, and outcome. Ironically, the internist or surgeon often employs similar reasoning to conceal the diagnosis of cancer: Why needlessly upset the patient when the disease may never recur or may be hopelessly malignant?

In most cases the patient, and perhaps his family, should be told what the psychiatrist concludes. If the diagnostic term is imperfect, it must be explained to the extent of the psychiatrist's knowledge; for example, "The schizophrenia is such that a relapse may occur within two years and the following symptoms should be watched for." The psychiatrist should do his best to warn the patient that "when you are stressed emotionally you have a tendency to confuse what is in your mind with what is real. Therefore, if a loved one were to die or if you were to move across country, you might be in danger of relapse." Perhaps out of an unwillingness to deemphasize the uniqueness of the individual and to view him statistically, psychiatrists collect little practical data of this kind. Surgeons know, for example, that if such and such a cancer has reached the lymph nodes or liver, the prognosis, on the average, is a certain number of months, which can be increased by a certain number of methods. Psychiatrists in American universities, however, do not tend to think that the schizophrenia of a 19-year-old with a good premorbid personality has "X" number of chances of recurring in five years, ten years, or never, and is subject to influence by "Y" number of means.

Psychiatrists have such strong feelings against supplying a diagnosis that they sometimes utter it out of despair. "You are borderline and will never be well," one analyst told his patient after three or four years of analysis. He thus avoided his medical obligation to cure her and at the same time released some of his frustration at being unable to do so.

THE PSYCHIATRIC MODEL

Another reason for withholding the diagnosis arises from the mistaken application of the psychiatric model, as opposed to the medical model. In the psychiatric model, the doctor allies himself with the healthy part of the patient's personality to observe and understand the causes of what both agree to be undesirable behavior or emotion. It is then up to the patient to change himself in the context of the psychiatric relationship. The medical patient submits his illness for diagnosis and is either told what to do or lets the doctor do something therapeutic to him.

Organically (biologically) oriented psychiatrists use the medical model. For example, they might say to a patient: "You have a depression with the following symptoms. Here is how to recognize it early and what to do about it." The analytic psychiatrist, predominant in the United States and especially in university centers, uses the psychiatric model and believes depression to be a "stance" to coerce help or love from a significant person. He does not regard his patient as having a depressive illness but regards him as not having abandoned the childlike expectation of being "given to" as opposed to the adult role of achieving for oneself. Even if this model is correct and if (as Thomas Szasz has stated) mental illness is a myth rather than a disease, schizophrenia does not exist, depression is a stance rather than a biochemical condition, and borderline means immaturity, I believe psychiatrists should nonetheless be sure to give the diagnosis, albeit in these "mythical" terms.

The word "diagnosis" means to distinguish or to know and refers in medicine to recognizing a disease from its symptoms. More than a mere label, it is the conclusion reached about causation from which therapeutic action is taken. The psychiatrist must tell the patient the result of his thinking. If he believes the patient's problems stem from misinterpretations of reality or from an unwillingness to put off the moment's pleasure for future reward, he ought to say so. If the physician believes that the patient is waiting in a depressed stance for others to take care of him, he should tell him. Being informed of his diagnosis helps the patient achieve the solution he desires; the doctor's thinking is also channeled more precisely. Once the diagnosis is stated, the patient may act immediately or, when he delays or forgets, his psychiatrist may remind him of it. In addition, a precise statement of the illness or problem helps the practitioner assess its outcome more accurately.

FEAR OF REINFORCEMENT

If full disclosure is such a good idea, then why do psychiatrists so often fail to give their patients the diagnosis? One reason is the psychiatrist's reluctance to repeat what angry families have been telling the patient for months or even years. "You want to be waited on. You won't take responsibility." Some psychiatrists are so troubled by members of their own families that they fear venting their anger and frustration on their patients and, as a result, go to the opposite extreme and say nothing at all. Others restrict themselves to obscure language for fear of producing the same reaction the patient has toward members of his family whom he either dislikes or mistrusts. If such reluctance represents true relationship-building attempts by the psychiatrist, it can be defended. For example, telling a paranoid that he is projecting (i.e., that his beliefs are unreal) is unwise if it alienates the therapist from the person he is trying to help. But if the psychiatrist's silence is due to fear of the patient's anger and results in avoiding transference reactions, it then defeats the whole purpose of the analytic therapist, which amounts to the analysis of the transference reaction itself. A fact frequently forgotten is that the patient will often listen to the trained and neutral physician when he will not listen to his wife or mother. Just because a patient's mother said something does not mean that it is necessarily wrong.

"But he won't listen," many of my colleagues would reply. Tell the patient what you think first, and if he does not listen, you can go on from there. Some psychiatrists believe that it is bad for the patient to know that he is schizophrenic because he may despair and stop trying. A diagnosis of schizophrenia is certainly depressing, and the patient may go through a stage of hopelessness. So does a newly diagnosed cancer patient. Psychiatrists and many medical doctors believe that most cancer patients know the nature of their illness without being told. Most schizophrenics do too, except for those too far out of contact. Telling a patient what he already knows has the added advantage of making him feel that the doctor is being honest.

The failure of psychiatrists to communicate with their patients has repeatedly come to my attention. In my clinic, psychiatric patients are given elaborate diagnostic exercises, including one-hour interviews but they are often denied a careful review of the physicians' clinical findings. A hospitalized patient recently called this to my attention when, after a conference lasting an hour and a half, she waited outside to ask me what was wrong and what she should do. This frequently happens and is usually followed by the conference chairman's hasty reply, "Ask your own doctor," as he rushes away. I decided that since this 60-year-old woman had patiently answered my questions in front of 35 colleagues, it was only fair to tell her what I thought. I did, and she was grateful and very much relieved.

A psychiatric resident whom I supervise presented the case of a 35-year-old virginal man who had been hospitalized with severe attacks of anxiety. The man repeatedly asked why he had palpitations and whether he was a homosexual. Doubt and fear prevented the doctor from answering these questions. He was uncertain whether the palpitations signaled suppressed aggression, he wanted the patient to develop his independence and a capacity for decision making, and he thought the patient, who liked to argue, would disagree.

Ironically, the resident shared the patient's concerns about himself. The resident believed that the patient's fear of becoming homosexual if he developed freedom of sexual expression was well founded. In spite of the therapist's silence, the patient thought he detected encouragement to ask a young woman for a date, "I didn't know you were interested in girls," the woman had said, refusing him, and the patient vowed never to invite another woman out. To this series of events, the resident showed no reaction. When the patient reported fantasizing a woman while masturbating for the first time in his life, he was greeted with more silence. As soon as the psychiatrist abandoned his uncertainty, took a stand, and openly encouraged his patient, the patient asked the young woman out again; this time she accepted.

A doctor ought not to allow himself to wait for complete certainty before giving his opinion, since this can become an excuse for silence. When a patient fears flying, the psychiatrist cannot guarantee that the plane will arrive safely but should, nonetheless, encourage him to try, especially if the physician has mastered his own fear. Some patients benefit by being told, "I worry in airplanes too. In fact 90 percent of all passengers are happier when the plane lands." Others require the assurance that the chances that one will die in a plane are less likely than in an automobile.

An important reason why psychiatrists withhold information, then, is doubt about really knowing the answers. The issue is one of epistemology: how do we know what we think we know, and when can we be sure we are right? Doctors are both intellectual and skeptical. They are aware of past medical certainties having turned into foolish relics, e.g., bloodletting, purgatives, and chaining the mentally ill. This leads them to shy away from being definite and risking an opinion that may later prove to be wrong.

But this cautious attitude can be harmful at times. This was manifested by an experiment in which psychiatrists were trained to give mood-elevating drugs to a group of depressed patients in two ways: (1) in a positive manner (this drug will help you and is very effective), and (2) in a scientific manner (this drug may or may not work, but try it and see). The cure rate for the first group was twice that of the second.

SUMMARY

Psychiatrists advocate honest and open communication by physicians with patients but too often do not practice what they preach. Their reasons for silence include uncertainty about the cause, treatment, and prognosis of psychiatric illnesses and unwillingness to depress, demoralize, anger, or alienate their patients.

If the psychiatrist can overcome his doubts and to the best of his ability honestly explain what is wrong with the patient and what is necessary to overcome the problem, then therapy will become more rapid and effective and its success or failure will be easier to evaluate. Giving the correct diagnosis and prescription may not make the psychiatrist popular with his listener, but this is not important as long as the patient can hear what is said and can learn to make use of it.

Changes in Physicians' Attitudes Toward Telling the Cancer Patient

Dennis H. Novack, MD, Robin Plumer,
Raymond L. Smith, Herbert Ochitill, MD,
Gary R. Morrow, PhD, and
John M. Bennett, MD

A number of surveys since 1953 have investigated the physician's approach to the cancer patient regarding the issue of disclosing the diagnosis.

Of 442 physicians surveyed through the mail in 1953, 31% said they always or usually tell the patient, while 69% said they usually do not or never tell the patient. Of those who generally did not make the diagnosis known, exception occurred when the patient refused treatment or needed to plan. Of those inclined to share the diagnosis, reluctance arose when they were discouraged by the family or afraid of the patient's response.[1] In 1960, of 5,000 physicians, 16% said that they always told the patient, and 22% responded that they never told the patient. The rest sometimes told the patient. Their deci-

sions were influenced by such factors as the stability of the patient, the insistence by the patient or family, the necessity for the patient to put affairs in order, and the unavailability of anyone else who could be told.[2]

In Oken's[3] survey of 219 physicians at Michael Reese Hospital, based on questionnaires and personal interviews, 90% generally did not inform the patient. Although more than three fourths of the group cited clinical experience as the major determinant of their policies, the data bore no relationship to length of experience or age. Many showed inconsistencies in attitudes, personal bias, and resistance to change and to further research, suggesting that emotion-laden a priori personal judgments were the real determinants of policy. Underlying were feelings of pessimism and futility about cancer.

By 1970 a questionnaire survey responded to by 178 physicians showed that 66%

Reprinted by permission of the authors and the American Medical Association from *JAMA*, vol. 241, no. 9, March 2, 1979, pp. 897-900. Copyright 1979, American Medical Association.

sometimes inform the patient, 25% always tell the patient, and only 9% never tell the patient.[4] This suggests a modification of previous practice. To assess whether this represents a genuine change, the present survey was undertaken.

METHODS

The survey population consisted of 699 physicians whose names appeared in the *Physician Staff Directory* of Strong Memorial Hospital. Only pathologists and psychiatrists were excluded.

All subjects received in 18-item structured questionnaire through the mail almost identical to Oken's questionnaire in 1961, which covered physicians' attitude and practice toward the cancer patient.

RESULTS

Two hundred seventy-eight, or 40% usable responses, were returned from a single mailing. Nine specialties were represented: internal medicine represented 35% of total returns; pediatrics, 7.5%; obstetrics and gynecology, 2.5%; surgery and neurosurgery, 10%; oncology, 11.7%; family practice, 2.1%; radiology, 2.1%; subspecialty, 18.7%; others, 7.9%; and specialty not indicated, 2.5%. The sample appeared to represent a cross section of specialties within the hospital's physician population, with the exceptions that oncology was slightly overrepresented, and surgery and obstetrics and gynecology were slightly underrepresented.

In comparing the 1977 and 1961 populations, the present sample had a mean age of 37

years and was 91% men, while the 1961 sample had a mean age of 50 years and was 97% men. Oken reported that the great bulk of physicians in the sample were in active private practice in addition to taking a regular part in the teaching program. Two thirds of our respondents were older than 31 years and were involved in the practice of their specialties. Many took an active role in the hospital's teaching program.

As shown in Table 1, 98% reported that their general policy is to tell the patient. Two thirds of this group say that they never or very rarely make exceptions to this rule. This stands in sharp contrast with Oken's 1961 data, which showed that 88% generally did not tell the patient, with 56% saying that they never or very rarely made exceptions to this rule.

No differences between specialties were found, with the exception that the pediatricians, while reporting that their usual policy is to tell the patient, make exceptions to this rule more frequently than other physicians. With minor exceptions this lack of specialty difference was a consistent finding for all questionnaire items.

The results seem to indicate that the many factors that went into the decision to tell the patient influenced not only whether a physician would tell the patient but also the manner in which he made the diagnosis known, perhaps influencing the timing or wording of the communication.

The four most frequent factors considered in the decision to tell the patient were age (56%), intelligence (44%), relative's wish about telling the patient (51%), and emotional stability (47%).

Four factors most frequently believed to be of special importance were the patient's expressed wish to be told (52%), emotional

TABLE 1   Physicians' Policies About Telling Cancer Patients

Exceptions	Do Not Tell, No. (%)		Tell, No. (%)	
	1977	1961	1977	1961
Never	1(0.4)	18(9)	17(7)	0(0)
Very rarely	2(0.8)	90(47)	152(61)	6(3)
Occasionally	1(0.4)	56(29)	71(28)	10(5)
Often	2(0.8)	5(3)	5(2)	8(4)
Usual policy	6(2)	169(88)	245(98)	24(12)

*1961 data from Oken.[3]

stability (21%), age (11%), and intelligence (10%).

Eighteen percent of the sample reported they were less likely to tell a child, while approximately 10% were inclined to tell a patient who was old or who had poor comprehension. Fourteen percent said that they would tell the patient less frequently or might delay telling if they thought the patient was prone to depression or suicide. Approximately 12% would tell the patient somewhat more frequently if personal affairs needed to be put in order.

The bases for policies in 1977 and 1961 are tabulated in Table 2.

The topic of communication with the cancer patient seems to be more frequently discussed now in medical schools and hospital training programs. Twenty-four percent of the 1977 sample vs 7% in the 1961 sample mention medical school teaching, and 53% of our sample vs 35% in 1961 mention hospital training as sources from which policies are acquired.

As before, clinical experience was given the major credit in both studies, with more than 90% citing it as a source and more than 70% citing it as a major source. As in Oken's data, analysis of the age of respondents citing clinical experience as a major policy determinant showed that younger physicians were just as likely to cite clinical experience as their seniors. Seventy-four percent of our group (and 86% of Oken's group) said that their policy had not changed in the past.

Thus, as in 1961, it appears that personal and emotional factors are of major importance in shaping policy, perhaps even more so in the present study. Subsequent to the general inquiry, "How did you acquire your policy?" it was specifically asked if personal issues were determinants. Seventy-one percent of the 1961 survey and 92% of the current survey reported that personal elements were involved. Again, as in 1961, these respondents were about equally divided as to whether these factors were most important. The physicians specializing in oncology (12% of total respondents) indicated that personal factors were less important in shaping their policies, suggesting that they believed there was some objective policy to be followed that was independent of personal considerations.

There is further evidences of the continuing importance of personal and emotional factors in shaping policy. Our sample evidences an even greater resistance to change and opposition to further research. Questioned about the likelihood of policy change in the future, our respondents show significantly less likelihood that they would change their policy in the future ($P < .01$). Five percent said that there was no possibility of change, 48% said that change was very unlikely, and 34% said that change was unlikely, although they were not sure. Only 9% said that change was probable, and 4% said that it was certain.

This resistance to change was also evident with 28% responding that their policy would not be swayed by research as opposed to 16% of Oken's sampling. Only 15% of our sample said that perhaps their policy would be changed; 29% responded this way in 1961. One of the comments seemed to sum up the general feeling: "I would not be swayed by research (but I think my opinion is correct)."

Responses to the last two survey questions are perhaps indicative of the conviction with

TABLE 2　Sources from which Policies Were Acquired

Source	Every Source, No. (%)		Major Source, No. (%)	
	1977	1961	1977	1961
Medical school teaching	59(24)	14(7)	7(3)	0(0)
Hospital training	128(53)	72(35)	33(15)	10(5)
Clinical experience	222(92)	191(94)	153(70)	146(77)
Illness in friends or family	89(37)	61(30)	15(7)	15(8)
Other	22(9)	24(12)	10(5)	17(9)
Total	520*	362*	218(100)†	188(100)†

*More than one answer can be given by respondent.

†Figures rounded to nearest percent.

which the present policies are held. One hundred percent (vs 60% of the 1961 sample) indicated a preference for being told if they themselves had cancer. One hundred percent thought that the patient has the right to know.

COMMENT

There appears to have been a major change in physicians' attitudes concerning telling patients their diagnosis of cancer. Even if only those physicians who believed strongly about telling the patient responded to our survey, there has still been a significant change since Oken's study. Indeed, there is some evidence that our results may be representative of more widely held views. In a recent study in which 50 patients undergoing radiotherapy were interviewed, 94% used the word "cancer" or "malignant tumor" to describe the reason for being treated. All patients were told their diagnosis by the physician who referred them for therapy.[5] How might we account for this change in attitude? Our respondents' written replies and additional comments suggest several explanations.

Therapy for many forms of cancer has notably improved in recent years. Oken's data suggested that the great majority of physicians believed that cancer connoted certain death. As many patients shared this pessimism, this common belief was often an effective deterrent to free communication. Today advances in therapy have brought longer survival, improved quality of life, and, in many cases, permanent cure. Physicians believe they can offer their cancer patients more hope.

There has been an increase in public awareness of cancer at many levels. The media are constantly presenting evidence of the ubiquity of carcinogens. Public figures such as Betty Ford and Happy Rockefeller spoke openly about their malignant neoplasms. The American Cancer Society publicizes the "Seven Danger Signals of Cancer." Perhaps all of this has led to a lesser stigmatization of cancer, a greater ease in talking about its reality, and a greater awareness of its signs and symptoms.

Oken suggested that most physicians thought that the diagnosis of cancer, with its expectation of death, deprived the patient of hope, and hence they were reluctant to tell cancer patients the diagnosis. Our data suggest that this attitude has also changed. Even when death is expected from the disease, physicians are nevertheless telling their patients the diagnosis. Perhaps improved therapy allows physicians to be overly optimistic with their patients. Perhaps some physicians feel more comfortable in relating to dying patients. At least, many understand better the dying process. This is certainly due, in part, to the recent upsurge of interest in death and dying. Good empirical studies have been done, and many authors have made important contributions to our knowledge in this field.[6-12] This knowledge may have led to more effective communication with dying patients, a reduction in the fear that the dying process necessarily engenders loss of hope, and a greater understanding of the concerns and needs of dying patients. Our data show that these issues are more frequently discussed in medical schools and hospital training programs.

Perhaps more patients are being told because more need to know. Many university hospitals are major clinical research centers, and patients who agree to participate in research protocols must be told their diagnosis to satisfy the legal requirements of informed consent. At the University of Rochester, in 1975, 15% of patients with all newly diagnosed cancer participated in national protocols.

It is impossible to know to what extent the literature on telling the cancer patient has shaped attitudes. If it has had any effect, however, it would be in the direction of encouraging frankness. Koenig[13] systematically reviewed 51 articles appearing in the professional journals between 1946 and 1966 that discussed the treatment of fatally ill patients. He concluded that the tendency of authors appears to be strongly in favor of informing fatally ill patients of their conditions. This has been more recently reaffirmed by Cassem and Stewart,[14] who, in suggesting a general policy of frankness, cite two sets of empirical studies. The first set includes those studies in which patients were asked whether or not they should be told. These indicate overwhelming positive favor for telling. The second set looks at the effects of telling on patients and their families. These studies dispelled the myth of the harm that telling the patient might engender.

The comments of some of our respondents indicate that the reason for the present reversal in attitude is due, in part, to more sweeping social changes. The rise in the consumerism movement and increasing public scrutiny of the medical profession have altered the physician-patient relationship. In this era of "patients' rights," an attitude of frankness feels right and, indeed, given the current disputatious atmosphere of medical practice, may be the safest one to adopt.

Many questions remain. Do physicians tell patients they have "cancer," or are euphemisms such as "tumor" or "growth" still widely used, and if so what does that mean for the communication process? Are changing attitudes on telling the patient accompanied by the emotional support that a patient's knowledge of his diagnosis may demand of a physician? Saunders[15] wrote, "The real question is not 'What do you tell your patients?' but rather, 'What do you let your patients tell you?'" Now that we tell our patients more, are we also listening more? Unfortunately one survey cannot answer these questions.

Is the present policy of telling the patient the best policy? The majority of our respondents cite clinical experience as shaping their present policy, even though most of them have never had experience with another policy. The majority of Oken's respondents also cited clinical experience in shaping the exact opposite policy. While not discounting the value of clinical experience, its use as a determinant of policy must be called into question.

Our data suggest that, as in Oken's study, the present policy is supported by strong belief and emotional investment in its being right. One hundred percent of our respondents stated that patients have a right to know. Yet in asserting this in a blanket manner, are physicians sometimes abdicating a responsibility to make subtle judgments in individual cases? Do patients also have a right not to know?

Is it possible to determine who should be told what, when, and how? What are the criterions by which we judge if telling is right? Patient evaluation in future studies on telling might include assessments of compliance with the medical regimen, quality of communication with physician and family members, ratings of adjustment to illness, or psychological tests of depression and anxiety.

Our respondents' written comments seem to indicate that the current policy of telling the patient is accompanied by increased sensitivity to patients' emotional needs. There is some evidence that telling is the best policy.[16] Yet how rational is the process of deciding what to tell the patient with cancer? Even though the policies have reversed, many physicians are still basing their communication with cancer patients on emotion-laden personal convictions. They are relying on honesty, sensitivity, and patients' rights rather than focusing on the following relevant scientific psychological question: Does telling the diagnosis of cancer help or harm (which) patients and how? Only further systematic research can answer these questions.

References

Fitts WT Jr, Ravdin IS: What Philadelphia physicians tell patients with cancer. *JAMA* 153:901–904, 1953.

Rennick D (ed): What should physicians tell cancer patients? *N Med Material* 2:51–53, 1960.

Oken D: What to tell cancer patients: A study of medical attitudes. *JAMA* 175:1120–1128, 1961.

Friedman HS: Physician management of dying patients: An exploration. *Psychiatry Med* 1:295–305, 1970.

Mitchell GW, Glicksman AS: Cancer patients: Knowledge and attitudes. *Cancer* 40:61–66, 1977.

Feifel H (ed): *The Meaning of Death.* New York, McGraw-Hill Book Co Inc, 1959.

Saunders C: Care of the dying. *Nursing Times* 55:960–961, 994–995, 1031–1032, 1067–1069, 1091–1092, 1129–1130, 1959.

Hinton JM: *Dying.* Baltimore, Penguin Books Ltd, 1967.

Glaser BG, Strauss AC: *Awareness of Dying.* Chicago, Aldine Publishing Co, 1965.

Kübler-Ross C: *On Death and Dying.* New York, MacMillan Co, 1969.

ENGEL GL: Psychological responses to major environmental stress, in *Psychological Development in Health and Disease*. Philadelphia, WB Saunders Co, 1962, pp 272-305.

GREENE WA: The physician and his dying patient, in Troupe SB, Greene WC (eds): *The Patient, Death and the Family*. New York, Charles Scribner's Sons, 1974, pp 85-99.

KOENIG RR: Anticipating death from cancer—physician and patient attitudes. *Mich Med* 68:899-905, 1969.

CASSEM NH, STEWART RS: Management and care of the dying patient. *Int J Psychiatry Med* 6:293-304, 1975.

SAUNDERS C: The moment of truth: Care of the dying person, in Pearson L (ed): *Death and Dying*. Cleveland, Case Western Reserve University Press, 1969, pp 49-78.

GERLE B, LANDEN G, SANDBLOM P: The patient with inoperable cancer from the psychiatric and social standpoint. *Cancer* 13:1206-1217, 1960.

From *Man, Mind, and Medicine*

Oliver M. Cope

DR. COPE: When I was a fourth-year student, William Sidney Thayer—the great professor of medicine at Hopkins, that wonderful understanding warm human being—came to Harvard and gave a *Care of the Patient* lecture. He described malignant disease and told how you handled it and how you always had to tell the patient the truth. This was a vivid experience for me. He described a patient who had come to him in Baltimore because he had been put off by physicians elsewhere. He knew he wasn't getting the answer, and so it was easy, I suppose, for Dr. Thayer to know that the thing to do was to tell him. The patient wanted it; that was why he came to Baltimore. So he told him. The fellow, of course, was upset; and his wife was angry with Dr. Thayer. He said she berated him: "What right did you have to tell him?" Then, two hours later, he got a telephone call. They had gone back to their hotel, and called Dr. Thayer to thank him for having told, because for the first time in several months, the two of them could sit down and talk.

That was a vivid model, and now I know of my mistakes. A woman had obvious

Reprinted with permission of author and publisher from *Man, Mind, and Medicine* (Philadelphia: J. B. Lippincott Co., 1968), pp. 28-29.

cancer of the thyroid, and knew it. She knew it because of the way her physicians dodged telling her; everybody was alarmed. Any fool could see that her doctors were alarmed; so she made me promise the night before the operation, religiously promise, that I would tell her the truth. She suspected the truth; she outlined to me the number of reasons she needed to know. She was a widow; her children were not quite launched and so on; and I had to tell her for very practical reasons. So it was. It was a rapidly growing, undifferentiated carcinoma, the type with a wretched prognosis, perhaps nine months or a year, and it would have to be treated by radiation.

So I waited until she was over the anesthetic, and the next morning I came in, pulled up a chair next to her, sat down by her bedside, and said: "I will now do what you asked me to do. You have a serious condition: we are going to give you x-ray treatment. There is no doubt that these treatments will help you. It is possible we will manage to eliminate the trouble completely, but just the same you had better do what you said about rearranging your estate and taking care of your children and so on." She thanked me very much, and I went out with great relief, thinking that I had carried it off. In the next two to three days, I was congratulating myself because she had taken it so well; I must have done a good job. On the fourth postoperative day, the nurse stopped me before I entered the room. "You know, Mrs. B is waiting. She wants to know when you are going to fulfill your promise and tell her what you found." I was younger then than I am now; I failed to take advantage of the broad hint offered me by the patient, namely, that she had shut out the bad news. So I went in and I said, "I hear from your nurse that I haven't told you. Don't you recall that the very day after operation I told you?" "Told me what?" So I went over it again. She, of course, went into a serious depression; and it was terrible. It ruined her life and, what is more, mistakes seem to be contagious. To make a long story short, the pathologist and I thought this was an undifferentiated carcinoma. It wasn't: it was one of those very peculiar tumors. The same type of tumor was found in the wall of her stomach four years later. She lived for 12 years after that to die of a coronary.

Most of us doctors don't have the understanding to manage these situations and we badly need to learn how.

DR. ZACHARIAS: Can you conceive of any kind of formal education that would have helped you with that?

DR. COPE: Yes, something, but certainly not what I had had. I acted on the single model given me, persuasively, by Dr. William Sidney Thayer.

DR. EISENBERG: Did you ever watch him do it instead of being told by him how to do it?

DR. COPE: No.

Placebos

Sissela Bok

The common practice of prescribing placebos to unwitting patients illustrates the two miscalculations so common to minor forms of deceit: ignoring possible harm and failing to see how gestures assumed to be trivial build up into collectively undesirable practices.[1] Placebos have been used since the beginning of medicine. They can be sugar pills, salt-water injections—in fact, any medical procedure which has no specific effect on a patient's condition, but which can have powerful psychological effects leading to relief from symptoms such as pain or depression.

Placebos are prescribed with great frequency. Exactly how often cannot be known, the less so as physicians do not ordinarily talk publicly about using them. At times, self-deception enters in on the part of physicians, so that they have unwarranted faith in the powers of what can work only as a placebo. As with salesmanship, medication often involves unjustified belief in the excellence of what is suggested to others. In the past, most remedies were of a kind that, unknown to the medical profession and their patients, could have only placebic benefits, if any.

The derivation of "placebo," from the Latin for "I shall please," gives the word a benevolent ring, somehow placing placebos beyond moral criticism and conjuring up images of hypochondriacs whose vague ailments are dispelled through adroit prescriptions of beneficient sugar pills. Physicians often give a humorous tinge to instructions for prescribing these substances, which helps to remove them from serious ethical concern. One authority wrote in a pharmacological journal that the placebo should be given a name previously unknown to the patient and preferably Latin and polysyllabic, and added:

> [I]t is wise if it be prescribed with some assurance and emphasis for psychotherapeutic effect. The older physicians each had his favorite placebic prescriptions—one chose tincture of Condurango, another the Fluidextract of *Cimicifuga nigra*.[2]

After all, health professionals argue, are not placebos far less dangerous than some genuine drugs? And more likely to produce a cure than if nothing at all is prescribed? Such a view was expressed in a letter to the *Lancet*:

> Whenever pain can be relieved with a ml of saline, why should we inject an opiate? Do anxieties or discomforts that are allayed with starch capsules require administration of a barbiturate, diazepam, or propoxphene?[3]

Such a simplistic view conceals the real costs of placebos, both to individuals and to the practice of medicine. First, the resort to placebos may actually prevent the treatment of an underlying, undiagnosed problem. And even if the placebo "works," the effect is often short-lived; the symptoms may recur, or crop up in other forms. Very often, the symptoms of which the patient complains are bound to go away by themselves, sometimes even from the mere contact with a health professional. In those cases, the placebo itself is unnecessary; having recourse to it merely reinforces a tendency to depend upon pills or treatments where none is needed.

In the aggregate, the costs of placebos are immense. Many millions of dollars are expended on drugs, diagnostic tests, and psychotherapies of a placebic nature. Even operations can be of this nature—a hysterectomy may thus be performed, not because the condition of the patient requires such surgery, but because she goes from one doctor to another seeking to have the surgery performed, or because she is judged to have a great fear of cancer which might be alleviated by the very fact of the operation.

Even apart from financial and emotional costs and the squandering of resources, the practice of giving placebos is wasteful of a very precious good: the trust on which so much in the medical relationship depends. The trust of those patients who find out they have been duped is lost, sometimes irretrievably. They may then lose confidence in physicians and even in bona fide medication which they may need in the future. They may obtain for themselves more harmful drugs or attach their hopes to debilitating fad cures.

The following description of a case[4] where a placebo was prescribed reflects a common approach.

A seventeen-year-old girl visited her pediatrician, who had been taking care of her since infancy. She went to his office without her parents, although her mother had made the appointment for her over the telephone. She told the pediatrician that she was very healthy, but that she thought she had some emotional problems. She stated that she was having trouble sleeping at night, that she was very nervous most of the day. She was a senior in high school and claimed she was doing quite poorly in most of her subjects. She was worried about what she was going to do next year. She was somewhat overweight. This, she felt, was part of her problem. She claimed she was not very attractive to the opposite sex and could not seem to "get boys interested in me." She had a few close friends of the same sex.

Her life at home was quite chaotic and stressful. There were frequent battles with her younger brother, who was fourteen, and with her parents. She claimed her parents were always "on my back." She described her mother as extremely rigid and her father as a disciplinarian, who was quite old-fashioned in his values.

In all, she spent about twenty minutes talking with her pediatrician. She told him that what she thought she really needed was tranquilizers, and that that was the reason she came. She felt that this was an extremely difficult year for her, and if she could have something to calm her nerves until she got over her current crises, everything would go better.

The pediatrician told her that he did not really believe in giving tranquilizers to a girl of her age. He said he thought it would be a bad precedent for her to establish. She was very insistent, however, and claimed that if he did not give her tranquilizers, she would "get them somehow." Finally, he agreed to call her pharmacy and order medication for her nerves. She accepted graciously. He suggested that she call him in a few days to let him know how things were going. He also called her parents to say that he had a talk with her and he was giving her some medicine that might help her nerves.

Five days later, the girl called the pediatrician back to say that the pills were really working well. She claimed that she had calmed down a great deal, that she was working things out better with her parents, and had a new outlook on life. He suggested that she keep taking them twice a day for the rest of the school year. She agreed.

A month later, the girl ran out of pills and called her pediatrician for a refill. She found that he was away on vacation. She was quite distraught at not having any medication left, so she called her uncle who was a surgeon in the next town. He called the pharmacy to renew her pills and, in speaking with the druggist, found out that they were only vitamins. He told the girl that the pills were only vitamins and that she could get them over the counter and didn't really need him to refill them. The girl became very distraught, feeling that she had been deceived and betrayed by her pediatrician. Her parents, when they heard, commented that they thought the pediatrician was "very clever."

The patients who do *not* discover the deception and are left believing that a placebic remedy has worked may continue to rely on it under the wrong circumstances. This is especially true with drugs such as antibiotics, which are sometimes used as placebos and sometimes for their specific action. Many parents, for example, come to believe that they must ask for the prescription of antibiotics every time their child has a fever or a cold. The fact that so many doctors accede to such requests perpetuates the dependence of these families on medical care they do not need and weakens their ability to cope with health problems. Worst of all, those children who cannot tolerate antibiotics may have severe reactions, sometimes fatal, to such unnecessary medication.[5]

Such deceptive practices, by their very nature, tend to escape the normal restraints of accountability and can therefore spread more easily than others. There are many instances in which an innocuous-seeming practice has grown to become a large-scale and more dangerous one. Although warnings against the "entering wedge" are often rhetorical devices, they can at times express justifiable caution; especially when there are great pressures to move along the undesirable path and when the safeguards are insufficient.

In this perspective, there is much reason for concern about placebos. The safeguards against this practice are few or nonexistent—both because it is secretive in nature and because it is condoned but rarely carefully discussed in the medical literature.[6] And the pressures are very great, and growing stronger, from drug companies, patients eager for cures, and busy physicians, for more medication, whether it is needed or not. Given this lack of safeguards and these strong pressures, the use of placebos can spread in a number of ways.

The clearest danger lies in the gradual shift from pharmacologically inert placebos to more active ones. It is not always easy to distinguish completely inert substances from somewhat active ones and these in turn from more active ones. It may be hard to distinguish between a quantity of an active substance so low that it has little or no effect and quantities that have some effect. It is not always clear to doctors whether patients require an inert placebo or possibly a more active one, and there can be the temptation to resort to an active one just in case it might also have a specific effect. It is also much easier to deceive a patient with a medication that is known to be "real" and to have power. One recent textbook in medicine goes so far as to advocate the use of small doses of effective compounds as placebos rather than inert substances—because it is important for both the doctor and the patient to believe in the treatment! This shift is made easier because the dangers and side effects of active agents are not always known or considered important by the physician.

Meanwhile, the number of patients receiving placebos increases as more and more people seek and receive medical care and as their desire for instant, push-button alleviation of symptoms is stimulated by drug advertising and by rising expectations of what science can do. The use of placebos for children grows as well, and the temptations to manipulate the truth are less easily resisted once such great inroads have already been made.

Deception by placebo can be spread from

therapy and diagnosis to experimentation. Much experimentation with placebos is honest and consented to by the experimental subjects, especially since the advent of strict rules governing such experimentation. But grievous abuses have taken place where placebos were given to unsuspecting subjects who believed they had received another substance. In 1971, for example, a number of Mexican-American women applied to a family-planning clinic for contraceptives. Some of them were given oral contraceptives and others were given placebos, or dummy pills that looked like the real thing. Without fully informed consent, the women were being used in an experiment to explore the side effects of various contraceptive pills. Some of those who were given placebos experienced a predictable side effect—they became pregnant. The investigators neither assumed financial responsibility for the babies nor indicated any concern about having bypassed the "informed consent" that is required in ethical experiments with human beings. One contented himself with the observation that if only the law had permitted it, he could have aborted the pregnant women!

The failure to think about the ethical problems in such a case stems at least in part from the innocent-seeming white lies so often told in giving placebos. The spread from therapy to experimentation and from harmlessness to its opposite often goes unnoticed in part *because* of the triviality believed to be connected with placebos as white lies. This lack of foresight and concern is most frequent when the subjects in the experiment are least likely to object or defend themselves; as with the poor, the institutionalized, and the very young.

In view of all these ways in which placebo usage can spread, it is not enough to look at each incident of manipulation in isolation, no matter how benevolent it may be. When the costs and benefits are weighed, not only the individual consequences must be considered, but also the cumulative ones. Reports of deceptive practices inevitably leak out, and the resulting

suspicion is heightened by the anxiety which threats to health always create. And so even the health professionals who do not mislead their patients are injured by those who do; the entire institution of medicine is threatened by practices lacking in candor, however harmless the results may appear in some individual cases.

This is not to say that all placebos must be ruled out; merely that they cannot be excused as innocuous. They should be prescribed but rarely, and only after a careful diagnosis and consideration of non-deceptive alternatives; they should be used in experimentation only after subjects have consented to their use.

Notes

1. This discussion draws on my two articles, "Paternalistic Deception in Medicine, and Rational Choice: The Use of Placebos," in Max Black, ed., *Problems of Choice and Decision* (Ithaca, N.Y.: Cornell University Program on Science, Technology and Society, 1975), pp. 73–107; and "The Ethics of Giving Placebos," *Scientific American* 231 (1974):17–23.
2. O. H. Pepper, "A Note on the Placebo," *American Journal of Pharmacy* 117 (1945):409–12.
3. J. Sice, "Letter to the Editor," *The Lancet* 2 (1972):651.
4. I am grateful to Dr. Melvin Levine for the permission to reproduce this case, used in the Ethics Rounds at the Children's Hospital in Boston.
5. C. M. Kunin, T. Tupasi, and W. Craig, "Use of Antibiotics," *Annals of Internal Medicine* 79 (October 1973):555–60.
6. In a sample of nineteen recent, commonly used textbooks, in medicine, pediatrics, surgery, anesthesia, obstetrics, and gynecology, only three even mention placebos, and none detail either medical or ethical dilemmas they pose. Four out of six textbooks on pharmacology mention them; only one mentions such problems. Only four out of eight textbooks on psychiatry even mention placebos; none takes up ethical problems. For references, see Bok, "Paternalistic Deception in Medicine and Rational Choice."

Some Moral Issues Concerning Current Ways of Dealing with Surgical Patients

Martin L. Kempner

It is now well known that surgical residents participate extensively in surgery performed on private patients. Their participation is extensive, both in number of operations in which they are involved and their role in any given operation. This involvement of the surgical resident raises a number of moral questions. Among them are questions as to what to tell the patient about who is doing the surgery, the risk to the patient when the resident performs the surgery, and the fee appropriate for the surgeon to charge when the resident is the primary operating surgeon. In this paper I am going to concentrate on the first question, though I shall have things to say about the last question as well. I shall be talking about surgery performed on private patients, not ward or service patients, though what will be said has implications for these patients also.

Interviews I have conducted with residents and attending physicians in several hospitals in New York City and the Lifflander Report on "ghost surgery" suggest that surgical patients are currently dealt with as follows. Patients are not directly and unequivocally told by their surgeons that a surgical resident (a surgeon-in-training) will participate, or participate extensively, in their operation. Instead, they are told that modern surgery is a team effort, that a team of surgeons will be involved, and that the surgeon they engaged will be the "responsible" surgeon. This does not change the belief of the patient that the surgeon engaged will perform, if not the entire operation, then at least the major or most serious part of it. In fact, in many instances, the chosen surgeon does very little or none of the surgery, but is involved rather in a supervisory and back-up capacity.

Thus, the patient does not get what he was led to believe he would get, the operative service of the surgeon he engaged. Further,

Reprinted by permission of the author and the *Bulletin of the New York Academy of Medicine*, Vol. 55, No. 1, January 1979.

although the patient's operation is performed by the resident, in many instances he is charged the surgeon's customary fee, the fee the surgeon does or would charge were he the primary operating surgeon.

This picture contains at least five elements that are open to criticism on moral grounds. The first questionable element concerns what patients are told about who will be involved in their operation. The main problem with the surgeon telling his patient that the surgery will be performed by a team is that it masks both the actual reason why residents operate and the true role of the surgeon in the operating room. Calling surgery a team effort makes it sound as if a group of already trained and experienced surgeons will operate. And, whereas a team approach is undoubtedly required for certain operations, the team concept, according to the Lifflander Report, is invoked for such procedures as herniorrhaphies, appendectomies, hysterectomies, colectomies, and cholecystectomies. It is disingenuous to say that such operations require a team approach. Moreover, even if it is granted that a team approach for these operations is in some sense better than a nonteam approach, to tell the patient that his operation is a team effort still masks the fact that the resident is on the team principally because he is in training, that he is trying to learn or to get better at the procedure in question. It still masks the fact that the surgeon's principal involvement with the operation is in the supervisory and back-up capacity. The patient, however, has the right to know the true roles of both resident and surgeon. This is extremely important information. It is information which could serve as a basis for the patient electing not to undergo the operation or deciding to look for an experienced surgeon to perform the entire operation. It must be remembered that morally the whole point of an informed consent requirement is to protect people from deception or from being misled so that they can form an accurate picture of the alternatives available and of the risks of each alternative. The purpose of providing an accurate picture is not simply to satisfy the patient's curiosity, thereby honoring his right to know. The purpose is to enable him to decide which alternative is the best given his own values and concerns, thereby honoring his right to choose. Indeed, if he is not provided with an accurate picture of the alternatives, in what sense has his autonomy, his right to determine what others should be allowed to do to him, been preserved?

In addition to (1) the deception involved in failing to clearly and unequivocally inform the patient about who participates in the operation and in what capacity, current practice has other morally objectionable elements. There is an implicit understanding (or contract) between the patient and the surgeon he engages, one component of which is that this surgeon will be the operating surgeon. But to substitute the operative services of the resident for those of the surgeon (2) violates this understanding. The patient understood that he would be receiving the surgeon's operative services, but received the operative services of someone else.[1] Further, the patient can complain that (3) he is being asked to pay for services which, though understood to be forthcoming, were not rendered. In effect, he is being asked to honor his end of the understanding between himself and the surgeon. The patient can also complain that (4) the operative services he received were inferior to those he understood he would get (more on this point below). Finally, the patient can complain that in paying the surgeon his customary fee, (5) he is being overcharged for the services he actually received, namely, those of the resident.

This last point requires some elaboration. Although there are other ways to make this point, I shall put it in terms of market considerations.[2] Consider what the patient would be willing to pay on the open market if given the opportunity to make a free and informed choice between the services of a surgeon and those of a resident or, to put the point in a slightly different way, if given a free and informed choice between the surgeon's participation as the primary operating surgeon and his participation in a supervisory and back-up capacity.

People quite naturally would purchase the operative services of the surgeon if the fee for those services and the fee for the services of the resident were the same. If they were to purchase the services of the resident at all, it would be for a smaller fee than they are willing to pay for the surgeon's operative services. But when patients are charged the surgeon's fee for surgery done primarily by the resident, they are being asked to pay a fee which they would have been unwilling to pay given a free and informed choice. From this perspective one can say that in being charged the surgeon's customary fee patients are charged more for the services of the resident than those services are worth to them. The residents' services are less attractive to the patient than the surgeons', in part because what the patient wants is the greater assurance of the desired result, i.e., successful surgery. Part of what a patient pays a more experienced surgeon for is the greater assurance of successful surgery. The patient does not have this when the resident performs the surgery. While the resident may be as successful in all phases of the surgery, he may not be, and the chances of obtaining the desired result are simply better with an experienced surgeon. Here it is not merely a question of what the resident can do, for one might be fortunate enough to get a top-flight resident. The whole idea here is that of proved success. What the person considering an operation wants to purchase is the services of the doctor with a proved track record, thereby maximizing his chances of a successful result.

Three responses are likely to be elicited by the preceding discussion. First, it may be said that residents, or most of them at any rate, are just as skilled as surgeons—if not in some instances better. So the substitution of the resident for the surgeon does not substitute operative services of lesser but comparable quality. Thus, the operative services of a resident are worth as much to the patient as the operative services of an experienced surgeon. Second, it may be said that the surgeon plays a vital role in the operation and it is for this role that he charges the patient. Thus, the surgeon does not charge for services he has not rendered. He renders important supervisory and back-up services, and clearly it is not wrong for him to charge the patient for these services.

Finally, it may be said that the current way of informing the patient about who will operate on him is morally justified. Many patients, it is maintained, would refuse surgery if told that their operation were to be performed by a resident, a surgeon-in-training, and that their own surgeon were to act primarily in a supervisory back-up capacity. If this is so, however, then the entire enterprise of training new surgeons would be brought to a halt, a disastrous consequence which would make all of us immeasurably worse off than we are now. The current way of informing the patient, which allows the training program to go forward, providing us with a new generation of very able surgeons, is therefore justified.

Consider the first point, regarding the claim that residents are as good as surgeons. Three points need to be made. First, no one can substantiate the claim that residents are as competent as experienced surgeons until extensive studies are done to compare the performance of supervised residents with the performance of surgeons in terms of morbidity and mortality.[3]

Second, it is simply not true that all residents at every stage of training are as good as experienced surgeons. This would deny the relevance of experience in developing competence as a surgeon—a claim contrary to what most surgeons say as well as to common knowledge about the achievement of competence of almost any skill (e.g., piano playing, bicycle riding, etc.). But third, suppose it were demonstrably true that residents are as proficient as experienced surgeons. Then we could say that when an equally good resident substitutes for the surgeon, the patient cannot complain that he has received operative services of a lesser quality. And perhaps we could say that the patient is not being overcharged. But notice that this would answer only (4) and (5) above. We are still left with points (3), (2), and especially (1)—the point that the substitution of a resident for an experienced surgeon has been concealed from the patient. On that point, the comparable quality of the resident and the surgeon serves as no defense at all. There the relevant consideration is what the patient was told or was led to believe he would get. It is the operative services of the surgeon and not those of the resident that the patient wants,

and it is those services he was told or led to believe he would get. The deception involved makes it wrong to substitute a resident for a surgeon, even if the resident is equally competent.

Consider the second point, namely, that it is for his supervisory and back-up role that the surgeon charges the patient. Here, too, several things need to be said. First, this is not made clear to the patient. The patient's understanding is that he is to receive the surgeon's operative services and not his supervisory and back-up services,[4] and it is for the operative services that the patient has agreed to pay. So the surgeon has violated the understanding between himself and his patient.

Second, I do not think it is appropriate to ask any one patient to bear the full cost of the supervisory and back-up role played by the surgeon. That role needs to be filled precisely because of the additional risks created for the patient by the resident's participation in his surgery. These are risks that the patient need not face because of his own medical condition. They are brought into existence by a social purpose (the training of new surgeons) extraneous to the patient's own medical needs. Someday it will benefit others that this patient agreed, by making himself "teaching material," to assume those additional risks. It will benefit all those future patients who will need the services of the next generation of surgeons. But, now, because this patient is not the only one to benefit from having made himself teaching material, because through this a social purpose is advanced, he alone should not have to bear the burdens which serving that purpose imposes. This implies, in regard to the burden of the expense for the supervisory and back-up role of the surgeon, that it is wrong for the present patient to shoulder the full cost of that role. Though it is appropriate to ask him to pay a part of that cost because he also benefits from that role, he alone should not be required to pay for all of it.

Consider finally the third point, that were patients told with complete candor who is involved in their surgery and in what capacity, the training program could not go forward. This argument might be persuasive if we could be sure that, in the face of the truth, there was absolutely no way to secure the participation of patients in surgical training. But is this so? Patients could be told by the surgeon they have engaged about how things are done at a teaching hospital and the many important advantages of care at a teaching hospital could be explained to them. They might then be told that it is a condition of entering such a hospital that patients allow residents to assume a large role in their care and to participate in their surgery—extensively if need be. People would then face the choice of whether to enter a teaching hospital or a nonteaching hospital. In the latter institution they would be assured the services of the surgeon they have engaged, but would be deprived of the advantages of care available at a teaching hospital. It seems to me that many people would choose to have their operation at a teaching hospital. If this is so, however, patients could be told the truth and training programs could nevertheless go forward.

It should be observed that this solution would avoid the first three morally objectionable elements of current practice noted at the beginning of this paper, but would still leave open the question of the surgeon's reimbursement, not merely the amount of reimbursement, but the way in which the surgeon should be paid for his actual role in the teaching hospital. This would involve such issues as whether the surgeon should be on salary at the hospital or whether, in light of the fact that surgical patients are a captive audience in no real position to negotiate, it is the hospital that should control the surgeon's fee. (This point was suggested to me by Professor Herman Somers.)

One final point: a situation similar to the one described in this paper regarding surgery may exist with regard to medicine in some teaching hospitals—a situation that may, to use Dr. Mack Lipkin's phrase, be appropriately described as "ghost medicine." Thus, some physicians have indicated that outside attending physicians are virtually excluded from the essential aspects of medical care for their patients once those patients are admitted to a teaching hospital. The patient then comes under the care of the chief of service and his house staff. Patients, however, are not informed of the situation—of the extensive role of the house staff in their care and of the very minor ancillary role of their own physicians. Nevertheless, the patient's physician, who may make daily visits, does charge his customary fee. With regard to this situation, I would suggest the same solution as the one proposed above.

Notes

1. I do not know whether this would constitute breach of contract legally.
2. This should not be taken to mean that I am committed to the marketplace as a morally ideal arrangement for the provision of health-care services. In this paper I am not addressing questions of what would be ideal. We already have a marketplace arrangement. Given that this is what we have, I here deal with how it can be made morally better than it is now.
3. Indeed, until such studies are done and their results made available, I do not see how it is possible reliably to inform the patient about the additional risks he confronts when the resident performs the surgery (risks over and above those present even when an experienced surgeon operates). The patient will not be able to form an accurate picture of the alternatives open to him without reliable information about the risks associated with each of those alternatives. But if this is so, then the patient will not be in a position to make an informed choice between those alternatives, and if he is not in a position to make such a choice he cannot give his informed consent to the proposed operation. It would seem to me, therefore, that if the patient's right to give informed consent is to be taken seriously, the profession has a duty to undertake the studies in question.
4. This was powerfully illustrated in a segment of one of the television programs in the CBS series entitled "Sixty Minutes."

PRIVACY AND CONFIDENTIALITY

From "Rights of Privacy in Medical Practice"

Leo J. Cass and William J. Curran

In discussing the relationship between physician and patient, we are brought back constantly to its basic foundations of mutual trust and confidentiality. In Anglo-American law, this is known as "a fiduciary relationship."[1]

In the United States there is a greater, perhaps excessive, interest in the subject of confidentiality: even so, perhaps more thought should be given to it in Britain.

The ethical and legal responsibilities of a confidential relationship for professional people have their narrowest application in what is called in America "a testimonial privilege." This privilege, which is statutory in about two-thirds of our States, allows a patient to prevent his physician from disclosing in court any information obtained as a result of the relationship.[2] In its broadest application, however, it is a part of the individual's *right of privacy*. This right is based on the idea that the details of a person's life are private and should be protected from intrusion; but that this right of privacy should be protected by law is a new concept. It is one of the few legal principles which the United States has *not* borrowed directly from English Common Law. It is a uniquely American doctrine. It had its origins in a paper by Warren and Brandeis.[3] (Louis D. Brandeis gained wide recognition through his service on the U.S. Supreme Court.) Despite the advocacy of these two lawyers, however, the American courts were slow to enforce the right. Even today, some of the American States still do not recognise its existence in a higher-court case.

A great surge forward in the enforcement of "privacy rights" may be expected soon, however, as a result of the recent decisions of

Reprinted, with deletions, from *The Lancet*. 2:783–785, October 16, 1965.

the U.S. Supreme Court in a series of far-reaching civil-rights cases.

Most important of all is the case, decided in June, 1965, where the court struck down as unconstitutional the Connecticut statute barring the *use* of contraceptive devices or drugs even by married couples. The court held that no law could be used to punish acts of intimacy in marriage. In this case[4] the Supreme Court recognised the right of privacy as a fundamental human right guaranteed by the Bill of Rights in the Constitution. . . .

PHYSICIAN AND PATIENT

In this paper we concentrate on those aspects of the right of privacy contained in the confidential relationship of physician and patient. The basic ethics of the advisory professions support this concept of confidentiality. The trust of patients rests upon this expected silence. Physicians cannot otherwise demand the truth of patients.

Damage is done to a patient, client, friend, or colleague more often as the result of a careless or boastful revelation than from the evil design or the demands of others outside our professions.

Furthermore the patient's permission to reveal information does not release the physician entirely from his responsibility. The patient's privacy must sometimes be protected in his own interest in spite of appearances to the contrary. The patient must have full knowledge of what he is doing when giving permission and he must do so without coercion. For the physician, there should be an implied limitation on the scope of any release of confidential information—that what is revealed would not be harmful to him. Legally he may be protected in revealing information even though it proves harmful but he will have broken his code of ethics and abused his professional position by permitting a patient to do harm to himself.

One of us (L. J. C.) had a case which caused some concern. A patient, seen at a consultation three years ago, was an alcoholic with cirrhosis and a drug addict. A few months later he sent a health form from a life-insurance company enclosing permission to reveal the findings of the examination. When informed that a full disclosure of his condition would be obligatory and that he should either withdraw permission or recognise the results of a full disclosure the patient sent, by return, a letter of thanks and withdrew his permission. A request from the same insurance company, with permission granted by the widow, revealed that the company were contesting payment of a $200,000 policy. On this request no action was taken since it was felt that a man should not be called upon to give testimony against himself after death when he refused with full knowledge of the consequences during life.

The individual is entitled at all times and under all circumstances to the protection of his confidences when he reveals them to professional advisers. He has even some rights if he reveals confidences to anyone. If confidences are disclosed it may be in violation of the person's right of privacy. If no damage results, there may be no grounds for legal action, even though a breach of ethics has occurred. If the revelation were made by a physician it is a greater infringement and the physician can be held actionable for any damage his patient may suffer, be it to his reputation or to his physical or mental health.

WHEN INFORMATION SHOULD BE REVEALED

When do physicians have a duty to reveal information? The physician may have an obligation to reveal medical facts to other members of the clinical service or to another person in whom there is a legitimate interest in the medical problem, when, by doing so, the best interests of the patient are served. The policy underlying confidentiality is the promotion of the health and welfare of the patient and the reputation of the profession by engendering certainty in the mind of the patient and the public that intimate details or derogatory factors will never be disclosed to the embarrassment or disgrace of a patient.

There are instances, however, when a higher purpose or good outweighs this obligation to the patient. The most obvious example is the duty to inform public officials of a dangerous, contagious disease in a patient which is a threat to the general public. In the United States, such cases come under the statutes called "the reporting laws." These laws are binding upon physicians, who have no choice but to reveal this information to the public authorities responsible. . . .

Papers given at medical meetings concerning the legal aspects of a university health-service have in the past too frequently stressed only one area—protection from the legal risks of malpractice suits. This is an understandable concern for physicians. Like other human beings they are interested in protecting themselves. It is regrettable, however, that so much time and space has been given to this subject. The practice of medicine is the pursuit of a profession. By definition, this means physicians are bound by a code of ethics to act at all times in the best interests of those they serve. The Law in America and in Britain enforces this responsibility in many aspects. One of the areas where the Law recognises and enforces this ethical imperative is that of keeping confidences by patients. Law and medicine therefore work together to assure what both desire to achieve—the maintenance of the highest standards of altruistic practice in the profession of medicine.

Notes

1. Prosser, W. L. The Law of Torts. St. Louis, 1958.
2. Dewitt, C. Privileged Communications between Physician and Patient. Springfield. 1958.
3. Warren, S. D., Brandeis, L. D. *Harvard Law Rev*. 1890, 4. 193.
4. Grisworld *v.* The State of Connecticut. *U.S. Law Week*, 1965, 33, 4587.

From "Confidentiality
and Privileged Communication"

Neil L. Chayet

The murder of 8 student nurses in Chicago and the slaughter of 15 persons in Dallas share many common elements, not the least of which is the significant involvement of the medical profession. In the nurses' case it was a physician who was responsible for the apprehension of Richard Speck, calling the police after he noticed a resemblance to the composite sketch of the suspected killer and the tattoo, "Born to Raise Hell." In Dallas a psychiatrist became the subject of a national discussion when he let it be known that Charles Whitman had given expression to a fantasy of going up to the tower and shooting people.

Both incidents raise the subject of confidentiality, the disclosure of confidential information that a physician has learned from or about his patient during the course of the doctor–patient relation.

What is the responsibility of the physician to inform the police that a past crime has occurred or that a future crime is contemplated? There is no question that the physician who noticed the tattoo acted properly in informing the police, who were conducting a widespread manhunt for the killer, and it is equally evident that the Texas psychiatrist had no clear duty to inform the authorities of Charles Whitman's statement because of the circumstances under which it was made.

The reasons for imposing confidentiality upon the doctor-patient relation go to the very heart of that relation, which, without complete trust in one's physician, is seriously impaired. With Richard Speck, however, it could well be said that no doctor-patient relation had yet arisen, for Speck was treated by the doctor as an emergency case while he was incoherent, and under circumstances that negated any understanding of the relation that he bore to the

Reprinted with permission of the author and *The New England Journal of Medicine* Vol. 275:18, 1009–10, November 3, 1966.

physician. Even if it could be argued that the doctor-patient relation was established, the doctor would have been justified in going to the police because of the danger to the community that existed while the killer was at large and because of the huge manhunt in progress. It is always permissible to inform the police of the whereabouts of a wanted criminal. The principle of confidentiality may protect medical findings, but it does not serve to prevent the police from finding their suspect.

It is clear that in most jurisdictions the physician is not saddled with the legal responsibility of reporting all crimes which may come to his attention. A few states, such as New Jersey, require that any person who has knowledge of any crime must report such knowledge to the authorities, otherwise he becomes guilty of a crime himself. However, there are no reported cases arising under this statute and it is thus doubtful if it, or statutes similar to it, have ever been enforced. Most states adhere to the more realistic standard of requiring the reporting of certain criminal acts such as gunshot and stab wounds.

The question of confidentiality is a more difficult one for the psychiatrist, particularly when he is confronted by a patient who openly contemplates a future crime. Successful psychotherapy is usually predicated on complete trust by the patient that his statements will be held in strictest confidence. When a future crime is discussed, it often signifies that the therapy is succeeding, and it would be untenable to ask the psychiatrist to rush to the authorities each time a patient revealed thoughts that could be considered criminal in nature. The only exception to this rule is that if the psychiatrist is convinced that his patient is in fact going to commit a crime that will result in injury or harm to persons or property, he must then take appropriate action and must go to the authorities if he is not able to discourage the criminal intent to his satisfaction. No patient has the moral right to convince his psychiatrist that he is going to commit a crime and then expect him to do nothing because of the principle of confidentiality.

Closely related to confidentiality is the question of privileged communication. Confidentiality and privileged communication are often spoken of together and have similar roots, but they are distinctly different concepts. Privileged communication refers only to in-court testimony. It arises when a doctor is asked a question on the witness stand, the answer to which involves the releasing of confidential information that is in the possession of the doctor because of his professional relation with his patient. If his state is one that has a statute that grants "privilege" to the doctor-patient relation he has a privilege not to answer the question. Actually, the privilege belongs to the patient, who may waive it if he wishes. If the privilege is not waived, the doctor is not permitted to answer the question. Statutes making the psychiatrist-patient relation privileged are becoming more common although lawyers and judges often argue that valuable information may be lost to them.

An interesting question would have been posed if Charles Whitman had lived to be tried for his crime. Would his statements to the psychiatrist prior to the crime have been admissible against him to prove his intent to commit the crime? Hopefully not, since the basic right which the criminal defendant has is the right not to testify against himself. Calling to the stand a psychiatrist to whom an admission or confession is made would circumvent this right which is so basic to our legal system. The law should not penalize those who seek psychiatric help by later forcing their psychiatrist to testify.

Tarasoff and the Psychotherapist's Duty to Warn

Dennis W. Daley

INTRODUCTION

The psychiatric profession has reacted with alarm to a recent California Supreme Court decision which it views as threatening the very basis of psychiatry—the psychiatrist–patient relationship.[1] The decision in *Tarasoff v. Regents of the University of California*[2] imposes on psychotherapists[3] who have reason to believe a patient may harm someone a duty to warn the potential victim. A strong dissent by Justice Clark claimed that the ruling will cripple the use of psychotherapy by destroying the confidentiality vital to the psychiatrist-patient relationship.

This Comment will highlight the issues of the therapist's duty to warn potential victims and the duty to confine dangerous patients. A more detailed emphasis is placed on confidentiality and privilege in the therapist-patient relationship and on the predictability of violence. These issues provide a background for an analysis of the potential effects of *Tarasoff* on the psychiatric profession and the practical problems arising from the decision.

Tarasoff v. Regents of the University of California

In 1967, Prosenjit Poddar, a Bengali Hindu of the Harijan (untouchable) caste, entered the University of California at Berkeley.[4] At folk dancing classes he met and fell in love with Tatiana Tarasoff. Poddar's attraction apparently was not shared by Tatiana who so informed him. A severe depression resulted from this rebuff manifesting itself in declining health and

Abridged from the *San Diego Law Review*, vol. 12, no. 4, July 1975, pp. 932–951. Reprinted with permission from the *San Diego Law Review*.

neglect of studies. After six months of languishing, Poddar sought psychiatric help as a voluntary out-patient at the Cowell Memorial Hospital at the University.

Plaintiffs alleged that during treatment with clinical psychologist Dr. Lawrence Moore, Poddar revealed his intent to kill Tatiana when she returned from a summer in Brazil. It was further alleged that two other doctors at the hospital concurred with Moore that Poddar was "at this point a danger to the welfare of other people and himself."[5] Moore wrote a letter of diagnosis to the campus police[6] requesting that they detain Poddar for a 72-hour emergency psychiatric detention for treatment and evaluation pursuant to Welfare and Institutions Code section 5150.[7] The campus police detained Poddar, but released him when he appeared rational and promised to stay away from Tatiana. Moore's superior, Dr. Powelson, then directed that no further action be taken against Poddar and that his records be destroyed. Two months later when Tatiana returned from Brazil, Poddar killed her with a butcher knife. No one had warned the girl or her parents of the threat. Plaintiffs, the victim's parents, brought a wrongful death action against the Regents, the campus police, and the hospital's doctors.

Justice Tobriner, writing for the majority, found that under the facts, plaintiffs could state a cause of action for negligent failure to warn. Addressing the issue of duty, the court stated:

> . . . we bear in mind that legal duties are not discoverable facts of nature, but merely conclusory expressions that, in cases of a particular type, liability should be imposed for damage done.[8]

The court recognized the general rule that there is ordinarily no duty to control the conduct of another or to warn those endangered by such conduct, but stated further that,

> . . . the courts have noted exceptions to this rule. In two classes of cases the courts have imposed a duty of care: (1) cases in which the defendant stands in some special relationship to either the person whose conduct needs to be controlled or in a relationship to the foreseeable victim of that

conduct and (2) cases in which the defendant has engaged, or undertaken to engage, in affirmative action to control the anticipated dangerous conduct or protect the prospective victim.[9]

With respect to the first exception, the supreme court, in direct opposition to the appellate court,[10] held that the psychiatrist-patient relationship in itself was sufficient to demonstrate the requisite special relationship between the defendant psychiatrist and Poddar. In addition, the court found the second exception to be applicable. Poddar was picked up as a result of Dr. Moore's letter to campus police. The bungled attempt to confine Poddar was found to have increased the danger to Tatiana. The court reasoned that as a result of the incident, Poddar discontinued the psychiatric treatment which could have prevented the murder.[11]

The defendant therapist's immunity from liability depended on the court's interpretation of what constitutes a "discretionary act" under section 820.2 of the Government Code.[12]

> Noting that virtually every public act admits of some element of discretion, we drew the line of *Johnson v. State*,[13] between discretionary policy decisions which enjoy statutory immunity and ministerial administrative acts which do not.[14]

The court concluded that failure to warn of latent dangers was not a basic policy decision and therefore falls outside the scope of discretionary omissions immunized by the Government Code.[15]

Plaintiff's cause of action for failure of the hospital's psychiatrists to confine Poddar was dismissed under Government Code section 856,[16] which insulates a defendant from liability. Although an exception is provided for "injury proximately caused by . . . negligent act[s] or omission[s] in carrying out or failing to carry out . . . a determination to confine or not to confine a person for mental illness,"[17] such was held not applicable to the circumstances present in *Tarasoff*. Dr. Moore did make a determination to confine Poddar, but countermand of the order by Dr. Powelson, Moore's superior, was deemed by the court to be a constructive decision not to confine.[18] Defendant police were also immune from liability for failure to continue detention of Poddar under section 5154 of the Welfare and Institutions Code which states:

> [t]he professional person in charge of the facility providing 72-hour treatment and evaluation, his designee, and the peace officer responsible for detainment of the person shall not be held civilly or criminally liable for any action by a person released at or before the end of 72 hours. . . . [19]

While *Tarasoff* imposes a new duty to warn upon doctors[20] and psychiatrists, the holding need not necessarily be viewed as a total departure from prior case law. In some respects it is merely an extension of principles expressed in previous cases.

The imposition of a legal duty depends upon policy considerations,[21] which policies are susceptible to influence by changing social mores and sentiments. Courts generally consider the moral blameworthiness of the defendant's conduct, the policy of preventing future harm, the burden on defendant of imposing a duty, and foreseeability of harm to the plaintiff.[22] The nonexistence of the duty to a third party effectively allows acts in careless disregard of that person's safety. The extent to which such an absence of duty offends the social conscience and notions of decency and fairness will determine its bounds.

It was thought[23] that the *Tarasoff* court might take the opportunity to further narrow the rule handed down in *Richards v. Stanley*[24] that, "in the absence of a special relationship between the parties, there is no duty to control the conduct of a third person so as to prevent him from causing harm to another."[25] Subsequent cases have indicated a trend away from the *Richards* principle.[26] *Hergenrether v. East*[27] held that an individual owes a duty of care to plaintiffs who are injured by the foreseeable negligent act of a third person when that individual has created the risk. In *Hergenrether* the act of leaving a truck parked on a skid row street with the keys in the ignition created a sufficiently foreseeable risk that a thief would steal the vehicle and negligently cause an accident. It could be said that *Tarasoff* expands this holding by imposing a duty not to create a risk to a plaintiff who is injured by the foreseeable *intentional* act of a third

person. *Hergenrether* uses a test for imposition of a duty of care depending on the foreseeability of serious injury and the burden of precautions. The same test would seem applicable in *Tarasoff*. In the face of a foreseeable injury and the inconsequential burden of giving warning, a balance would be struck in favor of an imposition of a duty to warn. The court, however, distinguished *Hergenrether* in that it requires the defendant only to take reasonable precautions to safeguard his own property.[28]

Another distinguishing characteristic of the *Hergenrether* line of cases[29] is that in each case there was an affirmative act by the defendant which created a foreseeable risk of harm to the plaintiff. These cases really discuss proximate cause issues. That is, assuming a breach of duty by defendant, is he to be held liable for the full extent of the injuries suffered by a plaintiff even though the injuries were brought about by the conduct (whether intentional, negligent, or innocent) of a third person? *Tarasoff* focuses on the question of duty rather than proximate cause. Simply hearing the patient say he intends to kill the plaintiff involves no conduct on the therapist's part which endangers a potential plaintiff.

In any event the court refused to reverse *Richards* but merely expanded the definition of the "special relationship" necessary to charge the defendant with a duty to control third persons. Whereas previously, a "special relationship" between plaintiff and defendant was necessary to establish a duty, now a "special relationship" between defendant and the third person will suffice. The psychiatrist-patient relationship now qualifies as a "special relationship" for purposes of establishing duty.

The moral question raised in *Tarasoff* is analogous to the highly criticized state of the law concerning the duty to rescue. There is generally no duty to come to the aid of another who is in danger.[30] Several morally revolting decisions have upheld this rule because of the "difficulties of setting any standards of unselfish service to fellow man, and of making any workable rule to cover possible situations where 50 people might fail to rescue one."[31] Rather than attempt to set up a rule with universal application, courts have focused on "special relationships" between people as a basis for whittling away at the disfavored general rule. Thus, one by one, carriers,[32] innkeepers,[33] shopkeepers,[34] social hosts[35] and jailers[36] have come under an affirmative duty to rescue. Though these situations are clearly distinguishable, *Tarasoff* may be an example of this whittling process and may represent another step toward turning moral duties into legal ones.

As previously noted,[37] a duty to warn may also be imposed when a defendant has voluntarily attempted to control the conduct of a third person. Once an attempt to control is undertaken, the defendant must act with reasonable care. If his conduct has contributed to a dangerous situation the defendant is under a duty to warn those who may be affected.[38] In California, statutory immunity protects state mental hospitals from liability for injury caused by the failure to control patients,[39] the release of patients,[40] or the escape of patients.[41] These immunities protect discretionary acts, but liability has been imposed for negligent execution of ministerial duties.[42] In *Johnson v. State*,[43] a teenaged parolee with homicidal tendencies was placed in a foster home without a warning being given to the foster parents. When the youth assaulted the foster mother, the state was held liable for breach of a duty to warn of the dangerous propensities. In accord is *Merchants National Bank & Trust Co. v. United States*,[44] in which the court found that the hospital had exercised no care in releasing a patient who had threatened to kill his wife and did so on release.[45]

Courts have rarely found open-door clinics liable for failure to control patients for several reasons. First, immunity statutes protect clinics in a number of states.[46] Second, because open-door therapy is somewhat experimental, courts have been loathe to stifle innovation by second guessing the decision to release, preferring initially to defer the decision to medical judgment. When therapists failed to predict suicidal,[47] homicidal or escapist tendencies which resulted in death or injuries, courts often found the violence to be unforeseeable.[48] Even if a diagnosis of dangerousness was made, but the patient was nevertheless treated under the open-door, courts have absolved hospitals from liability. In *Zilka v. State*,[49] under such circum-

stances, the court found no breach of the professional standard of care.

If these decisions are interpreted as implying or assuming that defendants owed a duty to plaintiffs, but that defendants were not liable because there was no breach (*Zilka*) or proximate causation[50] (*Bannon*), then *Tarasoff* does not seem to be a great departure from these holdings. However, since no previous case dealt with the specific issue of duty which was raised in *Tarasoff*, an attempt to discern an historical case law basis for imposing the duty may not prove fruitful.

RAMIFICATIONS

Tarasoff was greeted with a great deal of alarm by psychotherapists.[51] Three years earlier, the same court dealt the profession an initial blow by refusing to grant to therapists the absolute privilege of communication enjoyed by the clergy.[52] By upholding the patient-litigant exception[53] in *In re Lifschutz*,[54] the court denied the therapist the right to invoke the privilege against the will of the patient. The patient himself had raised the issue by claiming the defense of insanity. This well publicized case incurred a fair amount of criticism in the field of psychiatry, and a number of commentators called for remedial legislation.[55] The present case offers a much more severe threat to the previously favored position[56] of the psychotherapist.

The fear among psychiatrsts is that this case marks a trend toward further inroads on the profession's confidential relationship with patients and its statutory privileges.[57] There is a fear that the privilege may become so riddled with exceptions as to be meaningless, as is now the case with the physician–patient privilege.[58]

The dissenting opinion of Justice Clark in *Tarasoff* presents the basic argument of the profession. The opinion contends that the majority erred in basing a duty to warn on the existence of a psychiatrist-patient relationship for policy reasons because the decision destroys the guarantee of confidentiality, which is the basis of psychotherapy. Obviously, public policy favors treatment, but without guaranteed confidentiality fewer people will seek treatment. Those who do will be inhibited from making the full disclosure necessary for effective treatment.[59] The patient's trust in the therapist will be lessened by the possibility of disclosure, which will have a general detrimental effect on the relationship and the possibility for successful treatment.

Justice Clark contends that the inability of the profession to accurately predict violence will result in many more warnings than are necessary, since to avoid liability the therapist will resolve all doubts in favor of warning. Such warnings could have a much more widespread impact on the profession's reputation for secrecy than the majority anticipates.[60]

Must Psychiatrists Accurately Predict Violence?

Predicting violence in the individual is a task often undertaken by the psychiatric profession for use in judicial decision-making.[61] At least 17 states include a prediction of dangerousness as part of their civil commitment criteria.[62]

> [A]pproximately 50,000 mentally ill persons per year are predicted to be dangerous and preventively detained . . . . In addition, about 5% of the total mental . . . hospital population of the U.S. . . . are kept in maximum security sections on assessment of their potential dangerousness.[63]

The predictions affect those who have committed no crime as well as those who have committed crimes and are awaiting a judicial decision as to imprisonment, probation, or commitment.[64] Such predictions may also involve the length of detention of the individual. The ultimate deference to the predictive ability of psychiatrists is the indeterminate sentence.[65]

A satisfactory definition of dangerousness has been elusive.[66] Legislatures typically leave the term undefined in statutes[67] or list specific acts which are determined to constitute dangerous behavior.[68] Few cases provide clear meaning regarding interpretation of the term in the commitment process.[69] Many forms of offensive, eccentric, or nonconforming behavior may be considered dangerous, not because of threatened physical harm, but because of the unsettling impact of such behavior on the public. When construed so broadly, the concept becomes synonymous with mental illness.[70]

Despite society's heavy reliance on the psychiatric ability to predict dangerousness, it appears that such deference has been unwarranted.[71] Every study conducted to test the accuracy of such predictive ability has concluded that the prediction of dangerousness is difficult at best and largely guesswork.[72]

Three studies were reported by psychiatrists Wenk, Robinson, and Smith on predictions of dangerousness undertaken by the California Department of Corrections for use in parole decision-making.[73] In the first study in 1965, 86% of those identified by psychiatrists as potentially violent were not, in fact, charged with the commission of a violent act while on parole. In 1968, a second study revealed that of the group predicted to be dangerous, there were 326 incorrect identifications of violent individuals for every correct one during a one-year follow-up. The third study, using a history of actual violence as the sole predictor of future violence disclosed 19 false predictions out of every 20, based on the number of arrests of parolees during the follow-up period.

Over a longer follow-up period, violence predictions appear to have greater validity according to one study. Psychiatrists Kozol, Boucher, and Garofalo[74] conducted a five-year follow-up of 435 male offenders mostly convicted of violent sex crimes. As a result of intensive observation, analysis and diagnosis, the authors recommended the release of 386 prisoners as non-dangerous. Forty-nine others were released by the court contrary to the authors' recommendations. In a five-year follow-up period only 8% of the 386 predicted to be nondangerous, committed a serious assault. Almost 35% of those predicted to be dangerous committed such assaults. Clearly the psychiatrists demonstrated a much more accurate predictive ability than the court. However, viewed another way, 65% of those identified as dangerous did not, in fact, commit a dangerous act in the five-year follow-up period.[75]

that the patient is in such mental or emotional condition as to be dangerous to himself or to the person or property of another and that disclosure of the communication is necessary to prevent the threatened danger.[106]

The comments of the Law Revision Commission concerning the exception indicate that

[a]lthough the exception might inhibit the relationship between the patient and his psychotherapist to a limited extent, it is essential that appropriate action be taken if the psychotherapist becomes convinced during the course of treatment that the patient is a menace to himself and others and the patient refuses to permit the psychotherapist to make the disclosure necessary to prevent the threatened danger.[107]

The scope of the exception can be easily misconstrued. The language implies that confidential communications are privileged outside the courtroom and that therefore the dangerous patient exception also applies in a nonlegal setting. No doubt the term "appropriate action" in the comments contemplates commitment proceedings, but the statute is not very clear on this point. The prospective wording of the statute seems to imply that the sole use of the exception is in a courtroom during a commitment proceeding to determine the dangerousness of the patient. The psychiatrist's testimony would be used to determine the patient's threat to society. No duty is imposed by the exception despite the goal expressed in the comment that "it is essential that action be taken." It appears, then, that privileges and exceptions are relevant to a discussion of a tort duty only insofar as they are expressions of legislative policy.[108]

Confidentiality

The degree to which psychiatric disclosures become commonplace will determine the effects of this limited confidentiality. It may be true that people in a violent frame of mind do not read court decisions,[109] but one or two sensational cases of disclosure could destroy the profession's reputation for secrecy.[110]

What are the expectations of patients? Would they expect a psychiatrist to stand idly by after they have promised to kill someone? Would they actually be disappointed or surprised if the psychiatrist made an effort to stop them? Would other patients feel this was a breach of faith and be deterred from further treatment? Would the public be deterred from seeking treatment? One of the more outspoken defenders of the profession's need for confidentiality has opined:

The general public, prospective patients and patients in therapy will not lose faith in the psychiatrist as a keeper of secrets, when in cases of emergency, he acts contrary to strict and absolute confidentiality. Sooner or later the patient realizes that the psychiatrist has acted in his best interest. . . . However, situations of real emergencies necessitating disclosure are rare.[111]

Most arguments against requiring disclosure do not address themselves to a nonlegal setting.[112] This is probably because it is easier to find that confidentiality outweighs the benefit of having the therapist's testimony *after* a crime has been committed. A great deal more weight is added to arguments for disclosure where there is still a possibility of averting a tragedy.

There are numerous situations in other fields in which a duty to disclose is imposed by statute. "Battered Child Statutes"[113] require a doctor to report to police any evidence of child abuse. Doctors must report cases of venereal diseases which have been treated.[114] Prison psychiatrists must report knowledge of plans to commit crimes.[115] Apparently legislatures have decided that the public welfare outweighs any detriment to the confidential relationships in such circumstances.

It has been argued that when a therapist feels his patient is in such an emotional turmoil as to be likely to commit a dangerous act in the immediate future, the psychotherapist is in a unique position to treat the patient and eliminate the threat.[116] Many doubts have been raised concerning psychiatry's ability to prevent violence. Sedatives may temporarily reduce a patient's danger to society but no form of psychiatric treatment has yet been empirically demonstrated to have an enduring effect on reducing violent behavior.[117] In balancing the public's interest in effective therapy against its interest in being warned of potential danger, it is important to ascertain what degree of success psychotherapy has enjoyed. It is clear that psychotherapeutic "treatment is of no proven value in some types of emotional illness,"[118] for example, schizophrenia. More generally, the most authoritative research on the question[119] has shown that much of the success of consulting room type therapy is due to the passage of time rather than the therapy itself. This finding would seem to give more weight to the argument that a duty to warn will better serve the interest of the public safety than total deference to therapist-patient confidentiality.

Psychiatrists fear that *Tarasoff* may require them to disclose to potential victims all the innocuous threats made by the patient while under treatment. Certainly *Tarasoff* will require a judgment of some expertise. However, the standard of care required is that of the average, reasonable therapist under similar circumstances.[120] As the *Tarasoff* majority pointed out:

> The judgment of the therapist . . . is no more delicate or demanding than the judgment which doctors and professionals must regularly render under accepted rules of responsibility.[121]

A major unresolved problem with the *Tarasoff* decision is that the psychotherapist-patient privilege interferes with the ability of the plaintiff to offer proof at trial. For example, usually only two people know that the patient made a threat on someone's life during treatment, the patient himself and the therapist. The therapist is unlikely to simply admit the pivotal issue in his opponent's case, and even if he were so benign, the privilege may preclude such testimony unless the patient waives it.[122] The result may be that the patient decides whether or not his victim will be able to present evidence on the crucial issue of his case. In cases such as *Tarasoff*, where two psychotherapists and the police knew of the threats and corroborating office records and letters were available, the privilege may still prevent introduction of such evidence. The privilege extends to anyone who derived information on the confidential communication from any source other than the patient.[123] Therefore, in *Tarasoff*, unless the patient, Poddar, fails to invoke the privilege, any testimony derived from the therapist's statements concerning his consultation with Poddar must be excluded.

CONCLUSION

Duty is a matter of public policy subject to the influences of public statement. *Tarasoff* presented a compelling fact situation with an abuse of what heretofore was the discretion of the psychiatrist which so outraged the sensibilities of the court as to lead to the imposition of a new duty to warn potential victims of a dangerous patient.

For years society has deferred to psychiatric predictions of violence in determining the fate of numerous citizens charged with crimes or with mental illness. Psychiatrists failed to object to this use of their profession and, in fact, helped perpetuate the belief that their predictions had value. Psychiatrists probably possess no greater ability to predict violence in the individual than the layman.[124] But the psychiatrist's reputation for predictive ability may now be turned against him as a result of *Tarasoff*. Because of the reputation, juries may hold therapists to a higher degree of expertise than they actually possess.

It remains to be seen if the new duty to warn will result in an increase in warnings. A dramatic increase is unlikely simply because it is doubtful that the threat of financial liability adds a significantly greater incentive for action than saving a life, especially in a profession dedicated to humanitarian goals.

Lack of absolute confidentiality probably will not deter prospective patients to any great extent because of the unique nature of the therapist-patient relationship. "[T]he popularity of psychotherapy is perhaps not attributable to any notorious success but for the need in our society for a certain type of friendship."[125]

Notes

1. Time, Jan. 20, 1975, at 56.
2. 13 Cal. 3d 177, 529 P.2d 553, 118 Cal. Rptr. 129 (1974). This Comment is based on the California Supreme Court decision of Dec. 23,

1974. A rehearing was granted and oral arguments were heard on May 5, 1975.

3. Psychotherapists include psychiatrists, clinical psychologists, clinical social workers, school psychologists, and marriage counselors. CAL. EVID. CODE § 1010 (West Supp. 1974).

4. The criminal action against Poddar is People v. Poddar, 10 Cal. 3d 750, 518 P.2d 342, 111 Cal. Rptr. 910 (1974).

5. Dr. Gold, who initially examined Poddar, and Dr. Yandell, assistant to the director of the department of psychiatry. *See* Dr. Moore's letter to the Chief of Police, *infra* note 6.

6. Letter from Dr. Moore to William Beall, Chief of Police, Aug. 20, 1969 on file with Clerk of the Supreme Court of California, *cited in* brief for Respondent Moore at 168, Tarasoff v. Regents, 13 Cal. 3d 177, 529 P.2d 553, 118 Cal. Rptr. 129 (1974).

Mr. Poddar was first seen at Cowell Hospital by Dr. Stuart Gold June 5, 1969, on an emergency basis. After receiving medication he was referred to the outpatient psychiatry clinic for psychotherapy. Since then I have seen him here seven times.

His mental status varies considerably. At times he appears to be quite rational, at other times he appears quite psychotic. It is my impression that currently the appropriate diagnosis for him is paranoid schizophrenia reaction, acute and severe. He is at this point a danger to the welfare of other people and himself. That is, he has been threatening to kill an unnamed girl who he feels has betrayed him and has violated his honor. . . .

I have discussed this matter with Dr. Gold and we concur in the opinion that Mr. Poddar should be committed for observation in a mental hospital. I request the assistance of your department in this matter. *Id.*

7. Pursuant to the provisions of § 5150, a person may be detained for a period not exceeding 72 hours. A person detained for 72 hours under the provisions of § 5150 who has received an evaluation may be certified for not more than 14 days of involuntary intensive treatment under certain conditions. At the end of the 14-day period a person may be confined for an additional period not to exceed 90 days upon petition to the superior court when a person is a danger to himself or to others as a result of a mental disorder. CAL. WELF. & INST'NS CODE §§ 5150, 5250–54, 5300 (West 1972).

8. Tarasoff v. Regents, 13 Cal. 3d 177, 185, 529. P.2d 553, 557, 118 Cal. Rptr. 129, 133 (1974).

9. *Id.* at 186, 529 P.2d at 557, 118 Cal. Rptr. at 133 (citations omitted).

10. Tarasoff v. Regents, 33 Cal. App. 3d 275, 108 Cal. Rptr. 878 (1973).

11. Another issue raised in the opinion is whether the police have a duty to warn. Justice Tobriner wrote in brief and vague terms that the police had a duty to warn because the officer's attempt to control the anticipated dangerous conduct increased the risk of violence. As Justice Clark pointed out in his dissent, such a holding creates a new duty for police which could have broad implications. An adequate discussion of this issue, while significant, is beyond the scope of this Comment.

12. "[A] public employee is not liable for an injury resulting from his act or omission where the act or omission was the result of the exercise of the discretion vested in him, whether or not such discretion was abused." CAL. GOV'T CODE § 820.2 (West 1966).

13. 69 Cal. 2d 782, 447 P.2d 352, 73 Cal. Rptr. 240 (1968).

14. 13 Cal. 3d at 193, 529 P.2d at 562, 118 Cal. Rptr. at 138.

15. *See* Underwood v. United States, 356 F.2d 29 (1966).

16. "Neither a public entity or public employee acting within the scope of his employment is liable for any injury resulting from determining . . . (1) whether to confine a person for mental illness or addiction." CAL. GOV'T CODE § 856a (West 1966).

17. *Id.* §856c (1).

18. This argument seems weak in that the countermanding order wasn't made till the "negligent act . . . in failing to carry out a determination to confine" was made. A stronger argument would seem to be that there was no direct causation between the failure to confine and the death two months later. This argument is discussed by the appellate court. Tarasoff v. Regents, 33 Cal. App.3d 275, 279, 108 Cal. Rptr. 878, 884 (1973).

19. CAL. WELF. & INST'NS CODE § 5154 (West 1972).

20. The decision specifically applies to physicians, 13 Cal. 3d at 187, 529 P.2d at 558, 118 Cal. Rptr. at 134.

21. Dillon v. Legg, 68 Cal. 2d 728, 734, 441, P.2d 912, 917, 69 Cal. Rptr. 72, 77 (1968).

22. Rowland v. Christian, 69 Cal. 2d 108, 113 443 P.2d 561, 564, 70 Cal. Rptr. 97, 100 (1968).

23. Fleming & Maximov, *The Patient or His Victim: The Therapist's Dilemma*, 62 CALIF. L. REV. 1025 (1974).

24. 43 Cal. 2d 60, 271 P.2d 23 (1954).

25. *Id.* at 65, 271 P.2d at 27. *See also* Harper & Kime, *The Duty to Control the Conduct of Another*, 43 YALE L.J. 886 (1934).

26. *See* Vesely v. Sager, 5 Cal. 3d 153, 486 P.2d 151, 95 Cal. Rptr. 623 (1971); Brockett v. Kitchen Boyd Motor Co., 24 Cal. App. 3d 87, 100 Cal. Rptr. 752 (1972).

27. 61 Cal. 2d 440, 393 P.2d 164, 39 Cal. Rptr. 4 (1964).

28. 13 Cal. 3d at 186, 529 P.2d at 557, 118 Cal. Rptr. at 133.

29. Cases cited note 26 *supra.*

30. *See* W. PROSSER, LAW OF TORTS 340–41 (4th ed. 1971).

31. *Id.* at 341.

32. Yu v. New York, New Haven & Hart. R.R., 145 Conn. 451, 144 A.2d 56 (1958).

33. Dove v. Lowden, 47 F. Supp. 546 (W.D. Mo. 1942).

34. L.S. Ayres & Co. v. Hicks, 220 Ind. 86, 40 N.E.2d 334 (1942).

35. Hutchinson v. Dickie, 162 F.2d 103 (6th Cir. 1947).

36. Farmer v. State, 224 Miss. 96, 79 So. 2d 528 (1955).

37. *See* text accompanying note 9 *supra. See also* Morgan v. County of Yuba, 230 Cal. App. 2d 938, 41 Cal. Rptr. 508 (1964).

38. Johnson v. State, 69 Cal. 2d 782, 796–97, 447 P.2d 352, 362, 73 Cal. Rptr. 240, 252 (1968). *See also* United States v. Washington, 351 F.2d 913, 916 (9th Cir. 1965).

39. CAL. GOV'T CODE § 854.8 (West Supp. 1973).

40. *Id.* § 856.

41. *Id.* § 856.2.

42. *See* Greenberg v. Barbour, 322 F. Supp. 745 (D. Pa. 1971).

43. 69 Cal. 2d 782, 447 P.2d 352, 73 Cal. Rptr. 240 (1968).

44. 272 F. Supp. 409 (D.N.D. 1967).

45. *See also* Bullock v. Parkchester Gen. Hosp., 3 App. Div. 2d 254, 160 N.Y.S.2d 117 (1957).

46. In 1968 about 60% of the states still had such statutes. There has been a trend away from immunity statutes. Comment, *Liability of Mental Hospitals for Acts of Their Patients Under the Open Door Policy*, 57 VA. L. REV. 156 (1971). *See* Hernandez v. State, 11 Cal. App. 3d 895, 90 Cal. Rptr. 205 (1970); Santa Barbara County v. Superior Ct., 15 Cal. App. 3d 751, 93 Cal. Rptr. 406 (1971).

47. Goff v. County of Los Angeles, 254 Cal. App. 2d 45, 61 Cal. Rptr. 840 (1967).

48. Bannon v. United States, 293 F. Supp. 1050 (D.R.I. 1968).

49. 52 Misc. 2d 891, 277 N.Y.S.2d 312 (Ct. Cl. 1967).

50. *See also* Hicks v. United States, 357 F. Supp. 434 (D.D.C. 1973).

51. TIME, Jan. 20, 1975, at 56.

52. CAL EVID. CODE §§ 1030–34 (West 1966). The Clergyman-penitent privilege has no exceptions.

53. *Id.* § 1016.

There is no privilege under this article as to a communication relevant to an issue concerning the mental or emotional condition of the patient if such issue has been tendered by: (1) The patient; (b) Any party claiming through or under the patient. . . . *Id.*

54. 2 Cal. 3d 415, 467 P.2d 557, 85 Cal. Rptr. 829 (1970).

55. *See, e.g.,* Note, *Psychiatric Privilege*, 49 TEXAS L. REV 929 (1971).

56. *See* T. SZASZ, LAW, LIBERTY & PSYCHIATRY 79–80 (1963).

57. There are 11 exceptions to the psychotherapist-patient privilege already. CAL. EVID. CODE §§ 1016–26 (West 1966).

58. CAL. EVID. CODE § 994 (West 1966). There are 12 broad exceptions to the physician-patient privilege. *Id.* §§996–1007.

59. Many patients express hostility toward friends, relatives, and employers during therapy. If these hostilities were relayed by the therapist, it could have a severe impact on the patient's relationship with them thus exacerbating his problems.

60. 13 Cal. 3d at 201, 529 P.2d at 568, 118 Cal. Rptr. at 144.

61. A great deal of deference is given to psychiatric predictions by the judiciary. *See* Ennis & Litwack, *Psychiatry and the Presumption of Expertise: Flipping Coins in the Courtroom*, 62 CALIF. L. REV. 693, 694–95 (1974).

62. N. KITTRIE, THE RIGHT TO BE DIFFERENT (1971).

63. Rubin, *Prediction of Dangerousness in Mentally Ill Criminals*, 27 ARCH. GEN. PSYCHIAT. 397 (1972).

64. For arguments attacking this use of psychiatry, *see* T. SZASZ, IDEOLOGY AND INSANITY (1970).

65. Monahan, *The Prevention of Violence*, in COMMUNITY MENTAL HEALTH AND THE CRIMINAL JUSTICE SYSTEM (Monahan ed. in press).

66. *See* Goldstein & Katz, *Dangerousness and Mental*

Illness: Some Observations on the Decision to Release Persons Acquitted by Reason of Insanity, 70 YALE L.J. 225, 235 (1960).

67. *See. e.g.*, CAL. WELF. & INST'NS CODE § 5150 (West Supp. 1974). There would seem to be a constitutional argument that such statutes are void for vagueness.

68. If a person has "threatened, attempted or actually inflicted physical harm" on another before or after having been taken into custody and "as a result of a mental disorder, presents an imminent threat of substantial physical harm to others" the court may approve a petition for post-certification treatment for 90 days. CAL. WELF. & INST'NS CODE § 5304 (West Supp. 1974).

69. *See* United States v. Charnizon, 232 A.2d 586 (D.C. Cir. 1967) where the probability that defendant would issue checks drawn or insufficient funds rendered the defendant "dangerous."

70. Livermore, Malmquist & Meehl, *On the Justifications for Civil Commitment*, 117 U. PA. L. REV. 75 (1968).

71. *See generally* Roth, Dayley & Lerner, *Into the Abyss, Psychiatric Reliability*, 13 SANTA CLARA L. 400 (1973), and Ennis & Litwack, *supra* note 61.

72. Monahan, *supra* note 65.

73. Wenk, Robison & Smith, *Can Violence be Predicted?*, 18 CRIME AND DELINQUENCY 393 (1972).

74. Kozol, Boucher, & Garofalo, *The Diagnosis and Treatment of Dangerousness*, 18 CRIME AND DELINQUENCY 371 (1972).

75. Assume that one person out of a thousand will kill. Assume also that an exceptionally accurate test is created which differentiates with 95% effectiveness those who will kill from those who will not. If 100,000 people were tested, out of the 100 who would kill 95 would be isolated. Unfortunately, out of the 99,900 who would not kill, 4,995 people would also be isolated as potential killers. In these circumstances, it is clear that we could not justify incarcerating all 5,090 people. If, in the criminal law, it is better that ten guilty men go free than that one innocent man suffer, how can we say in the civil commitment area that it is better that fifty-four harmless people be incarcerated lest one dangerous man be free? Livermore, *supra* note 70, at 84.

76. Kozol, *supra* note 74, at 384 (emphasis added).

77. Fleming & Maximov, *supra* note 23, at 1036.

78. Wenk, *supra* note 73, at 402.

79. SZASZ, *supra* note 56, at 79.

80. Rouse v. Cameron, 387 F.2d 241 (D.C. Cir. 1967).

81. L.A. Times, Feb. 23, 1975, § 1, at 22, col. 1.

82. *In re* Lynch, 8 Cal. 3d 410, 503 P.2d 921, 105 Cal. Rptr. 217 (1972).

83. SZASZ, *supra* note 56, at 186.

84. On the other hand, it would seem unrealistic to require a showing that a person will be violent in the future beyond a reasonable doubt.

85. L.A. Times, *supra* note 81.

86. Ferleger, *Loosing the Chains: In Hospital Civil Liberties of Mental Patients*, 13 SANTA CLARA LAW: 447, 474 n.96 (1973).

87. Winters v. Miller, 446 F.2d 65 (2d Cir. 1971).

88. Gulevich & Bourne, *Mental Illness and Violence,* in VIOLENCE AND THE STRUGGLE FOR EXISTENCE 309 (Daniels, Gilula, & Ochberg eds. 1970).

89. Testimony by John Monahan, before the California Assembly Select Committee on Mentally Disordered Criminal Offenders, Dec. 13, 1973, in COMMUNITY MENTAL HEALTH AND THE CRIMINAL JUSTICE SYSTEM (Monahan ed. in press).

90. Tarasoff v. Regents, 13 Cal. 3d at 201, 529 P.2d at 567, 118 Cal. Rptr. at 143.

91. M. GUTTMACHER & H. WEIHOFEN, PSYCHIATRY AND THE LAW 272 (1952).

92. Comment, *Underprivileged Communications: Extension of the Psychotherapist-Patient Privilege to Patients of Psychiatric Social Workers,* 61 CALIF. L. REV 1050 (1973).

93. R. SLOVENKO, PSYCHOTHERAPY, CONFIDENTIALITY AND PRIVILEGED COMMUNICATION 3 (1966).

94. The term is defined in CAL. EVID. CODE § 901 (West 1966).

95. *Id.* § 1013.

96. *See* Broeder, *Silence and Perjury Before Police Officers,* 40 NEB. L. REV. 63 (1960).

97. The Hippocratic Oath states:
. . . whatever in connection with my professional practice . . . I see or hear in the life of man, which ought not to be spoken of abroad, I will not divulge, thinking that all such should be kept secret. *Reprinted in* SLOVENKO, *supra* note 93, at 198.

98. CAL. BUS & PROF. CODE § 2379 (West 1974).

99. Note, *Functional Overlap Between the Lawyer and Other Professionals: Its Implications for the Privileged Communication Doctrine,* 71 YALE L.J. 1226, 1256 (1962).

100. *See* Horne v. Patton, 291 Ala. 701, 709, 287 So. 2d 824, 830 (1974).

101. 29 Misc. 2d 791, 208 N.Y.S.2d 564 (Sup. Ct. 1960).

102. *Id.* at 794, 208 N.Y.S.2d at 568. *See also* Simon-

son v. Swenson, 104 Neb. 224, 177 N.W. 831 (1920).

103. 8 Utah 2d 191, 331 P.2d 814 (1958).

104. *Id.* at 198, 331 P.2d at 818.

105. Cal. Evid. Code §§ 1016-28 (West Supp. 1974).

106. Cal. Evid. Code § 1024 (West 1966).

107. *Id.* Comments of the Law Revision Commission.

108. *See* Fleming & Maximov, *supra* note 23, at 1063.

109. Time, Jan. 20, 1975, at 56.

110. Goldstein & Katz, *Psychiatrist-Patient Privilege: The GAP Proposal and the Connecticut Statute,* 36 Conn. B.J. 175, 183 (1962).

111. Slovenko, *supra* note 93, at 56.

112. An exception is Fleming & Maximov, *supra* note 23.

113. For a listing of each statute *see* Paulsen, *Child Abuse Reporting Laws: The Shape of the Legislation,* 67 Colum. L. Rev. 1 (1967); *see also* Brown, *Controlling Child Abuse: Reporting Laws,* 80 Case & Com. 10 (1975).

114. 53 Op. Cal. Att'y Gen. 10 (1970).

115. Slovenko, *supra* note 93, at 129.

116. *The GAP Proposal, supra* note 110, at 186-87.

117. Monahan, *Abolish the Insanity Defense?—Not Yet,* 26 Rutgers L. Rev. 719, 734 (1973).

118. Gunderson, *Controversies About the Psychotherapy of Schizophrenia,* 130 Am. J. Psychiat. 670, 677 (1973).

119. Bergin, *Some Implications of Psychotherapy Research for the Therapeutic Practice,* 71 J. Abnorm. Psychol. 235 (1966). *But see* Malan, *The Outcome Problem of Psychotherapy Research: A Historical Review* 29 Arch. Gen. Psychiat. 719 (1973).

120. Bardessono v. Michels, 3 Cal. 3d 780, 788, 478 P.2d 480, 484, 91 Cal. Rptr. 760, 764 (1970).

121. 13 Cal. 3d at 190, 529 P.2d at 560, 118 Cal. Rptr. at 136.

122. Cal. Evid. Code § 1014 (West 1968).

123. *Id.*

124. Ennis & Litwack, *supra* note 61, at 696.

125. Tarshis, *Liability for Psychotherapy,* 30 Fac. L. Rev. 75, 96 (1972).

Privacy and Social Control

Seymour L. Halleck

When an individual seeks help from a psychiatrist, he must usually reveal a great deal of embarrassing and potentially condemnatory information about himself. The patient has no alternative since almost all psychiatric techniques are ineffective unless he is willing to reveal himself honestly. Sometimes his honesty costs him dearly: information shared with the psychiatrist can be used to deny the patient important privileges and to deprive him of the ability to influence those around him.

Reprinted by permission of the author and publisher from *The Politics of Therapy,* pp. 119-28 (New York: Jason Aronson, Inc., 1971).

DOUBLE AGENT PROBLEMS

When a patient voluntarily contracts for the services of a physician, the physician is solely the patient's agent. In this role, he is likely to be vigilant in protecting his patient's privacy. The most serious breach of a patient's confidence occurs in situations where the physician's role is not clearly defined, that is, when he is employed by an agency and therefore has a dual allegiance—to the patient and to the agency. A patient does not always volunteer to see an agency-employed psychiatrist. He may be directed to submit to a psychiatric examination by the courts, or he may discover that he has to undergo an examination if he wishes to obtain a job or other privileges. If the patient assumes that he will be guaranteed the same degree of confidentiality from an agency-employed psychiatrist as he would from a psychiatrist whose services he sought voluntarily, he will probably be mistaken.

Many psychiatrists hold positions with the government and private agencies. Their employers may want them to help preserve stability in the particular community or organization as well as to help any clients referred to them. A patient, however, usually assumes that the doctor has no other purpose except to help him; he may not know or may easily forget that his psychiatrist also holds allegiance to an agency. Therefore, the patient may reveal things that can lead the psychiatrist to make decisions that result in denying the patient privileges.

If a student who is seeking admission to a university has a history of emotional illness, he might be asked to submit to an examination by a university-employed psychiatrist. If the student is honest in communicating his problems to the psychiatrist and if those problems are manifested by antisocial or deviant behavior, the psychiatrist may, on the basis of his examination, recommend that the student not be admitted. In this instance, the student's honesty would have been self-defeating. A prisoner who is being evaluated by a psychiatrist may tell him things that can result in an extension of his sentence. Either the psychiatrist participates directly in the restrictiveness by recommending that the patient be denied parole, or, more frequently, he provides the grounds for others to take restrictive action by putting adverse material into the patient's record. Thus, when the offender is eligible for parole, this information may be used by the paroling agency to justify continuing his sentence.

While a patient may certainly be victimized by a psychiatrist's dual allegiance, there are other important political consequences in using the double agent role to deny certain people privileges. Every agency, whether a university, a corporation, or a civil office of the army, wants to retain a degree of stability. Corporations and government agencies do not want to hire or promote anyone who might bring about drastic changes within the organization. Therefore, they are quite willing to use

psychiatrists to help maintain corporate or community stability. By helping to keep those who are different or deviant from achieving power or privileges, the psychiatrist serves as a protector of the status quo.

When I first began working as a student-health psychiatrist in 1958, I received many requests to examine students alleged to be emotionally disturbed in the various professional schools such as medicine, nursing, or education. In some instances these students were simply urged to see me; in others, they were told that failure to see me would jeopardize their academic status. Usually I was asked not only to try to help the disturbed student, but to advise the deans on whether that student should be allowed to remain in school. The latter request was usually phrased in terms of the student's danger to himself or others or in terms of his competence to fulfill his professional role. While I did not think that, as a psychiatrist, I had the skill to judge competence in any field other than my own, I believed I should see any students alleged to be dangerous. Some of the students I saw were seriously disturbed. A few were eager to accept my help, but many had borderline emotional problems, were not seeking help, and resented having to see me. This group also seemed to have serious grievances or ideological differences with their professors. Usually these professors had found something distasteful about the dissident students' personality, morality, or attitudes.

Whenever I confronted the professors and deans about the propriety of their referrals, they usually insisted that they only wanted reassurance that it was safe to allow the disturbed student to continue in school. Some maintained that the primary reason for referring a student was to ensure that he would receive help. For the most part, the professors and deans were sincere in making their referrals, but I suspect that in at least a few instances they were trying to use me to provide a convenient medical rationalization for weeding out troublemakers. During the past decade, I have tried to persuade administrators of professional schools that involuntary examination of disturbed students is, except in rare instances, an improper use of psychiatry. Still, I find myself occasionally in situations where my professional commitments require me to see a student whose professors would be happy to have a medical excuse for getting rid of a trouble-maker.

Several years ago a dean in the professional school of education asked me to evaluate a student who was threatening suicide. (I have selected this example because it occurred some time ago and the involved parties are no longer on campus. I could have described similar interactions with other professional departments on our campus.) He said that her professors were both worried about her condition and had serious doubts about her potential for being a satisfactory teacher. The dean maintained that he primarily wanted me to help the girl, but he also asked for my opinion on whether she was capable of continuing in school. I did not promise to give my opinion on the latter issue, but I felt I should see the girl since she was allegedly suicidal; the girl had been told that she could not continue her classes until she had been evaluated. The patient appeared in my office as an angry, resentful, and quite spirited young lady. She told me that she had been having a battle with one of her professors for several months; they had disagreed violently on the proper methods of teaching. She had taken a much more radical position on educational issues than was generally favored by her school. As their conflict escalated, the patient began to feel that her professor was giving her lower grades on examinations than she deserved. She argued with him about this but he insisted that she was being ''paranoid.'' When she talked to her adviser and her dean, they backed her professor and pointed out that she might be emotionally disturbed. During one session with the dean, the patient broke down, admitted that she had had extensive psychiatric treatment in the past, and said that the entire situation had so traumatized her that she was having suicidal thoughts.

I found the patient to be quite intelligent and aggressive. She had definite ideas about teaching her own classes which obviously conflicted with the views of her professional school. She seemed quite capable of carrying out her professional intentions if she were in an environment that would tolerate her views. The patient freely admitted that she had experienced considerable emotional distress in the past; as an adolescent she had indulged in a number of behaviors that are usually thought of as socially deviant. At the time I saw her, however, she seemed to be reasonably self-confident and comfortable; she was certainly not the type of individual who might injure others, and she gave no indication that her suicidal threat had been anything more than a hysterical and manipulative outburst. The patient also felt that, after ten years of psychotherapy with various therapists, it was important to her to break away from dependent relationships. She did not want to have me or any other psychiatrist help her.

I called the patient's dean and told him I could find no serious psychiatric disabilities in this girl and that the decision regarding her continuation in the professional school would have to be based on other than psychiatric criteria. He responded with disbelief. When I suggested that he was using psychiatric consultation in an inappropriate manner, he was skeptical. He accepted my recommendations with cool politeness but, from what I judged (perhaps in my own paranoia), with some annoyance at the stubbornness and intractability of certain psychiatrists.

Even in the enlightened setting of a university, the potential for using psychiatry repressively is enormous. If I had said that the patient was too sick to be a teacher or if I had informed the dean of the extent of her previous emotional disturbance, the patient could have been kept out of school without any opportunity to argue her case. Furthermore, an important ideological confrontation between a student and a professional school would have been avoided.

The role of double agent has troubled many psychiatrists. Thomas Szasz pointed out that if a psychiatrist tries to serve society and a patient simultaneously, society's needs generally take precedence and the patient's welfare is jeopardized.[1] He generally criticizes psychiatrists who accept positions with community or private agencies. However, I feel that there are enough instances in which both the patient's and the community's needs can be satisfied at the same time to justify the psychiatric double agent role.[2] If the student in the above example had told me that she wanted psychiatric treatment, I might have been able to help her with her internal problems as well as to stay in school. (Agencies are generally willing to tolerate troublesome individuals if they are receiving psychiatric treatment.) I also believe that if a psychiatrist assumes the double agent role, he must be completely honest in telling the patient how much confidentiality he can guarantee. If the patient knows before an examination starts exactly what is going to be said about him and to whom, he has at least some opportunity to protect himself.

Because our society is becoming more aware of infringements on individual liberty and because many people have heeded the cogent critiques of Dr. Szasz, both psychiatrists and their employers have become sensitive to the misuses of the double agent role. More and more psychiatrists are telling their patients what kind of information might be shared with an agency. And the employing agencies seem to be willing to give psychiatrists more freedom to help patients without requiring reports. In my prison work I have found that at least a few administrators now are more interested in having the psychiatric staff help inmates than in having them prepare reports that can be used to decide the inmates' futures. In my university work I now find that, except under extreme circumstances, the student can be guaranteed complete confidentiality. No administrator or professor can expect to receive information about a student unless there is a clear and immediate danger that he is homicidal or suicidal. There seems to be a similar trend developing in our community clinics. While these changes have helped to protect the patient, the psychiatrist who accepts the role of double agent still has substantial political influence. Unless he is constantly vigilant in protecting his patient's interest, he can easily lapse into the role of guardian of the status quo.

REQUESTS FOR INFORMATION

Unfortunately, the patient's privacy is threatened even in situations where his interactions with the psychiatrist are entirely voluntary and where the psychiatrist is not employed by an agency. Government agencies, corporations, and insurance companies are becoming interested in knowing the past psychiatric history of candidates for employment or insurance. Their application forms often ask the applicant whether he has ever received psychiatric treatment. If the applicant is honest (and perhaps unwise) enough to answer affirmatively, he is asked to provide the name of the physician or agency that treated him. He is also asked to sign a statement that he is willing to allow his physician to send information about him to his prospective employer or insurer. While the applicant seems to be signing such a form voluntarily, he has little choice—if he really wants the job or the insurance policy—but to allow those with power over his destiny to receive information that might reveal his greatest weaknesses.[3]

The psychiatrist who receives a request for information about a former patient (usually accompanied by a form saying that the patient has consented to have that information released) is in a difficult moral position. If the patient was not too disturbed and if the psychiatrist knows that he benefited from treatment, he can write some highly commendatory things about his client and there will be few complications. The psychiatrist's conscience will thus be clear and his patient will get his job or his policy. Usually, however, the situation is more equivocal. The psychiatrist frequently knows that some of the things he might reveal could prevent his former patient from getting a job or a policy. Sometimes there is very little the psychiatrist can say that would be favorable; if he responds honestly, the patient loses.

There is considerable reason to question the morality of agencies that snoop into people's past lives and of psychiatrists who cooperate with such ventures. Just because one has been a psychiatric patient usually has very little to do with whether or not he will be a good employee or a good insurance risk. Also, when a patient starts treatment he has no idea that his confessions to the psychiatrist may at some future time be used to hurt him. Furthermore, a patient's past problems are often unrelated to his present condition; his emotional state when he applies for a job or for insurance will probably be quite different from what it was when he was a patient.

The potential for using information repressively is especially great in clinics, where psychiatrists come and go rapidly, and where the doctor who is asked to provide information may not have been the one who treated the patient. In such instances, the doctor must obtain information from the patient's record. Psychiatrists have an unfortunate tendency to include information in their written records about homosexuality and other sexual peculiarities, drug usage, and even more serious forms of criminality. As I have previously noted, they are also inclined to diagnose people arbitrarily as schizophrenic or psychopathic and to enter these diagnoses in the patients' records; they rarely record information that reflects favorably upon patients. A doctor who knows the patient can usually say something good about him, but a doctor who knows only what the record says generally knows only bad things about the patient. The practice of sharing information obtained only from clinical records can be especially damaging to young people. The young patient is likely to experiment with a wide variety of behaviors; he may act unconventionally for a brief period of time and then settle down to more socially acceptable behavior. If his deviant behavior is noted in a psychiatric record, however, his future may be in jeopardy. . . .

By sharing information about patients who have deviant attitudes or behaviors, the psychiatrist also helps to keep provocative individuals from obtaining positions of power. "Peculiar" people who might want to change the system are weeded out. Obviously, none of the problems inherent in disclosing information about patients would arise if all psychiatrists agreed that such information would never be shared with prospective employers or insurers; if that were the case, there would be no further requests. Agencies, of course, would still have the right to screen applicants, but they would have to hire their own psychiatrists to do so. The agency-employed psychiatrist would thereby at least be identified as an individual whose primary loyalty was with the agency; the patient would know that he should be extremely careful in revealing anything about himself.

Notes

1. T. Szasz, *Law Liberty and Psychiatry* (New York: Macmillan, 1963).
2. S. L. Hallack, *Psychiatry and the Dilemmas of Crime* (New York: Harper & Row, 1967).
3. A. S. Mariner, "The Problem of Therapeutic Privacy," *Psychiatry* 30 (1967):60–73.

What's an FBI Poster Doing in a Nice Journal Like That?

Willard Gaylin

The pages of the *Archives of Dermatology*, with their full-color pictures of exotic skin diseases, are likely to strike the uninformed eye as bizarre and somewhat repellent. But even the best informed must have been startled by page 308 of the February 1972 issue. There, occupy-

Reprinted with permission from the author and *The Hastings Center Report*, April 1972. © Institute of Society, Ethics and the Life Sciences, 360 Broadway, Hastings-on-Hudson, N.Y. 10706.

ing almost the entire page, was an FBI wanted poster!

Appearing under the department heading, "News and Notes," the item looked identical to those appearing in police stations and post offices. But both of those are government agencies, and the *Archives* is an official publication of the American Medical Association. The graffiti that passes unnoticed in a subway station would outrage us if written on the wall of a church.

It seems ironic that the AMA, which has consistently opposed government intrusion into medical matters even where a legitimate public interest has been proved, should now have volunteered the services of organized medicine into a government function—and in an area so alien from the traditional medical mission as tracking down criminals.

Of course the thought occurs that it might not have been voluntary. The line between freedom and coercion is not so clearly drawn when the "petitioner" has the power of the Department of Justice. This thought, however, is only the first in the series of ethical and value questions inevitably raised by this eccentric utilization of a medical journal.

The notice, which also appeared in the *Archives of Internal Medicine*, described a 30-year-old woman indicted by a grand jury for "conspiring with another individual" in an act involving the interstate transportation of explosives. The alleged conspiracy violation occurred early in 1970. Along with the usual pictures in various poses, physical description, and biographical material, appeared the statement that she was known to be afflicted with an "acute and recurrent" skin condition. It further elaborates: "The recurrent aspect of this condition could necessitate treatment by a dermatologist." The reason for the FBI's wanting it in the *Archives of Dermatology* now becomes apparent. The reasons for the AMA's willingness to publish it are less immediately evident.

Before even the ethical questions, what is the legal responsibility of the physician reading this? Consultation with a professor of criminal law revealed that there were indeed open questions about liability and responsibility. If he had doubts—what of the average dermatologist?

The implications to the wanted person—who may or may not be a criminal—will also transcend ethical nicety. In this instance a fatal disease is not present—although it well might be in future cases, and it has been indicated that were the condition heart disease, diabetes, glaucoma, acute depression—the wanted notices would be referred to the appropriate journal. They would make it difficult, if not impossible, to get the necessary treatment.

The major question, however, seems to be whether medicine should be encouraged, or even allowed, to be an extension of the police functions of the society. There is no question that if this is seen as a legitimate function of medicine, it would represent a powerful and immense new ally for the police. In the files of physicians across the country are massive case records which would make an invaluable data bank (ready for computerization) of inestimable service in any police tracking function: the drugs one chronically uses, a tendency toward alcoholism, a hidden homosexual activity, proclivity for flirtations or other sexual idiosyncrasies, prescription glasses, specific allergies, dietary requirements, etc.

There is no question that all of this information would facilitate the police functions of the state. But is that the function of medicine? And in facilitating this other function *what would it do to the primary concern of medicine, which is relief of suffering, the treatment of illness, and the saving of life?* What happens to the tradition of confidentiality—so zealously protected over hundreds of years precisely because it has been seen as fundamental to the effective function of medicine? Such use of the profession by the police would represent the final destruction of the privacy, intimacy, and trust of a therapeutic relationship already seriously eroded.

It is conceivable that *in extremis* an institution must abandon its traditional role. The organized church has often supported the mass killing of war when it seemed essential for the survival of the state.

How are we to decide, however, *when* to violate our usual primary devotion and allegiance to the private person and his well-being, for the public purpose? How are we physicians to differentiate quantitatively amongst the various crimes and conditions of criminality in which we have no training? Are we prepared to assay indictment versus conviction, versus material witness, versus "wanted for questioning"? What are the relevant weights to be placed on conspiracy to blow up a heating system of the Pentagon, versus armed robbery of a bank, versus possession of marijuana, versus massive embezzlement? How do we weigh these public dangers against the health or survival of a patient? Ought we be making these decisions—or should they be left to public decision-making via the normal legislative processes which, for example, now dictates that gunshot wounds demand violation of confidentiality, but by implication of exclusion allows a host of other material the protection of confidentiality?

Which raises the question of how such significant decisions should be made. How, for example, are the power and responsibility which influence the whole balance of medicine and government distributed by a major organization such as the American Medical Association?

The Association is formed of elected delegates. These delegates, in turn, as an organization, elect a board. There is an executive secretary who administers the organization. There is a Judicial Council with its own legal counsel that acts as an ethical watchdog. At what area of this complex apparatus was the decision discussed, debated, considered, and finally decided? A call to the Editor of the *Archives of Dermatology* indicated that he had authority and responsibility only over the scientific articles, and no responsibility for this particular poster. A call to the Director, Division of Scientific Publications of the American Medical Association, confirmed that the editors of the specialty journal controlled only that localized aspect. The Chairman of the Judicial Council said the matter had never been brought to the Council, and, indeed, he was unaware of the publication of the posters when first consulted. He then suggested consulting the legal counsel of his committee who has had a long history of dealing with ethical issues and publication. *He* was unaware of the appearance of this FBI poster in the two publications until he was advised of the fact and, further, he could not recall its ever having been done before. He volunteered that when consulted in the past by various state journals, he had cautioned great prudence in publishing such material. Further calls to a variety of other sources in the American Medical Association (who must remain anonymous) indicate that it was "done somewhat experimentally" and spoke vaguely of "a great deal of pressure," having been exerted.

It was finally established that a request had been made in writing by the FBI to the Chief of the Division of Scientific Publication of the AMA, and that he made the decision, seeing no need to consult the Judicial Council, the representatives of the board of the American Medical Association, or the Executive Secretary of the American Medical Association and his full-time professional staff. He indicated that in his mind it was an "editorial decision" of no great moment and implied that it was a part of an ongoing tradition that preceded his assumption of office three years ago. But Dr. John Talbott, who formerly held the post, said that, to his memory, never under his tenure was an FBI poster replicated in either the *Journal of the American Medical Association* or any of its specialty journals. (This seems indeed true, although investigation shows that three brief excerpts from "wanted" notices did appear in JAMA early in Dr. Talbott's editorship—1961 and 1962. None, apparently, has appeared in the past ten years.)

Equally interesting was the gradual shift of the attitude of the staff of the Association when inquiries continued to indicate outside consternation. When they were first notified of the appearance of these pages, all seemed genuinely surprised, felt that the implications were of some moment, and suggested that, in a precedent-breaking move such as this, it seemed unlikely that one man, prudent though he be, would have initiated the action without extensive consultation.

But by the time this initial investigation was concluded, a new official profile was emerging, minimizing the innovation, suggesting it was a routine editorial-type decision, and denying even the presence of a problem. The man who made the decision stated that he would have no hesitation printing more such posters in the future, without advice or consultation, in whatever medical journals the AMA published, particularly when there was a specific medical potential for assisting the FBI, because "*no questions of medical ethics are involved.*"

The assumption that there are "no ethical issues involved" seems at this time to be the collective stance of the AMA. A formal statement read over the phone by the Secretary of the AMA Judicial Council also starts with the statement that no issue of ethics is here involved. This may represent the most distressing aspect of this entire episode. Whether the publication of such material by an official medical journal is "ethical" or "unethical" may be debatable (and should be debated). That major ethical issues are raised, however, is indisputable. It involves such basic traditional questions as confidentiality and trust, private needs versus public rights, professional values versus personal ethics, the special role of the healer and saver of life, and the power of the state.

For an individual to want to avoid recognition of error is understandable. For a group to underestimate the implications of any ethical question is certainly no crime. If, however, an entire organization such as the AMA proves so insensitive to questions of ethics as to deny their existence here—it could be disastrous.

Psychiatrists, Confidentiality, and Insurance Claims

Bennett L. Rosner

Most medical professionals, and especially psychiatrists, would agree on two basic principles of professional ethics: the confidentiality of the patient's medical record and the integrity of the therapeutic relationship. Yet a current pilot program, jointly organized by the national professional organization of psychiatrists and a major health insurance carrier, is chipping away at these tenets. And it is doing so with the tacit, if not willing, cooperation of the therapists.

In the summer of 1979, after several years of planning, the Aetna Life and Casualty Company of Hartford, Connecticut, and the American Psychiatric Association—both well known for their past sensitivity to the need for confidentiality of medical records—initiated a pilot program for peer review of outpatient psychiatric treatment covered by various Aetna health policies. A year and a half later, both partners in the project believe that the pilot program has been a success. Dr. William Guillette, Assistant Vice President and Medical Director of the Aetna, says "To date, the cooperation on the part of the mental health professionals has been outstanding. We have received and

Reprinted with permission from the author and The Hastings Center Report, December 1980, pp. 5-7. © Institute of Society, Ethics and the Life Sciences, 360 Broadway, Hastings-on-Hudson, N.Y. 10706.

reviewed over ten thousand completed Mental Health Treatment Reports.'' Although some APA members had expressed concern over potential abuses of the program, Norman Penner, Director of the Peer Review Project for the APA, reports: "Experience to date has proven these concerns unfounded."

Despite such positive reports, little is known generally, or even within the psychiatric profession, about this program. This being so, very little attention has been paid to the ethical problems that the program raises: issues of research design, confidentiality of medical records, the effect on the therapeutic relationship, and possible release of sensitive information to courts, law enforcement officials, employers, and others. In attempting to solve one acknowledged problem—the need for peer review of insurance claims—the APA and the Aetna have created several others. Before the pilot program is expanded to involve more patients and other insurance companies, these issues should be discussed more fully.

Three parties are legitimately interested in the issue of third-party reimbursement for psychiatric care—the insurance carrier, the physician, and the patient. Each party may have a number of concerns—sometimes shared, though in different degrees, and sometimes competing—about the effects of such a program. The stated goal of the APA and the Aetna has been to devise a reimbursement program for psychiatric care providing coverage that is both adequate and similar to coverage provided for other medical treatment. To date, most coverage for psychiatric care has entailed higher premiums and specific limitations, such as dollar amounts or number of visits. These penalties have been justified on the grounds that "psychiatric" disorders and treatments are much harder to define than "physical" ones. Psychotherapy for depression does not seem to be as concrete and documentable a treatment as insulin for diabetes. Whether this is true is immaterial. Insurance companies must document claims, or else premiums will escalate and make the insurance unmarketable. The consumer benefits when insurance is available at a reasonable cost.

The APA, representing the physician, is also interested in facilitating third-party reimbursement. Practitioners and the APA may also be concerned with the effect of such a program on the treatment process itself. That concern should be shared by the insurance carrier and patient as well, although the physician and patient may be more concerned than the insurance carrier.

Such a program raises many issues, which might be weighted according to each party's level of concern. At a minimum, the list should include: accountability for the need and type of treatment, noninterference with the treatment process, reasonable reimbursement to the patient for costs, consent of all parties involved, and assurance that the program does not jeopardize any of the parties involved in any way outside the treatment process. The merits of such a program should be measured on the basis of whether the program design considers these issues and whether its operation addresses them reliably and validly.

The pilot program designed by the APA and the Aetna for peer review operates in the following manner. The Aetna receives 2,000 claims every day for "mental and nervous conditions." Presently, 1,950 of these are routinely approved in field offices on the basis of industry-wide standard information received from the physician—essentially the patient's name, age, date of onset of disorder, diagnosis,

dates of treatment, and fees charged. Consent from the patient for this limited information is obtained on the benefit request form, which the patient must sign before filing. Above the patient's signature is the sentence: "I authorize the release of any medical information necessary to process this request." Below the patient's signature is the section to be completed by the physician, clearly showing the brief information being requested as previously described.

In the fifty remaining cases, which have been chosen for inclusion in the pilot program, treatment reports are required. The criteria for how these fifty cases are culled from the 2,000 are vague. Essentially these are deemed "suspicious" cases on the basis of information such as length of treatment, diagnosis, or type of treatment. What makes a case "suspicious" does not appear to be standard and it is likely that the designation varies in several field offices. In these fifty cases the following procedure is adopted:

The treating physician is sent a form stating that: "That Aetna Life and Casualty, following consultation with the American Psychiatric Association and the American Psychological Association, has developed procedures for special consultant review of requests for outpatient mental health benefits. This review requires that certain information in addition to that provided on the standard Aetna request for benefits form be obtained on those patients receiving mental health treatment." Dates of treatment are then noted and the completion of a "Mental Health Report" is requested.

A two-page form for the Mental Health Report is enclosed, including the following in the heading: patient's name, date of birth, address, sex, social security number, and name of employer. The form then provides space to write sentences or paragraphs responding to the following items: diagnosis, current problems including functional impairment (with examples); evidence of impairment (including mental status); duration and severity of impairment; when applicable, dates and results of physical examinations, including pertinent laboratory examinations (if the diagnosis is alcoholism, results of neurological, liver function, and chemical screening tests); modality, frequency, and length of psychotherapy sessions; medications, including name of drug, dosage, and dates prescribed; collateral contacts (including type, frequency, and duration); adjunctive therapies, if any; future treatment, including needs, goals, and estimated duration, and, if there are more than two sessions per week, a rationale for this need. In lieu of this two-page report the practitioner is informed that a narrative summary may be submitted, "provided it contains the specific material requested in this report." In addition the treating physician is advised of the following procedures:

> The basis of review will be the Mental Health Treatment Report (attached), submitted periodically by the provider. Since the Report will be the primary document used for review by peers, and will be the basis on which a decision is made regarding continuation of benefits, it is to the advantage of the patient and the provider that it be completed clearly and in sufficient detail to allow for a thorough review of services. The Report should include information on aspects of the case which may be unusual or which would be relevant to a judgment of adequacy and appropriateness of care. A lack of information necessary to make a decision may be grounds for denial of benefits.
>
> The information provided is for the purpose of the Aetna special review of outpatient psychiatric requests for benefits. None of this information will be microfilmed nor will it be copied, except for peer review. The copies submitted to peer review will be sterilized as to the names of the patient, provider and policyholder. None of the information will be disseminated to any other individual, agency, or organization nor will it be used for any other purpose.
>
> To insure confidentiality, the information you provide should be returned in the enclosed stamped, self-addressed envelope to William Guillette, M.D. Medical Director, Aetna Life and Casualty, Hartford, CT 06156.

The physician receives no further information, and the patient is not advised of any of the outlined procedures. If the insurance examiners feel that the report submitted does not contain sufficient information, they request an additional report. No one knows how many of the thousands of patients reviewed know that their reports are now on file in the Aetna offices.

The only way they could know is if their therapists informed them. Any answers to questions they might have regarding how the reports might be handled would, of necessity, be, limited to the sparse information outlined above.

What, in fact, does happen is the following. The Aetna staff alone reviews nine out of ten of the cases selected for Mental Health Reports and makes a decision about them. The remaining one report (or five out of the original 2,000 claims) is sent on for anonymous peer reivew; a decision about providing benefits in these cases is then based on this additional review. All reports are maintained in the Aetna files in their entirety until the completion of treatment, when they are destroyed.

How good is the program design? Some of the items that need to be taken into account seem to have been carefully addressed. For example, an attempt has been made to develop a comprehensive mechanism for accountability regarding the need for treatment, and reasonable reimbursement to the patient for costs has been considered, although there is still a percentage limitation on the amount reimbursed. However, other areas are poorly planned. Noninterference with the treatment process seems to be only a hope rather than part of a design. There is, for instance, no stated option for the therapist to respond that in a particular case participation in such a program would be deleterious to a sensitive treament process. (The nature of the doctor-patient relationship is often a major component in the progress of psychotherapy.)

An attempt has been made to assure confidentiality of the reports and thus avoid any jeopardy outside the treatment process. But the attempt seems to be directed toward the protection of the therapist as much as, if not more than, the patient. The peer reviewer does not have access to patient and therapist identity. However, sensitive information, with the patient fully identified, remains in the Aetna files and is reviewed by Aetna staff. Finally, although the Aetna acknowledges that there "should be an informed consent" they stated, a year after the inception of the program, that they were "currently working with the APA to achieve that goal." At present, well into the second year of the program, consent of patients is still not being obtained. With regard to involvement in the design of this program, it is reasonable to conclude that the balance of participation of the three interested parties weighs heavily in favor of the insurance carrier and the therapist (represented by the APA) in that order. There is essentially no input by the patient or a consumer advocate, and the design reflects that absence.

How will the effectiveness of this program be judged? Nothing has been published to date concerning this question. However, in presentations given at professional meetings, the Aetna and the APA seem to base their judgment on two issues: cost-effectiveness and the development of "problems." So far it appears that the program will be cost-effective and that no major "problems" have developed. The definition of "problems" seems to depend on whether mental health professionals and patients are cooperating with the program and whether any difficulties have arisen with regard to the therapeutic process or confidentiality. The lack of any major visible difficulties in these areas is taken as evidence that all is going well. No attempt has been made to investigate directly the reactions or concerns of the treating mental health professionals or their patients. It is hard to understand how the apparent lack of patient concern is taken as evidence of a smoothly running program since most patients do not even know they are participating.

The Aetna maintains that it will guarantee the confidentiality of the files in its possession. Although this sounds reassuring, what it really means is not exactly clear. When specifically questioned on this issue, the current medical director, Dr. William Guillette, stated that this guarantee means that he will not allow other divisions (such as life and casualty) of the Aetna access to his files. It is unclear whether this is a guaranteed company policy or whether such a policy would be subject to change. Clerical workers might well violate this guarantee in the case of a patient who is a public figure.

Furthermore, the medical director is noncommittal when it comes to the question of access to the files by parties outside the company. It is quite possible that, despite the company's disclaimer, files can be subject to subpoena in child custody suits, criminal actions (even if the patient is the victim of a crime and an astute defense attorney is attempting to discredit the patient's testimony), and a variety of other situations that have actually occurred in other settings. The response to such concerns has been that, "This hasn't happened yet," and that, "The doctor's files are subject to the same intrusion." This offers little solace. The individual therapist's file can be maintained with much more discretion since there is no outside pressure to write down extensive details. That files have not yet been subpoenaed only reflects that at this early stage not many people yet know of their existence. It is easy to imagine what will happen if such a program becomes widespread.

Other potential dangers are quite likely to come to fruition as the program progresses. Officials of the Mutual of Omaha Insurance Company have confirmed that when law enforcement officers approach the company requesting information, it is provided. State insurance departments can insist on access to files and indeed, Mutual officials have stated that as far as state and federal agencies are concerned, "We have no legal basis for denying the request."

What about the accuracy of the data being collected? In studies to determine the accuracy of mental health diagnostic information submitted to an insurance company in Washington, D.C., Steven S. Sharfstein, O.B. Towery, and Irvin D. Milowe concluded, "Diagnostic information submitted to insurance companies on claims forms is often inaccurate and therefore of little use for claims or peer review." (*American Journal of Psychiatry*, January 1980, pp. 70–73). They point out that "Most clinical practitioners have struggled with the fears and uncertainties about recording certain diagnoses on an insurance claims form; psychiatric diagnoses of schizophrenia or alcoholism are different in important ways from other types of medical diagnoses such as pneumonia or gout. The more consequential of these differences concern the social stigma attached to certain psychiatric diagnoses."

These studies concern *only* the submission of a *diagnosis*! The requirement of submission of an extensive and detailed mental health report would only increase the ambivalence of clinical practitioners over how "truthful" they should be. It is a very well known practice when submitting a diagnosis to translate labels such as homosexuality, impotence, pedophilia, suicidal ideation, and schizophrenia into identity confusion, situational reaction, depressive reaction, and anxiety reaction. In the evaluation of this current pilot program, there is no way to determine whether all that is being accomplished is a massive exercise in creative writing.

How might the legitimate need for a reliable, creditable, and ethical review system be met? Dr. Robert Gibson, past president of the APA, succinctly stated in the preface to the 1976 issue of the APA Manual of Psychiatric Peer Review: "In this age of public accountability it is no longer a question of whether psychiatric practice will be reviewed, it is simply a matter of by whom." Dr. Nancy Roeske, in recent testimony before the Senate Judiciary Subcommittee on the Constitution, expressed the APA's grave concern over the potential for serious violations of the principle of physician-patient privilege regarding privacy of communications inherent in the 1978 Supreme Court decision in *Zurcher* vs. *Stanford Daily*. In that decision the Supreme Court upheld the validity of a search warrant allowing local law enforcement officials to search the records of the *Stanford Daily News* for evidence concerning a crime involving a third party. Sheriff Zurcher had also received a warrant to search the records of a psychiatrist for evidence in an investigation involving one of the psychiatrist's patients. Roeske vehemently expressed the APA policy: "Patients have every right to expect that the intimate, personal information communicated to their physicians will remain private. . . . (*Psychiatric News*, May 16, 1980).

It is vital, therefore, that an effective peer review system have built-in provisions for maintaining the patient's complete anonymity and provisions for the patient's informed consent. Confidentiality is essential for both accurate reporting and protection from potentially disastrous abuse. This could be accomplished by assigning a code number to the patient and requesting that a report be forwarded *directly* to an anonymous peer review committee with the patient identified by code number only. A peer review opinion could then be forwarded to the insurance company under the code number and the report returned directly to the physician so that it will not be retained in the files of any third party. A system could be devised so that the physician would remain unknown to the reviewer and a guarantee made that the identity of the patient would never be revealed to anyone reading the report. This could be more truly a "peer review" program than the present system, which, in fact, is basically an internal company review since very few reports (121 as of mid-1980) are ever actually reviewed by peers.

Informed consent of the patient seems essential. Although it may not be the perfect model, the New York State Office of Mental Health Consent Form for release of information on psychiatric patients contains the basic components necessary for informed consent: (1) a description of the extent or nature of information to be disclosed; (2) the purpose and exact ways in which the information will and will *not* be used; (3) who will disclose the information; (4) to whom the information will be available; and (5) provisions for canceling the authorization and retrieval of the information. Since only the insurance company can provide the information needed for the statements required in such a consent form, it would be the company's responsibility to obtain the consent.

The Aetna and the APA have given considerable and serious thought to the issues involved. Yet, if one of the most responsible insurance companies in the country, in careful planning with a national professional organization which is fully aware and supportive of the important ethical considerations involved in psychiatric practice, can develop a plan which is so out of balance, what might we expect if that plan is adopted as the model for the industry by some 2,000 other insurance companies, some of which may be far less concerned about the issues involved? Would this peer review program, with such a casual research design and so many ethical problems, ever pass a stringent peer review?

Letters:
Psychiatrists, Insurance Companies, and Confidentiality

Dr. Bennett Rosner in his article, "Psychiatrists, Confidentiality, and Insurance Claims" (*Hastings Center Report,* December 1980, pp. 5–7) finds the program of professional oversight that the American Psychiatrist Association (APA) has been providing the Aetna Life and Casualty Company to be wanting in its attention to the therapeutic relationship in two essential ways. He claims that such a program interferes with the bond between doctor and patient and secondly, that the interests of this dyad are not sufficiently protected against intrusion by parties with ulterior interests.

As to the doctor-patient bond, while this issue has been debated extensively within psychiatry, I am unaware of any thorough research on the subject. However, the reality is that both doctor and patient often tacitly admit another party—an insurance carrier—into that relationship as a payer of services. The payer's involvement under such circumstances is regulated by a contract designed to protect the carrier's interests as well as to promote those of the patient (who might otherwise be unable to afford treatment). The APA Peer Review Project merely establishes for the carrier that services provided under contract are being delivered and delivered in a way that is sanctioned by the professional's collegial community. Neither the patient nor the physician is unaware of the tacit participation of the payer, and all but the most naive among these groups are quite aware that insurance companies may obtain such additional medical information as may be necessary to properly adjudicate any and all claims, be they in surgery, gynecology, dermatology, or psychiatry.

As to the vulnerability of the information compelled by such a review, we can only point to a general trend of intrusion by law enforce-

ment and other entities into the all-too-violable confidences exchanged between doctor and patient. However, in no case that we can foresee could coercive forces make greater inroads into the privacy of the therapeutic relationship by information culled from this program's records than by means already available to them.

To state the case in this manner, however, gives a negative construction to a positive program of information control. The procedures we have designed for the transmission of clinical information on psychiatric patients will greatly reduce the volume of information now routinely transmitted to third parties by hospitals and mitigate against its arbitrary use. Criteria for case selection reduce the number of cases considered. Review procedures minimize abuse of the information collected because in order to enter into agreement with the APA for review services Aetna and other insurance carriers actually waive their contractual right to process and store information collected through legitimate means in ways that they alone might otherwise choose. Aetna and other carriers must now guarantee that such information will be subject to processes of review and eventual destruction of documentation that scrupulously protect against interference from outside parties and from other lines of business within the insurance company itself. Aetna had for 17 years required the completion of a treatment report which asked for much the same data now requested on our own Mental Health Treatment Report. These data did not enjoy the protection now afforded by virtue of the procedures stipulated in the APA-Aetna program.

Certainly, no system of checks and balances is perfect, though we in psychiatry, as those in other fields of endeavor, strive for programs that serve our best ideals. It should be noted, though, that the present program of oversight is not an agglomeration of procedures fashioned into a system with only slight regard to their ultimate consequences, as Dr. Rosner might have us believe. The program was designed by a committee of nine psychiatrists. It has been subjected to slow, careful, painstaking review by a broad spectrum of the APA's constitutional entities, and it has been the topic of open discussion at various APA-sponsored forums. The final decision to enter into the agreement with Aetna was made by the Board of Trustees of the Association after careful consideration of the issues that Dr. Rosner now raises in his article.

All parties involved in such a review process gain from the agreements forged in this manner. The insurance carrier gains by being able to base payment decisions on standards relevant to the correct and competent delivery of psychiatric services. The consumer (i.e., the patient) gains by the protection afforded by the review process against improper or inadequate delivery of services. The profession, through the offices of the APA, gains by furthering at least two of its constitutional goals: promoting professional competence and maintaining the integrity of the doctor-patient relationship. The overall benefit of such a system comes in its potential for encouraging the insurance company to restructure its mental health benefits, allowing the removal of arbitrary limitations on psychiatric benefits and permitting more insurance money to flow to those patients who need it the most, without arbitrary ceilings or exclusions.

Norman R. Penner

Director, Office of Peer Review
American Psychiatric Association

Dr. Rosner states that any program should, at a minimum, include: (1) accountability for the need and type of treatment; (2) noninterference with treatment process; (3) reasonable reimbursement to the patient for costs; (4) consent of all parties involved; (5) assurance that the program does not jeopardize any of the parties involved in any way outside the treatment process.

Dr. Rosner apparently feels that the program is acceptable with respect to objectives 1 and 3. He states that "noninterference with the treatment process seems to be only a hope rather than a design." He then goes on to a long

description of how we handle claims and the "potential dangers" that exist. Dr. Rosner concludes by stating, "Would this peer review program, with such a casual research design and so many ethical problems, ever pass a stringent peer review?" Why would the insurance industry want to participate in such a project and subject itself to criticism by providers such as Dr. Rosner? To answer that question, one has to look at the history of mental health insurance.

The treatment of mental illness has been discriminated against since Hippocrates, and the vast majority of group health policies still limit mental health benefits. In addition, these policies only reimburse for the treatment of a disease or accidental injury, providing the treatment is reasonable and customary, *medically necessary* and *generally accepted.* Thus, health insurance is only intended to cover medical mental disorders, not the problems of living such as floundering marriages, child rearing problems, or the difficulties in finding a meaning in life. Insurance is meant to pay for the sick, not the discontented who are seeking an improved lifestyle. Another problem, from the insurance industry's viewpoint, is the inability of psychiatrists to agree on the types of therapies that can be considered usual and customary for a particular condition. There are so many different therapies, each with its own proponents and wide variations in cost, that to the outsider, it looks like the Therapy of the Month Club.

Insurance carriers respond to consumer demand. In order to appeal to the buying groups, we must have an attractive benefit structure, competitive cost, and satisfactory handling of claims. At the present time, the consumers are not demanding better mental health benefits, rather they want dental and vision care benefits. These benefits have built in control mechanisms that are accepted by the providers. Dr. Rosner either doesn't want any controls or wants the system to allow the psychotherapist to "mind the shop." That's where we have come from and, based on our experience, it doesn't work.

On April 10, 1979, the *Washington Post* carried an article on the liberal mental health benefits provided by the Blues to government employees. They stated, "Insurers seek accountability but patients want privacy." You can't have it both ways. The day of the double standard has passed and if patients and the providers want insurance coverage, they must understand that they are going to have to provide what is considered by their peers as a reasonable amount of information in order to resolve questions of necessity, appropriateness, and quality.

Dr. Rosner quotes Dr. Gibson correctly. Unfortunately, he then goes on to recommend a review process that has been thoroughly discussed by the experts and discarded as unworkable.

Contrary to the impression conveyed by Dr. Rosner, this program was not developed by the insurance industry but, rather, by the American Psychiatric Association. It was the result of many years of work by highly motivated and qualified psychiatrists who recognized the problems and realized that the profession must be accountable to their patients, assuring them that they receive quality care that is medically necessary. That was and will remain the primary goal. Any savings to the policyholder would be incidental to that goal.

It is not perfect and there will continue to be improvements, but it is long overdue and it is a major step forward.

William Guillette, M.D.
Assistant Vice President and Medical Director
Aetna Life & Casualty

Dr. Bennett Rosner levels very serious criticisms at the APA-Aetna program, which if true reflect badly on the offices and staff of the APA. Since I was in turn vice-president, president elect, and president of the APA during the time this program came into being, it seems appropriate that I respond.

Most painful to me is Dr. Rosner's allegation that the APA-Aetna project creates ethical problems. Unfortunately, he never makes a clear statement about the nature of these ethical problems; indeed, there is no ethical analysis to be found in his account. One can think of ethical problems in two ways. First there is a formulated canon of ethics that sets out correct behavior. Violation of these canons is unethical. I can assure Dr. Rosner and your

readers that the APA-Aetna review program does not violate the canons of ethics for psychiatry. It may be that Dr. Rosner is invoking the radical canon that psychiatric confidentiality should be absolute. If so I simply disagree. Confidentiality is important for psychiatry, but it does not trump all other values.

Here we come to the second, and what I consider the real, ethical problem: What to do when two values conflict. A patient leaves Dr. Rosner's office after announcing that he is going to kill Dr. Rosner's wife and children. Would Dr. Rosner place confidentiality above the protection of life? Dr. Rosner presides over an outpatient clinic in a teaching hospital; how often does he sacrifice patient confidentiality on the altar of education? What about the secretaries, filing clerks, typing pool, and record room at his hospital—does that system preserve patient confidentiality better than Aetna does?

The potential abuses of confidentiality that the APA-Aetna program might in fact permit (and I claim that Dr. Rosner has grossly exaggerated the possibilities) must be balanced against the actual abuses of third party payment perpetrated by health care providers. Indeed the APA's involvement in this kind of program began not with Aetna but in response to the highly publicized, scandalous exploitation and fraud by health providers of the CHAMPUS (Civilian Health and Medical Program of the Uniformed Services) program run by the Department of Defense. The scandal involved not only unjustified enrichment of providers but horrible treatment of patients, particularly children. The future of mental health benefits under CHAMPUS was in question and the APA participated with NIMH in negotiating a system of peer review that would involve some greater degree of accountability and would reassure the fiscal decision makers that tax dollars were being used in a justifiable fashion. The APA in my judgment succeeded; it brought some measure of respectability to a program with generous psychiatric benefits that was on the brink of disaster.

When the crisis was over the APA became concerned about whether accountability could be preserved, with even greater protection of confidentiality. The details of the system that had been devised were scrutinized by various components of the APA and suggestions were made particularly by our Committee on Confidentiality. My own position was that any innovation that would improve confidentiality and would not sacrifice accountability should be supported. I make no claim that the APA's peer review system actually works to control unnecessary medical treatment or even fraud. But I do not think Dr. Rosner's scheme for peer review would guarantee more accountability.

The APA has tried to be an advocate for patients. Without public or private insurance benefits there would be no treatment for the majority of our patients and no opportunity for Dr. Rosner to worry about confidentiality.

All that I have described occurred before what Dr. Rosner presents as the "pilot" APA-Aetna program. Indeed it was the success of the CHAMPUS program that prompted Aetna to consider an APA involvement in peer review. This entire scenario took place against a background in which National Health Insurance seemed imminent. Inflationary impact of the health sector on the national economy was front page news, and the APA was deeply concerned that once again the mentally ill were to be abandoned by the federal government. The challenge to the APA was to press for equal coverage of psychiatric treatment and to accept systems of accountability equivalent to those imposed on the rest of the medical profession. Dr. Rosner writes about "casual research design." No one who was involved thought research was being done. We were negotiating in the real world in an attempt to demonstrate to the public and private decision makers in the health insurance field that psychiatrists, like the rest of medicine, could accept responsible peer review and that our patients should get equal or at least better psychiatric coverage.

The decision to embark on the Aetna project produced considerable controversy within the APA, much of it around the provisions for confidentiality. Most of the arguments were debated in great detail. That debate was brought to the floor of the Assembly of District Branches and several times pursued as the major business on the agenda of the Board of Trustees, which brought together the chairs of the APA Committee on Confidentiality and Commission on Standards of Practice and Third-Party Payment. The patient's interest in confidentiality was pursued with an intensity that at times bordered on fanaticism. The resulting decisions and arrangements were a negotiated settlement, not a "casual research design."

It is disappointing to find a psychiatrist like Dr. Rosner insinuating that the interests of patients in confidentiality were not adequately represented and suggesting that a "consumer advocate" would have done better. Dr. Rosner should know that the elected officers of the APA include many who are "experienced" patients. Having spent many years revealing the most intimate details of our own lives to our psychiatrists, are we unable to recognize the importance of patient confidentiality?

Finally, I am never sure what the term consumer advocate means. Typically in psychiatry it has meant a lawyer who has an interest in civil liberties. If that is what Dr. Rosner meant, then the record will prove that the APA has consistently been a stronger advocate of patient confidentiality than has the American Civil Liberties Union. Having subjected the reader and Dr. Rosner to all this, I shall pour salt on the wounds by reporting that I was perhaps the only officer of the association who consistently raised questions about the wisdom of the APA-Aetna project. My objections, however, were quite different from those raised by Dr. Rosner's article.

Alan A. Stone, M.D.
Center for Advanced Study
in the Behavioral Sciences

Bennett Rosner replies:

I am saddened by what appears to be the total lack of understanding demonstrated by the comments of Mr. Penner and Drs. Stone and Guillette. In their zeal to defend the Aetna-APA program they have launched into a sales pitch rather than a concerned analysis of the simple, self-evident truths that are basic to the article. These are: (1) No informed consent is sought from patients; (2) the program as constituted is an insurance company review with a minuscule component of peer review to legitimate it; (3) there is every reason to believe that much of the data collected without anonymity are false data; (4) no attempt is being made to determine what the consumers (patients and their therapists) think about the success or failure of the program; (5) a more effective program is possible. None of these issues is addressed in the comments on the article. Rather, I am accused of a blind diatribe on patient confidentiality.

Shame on Dr. Stone (also a professor of law at Harvard University) who sees no ethical issue involved in the amassing of extensive, detailed personal files on patients without their consent or, in most cases, knowledge. The "consent" obtained is not only uninformed; it deceptively implies that only a diagnosis is being submitted. Mr. Penner misleads us when he says that for seventeen years "much the same data" were asked for.

While the article was in press a request for informed consent involving a patient of mine was "honored" by the Aetna with a letter threatening discontinuation of benefits. An additional request and numerous telephone calls through the bureaucracy resulted in swift implementation of the threat. Finally a call to Dr. Guillette did set the matter straight. But what happens when Dr. Guillette retires or when the therapist does not know him personally?

Dr. Stone knows better than to confuse us with the abused, trite, and misleading "example" of "what-do-you-do-when-Jack-the-Ripper-is your patient." Let's not confuse dragons and sheep. We are not talking about Jack the Ripper but thousands of patients who unknowingly have thousands of dossiers on file about themselves. Patients in public hospitals and public clincs *know* that such files exist, and in the clinical services for which I am responsible they are fully informed about how their records will be used. If they then choose to have their

treatment in this setting there is nothing unethical about that. If in other such settings patients are not fully informed (and I am sure this happens), that is not a rationale for extending the abuse of patients' rights to the private sector.

I am not reassured to learn that Dr. Guillette (who is not a psychiatrist and reviews the vast majority of treatment reports) is able to distinguish between "medical mental disorders" and the symptoms he gratuitously lists as not indicative of illness. I know of no trained psychiatrist who is so glibly capable of separating out such complicated issues.

Finally, we are assured about the extensive thought and consideration that went into the design of this program. The seniority and stature of the numerous committees cited do not impress me any more than the degrees held by the aeronautical engineers who designed the engine mounts and cargo door locks of the DC-10. Administrators and committees can get out of touch with patients and therapists even if they themselves were former patients and therapists. They haven't talked lately to many patients or practicing therapists who see patients daily. I have, and the patients and therapists "in the field" view this program with abhorrence even if the experts think "it is good for them."

Recent articles in the APA's *Psychiatric News* state with confidence that the program is a success and will be expanded. Yet the APA has refused to publish dissenting views. With this in mind I am currently conducting a random study of practitioners to determine their views on the program (an item the APA has neglected). Will the APA publish the study results?

The Urban Emergency Department:
The Issue of Professional Responsibility

Natalie Abrams, Michael D. Buckner,
and Richard I. Levin

INTRODUCTION

The concept of an "emergency room" was born in armed conflict. It was apparently first described in Homer's *Iliad,* which tells of the wounded being carried from the field to be tended in special barracks, the *Klisiai.*[1] During the centuries when therapeutics for massive trauma and agonal states remained undeveloped, there was no need for hospitals to set aside a room for emergencies; indeed, for the first 200 years of this country's history, in emergency circumstances the doctor came to the patient.[2]

Several critical changes in the practice and organization of medicine have completely altered this situation in less than 30 years. At the conclusion of World War II, most hospitals were equipped with an "accident room" where trauma patients could be evaluated and fractures set.[3] A marked increase in public demand for treatment, matched by the extraordinary advances in medical science in providing it, created a need for expanded services.

While the traditional definition of an emergency had been the ultimate threat to life or limb, the current *de facto* definition is any condition for which the patient seeks immediate medical attention.[4] This radical alteration in concept, coupled with such advances as defibrillation,[5] closed-chest cardiac massage,[6] and the surgical management of massive trauma, has led to increases of up to 600% in emergency visits in some hospitals since 1945, while a 10% yearly increment is noted as the national average.[4] Further, legal precedent such as that of the Manlove case (*Wilmington General Hospital vs Manlove,* 174 A 2nd 135, S Ct, Delaware, 1961), the recognition of responsibility for the indigent under the Hill-Burton

Reprinted with permission from the authors and *Annals of Emergency Medicine,* 11:2, February 1982, pp. 86–90.

Act, and the adoption of various guidelines and codes by licensing agencies, has mandated that general hospitals treat all who seek help.[2,4] These pressures have wrought a new discipline: the accident room became an emergency room, which evolved to the emergency department, which became subdivided to handle the vast array of patient-defined exigencies.

The spectrum of complaints encountered in an urban emergency facility is all-encompassing. The mix of peoples of vastly different backgrounds, the fervid life of the city, and the telescoping of all conceivable socioeconomic difficulties into a small geographical area conspire to make the emergency department experience rich but unnerving in its complexity. The emergency service routinely manages a variety of social emergencies because of default by other agencies which, by budgetary constraint or other circumstances, cannot provide 24-hour coverage. These conditions often result in moral, ethical, and legal problems which are as difficult as the formulation of a diagnosis, if, in fact, any illness is present at all.

The basic tenet of the therapeutic relationship is mutual trust. The only way that a correct diagnosis and subsequent proper therapy can be achieved is by the patient truthfully describing his medical history. The patient's complaint is the truth, or is firmly conceived by the patient as the truth, in all sustained doctor-patient relationships. However, in the emergency department, because of the mix of problems which people bring to the hospital (as the agency of only resort), complaints are occasionally fabrications designed not to mislead per se, but to gain access to help of a different kind. The recognition, by emergency physicians and other health workers, of this possibility of manufactured illness may drastically alter the course of a patient encounter. The case described, while by no means ordinary or representative, allows a discussion of some of these issues arising from the centripetal action of the metropolitan emergency department.

CASE REPORT

A 36-year-old white man was brought by ambulance to Bellevue Hospital Center from a department store where he claimed to have had a seizure. On initial interview by the triage nurse, the patient indicated that he was a Major in the United States Army, on leave from his post as a recruiting officer at Fort Sheridan in Chicago.

On the previous night the patient had been assaulted and robbed of all his possessions, including identification. He had been hit on the forehead, had lost conciousness, and awakened some time later. He had a headache and was slightly dizzy, but was able to return to his hotel and notify his base of the situation. Military transportation was being arranged for the next day.

On the day of admission, the patient claimed to have been browsing in a department store when he suddenly "blacked out and fell down and started shaking." The store nurse called an ambulance, and the patient was taken to another hospital. His memory for events at that hospital was very poor: he could not recall how long he was there, whether radiographs had been taken, what advice or explanation had been rendered, or how he came to be released. He returned to the original store to continue browsing. On questioning, he indicated he had had a single alcoholic drink at approximately 3:00 pm. Some time later, while still in the same department store, he "flipped-out" and became unconscious once again. He claimed that store personnel told him afterward that he had had another seizure and was unconscious for several minutes. He denied urinary or fecal incontinence, and any history of epilepsy, meningitis, or head trauma. He offered no additional complaints and denied any prior major illness or hospitalization. The review of systems was unremarkable. He denied heavy alcohol consumption, the use of drugs, smoking, or other habits to excess.

Physical examination revealed a well-developed man in no apparent distress. Pulse was 100 beats/min; blood pressure, 140/90 mm Hg; respirations, 20/min; and temperature, 37.1 C. There was a hematoma on the forehead over the left eye; there was no evidence of depression or crepitus. The right pupil was 2 mm larger than the left, but both were concentric, round, and reactive to light and accommodation. The extra-ocular muscles were intact; the conjuctivae and sclerae were normal. Both ear canals were free of blood.

On neurological examination, the patient was oriented to time, place, and person. Distant memory was intact; general information was excellent. He remained extremely vague about only two items: the events at the other hospital, and the arrangements for surviving in New York City for two days without funds while the military arranged for his transportation. Reasoning capacity judged by proverb and analogy testing was normal. Alcohol was noted on the patient's breath. Anisocoria was present; the cranial nerves were intact. Strength was excellent. A fine tremor on extension was noted. The reflexes were equal and symmetrical; no nystagmus, dysmetria, or ataxia were present. Sensation was intact. There was no nuchal rigidity.

DISCUSSION

Decision-Stage 1: Confidentiality

At this point, on the basis of the abnormal findings and the apparent altered memory, the examining physician was concerned about the possibility of neurologic damage, but was suspicious of the history because of the particular selectivity of the memory defect and certain details which seemed rather bizarre. Therefore, a consultation with a neurologist and skull films were ordered, and the patient was told of these plans for his evaluation.

Feeling that it was important to verify the patient's history as contributory to the definition of neurologic injury, the physician sought corroboration. The patient refused permission to contact his family, and therefore other sources were pursued; two were contacted. The local hotel had no record of his registration. The duty officer at Fort Sheridan was contacted and asked, on the basis of medical necessity, to verify that the patient was a recruitment officer. No such person was stationed at that base, and it was suggested that a call to Washington be made to determine whether the patient was in the military.

The decision to seek corroboration of the history is the first point at which an ethical issue arises. This is the first of a series of discrete "decision stages" during which the decisions made by the physician confront new information or require a new course of action.

A doctor-patient relationship was established when the man presented with complaints of head trauma and the new onset of seizures. At this point, the physician treated the situation as any other emergency encounter. A medical history was taken, the patient was sent for tests, and a referral was made to the neurologist. The first ethical question is whether there were medical grounds for seeking external corroboration of the patient's story.

While many might argue that the house officer was merely "staying on top of the situation" by making outside calls, these calls threatened confidentiality and raised several other ethical issues. The physician's curiosity was clearly heightened by the inconsistencies in the patient's history, but mere inquisitiveness is insufficient (at least on professional grounds) to justify the breach of what would, under normal circumstances, be a confidential encounter between patient and physician. However, can any adequate justification be given for proceeding to place calls to the hotel and the Army when the patient had denied permission to speak to his own family?

A patient has the right to request that physicians concern themselves with diagnosis and treatment; but supposing a serious case of amnesia and disorientation or a fabrication of illness, one could question the validity of this right. It might even be claimed that the physician should verify a patient's biographical information as an integral part of diagnosis. Therefore, to the extent that corroboration of the patient's history was necessary to the definition of neurologic injury, the inquiry was permissible, and perhaps obligatory.

The urban emergency department context presents added justification for seeking outside corroboration, because the presenting complaint is commonly not a true statement of the problem when the aid sought is nonmedical. When psychiatric, social, or legal assistance is required and the patient knows of no recourse other than the emergency facility, feigned illness will allow entry into the system which the patient perceives as helpful in a much broader context than purely medical. On this basis, the seeking of corroboration can also be seen as justifiable. Thus, through this point, we believe there was sufficient justification for the physician's approach. A more serious question is raised subsequently.

Decision-Stage II: Harm

When he was not able to verify the facts of the patient's residence and occupation, as well as the recent history of seizures at a well-known midtown department store, the physician naturally found himself attempting to establish reliable information. A discussion ensued with other members of the staff regarding whether a call to the Pentagon might potentially lead to harm for the patient. Although the patient might have been a deserter, and contacting the military might have resulted in his arrest or punishment, the decision was made to place the call.

Defense operator 13 apologized for the difficulty in verifying the patient's identity and gave the number for the Universal Locator (UL) in Indiana. The UL was called, and after listening to a brief description of the problem, the operator consulted his computer. He asked the physician to verify his name, hospital, and telephone number, and then informed him that the patient had deserted 48 hours earlier from Fort Benning, Georgia, where he was undergoing psychiatric evaluation. Further, a federal warrant had been issued for the patient's arrest.

The question of potential harm which had been raised in the physician's mind was now instantly crystallized. On the one hand, confidentiality could be justified solely by a patient's right to keep certain information private, regardless of the benefit or harm produced by revealing the information. On the other, maintaining confidentiality could be justified by the expected consequences: if beneficial consequences are to be produced by revealing or maintaining information, then it is the consequences, rather than individual rights, that should guide conduct.

Based on the physician's assessment of the patient as not dangerous to himself or to society, calling the UL and thus revealing confidential information (namely, that a physician-patient relationship had been established and the whereabouts of the patient) was not justified according to either interpretation of the principle of confidentiality: it violated the patient's rights and was not likely to produce beneficial consequences for the patient or for society. Furthermore, such a course of action was clearly in violation of the physician's pledge to "above all, do no harm." Such a pledge should not be seen as restricted to avoiding physical injury, but should also include the avoidance of social harm, except in those few cases in which such harm is an inevitable consequence of actions which the physician is legally obligated to take. In retrospect, the physician felt it would have been a much better course to approach the patient rather than the UL with his concerns.

Decision-Stage III: Detention

The final stage of this encounter developed when the UL informed the physician of the patient's deserter status, his status as a psychiatric patient at his base, and the existence of a federal warrant. At this point, the physician was asked by the armed forces operator to detain this patient. The physician indicated that he did not think this was legally permissible, but that he would check with hospital administration.

In the meantime, the UL notified the local Armed Forces Police (AFP). They, in turn, called and indicated that they did not have the manpower to come and arrest the patient; however, they would call the local precinct of the New York Police Department and ask them to make the arrest. The precinct declined (no reason was given), and a more distant AFP unit ultimately called to say that if the patient could be detained until 7 am, someone would arrive to transport him. The AFP was queried about liability if the patient, for whom a federal warrant had been issued, was allowed to go; the officer stated that all that was necessary had been

done, but that this was merely his opinion. The hospital administrator was fully informed and suggested that the physician proceed with the course dictated by his best judgment, and that the administrator would involve counsel if necessary.

During these conversations, the results of the skull series, the neurology consultation, and a lumbar puncture were reported as normal. At this point, the physician elected to inform the patient of the new knowledge that had been gathered and to advise him that he could not be held in the hospital, but that a psychiatric consultation was strongly recommended. Accompanied by the hospital police at a distance, the physician told the patient of the new data and recommendations. The patient calmly stated that he would like to see the psychiatrist. He was then evaluated in the psychiatric emergency department, where he remained until the AFP arrived. The subsequent history is unknown.

Legal Issues

The first question raised at this stage regards the nature of the UL operator's request to the physician. The operator's status and authority for such a request are clearly suspect. Furthermore, what are the physician's legal obligations in light of the knowledge that the patient is a member of the military who is being sought under a federal warrant, ie, by the law?

Although the legal status of such a request was not known at the time and was not immediately ascertained, it was subsequently learned that under New York Criminal Procedure Law (120.10) a warrant is addressed to the police, and therefore there is no legal obligation for a citizen to act on such a warrant. While unreasonable refusal to aid a police officer in the course of performing his duties (e.g., arresting a person) is a misdemeanor (NY Penal Law 195.10), this seems to apply only when a police officer asks a specific person for help at the scene of a crime. Thus the physician was under no legal obligation to detain the patient.

Furthermore, it probably would not have been legally permissible for the physician to detain the patient. Because the patient's behavior did not provide any grounds for an involuntary referral to psychiatric admitting, and because the patient would not have had to consent voluntarily to visiting the psychiatric unit, the physician, in order to detain, would have had to choose candor, subterfuge, or an explicit use of compulsion on what he deemed medically insufficient grounds. Although according to New York Penal Law, article 35.10,[5] a physician is justified in using force to administer necessary treatment, the term "necessary" is usually interpreted in a narrow sense; in this case, detention would probably not be legally justifiable.

Ethics Issues

A second question raised is whether there is a moral obligation for truth-telling in such a doctor-patient relationship. Was it obligatory for the physician to tell the patient that he could not be held against his will nor forced to see a psychiatrist? It is interesting to note that the Hippocratic Oath, the Declaration of Geneva by the World Medical Association (1948), and the Principles of Medical Ethics of the AMA do not view veracity as an absolute or even clear obligation.

While there are recognized circumstances in which truth may not be beneficial to a patient, this situation does not appear to be one of them. Four arguments are typically offered for nondisclosure and deception in a therapeutic context.[7] One argument is that some forms of nondisclosure actually constitute "benevolent deception" in that the patient would be better off not knowing the information. A second is that in some situations, truth-telling is not appropriate because the patient could not comprehend the information. A third is that some patients do not really want to know the truth, especially a bad prognosis. Lastly, it is argued that in some situations, coercing an individual by means of deception to obtain needed care is desirable because such deception would actually be in the patient's best interest.

Only the last argument is applicable to the situation presented by our case. The question is whether the traditional paternalistic stance of medicine can be justified in this instance. Would it be justifiable to deceive the patient in order to ensure that he receives what the physician believes is necessary psychiatric care?

Because the patient did not appear danger-ous to himself or to society, the physician did not feel justified in using deception to detain him or to force him to seek psychiatric care. Enough had taken place between the physician and the patient for the physician to be relatively confident that the patient would not leave and would voluntarily agree to see a psychiatrist. If the physician did not really believe this would be the case, or if he feared that the patient would have reacted violently to the discovery about his false statements, it is not clear whether the physician would have told the patient the truth and given him the option of leaving. Truth-telling was made considerably easier by the realities of this case.

The paramount and most controversial issue presented by this stage, and the entire case, is the question of detention. This question is so difficult that, in practical terms, it is frequently left unasked in the urban emergency department. When can it be said that a physician has either the right or the obligation to detain an individual? In our society, there is a generally recognized presumption in favor of freedom. The burden of proof therefore rests on those who would want to detain; the question becomes what are the conditions under which the presumption of liberty can legitimately be overridden.

Traditionally, social and legal philosophy recognize a number of alternative justifications for restricting an individual's liberty.[8-10] The most widely accepted justification is the prevention of harm to others, whether it be individual persons (the private harm principle) or "impairment of institutional practices that are in the public interest" (the public harm principle).[11] Based on the physician's assessment of the patient's mental status and his belief that the patient was not dangerous to others, the private harm principle would not be applicable. It would not be possible for the physician to detain based on the belief that harm to others is thereby being prevented or would be prevented in the future. There is also legal precedent on this issue. The court found in *Nance vs James Arthur Smith Hospital, Inc* (329 So. 2d 377, Fla App, 1976) that the hospital could not be held liable for the subsequent violent actions of a patient discharged from the emergency department when no evidence of a violent psychiatric state was found to be present during their examination.[12] This suggests the legal impropriety of holding a patient for the possibility of future psychiatric disturbances.

Whether the emergency physician was justified in making such an assessment is, however, a separate issue. Assuming the availability of a psychiatric consultant, as well as the fact that other psychiatrists at the base from which the patient escaped were currently evaluating him, it might have been more appropriate for the determination of danger to self or others to have been made by a psychiatrist.

The public harm principle poses a more difficult challenge. Can it be said that the physician, by not aiding the involved social institutions (namely the police and the military), was undermining their authority and weakening their ability to perform necessary functions on which we all depend? The facts of the case do not seem to support this interpretation. The police were, in fact, notified, but refused to assume any responsibility and provided no reasons for their lack of involvement despite the federal warrant for the patient. Furthermore, by reporting the patient's presence, the physician was attempting to utilize, rather than undermine, the appropriate authorities. A new question was raised, however, by the authorities' failure to act appropriately. If returning the patient to the original psychiatric institution was the goal, can it be said that the physician's responsibility was fulfilled by simply reporting the patient's whereabouts?

Assuming that, in order to successfully bring about a certain goal, there is a need for cooperation among individuals in different capacities, if a "link in the chain" fails, can one rest content with the knowledge that he did his part? In other words, did it become the physician's moral responsibility to detain the patient until the authorities arrived, simply by virtue of the fact that the police failed to fulfill their responsibilities? Are there grounds for such a moral obligation to detain regardless of whether there was a medical justification for such detention? If there were such a moral obligation, does its satisfaction require the physician to use various delaying tactics (tests, further examinations, etc) or, perhaps, overt coercion in order to detain the patient? If there were not such an

obligation, would it even be permissible as a matter of professional discretion for the physician to detain the patient? In essence, the question is whether social functions with obligations beyond patient care should be seen as part of the physician's role. We think, in general, they should not.

A third principle cited as a justification for limiting liberty is the prevention of self-harm (principle of paternalism).[11-13] Again, this principle does not seem applicable. According to the physician's evaluation, the patient was not likely to harm himself and therefore could not be detained on this basis.

A fourth principle which is frequently cited in medical contexts involves the production of benefit for the individual (extreme paternalism) or for others (the welfare principle).[11] According to the principle of extreme paternalism, it is permissible to limit freedom not only to prevent harm to the person, but also to benefit the individual. If the physician believed that the patient would benefit from medical or psychiatric care, this would be a legitimate basis for detaining him. Arguments based on the right to self-determination and autonomy are, however, usually employed to preclude such extreme paternalism, and certainly preclude the violation of individual liberties for the public benefit.

Based on the above, it is difficult to find an acceptable reason for detaining the patient. The situation would have been different if the emergency physician had known the basis for the patient's original institutionalization, eg, if the patient were a known convict or known to be dangerous to himself or others. This information would place an additional burden on the attending physician.

Modifying the case by presuming the patient dangerous to the community in a different way, eg, if he were a known carrier of a lethal virus and would, therefore, adversely affect public health, highlights a most important question. Is detention of the patient inappropriate because of the presumption of liberty and the belief that no harm would result from the patient's freedom, or is detention of the patient inappropriate because of the nature of the physician's role and the belief that it is not part of the responsibility of a physician to violate the trust implicit in the physician-patient relationship except in those instances in which the health of the community is at stake? In other words, even if the patient were thought to be potentially dangerous to others in ways unrelated to health, or were a known convict, should these factors warrant detention?

It is our contention that functioning in such a capacity would, in fact, run counter to the professional role of a physician and the fiduciary relationship between physician and patient. Except for purposes of protecting the health of the community, or perhaps of the patient himself in certain cases, the physician may not act against the wishes of the individual patient. Certainly any physician behavior which is motivated by concerns other than the best interest of the patient would be a violation of this fiduciary relationship, and functioning in such a capacity would therefore have to be made explicit to the patient. According to Fried,[14] a fiduciary "may not pursue activities that either do in fact conflict with or influence his judgment, or might appear to do so, without the explicit consent of the client."

Assuming that detention of a potentially dangerous individual, though perhaps permissible, is not an obligation of an ordinary citizen, there would have to be something particular about the physician's role that would mandate such a duty. Simply the ability to detain, by either force or deception, would not seem sufficient. In addition, the role definition itself (ie, as a fiduciary) argues against detention and possibly against even reporting the patient's presence, for this might well be seen as a breach of confidentiality. Based on the obligation to inform the patient of any conflicting responsibilities, incorporating such duties into the overall responsibilities of health care professionals might well risk deterring individuals who might need health care from seeking it.

CONCLUSION

Balancing the risks of detaining and breaching confidentiality versus not detaining and maintaining confidentiality is a difficult and controversial task. However, if physicians are not considered exempt from such functions, there is an additional risk that the whole health care establishment might be seen as a vehicle for, or a means toward, social control. We believe that the physician-patient relationship and the concept of personal care should be held inviolate, other than in the most exceptional of circumstances. The circumstances described in this case do not provide such an exception.

References

1. MAJNO G: *The Healing Hand. Man and Wound in the Ancient World.* Boston, Harvard University Press, 1975, p 124.
2. DALEN JE: Medicolegal aspects of on-the-scene emergency medical care: Scope of the problems, in *Proceedings of the First National Conference on the Medicolegal Implications of Emergency Medical Care.* Dallas, American Heart Association, 1976.
3. LURIA MN, MORTON JH: The function and administration of a university emergency department, in Jelenko C, Frey CF (eds): *Emergency Medical Services: An Overview.* Bowie, Maryland, Robert J. Brandy, Co, 1976.
4. MILLS JD: Introduction: Overview of field of emergency medicine, in Jenkins AL (ed): *Emergency Department Organization and Management.* St. Louis, CV Mosby Co, 1978.
5. BECK CS, PRITCHARD WH, FEIL H: Ventricular fibrillation of prolonged duration abolished by electric shock. *JAMA* 173:1064, 1960.
6. KOUWENHOUVEN WB, JUDE JR, KNICKERBOCKER GG: Closed chest cardiac massage. *JAMA* 173: 1064, 1960.
7. BEAUCHAMP T, CHILDRESS J: *Principles of Biomedical Ethics.* New York, Oxford University Press, 1979, pp 205–209.
8. DWORKIN G: Paternalism. *Monist* 56:1, 1972.
9. HART HLA: *Law, Liberty and Morality.* Stanford, Stanford University Press, 1963
10. MILL JS: *On Liberty.* New York, Liberal Arts Press, 1956.
11. FEINBERG J: *Social Philosophy.* Englewood Cliffs, New Jersey, Prentice Hall, 1973, p 33.
12. BERNSTEIN AH: Hospital emergency services and the law. *Hospitals* 51:100, 1977.
13. TAIT BS, WINSLOW G: Beyond consent—The ethics of decision-making in emergency medicine. *West J Med* 126:156–159, 1979.
14. FRIED C: *Medical Experimentation: Personal Integrity and Social Policy.* New York, American Elsevier Pub, 1974, p 34.

Chapter 4

BIRTH AND DEATH

INTRODUCTION

Conception, birth, and death constitute the limits of human experience and existence and thus play a major role in any moral theory. By and large, life is viewed as being of very high value, and nonlife, or death, is of negative value for each person. Medicine has a major role to play in all three events. Health professionals can now facilitate conception and birth in many cases where physiology previously prevented them; conversely, medical practitioners can also prevent either event, or both, and determine facts which will make some prospective parents wonder about the moral desirability of bearing children for themselves. At the other end of the scale, health professionals can also postpone death almost indefinitely in a great many cases, although they cannot always return their patients to health.

Such power creates serious moral qualms about its best uses. In this chapter, we look at some of the troubling issues advanced knowledge raises in the areas of birth and death. Underlying all the particular problems is the

ultimate value decision: Is life always preferable to death, and if not, what kinds of criteria make life likely to be intolerable?

The ability to postpone or hasten death carries with it a profound responsibility. The costs of moral error are high. There is a strong social taboo against causing death, which is reflected in virtually every moral theory. In fact, we can see that every serious moral theory places a high value on life, supporting a *prima facie* duty to preserve life. None permits termination of life without strong moral justification. For instance, in Kant's theory, life is argued to be among each person's set of fundamental ends; utilitarians recognize that most persons want to live and that it is in the greatest general interest to protect this desire; and religious theories generally claim that there is a sanctity associated with life.

Nonetheless, on examination we notice that our attitudes about morally acceptable behavior in regard to causing death are really rather muddled. The articles in the section "Killing and Letting Die'' expose some of these confusions.

Timothy Goodrich demonstrates the inadequacy of holding the most straightforward position against killing, namely, opposing it absolutely. Since everyone believes that some forms of killing are actually worse than others —for example, killing people is always viewed more seriously than killing insects—we must develop a theory to account for these complexities. We must, for instance, develop a theoretical justification for placing a higher value on human life. Further, although nearly everyone is likely to allow that there are some circumstances in which the value of a particular human life is to be overridden, it is difficult to formulate precise principles governing the termination of life.

Thus, it is not adequate to rely on an appeal to an unqualified right to life. Any defense of a right to life for some must also provide criteria by which to distinguish between those circumstances in which life must be protected and those in which it may be terminated. The problems Goodrich describes are elaborated on at length throughout the chapter, and they present a challenge for all moral theories. An adequate ethical theory must be able to account for the moral distinctions we are called on to make in this area and must also give guidance in situations in which the value of life is challenged by other values.

In medical contexts, we frequently encounter some standard concerning the quality of life challenging the notion of an absolute human right to life. Many people believe that if a life is of poor quality, it may not be worth living and that no individual should be made to continue living under such circumstances. It is argued that life is desirable only as long as it meets some standard of acceptable quality. And even though many persons choose to continue living when the quality of their lives seems to fall below any such minimal level, this evidence is not necessarily proof that they still view life as desirable, because their decision may be based on a feeling that it is wrong deliberately to end their lives.

In those circumstances where expected quality of life is so poor that we feel confident death is the best outcome for a patient, we are confronted with the problem of whether it matters how death is brought about. James Rachels and Bonnie Steinbock discuss whether or not there is any moral difference between acts of killing and acts of allowing someone to die, such that one is more reprehensible than the other. The question is made even more confusing by the difficulty of drawing a clear conceptual distinction between the two kinds of cases so that we can readily recognize an act as one or the other. For instance, is turning off a respirator an act of killing or of letting die? How about withholding insulin from a diabetic or antibiotics from someone with treatable pneumonia?

Rachels argues that there is no moral difference between killing and letting die per se, and hence each is permissible in the appropriate circumstances. Steinbock agrees that there may be no moral difference, but she concludes that both kinds of acts are wrong insofar as they constitute intentional terminations of life. Nonetheless, she is willing to acknowledge that it may still be morally permissible to cease active treatment (but not ''ordinary care'') for a patient when it is a burden to him or her and unlikely to do much good, even if it is known that a hastened death may result.

Philippa Foot investigates the question of a moral distinction between killing and letting die by examining the doctrine of the double effect. Under this doctrine, an undesirable consequence such as death makes an action wrong if it is intended, as in a killing, but it may also arise from an action that is permissible if it is merely foreseen but not directly intended. Although she finds the double effect inadequate to bear the moral weight of this issue, she proposes an alternative distinction. She argues that there is a moral difference between negative duties, that is, not causing injury, and positive duties, that is, actually rendering aid. In this model, actions specifically intended to end a life are always wrong, but stopping treatment (not providing aid) may sometimes be justified even if death results. However, this conclusion depends on the assumption that death is a harm, and there are some circumstances in which that is not so.

The problem of justifying killing or letting a patient die arises for health professionals when they are dealing with very ill patients who are beyond the reach of medical cures. In the section "Reproduction" we consider some other moral questions of medical intervention with human life which arise in connection with initial decisions about having children. Medical expertise can now control a great many aspects of reproduction, and moral questions abound about the morally proper use of medical intervention in the stages of human reproduction.

Of these many moral problems, abortion has long been the most controversial from the public perspective. Thus we begin with a look at some of the views associated with this issue.

John T. Noonan considers the problem from the perspective from which it has been most frequently discussed, that of historical religious tradition. In this framework, he views the problem to be that of determining the humanity of a being. He claims that if the fetus is human, it deserves love, since religion stresses the love of humanity; and hence, it would follow that abortion is wrong. Noonan's problem, then, is deciding at what point an organism becomes human and entitled to love and respect. He is concerned with finding some objectively identifiable criterion by which we may distinguish life deserving of full human rights from other life. His conclusion is stated in biological terms: Whatever is conceived of human parents is human, and alternatively, "a being with a human genetic code is man"; hence a fetus is human from the time of conception.

Michael Tooley is also concerned with providing a sound, morally significant criterion for determining who has a right to life. Tooley grants that a fetus is human but not that this biological feature has moral significance. The relevant criterion, rather, is that we have a right to life if we desire life or are at least "capable of desiring to continue existing as a subject of experiences and other mental states." Tooley argues that being a person, rather than simply being genetically human, is the significant feature. Neither fetuses nor very young infants fulfill this criterion, and hence, Tooley claims, they have no serious right to life. The point up to which we can morally kill human beings is, then, not conception, viability, or even birth, but some time after birth when self-awareness develops.

Jane English objects to both these approaches. She argues that our concept of being a person is complex and ambiguous; since there is no single set of criteria by which we judge whether something is a person, there is no way of resolving the question of whether or not the fetus is a person. This does not trouble her, though, since she also argues that the morality of abortion rests on factors other than the personhood status of the fetus. Her view is that even if we knew that the fetus is not a person we could still identify circumstances in which abortion is wrong, and conversely, even if we agreed the fetus is a person, abortion would be morally correct in some other cases. Hence the morality of abortion cannot be resolved by settling the question of personhood.

Martha Brandt Bolton also steers a middle course on abortion, rejecting both the conservative approach represented by Noonan and the opposite extreme defended by Tooley. To her the issue of abortion does not just involve the question of whether or not it is acceptable to kill a fetus; to refrain from aborting also entails that the woman provide a great deal of positive aid (nurturance) to the fetus. In Foot's terms we could say that the abortion question has been miscast as solely a question of honoring negative duties, when in fact a decision against abortion entails a commitment toward positive duties. Bolton argues that such duties must be examined in the context of other duties the woman may have that conflict with her duties to the fetus. Pregnancy is not an isolated, independent action; the obligation a woman has to a fetus should be weighed against any other duties she may have with which it cannot be made compatible.

Daniel I. Wikler does not address the moral legitimacy of abortion but begins with the fact that right or wrong, women do have abortions and this practice occasionally results in a further moral dilemma. In mid- or late term abortions, the fetus is sometimes alive when removed from the womb. Wikler asks what obligations are owed to these abortuses. Does morality demand that we treat them as very ill newborns and try to preserve their lives, or is it permissible to kill them or allow them to die, given that their death was the expected outcome of the abortion? He proposes that we owe them the same treatment as other patients in similar circumstances. Clearly this recommendation, if correct, requires further analysis before it can be used to offer specific direction in actual cases.

The other essays concentrate on problems associated with the biologically prior decision of whether it is proper even to take steps to conceive a fetus under some circumstances. Leon R. Kass and Samuel Gorovitz offer conflicting views about the acceptability of using the newly developed technologies associated with conception, focusing on *in vitro* fertilization. Their positions reveal a disagreement about the substantive practice at issue and also about the appropriate methodology of deciding such cases. They differ about which facts are relevant to the moral issue and even what the facts are. Kass warns of dangers these practices pose to social attitudes about being human, to family relations, and to social structure. Gorovitz finds that the causal connection Kass and others point to between such use of technology in reproduction and a resulting collapse of social values is unproven and likely to be quite weak, at best. He argues that reproductive technology cannot be rejected on vague abstract grounds, but rather each particular practice must be evaluated for its moral acceptability according to the relevant facts of the actual case. Thus, he does not establish that all possible uses of technology in reproduction and elsewhere in medicine are good, but rather that they cannot be judged bad merely in terms of their newness.

In vitro fertilization is part of a technique for achieving conception in cases where there is a blockage in the potential mother's fallopian tubes. Further dilemmas of reproduction arise in considering decisions about the desirability of conception by prospective parents in the face of worrisome genetic knowledge. Oliver Wendell Holmes offers a succinct defense of involuntary negative eugenics in the famous passage quoted here from his decision in *Buck* v. *Bell*. Ruth Macklin, Neil Holtzman, and L. M.

Purdy offer more complex analyses of genetic problems.

Macklin concentrates on the roles of genetic counselors and legislators in genetic planning. Although she acknowledges grounds for public concern about the outcome of childbearing for carriers of certain diseases, she argues for individual autonomy in reproductive decisions. It is her view that morality demands that genetic information be a voluntary tool of clients and not a means for social control.

Holtzman and Purdy discuss some possible effects and uses of genetic information by the recipients. Holtzman offers a warning against mass screening programs for carriers of genetic disease by citing some dangers such programs have encountered. Since stigmatization and anxiety plague some people when informed of their carrier status, mass screening must not be initiated lightly. He argues for better public education on genetics and voluntary participation in any established screening program. From a different perspective, Purdy presents arguments to be considered by potential parents who know themselves to be carriers of serious genetic disease. She argues that if there is a significant likelihood of passing on the disease (say greater than a 10 percent chance) and if the disease is serious, like Huntington's Disease, it is immoral to have children.

In the section "Birth Defects," we consider some problems posed by the birth of seriously defective infants. Some of these defects can be anticipated through genetic and prenatal screening, but many are first identified on the birth of the child. A child born with serious birth defects confronts all concerned with difficult questions about the probable quality of the child's life.

There are several different questions to be resolved if we grant that the quality of a life may affect the value of that life. Under what circumstances can such considerations overrule the fundamental value placed on human life? Are we morally permitted to terminate our lives when it seems to us that we can no longer achieve the minimal acceptable quality? When, if ever, is a person justified in deciding for another that the latter's life should be ended?

There are serious problems in allowing

quality of life to be a criterion in decisions between life and death. With it, we seem to be moving from the realm of moral values into that of tastes and preferences. Although we cannot provide empirical proofs for our ethical views, we can and do provide reasons and arguments on their behalf. Preferences, however, do not require defense. Deciding what constitutes a high or low quality of life may be just such a matter of taste. Many people uncomplainingly pursue life patterns others view as intolerable. Some take pleasure in ways of life that horrify and repulse others. How can we hope to make judgments on some general, universal standards of quality of life when we have such fundamental disagreements on the best ways to live?

It is important to move cautiously in such investigations. In decisions to end human life we must be certain that the criteria on which judgment is based are ethically relevant, that is, that we have ethically valid reasons for treating these cases differently from those in which life is protected.

The presence of two different sorts of conditions may lead us to judge lives as being of such poor quality that it is questionable whether they are worth living, and hence, worth sustaining. The first is the criterion of pain: If a life is devoid of any reasonable hope for happiness because of an incapacitating, misery-inducing condition, the individual in question may want to cease living. Uncontrollable suffering seems always at least to call into question the value of the suffering life. The second criterion is some standard of awareness: The human being who is unconscious or unaware of his or her surroundings, who engages in no activity, and for whom there is no prospect of change in these respects also challenges our notions of the absolute value of human life. Such a life seems scarcely human to us at all.

When infants are born with such severe defects that there is little or no hope of their achieving even a tolerable quality of life, it seems cruel to keep them alive. For many of these children, life seems to offer nothing but pain and suffering or perhaps permanent unconsciousness; for their families it may mean enormous emotional and financial hardship. In such cases, their speedy death seems to be in the interest of all, and yet there is a general prohibition against killing. Further, it is seldom possible to predict with perfect accuracy what any person's quality of life will actually be: Down's syndrome (once referred to as *mongolism*), for example, can be identified even before birth, but the degree of retardation and particular personality features relating to the afflicted individual's chances of happiness cannot be known for years. Anthony Shaw and Iris Shaw, based on their personal experiences, bring out the problems such children pose and the awesome responsibility any decision entails.

Further direct testimony is provided by Raymond S. Duff and A. G. M. Campbell, who describe their experience over a two-and-a-half-year period in a special-care nursery with very seriously ill newborns. They focus on the 299 deaths that occurred in this period, paying special attention to the 43 cases in which death was associated with withdrawal or discontinuance of treatment because of severe impairment. They explain how the decision to stop treatment was arrived at—who was involved and what sorts of considerations were raised. Like Shaw and Shaw, Duff and Campbell wish to focus professional and public attention on the fact that such decisions are being made in the hope that some consensus may be reached about how comparable decisions ought to be made in the future. Both sets of authors are certain that there are circumstances that justify withholding treatment in the knowledge that the infant's early death will result.

Richard A. McCormick offers a criterion by which to judge when medical efforts ought to be made to try to preserve life and when they ought to be suspended. The criterion he recommends is that of having the potential for human relationships. He considers this condition central to human life and argues that life without human relationships is not really human at all. Thus, any infant so damaged as to have no capacity for human relationships, or to be likely to be so absorbed with his or her personal suffering as to be incapable of relating to others, need not be kept alive.

The rest of the readings on birth defects focus on one particular sort, spina bifida.

Children born with this condition often either die within their first year or survive to experience a very unhappy life. Hence, the question arises, should we approve vigorous medical treatment of such infants to improve their chances of survival? The problem is made more difficult by the uncertainty at birth of the individual's future quality of life. Spina bifida victims are physically handicapped, many are retarded, and almost all have social difficulties; yet a few overcome these obstacles to live very worthwhile lives.

R. B. Zachary, Eliot Slater, John M. Freeman, and Robert E. Cooke are all physicians who have been involved in the treatment of spina bifida. The discussion among them concerns the nature of the responsibility of the physician and of society toward these children. Slater and Freeman argue that the humane and rational course is to help the hopeless among these infants to die quickly to save them from suffering. Zachary and Cooke argue that there is indeed a responsibility to ease suffering, but that it should be fulfilled by more vigorous research and treatment rather than by the negative solution of death. All agree that at present, keeping all such infants alive will result in serious suffering for most of them.

The next article is a personal account of living with a severe birth defect. Karen Metzler was born with multiple birth defects, including spina bifida; because of the severity of her handicaps, she has a special perspective on societal response to handicapped persons. Her essay is the transcript of a talk to a class on moral problems in medicine.

Medical decisions about seriously ill patients of all ages inevitably provoke questions about the meaning and value of death. Health professionals, especially those working in acute-care facilities, are frequently brought face-to-face with these numerous conceptual and moral puzzles. Many of these dilemmas arise throughout the book. In the section entitled "Death," we concentrate on two kinds of problems, how death is to be identified and the moral questions associated with suicide.

Modern science and technology have complicated our conceptual options for defining death. We now know that some parts of an organism may stop functioning while others continue, as for instance bodily cells continue to live for a time after respiration ceases. More problematically, we have also acquired the technology to maintain respiration and circulation artifically in many cases for years after they stop functioning independently. When there is no brain function associated with such existence, it is difficult to view the person as alive even though the heart continues its assisted beating. Also there is a huge expense attached to these procedures and the associated care for the recipients; legal arrangements, such as when to execute the patients' wills, are confused since the ambiguous state of these patients leaves such affairs in limbo; and further, if such life support systems were to be turned off, there is a vital role which many of the undamaged organs of these patients could play for other critically ill patients who would have a good prognosis if transplants could be arranged. Hence, pressure mounts to view as already dead the bodies of patients with no brain function and cardiovascular functioning dependent on machines.

The Ad Hoc Committee of the Harvard Medical School proposes this solution in its influential report. Although the report has been widely relied on in clinical practice, it reflects some underlying conceptual confusions. Essentially, the committee assumes without argument that death should be equated with brain death, which in turn is equated with the clinical condition of irreversible coma. The substantial part of the argument is concerned with providing criteria for recognition of irreversible coma so that death can be declared whenever the tests are satisfied. R. B. Schiffer explains the confusions inherent in this procedure and also offers a definition oriented around the central nervous system as an alternative. In particular, Schiffer points out that any definition of death is part of a general conceptual framework and hence must fit into existing notions we have regarding personal life.

The problem of defining death is primarily a conceptual rather than a moral puzzle, although many moral decisions rest on it (since our duties to dead bodies are different from our duties to live people). With the excerpt from the ancient writer Seneca, the readings move back into the area of direct moral problems. The relation between quality of life and the value of life is again at issue, but with a significant difference. Now we are concerned with an individual's decision that his or her own life is not worth living, whereas the preceding section was concerned with making that decision for another. It is often argued that individuals have a special proprietorship over their own bodies —that they own them and can do with them as they please. But others argue that persons have special responsibilities toward their own bodies —that they have duties toward themselves that require protection of their bodies. Under what circumstances, if any, is a person justified in bringing about his or her own death?

Suicide has been a subject of special interest to physicians and philosophers throughout the ages. The section begins with a sampling of the philosophical literature on suicide going back to Seneca, who wrote in the first century A.D. Seneca addresses the question that has been central to this entire chapter: Is it living that matters or living well? Kant objects to this line of reasoning, for he thinks that it is a mistake to view happiness as the purpose of life. Such pursuit of pleasure, when frustrated, naturally leads to thoughts of suicide, but Kant argues that we have no license to take our own lives. Suicide is not an act we could consistently will to be governed by a universal law, and hence it is not acceptable under the categorical imperative.

David Hume believes that persons naturally cherish life and only incline to suicide under desperate conditions. Further, he argues that there is nothing wrong with suicide even if it should be chosen: It is not a crime against God, other persons, or oneself. Of course, the question of whether suicide is wrong is separable from the question of whether the state can justifiably treat it as a crime, for the state can define as criminal acts that are otherwise morally neutral (for example, traveling at sixty miles per hour), and it can choose not to outlaw acts that are morally wrong (for example, being gratuitously insulting).

In the contemporary literature that follows we can perceive a radical change in emphasis.

Classically, the debate has focused on whether or not the individual has a right to commit suicide, but now the issue has become whether or not it is rational to commit suicide. The underlying assumption is that if suicide is not rational, it should be prevented.

George Murphy, a psychiatrist, takes the position that most people who attempt suicide are psychiatrically ill and seeking treatment, and hence all should be treated. Jerome Motto takes a more moderate position, allowing that suicide might well be a rational choice, and when it is a result of a rational decision, it ought to be allowed. He proposes some criteria by which to identify both those who are properly (that is reasonably) exercising their right to suicide and those who are acting irrationally and should be prevented. Yet even when we decide persons are acting irrationally, there are serious moral questions about the degree of interference with their behavior that can be justified, as we saw in Chapter Two in the discussion of paternalism.

Voluntary euthanasia is closely related to suicide, for both share the necessary condition that the desirability of death is to be determined by the person who is to die. However, it differs from suicide in that it demands that the person be suffering from some physical condition which cannot be easily cured, and further, euthanasia requires the active participation of another person (usually the patient's physician; less frequently, it is the patient's nurse). Most people are especially sympathetic to the very ill and able to empathize to some degree at least with their desire to die, so euthanasia tends to be viewed with more popular tolerance than suicide. The fact that patients must solicit the cooperation of another person in order to die makes their situation seem even more desperate and makes the prospects of success more difficult, especially as euthanasia is not sanctioned by the law. Even defining euthanasia is difficult, though, and Tom Beauchamp and Arnold Davidson reveal the complexities in "The Definition of Euthanasia."

Yale Kamisar and Glanville Williams debate what the law ought to prescribe with regard to euthanasia. Recognizing that we do not and should not legislate against all and only those activities we recognize as immoral, Kamisar and Williams keep the issue of whether euthanasia is morally permissible distinct from that of whether it should be legally permissible. Kamisar allows that euthanasia may be morally justified in some circumstances but fears the implications of a formal policy condoning it. He argues that any legislative attempt to authorize euthanasia in appropriate circumstances is certain to lead to abuse in other cases. However, Williams sees no grounds for legally prohibiting euthanasia in those circumstances in which it is morally permissible. He does not foresee widespread abuse if the legislation is carefully drafted, and hence he can see no ground for restricting individual autonomy in such choices.

The remaining articles convey a sense of the kinds of cases in which euthanasia decisions arise. To decide on the moral acceptability of euthanasia, we must have a concrete sense of what sorts of situations the abstract discussions are meant to embrace. Mary Rose Barrington presents several examples of extreme suffering. How, she asks, can any humane person insist on keeping another alive under such circumstances? Our duty to respect life comes into conflict with duties to minimize suffering and to respect autonomy, as can be seen in the case studies documented by John E. Schowalter *et al.* and Sharon H. Imbus and Bruce Zawacki. The letters following the latter example vividly show that moral issues tend to be mixed. Euthanasia decisions reflect commitment to the patients' best interests and personal choices, but they are also influenced by questions of paternalism and fair distribution of resources and a multitude of other duties, making them even more complex and difficult.

Susan Sherwin

KILLING AND LETTING DIE

From "The Morality of Killing"

Timothy Goodrich

At first sight there doesn't seem to be any problem about killing. Most people would say that it is wrong to kill and that's all there is to it. The same opinion is proclaimed by many members of the Christian religion. They say that "Thou shalt not kill" is an absolute command. But there are several issues involving the morality of killing where ordinary men, secular and religious alike, make judgements or evince perplexity which reveals that common sense mor-

Reprinted with permission of the author and publisher from *Philosophy* 44:168, 127–39, 1969. Copyright, the Royal Institute of Philosophy.

ality is less clear about killing than it at first appears.

I want to elucidate these issues and to show that the usual ways of settling them are fallacious. At the same time I want to show how attention to these issues reveals the inadequacies of many philosophical theories about morals.

First of all there is a difficulty which frequently comes up in discussions of pacifism. Sometimes people object to military service just on the grounds that it is wrong to kill. (There are other grounds, but these are beside the point.) Against this the reply is often as follows. Suppose that by killing one person you can prevent more people being killed in the long run. Thus, if Hitlers' assassins had succeeded, they might, in the long run, have prevented a great many other people from being killed. Are we to reproach them on the grounds that "It is wrong to kill"? Likewise the killings involved in the 1939–45 war were probably fewer than would have occurred if Hitler and his allies had gone unopposed. So, surely, "Killing is wrong" cannot be a valid reason for objecting to *any* sort of military service (although it might to some, depending on the nature of the action to be fought). How the difficulty is formulated will depend on whether we regard killing as just a physical act like shooting or stabbing or as also including actions which have as remote but foreseeable consequences that people will die. If we say that killing is just a physical act, then it follows at once that "killing is wrong" is not an absolute rule; the killing of Hitler is, e.g., an exception to it. If, on the other hand, we say that it includes actions which (knowingly) cause deaths in the long run, then it follows that there are moral questions about killing which "killing is wrong" does not cover. For, on this view, anyone who could have assassinated Hitler was a killer whatever he did—if he didn't kill Hitler then he killed the people who were killed as a result of Hitler's continuing to live. But if whatever a man does he is a killer, "killing is wrong" gives no guidance to action—yet most people would hold that in such a situation it is still true that some actions are better than others. Hence whichever view we take about the nature of killing, the common sense morality of killing cannot be summed up in the pristine simplicity of "killing is (absolutely) wrong."

The obvious next step is to say that, where there is an alternative, killing is wrong, but otherwise we should minimise the number of individuals killed. But so far the difficulties have only begun.

How far is this principle to be applied to animals? If we were to apply it completely to animals and there was a choice between the death of two animals and one man, then we would have to choose the death of the man, since the death of one man is a smaller number of deaths that the death of two animals. But few people would accept this consequence, so that

common sense cannot regard animals as falling straightforwardly under the rule "minimise killing." If fact it seems generally to be held that human life is infinitely more valuable than animal life: there is no number of animals, however great, that is worth the sacrifice of even one human being.

But on what grounds is this huge bias in favour of human life based? Some say that the basis of the distinction is man's rationality. But it is certain that there are some human beings in mental institutions whose mental powers are inferior to those of an ape, so that rationality will not do as a defence of an absolute distinction between men and animals. Others say that what makes man special is the possession of a soul. But how can we tell if a creature has a soul? If the presence of a soul is signified by the possession of mental powers, then this is open to exactly the same objection as the first suggestion: some men have mental powers inferior to those of some animals, so either some men do not have souls or some animals do, and in either case we have not been provided with a basis for an absolute distinction between men and animals. If, on the other hand, the presence of a soul is not signified by the mental powers of its possessor, it is not clear how we are to discover whether a creature has a soul, and until some method is proposed, this suggestion is just useless. A third suggestion is that we regard all human life as sacred because unless we can be sure that *every* human life is regarded as equally valuable, no human being will feel safe. But this is to give up completely the idea that killing people is *just* wrong. It is now claimed to be wrong only in so far as it leads to insecurity. Killing is wrong not in itself but because of its consequences. Most men would be morally repelled by such a view. In any case, it is just false that unless every human life is respected no-one will feel safe. Evidently no-one feels insecure because the lives of animals are often held to be of little account. Likewise in slave-owning societies the slave-owning class felt no insecurity even though they held the lives of their slaves to be of little account. All that is necessary for security is that there should be respect for life in some class of individuals of which you are a member, and this need not be the class of human beings.

So it looks as if common sense knows of no grounds for the grand distinction it makes between men and animals.

Yet on the other hand people do on the whole seem to hold that we have *some* duties to animals.

Two kinds of view appear here. One is that it is wrong to kill animals, or at any rate some kinds of animals, as far as this is compatible with human life. The other is that we have a duty to prevent animal suffering. Where these seem to conflict—where an animal is suffering from an incurable disease, say, it is usually assumed that our duty to prevent the suffering outweighs our duty not to kill, and we should in fact kill it (i.e., have it "put to sleep").[1]

But there is a lot of moral diversity on this. Some people think that it is wrong to inflict suffering on animals, but not wrong to kill them. So they object to bullfighting, but not to the "putting down" of racehorses; to hunting, but not to the "humane killing" of cattle. (This shatters the notion that "common sense" says it is *always* wrong to kill.)

On the other hand there are some people who believe that *all* life should be respected (e.g., Dr. Schweitzer) and certainly most people seem to hold that we should have at least *some* respect for the lives of *some* animals.

Can any rational defence be put forward for any of these views? The one most frequently cited goes something like this: How would you like it if you were hunted by a pack of bloodthirsty hounds? According to Professor Hare, who is an influential philosopher, we must hold that this sort of question is made relevant by the very nature of moral language. Those who say that foxhunting is all right are committed to the universal judgment that anyone who inflicts suffering and death on another creature in this way is doing what is all right, and hence that, even if he were the creature in question, it would be all right. As Kant said: "So act that you may will the maxim of your action to the universal law." According to Hare, those who indulged in bear-baiting should have reasoned thus: "If we were bears we should suffer horribly if treated thus: therefore we cannot accept any maxim which permits bears to be treated thus; therefore we cannot say that it is all right to treat bears thus" ("Freedom and Reason").

But there is an obvious difficulty with this argument. I could conceive of myself as being considerably different from what I am while still being the same person. But could I be a bear or a fox and still be me? Does it make sense to say "What if you were the fox?" What could there be here to preserve my personal identity? This comes out even more clearly for those who believe that we should respect *all* (animal?) life. Could I conceive of myself as being a fly or a worm or an amoeba? It is difficult to see what sense there could be in saying "I happen to be a human, but I might have been a worm."

It might be suggested that I need only respect those individuals whom I could conceive myself as being. But this is far from self-evident. It certainly seems to make sense to say that I ought not to inflict suffering on a bear, even though I couldn't conceivably *be* a bear (Kant did indeed say that his principle entailed (only) that we should treat *humanity* as an end. This was because he held that it was just humans (and angels) who were endowed with rationality. I hope I have shown that this view is doubly inadequate.)

A further difficulty with this argument is that, as far as killing goes, the question "How would you like it?" is not always a sensible one. To be able to like or dislike something, you must be aware of it. But sometimes animals may be killed without their knowing it: the household pet may be a nuisance and be taken to the vet where it is put in a comfortable basket and immersed in odourless lethal gas. If someone said "How would you like it, if you were that animal?" I could reply that the question did not arise, since if I were the animal, I wouldn't know anything about it.

This attempt to justify a certain moral attitude to animals fails, therefore—showing also, incidentally, an inadequacy of the philosophical theory associated with it.

There is another consequence of this way of justifying our attitudes to animals which is very curious. If it is said that "How would you like it, if you were that individual?" is just as relevant for animals as for men, then it seems to follow that animals are just as important as men, and this is in conflict with the common conviction that the lives of men are infinitely more valuable than the lives of animals.

If this consequence is accepted by those who advocate "respect for life," they will have to grapple with another. Is all non-human life equally valuable? Is the cow as important as the flies that buzz round its nose? If not, the animal kingdom will have to be graded in order of importance. Will this grading be done by species, or by the level of mental complexity, or what? What are the relevant grading criteria? If it is replied that animal life as such is valuable, irrespective of what kind of life, it will have to be conceded that the death of a monkey is to be preferred to the death of two earwigs. Furthermore, there is a smooth gradation of characteristics from the most complex forms of animal life, to the simple unicellular organisms and even to the bacteria and viruses. Where is "respect for life" to stop?

Clearly, then, there is *no* obviously correct moral attitude to the killing of animals. Again, common sense is less straightforward than it thinks it is.

Now I want to raise a number of new difficulties which come out particularly clearly in our consideration of animals, but, as we shall see, arise similarly for humans. If we say that we have duties to animals, or that we must respect their lives, this assumes that there are animals there to whom we have duties or whose lives must be respectd. But if, say, we all decided to become vegetarians, the result would not be that all the livestock that we might have eaten would live long and happy lives and die at a ripe old age. Rather, farmers would simply cease to raise livestock. All those animals that we now feel sorry for would just never come into existence at all. Is it fulfilling our duty to these potential animals to prevent them from coming into existence? But we said just now that having a duty to an individual assumes that he exists. There is a logical objection to talking about a duty to a non-existent individual (which I shall go into later). We might try to overcome the difficulty by saying that our duties are to the animals that exist now, and we cannot start having duties to future animals until they are born. But this ignores the fact that, with farm animals, we can decide whether they reproduce or not, and the question is: Does the rule that we should minimise killing entail that,

if we know for certain that an individual yet to be born will be killed, it is better that he should not be born?

We get similar puzzles if we introduce the idea of suffering. It is conceivable that we could know for certain that if an animal were born in certain circumstances, it would suffer all its life. In fact it may be that we can actually say this of animals born in some factory farms. We can ask, just as we did about killing: Does the rule that we should minimise suffering entail that, if we know for certain that an individual yet to be born will suffer all its life, it is better that it should not be born? Again, very often people even say that it is cruel to keep a suffering animal alive. We are thinking of ourselves, they say, not of the good of the animal, if we keep a pet with a painful and incurable disease instead of having it destroyed. But there is something odd in the idea that it is a kindness to an animal to end its existence. Just as it seems odd to say that it can be in an animal's interest not to begin to exist, so it seems odd to say that it can be in its interests to cease to exist.

These are logical puzzles, not moral ones. But logical confusion can lead to great moral confusion. Here the philosopher may make a humble contribution to enlightening the morals of our time. For these puzzles arise in a more exciting context. The questions we have just been considering in relation to animals reappear in relation to humans as questions about euthanasia, abortion and population control.

Consider euthanasia. Supporters of euthanasia sometimes say that it is cruel to keep an incurable and suffering person alive; that it would be an act of charity to end his life.

Yet while it seems obvious to the man of common sense that we should painlessly destroy animals suffering from incurable painful diseases, it does not seem equally obvious to him that this should be done to human beings. But he seems to have as much reason in the one case as the other. For it is generally held that we have a duty to minimise suffering among humans even more than among animals. However, there is a further factor in the case of humans which does not arise with animals. A man can give or withhold his assent to what is done to him. Common sense seems to recognize yet a third principle here: that a man should be free to make up his own mind about what concerns him alone (liberalism). And if anything concerns a man alone surely it is the question whether he should die. We might think, then, that the common sense view must be that the question of his death should be entirely up to the suffering man. This again would depart from the view that killing is always wrong. But matters are more complicated than this. Consider other kinds of suicide. Most people would think it their duty to try to stop a healthy person from committing suicide. So it seems that common sense does not hold that we have an absolute duty to leave people alone in all matters which concern themselves. Thus the relevance of the rule against interference in a man's private decision does not automatically decide the issue of euthanasia. We find, then, at least three rules that are considered to apply to euthanasia: minimise killing, minimise suffering ((Negative) Utilitarianism), and don't interfere in a man's private decisions(liberalism). But common sense does not obviously come down in favour of one rather than another. There does not seem to be any common sense view here at all. The Deontologist would say that we have to consider each situation on its merits with all of these rules in mind. ''All we can do is consider all the appreciable advantages and disadvantages of which we can think in regard to each of the alternative actions between which we choose, and having done this see what the total impression is on our mind'' (Ewing, *Ethics*). But, if we are to judge by the reports of doctors and nurses, the total impression produced by this exercise does not lead to any decisive result at all, and there seems no reason why it should. If the Deontologist holds that by bearing in mind all the morally significant features of a situation we will necessarily come to a decision about what is the right course of action, it is obvious that his is a false theory.

But perhaps the choice between killing and minimising suffering is not quite of the form that this view takes it to be. I have already claimed that there is something odd about saying that it is cruel to keep a suffering animal alive. The same, of course, will go for humans. It is a difficult logical problem whether it can make sense to say that it is in a man's interests to die. But this is better considered together with the questions of abortion and population control.

Perhaps it is worth pointing out that, again, appeal to the question ''How would *you* like it?'' will not settle this issue. Proponents of euthanasia are usually prepared to apply their prescriptions to themselves, and so are their opponents prepared to apply *their* prescription to *themselves.* And there hardly seems any ground for labelling one of these sides ''fanatics.''

A convenient way to start our discussion of the moral issue of abortion is by considering the conditions under which the bill to amend the law about abortion would make abortion permissible. They are:

(a) that the continuance of the pregnancy would involve serious risk to the life or of grave injury to the health, whether physical or mental, of the pregnant woman whether before, at or after the birth of the child; or

(b) that there is a substantial risk that if the child were born it would suffer from such physical or mental abnormalities as to be seriously handicapped; or

(c) that the pregnant woman's capacity as a mother will be severely overstrained by the care of a child or of another child as the case may be (the 'Social clause'); or

(d) that the pregnant woman is a defective or became pregnant while under the age of sixteen or became pregnant as a result of rape.[2]

In one case the reason for killing the foetus (= the human embryo) is that otherwise the mother is likely to die. If we say that the foetus is a living thing, this is a case where a man, the doctor, will cause a death whatever he does. If he does not kill the foetus, he kills the mother. This is a situation of the sort I mentioned first. Here again, ''Killing is wrong'' is not adequate to the situation. But we cannot make this choice on the basis of numbers, so even ''Minimise killing'' is inadequate. Most people think that in this situation, the foetus is to be killed. Why they think this is unclear. If it is because they think the mother, but not the foetus, deserves the title of ''person,'' this should be borne in mind when we consider the view that abortion is murder. In all the other cases the reasons suggested for ending the existence of the embryo are connected with human suffering, either that of the mother or that of the potential child. Now we find that all the puzzles which seemed somewhat strained and ridiculous in our consideration of animals are actually propounded when people talk about abortion. It is reasonable to suppose that a child suffering from severe mental or physical abnormalities, or who is the unwanted child of a young girl, will be unhappy, to say the least. It is quite possible that it will suffer for the whole of its life. But is it obvious, as some people say it is, that, because we should minimise suffering, we should prevent these children from coming into existence? Some people say that we actually have the duty to these potential human beings, if we know they will suffer when they come into the world, of stopping them entirely from beginning their life. You will recognize these as essentially the same problems as we had before: ''Can we have duties to non-existent individuals?'' and ''Does the rule that we should minimise suffering entail that, if we know an individual will suffer all its life, it is better that it should not be born?'' Then again, some people say that it is actually in the interests of the unborn, sometimes, not to be born. This is of the same type as the problem about euthanasia: just as there is something logically odd about saying that it is being kind to someone, or in his interests, to cease to exist, so it seems odd to say that it is kind to him or in his interests not to let him begin to exist.

As a matter of fact, these questions are not special to abortion. They arise whenever we consider the question of controlling the number of people to be born. What makes the question of abortion specially difficult is that some people claim that the human embryo is a person and therefore that to kill it is to commit murder. But let us consider the *general* problem first.

There are a great many miserable people in the world, and one of the chief sources of misery is a lack of the basic necessities of life; food, drink, clothing and shelter and so on. A great deal is done by charitable institutions in providing these things, but, in spite of this, the problem gets no better. This is because the population of the poor parts of the world, as a result of the better life expectancy brought about by modern medicine, is expanding at a colossal rate. By the end of the century, the population of the world will have more than doubled. But the production of the material necessities of life will scarcely have kept pace, even with all the help from such bodies as Oxfam and Christian Aid. It is suggested, therefore, that the obvious thing to do is to control the increase in population by the widespread application of some form of contraception. And so it is. But it is worth asking on what principle this suggestion is made. If the principle is that we should minimise human suffering, are we saying that since we know that these individuals will suffer all their lives, it is better that they should not be born? Are we saying that we have duties to them, and that it is in their best interest not to exist?

The best way to sort out these puzzles is to go via a general consideration of utilitarianism. I will consider positive as well as negative utilitarianism; the same argument applies to both.[3]

Positive utilitarianism says that we should maximise happiness. It is often held that this entails that we should produce as many children as possible, so long as their happiness would exceed their misery, since this increases the amount of happiness in the world. This assumes that we can talk about a grand total of happiness. Now we certainly can say that a person is not very happy, quite happy or very happy, so in a rough and ready way we can talk about the amount of happiness of an individual. But can we talk about the amount of happiness of a group? i.e., can we add up their individual happiness to make a sum total? If we put two pound weights together we get a collection which has a weight of two pounds. But if we put two equally happy people together, do we get a group with twice their individual happiness? The same with suffering. If a room contains a miserable man, and he's joined by another equally miserable man, is there twice as much misery in the room? And if we put one fairly happy and one fairly miserable man together, do we have a collection that is neither miserable nor happy? Again, how happy would a man have to be for his happiness to equal the happiness of five slightly happy people together? Clearly it is just senseless to talk of adding up happiness as we add up weight or length. It follows, then, that there is no such thing as a grand total of happiness, and so we cannot sensibly be told to make this total as big as possible. Thus it makes no sense either to say that the more non-suffering people there are in the world, the more happiness there is in it. Nor does it make sense to say that the fewer suffering people there are in the world, the less suffering there is in it.

We can see then, that it is absurd to say, as so many philosophers have done, that "Happiness is good and suffering evil"—just so—since happiness and suffering cannot be talked about apart from individual people's experiencing them.[4] If utilitarianism is to make sense, it must include in it some reference to *whose* happiness is to be maximised. Let us take Bentham's "Everyone to count for one and no one for more than one" as our cue. We could reformulate utilitarianism now as "Everyone equally should be as happy as possible." Once we have said this, however, it follows that utilitarianism tells us nothing about how many individuals there should be. For "everyone" presupposes that we already have a class of humans, about which the principle goes on to assert something. Nothing can be made to follow from this about the number of members this class ought to contain; the class, i.e., the class with however many members it contains, is pre-supposed from the start. It may be that the mistaken impression that this inference is valid has been fostered by an indecisive rendering of "the class of men." Suppose a radical reformer says: "There are now so many people that everyone is unhappy. So let us liquidate half the human population and then everyone will be happy." It is impossible to infer that the purge should be made via "Everyone should be happy." For "everyone" (i.e., the class of men) is not used univocally here: the first "everyone" may be expanded to "everyone now" and the second to "everyone after the purge." If "everyone" in the principle consists of the chosen people, then the fact about the first "everyone" is irrelevant to applying it. If it really means everyone, then so is the fact about the second "everyone." I think utilitarians have usually intended "everyone" in their principle to be what it says: everyone past, present and future. We may, indeed, raise a problem about "The class of men" since if it is in our choice how many men there are to be, the class, it might be said, is not well formed, because it has no definite number of members. But all this would show is not that utilitarianism can tell us how many members it should have, but that "All men should be as happy as possible" is not a significant proposition.[5]

The upshot, then, is that decisions about population control cannot be based on the principle that we should maximise happiness (or at least minimise suffering). Now let us go back to our problems. One of our problems was this: "Does the rule that we should minimise suffering entail, if we know an individual will suffer all its life, it is better that it should not be born?" We can now see that the answer is "No." The rule "Minimise suffering" has to be formulated as "Everyone should suffer as little as possible," and nothing follows from this about how many people there should be. We may well want to adopt a further principle to the effect that the number of individuals should be such that each suffers as little as possible, or perhaps that the number of individuals should be such that each is as happy as possible. But it is important to see that these are completely different from the utilitarian principle and do not follow from it. Perhaps it is worth pointing out, by the way, that if we did adopt the latter principle, we would probably be committed to a very drastic reduction in the world's population indeed. It might be concluded, for instance, that the maximum happiness could only be obtained in a very few places, e.g., the South Sea Isles, so that ideally the population of the world should be scaled down to nothing elsewhere....

Of course, once again we can say it would be a good thing if a couple had a child or if a man were to die. All I say is that these things cannot follow from saying that we should act benevolently to people. In particular, we cannot say that it would be *cruel* to bring an individual into the world, or that it would be *cruel* not to kill him. The concept of cruelty presupposes the applicability of utilitarian criteria, and this requirement is not met where the existence of an individual is in question.

To get back to abortion. I have considered the questions of suffering, but those who oppose abortion usually say this is not all there is to it. Abortion is (really) killing. So, in a Commons debate on the subject, Mrs. Jill Knight (M. P. for Edgbaston) said: ''Babies are not like bad teeth to be jerked out just because they cause suffering. An unborn baby is a baby nevertheless. Would the sponsors of the Bill think it right to kill a baby they can see? Of course they would not. Why then do they think it right to kill one they cannot see?. . . I have come to believe that those who support abortion on demand do so because in all sincerity they cannot accept that an unborn baby is a human being. Yet surely it is. Its heart beats, it moves, it sleeps, it eats. Uninterfered with, it has a potential life ahead of it of 70 years or more; it may be a happy life, or a sad life; it may be a genius, or it may be just plain average; but surely as a healthy, living baby it has a right not to be killed simply because it may be inconvenient for a year or so to its mother.'' (Commons Debate, 22nd July, 1966.)

Is the foetus a person? The criteria offered by Mrs. Knight are that its heart beats, it moves, it sleeps and it eats. (The last two seem a bit doubtful.) But obviously these are very far from constituting *all* the criteria we use in applying the concept of ''person.'' Mrs. Knight's criteria apply to a great many animals, which we do not normally describe as ''people''—if we did, we could be charged with the grossest immorality in our actions towards them, since, as I observed earlier, we do not regard their lives as sacred.

Some people think that foetuses are people because they have souls. Actually, some of these people claim to know that God creates the soul just at the moment when the sperm fertilizes the ovum. But, as with animals, we may ask how we are to tell whether something has a soul? Doubtless I must accept this on faith. But how do I go about doing this? Either ''soul'' means ''mind,'' or its meaning has not been explained. As to the second, I might as well be told to believe that the mome raths outgrabe. As to the first, all the normal tests for souls: thought, sensation, etc., fail, as far as we know, when applied to foetuses.

Now, contrary to these last two views of the matter, I maintain that the difficulty in deciding whether the foetus is a person is not that of hunting round till we find one crucial characteristic which will decide the question,

for there is no such characteristic. The concept of a person is not that sort of concept. I will not be so adventurous as to say anything positive about ''person''; I think it is enough to say that it is a concept with decidedly fuzzy edges, and that the foetus finds itself in the fuzz. The question ''Is the foetus a person?'' is like all those other borderline questions that philosophers have cited in the last 20 years: ''Is a tomato a fruit or a vegetable?'' Is medicine a science?'' ''Are viruses living things?''

Supposing that what I have just said is correct, what follows about the rightness or wrongness of abortion? This depends on what view we take about how we establish the rightness or wrongness of *anything*. On the two most widely canvassed of such views, by intellectual apprehension and by committal, i.e., intuitionism and ''existentialism,'' the results are extremely curious.

On the ''existentialist'' view we establish our moral principles by bare choice, by just committing ourselves to one principle rather than another. We are ''self-legislating subjects in a kingdom of ends.'' But if this is so, our anxiety over whether the foetus is a person reveals a misunderstanding of our true position as moral agents. For to take it that the rule against killing people is already laid down and that our function is only to interpret this rule is to put ourselves in the position of judges applying an already promulgated law. Whereas, if we ourselves are the legislators there is no question of interpretation. If we laid down the law, we must have known what we intended by it—it would be absurd to say that someone said something and only later found out what he intended by it. If in some unclear case we want to legislate further, of course we *can*. But there is no question of agonising about it; there cannot be anything to agonise *about*. ''To describe such ultimate decisions as arbitrary, because *ex hypothesi* everything which could be used to justify them has already been included in the decision, would be like saying that a complete description of the universe was utterly unfounded, because no further fact could be called upon in corroboration of it.''[6]

The objection that may be felt here is that, after all, we *do* agonise. We know the effect of deciding one way or the other, but we still feel unable to make the *right* decision, or, as used to be said about Attitude Theories, we do not want merely to find out what *in fact* we approve of, but what is *worthy* of approval. The point is not that we lack feelings about the issue one way or the other. We feel that *some* attitude is appropriate, that some kind of behaviour is worthy of approval, but are unsure what it is.

Intuitionism does no better. Intuitionism claims that we know some moral statements just in the same way as we know some empirical statements. So "Abortion is wrong" is not merely rather like "Viruses are living creatures"; it is simply another example illustrating exactly the same thing—the only difference is that the one is about the moral world while the other is about the empirical world.

But in that case we must say exactly the same thing about both of them. We cannot straightforwardly answer the question "Are viruses living things?" We do not say: they *must* be either living or non-living, though perhaps we'll never know which. All we can say is: viruses satisfy *some* of the tests for living things, but not enough to make it unmisleading to say they *are* living things: "Say what you like." On analogy with this, the intuitionist is obliged to say that abortion is wrongish, though not wrong, and allrightish, though not all right. If we *decide* to say that abortion is wrong, our decision is as arbitrary as the decision to say that viruses are living creatures. We are no longer making a simple report on the world of values. If someone says "We have *got* to decide, because we have to decide what to *do*," the intuitionist presumably replies that making a moral judgment is reporting on the world of values, what people *do* is another question. This is a neat example of that feature of intuitionism that prescriptivists have so long complained about.[7]

All this is rather unsettling. I would like now to give all the correct answers. Unfortunately I don't know them. However, it is something to have shown that arguments usually taken as valid are in fact fallacious. "We are in a better position in relation to a question if we not only do not know the answer, but do not even think we know."

Notes

1. But this is not the correct way of formulating the conflict. Cf. my conclusions on euthanasia.
2. "Medical Termination of Pregnancy Bill," 1966, presented by Mr. David Steel, M.P. (in its original form.
3. Jan Narveson deals with this subject in his "Utilitarianism and New Generations" in *Mind* 1967. It will be seen that I do not follow his treatment. This is because he seems to accept that we can talk of a sum of happiness or suffering. He is led to say that utilitarianism forbids the bringing into the world of children who will on the whole suffer, but does not prescribe bringing into the world children who will on the whole be happy. On my view utilitarianism says nothing about either. It is very difficult to see how it can say something about the one and not the other.
4. Cp. G. E. Moore on pleasure: "Our question is: Is it the pleasure, as distinct from the consciousness of it, that we set value on? Do we think the pleasure valuable in itself, or must we insist that, if we are to think the pleasure good, we must have consciousness of it too?" (*Principia Ethica,* p. 88).
5. The point in this paragraph has, of course nothing to do with the question of existential import. When I say that "All men should be as happy as possible" presupposes a class of men, I offer no opinion about what should be said if there were no men. Happily we do not have to consider this question, since the class of men is not the null class.
6. *Language of Morals,* p. 69.
7. In case anyone should think that this difficulty can be surmounted by talking of "prima facie" duties, I should point out that this is not a conflict of duties but a doubtful application of one single duty.

Active and Passive Euthanasia

James Rachels

The distinction between active and passive euthanasia is thought to be crucial for medical ethics. The idea is that it is permissible, at least in some cases, to withhold treatment and allow a patient to die, but it is never permissible to take any direct action designed to kill the patient. This doctrine seems to be accepted by most doctors, and it endorsed in a statement adopted by the House of Delegates of the American Medical Association on December 4, 1973:

> The intentional termination of the life of one human being by another—mercy killing—is contrary to that for which the medical profession stands and is contrary to the policy of the American Medical Association.

> The cessation of the employment of extraordinary means to prolong the life of the body when there is irrefutable evidence that biological death is imminent is the decision of the patient and or his immediate family. The advice and judgment of the physician should be freely available to the patient and or his immediate family.

However, a strong case can be made against this doctrine. In what follows I will set out some of the relevant arguments, and urge doctors to reconsider their views on this matter.

To begin with a familiar type of situation, a patient who is dying of incurable cancer of the throat is in terrible pain, which can no longer be satisfactorily alleviated. He is certain to die within a few days, even if present treatment is continued, but he does not want to go on living for those days since the pain is unbearable. So he asks the doctor for an end to it, and his family joins in the request.

Suppose the doctor agrees to withhold treatment, as the conventional doctrine says he may. The justification for his doing so is that the patient is in terrible agony, and since he is

Reprinted by permission of the author and *The New England Journal of Medicine,* vol. 292, no. 2, January 9, 1975, pp. 78–80.

going to die anyway, it would be wrong to prolong his suffering needlessly. But now notice this. If one simply withholds treatment it may take the patient longer to die, and so he may suffer more than he would if more direct action were taken and a lethal injection given. This fact provides strong reason for thinking that, once the initial decision not to prolong his agony has been made, active euthanasia is actually preferable to passive euthanasia, rather than the reverse. To say otherwise is to endorse the option that leads to more suffering rather than less, and is contrary to the humanitarian impulse that prompts the decision not to prolong his life in the first place.

Part of my point is that the process of being "allowed to die" can be relatively slow and painful, whereas being given a lethal injection is relatively quick and painless. Let me give a different sort of example. In the United States about one in 600 babies is born with Down's syndrome. Most of these babies are otherwise healthy—that is, with only the usual pediatric care, they will proceed to an otherwise normal infancy. Some, however, are born with congenital defects such as intestinal obstructions that require operations if they are to live. Sometimes, the parents and the doctor will decide not to operate, and let the infant die. Anthony Shaw describes what happens then.

> . . . When surgery is denied (the doctor) must try to keep the infant from suffering while natural forces sap the baby's life away. As a surgeon whose natural inclination is to use the scalpel to fight off death, standing by and watching a salvageable baby die is the most emotionally exhausting experience I know. It is easy at a conference, in a theoretical discussion, to decide that such infants should be allowed to die. It is altogether different to stand by in the nursery and watch as dehydration and infection wither a tiny being over hours and days. This is a terrible ordeal for me and the hospital staff—much more so than for the parents who never set foot in the nursery.[1]

I can understand why some people are opposed to all euthanasia, and insist that such infants must be allowed to live. I think I can also understand why other people favor destroying these babies quickly and painlessly. But why should anyone favor letting "dehydration and infection wither a tiny being over hours and days?" The doctrine that says that a baby may be allowed to dehydrate and wither, but may not be given an injection that would end its life without suffering, seems so patently cruel as to require no further refutation. The strong language is not intended to offend, but only to put the point in the clearest possible way.

My second argument is that the conventional doctrine leads to decisions concerning life and death made on irrelevant grounds.

Consider again the case of the infants with Down's syndrome who need operations for congenital defects unrelated to the syndrome to live. Sometimes, there is no operation, and the baby dies, but when there is no such defect, the baby lives on. Now, an operation such as that to remove an intestinal obstruction is not prohibitively difficult. The reason why such operations are not performed in these cases is, clearly, that the child has Down's syndrome and the parents and doctor judge that because of that fact it is better for the child to die.

But notice that this situation is absurd, no matter what view one takes of the lives and potentials of such babies. If the life of such an infant is worth preserving, what does it matter if it needs a simple operation? Or, if one thinks it better that such a baby should not live on, what difference does it make that it happens to have an unobstructed intestinal tract? In either case, the matter of life and death is being decided on irrelevant grounds. It is the Down's syndrome, and not the intestines, that is the issue. The matter should be decided, if at all, on that basis, and not be allowed to depend on the essentially irrelevant question of whether the intestinal tract is blocked.

What makes this situation possible, of course, is the idea that when there is an intestinal blockage, one can "let the baby die," but when there is no such defect there is nothing that can be done, for one must not "kill" it. The fact that this idea leads to such results as

deciding life or death on irrelevant grounds is another good reason why the doctrine should be rejected.

One reason why so many people think that there is an important moral difference between active and passive euthanasia is that they think killing someone is morally worse than letting someone die. But is it? Is killing, in itself, worse than letting die? To investigate this issue, two cases may be considered that are exactly alike except that one involves killing whereas the other involves letting someone die. Then, it can be asked whether this difference makes any difference to the moral assessments. It is important that the cases be exactly alike, except for this one difference, since otherwise one cannot be confident that it is this difference and not some other that accounts for any variation in the assessments of the two cases. So, let us consider this pair of cases:

In the first, Smith stands to gain a large inheritance if anything should happen to his six-year-old cousin. One evening while the child is taking his bath, Smith sneaks into the bathroom and drowns the child, and then arranges things so that it will look like an accident.

In the second, Jones also stands to gain if anything should happen to his six-year-old cousin. Like Smith, Jones sneaks in planning to drown the child in his bath. However, just as he enters the bathroom Jones sees the child slip and hit his head, and fall face down in the water. Jones is delighted; he stands by, ready to push the child's head back under if it is necessary, but it is not necessary. With only a little thrashing about, the child drowns all by himself, "accidentally," as Jones watches and does nothing.

Now Smith killed the child, whereas Jones "merely" let the child die. That is the only difference between them. Did either man behave better, from a moral point of view? If the difference between killing and letting die were in itself a morally important matter, one should say that Jones's behavior was less reprehensible than Smith's. But does one really want to say that? I think not. In the first place, both men acted from the same motive, personal gain, and both had exactly the same end in view when they acted. It may be inferred from Smith's conduct that he is a bad man, although that judgment may be withdrawn or modified if certain further facts are learned about him—for example, that he is mentally deranged. But would not the very same thing be inferred about Jones from his conduct? And would not the same further considerations also be relevant to any modification of this judgment? Moreover, suppose Jones pleaded, in his own defense, "After all, I didn't do anything except just stand there and watch the child drown. I didn't kill him; I only let him die." Again, if letting die were in itself less bad than killing, this defense should have at least some weight. But it does not. Such a "defense" can only be regarded as a grotesque perversion of moral reasoning. Morally speaking, it is no defense at all.

Now it may be pointed out, quite properly, that the cases of euthanasia with which doctors are concerned are not like this at all. They do not involve personal gain or the destruction of normal healthy children. Doctors are concerned only with cases in which the patient's life is of no further use to him, or in which the patient's life has become or will soon become a terrible burden. However, the point is the same in these cases: the bare difference between killing and letting die does not, in itself, make a moral difference. If a doctor lets a patient die, for humane reasons, he is in the same moral position as if he had given the patient a lethal injection for humane reasons. If his decision was wrong—if, for example, the patient's illness was in fact curable—the decision would be equally regrettable no matter which method was used to carry it out. And if the doctor's decision was the right one, the method used is not in itself important.

The AMA policy statement isolates the crucial issue very well; the crucial issue is "the intentional termination of the life of one human being by another." But after identifying this issue, and forbidding "mercy killing," the statement goes on to deny that the cessation of treatment is the intentional termination of a life. This is where the mistake comes in, for what is the cessation of treatment, in these circumstances, if it is not "the intentional termination of the life of one human being by another?" Of course it is exactly that, and if it were not, there would be no point to it.

Many people will find this judgment hard to accept. One reason, I think, is that it is very easy to conflate the question of whether killing is, in itself, worse than letting die, with the very different question of whether most actual cases of killing are more reprehensible than most actual cases of letting die. Most actual cases of killing are clearly terrible (think, for example, of all the murders reported in the newspapers), and one hears of such cases every day. On the other hand, one hardly ever hears of a case of letting die, except for the actions of doctors who are motivated by humanitarian reasons. So one learns to think of killing in a much worse light than of letting die. But this does not mean that there is something about killing that makes it in itself worse than letting die, for it is not the bare difference between killing and letting die that makes the difference in these cases. Rather, the other factors—the murderer's motive of personal gain, for example, contrasted with the doctor's humanitarian motivation—account for different reactions to the different cases.

I have argued that killing is not in itself any worse than letting die; if my contention is right, it follows that active euthanasia is not any worse than passive euthanasia. What arguments can be given on the other side? The most common, I believe, is the following:

"The important difference between active and passive euthanasia is that, in passive euthanasia, the doctor does not do anything to bring about the patient's death. The doctor does nothing, and the patient dies of whatever ills already afflict him. In active euthanasia, however, the doctor does something to bring about the patient's death: he kills him. The doctor who gives the patient with cancer a lethal injection has himself caused his patient's death; whereas if he merely ceases treatment, the cancer is the cause of death."

A number of points need to be made here. The first is that it is not exactly correct to say that in passive euthanasia the doctor does nothing, for he does do one thing that is very important: he lets the patient die. "Letting someone die" is certainly different, in some respects, from other types of action—mainly in that it is a kind of action that one may perform by way of not performing certain other actions. For example, one may let a patient die by way of not giving medication, just as one may insult someone by way of not shaking his hand. But for any purpose of moral assessment, it is a type of action nonetheless. The decision to let a patient die is subject to moral appraisal in the same way that a decision to kill him would be subject to moral appraisal: it may be assessed as wise or unwise, compassionate or sadistic, right or wrong. If a doctor deliberately let a patient die who was suffering from a routinely curable illness, the doctor would certainly be to blame for what he had done, just as he would be to blame if he had needlessly killed the patient. Charges against him would then be appropriate. If so, it would be no defense at all for him to insist that he didn't "do anything." He would have done something very serious indeed, for he let his patient die.

Fixing the cause of death may be very important from a legal point of view, for it may determine whether criminal charges are brought against the doctor. But I do not think that this notion can be used to show a moral difference between active and passive euthanasia. The reason why it is considered bad to be the cause of someone's death is that death is regarded as a great evil—and so it is. However, if it has been decided that euthanasia—even passive euthanasia—is desirable in a given case, it has also been decided that in this instance death is no greater an evil than the patient's continued existence. And if this is true, the usual reason for not wanting to be the cause of someone's death simply does not apply.

Finally, doctors may think that all of this is only of academic interest—the sort of thing that philosophers may worry about but that has no practical bearing on their own work. After all,

doctors must be concerned about the legal consequences of what they do, and active euthanasia is clearly forbidden by the law. But even so, doctors should also be concerned with the fact that the law is forcing upon them a moral doctrine that may well be indefensible, and has a considerable effect on their practices. Of course, most doctors are not now in the position of being coerced in this matter, for they do not regard themselves as merely going along with what the law requires. Rather, in statements such as the AMA policy statement that I have quoted, they are endorsing this doctrine as a central point of medical ethics. In that statement, active euthanasia is condemned not merely as illegal but as "contrary to that for which the medical profession stands," whereas passive euthanasia is approved. However, the preceding considerations suggest that there is really no moral difference between the two, considered in themselves (there may be important moral differences in some cases in their *consequences,* but, as I pointed out, these differences may make active euthanasia, and not passive euthanasia, the morally preferable option). So, whereas doctors may have to discriminate between active and passive euthanasia to satisfy the law, they should not do any more than that. In particular, they should not give the distinction any added authority and weight by writing it into official statements of medical ethics.

Notes

1. Shaw A.: 'Doctor, Do We Have a Choice?' *The New York Times Magazine,* January 30, 1972, p. 54.

The Intentional Termination Of Life

Bonnie Steinbock

According to James Rachels and Michael Tooley, whose articles immediately precede this, a common mistake in medical ethics is the belief that there is a moral difference between active and passive euthanasia. This is a mistake, they argue, because the rationale underlying the distinction between active and passive euthanasia is the idea that there is a significant moral difference between intentionally killing and intentionally letting die. "This idea," Tooley says, "is admittedly very common. But I believe that it can be shown to reflect either confused thinking or a moral point of view unrelated to the interests of individuals." Whether or not the belief that there is a significant moral difference is mistaken is not my concern here. For it is far from clear that this distinction *is* the basis of the doctrine of the American Medical Association which Rachels attacks. And if the killing/letting die distinction is not the basis of the AMA doctrine, then arguments showing that the distinction has no moral force do not, in themselves, reveal in the doctrine's adherents either "confused thinking" or "a moral point of view unrelated to the interests of individuals." Indeed, as we examine the AMA doctrine, I think it will become clear that it appeals to and makes use of a number of overlapping distinctions, which may have moral significance in particular cases, such as the distinction between intending and foreseeing, or between ordinary and extraordinary care. Let us then turn to the 1973 statement, from the House of Delegates of the American Medical Association, which Rachels cites:

> The intentional termination of the life of one human being by another—mercy killing—is contrary to that for which the medical profession stands and is contrary to the policy of the American Medical Association.
>
> The cessation of the employment of extraor-

Reprinted with permission from the author and *Ethics in Science and Medicine*, vol. 6, no. 1, 1979, pp. 59–64. Copyright 1979, Pergamon Press, Ltd.

dinary means to prolong the life of the body when there is irrefutable evidence that biological death is imminent is the decision of the patient and/or his immediate family. The advice and judgment of the physician should be freely available to the patient and/or his immediate family.

Rachels attacks this statement because he believes that it contains a moral distinction between active and passive euthanasia. Tooley also believes this to be the position of the AMA, saying:

> Many people hold that there is an important moral distinction between passive euthanasia and active euthanasia. Thus, while the AMA maintains that people have a right "to die with dignity," so that it is morally permissible for a doctor to allow someone to die if that person wants to and is suffering from an incurable illness causing pain that cannot be sufficiently alleviated, the AMA is unwilling to countenance active euthanasia for a person who is in similar straits, but who has the misfortune not to be suffering from an illness that will result in a speedy death.

Both men, then, take the AMA position to prohibit active euthanasia, while allowing, under certain conditions, passive euthanasia.

I intend to show that the AMA statement does not imply support of the active/passive euthanasia distinction. In forbidding the intentional termination of life, the statement rejects both active and passive euthanasia. It does allow for "the cessation of the employment of extraordinary means" to prolong life. The mistake Rachels and Tooley make is in identifying the cessation of life-prolonging treatment with passive euthanasia, or intentionally letting die. If it were right to equate the two, then the AMA statement would be self-contradictory, for it would begin by condemning, and end by allowing, the intentional termination of life. But if the cessation of life-prolonging treatment is not always or necessarily passive euthanasia, then there is no confusion and no contradiction.

Why does Rachels think that the cessation of

life-prolonging treatment is the intentional termination of life? He says:

> The AMA policy statement isolates the crucial issue very well: the crucial issue is "the intentional termination of the life of one human being by another." But after identifying this issue, and forbidding "mercy killing," the statement goes on to deny that the cessation of treatment is the intentional termination of a life. This is where the mistake comes in, for what is the cessation of treatment, in these circumstances, if it is not "the intentional termination of the life of one human being of another"? Of course it is exactly that, and if it were not, there would be no point to it.

However, there *can* be a point (to the cessation of life-prolonging treatment) other than an endeavor to bring about the patient's death, and so the blanket identification of cessation of treatment with the intentional termination of a life is inaccurate. There are at least two situations in which the termination of life-prolonging treatment cannot be identified with the intentional termination of the life of one human being by another.

The first situation concerns the patient's right to refuse treatment. Both Tooley and Rachels give the example of a patient dying of an incurable disease, accompanied by unrelievable pain, who wants to end the treatment which cannot cure him but can only prolong his miserable existence. Why, they ask, may a doctor accede to the patient's request to stop treatment, but not provide a patient in a similar situation with a lethal dose? The answer lies in the patient's right to refuse treatment. In general, a competent adult has the right to refuse treatment, even where such treatment is necessary to prolong life. Indeed, the right to refuse treatment has been upheld even when the patient's reason for refusing treatment is generally agreed to be inadequate.[1] This right can be overridden (if, for example, the patient has dependent children) but, in general, no one may legally compel you to undergo treatment to which you have not consented. "Historically, surgical intrusion has always been considered a technical battery upon the person and one to be excused or justified by consent of the patient or justified by necessity created by the circumstances of the moment. . . ."[2]

At this point, an objection might be raised that if one has the right to refuse life-prolonging treatment, then consistency demands that one have the right to decide to end his or her life, and to obtain help in doing so. The idea is that the right to refuse treatment somehow implies a right to voluntary euthanasia, and we need to see why someone might think this. The right to refuse treatment has been considered by legal writers as an example of the right to privacy or, better, the right to bodily self-determination. You have the right to decide what happens to your own body, and the right to refuse treatment is an instance of that right. But if you have the right to determine what happens to your own body, then should you not have the right to choose to end your life, and even a right to get help in doing so?

However, it is important to see that the right to refuse treatment is not the same as, nor does it entail, a right to voluntary euthanasia, even if both can be derived from the right to bodily self-determination. The right to refuse treatment is not itself a "right to die"; that one may choose to exercise this right even at the risk of death, or even *in order to die,* is irrelevant. The purpose of the right to refuse medical treatment is not to give persons a right to decide whether to live or die, but to protect them from the unwanted interferences of others. Perhaps we ought to interpret the right to bodily self-determination more broadly, so as to include a right to die; but this would be a substantial extension of our present understanding of the right to bodily self-determination, and not a consequence of it. If we were to recognize a right to voluntary euthanasia, we would have to agree that people have the right not merely to be left alone but also the right to be killed. I leave to one side that substantive moral issue. My claim is simply that there can be a reason for terminating life-prolonging treatment other than "to bring about the patient's death."

The second case in which termination of treatment cannot be identified with intentional termination of life is where continued treatment has little chance of improving the patient's condition and brings greater discomfort than relief.

The question here is what treatment is appropriate to the particular case. A cancer specialist describes it in this way:

My general rule is to administer therapy as long as a patient responds well and has the potential for a reasonably good quality of life. But when all feasible therapies have been administered and a patient shows signs of rapid deterioration, the continuation of therapy can cause more discomfort than the cancer. From that time I recommend surgery, radiotherapy, or chemotherapy only as a means of relieving pain. But if a patient's condition should once again stabilize after the withdrawal of active therapy and if it should appear that he could still gain some good time, I would immediately reinstitute active therapy. The decision to cease anticancer treatment is never irrevocable, and often the desire to live will push a patient to try for another remission, or even a few more days of life.[3]

The decision here to cease anticancer treatment cannot be construed as a decision that the patient die, or as the intentional termination of life. It is a decision to provide the most appropriate treatment for that patient at that time. Rachels suggests that the point of the cessation of treatment is the intentional termination of life. But here the point of discontinuing treatment is not to bring about the patient's death but to avoid treatment that will cause more discomfort than the cancer and has little hope of benefiting the patient. Treatment that meets this description is often called "extraordinary."[4] The concept is flexible, and what might be considered "extraordinary" in one situation might be ordinary in another. The use of a respirator to sustain a patient through a severe bout with a respiratory disease would be considered ordinary; its use to sustain the life of a severely brain-damaged person in an irreversible coma would be considered extraordinary.

Contrasted with extraordinary treatment is ordinary treatment, the care a doctor would normally be expected to provide. Failure to provide ordinary care constitutes neglect, and can even be construed as the intentional infliction of harm, where there is a legal obligation to provide care. The importance of the ordinary/extraordinary care distinction lies partly in its connection to the doctor's intention. The withholding of extraordinary care should be seen as a decision not to inflict painful treatment on a patient without reasonable hope of success. The withholding of ordinary care, by contrast, must be seen as neglect. Thus, one doctor says, "We have to draw a distinction between ordinary and extraordinary means. We never withdraw what's needed to make a baby comfortable, we would never withdraw the care a parent would provide. We never kill a baby. . . . But we may decide certain heroic intervention is not worthwhile"[5]

We should keep in mind the ordinary/extraordinary care distinction when considering an example given by both Tooley and Rachels to show the irrationality of the active/passive distinction with regard to infanticide. The example is this: a child is born with Down's syndrome and also has an intestinal obstruction that requires corrective surgery. If the surgery is not performed, the infant will starve to death, since it cannot take food orally. This may take days or even weeks, as dehydration and infection set in. Commenting on this situation in his article in this book, Rachels says:

> I can understand why some people are opposed to all euthanasia, and insist that such infants must be allowed to live. I think I can also understand why other people favor destroying these babies quickly and painlessly. But why should anyone favor letting "dehydration and infection wither a tiny being over hours and days"? The doctrine that says that a baby may be allowed to dehydrate and wither, but may not be given an injection that would end its life without suffering, seems so patently cruel as to require no further refutation.

Such a doctrine perhaps does not need further refutation; but this is not the AMA doctrine. The AMA statement criticized by Rachels allows only for the cessation of extraordinary means to prolong life when death is imminent. Neither of these conditions is satisfied in this example. Death is not imminent in this situation, any more than it would be if a normal child had an attack of appendicitis. Neither the corrective surgery to remove the intestinal obstruction nor the intravenous feeding required to keep the infant alive until such surgery is performed can be regarded as extraordinary means, for neither is particularly expensive, nor does either place an overwhelming burden on the patient or others. (The continued existence of the child might be thought to place an overwhelming burden on its parents, but that has nothing to do with the characterization of the means to prolong its life as extraordinary. If it had, then *feeding* a severely defective child who required a great deal of care could be regarded as extraordinary.) The chances of success if the operation is undertaken are quite good, though there is always a risk in operating on infants. Though the Down's syndrome will not be alleviated, the child will proceed to an otherwise normal infancy.

It cannot be argued that the treatment is withheld for the infant's sake, unless one is prepared to argue that all mentally retarded babies are better off dead. This is particularly implausible in the case of Down's syndrome babies, who generally do not suffer and are capable of giving and receiving love, of learning and playing, to varying degrees.

In a film on this subject entitled, "Who Should Survive?", a doctor defended a decision not to operate, saying that since the parents did not consent to the operation, the doctors' hands were tied. As we have seen, surgical intrusion requires consent, and in the case of infants, consent would normally come from the parents. But, as legal guardians, parents are required to provide medical care for their children, and failure to do so can constitute criminal neglect or even homicide. In general, courts have been understandably reluctant to recognize a parental right to terminate life-prolonging treatment.[6] Although prosecution is unlikely, physicians who comply with invalid instructions from the parents and permit the infant's death could be liable for aiding and abetting, failure to report child neglect, or even homicide. So it is not true that, in this situation, doctors are legally bound to do as the parents wish.

To sum up, I think that Rachels is right to regard the decision not to operate in the Down's syndrome example as the intentional termination of life. But there is no reason to believe that either the law or the AMA would regard it otherwise. Certainly the decision to withhold treatment is not justified by the AMA statement. That such infants have been allowed to die cannot be denied; but this, I think, is the result of doctors misunderstanding the law and the AMA position.

Withholding treatment in this case is the intentional termination of life because the infant is deliberately allowed to die; that is the point of not operating. But there are other cases in which that is not the point. If the point is to avoid inflicting painful treatment on a patient with little or no reasonable hope of success, this is not the intentional termination of life. The permissibility of such withholding of treatment, then, would have no implications for the permissibility of euthanasia, active or passive.

The decision whether or not to operate, or to institute vigorous treatment, is particularly agonizing in the case of children born with spina bifida, an opening in the base of the spine usually accompanied by hydrocephalus and mental retardation. If left unoperated, these children usually die of meningitis or kidney failure within the first few years of life. Even if they survive, all affected children face a lifetime of illness, operations, and varying degrees of disability. The policy used to be to save as many as possible, but the trend now is toward selective treatment, based on the physician's estimate of the chances of success. If operating is not likely to improve significantly the child's condition, parents and doctors may agree not to operate. This is not the intentional termination of life, for again the purpose is not the termination of the child's life but the avoidance of painful and pointless treatment. Thus, the fact that withholding treatment is justified does not imply that killing the child would be equally justified.

Throughout the discussion, I have claimed that intentionally ceasing life-prolonging treatment is not the intentional termination of life unless the doctor has, as his or her purpose in stopping treatment, the patient's death.

It may be objected that I have incorrectly characterized the conditions for the intentional termination of life. Perhaps it is enough that the doctor intentionally ceases treatment, foreseeing that the patient will die.

In many cases, if one acts intentionally, foreseeing that a particular result will occur, one can be said to have brought about that result intentionally. Indeed, this is the general legal rule. Why, then, am I not willing to call the cessation of life-prolonging treatment, in compliance with the patient's right to refuse treatment, the intentional termination of life? It is not because such an *identification* is necessarily opprobrious; for we could go on to *discuss* whether such cessation of treatment is a *justifiable* intentional termination of life. Even in the law, some cases of homicide are justifiable; e.g., homicide in self-defense.

However, the cessation of life-prolonging treatment, in the cases which I have discussed, is not regarded in law as being justifiable homicide, because it is not homicide at all. Why is this? Is it because the doctor "doesn't do anything," and so cannot be guilty of homicide? Surely not, since, as I have indicated, the law sometimes treats an omission as the cause of death. A better explanation, I think, has to do with the fact that in the context of the patient's right to refuse treatment, a doctor is not at liberty to continue treatment. It seems a necessary ingredient of intentionally letting die that one could have done something to prevent the death. In this situation, of course the doctor can physically prevent the patient's death, but since we do not regard the doctor as *free* to continue treatment, we say that there is "nothing he can do." Therefore he does not intentionally let the patient die.

To discuss this suggestion fully, I would need to present a full-scale theory of intentional action. However, at least I have shown, through the discussion of the above examples, that such a theory will be very complex, and that one of the complexities concerns the agent's reason for acting. The reason why an agent acted (or failed to act) may affect the characterization of what he did intentionally. The mere fact that he did *something* intentionally, foreseeing a certain result, does not necessarily mean that he brought about that *result* intentionally.

In order to show that the cessation of life-prolonging treatment, in the cases I've discussed, is the intentional termination of life, one would either have to show that treatment was stopped in order to bring about the patient's death, or provide a theory of intentional action according to which the reason for ceasing treatment is irrelevant to its characterization as the intentional termination of life. I find this suggestion implausible, but am willing to consider arguments for it. Rachels has pro-

vided no such arguments: indeed, he apparently shares my view about the intentional termination of life. For when he claims that the cessation of life-prolonging treatment *is* the intentional termination of life, his reason for making the claim is that "if it were not, there would be no point to it." Rachels believes that the point of ceasing treatment, "in these cases," is to bring about the patient's death. If that were not the point, he suggests, why would the doctor cease treatment? I have shown, however, that there can be a point to ceasing treatment which is not the death of the patient. In showing this, I have refuted Rachels' reason for identifying the cessation of life-prolonging treatment with the intentional termination of life, and thus his argument against the AMA doctrine.

Here someone might say: Even if the withholding of treatment is not the intentional termination of life, does that make a difference, morally speaking? If life-prolonging treatment may be withheld, for the sake of the child, may not an easy death be provided, for the sake of the child, as well? The unoperated child with spina bifida may take months or even years to die. Distressed by the spectacle of children "lying around, waiting to die," one doctor has written, "It is time that society and medicine stopped perpetuating the fiction that withholding treatment is ethically different from terminating a life. It is time that society began to discuss mechanisms by which we can alleviate the pain and suffering for those individuals whom we cannot help."[7]

I do not deny that there may be cases in which death is in the best interests of the patient. In such cases, a quick and painless death may be the best thing. However, I do not think that, once active or vigorous treatment is stopped, a quick death is always preferable to a lingering one. We must be cautious about attributing to defective children *our* distress at seeing them linger. Waiting for them to die may be tough on parents, doctors, and nurses—it isn't necessarily tough on the child. The decision not to operate need not mean a decision to neglect, and it may be possible to make the remaining months of the child's life comfortable, pleasant, and filled with love. If this alternative is possible, surely it is more decent and humane than killing the child. In such a situation, withholding treatment, foreseeing the child's death, is not ethically equivalent to killing the child, and we cannot move from the permissibility of the former to that of the latter. I am worried that there will be a tendency to do precisely that if active euthanasia is regarded as morally equivalent to the withholding of life-prolonging treatment.

necessarily the intentional termination of life, so that if it is permissible to withhold life-prolonging treatment it does not follow that, other things being equal, it is permissible to kill. Furthermore, most of the time, other things are not equal. In many of the cases in which it would be right to cease treatment, I do not think that it would also be right to kill.

CONCLUSION

The AMA statement does not make the distinction Rachels and Tooley wish to attack, that between active and passive euthanasia. Instead, the statement draws a distinction between the intentional termination of life, on the one hand, and the cessation of the employment of extraordinary means to prolong life, on the other. Nothing said by Rachels and Tooley shows that this distinction is confused. It may be that doctors have misinterpreted the AMA statement, and that this has led, for example, to decisions to allow defective infants to starve slowly to death. I quite agree with Rachels and Tooley that the decisions to which they allude were cruel and made an irrelevant grounds. Certainly it is worth pointing out that allowing someone to die *can* be the intentional termination of life, and that it can be just as bad as, or worse than, killing someone. However, the withholding of life-prolonging treatment is not

Notes

1. For example, *In re Yetter,* 62 Pa. D. & C. 2d 619 (C.P., Northampton County Ct. 1974).
2. David W. Meyers, "Legal Aspects of Voluntary Euthanasia," in *Dilemmas of Euthanasia,* ed. John Behnke and Sissela Bok (New York: Anchor Books, 1975), p. 56.
3. Ernest H. Rosenbaum, M.D., *Living With Cancer* (New York: Praeger, 1975), p. 27.
4. See Tristram Engelhardt, Jr., "Ethical Issues in Aiding the Death of Young Children," in *Beneficent Euthanasia,* ed. Marvin Kohl (Buffalo, N.Y.: Prometheus Books, 1975); in this volume, pp. 81–91.
5. B. D. Colen, *Karen Ann Quinlan: Living and Dying in the Age of Eternal Life* (Los Angeles: Nash, 1976), p. 115.
6. See Norman L. Cantor, "Law and the Termination of an Incompetent Patient's Life-Preserving Care," in *Dilemmas of Euthanasia,* pp. 69–105.
7. John Freeman, "Is There a Right to Die—Quickly?" *Journal of Pediatrics,* 80, no. 5 (1972), 904–905.

The Problem of Abortion and the Doctrine of the Double Effect

Philippa Foot

One of the reasons why most of us feel puzzled about the problem of abortion is that we want, and do not want, to allow to the unborn child the rights that belong to adults and children.

Reprinted with the author's permission from the Oxford Review, No. 5, 5–15, (1967).

When we think of a baby about to be born it seems absurd to think that the next few minutes or even hours could make so radical a difference to its status; yet as we go back in the life of the foetus we are more and more reluctant to say that this is a human being and must be treated as such. No doubt this is the deepest source of our dilemma, but it is not the only one. For we are also confused about the general question of what we may and may not do where the interests of human beings conflict. We have strong intuitions about certain cases; saying for instance, that it is all right to raise the level of education in our country, though statistics allow us to predict that a rise in the suicide rate will follow, while it is not all right to kill the feeble-minded to aid cancer research. It is not easy, however, to see the principles involved, and one way of throwing light on the abortion issue will be by setting up parallels involving adults or children once born. So we will be able to isolate the "equal rights" issue, and should be able to make some advance.

I shall not, of course, discuss all the principles that may be used in deciding what to do where the interest or rights of human beings conflict. What I want to do is to look at one particular theory, known as the "doctrine of the double effect" which is invoked by Catholics in support of their views on abortion but supposed by them to apply elsewhere. As used in the abortion argument this doctrine has often seemed to non-Catholics to be a piece of complete sophistry. In the last number of the *Oxford Review* it was given short shrift by Professor Hart.[1] And yet this principle has seemed to some non-Catholics as well as to Catholics to stand as the only defence against decisions on other issues that are quite unacceptable. It will help us in our difficulty about abortion if this conflict can be resolved.

The doctrine of the double effect is based on a distinction between what a man foresees as a result of his voluntary action and what, in the strict sense, he intends. He intends in the strictest sense both those things that he aims at as ends and those that he aims at as means to his ends. The latter may be regretted in themselves but nevertheless desired for the sake of the end, as we may intend to keep dangerous lunatics confined for the sake of our safety. By contrast a man is said not strictly, or directly, to intend the foreseen consequences of his voluntary actions where these are neither the end at which he is aiming nor the means to this end. Whether the word "intention" should be applied in both cases is not of course what matters: Bentham spoke of "oblique intention," contrasting it

with the "direct intention" of ends and means, and we may as well follow his terminology. Everyone must recognize that some such distinction can be made, though it may be made in a number of different ways, and it is the distinction that is crucial to the doctrine of the double effect. The words "double effect" refer to the two effects that an action may produce: the one aimed at, and the one foreseen but in no way desired. By "the doctrine of the double effect" I mean the thesis that it is sometimes permissible to bring about by oblique intention what one may not directly intend. Thus the distinction is held to be relevant to moral decision in certain difficult cases. It is said for instance that the operation of hysterectomy involves the death of the foetus as the foreseen but not strictly or directly intended consequence of the surgeon's act, while other operations kill the child and count as the direct intention of taking an innocent life, a distinction that has evoked particularly bitter reactions on the part of non-Catholics. If you are permitted to bring about the death of the child, what does it matter how it is done? The doctrine of the double effect is also used to show why in another case, where a woman in labour will die unless a craniotomy operation is performed, the intervention is not to be condoned. There, it is said, we may not operate but must let the mother die. We foresee her death but do not directly intend it, whereas to crush the skull of the child would count as direct intention of its death.[2]

This last application of the doctrine has been queried by Professor Hart on the ground that the child's death is not strictly a means to saving the mother's life and should logically be treated as an unwanted but foreseen consequence by those who make use of the distinction between direct and oblique intention. To interpret the doctrine in this way is perfectly reasonable given the language that has been used; it would, however, make nonsense of it from the beginning. A certain event may be desired under one of its descriptions, unwanted under another, but we cannot treat these as two different events, one of which is aimed at and the other not. And even if it be argued that there are here two different events—the crushing of the child's skull and its death—the two are obviously much too close for an application of the doctrine of the double effect. To see how odd it would be to apply the principle like this we may consider the story, well known to philosophers, of the fat man stuck in the mouth of the cave. A party of potholers have imprudently allowed the fat man to lead them as they make their way out of the cave, and he gets stuck, trapping the others behind him. Obviously the right thing to do is to sit down and wait until the fat man grows thin; but philosophers have arranged that flood waters should be rising within the cave. Luckily (luckily?) the trapped party have with them a stick of dynamite with which they can blast the fat man out of the mouth of the cave. Either they use the dynamite or they drown. In one version the fat man, whose head is *in* the cave, will drown with them; in the other he will be rescued in due course.[3] Problem: may they use the dynamite or not? Later we will find parallels to this example. Here it is introduced for light relief and because it will serve to show how ridiculous one version of the doctrine of the double effect would be. For suppose that the trapped explorers were to argue that the death of the fat man might be taken as a merely foreseen consequence of the act of blowing him up. (''We didn't want to kill him . . . only to blow him into small pieces'' or even ''. . . only to blast him out of the mouth of the cave.'') I believe that those who use the doctrine of the double effect would rightly reject such a suggestion, though they will, of course, have considerable difficulty in explaining where the line is to be drawn. What is to be the criterion of ''closeness'' if we say that anything very close to what we are literally aiming at counts as if part of our aim?

Let us leave this difficulty aside and return to the arguments for and against the doctrine, supposing it to be formulated in the way considered most effective by its supporters, and ourselves bypassing the trouble by taking what must on any reasonable definition be clear cases of ''direct'' or ''oblique'' intention.

The first point that should be made clear, in fairness to the theory, is that no one is suggesting that it does not matter what you bring about as long as you merely foresee and do not strictly intend the evil that follows. We might think, for instance, of the (actual) case of wicked merchants selling, for cooking, oil they knew to be poisonous and thereby killing a number of innocent people, comparing and contrasting it with that of some unemployed gravediggers, desperate for custom, who got hold of this same oil and sold it (or perhaps *they* secretly gave it away) in order to create orders for graves. They strictly (directly) intend the deaths they cause, while the merchants could say that it was not part of their *plan* that anyone should die. In morality, as in law, the merchants, like the gravediggers, would be considered as murderers; nor are the supporters of the doctrine of the double effect bound to say that there is the least difference between them in respect of moral turpitude. What they are committed to is the thesis that *sometimes* it makes a difference to the permissibility of an action involving harm to others that this harm, although foreseen, is not part of the agent's direct intention. An end such as earning one's living is clearly not such as to justify *either* the direct or oblique intention of the death of innocent people, but in certain cases one is justified in bringing about knowingly what one could not directly intend.

It is now time to say why this doctrine should be taken seriously in spite of the fact that it sounds rather odd, that there are difficulties about the distinction on which it depends, and that it seemed to yield one sophistical conclusion when applied to the problem of abortion. The reason for its appeal is that its opponents have often *seemed* to be committed to quite indefensible views. Thus the controversy has raged around examples such as the following. Suppose that a judge or magistrate is faced with rioters demanding that a culprit be found for a certain crime and threatening otherwise to take their own bloody revenge on a particular section of the community. The real culprit being unknown, the judge sees himself as able to prevent the bloodshed only by framing some innocent person and having him executed. Beside this example is placed another in which a pilot whose aeroplane is about to crash is deciding whether to steer from a more to a less inhabited area. To make the parallel as close as possible it may rather be supposed that he is the driver of a runaway tram which he can only steer from one narrow track on to another; five men are working on one track and one man on the other;

anyone on the track he enters is bounded to be killed. In the case of the riots the mob have five hostages, so that in both the exchange is supposed to be one man's life for the lives of five. The question is why we should say, without hesitation, that the driver should steer for the less occupied track, while most of us would be appalled at the idea that the innocent man could be framed. It may be suggested that the special feature of the latter case is that it involves the corruption of justice, and this is, of course, very important indeed. But if we remove that special feature, supposing that some private individual is to kill an innocent person and pass him off as the criminal we still find ourselves horrified by the idea. The doctrine of the double effect offers us a way out of the difficulty, insisting that it is one thing to steer towards someone foreseeing that you will kill him and another to aim at his death as part of your plan. Moreover there is one very important element of good in what is here insisted. In real life it would hardly ever be certain that the man on the narrow track would be killed. Perhaps he might find a foothold on the side of the tunnel and cling on as the vehicle hurtled by. The driver of the tram does not then leap off and brain him with a crowbar. This judge, however, needs the death of the innocent man for his (good) purposes. If the victim proves hard to hang he must see to it that he dies another way. To choose to execute him is to choose that this evil *shall come about,* and this must therefore count as a *certainty* in weighing up the good and evil involved. The distinction between direct and oblique intention is crucial here, and is of great importance in an uncertain world. Nevertheless this is no way to defend the doctrine of the double effect. For the question is whether the difference between aiming at something and obliquely intending it is *in itself* relevant to moral decisions; not whether it is important when correlated with a difference of certainty in the balance of good and evil. Moreover we are particularly interested in the application of the doctrine of the double effect to the question of abortion, and no one can deny that in medicine there are sometimes certainties so complete that it would be a mere quibble to speak of the "probable outcome" of this course of action or that. It is not, therefore, with a merely philosophical interest that we should

put aside the uncertainty and scrutinize the examples to test the doctrine of the double effect. Why can we not argue from the case of the steering driver to that of the judge?

Another pair of examples poses a similar problem. We are about to give to a patient who needs it to save his life a massive dose of a certain drug in short supply. There arrive, however, five other patients each of whom could be saved by one-fifth of that dose. We say with regret that we cannot spare our whole supply of the drug for a single patient, just as we should say that we could not spare the whole resources of a ward for one dangerously ill individual when ambulances arrive bringing in the victims of a multiple crash. We feel bound to let one man die rather than many if that is our only choice. Why then do we not feel justified in killing people in the interests of cancer research or to obtain, let us say, spare parts for grafting on to those who need them? We can suppose, similarly, that several dangerously ill people can be saved only if we kill a certain individual and make a serum from his dead body. (These examples are not over fanciful considering present controversies about prolonging the life of mortally ill patients whose eyes or kidneys are to be used for others.) Why cannot we argue from the case of the scarce drug to that of the body needed for medical purposes? Once again the doctrine of the double effect comes up with an explanation. In one kind of case but not the other we aim at the death of the innocent man.

A further argument suggests that if the doctrine of the double effect is rejected this has the consequence of putting us hopelessly in the power of bad men. Suppose for example that some tyrant should threaten to torture five men if we ourselves would not torture one. Would it be our duty to do so, supposing we believed him, because this would be no different from choosing to rescue five men from his tortures rather than one? If so anyone who wants us to do something we think wrong has only to threaten that otherwise he himself will do something we think worse. A mad murderer, known to keep his promises, could thus make it our duty to kill some innocent citizen to prevent him from killing two. From this conclusion we are again rescued by the doctrine of the double effect. If we refuse, we foresee that the greater number will be killed but we do not intend it: it is he who intends (that is strictly or directly intends) the death of innocent persons; we do not.

At one time I thought that these arguments in favour of the doctrine of the double effect were conclusive, but I now believe that the conflict should be solved in another way. The clue that we should follow is that the strength of the doctrine seems to lie in the distinction it makes between what we do (equated with direct intention) and what we allow (thought of as obliquely intended). Indeed it is interesting that the disputants tend to argue about whether we are to be held responsible for what we allow as we are for what we do.[4] Yet it is not obvious that this is what they should be discussing, since the distinction between what one does and what one allows to happen is not the same as that between direct and oblique intention. To see this one has only to consider that it is possible *deliberately* to allow something to happen, aiming at it either for its own sake or as part of one's plan for obtaining something else. So one person might want another person dead, and deliberately allow him to die. And again one may be said to *do* things that one does not aim at, as the steering driver would kill the man on the track. Moreover there is a large class of things said to be brought about rather than either done or allowed, and either kind of intention is possible. So it is possible to *bring about* a man's death by getting him to go to sea in a leaky boat, and the intention of his death may be either direct or oblique.

Whatever it may, or may not, have to do with the doctrine of the double effect, the idea of *allowing* is worth looking into in this context. I shall leave aside the special case of giving permission, which involves the idea of authority, and consider the two main divisions into which cases of allowing seem to fall. There is firstly the allowing which is forbearing to prevent. For this we need a sequence thought of as somehow already in train, and something that the agent could do to intervene. (The agent must be able to intervene, but does not do so.) So, for instance, he could warn someone, but *allows* him to walk into a trap. He could feed an animal but *allows* it to die for lack of food. He could stop a leaking tap but *allows* the water to go on flowing. This is the case of allowing with which we

shall be concerned, but the other should be mentioned. It is the kind of allowing which is roughly equivalent to *enabling;* the root idea being the removal of some obstacle which is, as it were, holding back a train of events. So someone may remove a plug and *allow* water to flow; open a door and *allow* an animal to get out; or give someone money and *allow* him to get back on his feet.

The first kind of allowing requires an a omission, but there is no other general correlation between omission and allowing, commission and bringing about or doing. An actor who fails to turn up for a performance will generally spoil it rather than allow it to be spoiled. I mention the distinction between omission and commission only to set it aside.

Thinking of the first kind of allowing (forbearing to prevent), we should ask whether there is any difference, from the moral point of view, between what one does or causes and what one merely allows. It seems clear that on occasions one is just as bad as the other, as is recognized in both morality and law. A man may murder his child or his aged relatives, by allowing them to die of starvation as well as by giving poison; he may also be convicted of murder on either account. In another case we would, however, make a distinction. Most of us allow people to die of starvation in India and Africa, and there is surely something wrong with us that we do; it would be nonsense, however, to pretend that it is only in law that we make a distinction between allowing people in the underdeveloped countries to die of starvation and sending them poisoned food. There is worked into our moral system a distinction between what we owe people in the form of aid and what we owe them in the way of non-interference. Salmond, in his *Jurisprudence,* expressed as follows the distinction between the two.

A positive right corresponds to a positive duty, and is a right that he on whom the duty lies shall do some positive act on behalf of the person entitled. A negative right corresponds to a negative duty, and is a right that the person bound shall refrain from some act which would operate to the prejudice of the person entitled. The former is a right to be positively benefited; the latter is merely a right not to be harmed."[5]

As a general account of rights and duties this is defective, since not all are so closely connected with benefit and harm. Nevertheless for our purposes it will do well. Let us speak of negative duties when thinking of the obligation to refrain from such things as killing or robbing, and of the positive duty, e.g., to look after children or aged parents. It will be useful, however, to extend the notion of positive duty beyond the range of things that are strictly called duties, bringing acts of charity under this heading. These are owed only in a rather loose sense, and some acts of charity could hardly be said to be *owed* at all, so I am not following ordinary usage at this point.

Let us now see whether the distinction of negative and positive duties explains why we see differently the action of the steering driver and that of the judge, of the doctors who withhold the scarce drug and those who obtain a body for medical purposes, of those who choose to rescue the five men rather than one man from torture and those who are ready to torture the one man themselves in order to save five. In each case we have a conflict of duties, but what kind of duties are they? Are we, in each case, weighing positive duties against positive, negative against negative, or one against the other? Is the duty to refrain from injury, or rather to bring aid?

The steering driver faces a conflict of negative duties, since it is his duty to avoid injuring five men and also his duty to avoid injuring one. In the circumstances he is not able to avoid both, and it seems clear that he should do the least injury he can. The judge, however, is weighing the duty of not inflicting injury against the duty of bringing aid. He wants to rescue the innocent people threatened with death but can do so only by inflicting injury himself. Since one does not *in general* have the same duty to help people as to refrain from injuring them, it is not possible to argue to a conclusion about what he should do from the steering driver case. It is interesting that, even where the strictest duty of positive aid exists, still does not weigh as if a negative duty were involved. It is not, for instance, permissible to commit a murder to bring one's starving children food. If the choice is between inflicting injury on one or many there seems only one rational course of action; if the choice is between aid to some at the cost of injury to others, and refusing to inflict the injury to bring the aid, the whole matter is open to dispute. So it is not inconsistent of us to think that the driver must steer for the road on which only one man stands while the judge (or his equivalent) may not kill the innocent person in order to stop the riots. Let us now consider the second pair of examples, which concern the scarce drug on the one hand and on the other the body needed to save lives. Once again we find a difference based on the distinction between the duty to avoid injury and the duty to provide aid. Where one man needs a massive dose of the drug and we withhold it from him in order to save five men, we are weighing aid against aid. But if we consider killing a man in order to use his body to save others, we are thinking of doing him injury to bring others aid. In an interesting variant of the model, we may suppose that instead of killing someone we deliberately let him die. (Perhaps he is a beggar to whom we are thinking of giving food, but then we say "No, they need bodies for medical research.") Here it does seem relevant that in allowing him to die we are aiming at his death, but presumably we are inclined to see this as a violation of negative rather than positive duty. If this is right, we see why we are unable in either case to argue to a conclusion from the case of the scarce drug.

In the examples involving the torture of one man or five men, the principle seems to be the same as for the last pair. If we are bringing aid (rescuing people about to be tortured by the tyrant), we must obviously rescue the larger rather than the smaller group. It does not follow, however, that we would be justified in inflicting the injury, or getting a third person to do so, in order to save the five. We may therefore refuse to be forced into acting by the threats of bad men. To refrain from inflicting injury ourselves is a stricter duty than to prevent other people from inflicting injury, which is not to say that the other is not a very strict duty indeed.

So far the conclusions are the same as those at which we might arrive following the doctrine of the double effect, but in others they will be different, and the advantage seems to be all on the side of the alternative. Suppose, for instance, that there are five patients in a hospital whose lives could be saved by the manufacture of a certain gas, but that this inevitably releases lethal fumes into the room of another patient whom for some reason we are unable to move. His death, being of no use to us, is clearly a side effect, and not directly intended. Why then is the case different from that of the scarce drug, if the point about that is that we foresaw but did not strictly intend the death of the single patient? Yet it surely is different. The relatives of the gassed patient would presumably be successful if they sued the hospital and the whole story came out. We may find it particularly revolting that someone should be *used* as in the case where he is killed or allowed to die in the interest of medical research, and the fact of *using* may even determine what we would decide to do in some cases, but the principle seems unimportant compared with our reluctance to bring such injury for the sake of giving aid.

My conclusion is that the distinction between direct and oblique intention plays only a quite subsidiary role in determining what we say in these cases, while the distinction between avoiding injury and bringing aid is very important indeed. I have not, of course, argued that there are no other principles. For instance it clearly makes a difference whether our positive duty is a strict duty or rather an act of charity: feeding our own children or feeding those in far away countries. It may also make a difference whether the person about to suffer is one thought of as uninvolved in the threatened disaster, and whether it is his presence that constitutes the threat to the others. In many cases we find it very hard to know what to say, and I have not been arguing for any general conclusion such as that we may never, whatever the balance of good and evil, bring injury to one for the sake of aid to others, even when this injury amounts to death. I have only tried to show that even if we reject the doctrine of the double effect we are not forced to the conclusion that the size of the evil must always be our guide.

Let us now return to the problem of abortion, carrying out our plan of finding parallels involving adults or children rather than the unborn. We must say something about the different cases in which abortion might be considered on medical grounds.

First of all there is the situation in which nothing that can be done will save the life of child and mother, but where the life of the mother can be saved by killing the child. This is parallel to the case of the fat man in the mouth of the cave who is bound to be drowned with the others if nothing is done. Given the certainty of the outcome, as it was postulated, there is no serious conflict of interests here, since the fat man will perish in either case, and it is reasonable that the action that will save someone should be done. It is a great objection to those who argue that the direct intention of the death of an innocent person is never justifiable that the edict will apply even in this case. The Catholic doctrine on abortion must here conflict with that of most reasonable men. Moreover we would be justified in performing the operation whatever the method used, and it is neither a necessary nor a good justification of the special case of hysterectomy that the child's death is not directly intended, being rather a foreseen consequence of what is done. What difference could it make as to how the death is brought about?

Secondly we have the case in which it is possible to perform an operation which will save the mother and kill the child or kill the mother and save the child. This is parallel to the famous case of the shipwrecked mariners who believed that they must throw someone overboard if their boat was not to founder in a storm, and to the other famous case of the two sailors, Dudley and Stephens, who killed and ate the cabin boy when adrift on the sea without food. Here again there is no conflict of interests so far as the decision to act is concerned; only in deciding whom to save. Once again it would be reasonable to act, though one would respect someone who held back from the appalling action either because he preferred to perish rather than do such a thing or because he held on past the limits of reasonable hope. In real life the certainties postulated by philosophers hardly ever exist, and Dudley and Stephens were rescued not long after their ghastly meal. Nevertheless if the certainty were absolute, as it might be in the abortion case, it would seem better to save one than none. Probably we should decide in favour of the mother when weighing her life against that of the unborn child, but it is interesting that, a few years later, we might easily decide it the other way.

The worst dilemma comes in the third kind of example where to save the mother we must kill the child, say by crushing its skull, while if nothing is done the mother will perish but the child can be safely delivered after her death. Here the doctrine of the double effect has been invoked to show that we may not intervene, since the child's death would be directly intended while the mother's would not. On a strict parallel with cases not involving the unborn we might find the conclusion correct though the reason given was wrong. Suppose, for instance, that in later life the presence of a child was certain to bring death to the mother. We would surely not think ourselves justified in ridding her of it by a process that involved its death. For in general we do not think that we can kill one innocent person to rescue another, quite apart from the special care that we feel is due to children once they have prudently got themselves born. What we would be prepared to do when a great many people were involved is another matter, and this is probably the key to one quite common view of abortion on the part of those who take quite seriously the rights of the unborn child. They probably feel that if *enough* people are involved one must be sacri-

ficed, and they think of the mother's life against the unborn child's life as if it were many against one. But of course many people do not view it like this at all, having no inclination to accord to the foetus or unborn child anything like ordinary human status in the matter of rights. I have not been arguing for or against these points of view but only trying to discern some of the currents that are pulling us back and forth. The levity of the examples is not meant to offend.

Notes

1. H. L. A. Hart, "Intention and Punishment," *Oxford Review,* Number 4, Hilary 1967. I owe much to this article and to a conversation with Professor Hart, though I do not know whether he will approve of what follows.
2. For discussions of the Catholic doctrine on abortion see Glanville Williams, *The Sanctity of Life and the Criminal Law* (New York, 1957); also N. St. John Stevas, *The Right to Life* (London, 1963).
3. It was Professor Hart who drew my attention to this distinction.
4. See, e.g., J. Bennett, "Whatever the Consequences," *Analysis,* January 1966, and G. E. M. Anscombe's reply in *Analysis,* June 1966. See also Miss Anscombe's "Modern Moral Philosophy" in *Philosophy,* January 1958.
5. J. Salmond, *Jurisprudence,* 11th edition, p. 283.

REPRODUCTION

From "An Almost Absolute Value in History"

John T. Noonan, Jr.

What determines when a being is human? When is it lawful to kill? These questions are linked in any consideration of the morality of abortion. They are questions central to any morality for man.

In answering such moral questions the temptation to invoke historical determinism is not unknown. A species of behavior is said to be right because it inevitably will be practiced and accepted in the future. "Trends" are hypostatized into forces like older theological conceptions of the divine will; they are supposed to exist independently of human volition and to legitimate by necessity the human acts which they require.

Such use of history, I suppose, appears exploitative and dishonest to most men who have tried to discern the thought of the past. In looking at the data and documents of another age, one does not encounter irresistible trends moving with mysterious authority to foreordained results. Order in human history is the pattern made by the historian in his choice of categories and selection of events. What he encounters is a record of human thought with no greater necessity to it than the result of any meeting of human minds.

The rejection of necessity in human development is not a rejection of continuity, recurrences, and even direction in human experience. These philosophical notions, or something like them, appear as preconditions for the perception and organization of historical "facts." Something like organic behavior may be postulated in the experience of groups of men. Ideas do have implications which are sometimes worked out. No value can be pur-

sued alone without its single-minded pursuit endangering other values, so that balance is the condition of stable phases. Human groups mature. To suppose that these characteristics of human behavior constitute suprahuman forces is to replace history with ideology. To ignore the organic character of human experience is to reduce history to chronology.

History can record insights gained by human beings, insights which once generalized by education are taken as a part of the mental outlook of the persons subject to such education. Such is the insight into the connection between being human and being free. Once men have seen that the determination of their own potential humanity can be injured by the domination of others, they insist on their freedom of action and of thought. The pursuit of freedom as a single absolute, however, is unworkable because the maximum conceivable freedom of action for one man necessarily involves the right to dispose of other men; and any society committed to freedom as a human good must move dynamically toward a balance where freedom for one man is not achieved at the expense of freedom for another.

In the conflict over abortion, the desire of many women to be free from restraints imposed by men and the desire of many contemporary human beings to be free from the domination of sexual codes established by others give dynamic power to any proposal to reject all limitations on abortion. In a society peculiarly conscious of the difference made by age, it is easy to define one class by age so that it is not regarded as even human, so that then there can be no objection to elimination of members of the class whenever a member of it interferes with the freedom of those who are human. In this case, then, there is no need to balance the gain in freedom of some humans by the loss to other humans.

The question remains, Can age be the determinant of humanity? Behind this question, the questions are repeated, What determines when a being is human? When can human freedom be vindicated by killing other human beings? In this chapter I propose to examine these questions as they have been answered in the context of a religious tradition concerned with them since its inception.

The impatience expressed by proponents of abortion with a view asserting the humanity of the fetus sometimes incorporates an elitism which assumes that everyone—that is, every enlightened person, everyone in the ruling group—knows who is human. The elite may become franker and say, Even if the embryo is human, we can distinguish between human lives. Some lives are more valuable than others. To sacrifice a poor, undeveloped life for a rich developed life is a decision which morally can and should be made. More probably, the expedient of the rulers of *Animal Farm* will be adopted, and some lives will be recognized as more equal than others. To any variety of this viewpoint, a religious teaching which asserts the basic equality of men must seem irrelevant; but it is difficult to extricate the aspirations of the modern world from the assumption of basic equality. A teaching anchored in this assumption may be stronger than the very strong attraction to believe that some lives are more valuable than others.

The teaching of a religious body may invoke revelation, claim authority, employ symbolism, which make the moral doctrine it teaches binding for believers in the religion but of academic concern to those outside its boundaries. The moral teaching of a religious body may also embody insights, protect perceptions, exemplify values, which concern humanity. The teaching of the moralists of the Catholic Church on abortion is particularly rich in interaction between specifically supernatural themes—for example, the Nativity of the Lord and the Immaculate Conception of Mary—and principles of a general ethical applicability. In its full extent, the teaching depends on the self-sacrificing example of the Lord—to the Greeks, foolishness. In its basic assumption of the equality of human lives, it depends on a stoic, democratic contention which any man might embrace and Western humanism has hitherto embraced. In its reliance on ecclesiastical authority to draw a line, it withdraws from the sphere of debate with all men of goodwill; in its casuistic examination of principle, it offers instances where the common tools of moral analysis may be observed industriously employed. The teaching in its totality cannot be detached from the religious tradition which has borne it. The teaching in its fundamental questions about the meaning of love and humanity cannot be disregarded by those who would meet the needs of man humanly. . . .

The most fundamental question involved in the long history of thought on abortion is: How do you determine the humanity of a being? To phrase the question that way is to put in comprehensive humanistic terms what the theologians either dealt with as an explicitly theological question under the heading of "ensoulment" or dealt with implicitly in their treatment of abortion. The Christian position as it originated did not depend on a narrow theological or philosophical concept. It had no relation to theories of infant baptism. It appealed to no special theory of instantaneous ensoulment. It took the world's view on ensoulment as that view changed from Aristotle to Zacchia. There was, indeed, theological influence affecting the theory of ensoulment finally adopted, and, of course, ensoulment itself was a theological concept, so that the position was always explained in theological terms. But the theological notion of ensoulment could easily be translated into humanistic language by substituting "human" for "rational soul"; the problem of knowing when a man is a man is common to theology and humanism.

If one steps outside the specific categories used by the theologians, the answer they gave can be analyzed as a refusal to discriminate among human beings on the basis of their varying potentialities. Once conceived, the being was recognized as man because he had man's potential. The criterion for humanity, thus, was simple and all-embracing: if you are conceived by human parents, you are human.

The strength of this position may be tested by a review of some of the other distinctions offered in the contemporary controversy over legalizing abortion. Perhaps the most popular distinction is in terms of viability. Before an age of so many months, the fetus is not viable, that is, it cannot be removed from the mother's womb and live apart from her. To that extent, the life of the fetus is absolutely dependent on the life of the mother. This dependence is made the basis of denying recognition to its humanity.

There are difficulties with this distinction. One is that the perfection of artificial incubation may make the fetus viable at any time: it may be removed and artificially sustained. Experiments with animals already show that such a procedure is possible. This hypothetical extreme case relates to an actual difficulty: there is considerable elasticity to the idea of viability. Mere length of life is not an exact measure. The viability of the fetus depends on the extent of its anatomical and functional development. The weight and length of the fetus are better guides to the state of its development than age, but weight and length vary. Moreover, different racial groups have different ages at which their fetuses are viable. Some evidence, for example, suggests that Negro fetuses mature more quickly than white fetuses. If viability is the norm, the standard would vary with race and with many individual circumstances.

The most important objection to this approach is that dependence is not ended by viability. The fetus is still absolutely dependent on someone's care in order to continue existence; indeed a child of one or three or even five years of age is absolutely dependent on another's care for existence; uncared for, the older fetus or the younger child will die as surely as the early fetus detached from the mother. The unsubstantial lessening in dependence at viability does not seem to signify any special acquisition of humanity.

A second distinction has been attempted in terms of experience. A being who has had experience, has lived and suffered, who possesses memories, is more human than one who has not. Humanity depends on formation by experience. The fetus is thus "unformed" in the most basic human sense.

This distinction is not serviceable for the embryo which is already experiencing and reacting. The embryo is responsive to touch after eight weeks and at least at that point is experiencing. At an earlier stage the zygote is certainly alive and responding to its environment. The distinction may also be challenged by the rare case where aphasia has erased adult memory: has it erased humanity? More fundamentally, this distinction leaves even the older fetus or the younger child to be treated as an unformed inhuman thing. Finally, it is not clear why experience as such confers humanity. It could be argued that certain central experiences such as loving or learning are necessary to make a man human. But then human beings who have failed to love or to learn might be excluded from the class called man.

A third distinction is made by appeal to the sentiments of adults. If a fetus dies, the grief of the parents is not the grief they would have for a living child. The fetus is an unnamed "it" till birth, and is not perceived as personality until at least the fourth month of existence when movements in the womb manifest a vigorous presence demanding joyful recognition by the parents.

Yet feeling is notoriously an unsure guide to the humanity of others. Many groups of humans have had difficulty in feeling that persons of another tongue, color, religion, sex, are as human as they. Apart from reactions to alien groups, we mourn the loss of a 10-year-old boy more than the loss of his one-day-old brother or his 90-year-old grandfather. The difference felt and the grief expressed vary with the potentialities extinguished, or the experience wiped out; they do not seem to point to any substantial difference in the humanity of baby, boy, or grandfather.

Distinctions are also made in terms of sensation by the parents. The embryo is felt within the womb only after about the fourth month. The embryo is seen only at birth. What can be neither seen nor felt is different from what is tangible. If the fetus cannot be seen or touched at all, it cannot be perceived as man.

Yet experience shows that sight is even more untrustworthy than feeling in determining humanity. By sight, color became an appropriate index for saying who was a man, and the evil of racial discrimination was given foundation. Nor can touch provide the test; a being confined by sickness, "out of touch" with others, does not thereby seem to lose his humanity. To the extent that touch still has appeal as a criterion, it appears to be a survival of the old English idea of "quickening"—a possible mistranslation of the Latin *animatus* used in the canon law. To that extent touch as a criterion seems to be dependent on the Aristotelian notion of ensoulment, and to fall when this notion is discarded.

Finally, a distinction is sought in social visibility. The fetus is not socially perceived as human. It cannot communicate with others. Thus, both subjectively and objectively, it is not a member of society. As moral rules are rules for the behavior of members of society to each other, they cannot be made for behavior toward what is not yet a member. Excluded from the society of men, the fetus is excluded from the humanity of men.

By force of the argument from the consequences, this distinction is to be rejected. It is more subtle than that founded on an appeal to physical sensation, but it is equally dangerous in its implications. If humanity depends on social recognition, individuals or whole groups may be dehumanized by being denied any status in their society. Such a fate is fictionally portrayed in *1984* and has actually been the lot of many men in many societies. In the Roman empire, for example, condemnation to slavery meant the practical denial of most human rights; in the Chinese Communist world, landlords have been classified as enemies of the people and so treated as nonpersons by the state. Humanity does not depend on social recognition, though often the failure of society to recognize the prisoner, the alien, the heterodox as human has led to the destruction of human beings. Anyone conceived by a man and a woman is human. Recognition of this condition by society follows a real event in the objective order, however imperfect and halting the recognition. Any attempt to limit humanity to exclude some group runs the risk of furnishing authority and precedent for excluding other groups in the name of the consciousness or perception of the controlling group in the society.

A philosopher may reject the appeal to the humanity of the fetus because he views "humanity" as a secular view of the soul and because he doubts the existence of anything real and objective which can be identified as humanity. One answer to such a philosopher is to ask how he reasons about moral questions without supposing that there is a sense in which he and the others of whom he speaks are human. Whatever group is taken as the society which determines who may be killed is thereby taken as human. A second answer is to ask if he does not believe that there is a right and wrong way of deciding moral questions. If there is such a difference, experience may be appealed to; to decide who is human on the basis of the sentiment of a given society has led to consequences which rational men would characterize as monstrous.

The rejection of the attempted distinctions based on viability and visibility, experience and feeling, may be buttressed by the following considerations: Moral judgments often rest on distinctions, but if the distinctions are not to appear arbitrary fiat, they should relate to some real difference in probabilities. There is a kind of continuity in all life, but the earlier stages of the elements of human life possess tiny probabilites of development. Consider for example, the spermatozoa in any normal ejaculate: There are about 200,000,000 in any single ejaculate, of which one has a chance of developing into a zygote. Consider the oocytes which may become ova: there are 100,000 to 1,000,000 oocytes in a female infant, of which a maximum of 390 are ovulated. But once spermatozoon and ovum meet and the conceptus is formed, such studies as have been made show that roughly in only 20 percent of the cases will spontaneous abortion occur. In other words, the chances are about 4 out of 5 that this new being will develop. At this stage in the life of the being there is a sharp shift in probabilities, an immense jump in potentialities. To make a distinction between the rights of spermatozoa and the rights of the fertilized ovum is to respond to an enormous shift in possibilities. For about twenty days after conception the egg may split to form twins or combine with another egg to form a chimera, but the probability of either event happening is very small.

It may be asked, What does a change in biological probabilities have to do with establishing humanity? The argument from probabilities is not aimed at establishing humanity but at establishing an objective discontinuity which may be taken into account in moral discourse. As life itself is a matter of probabilities, as most moral reasoning is an estimate of probabilities, so it seems in accord with the structure of reality and the nature of moral thought to found a moral judgment on the change in probabilities at conception. The appeal to probabilities is the most commonsensical of arguments, to a greater or smaller degree all of us base our actions on probabilities, and in morals, as in law, prudence and negligence are often measured by the account one has taken of the probabilities. If the chance is 200,000,000 to 1 that the movement in the bushes into which you shoot is a man's, I doubt if many persons would hold you careless in shooting; but if the chances are 4 out of 5 that the movement is a human being's, few would acquit you of blame. Would the argument be different if only one out of ten children conceived came to term? Of course this argument would be different. This argument is an appeal to probabilities that actually exist, not to any and all states of affairs which may be imagined.

The probabilities as they do exist do not show the humanity of the embryo in the sense of a demonstration in logic any more than the probabilities of the movement in the bush being a man demonstrate beyond all doubt that the being is a man. The appeal is a "buttressing" consideration, showing the plausibility of the standard adopted. The argument focuses on the decisional factor in any moral judgment and assumes that part of the business of a moralist is drawing lines. One evidence of the nonarbitrary character of the line drawn is the difference of probabilities on either side of it. If a spermatozoon is destroyed, one destroys a being which had a chance of far less than 1 in 200 million of developing into a reasoning being, possessed of the genetic code, a heart and other organs, and capable of pain. If a fetus is destroyed, one destroys a being already possessed of the genetic code, organs, and sensitivity to pain, and one which had an 80 percent chance of developing further into a baby outside the womb who, in time, would reason.

The positive argument for conception as the decisive moment of humanization is that at conception the new being receives the genetic code. It is this genetic information which determines his characteristics, which is the biological carrier of the possibility of human wisdom, which makes him a self-evolving being. A being with a human genetic code is man.

This review of current controversy over the humanity of the fetus emphasizes what a fundamental question the theologians resolved in asserting the inviolability of the fetus. To regard the fetus as possessed of equal rights with other humans was not, however, to decide every case where abortion might be employed. It did decide the case where the argument was that the fetus should be aborted for its own good. To say a being was human was to say it had a destiny to decide for itself which could not be taken from it by another man's decision. But human beings with equal rights often come in conflict with each other, and some decision must be made as whose claims are to prevail. Cases of conflict involving the fetus are different only in two respects: the total inability of the fetus to speak for itself and the fact that the right of the fetus regularly at stake is the right to life itself.

The approach taken by the theologians to these conflicts was articulated in terms of "direct" and "indirect." Again, to look at what they were doing from outside their categories, they may be said to have been drawing lines or "balancing values." "Direct" and "indirect" are spatial metaphors; "line-drawing" is another. "To weigh" or "to balance" values is a metaphor of a more complicated mathematical sort hinting at the process which goes on in moral judgments. All the metaphors suggest that, in the moral judgments made, comparisons were necessary, that no value completely controlled. The principle of double effect was no doctrine fallen from heaven, but a method of analysis appropriate where two relative values were being compared. In Catholic moral theology, as it developed, life even of the innocent was not taken as an absolute. Judgments on acts affecting life issued from a process of weighing. In the weighing, the fetus was always given a value greater than zero, always a value separate and independent from its parents. This valuation was crucial and fundamental in all Christian thought on the subject and marked it off from any approach which considered that only the parents' interests needed to be considered.

Even with the fetus weighed as human, one interest could be weighed as equal or superior: that of the mother in her own life. The casuists between 1450 and 1895 were willing to weigh this interest as superior. Since 1895, that interest was given decisive weight only in the two special cases of the cancerous uterus and the ectopic pregnancy. In both of these cases the fetus itself had little chance of survival even if the abortion were not performed. As the balance was once struck in favor of the mother whenever her life was endangered, it could be so struck again. The balance reached between 1895 and 1930 attempted prudentially and pastorally to forestall a multitude of exceptions for interests less than life.

The perception of the humanity of the fetus and the weighing of fetal rights against other human rights constituted the work of the moral analysts. But what spirit animated their abstract judgments? For the Christian community it was the injunction of Scripture to love your neighbor as yourself. The fetus as human was a neighbor; his life had parity with one's own. The commandment gave life to what otherwise would have been only rational calculation.

The commandment could be put in humanistic as well as theological terms: Do not injure your fellow man without reason. In these terms, once the humanity of the fetus is perceived, abortion is never right except in self-defense. When life must be taken to save life, reason alone cannot say that a mother must prefer a child's life to her own. With this exception, now of great rarity, abortion violates the rational humanist tenet of the equality of human lives.

For Christians the commandment to love had received a special imprint in that the exemplar proposed of love was the love of the Lord for his disciples. In the light given by this example, self-sacrifice carried to the point of death seemed in the extreme situations not without meaning. In the less extreme cases, preference for one's own interests to the life of another seemed to express cruelty or selfishness irreconcilable with the demands of love.

Abortion and Infanticide[1]

Michael Tooley

This essay deals with the question of the morality of abortion and infanticide. The fundamental ethical objection traditionally advanced against these practices rests on the contention that human fetuses and infants have a right to life. It is this claim which will be the focus of attention here. The basic issue to be discussed, then, is what properties a thing must possess in order to have a serious right to life. My ap-

From *Philosophy & Public Affairs*, Vol. 2, No. 1 (Fall 1972). Copyright © 1972 by Princeton University Press. Reprinted by permission of Princeton University Press and the author.

proach will be to set out and defend a basic moral principle specifying a condition an organism must satisfy if it is to have a serious right to life. It will be seen that this condition is not satisfied by human fetuses and infants, and thus that they do not have a right to life. So unless there are other substantial objections to abortion and infanticide, one is forced to conclude that these practices are morally acceptable ones. In contrast, it may turn out that our treatment of adult members of other species— cats, dogs, polar bears—is morally indefensible. For it is quite possible that such animals do possess properties that endow them with a right to life.

I. ABORTION AND INFANTICIDE

One reason the question of the morality of infanticide is worth examining is that it seems very difficult to formulate a completely satisfactory liberal position on abortion without coming to grips with the infanticide issue. The problem the liberal encounters is essentially that of specifying a cutoff point which is not arbitrary: at what stage in the development of a human being does it cease to be morally permissible to destroy it? It is important to be clear about the difficulty here. The conservative's objection is not that since there is a continuous line of development from zygote to a newborn baby, one must conclude that if it is seriously wrong to destroy a newborn baby it is also seriously wrong to destroy a zygote or any intermediate stage in the development of a human being. His point is rather that if one says it is wrong to destroy a newborn baby but not a zygote or some intermediate stage in the development of a human being, one should be prepared to point to a *morally relevant* difference between a newborn baby and the earlier stage in the development of a human being.

Precisely the same difficulty can, of course, be raised for a person who holds that infanticide is morally permissible. The conservative will ask what morally relevant differences there are between an adult human being and a newborn baby. What makes it morally permissible to destroy a baby, but wrong to kill an adult? So the challenge remains. But I will argue that in this case there is an extremely plausible answer.

Reflecting on the morality of infanticide forces one to face up to this challenge. In the case of abortion a number of events—quickening or viability, for instance—might be taken as cutoff points, and it is easy to overlook the fact that none of these events involves any morally significant change in the developing human. In contrast, if one is going to defend infanticide, one has to get very clear about what makes something a person, what gives something a right to life.

One of the interesting ways in which the abortion issue differs from most other moral issues is that the plausible positions on abortion appear to be extreme positions. For if a human fetus is a person, one is inclined to say that, in general, one would be justified in killing it only to save the life of the mother.[2] Such is the extreme conservative position.[3] On the other hand, if the fetus is not a person, how can it be seriously wrong to destroy it? Why would one need to point to special circumstances to justify such action? The upshot is that there is no room for a moderate position on the issue of abortion such as one finds, for example, in the Model Penal Code recommendations.[4]

Aside from the light it may shed on the abortion question, the issue of infanticide is both interesting and important in its own right. The theoretical interest has been mentioned: it forces one to face up to the question of what makes something a person. The practical importance need not be labored. Most people would prefer to raise children who do not suffer from gross deformities or from severe physical, emotional, or intellectual handicaps. If it could be shown that there is no moral objection to infanticide the happiness of society could be significantly and justifiably increased.

Infanticide is also of interest because of the strong emotions it arouses. The typical reaction to infanticide is like the reaction to incest or cannibalism, or the reaction of previous generations to masturbation or oral sex. The response, rather than appealing to carefully formulated moral principles, is primarily visceral. When philosophers themselves respond in this way, offering no arguments, and dismissing infanticide out of hand, it is reasonable to suspect that one is dealing with a taboo rather than with a rational prohibition.[5] I shall attempt to show that this is in fact the case.

II. TERMINOLOGY: "PERSON" VERSUS "HUMAN BEING"

How is the term "person" to be interpreted? I shall treat the concept of a person as a purely moral concept, free of all descriptive content. Specifically, in my usage the sentence "X is a person" will be synonymous with the sentence "X has a (serious) moral right to life."

This usage diverges slightly from what is perhaps the more common way of interpreting the term "person" when it is employed as a purely moral term, where to say that X is a person is to say that X has rights. If everything that had rights had a right to life, these interpretations would be extensionally equivalent. But I am inclined to think that it does not follow from acceptable moral principles that whatever has any rights at all has a right to life. My reason is this. Given the choice between being killed and being tortured for an hour, most adult humans would surely choose the latter. So it seems plausible to say it is worse to kill an adult human being than it is to torture him for an hour. In contrast, it seems to me that while it is not seriously wrong to kill a newborn kitten, it is seriously wrong to torture one for an hour. This *suggests* that newborn kittens may have a right not to be tortured without having a serious right to life. For it seems to be true that an individual has a right to something whenever it is the case that, if he wants that thing, it would be wrong for others to deprive him of it. Then if it is wrong to inflict a certain sensation upon a kitten if it doesn't want to experience that sensation, it will follow that the kitten has a right not to have that sensation inflicted upon it.[6] I shall return to this example later. My point here is merely that it provides some reason for holding that it does not follow from acceptable moral principles that if something has any rights at all, it has a serious right to life.

There has been a tendency in recent discussions of abortion to use expressions such as "person" and "human being" interchangeably. B. A. Brody, for example, refers to the difficulty of determining "whether destroying the foetus constitutes the taking of a human life," and suggests it is very plausible that "the taking of a human life is an action that has bad consequences for him whose life is being taken."[7] When Brody refers to something as a human life he apparently construes this as entailing that the thing is a person. For if every living organism belonging to the species homo sapiens counted as a human life, there would be no difficulty in determining whether a fetus inside a human mother was a human life.

The same tendency is found in Judith Jarvis Thomson's article, which opens with the statement: "Most opposition to abortion relies on the premise that the fetus is a human being, a person, from the moment of conception."[8] The same is true of Roger Wertheimer, who explicitly says: "First off I should note that the expression 'a human life,' 'a human being,' 'a person' are virtually interchangeable in this context."[9]

The tendency to use expressions like "person" and "human being" interchangeably is an unfortunate one. For one thing, it tends to lend covert support to antiabortionist positions. Given such usage, one who holds a liberal view of abortion is put in the position of maintaining that fetuses, at least up to a certain point, are not human beings. Even philosophers are led astray by this usage. Thus Wertheimer says that "except for monstrosities, every member of our species is indubitably a person, a human being, at the very latest at birth."[10] Is it really *indubitable* that newborn babies are persons? Surely this is a wild contention. Wertheimer is falling prey to the confusion naturally engendered by the practice of using "person" and "human being" interchangeably. Another example of this is provided by Thomson: "I am inclined to think also that we shall probably have to agree that the fetus has already become a human person well before birth. Indeed, it comes as a surprise when one first learns how early in its life it begins to acquire human characteristics. By the tenth week, for example, it already has a face, arms and legs, fingers and toes; it has internal organs, and brain activity is detectable."[11] But what do such physiological characteristics have to do with the question of whether the organism is a person? Thomson, partly, I think, because of the unfortunate use of terminology, does not even raise this question. As a result she virtually takes it for granted that there are some cases in which abortion is "positively indecent."[12]

There is a second reason why using "person" and "human being" interchangeably is unhappy philosophically. If one says that the dispute between pro- and anti-abortionists centers on whether the fetus is a human, it is natural to conclude that it is essentially a disagreement about certain facts, a disagreement about what properties a fetus possesses. Thus Wertheimer says that "if one insists on using the raggy fact-value distinction, then one ought to say that the dispute is over a matter of fact in the sense in which it is a fact that the Negro slaves were human beings."[13] I shall argue that the two cases are not parallel, and that in the case of abortion what is primarily at stake is what moral principles one should accept. If one says that the central issue between conservatives and liberals in the abortion question is whether the fetus is a person, it is clear that the dispute may be either about what properties a thing must have in order to be a person, in order to have a right to life—a moral question—or about whether a fetus at a given stage of development as a matter of fact possesses the properties in question. The temptation to suppose that the disagreement must be a factual one is removed.

It should now be clear why the common practice of using expressions such as "person" and "human being" interchangeably in discussions of abortion is unfortunate. It would perhaps be best to avoid the term "human" altogether, employing instead some expression that is more naturally interpreted as referring to a certain type of biological organism characterized in physiological terms, such as "member of the species Homo sapiens." My own approach will be to use the term "human" only in contexts where it is not philosophically dangerous.

III. THE BASIC ISSUE: WHEN IS A MEMBER OF THE SPECIES HOMO SAPIENS A PERSON?

Settling the issue of the morality of abortion and infanticide will involve answering the following questions: What properties must something have to be a person, i.e., to have a serious right to life? At what point in the development of a member of the species Homo sapiens does the organism possess the properties that make it a person? The first question raises a moral issue. To answer it is to decide what basic[14] moral principles involving the ascription of a right to life one ought to accept. The second question raises a purely factual issue, since the properties in question are properties of a purely descriptive sort.

Some writers seem quite pessimistic about the possibility of resolving the question of the morality of abortion. Indeed, some have gone so far as to suggest that the question of whether the fetus is a person is in principle unanswerable: "we seem to be stuck with the indeterminateness of the fetus' humanity."[15] An understanding of some of the sources of this pessimism will, I think, help us to tackle the problem. Let us begin by considering the similarity a number of people have noted between the issue of abortion and the issue of Negro slavery. The question here is why it should be more difficult to decide whether abortion and infanticide are acceptable than it was to decide whether slavery was acceptable. The answer seems to be that in the case of slavery there are moral principles of a quite uncontroversial sort that settle the issue. Thus most people would agree to some such principle as the following: No organism that has experiences, that is capable of thought and of using language, and that has harmed no one, should be made a slave. In the case of abortion, on the other hand, conditions that are generally agreed to be sufficient grounds for ascribing a right to life to something do not suffice to settle the issue. It is easy to specify other, purportedly sufficient conditions that will settle the issue, but no one has been successful in putting forward considerations that will convince others to accept those additional moral principles.

I do not share the general pessimism about the possibility of resolving the issue of abortion and infanticide because I believe it is possible to point to a very plausible moral principle dealing with the question of *necessary* conditions for something's having a right to life, where the conditions in question will provide an answer to the question of the permissibility of abortion and infanticide.

There is a second cause of pessimism that should be noted before proceeding. It is tied up with the fact that the development of an organism is one of gradual and continuous change. Given this continuity, how is one to draw a line at one point and declare it permissible to destroy a member of Homo sapiens up to, but not beyond, that point? Won't there be an arbitrariness about any point that is chosen? I will return to this worry shortly. It does not present a serious difficulty once the basic moral principles relevant to the ascription of a right to life to an individual are established.

Let us turn now to the first and most fundamental question: What properties must something have in order to be a person, i.e., to have a serious right to life? The claim I wish to defend is this: An organism possesses a serious right to life only if it possesses the concept of a self as a continuing subject of experiences and other mental states, and believes that it is itself such a continuing entity.

My basic argument in support of this claim, which I will call the self-consciousness requirement, will be clearest, I think, if I first offer a simplified version of the argument, and then consider a modification that seems desirable. The simplified version of my argument is this. To ascribe a right to an individual is to assert something about the prima facie obligations of other individuals to act, or to refrain from acting, in certain ways. However, the obligations in question are conditional ones, being dependent upon the existence of certain desires of the individual to whom the right is ascribed. Thus if an individual asks one to destroy something to which he has a right, one does not violate his right to that thing if one proceeds to destroy it. This suggests the following analysis: "A has a right to X" is roughly synonymous with "If A desires X, then others are under a prima facie obligation to refrain from actions that would deprive him of it."[16]

Although this analysis is initially plausible, there are reasons for thinking it not entirely correct. I will consider these later. Even here, however, some expansion is necessary, since there are features of the concept of a right that are important in the present context, and that ought to be dealt with more explicitly. In particular, it seems to be a conceptual truth that things that lack consciousness, such as ordinary machines, cannot have rights. Does this conceptual truth follow from the above analysis of the concept of a right? The answer depends on how the term "desire" is interpreted. If one adopts a completely behavioristic interpretation of "desire," so that a machine that searches for an electrical outlet in order to get its batteries recharged is described as having a desire to be recharged, then it will not follow

from this analysis that objects that lack consciousness cannot have rights. On the other hand, if "desire" is interpreted in such a way that desires are states necessarily standing in some sort of relationship to states of consciousness, it will follow from the analysis that a machine that is not capable of being conscious, and consequently of having desires, cannot have any rights. I think those who defend analyses of the concept of a right along the lines of this one do have in mind an interpretation of the term "desire" that involves reference to something more than behavioral dispositions. However, rather than relying on this, it seems preferable to make such an interpretation explicit. The following analysis is a natural way of doing that: "A has a right to X" is roughly synonymous with "A is the sort of thing that is a subject of experiences and other mental states, A is capable of desiring X, and if A does desire X, then others are under a prima facie obligation to refrain from actions that would deprive him of it."

The next step in the argument is basically a matter of applying this analysis to the concept of a right to life. Unfortunately the expression "right to life" is not entirely a happy one, since it suggests that the right in question concerns the continued existence of a biological organism. That this is incorrect can be brought out by considering possible ways of violating an individual's right to life. Suppose, for example, that by some technology of the future the brain of an adult human were to be completely reprogrammed, so that the organism wound up with memories (or rather, apparent memories), beliefs, attitudes, and personality traits completely different from those associated with it before it was subjected to reprogramming. In such a case one would surely say that an individual had been destroyed, that an adult human's right to life had been violated, even though no biological organism had been killed. This example shows that the expression "right to life" is misleading, since what one is really concerned about is not just the continued existence of a biological organism, but the right of a subject of experiences and other mental states to continue to exist.

Given this more precise description of the right with which we are here concerned, we are now in a position to apply the analysis of the concept of a right stated above. When we do so we find that the statement ''A has a right to continue to exist as a subject of experiences and other mental states'' is roughly synonymous with the statement ''A is a subject of experiences and other mental states, A is capable of desiring to continue to exist as a subject of experiences and other mental states, and if A does desire to continue to exist as such an entity, then others are under a prima facie obligation not to prevent him from doing so.''

The final stage in the argument is simply a matter of asking what must be the case if something is to be capable of having a desire to continue existing as a subject of experiences and other mental states. The basic point here is that the desires a thing can have are limited by the concepts it possesses. For the fundamental way of describing a given desire is as a desire that a certain proposition be true.[17] Then, since one cannot desire that a certain proposition be true unless one understands it, and since one cannot understand it without possessing the concepts involved in it, it follows that the desires one can have are limited by the concepts one possesses. Applying this to the present case results in the conclusion that an entity cannot be the sort of thing that can desire that a subject of experiences and other mental states exist unless it possesses the concept of such a subject. Moreover, an entity cannot desire that it itself *continue* existing as a subject of experiences and other mental states unless it believes that it is now such a subject. This completes the justification of the claim that it is a necessary condition of something's having a serious right to life that it possess the concept of a self as a continuing subject of experiences, and that it believe that it is itself such an entity.

Let us now consider a modification in the above argument that seems desirable. This modification concerns the crucial conceptual claim advanced about the relationship between ascription of rights and ascription of the corresponding desires. Certain situations suggest that there may be exceptions to the claim that if a person doesn't desire something, one cannot violate his right to it. There are three types of situations that call this claim into question: (i) situations in which an individual's desires

reflect a state of emotional disturbance; (ii) situations in which a previously conscious individual is temporarily unconscious; (iii) situations in which an individual's desires have been distorted by conditioning or by indoctrination.

As an example of the first, consider a case in which an adult human falls into a state of depression which his psychiatrist recognizes as temporary. While in the state he tells people he wishes he were dead. His psychiatrist, accepting the view that there can be no violation of an individual's right to life unless the individual has a desire to live, decides to let his patient have his way and kills him. Or consider a related case in which one person gives another a drug that produces a state of temporary depression; the recipient expresses a wish that he were dead. The person who administered the drug then kills him. Doesn't one want to say in both these cases that the agent did something seriously wrong in killing the other person? And isn't the reason the action was seriously wrong in each case the fact that it violated the individual's right to life? If so, the right to life cannot be linked with a desire to live in the way claimed above.

The second set of situations are ones in which an individual is unconscious for some reason—that is, he is sleeping, or drugged, or in a temporary coma. Does an individual in such a state have any desires? People do sometimes say that an unconscious individual wants something, but it might be argued that if such talk is not to be simply false it must be interpreted as actually referring to the desires the individual *would* have if he were now conscious. Consequently, if the analysis of the concept of a right proposed above were correct, it would follow that one does not violate an individual's right if one takes his car, or kills him, while he is asleep.

Finally, consider situations in which an individual's desires have been distorted, either by inculcation or irrational beliefs or by direct conditioning. Thus an individual may permit someone to kill him because he has been convinced that if he allows himself to be sacrificed to the gods he will be gloriously rewarded in a life to come. Or an individual may be enslaved after first having been conditioned to desire a life of slavery. Doesn't one want to say that in the former case an individual's right to life has been violated, and in the latter his right to freedom?

Situations such as these strongly suggest that even if an individual doesn't want something, it is still possible to violate his right to it. Some modification of the earlier account of the concept of a right thus seems in order. The analysis given covers, I believe, the paradigmatic cases of violation of an individual's rights, but there are other, secondary cases where one also wants to say that someone's right has been violated which are not included.

Precisely how the revised analysis should be formulated is unclear. Here it will be sufficient merely to say that, in view of the above, an individual's right to X can be violated not only when he desires X, but also when he *would* now desire X were it not for one of the following: (i) he is in an emotionally unbalanced state; (ii) he is temporarily unconscious; (iii) he has been conditioned to desire the absence of X.

The critical point now is that, even given this extension of the conditions under which an individual's right to something can be violated, it is still true that one's right to something can be violated only when one has the conceptual capability of desiring the thing in question. For example, an individual who would now desire not to be a slave if he weren't emotionally unbalanced, or if he weren't temporarily unconscious, or if he hadn't previously been conditioned to want to be a slave, must possess the concepts involved in the desire not to be a slave. Since it is really only the conceptual capability presupposed by the desire to continue existing as a subject of experiences and other mental states, and not the desire itself, that enters into the above argument, the modification required in the account of the conditions under which an individual's rights can be violated does not undercut my defense of the self-consciousness requirement.[18]

To sum up, my argument has been that having a right to life presupposes that one is capable of desiring to continue existing as a subject of experiences and other mental states. This in turn presupposes both that one has the concept of such a continuing entity and that one believes that one is oneself such an entity. So an entity that lacks such a consciousness of itself as a con-

tinuing subject of mental states does not have a right to life.

It would be natural to ask at this point whether satisfaction of this requirement is not only necessary but also sufficient to ensure that a thing has a right to life. I am inclined to an affirmative answer. However, the issue is not urgent in the present context, since as long as the requirement is in fact a necessary one we have the basis of an adequate defense of abortion and infanticide. If an organism must satisfy some other condition before it has a serious right to life, the result will merely be that the interval during which infanticide is morally permissible may be somewhat longer. Although the point at which an organism first achieves self-consciousness and hence the capacity of desiring to continue existing as a subject of experiences and other mental states may be a theoretically incorrect cutoff point, it is at least a morally safe one: any error it involves is on the side of caution.

IV. SOME CRITICAL COMMENTS ON ALTERNATIVE PROPOSALS

I now want to compare the line of demarcation I am proposing with the cutoff points traditionally advanced in discussions of abortion. My fundamental claim will be that none of these cutoff points can be defended by appeal to plausible, basic moral principles. The main suggestions as to the point past which it is seriously wrong to destroy something that will develop into an adult member of the species Homo sapiens are these: (a) conception; (b) the attainment of human form; (c) the achievement of the ability to move about spontaneously; (d) viability; (e) birth.[19] The corresponding moral principles suggested by these cutoff points are as follows: (1) It is seriously wrong to kill an organism, from a zygote on, that belongs to the species Homo sapiens. (2) It is seriously wrong to kill an organism that belongs to Homo sapiens and that has achieved human form. (3) It is seriously wrong to kill an organism that is a member of Homo sapiens and that is capable of spontaneous movement. (4) It is seriously wrong to kill an organism that belongs to Homo sapiens and that is capable of existing outside the womb. (5) It is seriously wrong to kill an organism that is a member of Homo sapiens that is no longer in the womb.

My first comment is that it would not do *simply* to omit the reference to membership in the species Homo sapiens from the above principles, with the exception of principle (2). For then the principles would be applicable to animals in general, and one would be forced to conclude that it was seriously wrong to abort a cat fetus, or that it was seriously wrong to abort a motile cat fetus, and so on.

The second and crucial comment is that none of the five principles given above can plausibly be viewed as a *basic* moral principle. To accept any of them as such would be akin to accepting as a basic moral principle the proposition that it is morally permissible to enslave black members of the species Homo sapiens but not white members. Why should it be seriously wrong to kill an unborn member of the species Homo sapiens but not seriously wrong to kill an unborn kitten? Difference in species is not per se a morally relevant difference. If one holds that it is seriously wrong to kill an unborn member of the species Homo sapiens but not an unborn kitten, one should be prepared to point to some property that is morally significant and that is possessed by unborn members of Homo sapiens but not by unborn kittens. Similarly, such a property must be identified if one believes it seriously wrong to kill unborn members of Homo sapiens that have achieved viability but not seriously wrong to kill unborn kittens that have achieved that state.

What property might account for such a difference? That is to say, what *basic* moral principles might a person who accepts one of these five principles appeal to in support of his secondary moral judgment? Why should events such as the achievement of human form, or the achievement of the ability to move about, or the achievement of viability, or birth serve to endow something with a right to life? What the liberal must do is to show that these events involve changes, or are associated with changes, that are morally relevant.

Let us now consider reasons why the events involved in cutoff points (b) through (e) are not morally relevant, beginning with the last two: viability and birth. The fact that an organism is not physiologically dependent upon another organism, or is capable of such physiological independence, is surely irrelevant to whether the organism has a right to life. In defense of this contention, consider a speculative case where a fetus is able to learn a language while in the womb. One would surely not say that the fetus had no right to life until it emerged from the womb, or until it was capable of existing outside the womb. A less speculative example is the case of Siamese twins who have learned to speak. One doesn't want to say that since one of the twins would die were the two to be separated, it therefore has no right to life. Consequently it seems difficult to disagree with the conservative's claim that an organism which lacks a right to life before birth or before becoming viable cannot acquire this right immediately upon birth or upon becoming viable.

This does not, however, completely rule out viability as a line of demarcation. For instead of defending viability as a cutoff point on the ground that only then does a fetus acquire a right to life, it is possible to argue rather that when when one organism is physiologically dependent upon another, the former's right to life may conflict with the latter's right to use its body as it will, and moreover, that the latter's right to do what it wants with its body may often take precedence over the other organism's right to life. Thomson has defended this view: "I am arguing only that having a right to life does not guarantee having either a right to the use of or a right to be allowed continued use of another person's body—even if one needs it for life itself. So the right to life will not serve the opponents of abortion in the very simple and clear way in which they seem to have thought it would."[20] I believe that Thomson is right in contending that philosophers have been altogether too casual in assuming that if one grants the fetus a serious right to life, one must accept a conservative position on abortion.[21] I also think the only defense of viability as a cutoff point which has any hope of success at all is one based on the considerations she advances. I doubt very much, however, that this defense of abortion is ultimately tenable. I think that one can grant even stronger assumptions than those made by Thomson and still argue persuasively for a semiconservative view. What I have in mind is this. Let it be granted, for the sake of argument, that a woman's right to free her body of parasites which will inhibit her freedom of action and possibly impair her health is stronger than the parasite's right to life, and is so even if the parasite has as much right to life as an adult human. One can still argue that abortion ought not to be permitted. For if A's right is stronger than B's, and it is impossible to satisfy both, it does not follow that A's should be satisfied rather than B's. It may be possible to compensate A if his right isn't satisfied, but impossible to compensate B if his right isn't satisfied. In such a case the best thing to do may be to satisfy B's claim and to compensate A. Abortion may be a case in point. If the fetus has a right to life and the right is not satisfied, there is certainly no way the fetus can be compensated. On the other hand, if the woman's right to rid her body of harmful and annoying parasites is not satisfied, she can be compensated. Thus it would seem that the just thing to do would be to prohibit abortion, but to compensate women for the burden of carrying a parasite to term. Then, however, we are back at a (modified) conservative position.[22] Our conclusion must be that it appears unlikely there is any satisfactory defense either of viability or of birth as cutoff points.

Let us now consider the third suggested line of demarcation, the achievement of the power to move about spontaneously. It might be argued that acquiring this power is a morally relevant event on the grounds that there is a connection between the concept of an agent and the concept of a person, and being motile is an indication that a thing is an agent.[23]

It is difficult to respond to this suggestion unless it is made more specific. Given that one's interest here is in defending a certain cutoff point, it is natural to interpret the proposal as suggesting that motility is a necessary condition of an organism's having a right to life. But this won't do, because one certainly wants to ascribe a right to life to adult humans who are completely paralyzed. Maybe the suggestion is rather that motility is a sufficient condition of something's having a right to life. However, it is clear that motility alone is not sufficient, since this would imply that all animals, and also certain machines, have a right to life. Perhaps,

then, the most reasonable interpretation of the claim is that motility together with some other property is a sufficient condition of something's having a right to life, where the other property will have to be a property possessed by unborn members of the species Homo sapiens but not by unborn members of other familiar species.

The central question, then, is what this other property is. Until one is told, it is very difficult to evaluate either the moral claim that motility together with that property is a sufficient basis for ascribing to an organism a right to life or the factual claim that a motile human fetus possesses that property while a motile fetus belonging to some other species does not. A conservative would presumably reject motility as a cutoff point by arguing that whether an organism has a right to life depends only upon its potentialities, which are of course not changed by its becoming motile. If, on the other hand, one favors a liberal view of abortion, I think that one can attack this third suggested cutoff point, in its unspecified form, only by determining what properties are necessary, or what properties sufficient, for an individual to have a right to life. Thus I would base my rejection of motility as a cutoff point on my claim, defended above, that a necessary condition of an organism's possessing a right to life is that it conceive of itself as a continuing subject of experiences and other mental states.

The second suggested cutoff point—the development of a recognizably human form— can be dismissed fairly quickly. I have already remarked that membership in a particular species is not itself a morally relevant property. For it is obvious that if we encountered other "rational animals," such as Martians, the fact that their physiological makeup was very different from our own would not be grounds for denying them a right to life.[24] Similarly, it is clear that the development of human form is not in itself a morally relevant event. Nor do there seem to be any grounds for holding that there is some other change, associated with this event, that is morally relevant. The appeal of this second cutoff point is, I think, purely emotional.

The overall conclusion seems to be that it is very difficult to defend the cutoff points traditionally advanced by those who advocate either a moderate or a liberal position on abortion. The reason is that there do not seem to be any basic moral principles one can appeal to in support of the cutoff points in question. We must now consider whether the conservative is any better off.

V. REFUTATION OF THE CONSERVATIVE POSITION

Many have felt that the conservative's position is more defensible than the liberal's because the conservative can point to the gradual and continuous development of an organism as it changes from a zygote to an adult human being. He is then in a position to argue that it is morally arbitrary for the liberal to draw a line at some point in this continuous process and to say that abortion is permissible before, but not after, that particular point. The liberal's reply would presumably be that the emphasis upon the continuity of the process is misleading. What the conservative is really doing is simply challenging the liberal to specify the properties a thing must have in order to be a person, and to show that the developing organism does acquire the properties at the point selected by the liberal. The liberal may then reply that the difficulty he has meeting this challenge should not be taken as grounds for rejecting his position. For the conservative cannot meet this challenge either; the conservative is equally unable to say what properties something must have if it is to have a right to life.

Although this rejoinder does not dispose of the conservative's argument, it is not without bite. For defenders of the view that abortion is always wrong have failed to face up to the question of the basic moral principles on which their position rests. They have been content to assert the wrongness of killing any organism, from a zygote on, if that organism is a member of the species Homo sapiens. But they have overlooked the point that this cannot be an acceptable *basic* moral principle, since differences in species is not in itself a morally relevant difference. The conservative can reply, however, that it is possible to defend his position—but not the liberal's—*without* getting clear about the properties a thing must possess if it is to have a

right to life. The conservative's defense will rest upon the following two claims: first, that there is a property, even if one is unable to specify what it is, that (i) is possessed by adult humans, and (ii) endows any organism possessing it with a serious right to life. Second that if there are properties which satisfy (i) and (ii) above, at least one of those properties will be such that any organism potentially possessing that property has a serious right to life even now, simply by virtue of that potentiality, where an organism possesses a property potentially if it will come to have that property in the normal course of its development. The second claim— which I shall refer to as the potentiality principle—is critical to the conservative's defense. Because of it he is able to defend his position without deciding what properties a thing must possess in order to have a right to life. It is enough to know that adult members of Homo sapiens do have such a right. For then one can conclude that any organism which belongs to the species Homo sapiens, from a zygote on, must also have a right to life by virtue of the potentiality principle.

The liberal, by contrast, cannot mount a comparable argument. He cannot defend his position without offering at least a partial answer to the question of what properties a thing must possess in order to have a right to life.

The importance of the potentiality principle, however, goes beyond the fact that it provides support for the conservative's position. If the principle is unacceptable, then so is his position. For if the conservative cannot defend the view that an organism's having certain potentialities is sufficient grounds for ascribing to it a right to life, his claim that a fetus which is a member of Homo sapiens has a right to life can be attacked as follows. The reason an adult member of Homo sapiens has a right to life, but an infant ape does not, is that there are certain psychological properties which the former possesses and the latter lacks. Now, even if one is unsure exactly what these psychological properties are, it is clear that an organism in the early stages of development from a zygote into an adult member of Homo sapiens does not possess these properties. One need merely compare a human fetus with an ape fetus. What mental states does the former enjoy that the latter does not? Surely it is reasonable to hold that there are no significant differences in their respective mental lives—assuming that one wishes to ascribe any mental states at all to such organisms. (Does a zygote have a mental life? Does it have experiences? Or beliefs? Or desires?) There are, of course, physiological differences, but these are not in themselves morally significant. *If* one held that potentialities were relevant to the ascription of a right to life, one could argue that the physiological differences, though not morally significant in themselves, are morally significant by virtue of their causal consequences they will lead to later psychological differences that are morally relevant, and for this reason the physiological differences are themselves morally significant. But if the potentiality principle is not available, this line of argument cannot be used, and there will then be no differences between a human fetus and an ape fetus that the conservative can use as grounds for ascribing a serious right to life to the former but not to the latter.

It is therefore tempting to conclude that the conservative view of abortion is acceptable if and only if the potentiality principle is acceptable. But to say that the conservative position can be defended if the potentiality principle is acceptable is to assume that the argument is over once it is granted that the fetus has a right to life, and, as was noted above, Thomson has shown that there are serious grounds for questioning this assumption. In any case, the important point here is that the conservative position on abortion is acceptable *only if* the potentiality principle is sound.

One way to attack the potentiality principle is simply to argue in support of the self-consciousness requirement—the claim that only an organism that conceives of itself as a continuing subject of experiences has a right to life. For this requirement, when taken together with the claim that there is at least one property, possessed by adult humans, such that any organism possessing it has a serious right to life, entails the denial of the potentiality principle. Or at least this is so if we add the uncontroversial empirical claim that an organism that will in the normal course of events develop into an

adult human does not from the very beginning of its existence possess a concept of a continuing subject of experiences together with a belief that it is itself such an entity.

I think it best, however, to scrutinize the potentiality principle itself, and not to base one's case against it simply on the self-consciousness requirement. Perhaps the first point to note is that the potentiality principle should not be confused with principles such as the following: the value of an object is related to the value of the things into which it can develop. This "valuation principle" is rather vague. There are ways of making it more precise, but we need not consider these here. Suppose now that one were to speak not of a right to life, but of the value of life. It would then be easy to make the mistake of thinking that the valuation principle was relevant to the potentiality principle—indeed, that it entailed it. But an individual's right to life is not based on the value of his life. To say that the world would be better off if it contained fewer people is not to say that it would be right to achieve such a better world by killing some of the present inhabitants. *If* having a right to life were a matter of a thing's value, then a thing's potentialities, being connected with its expected value, would clearly be relevant to the question of what rights it had. Conversely, once one realizes that a thing's rights are not a matter of its value, I think it becomes clear that an organism's potentialities are irrelevant to the question of whether it has a right to life.

But let us now turn to the task of finding a direct refutation of the potentiality principle. The basic issue is this. Is there any property J which satisfies the following conditions: (1) There is a property K such that any individual possessing property K has a right to life, and there is a scientific law L to the effect that any organism possessing property J will in the normal course of events come to possess property K at some later time. (2) Given the relationship between property J and property K just described, anything possessing property J has a right to life. (3) If property J were not related to property K in the way indicated, it would not be the case that anything possessing property J thereby had a right to life. In short, the question is whether there is a property J that bestows a right to life on an organism *only because* J stands in a certain causal relationship to a second property K, which is such that anything possessing that property ipso facto has a right to life.

My argument turns upon the following critical principle: Let C be a causal process that normally leads to outcome E. Let A be an action that initiates process C, and B be an action involving a minimal expenditure of energy that stops process C before outcome E occurs. Assume further that actions A and B do not have any other consequences, and that E is the only morally significant outcome of process C. Then there is no moral difference between intentionally performing action B and intentionally refraining from performing action A, assuming identical motivation in both cases. This principle, which I shall refer to as the moral symmetry principle with respect to action and inaction, would be rejected by some philosophers. They would argue that there is an important distinction to be drawn between "what we owe people in the form of aid and what we owe them in the way of noninterference."[25] and that the latter, "negative duties," are duties that it is more serious to neglect than the former, "positive" ones. This view arises from an intuitive response to examples such as the following. Even if it is wrong not to send food to starving people in other parts of the world, it is more wrong still to kill someone. And isn't the conclusion, then, that one's obligation to refrain from killing someone is a more serious obligation than one's obligation to save lives?

I want to argue that this is not the correct conclusion. I think it is tempting to draw this conclusion if one fails to consider the motivation that is likely to be associated with the respective actions. If someone performs an action he knows will kill someone else, this will usually be grounds for concluding that he wanted to kill the person in question. In contrast, failing to help someone may indicate only apathy, laziness, selfishness, or an amoral outlook: the fact that a person knowingly allows another to die will not normally be grounds for concluding that he desired that person's death.

Someone who knowingly kills another is more likely to be seriously defective from a moral point of view than someone who fails to save another's life.

If we are not to be led to false conclusions by our intuitions about certain cases, we must explicitly assume identical motivations in the two situations. Compare, for example, the following: (1) Jones sees that Smith will be killed by a bomb unless he warns him. Jones's reaction is: "How lucky, it will save me the trouble of killing Smith myself." So Jones allows Smith to be killed by the bomb, even though he could easily have warned him. (2) Jones wants Smith dead, and therefore shoots him. Is one to say there is a significant difference between the wrongness of Jones's behavior in these two cases? Surely not. This shows the mistake of drawing a distinction between positive duties and negative duties and holding that the latter impose stricter obligations than the former. The difference in our intuitions about situations that involve giving aid to others and corresponding situations that involve not interfering with others is to be explained by reference to probable differences in the motivations operating in the two situations, and not by reference to a distinction between positive and negative duties. For once it is specified that the motivation is the same in the two situations, we realize that inaction is as wrong in the one case as action is in the other.

There is another point that may be relevant. Action involves effort, while inaction usually does not. It usually does not require any effort on my part to refrain from killing someone, but saving someone's life will require an expenditure of energy. One must then ask how large a sacrifice a person is morally required to make to save the life of another. If the sacrifice of time and energy is quite large it may be that one is not morally obliged to save the life of another in that situation. Superficial reflection upon such cases might easily lead us to introduce the distinction between positive and negative duties, but again it is clear that this would be a mistake. The point is not that one has a greater duty to refrain from killing others than to perform positive actions that will save them. It is rather that positive actions require effort, and this means that in deciding what to do a person has to take into account his own right to do what he wants with his life, and not only the other person's right to life. To avoid this confusion, we should confine ourselves to comparisons between situations in which the positive action involves minimal effort.

The moral symmetry principle, as formulated above, explicitly takes these two factors into account. It applies only to pairs of situations in which the motivations are identical and the positive action involves minimal effort. Without these restrictions, the principle would be open to serious objection; with them, it seems perfectly acceptable. For the central objection to it rests on the claim that we must distinguish positive from negative duties and recognize that negative duties impose stronger obligations than positive ones. I have tried to show how this claim derives from an unsound account of our moral intuitions about certain situations.

My argument against the potentiality principle can now be stated. Suppose at some future time a chemical were to be discovered which when injected into the brain of a kitten would cause the kitten to develop into a cat possessing a brain of the sort possessed by humans, and consequently into a cat having all the psychological capabilities characteristic of adult humans. Such cats would be able to think, to use language, and so on. Now it would surely be morally indefensible in such a situation to ascribe a serious right to life to members of the species Homo sapiens without also ascribing it to cats that have undergone such a process of development: there would be no morally significant differences.

Secondly, it would not be seriously wrong to refrain from injecting a newborn kitten with the special chemical, and to kill it instead. The fact that one could initiate a causal process that would transform a kitten into an entity that would eventually possess properties such that anything possessing them ipso facto has a serious right to life does not mean that the kitten has a serious right to life even before it has been subjected to the process of injection and transformation. The possibility of transforming kittens into persons will not make it any more wrong to kill newborn kittens than it is now.

Thirdly, in view of the symmetry principle,

if it is not seriously wrong to refrain from initiating such a causal process, neither is it seriously wrong to interfere with such a process. Suppose a kitten is accidentally injected with a chemical. As long as it has not yet developed those properties that in themselves endow something with a right to life, there cannot be anything wrong with interfering with the causal process and preventing the development of the properties in question. Such interference might be accomplished either by injecting the kitten with some "neutralizing" chemical or simply by killing it.

But if it is not seriously wrong to destroy an injected kitten which will naturally develop the properties that bestow a right to life, neither can it be seriously wrong to destroy a member of Homo sapiens which lacks such properties, but will naturally come to have them. The potentialities are the same in both cases. The only difference is that in the case of a human fetus the potentialities have been present from the beginning of the organism's development, while in the case of the kitten they have been present only from the time it was injected with the special chemical. This difference in the time at which the potentialities were acquired is a morally irrelevant difference.

It should be emphasized that I am not here assuming that a human fetus does not possess properties which in themselves, and irrespective of their causal relationships to other properties, provide grounds for ascribing a right to life to whatever possesses them. The point is merely that if it is seriously wrong to kill something, the reason cannot be that the thing will later acquire properties that in themselves provide something with a right to life.

Finally, it is reasonable to believe that there are properties possessed by adult members of Homo sapiens which establish their right to life, and also that any normal human fetus will come to possess those properties shared by adult humans. But it has just been shown that if it is wrong to kill a human fetus, it cannot be because of its potentialities. One is therefore forced to conclude that the conservative's potentiality principle is false.

In short, anyone who wants to defend the potentiality principle must either argue against the moral symmetry principle or hold that in a world in which kittens could be transformed into ''rational animals'' it would be seriously wrong to kill newborn kittens. It is hard to believe there is much to be said for the latter moral claim. Consequently one expects the conservative's rejoinder to be directed against the symmetry principle. While I have not attempted to provide a thorough defense of that principle, I have tried to show that what seems to be the most important objection to it—the one that appeals to a distinction between positive and negative duties—is based on a superficial analysis of our moral intuitions. I believe that a more thorough examination of the symmetry principle would show it to be sound. If so, we should reject the potentiality principle, and the conservative position on abortion as well.

VI. SUMMARY AND CONCLUSIONS

Let us return now to my basic claim, the self-consciousness requirement: An organism possesses a serious right to life only if it possesses the concept of a self as a continuing subject of experiences and other mental states, and believes that it is itself such a continuing entity. My defense of this claim has been twofold. I have offered a direct argument in support of it, and I have tried to show that traditional conservative and liberal views on abortion and infanticide, which involve a rejection of it, are unsound. I now want to mention one final reason why my claim should be accepted. Consider the example mentioned in section II—that of killing, as opposed to torturing, newborn kittens. I suggested there that while in the case of adult humans most people would consider it worse to kill an individual than to torture him for an hour, we do not usually view the killing of a newborn kitten as morally outrageous, although we would regard someone who tortured a newborn kitten for an hour as heinously evil. I pointed out that a possible conclusion that might be drawn from this is that newborn kittens have a right not to be tortured, but do not have a serious right to life. If this is the correct conclusion, how is one to explain it? One merit of the self-consciousness requirement is that it provides an explanation of this situation. The

reason a newborn kitten does not have a right to life is explained by the fact that it does not possess the concept of a self. But how is one to explain the kitten's having a right not to be tortured? The answer is that a desire not to suffer pain can be ascribed to something without assuming that it has any concept of a continuing self. For while something that lacks the concept of a self cannot desire that a self not suffer, it can desire that a given sensation not exist. The state desired—the absence of a particular sensation, or of sensations of a certain sort—can be described in a purely phenomenalistic language, and hence without the concept of a continuing self. So long as the newborn kitten possesses the relevant phenomenal concepts, it can truly be said to desire that a certain sensation not exist. So we can ascribe to it a right not to be tortured even though, since it lacks the concept of a continuing self, we cannot ascribe to it a right to life.

This completes my discussion of the basic moral principles involved in the issue of abortion and infanticide. But I want to comment upon an important factual question, namely, at what point an organism comes to possess the concept of a self as a continuing subject of experiences and other mental states, together with the belief that it is itself such a continuing entity. This is obviously a matter for detailed psychological investigation, but everyday observation makes it perfectly clear, I believe, that a newborn baby does not possess the concept of a continuing self, any more than a newborn kitten possesses such a concept. If so, infanticide during a time interval shortly after birth must be morally acceptable.

But where is the line to be drawn? What is the cutoff point? If one maintained, as some philosophers have, that an individual possesses concepts only if he can express these concepts in language, it would be a matter of everyday observation whether or not a given organism possessed the concept of a continuing self. Infanticide would then be permissible up to the time an organism learned how to use certain expressions. However, I think the claim that acquisition of concepts is dependent on acquisition of language is mistaken. For example, one wants to ascribe mental states of a conceptual sort—such as beliefs and desires—to organisms that are incapable of learning a language. This issue of prelinguistic understanding is clearly outside the scope of this discussion. My point is simply that *if* an organism can acquire concepts without thereby acquiring a way of expressing those concepts linguistically, the question of whether a given organism possesses the concept of a self as a continuing subject of experiences and other mental states, together with the belief that it is itself such a continuing entity, may be a question that requires fairly subtle experimental techniques to answer.

If this view of the matter is roughly correct, there are two worries one is left with at the level of practical moral decisions, one of which may turn out to be deeply disturbing. The lesser worry is where the line is to be drawn in the case of infanticide. It is not troubling because there is no serious need to know the exact point at which a human infant acquires a right to life. For in the vast majority of cases in which infanticide is desirable, its desirability will be apparent within a short time after birth. Since it is virtually certain that an infant at such a stage of its development does not possess the concept of a continuing self, and thus does not possess a serious right to life, there is excellent reason to believe that infanticide is morally permissible in most cases where it is otherwise desirable. The practical moral problem can thus be satisfactorily handled by choosing some period of time, such as a week after birth, as the interval during which infanticide will be permitted. This interval could then be modified once psychologists have established the point at which a human organism comes to believe that it is a continuing subject of experiences and other mental states.

The troubling worry is whether adult animals belonging to species other than Homo sapiens may not also possess a serious right to life. For once one says that an organism can possess the concept of a continuing self, together with the belief that it is itself such an entity, without having any way of expressing that concept and that belief linguistically, one has to face up to the question of whether animals may not possess properties that bestow a serious right to life upon them. The suggestion itself is a familiar one, and one that most of us are accustomed to dismiss very casually. The

line of thought advanced here suggests that this attitude may turn out to be tragically mistaken. Once one reflects upon the question of the *basic* moral principles involved in the ascription of a right to life to organisms, one may find himself driven to conclude that our everyday treatment of animals is morally indefensible, and that we are in fact murdering innocent persons.

Notes

1. I am grateful to a number of people, particularly the Editors of *Philosophy & Public Affairs,* Rodelia Hapke, and Walter Kaufmann, for their helpful comments. It should not, of course, be inferred that they share the views expressed in this paper.
2. Judith Jarvis Thomson, in her article "A Defense of Abortion," *Philosophy & Public Affairs* 1, no. 1 (Fall 1971): 47–66, has argued with great force and ingenuity that this conclusion is mistaken. I will comment on her argument later in this paper.
3. While this is the position conservatives tend to hold, it is not clear that it is the position they ought to hold. For if the fetus is a person it is far from clear that it is permissible to destroy it to save the mother. Two moral principles lend support to the view that it is the fetus which should live. First, other things being equal, should not one give something to a person who has had less rather than to a person who has had more? The mother has had a chance to live, while the fetus has not. The choice is thus between giving the fetus an opportunity to enjoy life while not giving the mother a further opportunity to do so. Surely fairness requires the latter. Secondly, since the fetus has a greater life expectancy than the mother, one is in effect distributing more goods by choosing the life of the fetus over the life of the mother.

  The position I am here recommending to the conservative should not be confused with the official Catholic position. The Catholic Church holds that it is seriously wrong to kill a fetus directly even if failure to do so will result in the death of *both* the mother and the fetus. This perverse value judgment is not part of the conservative's position.
4. Section 230.3 of the American Law Institute's *Model Penal Code* (Philadelphia, 1962). There is some interesting, though at times confused, discussion of the proposed code in *Model Penal*

Code—Tentative Draft No. 9 (Philadelphia, 1959), pp. 146–162.

5. A clear example of such an unwillingness to entertain seriously the possibility that moral judgments widely accepted in one's own society may nevertheless be incorrect is provided by Roger Wertheimer's superficial dismissal of infanticide on pages 69–70 of his article "Understanding the Abortion Argument," *Philosophy & Public Affairs 1,* no. 1 (Fall 1971): 67–95.

6. Compare the discussion of the concept of a right offered by Richard B. Brandt in his *Ethical Theory* (Englewood Cliffs, N.J., 1959), pp. 434–441. As Brandt points out, some philosophers have maintained that only things that can *claim* rights can have rights. I agree with Brandt's view that "inability to claim does not destroy the right" (p. 440).

7. B. A. Brody, "Abortion and the Law," *Journal of Philosophy.* LXVIII, no. 12 (17 June 1971): 357–369. See pp. 357–358.

8. Thomson, "A Defense of Abortion," p. 47.

9. Wertheimer, "Understanding the Abortion Argument," p. 69.

10. *Ibid.*

11. Thomson, "A Defense of Abortion," pp. 47–48.

12. *Ibid.,* p. 65.

13. Wertheimer, "Understanding the Abortion Argument," p. 78.

14. A moral principle accepted by a person is *basic for him* if and only if his acceptance of it is not dependent upon any of his (nonmoral) factual beliefs. That is, no change in his factual beliefs would cause him to abandon the principle in question.

15. Wertheimer, "Understanding the Abortion Argument," p. 88.

16. Again, compare the analysis defended by Brandt in *Ethical Theory,* pp. 434–441.

17. In everyday life one often speaks of desiring things, such as an apple or a newspaper. Such talk is elliptical, the context together with one's ordinary beliefs serving to make it clear that one wants to eat the apple and read the newspaper. To say that what one desires is that a certain proposition be true should not be construed as involving any particular ontological commitment. The point is merely that it is sentences such as "John wants it to be the case that he is eating an apple in the next few minutes" that

provide a completely explicit description of a person's desires. If one fails to use such sentences one can be badly misled about what concepts are presupposed by a particular desire.

18. There are, however, situations other than those discussed here which might seem to count against the claim that a person cannot have a right unless he is conceptually capable of having the corresponding desire. Can't a young child, for example, have a right to an estate, even though he may not be conceptually capable of wanting the estate? It is clear that such situations have to be carefully considered if one is to arrive at a satisfactory account of the concept of right. My inclination is to say that the correct description is not that the child now has a right to the estate, but that he will come to have such a right when he is mature, and that in the meantime no one else has a right to the estate. My reason for saying that the child does not now have a right to the estate is that he cannot now do things with the estate, such as selling it or giving it away, that he will be able to do later on.

19. Another frequent suggestion as to the cutoff point not listed here is quickening. I omit it because it seems clear that if abortion after quickening is wrong, its wrongness must be tied up with the motility of the fetus, not with the mother's awareness of the fetus' ability to move about.

20. Thomson, "A Defense of Abortion," p. 56.

21. A good example of a failure to probe this issue is provided by Brody's "Abortion and the Law."

22. Admittedly the modification is a substantial one, since given a society that refused to compensate women, a woman who had an abortion would not be doing anything wrong.

23. Compare Wertheimer's remarks, "Understanding the Abortion Argument," p. 79.

24. This requires qualification. If their central nervous systems were radically different from ours, it might be thought that one would not be justified in ascribing to them mental states of an experiential sort. And then, since it seems to be a conceptual truth that only things having experiential states can have rights, one would be forced to conclude that one was not justified in ascribing any rights to them.

25. Philippa Foot, "The Problem of Abortion and the Doctrine of the Double Effect," *The Oxford Review* 5 (1967): 5–15.

Abortion and the Concept of a Person

Jane English

The abortion debate rages on. Yet the two most popular positions seem to be clearly mistaken. Conservatives maintain that a human life begins at conception and that therefore abortion must be wrong because it is murder. But not all killings of humans are murders. Most notably, self defense may justify even the killing of an innocent person.

Liberals, on the other hand, are just as mistaken in their argument that since a fetus does not become a person until birth, a woman may do whatever she pleases in and to her own body. First, you cannot do as you please with your own body if it affects other people adversely.[1] Second, if a fetus is not a person, that does not imply that you can do to it anything you wish. Animals, for example, are not persons, yet to kill or torture them for no reason at all is wrong.

At the center of the storm has been the issue of just when it is between ovulation and adulthood that a person appears on the scene. Conservatives draw the line at conception, liberals at birth. In this paper I first examine our concept of a person and conclude that no single criterion can capture the concept of a person and no sharp line can be drawn. Next I argue that if a fetus is a person, abortion is still justifiable in many cases; and if a fetus is not a person, killing it is still wrong in many cases. To a large extent, these two solutions are in agreement. I conclude that our concept of a person cannot and need not bear the weight that the abortion controversy has thrust upon it.

I

The several factions in the abortion argument have drawn battle lines around various proposed criteria for determining what is and what is not a person. For example, Mary Anne Warren[2] lists five features (capacities for reasoning,

Reprinted by permission of the Canadian Association for Publishing in Philosophy from the *Canadian Journal of Philosophy* 5 No. 2, October 1975.

self-awareness, complex communication, etc.) as her criteria for personhood and argues for the permissibility of abortion because a fetus falls outside this concept. Baruch Brody[3] uses brain waves. Michael Tooley[4] picks having-a-concept-of-self as his criterion and concludes that infanticide and abortion are justifiable, while the killing of adult animals is not. On the other side, Paul Ramsey[5] claims a certain gene structure is the defining characteristic. John Noonan[6] prefers conceived-of-humans and presents counterexamples to various other candidate criteria. For instance, he argues against viability as the criterion because the newborn and infirm would then be non-persons, since they cannot live without the aid of others. He rejects any criterion that calls upon the sorts of sentiments a being can evoke in adults on the grounds that this would allow us to exclude other races as non-persons if we could just view them sufficiently unsentimentally.

These approaches are typical: foes of abortion propose sufficient conditions for personhood which fetuses satisfy, while friends of abortion counter with necessary conditions for personhood which fetuses lack. But these both presuppose that the concept of a person can be captured in a straightjacket of necessary and/or sufficient conditions.[7] Rather, 'person' is a cluster of features, of which rationality, having a self-concept and being conceived of humans are only part.

What is typical of persons? Within our concept of a person we include, first, certain biological factors: descended from humans, having a certain genetic make-up, having a head, hands, arms, eyes, capable of locomotion, breathing, eating, sleeping. There are psychological factors: sentience, perception, having a concept of self and of one's own interests and desires, the ability to use tools, the ability to use language or symbol systems, the ability to joke, to be angry, to doubt. There are rationality factors: the ability to reason and draw conclusions, the ability to generalize and to learn from past experience, the ability to sacrifice present interests for greater gains in the future. There are social factors: the ability to work in groups and respond to peer pressures, the ability to recognize and consider as valuable the interests of others, seeing oneself as one among "other minds," the ability to sympathize, encourage, love, the ability to evoke from others the responses of sympathy, encouragement, love, the ability to work with others for mutual advantage. Then there are legal factors: being subject to the law and protected by it, having the ability to sue and enter contracts, being counted in the census, having a name and citizenship, the ability to own property, inherit, and so forth.

Now the point is not that this list is incomplete, or that you can find counterinstances to each of its points. People typically exhibit rationality, for instance, but someone who was irrational would not thereby fail to qualify as a person. On the other hand, something could exhibit the majority of these features and still fail to be a person, as an advanced robot might. There is no single core of necessary and sufficient features which we can draw upon with the assurance that they constitute what really makes a person; there are only features that are more or less typical.

This is not to say that no necessary or sufficient conditions can be given. Being alive is a necessary condition for being a person, and being a U.S. Senator is sufficient. But rather than falling inside a sufficient condition or outside a necessary one, a fetus lies in the penumbra region where our concept of a person is not so simple. For this reason I think a conclusive answer to the question whether a fetus is a person is unattainable.

Here we might note a family of simple fallacies that proceed by stating a necessary condition for personhood and showing that a fetus has that characteristic. This is a form of the fallacy of affirming the consequent. For example, some have mistakenly reasoned from the premise that a fetus is human (after all, it is a human fetus rather than, say, a canine fetus), to the conclusion that it is a human. Adding an equivocation on 'being', we get the fallacious argument that since a fetus is something both living and human, it is a human being.

Nonetheless, it does seem clear that a fetus has very few of the above family of characteristics, whereas a newborn baby exhibits a much larger proportion of them—and a two-year-old has even more. Note that one traditional anti-abortion argument has centered on pointing out the many ways in which a fetus resembles a baby. They emphasize its development ("It already has ten fingers . . .") without mentioning its dissimilarities to adults (it still has gills and a tail). They also try to evoke the sort of sympathy on our part that we only feel toward other persons ("Never to laugh . . . or feel the sunshine?"). This all seems to be a relevant way to argue, since its purpose is to persuade us that a fetus satisfies so many of the important features on the list that it ought to be treated as a person. Also note that a fetus near the time of birth satisfies many more of these factors than a fetus in the early months of development. This could provide reason for making distinctions among the different stages of pregnancy, as the U.S. Supreme Court has done.[8]

Historically, the time at which a person has been said to come into existence has varied widely. Muslims date personhood from fourteen days after conception. Some medievals followed Aristotle in placing ensoulment at forty days after conception for a male fetus and eighty days for a female fetus.[9] In European common law since the Seventeenth Century, abortion was considered the killing of a person only after quickening, the time when a pregnant woman first feels the fetus move on its own. Nor is this variety of opinions surprising. Biologically, a human being develops gradually. We shouldn't expect there to be any specific time or sharp dividing point when a person appears on the scene.

For these reasons I believe our concept of a person is not sharp or decisive enough to bear the weight of a solution to the abortion controversy. To use it to solve that problem is to clarify *obscurum per obscurius.*

II

Next let us consider what follows if a fetus is a person after all. Judith Jarvis Thomson's landmark article, "A Defense of Abortion,"[10] correctly points out that some additional argumentation is needed at this point in the conservative argument to bridge the gap between the premise that a fetus is an innocent person and the conclusion that killing it is always wrong. To arrive at this conclusion, we would need the additional premise that killing an innocent person is always wrong. But killing an innocent person is sometimes permissible, most notably in self defense. Some examples may help draw out our intuitions or ordinary judgments about self defense.

Suppose a mad scientist, for instance, hypnotized innocent people to jump out of the bushes and attack innocent passers-by with knives. If you are so attacked, we agree you have a right to kill the attacker in self defense, if killing him is the only way to protect your life or to save yourself from serious injury. It does not seem to matter here that the attacker is not malicious but himself an innocent pawn, for your killing of him is not done in a spirit of retribution but only in self defense.

How severe an injury may you inflict in self defense? In part this depends upon the severity of the injury to be avoided: you may not shoot someone merely to avoid having your clothes torn. This might lead one to the mistaken conclusion that the defense may only equal the threatened injury in severity; that to avoid death you may kill, but to avoid a black eye you may only inflict a black eye or the equivalent. Rather, our laws and customs seem to say that you may create an injury somewhat, but not enormously, greater than the injury to be avoided. To fend off an attack whose outcome would be as serious as rape, a severe beating or the loss of a finger, you may shoot; to avoid having your clothes torn, you may blacken an eye.

Aside from this, the injury you may inflict should only be the minimum necessary to deter or incapacitate the attacker. Even if you know he intends to kill you, you are not justified in shooting him if you could equally well save yourself by the simple expedient of running away. Self defense is for the purpose of avoiding harms rather than equalizing harms.

Some cases of pregnancy present a parallel situation. Though the fetus is itself innocent, it may pose a threat to the pregnant woman's well-being, life prospects or health, mental or physical. If the pregnancy presents a slight threat to her interests, it seems self defense cannot justify abortion. But if the threat is on a par with a serious beating or the loss of a finger, she may kill the fetus that poses such a threat, even if it is an innocent person. If a lesser harm to the fetus could have the same defensive effect, killing it would not be justified. It is unfortunate that the only way to free the woman from the pregnancy entails the death of the fetus (except in very late stages of pregnancy). Thus a self defense model supports Thomson's point that the woman has a right only to be freed from the fetus, not a right to demand its death.[11]

The self defense model is most helpful when we take the pregnant woman's point of view. In the pre-Thomson literature, abortion is often framed as a question for a third party: do you, a doctor, have a right to choose between the life of the woman and that of the fetus? Some have claimed that if you were a passer-by who witnessed a struggle between the innocent hypnotized attacker and his equally innocent victim, you would have no reason to kill either in defense of the other. They have concluded that the self defense model implies that a woman may attempt to abort herself, but that a doctor should not assist her. I think the position of the third party is somewhat more complex. We do feel some inclination to intervene on behalf of the victim rather than the attacker, other things equal. But if both parties are innocent, other factors come into consideration. You would rush to the aid of your husband whether he was attacker or attackee. If a hypnotized famous violinist were attacking a skid row bum, we would try to save the individual who is of more value to society. These considerations would tend to support abortion in some cases.

But suppose you are a frail senior citizen who wishes to avoid being knifed by one of these innocent hypnotics, so you have hired a bodyguard to accompany you. If you are attacked, it is clear we believe that the bodyguard, acting as your agent, has a right to kill the attacker to save you from a serious beating. Your rights of self defense are transferred to your agent. I suggest that we should similarly view the doctor as the pregnant woman's agent in carrying out a defense she is physically incapable of accomplishing herself.

Thanks to modern technology, the cases are

rare in which a pregnancy poses as clear a threat to a woman's bodily health as an attacker brandishing a switchblade. How does self defense fare when more subtle, complex and long-range harms are involved?

To consider a somewhat fanciful example, suppose you are a highly trained surgeon when you are kidnapped by the hypnotic attacker. He says he does not intend to harm you but to take you back to the mad scientist who, it turns out, plans to hypnotize you to have a permanent mental block against all your knowledge of medicine. This would automatically destroy your career which would in turn have a serious adverse impact on your family, your personal relationships and your happiness. It seems to me that if the only way you can avoid this outcome is to shoot the innocent attacker, you are justified in so doing. You are defending yourself from a drastic injury to your life prospects. I think it is no exaggeration to claim that unwanted pregnancies (most obviously among teenagers) often have such adverse life-long consequences as the surgeon's loss of livelihood.

Several parallels arise between various views on abortion and the self defense model. Let's suppose further that these hypnotized attackers only operate at night, so that it is well known that they can be avoided completely by the considerable inconvenience of never leaving your house after dark. One view is that since you could stay home at night, therefore if you go out and are selected by one of these hypnotized people, you have no right to defend yourself. This parallels the view that abstinence is the only acceptable way to avoid pregnancy. Others might hold that you ought to take along some defense such as Mace which will deter the hypnotized person without killing him, but that if this defense fails, you are obliged to submit to the resulting injury, no matter how severe it is. This parallels the view that contraception is all right but abortion is always wrong, even in cases of contraceptive failure.

A third view is that you may kill the hypnotized person only if he will actually kill you, but not if he will only injure you. This is like the position that abortion is permissible only if it is required to save a woman's life. Finally we have the view that it is all right to kill the attacker, even if only to avoid a very slight inconvenience to yourself and even if you knowingly walked down the very street where all these incidents have been taking place without taking along any Mace or protective escort. If we assume that a fetus is a person, this is the analogue of the view that abortion is always justifiable, ''on demand.''

The self defense model allows us to see an important differrence that exists between abortion and infanticide, even if a fetus is a person from conception. Many have argued that the only way to justify abortion without justifying infanticide would be to find some characteristic of personhood that is acquired at birth. Michael Tooley, for one, claims infanticide is justifiable because the really significant characteristics of person are acquired some time after birth. But all such approaches look to characteristics of the developing human and ignore the relation between the fetus and the woman. What if, after birth, the presence of an infant or the need to support it posed a grave threat to the woman's sanity or life prospects? She could escape this threat by the simple expedient of running away. So a solution that does not entail the death of the infant is available. Before birth, such solutions are not available because of the biological dependence of the fetus on the woman. Birth is the crucial point not because of any characteristics the fetus gains, but because after birth the woman can defend herself by a means less drastic than killing the infant. Hence self defense can be used to justify abortion without necessarily thereby justifying infanticide.

III

On the other hand, supposing a fetus is not after all a person, would abortion always be morally permissible? Some opponents of abortion seem worried that if a fetus is not a full-fledged person, then we are justified in treating it in any way at all. However, this does not follow. Nonpersons do get some consideration in our moral code, though of course they do not have the same rights as persons have (and in general they do not have moral responsibilities), and though their interests may be overridden by the interests of persons. Still, we cannot just treat them in any way at all.

Treatment of animals is a case in point. It is wrong to torture dogs for fun or to kill wild birds for no reason at all. It is wrong Period, even though dogs and birds do not have the same rights persons do. However, few people think it is wrong to use dogs as experimental animals, causing them considerable suffering in some cases, provided that the resulting research will probably bring discoveries of great benefit to people. And most of us think it all right to kill birds for food or to protect our crops. People's rights are different from the consideration we give to animals, then, for it is wrong to experiment on people, even if others might later benefit a great deal as a result of their suffering. You might volunteer to be a subject, but this would be supererogatory; you certainly have a right to refuse to be a medical guinea pig.

But how do we decide what you may or may not do to non-persons? This is a difficult problem, one for which I believe no adequate account exists. You do not want to say, for instance, that torturing dogs is all right whenever the sum of its effects on people is good—when it doesn't warp the sensibilities of the torturer so much that he mistreats people. If that were the case, it would be all right to torture dogs if you did it in private, or if the torturer lived on a desert island or died soon afterward, so that his actions had no effect on people. This is an inadequate account, because whatever moral consideration animals get, it has to be indefeasible, too. It will have to be a general proscription of certain actions, not merely a weighing of the impact on people on a case-by-case basis.

Rather, we need to distinguish two levels on which consequences of actions can be taken into account in moral reasoning. The traditional objections to Utilitarianism focus on the fact that it operates solely on the first level, taking all the consequences into account in particular cases only. Thus Utilitarianism is open to "desert island" and "lifeboat" counterexamples because these cases are rigged to make the consequences of actions severely limited.

Rawls' theory could be described as a teleological sort of theory, but with teleology operating on a higher level.[12] In choosing the principles to regulate society from the original position, his hypothetical choosers make their decision on the basis of the total consequences of various systems. Furthermore, they are constrained to choose a general set of rules which people can readily learn and apply. An ethical theory must operate by generating a set of sympathies and attitudes toward others which reinforces the functioning of that set of moral principles. Our prohibition against killing people operates by means of certain moral sentiments including sympathy, compassion and guilt. But if these attitudes are to form a coherent set, they carry us further: we tend to perform supererogatory actions, and we tend to feel similar compassion toward person-like non-persons.

It is crucial that psychological facts play a role here. Our psychological constitution makes it the case that for our ethical theory to work, it must prohibit certain treatment of nonpersons which are significantly person-like. If our moral rules allowed people to treat some person-like nonpersons in ways we do not want people to be treated, this would undermine the system of sympathies and attitudes that makes the ethical system work. For this reason, we would choose in the original position to make mistreatment of some sorts of animals wrong in general (not just wrong in the cases with public impact), even though animals are not themselves parties in the original position. Thus it makes sense that it is those animals whose appearance and behavior are most like those of people that get the most consideration in our moral scheme.

It is because of "coherence of attitudes," I think, that the similarity of a fetus to a baby is very significant. A fetus one week before birth is so much like a newborn baby in our psychological space that we cannot allow any cavalier treatment of the former while expecting full sympathy and nurturative support for the latter. Thus, I think that anti-abortion forces are indeed giving their strongest arguments when they point to the similarities between a fetus and a baby, and when they try to evoke our emotional attachment to and sympathy for the fetus. An early horror story from New York about nurses who were expected to alternate between caring for six-week premature infants and disposing of viable 24-week aborted fetuses is just that—a horror story. These beings are so much alike that no one can be asked to draw a distinction and treat them so very differently.

Remember, however, that in the early weeks after conception, a fetus is very much unlike a person. It is hard to develop these feelings for a set of genes which doesn't yet have a head, hands, beating heart, response to touch or the ability to move by itself. Thus it seems to me that the alleged "slippery slope" between conception and birth is not so very slippery. In the early stages of pregnancy, abortion can hardly be compared to murder for psychological reasons, but in the latest stages it is psychologically akin to murder.

Another source of similarity is the bodily continuity between fetus and adult. Bodies play a surprisingly central role in our attitudes toward persons. One has only to think of the philosophical literature on how far physical identity suffices for personal identity or Wittgenstein's remark that the best picture of the human soul is the human body. Even after death, when all agree the body is no longer a person, we still observe elaborate customs of respect for the human body; like people who torture dogs, necrophiliacs are not to be trusted with people.[13] So it is appropriate that we show respect to a fetus as the body continuous with the body of a person. This is a degree of resemblance to persons that animals cannot rival.

Michael Tooley also utilizes a parallel with animals. He claims that it is always permissible to drown newborn kittens and draws conclusions about infanticide.[14] But it is only permissible to drown kittens when their survival would cause some hardship. Perhaps it would be a burden to feed and house six more cats or to find other homes for them. The alternative of letting them starve produces even more suffering than the drowning. Since the kittens get their rights secondhand, so to speak, *via* the need for coherence in our attitudes, their interests are often overriden by the interests of full-fledged persons. But if their survival would be no inconvenience to people at all, then it is wrong to drown them, *contra* Tooley.

Tooley's conclusions about abortion are wrong for the same reason. Even if a fetus is not a person, abortion is not always permissible, because of the resemblance of a fetus to a per-

son. I agree with Thomson that it would be wrong for a woman who is seven months pregnant to have an abortion just to avoid having to postpone a trip to Europe. In the early months of pregnancy when the fetus hardly resembles a baby at all, then, abortion is permissible whenever it is in the interests of the pregnant woman or her family. The reasons would only need to outweigh the pain and inconvenience of the abortion itself. In the middle months, when the fetus comes to resemble a person, abortion would be justifiable only when the continuation of the pregnancy or the birth of the child would cause harms—physical, psychological, economic or social—to the woman. In the late months of pregnancy, even on our current assumption that a fetus is not a person, abortion seems to be wrong except to save a woman from significant injury or death.

The Supreme Court has recognized similar gradations in the alleged slippery slope stretching between conception and birth. To this point, the present paper has been a discussion of the moral status of abortion only, not its legal status. In view of the great physical, financial and sometimes psychological costs of abortion, perhaps the legal arrangement most compatible with the proposed moral solution would be the absence of restrictions, that is, so-called abortion "on demand."

So I conclude, first, that application of our concept of a person will not suffice to settle the abortion issue. After all, the biological development of a human being is gradual. Second, whether a fetus is a person or not, abortion is justifiable early in pregnancy to avoid modest harms and seldom justifiable late in pregnancy except to avoid significant injury or death.

Notes

1. We also have paternalistic laws which keep us from harming our own bodies even when no one else is affected. Ironically, anti-abortion laws were originally designed to protect pregnant women from a dangerous but tempting procedure.
2. Mary Anne Warren, "On the Moral and Legal Status of Abortion," *Monist* 5 (1973), p. 55.
3. Baruch Brody, "Fetal Humanity and the

Theory of Essentialism,'' in Robert Baker and Frederick Elliston (eds.), *Philosophy and Sex* (Buffalo, N.Y., 1975).

4. Michael Tooley, ''Abortion and Infanticide,'' *Philosophy and Public Affairs* 1 (1971). [See above, pp. 60–77.]

5. Paul Ramsey, ''The Morality of Abortion,'' in James Rachels, ed., *Moral Problems* (New York, 1971).

6. John Noonan, ''Abortion and the Catholic Church: a Summary History,'' *Natural Law Forum* 12 (1967), pp. 125–131.

7. Wittgenstein has argued against the possibility of so capturing the concept of a game, *Philosophical Investigations* (New York, 1958), §66–71.

8. Not because the fetus is partly a person and so has some of the rights of persons but rather because of the rights of person-like non-persons. This I discuss in part III below.

9. Aristotle himself was concerned, however, with the different question of when the soul takes form. For historical data, see Jimmye Kimmey, ''How the Abortion Laws Happened,'' *Ms* 1 (April, 1973), pp. 48ff and John Noonan, *loc. cit.*

10. J.J. Thomson, ''A Defense of Abortion,'' *Philosophy and Public Affairs* 1 (1971).

11. *Ibid.,* p. 52.

12. John Rawls, *A Theory of Justice* (Cambridge, Mass., 1971), §§ 3–4.

13. On the other hand, if they can be trusted with people, then our moral customs are mistaken. It all depends on the facts of psychology.

14. *Op. cit.,* pp. 40, 60–61.

Responsible Women and Abortion Decisions

Martha Brandt Bolton

I

When a pregnant woman considers whether or not to seek an abortion, is she facing a choice between doing what is morally wrong and doing what is morally right, or is her choice without moral significance? There are two answers to this question which have become familiar to all of us, and I want to argue that both of them are wrong.

One answer comes from those who hold that the fetus is already a living human being and a person; they hold that a fetus, like every other person, has a right not to be deliberately killed. Some who hold this view allow that circumstances may permit the killing of the fetus—for example, when it is necessary to save the life of the pregnant woman. Generally speaking, however, according to those who advocate the fetus' ''right to life,'' the decision to have an abortion is comparable to the decision to mur-

Reprinted with permission from *Having Children,* Onora O'Neill and William Ruddick, eds. (New York: Oxford University Press, 1979).

der. Thus, they hold that in general, abortions are morally wrong.

The second familiar answer to our question is that, in general, an abortion has no moral significance; it is not morally wrong, but neither is it morally permissible or right. It is a personal and private decision comparable to the decision to have an abscessed tooth pulled or a bothersome tumor removed. According to this view, neither the fetus nor anyone else has rights which are violated by abortion. A woman is free to have, or not to have, an abortion as she chooses. I should clarify at once a point about this position that abortion is morally insignificant. It must be distinguished from that taken by a majority of the Supreme Court in the 1973 decision that laws prohibiting abortion during the first three months of pregnancy are unconstitutional. The Court found that abortion does not violate anyone's *constitutional* rights, and it is not the sort of action which the *state* has an interest in prohibiting. The position with which I am concerned has it that abortion violates no one's *moral* rights and cannot be prohibited, or required, on *moral* grounds.

As I have said, I think that both of these familiar views about the morality of abortion are wrong. Let me begin with the anti-abortionists, who claim that a fetus has a right not to be killed comparable to that of any person. Anti-abortionists make this claim, in part, because they hold that a fetus is already a person.[1] The thought that a newly conceived fetus is a person seems absurd to some, but it seems credible to others. The reason is that there is no readily available or widely accepted view about exactly what a person is.

One distinctive characteristic of persons is that they are entitled to special consideration. We are obligated to treat the lives, needs, and desires of other *persons* with consideration equal to that we think should be given to our own. For instance, conflicts between my needs and wants and those of other persons cannot automatically be decided in favor of me; the others have rights against my actions, and I am morally obligated to respect them. It is true that I may have moral obligations to animals, which are clearly not persons. But the point about persons is that I have *special* obligations to them, and they have *particular* rights that limit what it is morally permissible for me to do. The category of persons is in part a moral one; having certain rights and participating in a certain network of obligations is at least part of what it is to be a person.

The problem is that we do not know how to describe, in a general way, what creatures entitled to this special consideration must be like. We all agree about most cases we confront (although historically there has been debate about black people and women, in general). But even the most sensitive and honest of us can conceive of cases in which we would not know what to think.

One sort of puzzling case concerns creatures that are clearly not biological humans or *homo sapiens*. Imagine the moral questions that might arise if we encountered highly developed forms of life on other planets, or if we discovered creatures who are the ''missing link'' in the evolution of humans from apes. Should we force such creatures to work for us? Should we eat them? What about cross-breeding? Non-fictional cases may actually be at hand. Does the gorilla from the San Francisco Zoo, who is able to use language, have any of the rights of a person? The biological facts do not provide answers to these questions. Creatures that are indisputably not *homo sapiens* may nevertheless be entitled to the special consideration we owe to *persons*. By the same token, the fact that a creature *is* a biological human being does not settle such questions either. Consider cases of extreme criminal insanity or humans deep in coma with no hope of regaining consciousness. No doubt, we do have certain obligations to these humans, but we probably do not have the full range of obligations that we have to others in our community. If so, then a human being may be a person at one stage of his/her biological life and a non-person at other stages. Whether or not this is the case, and which stages of development are person-stages, will not be settled by biological facts about us.

II

Anti-abortionists begin the discussion of the morality of abortion with the claim that a fetus is a person. Most base this claim on biological facts, but as I have said, such facts do not settle the question. Others, recognizing that there is legitimate doubt that a fetus is a person, reason that the fetus should be given the benefit of the doubt. From there, anti-abortionists argue that it is a fundamental right of a person not to be deliberately killed.[2] This right is forfeited in certain circumstances where killing is justified, most notably in self-defense.[3] But the fact is that these circumstances rarely arise in pregnancy; they are confined to cases in which the life or health of the pregnant woman is seriously threatened by the presence of the fetus. Thus, a fetus cannot be killed (or can only very rarely be killed) if the fetus has the rights of a person.

I have already said that the assumption that a fetus is a person is unfounded, but I think that the anti-abortionist has a more serious problem. I think the claim that the fetus has the *same* rights as an undisputed person does can be shown to be clearly wrong.[4] If I am correct in thinking that a fetus cannot have the same right not to be killed as an undisputed person has, then the anti-abortionists are wrong when they prohibit abortion on grounds that persons as such have a right not to be killed.

To see the incoherence in the anti-abortionists' argument, we need to look at the gaps in their account of what is at stake in an abortion. They emphasize the fetus' alleged "right to life." They do not emphasize a matter which is equally important. This is that if a pregnant woman is obligated not to kill a fetus, then she is obligated to do a great deal more than that. She can meet the alleged obligation not to kill only if she takes on the various obligations involved in bearing and having a child. At the least, she must nurture the fetus, carry it to term, and give it birth; she must then care for the infant or make alternative arrangements for its care. Of course, there may be others willing to adopt the infant and raise the child; but we should not lose sight of the fact that for some babies there are not likely to be adoptive parents. For pregnant women whose potential babies will not be accepted for adoption, the responsibilities involved in caring for the fetus loom very large. For any pregnant woman, the only way to avoid killing a fetus is to take responsibility for nurturing and giving birth to it; for some, the alternative is undertaking to care for and raise a child. Anti-abortionists insist on the fetus' right not to be killed; they discount the fact that a fetus has the right *only if* it also has a right to be nurtured by the pregnant woman and raised by her or someone else.

It is important to describe the fetus' alleged right in this way, rather than in the way in which anti-abortionists typically do. Respecting the right of another person not to be killed is relatively simple. It is a matter of refraining from doing something. But respecting a fetus' right to be nurtured and developed involves a complex pattern of activities which form a prominent, demanding, and (in some cases) permanent part of one's life. It is relatively easy to live without deliberately killing someone; but it may require an indefinitely large commitment of time, energy, emotion, and physical resources to nurture and care for a child. Furthermore, the obligation not to kill is conceptually simple; it extends to *all* other persons, and the situations in which it is forfeited are familiar (for instance, self-defense). In contrast, the obligation to nurture and develop others is con-

ceptually complex. It is not entirely clear how much of one's resources such obligations demand, nor is it clear how far they extend. Surely they do not extend to *all* other persons, for anyone's personal resources are too slight to meet such massive demands. By the same token, the limitations on any one person's resources make it inevitable that obligations to help different persons will conflict; some will have to be chosen over others. When anti-abortionists emphasize the obligation not to kill a fetus, they make it seem as if our obligations to fetuses were as simple as our obligations not to kill other persons. But this is seriously misleading. Fetuses differ from persons in that a pregnant woman cannot avoid killing a fetus unless she undertakes to nurture and develop it. Her obligations to a fetus cannot be any more simple than her obligations to help in the growth and development of others who may need it; and I have suggested that these obligations are complex and limited.

Let me illustrate what I mean when I say that obligations to aid the development and growth of others are limited and complex. Consider a mother with several children, one of whom has a disability which retards normal development. Suppose that with expensive treatment and patient training, the retarded child will slowly develop many capacities that other children acquire rapidly and without special help. The woman's resources are limited; her money, time, physical strength, and emotional capacity are not inexhaustible. Developing a certain capacity in the retarded child—say, the ability to make short unaccompanied trips outside the house—may put a severe strain on her resources. Her time and energy are needed to support the family, and she hasn't the money to engage someone else to work with the special child. There is a point beyond which she is not morally required to devote resources to the growth and development of the special child. Because her resources are limited, she must choose how they will be used. Her obligations to aid the special child are limited not only by her own strength and resources but also by her obligations to the other children. The mere fact that a child needs help in order to develop does not always establish an overriding obligation for the mother to meet the need.

So far, I have been considering limitations on the mother's obligation to supply what is needed for the child to develop a specific skill. This affects the child's prospects for a satisfying life, but not the child's life itself. But clearly, similar considerations bear on the resources required to sustain the child's basic care. If resources are severely strained, the mother may have to relinquish all care of the child. Usually, she can make satisfactory alternative arrangements, and there is surely nothing morally wrong about her doing so. Even if alternative arrangements are not available, she may be forced to stop caring for the child if her resources are sufficiently strained. The point is that her obligations to support the development of a particular child are limited by her situation, and they are complex. Both her resources and her other obligations determine their extent.

I have been saying that a mother does not have *limitless* obligations to aid in the development of a child, or even to sustain a child's life. The same holds for any one person's obligations to support the growth, or even the life, of any other person. The basic fact that any one person's time, energy, and other resources have limits makes it absurd to suggest otherwise.

There are, then, *two* features of a person's rights and obligations which are relevant to the issue of abortion, and the anti-abortionists' insistence on one of them obscures the other. The features are: first, that a person has a right not to be killed which extends to virtually all circumstances except those of self-defense; and second, that any one person's obligations to aid another's growth or sustain another's life must, in the nature of the case, have limits.

Where the rights and obligations of undisputed persons are concerned, these fundamental features are fully compatible. One person's obligation to sustain the life of another stops at a certain point; at that point, the other's requirements may not be fully met and he/she may die. In refusing further aid, a person does not violate the other's right not to be killed; he/she may only be acting responsibly given his/her other commitments and in any case, there are limits to the extent to which anyone is obligated to sustain the life of another. Let us see how this works in a couple of cases. Consider a family supporting an elderly member who needs expensive medical care; suppose the medical situation worsens, and care becomes prohibitively expensive for the family. To reserve enough money to supply other basic needs, they must withdraw financial support for the medical care and, as a result, the elderly person dies. The withdrawal of support is regrettable, but not morally wrong; surely the elderly person's right not to be killed has not been violated. The elderly person is simply left to his/her own resources; when they do not suffice, the person is allowed to die. Or, consider a situation in which one person rescues another from nearly drowning and administers artificial respiration. For a while, the artificially provided oxygen sustains the victim's life, but the life-sustaining activity of the rescuer cannot be continued indefinitely. At some point, the person must be returned to his/her own means of sustaining life and, if they are inadequate, the person must be allowed to die. The death is by drowning; no one would suggest that the person was killed by the one who attempted to save his/her life. No one would think that the victim's right not to be killed had been violated. In cases like these, where one person's life is sustained by the activities or resources of another, we can distinguish between two sorts of actions: (i) the one person's ceasing the activity which sustains the other's life and (ii) the one person's deliberately killing the other. Actions of the first sort do not violate a person's right not to be the victim of actions of the second sort.

I suggest that what enables us to make this important distinction is that persons typically have resources of *their own* for sustaining their lives. At some time in their lives, undisputed persons have carried on their own life functions without direct dependence upon others. When such a person's life functions are later sustained by someone else, we suppose the person has (currently inadequate) resources to which he/she can be returned.

However, a fetus is importantly different from an undisputed person. We cannot distinguish between the pregnant woman's withdrawing her support for its life functions and her killing it.[5] I suggest that the reason is that a fetus, or at least one not yet viable, has no resources of its *own* for carrying on life functions.[6] A fetus cannot be returned to its own resources and allowed to die. If the woman ceases her support for its life, we seem forced to say that the fetus has been killed. So, whereas we can reconcile the limits on our obligations to sustain the life of an undisputed person with our obligation not to kill such a person, we *cannot* do so in the case of a (previable) fetus. It is this that convinces me that a fetus cannot have the *same* right not to be killed that an undisputed person has.

Let me summarize. An undisputed person has a right not to be deliberately killed and (at best) a right to limited aid in growth and sustaining his/her life from a particular other person. Now consider a fetus. If a fetus has a right not to be deliberately killed (except in self-defense), then it has a right to be nurtured by the pregnant woman, and this is *not* a limited claim on her resources. Thus, a fetus has a right to demand more than an undisputed person does, and so its rights are not *the same* as such a person's are. On the other hand, if a fetus has only the same right to help from the pregnant woman that an undisputed person has, then there are limits to her obligations to it. Then, there will be a point at which the woman's obligations cease and the fetus can be killed, even though the killing is not done in self-defense. It follows, again, that a fetus does not have *the same* rights that an undisputed person does. A fetus cannot be accorded one of the relevant rights which undisputed persons have without also being given either a stronger right to help or a weaker right not to be killed than we accord to such persons.[7] Thus, a fetus cannot have the same right not to be killed that undisputed persons have.

III

If my view so far is correct, anti-abortionists cannot coherently support a general prohibition against abortion by appeal to the claim that a fetus has the rights of a person. Their response may be that, in fact, a pregnant woman's obligations to a fetus are *stronger* than her obligations to a person.[8] Anti-abortionists may claim she has a special duty to care for the fetus, so that her obligations to it are not limited in the ways obligations to other persons are. Accordingly, an anti-abortionist might persist in maintaining that aborting a fetus is generally morally wrong.

I think that this anti-abortionist position also is untenable. In particular, it distorts the situation of a woman as a morally responsible agent. It appeals, on the one hand, to the pregnant woman's ability to choose to do what is morally right (concerning abortion); on the other, it implies that she cannot be a responsible participant in a full moral life. Let me explain why I think that this is so.

The important fact about a pregnant woman's moral situation is the one I have been emphasizing: if she does not have an abortion, she must shoulder the more or less extensive and demanding responsibility of caring for the fetus. Now, many women have the various resources required to nurture the fetus and care for the potential child, or at least to make arrangements for its care. But many other women *do not,* and we need to be particularly concerned about their situation. Suppose that a pregnant woman knows that she cannot properly care for the fetus, or that the needs of the potential child will not be met. To undertake to nurture the fetus and give birth to a child, given her situation, would be morally irresponsible; it would be to accept obligations which she *knows* she cannot meet. No coherent moral rule requires a person to accept obligations which he/she knows cannot be fulfilled. Yet this is precisely what the anti-abortionists' moral stance requires of a pregnant woman in this situation. It requires that she refrain from abortion, and she cannot do so without incurring obligations to care for the fetus; in the sorts of circumstances with which I am concerned, she knows she must fail to meet them.[9]

Situations of the sort in question are, unfortunately, not merely hypothetical. Consider a case in which there is extreme emotional trauma connected with the woman's pregnancy, so that she is deeply ambivalent about the fetus. Such emotional ambivalence could be the result of her having been the victim of rape, or it could result from the unexpected death of the father of the fetus, or from the extreme youth and immaturity of the mother. The woman may recognize that her emotional ambivalence will keep her from providing adequate care for the fetus. It is important to realize that her inability to care for the fetus may be a genuine one which would be impossible to overcome. In another sort of case, she may know that she will be unable to provide adequate care for the fetus, either because she is addicted to alcohol or other harmful drugs or because she does not have access to the proper food or medical care. Or, she may know that she will be unable to care for the potential child and, further, that no one else in her community will be willing or able to do so.[10] Of course, pregnant women who face grave difficulties of these sorts are sometimes able to overcome them, especially if help from others in the community is available. But there will inevitably be cases in which it would be unreasonable, even irresponsible, to think that the difficulties could be overcome. Sometimes the resources required to nurture a fetus and care for a child are simply not available to a particular pregnant woman. For a woman in such a situation, the anti-abortionists' position has absurd implications. It implies that she is morally obligated to undertake responsibilities which she knows she must fail to meet. In brief, it places on her a moral responsibility to do what is morally irresponsible.

In less dire circumstances, a pregnant woman is still placed in an anomalous moral situation by the anti-abortionists' position. That position gives her an overriding obligation to care for the fetus. Now, what if the woman has already made important commitments which conflict with her developing the fetus? What if others are depending upon her? She has a responsibility to take reasonable precautions against conception, but responsible action of this sort is not a guarantee against pregnancy. If her obligation to the fetus takes precedence, she must fail to follow through on her commitments. But then, she should never have taken them on. Knowing that she might become pregnant, she should have recognized that she might be unable to fulfill her commitments. Accepting them was irresponsible. She should have avoided projects of helping others in which they could come to depend upon her, because she was liable to incur over-

riding obligations to a fetus. Thus, throughout child-bearing years, a woman can act responsibly only by truncating her participation in activities in which others come to depend upon her. But I think this is untenable, for it is central to the life of a morally responsible person to aspire to projects of this sort.

I think it is also central to the life of a morally responsible person that he/she develop abilities which make him/her a useful, productive, contributing member of the community.[11] Doing so often requires large commitments of a person's time, thought, and other personal resources; such commitments are liable to conflict with the activity of nurturing a fetus and raising a child. So, while moral responsibility generally involves a more or less demanding program of developing one's contribution to the community, the anti-abortionists' view requires that a woman refrain from that sort of program. I think that this account of the moral situation of a woman is untenable.

IV

I have argued that the anti-abortionist position that abortion is virtually always wrong is untenable, but I think the other extreme position—that abortion is morally neutral—is equally mistaken. As I have said, I do not think that a fetus can usefully be regarded as a person in discussions of abortion. But it seems to me that the mere fact that it will become a human being, if properly nurtured, indicates that it is entitled to some sort of consideration.[12] I am inclined to think that a pregnant woman has some obligation to nurture a fetus although her obligation is far from absolute.

Further, it is clear that the decision to have, or *not* to have, an abortion does not affect the pregnant woman, alone. It determines whether or not a new member will be brought into the woman's family, her living situation, and her community. Its outcome stands to affect a wide range of others, favorably or unfavorably; their welfare and interests are at stake. Moreover, decisions concerning abortions often occur in situations where there are conflictng commitments and obligations. So, the decision to have an abortion, or not to have one, is not a purely personal matter without moral significance.[13]

I now want to say something about what sorts of considerations generally seem to bear upon the problem of the moral value of a particular abortion.[14] There seem to me to be (at least) three sorts of considerations relevant to the decision. The first is that as a potential human being, a fetus has some claim to be nurtured; like other claims on her aid, this one can be overridden by other factors in a particular woman's situation. The second relevant consideration is the way in which bearing a child, and possibly raising it, fits into the life of the pregnant woman; she must be able to plan a morally coherent life. Will nurturing the fetus prevent her from fulfilling important obligations to others? Will it prevent her from pursuing her plans for becoming a productive and useful member of her community? Is she in a situation in which she can successfully meet her responsibility to the fetus, if she undertakes to nurture it? It seems to me that the answers to these questions are critical. They may indicate that abortion is morally permissible, and they may even indicate that it is morally required. The third relevant consideration is the way in which having a child will affect others in the woman's family, living situation, and the larger community with which she identifies. If their welfare would be severely diminished by her child-raising activity, then I think she ought not to engage in it. On the other hand, if the welfare of others in her community would be enhanced by her having the child, then I think this is relevant. She then has some obligation to have the child, just as she has some obligation to undertake other projects which contribute to the well-being of others. As a morally sensitive person, she ought to pursue some projects of this sort, but there are limits to her obligations to pursue any one in particular. Let me fill in some of the details.

I believe the most important consideration is how bearing and raising a child would fit into the pregnant woman's life. As I have said, nurturing and developing a child requires a major commitment of one's mental and physical resources. A fetus has some claim on these resources, but it does not take precedence over the claims of others to whom the woman has conflicting obligations. She must choose those projects for helping others and strengthening her productive capability which she will pursue. Projects which interest her, engage her particular skills and talents, and those she will find especially rewarding may be given preference over others. If these factors suggest that she is better suited to other projects, then I think she is not morally obligated to nurture the fetus instead; in such cases, abortion is permissible. I am not suggesting that it is morally permissible to ignore all projects of helping others or contributing to their welfare. It is just that it must be permissible to exercise some control over the projects one undertakes; otherwise, it would be impossible to lead a coherent, morally responsible life.[15]

Consider a couple of examples. Take a young woman in college studying to go to medical school and looking forward to the practice of medicine. If she decides to give birth to a child, and especially if she decides to raise it, she is unlikely to complete her studies.[16] She must choose between nurturing the fetus and preparing herself to help her community in other ways. I see no reason why she should be obligated to choose one project rather than the other. It is a question of which she is more interested in, which she considers more important, which she finds herself better suited to pursue. What about a teen-aged woman who is emotionally immature and, in addition, has no means of supporting herself? If she cannot successfully meet the obligations involved in nurturing the fetus—say, because of her immaturity or the ridicule to which she is subject in her community—then I think it is absurd to suggest that she is morally required to do so. In another sort of case, a pregnant woman may already have begun projects which make large demands on her resources. They may be projects of raising other children, working with the elderly in her community, or employment in which others are counting on her continued participation. She may face a choice between failing to meet her obligations to others (in case she bears the child) and seeking an abortion. I think she is permitted to choose abortion. In extreme cases of dependence of others on her, she may even be required to seek abortion.

The final consideration relevant to the decision to have an abortion is the welfare of the pregnant woman's family, living companions, and the members of the larger community with which she identifies. Situations in which the welfare of these persons is endangered by her having a child are rare; but suppose, for example, that the family or community does not have resources to feed or care for an additional member, or that the fetus will have a tendency to infection or to socially destructive acts which the community is unable to control. In such cases, the interest of others in preserving their lives or health is violated by admitting the child into their community, and it seems to me that the woman ought not to bear the child (at least in that community). In most such cases, I think the woman would not want to bear the child, since she identifies with the community. Even if she does want to bear the child, I think she ought not to endanger others by doing so.

There are also cases in which others stand to benefit from the pregnant woman's bearing a child. Suppose, for example, that her family needs additional members to help with the production of food, to protect itself, or to carry on some other activity of value to them. Or, there may be those in the woman's community anxious to adopt the child. Another case is found among certain American Indian tribes; they have so few members that there is danger that the gene pool will become too small to sustain a healthy population. Now, the pregnant woman is in a position to benefit these others by having the child, and I think she ought to choose some projects which benefit others. The relevant factors are by now familiar: does she have conflicting prior obligations? Is the strain on her resources excessive? Does she strongly prefer alternative projects for contributing to the welfare of others?[17] If so, her obligation to have the child is overridden. If not, then she ought to have it. The (possible) benefit to others functions like the background claim of the fetus to be nurtured. Both provide reasons why a pregnant woman should decide against abortion and choose to nurture the fetus. But other facts about her situation are also relevant, and the reasons against nurturing the child may outweigh these reasons for it. In a wide variety of situations, abortion may be morally permitted, and in some it is morally required.[18]

Notes

1. For an account of the anti-abortionist position, see Roger Wertheimer, "Understanding the Abortion Argument," *Philosophy and Public Affairs,* 1, 1971. The official Roman Catholic stance on abortion is more complex, and elusive, than the ones discussed here; see Susan T. Nicholson, "The Roman Catholic Doctrine of Therapeutic Abortion," in *Feminism and Philosophy,* ed. by Mary Vetterling-Braggin, Frederick A. Elliston, and Jane English (Totowa, N.J.: Littlefield, Adams, 1977).

2. This argument has most fully and forcefully been made by Baruch Brody in *Abortion and the Sanctity of Human Life* (Cambridge, Mass.: M.I.T. Press, 1975); also see John Finnis, "The Rights and Wrongs of Abortion," *Philosophy and Public Affairs,* 2, 1973.

3. It is difficult to say whether there are other circumstances in which killing is justified—e.g., in cases of capital punishment, or where many lives may be saved by killing a few. It is also difficult to say precisely what sorts of self-defense justify killing—e.g., how immediate and violent the threat must be, how severe the threatened bodily harm must be. Some of these issues are discussed in Brody, op. cit.

4. Of course, no one claims that a fetus has all the rights of a mature person. The fetus is claimed to have the same right as an undisputed person not to be killed, and it is this claim that I want to dispute.

5. Some defenses of the morality of abortion in a fairly wide range of cases depend upon a distinction between removing the fetus and killing it. The general argument is that the pregnant woman may have a right to have the fetus removed, even though she has no right to have killed. See Judith Jarvis Thomson, "A Defense of Abortion," *Philosophy and Public Affairs,* 1, 1971, and Nicholson, op. cit. My view is that where a previable fetus is concerned, the distinction will not bear this weight.

6. Strictly speaking, this is true only of a fetus prior to the time at which it becomes viable (sometime after the twenty-fourth week, as things now stand). My claim is that as long as no distinction can be made between withdrawing support of the fetus and killing it, the fetus cannot have the same rights that undisputed persons do. In cases where this distinction can be made, I offer no reason to think that fetuses cannot be treated as undisputed persons.

7. In some of the most interesting discussions of abortion, this point is ignored. Having decided

to treat a fetus as a person, the discussants must proceed to make dubious claims about the rights undisputed persons would have in situations comparable to those of fetuses. Thus, Thomson, op. cit., maintains that you are not morally obligated to refrain from killing another person by refusing him/her "the use of your body" when granting it is excessively burdensome. But Brody, op. cit., counters that a person has a right not to be killed, no matter what burdens this restraint places on others (including use of their bodies). Thomson begins with (something like) the point that a person's obligations to aid another are limited and ends by distorting the other's right not to be killed. Brody begins with a person's right not to be killed and ends by distorting another's obligations to aid the person. There appears to be no way to resolve this dispute. The problem, I think, is that the conflict concerns the rights persons are supposed to have in a sort of situation in which undisputed persons are *never found;* and the fact that they are never found in such situations is an indispensable condition of their having the rights they do. In the crucial case, undisputed persons are simply *dis*analogous to fetuses.

8. This would seem to be a better strategy, in any case. For our paradigms of persons are mature, capable, and relatively autonomous adults. Fetuses are much more like very young children than paradigmatic persons. Moreover, it would generally be conceded that a parent's obligations to care for his/her children are much stronger than his/her obligations to help other persons in general.

9. At the same time, a woman who recognizes that she would be unable to fulfill obligations to a fetus or child should take reasonable measures to prevent conception. A pregnant woman in this situation may, or may not, have accepted the responsibility to use whatever safe, effective, and humane means of contraception are available to her. However, in either case, I think that she cannot be morally required to bear responsibilities she knows she cannot meet.

10. The extent to which a woman's activities must be curtailed to meet the obligations involved in nurturing a fetus obviously depends upon the degree to which her community supports her activity. Thus, the absurdity of the anti-abortionists' position, whether it makes reasonable development of a full moral life more or less compatible with meeting one's obligations to fetuses, depends upon the arrangments in any particular community. This, in itself, is reason to be suspicious of the view that abortion, in itself and regardless of the circumstances of the pregnant woman, is morally wrong.

11. There is not space here to argue for the connection between development of one's capacities and a fully moral life; for one interesting treatment, see Larry Blum et al., "Altruism and Women's Oppression," *Philosophical Forum,* 5, 1973–74.

12. This consideration does not seem to me to extend to human eggs or sperms, or other substances which could be developed into human beings. The ovum and sperm are "ingredients" that yield a human being, whereas it is the fetus that becomes a human being. Further, the fact that the genetic makeup of the fetus is determined, whereas that of an egg or sperm is not, seems to be relevant.

13. Different arguments for a similar view are given by Jane English, "Abortion and the Concept of a Person," *Canadian Journal of Philosophy,* 5, 1975.

14. I will consider only women who did not choose to become pregnant. It is important to remember that a woman may well have accepted the responsibility to use reasonable contraception techniques and still have become pregnant.

15. For a discussion of the role of abortion in exercising responsible control over one's life, see Howard Cohen, "Abortion and the Quality of Life," in *Philosophy and Feminism,* op. cit.

16. If her community provides far-reaching support for child-bearing and rearing-activity, the conflict between having a child and other sorts of useful activity can be greatly diminished. The support provided by public institutions, or other agencies, bears on the decision to have an abortion in almost every case. It is an unfortunate consequence that those who receive least support from their society (the poor and disadvantaged) will be morally required to seek abortion more frequently than those who receive more support. This injustice results from injustice elsewhere in the society.

17. For discussion of the obligations a black woman has to contribute to her community by bearing children, see Toni Cade, "On the Issue of Roles," in *The Black Woman,* ed. by Toni Cade (New York: New American Library, 1970).

18. Thanks are due to Amèlie Rorty, Martin Bunzl, and Onora O'Neill for useful comments on various versions of this paper which began as a talk to undergraduates.

Ought We to Try to Save Aborted Fetuses?

Daniel I. Wikler

Abortions performed during the second and third trimesters of pregnancy sometimes result in abortuses (aborted fetuses) which might be saved if given vigorous medical care. Does morality require that they receive it? Is their death precisely as acceptable on moral grounds as the abortion itself? The issue is now raised only occasionally, for abortions which might produce living fetuses are not commonly performed. As the age of viability continues to decrease, however, we can expect more such cases. Indeed, in the very long run the problem may be posed by all abortions, if medical technology succeeds in producing an artificial womb capable of salvaging embryos and fetuses from the moment of conception.

It may seem that controversy over the fate of the abortus is merely one skirmish in the larger battle over abortion. Socially and politically this may well be the case. Persons opposing the recent relaxation of prohibitions on abortion may raise the question of the abortus's fate in order to keep the abortion controversy alive and to engender sympathy for fetuses.[1] The general strategy here might be to soften up the opposition by focusing on peripheral issues—public funding of abortions, fetal research, and other topics in addition to resuscitation of abortuses—as preparation for a campaign against abortion itself. Feminists and others who prize newly won abortion rights may be put on guard by this tactic and refuse to grant any moral standing to the abortus, insisting rather that the mother must retain full control over its fate after abortion as she now does beforehand. It would become easy to predict a person's stand on rescuing abortuses once the person's view of abortion became known: pro-abortion, anti-resuscitation; anti-abortion, pro-resuscitation.

To some, these pairings might appear sound not only strategically but also theoretically: They are the positions one would expect even if

From *Ethics,* 90 (October 1979), pp. 58–65. Reprinted by permission of the author and the University of Chicago Press. © 1979 by the University of Chicago.

there were no ideological or political struggle in the background. This, I will argue, is mistaken. The logic of pro- and anti-abortion views, respectively, does not necessarily bind one to the corresponding anti- or pro-resuscitation position. In the analysis which follows, I attempt to show that all combinations of these views could be (internally) consistent. This is not because the two questions are wholly independent of each other conceptually, but because different grounds for the same position on abortion may dictate opposite conclusions on the rights of the abortus. I will be content here to sketch the connections between these views. The "correct" solution to the problem of the abortus's fate depends on answers to the larger issues of abortion and the right to medical care, neither of which I will attempt to resolve here.

ANTI-ABORTION VIEWS

Do abortuses, then, deserve the same treatment as other patients in need of care? Those who find abortion morally repugnant generally will answer in the affirmative. Though one might oppose abortion out of a desire for population growth or for a variety of other reasons, the standard moral consideration is concern for the welfare of the fetus. Few persons who oppose abortion on this ground will have reason to cease being concerned when the fetus leaves the womb; abortion would be, for these purposes, merely one sort of premature delivery.

Some opponents of abortion, however, do have cause to refrain from advocacy of resuscitation of aborted fetuses. Abortion is found morally unacceptable by these persons because it is seen as taking a life, an act which, in their view, cannot be justified by the resulting enhancement of the pregnant woman's welfare. Indeed, as is well known, some oppose abortion for this reason even when the failure to abort results in the mother's death.[2] As Roman Catholic theologians must tire of explaining, the choice for the fetus over the mother in this situation does not derive from callousness or antipathy to adult women. It is based—in theory, at least—upon the difference in character between the acts of killing the fetus and allowing the mother to die. The former is said to be an act "against life" and the latter not, although, to my mind, the point thus expressed is obscure and unconvincing. Clearer and more intuitive is the related distinction between a right not to be killed versus a right to have one's life saved. It is reasonable (though controversial) to posit natural right to the first but not the second (and to believe that the distinction between killing and allowing to die is there to make). A conscientious holder of these views might oppose abortion even when all of his or her sympathies are with the endangered mother, simply because the fetus's protection is due it by right. Once aborted, however, the tables turn: Though actual killing of the abortus would be ruled out, there may be no imperative to provide the care it needs to survive. Of course, the fact that these two positions are consistent with each other does not show that either is correct or that many would be (psychologically) likely to hold them in conjunction. Further, the abortus's right to medical care might exist by virtue of specific duties to provide aid on the part of the parent, the doctor, or the state.

A more likely reason for an opponent of abortion to stand against aid to the fetus would be a belief that the abortion in some way robbed the fetus of its claim to rights of all sorts. In particular, some opponents of abortion insist that the fetus's right to be brought to term in utero derives not from its already being a "person" with the rights attendant thereto but by virtue of its potential to become one. If the fetus has rights only qua potential person—"person" understood as conscious being with ability to reason—then the abortus which suffers brain damage or other serious injury during or as a result of an abortion will be ascribed no rights. And this potential is often lost during abortions. Most mid-trimester abortuses do not live for long, even with maximum care; and some of those which do suffer from mental deficits so

great that the ability to reason is never acquired. Still, a person who opposed abortion out of regard for the fetus's potential must, it seems, accord to the abortus with good prognosis the same status as that of other patients in need.

PRO-ABORTION VIEWS

It is preposterous to many advocates of legalized abortion that the state should simultaneously permit abortions and require resuscitation of abortuses. The very purpose of many of these abortions is the destruction of the fetus, and this act seemingly is endorsed socially by the legal right to seek abortion. The fact of expulsion from the womb seems insufficiently significant to change permission to kill into a duty to save. Requiring a lifesaving medical team to be prepared to rush into the operating clinic in the event that the abortion team fails to achieve the fetus's death seems to betray at best a serious ambivalence in the concern for the fetus and in the attitude to abortion.

Yet, despite appearances, it can be perfectly consistent to insist on the woman's right to abortion and at the same time to require that any live abortuses be saved, even if contrary to the wishes of the mother. Again, the variable here is the ground upon which approval of abortion rests. Two kinds of justifications for abortion are most important: first, that the fetus, being insufficiently "human" or not a person,[3] lacks a right to life; and second, that a mother's right to do as she wishes with her own body overrides any rights the fetus may have. Each for these views admits of variants from which one might deduce both support for abortion and insistence on care of the abortus.

THE ABORTUS AS A PERSON

The first of these pro-abortion views is actually several: What distinguishes them is the stage of development during pregnancy at which the fetus is thought to gain moral status. The candidates are numerous, ranging from conception to implantation to the appearance of brainwaves[4] or from recognizably human form[5] to viability[6] to birth. The choice of one of these as the moment at which the fetus acquires rights, including the right to life, depends in turn upon one's conception of personhood and choice of moral theory. We need not concern ourselves here with these arguments. It will be helpful, however, to sort these developmental milestones into two categories: those whose occurrence is causally and/or conceptually independent of abortion, and those whose occurrence is not. In the former category are many of the stages most often mentioned as the point of "personhood": conception, development of human form, and beginnings of consciousness. These are independent of abortion in the sense that whether a fetus has reached these stages by the time of abortion is strictly a matter of its developmental schedule. Abortion does not cause them to occur (though, of course, the peril in which the fetus is placed during and after abortion could cause it to lose what it once had). If, at any one of these stages, the abortion is thought to be morally justified, then the fetus will (in this view) have failed to develop whatever characteristics are held to be constitutive of being a person. The abortus, being no further advanced than the fetus was with respect to any of the milestones in this category, will also lack moral status and will not command the same medical care as other patients in need. Mother or doctor will be justified in taking steps to end the abortus's life, in this view, just as both were when the fetus was in utero. Of course, the mother might ask that the abortus be rescued, just as she might have decided to bring the baby to term and then deliver normally. But if she does not, there is no more reason to condemn her in the one case than in the other; it is her decision whether to save, let die, or kill.

The situation is quite different, however, for milestones in the second category, those linked to the abortion process. Abortion causes certain changes to take place; and, if it should happen that a person's conception of "humanness" or personhood involved characteristics which a fetus thus acquires by these changes, the abortus might be accorded a different fate.

Before stating a plausible example, however, I want to consider a possible indicator of humanness which, while it does not belong in this group, may at first appear to. This is the at-

tainment of viability, which, besides having historical prominence, is the only criterion of personhood (other than the membership in our species) with significance in current American law.[7] This milestone might figure in the debate as part of the following argument: The fetus becomes a person and acquires human rights upon viability; if the fetus survives the abortion and promises to respond to medical resuscitation, its viability is established. Hence, a living abortus has the same moral status and rights as other patients, at least those with similar prognosis; and it acquires these rights in the process of (surviving) the abortion.

This argument does not go through. It is true that if an abortus has a good chance for survival, its viability is established; this is a matter of definition. But the viability is not brought about by the abortion. Viability is the capacity for independent existence, not the performance thereof. The capacity can, of course, be present in utero. An abortus's good prognosis shows that the fetus/abortus was viable not only after leaving the womb but also before. And this shows not only that the abortus has a right to the same treatment as other patients, but that it had a right not to be aborted—provided, as here by hypothesis, that viability marks the time at which abortion becomes immoral. Those who use viability as a standard for personhood, then, would have no reason to support resuscitation of survivors of abortions of which they approve.

There is, however, at least one milestone in the fetal career which is achieved upon abortion, namely, physical separation. Separation, and actual independent existence, seems to be the criterion of personhood for many who find nothing wrong with abortion even in the last weeks of pregnancy but who find infanticide morally repugnant. That a fetus *could* live independently, in this view, is no reason to count the fetus as an individual distinct from its mother; viability, like all other stages of fetal development, is morally inconsequential. The removal of the fetus from the womb, however, would by this standard create a person, whether this occurs in abortion or in birth. Ending the life of a viable abortus, then, will be counted as infanticide and be subject to moral condemnation, while ending the life of even a viable fetus violates no right to life. It may seem improbable that a person could be led by these considerations to the position of approving of abortion and requiring resuscitation, but no more improbable than the widely accepted criterion of separation itself.

FETAL RIGHTS AND MOTHER'S RIGHTS

The justification for abortion which, most naturally extends to support for the abortus makes no mention of personhood criteria.[8] It begins by conceding (perhaps only for purposes of argument) that the fetus is as human as adults are, possessing the same set of natural rights. Abortion is morally acceptable in this view because the right to life does not guarantee the unconsented use of another's body, even if necessary for survival. The pregnant woman's right to do as she pleases with her body is held to allow her to refuse her womb's protective environment to a fully human fetus, the latter's right to life notwithstanding. There is no pretending, of course, that the discomfort and inconvenience of the average pregnancy is as detrimental to the mother's well-being as death would be to the fetus's. But concern for the fetus's welfare is not seen to require sacrifice by an unwilling mother, any more than one would require a healthy person unwillingly to surrender a kidney to save the life of another person dying of end-stage renal disease. We may urge the mother to refrain from abortion, but if this account of the several rights involved is correct we cannot require her to do so.

Once the fetus has been expelled from the mother's body, however, its moral status is in no way denied by this sort of argument. What is striking about this defense of abortion is that it concedes at the outset what most have thought to be the basic anti-abortion premise, namely, that the fetus is a person with a right to life. The act of abortion does nothing to strip the fetus of this right (provided that the abortus has a favorable prognosis). There is no reason, then, for one who supports a right to abort on these grounds to see the abortus as having less right to treatment than other patients in similar circumstances: certainly the abortus's right is not overridden by the mother's right to do as she wants with her body. This view will support the mother's right to abort as a necessary evil, one which must be accepted in order to respect the mother's rights. Denying the same care to the abortus that other patients would receive, however, would simply be an evil.

In the view under discussion, the mother has a right to seek an abortion because of her rights over her body. A related view might support the mother's abortion on the grounds of a putative right to determine whether she is to be a mother. Indeed, it is reasonable to suppose that many more women seeking abortions do so in order to avoid bearing and raising the child than to avoid the inconvenience and discomfort of pregnancy. A right protecting this interest would not only legitimate abortion but, it might be argued, would also allow a mother to demand that the living product of that abortion not be given medical care. The abortion itself would be one exercise of that right, but if the fetus survived it the exercise would have to be counted as unsuccessful. Letting the abortus die, or even killing it, would represent a second exercise of that same right. And, were there such a right, letting the abortus die would be just as legitimate as the abortion itself, for in both cases the alleged right to decide whether to be a mother is held to override the right to life of the fetus/abortus. Of course, the "right not to be a mother" is a dubious one. It would license infanticide as well and even the killing of older children. Those who support a right to seek abortion out of concern for a woman's being able to decide whether to be a mother need not recognize any right to the latter. They can try to justify abortion by reference to rights over the body or to the fetus's lack of personhood, each of which (it is argued) would make abortion morally defensible even when the sole motive is avoidance of being a mother. These distinct justifications for abortion have much the same effect when, as in the usual case, abortion results in the death of the fetus. When the product of abortion is living and viable, their import is different. Abortion qua termination of pregnancy satisfies the woman's rights over her body but not any right to decide on motherhood. That termination of pregnancy and termination of fetal life have for so long nearly always occurred together has obscured the need to clarify the nature of the mother's rights involved. This, in turn, has perhaps made it less clear what sort of treatment of the abortus must be favored by one who supports, on these grounds, the mother's right to seek an abortion.

CONCLUSION

There are, then, conceptual links between views on abortion and on the right of a live abortus to medical care, but the relationships need not be the simple correlations which are most commonly held. Though most opponents of abortion may be those most concerned over the fate of the viable abortus, there are possible grounds for opposition to abortion which do not imply support for treatment of abortuses. Similarly, some of the arguments commonly given in support of a woman's right to seek an abortion do not support a mother's or doctor's effort to "finish the job" and see to it that the fetus dies. Some of these pro-abortion arguments seem, rather, to require that the fetus receive the same care as others in like circumstances.

What sort of care ought the abortus to receive if it deserves the same treatment as other patients in similar circumstances? The answer does not issue from any of the arguments considered above. A right to equal treatment establishes only that the infant's being an abortus is not to be taken into account in determining its rights. It is still appropriate to take note of several aspects of its situation which might not have been present had it been brought to term. Among these are the facts that it is unwanted; that no one will have contracted with a doctor to provide it medical services; that it is indigent; and, in some cases, that its prognosis is poor. I believe that most of us would recognize a maternal or societal duty to provide care for most patients in this category (with the possible exception of those with poor prognoses),[9] but this is a question to be decided only on the basis of a comprehensive theory of distributive justice.

Notes

1. Current American law seems to support this position. Though late-term abortions are legal in many states, killing an abortus has been branded a felony. Mothers who do not allow (even those who fail to request) medical care for offspring could be charged with neglect, and medical staff who acquiesce may be guilty of conspiracy and of failing to report child abuse. See *Commonwealth v. Edelin*, 359 N.E., 2d 4, and Robertson, *Involuntary Euthanasia of Defective Newborns: A Legal Analysis*, 27 STAN. L. REV. 237 (1975).

2. Here, as throughout the paper, I use the term 'mother' as an abbreviation for 'presently or formerly pregnant woman.' I do not mean to beg the question of which obligations the woman may have regarding the child, despite the suggestiveness of the connotations of mother in ordinary speech.

3. I will use 'person,' 'human being,' and 'being with moral status' interchangeably, though were I discussing abortion itself I would have good reason not to. The idea I want to capture with this loose terminology is that an entity acquires the standard set of natural rights and/or is entitled to the same sorts of treatment which moral rules require others receive if and only if it has certain properties or a certain kind of nature.

4. Baruch Brody, "On the Humanity of the Foetus," in *Abortion: Pro and Con*, ed. Robert L. Perkins (Cambridge, Mass.: Schenkman Publishing Co., 1974).

5. Lawrence Becker, "Human Being: The Boundaries of the Concept," *Philosophy and Public Affairs* 4, no. 4 (Summer 1975): 334–59.

6. In *Roe* v. *Wade*, the U.S. Supreme Court forbade states to pass laws restricting abortions before viability. States may ban abortions after viability. At the same time, the Court insisted that it would take no position on the question of when life began.

7. It may occur to the reader that if the fetus has a good chance to live on its own, abortion will be little or no offense to it: hence, one who holds viability to be the point at which the fetus acquires rights might not oppose abortion thereafter. This shows the oddity of the Supreme Court ruling, which makes it possible for the states to allow abortion during the period in which abortion will be fatal to the fetus but to forbid it during the period in which it would not. Of course, the fact that abortions are usually harmful even to viable fetuses may have been a factor in the decision.

This point was made by my colleague, John Robertson, J.D.

8. See Judith Thomson, ''A Defense of Abortion'' (*Philosophy and Public Affairs* 1, no. 1 [Fall 1971]:

47–66) for an exposition of this view. Thomson, incidentally, specifically denies that a mother may order a surviving abortus killed.

9. See Robertson.

From "Making Babies" Revisited

Leon R. Kass

And the man knew not Eve his wife; but she conceived without him and bore Cain, and said: I have gotten a man with the help of Dr. Steptoe.
Ectogenesis IV, 1

And Isaac entreated the NIH for his wife, because she was barren; and the NIH let Itself be entreated of him, and Rebekah his wife conceived.
Ectogenesis XXV, 21

Seven years ago in the pages of this journal, in an article entitled ''Making Babies—the New Biology and the 'Old' Morality'' (Number 26, Winter 1972), I explored some of the moral and political questions raised by projected new powers to intervene in the processes of human reproduction. I concluded that it would be foolish to acquire and use these powers. The questions have since been debated in ''bioethical'' circles and in college classrooms, and they have received intermittent attention in the popular press and in sensational novels and movies. This past year they have gained the media limelight with the Del Zio suit against Columbia University, and more especially with the birth last summer in Britain of Louise Brown, the first identified human baby born following conception in the laboratory. . . .

I was asked by the [Ethics Advisory] Board to discuss the ethical issues raised by the proposed research on human *in vitro* fertilization, laboratory cultures of—and experimentation with—human embryos, and the intra-uterine transfer of such embryos for the purpose of assisting human generation. . . .

Reprinted (with deletions) with permission of the author from *The Public Interest,* no. 54 (Winter, 1979), pp. 32–60. © 1979 by National Affairs, Inc.

II

How should one think about the ethical issues, here and in general? There are many possible ways, and it is not altogether clear which way is best. For some people ethical issues are immediately matters of right and wrong, of purity and sin, of good and evil. For others, the critical terms are benefits and harms, risks and promises, gains and costs. Some will focus on so-called rights of individuals or groups, e.g., a right of life or childbirth; still others will emphasize so-called goods for society and its members, such as the advancement of knowledge and the prevention and cure of disease.

My own orientation here is somewhat different. I wish to suggest that before deciding what to do, one should try to understand the implications of doing or not doing. The first task, it seems to me, is not to ask ''moral or immoral?'' ''right or wrong?'' but to try to understand fully the meaning and significance of the proposed actions.

This concern with significance leads me to take a broad view of the matter. For we are concerned here not only with the proposed research of Dr. Soupart,* and the narrow issues of safety and informed consent it immediately raises, but also with a whole range of implications including many that are tied to definitely foreseeable consequences of this research and its pre-

* *Editor's Note:* Kass's remarks are addressed to an Ethics Advisory Board established by the Secretary of HEW to provide recommendations on principles of funding research proposals involving *in vitro* fertilization. Dr. Soupart submitted a research proposal to investigate possible genetic risk for certain procedures used in *in vitro* fertilization.

dictable extensions—and touching even our common conception of our own humnaity. The very establishment of a special Ethics Advisory Board testifies that we are at least tacitly aware that more is at stake than in ordinary biomedical research, or in experimenting with human subjects at risk of bodily harm. At stake is the *idea* of the *humanness* of our human life and the meaning of our embodiment, our sexual being, and our relation to ancestors and descendants. In reaching the necessarily particular and immediate decision in the case at hand, we must be mindful of the larger picture and must avoid the great danger of trivializing this matter for the sake of rendering it manageable.

III

What is the status of a fertilized human egg (i.e., a human zygote) and the embryo that develops from it? How are we to regard its being? How are we to regard it morally, i.e., how are we to behave toward it? These are, alas, all-too-familiar questions. At least analogous, if not identical, questions are central to the abortion controversy and are also crucial in considering whether and what sort of experimentation is properly conducted on living but aborted fetuses. Would that it were possible to say that the matter is simple and obvious, and that it has been resolved to everyone's satisfaction!

But the controversy about the morality of abortion continues to rage and divide our nation. Moreover, many who favor or do not oppose abortion do so despite the fact that they regard the pre-viable fetus as a living human organism, even if less worthy of protection than a woman's desire not to give it birth. Almost everyone senses the importance of this matter for the decision about laboratory culture of, and experimentation with, human embryos. Thus, we are obliged to take up the question of the status of the embryos, in a search for the outlines of some common ground on which many of us can stand. To the best of my knowledge, the discussion which follows is not informed by any particular sectarian or religious teaching, though it may perhaps reveal that I am a person not devoid of reverence and the capacity for awe and wonder, said by some to be the core of the "religious" sentiment.

I begin by noting that the circumstances of laboratory-grown blastocysts (i.e., 3-to-6-day-old embryos) and embryos are not identical with those of the analogous cases of 1) living fetuses facing abortion and 2) living aborted fetuses used in research. First, the fetuses whose fates are at issue in abortion are unwanted, usually the result of "accidental" conception. Here, the embryos are wanted, and deliberately created, despite certain knowledge that many of them will be destroyed or discarded.[1] Moreover, the fate of these embryos is not in conflict with the wishes, interests, or alleged rights of the pregnant women. Second, though the HEW guidelines governing fetal research permit studies conducted on the not-at-all-viable aborted fetus, such research merely takes advantage of available "products" of abortions not themselves undertaken for the sake of the research. No one has proposed and no one would sanction the deliberate production of live fetuses to be aborted for the sake of research, even very beneficial research.[2] In contrast, we are here considering the deliberate production of embryos for the express purpose of experimentation.

The cases may also differ in other ways. Given the present state of the art, the largest embryo under discussion is the blastocyst, a spherical, relatively undifferentiated mass of cells, barely visible to the naked eye. In appearance it does not look human; indeed, only the most careful scrutiny by the most experienced scientist might distinguish it from similar blastocysts of other mammals. If the human zygote and blastocyst are more like the animal zygote and blastocyst than they are like the 12-week-old human fetus (which already has a humanoid appearance, differentiated organs, and electrical activity of the brain), then there would be a much-diminished ethical dilemma regarding their deliberate creation and experimental use. Needless to say, there are articulate and passionate defenders of all points of view. Let us try, however, to consider the matter afresh.

First of all, the zygote and early embryonic stages are clearly alive. They metabolize, respire, and respond to changes in the environment; they grow and divide. Second, though not yet organized into distinctive parts or organs, the blastocyst is an organic whole, self-developing, genetically unique and distinct from the egg and sperm whose union marked the beginning of its career as a discrete, unfolding being. While the egg and sperm are alive as cells, something new and alive *in a different sense* comes into being with fertilization. The truth of this is unaffected by the fact that fertilization takes time and is not an instantaneous event. For after fertilization is *complete,* there exists a new individual, with its unique genetic identity, fully potent for the self-initiated development into a mature human being, if circumstances are cooperative. Though there is some sense in which the lives of egg and sperm are continuous with the life of the new organism-to-be (or, in human terms, that the parents live on in the child or child-to-be), in the decisive sense there is a discontinuity, a new beginning, with fertilization. *After* fertilization, there is continuity of subsequent development, even if the locus of the embryo alters with implantation (or birth). Any honest biologist must be impressed by these facts, and must be inclined, at least on first glance, to the view that a human life begins at fertilization. Even Dr. Robert Edwards has apparently stumbled over this truth, perhaps inadvertently, in the remark about Louise Brown attributed to him in an article by Peter Gwynne in *Science Digest:* "The last time I saw *her, she* was just eight cells in a test-tube. *She* was beautiful *then,* and she's still beautiful *now!*"[3]

But granting that a human life begins at fertilization, and comes-to-be via a continuous process thereafter, surely—one might say—the blastocyst itself is hardly a human being. I myself would agree that a blastocyst is not, in a *full* sense, a human being—or what the current fashion calls, rather arbitrarily and without clear definition, a person. It does not look like a human being nor can it do very much of what human beings do. Yet, at the same time, I must acknowledge that the human blastocyst is 1) human in origin and 2) *potentially* a mature human being, if all goes well. This too is beyond dispute; indeed it is precisely because of its peculiarly human potentialities that people propose to study *it* rather than the embryos of other mammals. The human blastocyst, even the human blastocyst *in vitro,* is not humanly

nothing; it possesses a power to become what everyone will agree is a human being.

Here it may be objected that the blastocyst *in vitro* has today no such power, because there is now no way *in vitro* to bring the blastocyst to that much later fetal stage at which it might survive on its own. There are no published reports of culture of human embryos past the blastocyst stage (though this has been reported for mice). The *in vitro* blastocyst, like the 12-week-old aborted fetus, is *in this sense* not viable (i.e., it is at a stage of maturation before the stage of possible independent existence). But if we distinguish, among the *not*-viable embryos, between the *pre*-viable and the *not-at-all* viable—on the basis that the former, though not yet viable is capable of *becoming or being made* viable[4]—we note a crucial difference between the blastocyst and the 12-week abortus. Unlike an aborted fetus, the blastocyst is possibly salvageable, and hence *potentially* viable *if it is transferred to a woman for implantation.* It is not strictly true that the *in vitro* blastocyst is *necessarily* not-viable. Until proven otherwise, by embryo transfer and attempted implantation, we are right to consider the human blastocyst *in vitro* as potentially a human being and, in this respect, not fundamentally different from a blastocyst *in utero.* Too put the matter more forcefully, the blastocyst *in vitro* is *more* "viable," in the sense of more salvageable, than aborted fetuses at most later stages, up to say 20 weeks.

This is not to say that such a blastocyst is therefore endowed with a so-called right to life, that failure to implant it is negligent homicide, or that experimental touchings of such blastocysts constitute assault and battery. (I myself tend to reject such claims, and indeed think that the ethical questions are not best posed in terms of "rights.") But the blastocyst is not nothing; it is *as least* potential humanity, and as such it elicits, or ought to elicit, our feelings of awe and respect. In the blastocyst, even in the zygote, we face a mysterious and awesome power, a power governed by an immanent plan that may produce an indisputably and fully human being. It deserves our respect not because it has rights or claims or sentience (which it does not have at this stage), but because of what it is, now *and* prospectively.

Let us test this provisional conclusion by considering intuitively our response to two possible fates of such zygotes, blastocysts, and early embryos. First, should such an embryo die, will we be inclined to mourn its passing? When a woman we know miscarries, we are sad—largely for *her* loss and disappointment, but perhaps also at the premature death of a life that might have been. But we do not mourn the departed fetus, nor do we seek ritually to dispose of the remains. In this respect, we do not treat even the fetus as fully one of us.

On the other hand, we would I suppose recoil even from the thought, let alone the practice—I apologize for forcing it upon the reader—of eating such embryos, should someone discover that they would provide a great delicacy, a "human caviar." The human blastocyst would be protected by our taboo against cannibalism, which insists on the humanness of human flesh and which does not permit us to treat even the flesh of the dead as if it were mere meat. *The human embryo is not mere meat; it is not just stuff; it is not a thing.*[5] Because of its origin and because of its capacity, it commands a higher respect.

How much more respect? As much as for a fully developed human being? My own inclination is to say "probably not," but who can be certain? Indeed, there might be prudential and reasonable grounds for an affirmative answer, partly because the presumption of ignorance ought to err in the direction of never underestimating the basis for respect of human life, partly because so many people feel very strongly that even the blastocyst is protectably human. As a first approximation, I would analogize the early embryo *in vitro* to the early embryo *in utero* (because both are potentially viable and human). On this ground alone, *the most sensible policy is to treat the early embryo as a pre-viable fetus, with constraints imposed on early embryo research at least as great as those on fetal research.*

To some this may seem excessively scrupulous. They will argue for the importance of the absence of distinctive humanoid appearance or the absence of sentience. To be sure, we would feel more restraint in invasive procedures conducted on a five-month-old or even 12-week-old living fetus than on a blastocyst. But this added restraint on inflicting suffering on a "look-alike," feeling creature in no way denies the propriety of a prior restraint, grounded in respect for individuated, living, potential humanity. Before I would be persuaded to treat early embryos differently from later ones, I would insist on the establishment of a reasonably clear, naturally grounded boundary that separates "early" and "late," and which provides the basis for respecting "the early" less than "the late." This burden *must* be accepted by proponents of experimentation with human embryos *in vitro* if a decision to permit creating embryos for such experimentation is to be treated as ethically responsible.

IV

Where does the above analysis lead in thinking about treatment of *in vitro* human embryos? I shall indicate, very briefly, the lines toward a possible policy, though that is not my major intent.

The *in vitro* fertilized embryo has four possible fates: 1) *implantation,* in the hope of producing from it a child; 2) *death,* by active "killing" or disaggregation, or by a "natural" demise; 3) use in *manipulative experimentation*—embryological, genetic, etc.; 4) use in attempts at *perpetuation in vitro* beyond the blastocyst stage, ultimately, perhaps, to viability. I will not now consider this fourth and future possibility, though I would suggest that full laboratory growth of an embryo into a viable human being (i.e., ectogenesis), while perfectly compatible with respect owed to its potential humanity as an individual, may be incompatible with the kind of respect owed to its humanity that is grounded in the bonds of lineage and the nature of parenthood.

On the strength of my analysis of the status of the embryo, and the respect due it, no objection would be raised to implantation. *In vitro* fertilization and embryo transfer to treat infertility, as in the case of Mr. and Mrs. Brown, is perfectly compatible with a respect and reverence for human life, including potential human life. Moreover, no disrespect is intended or practiced by the mere fact that several eggs are removed for fertilization, to increase the chance of success. Were it possible to guarantee successful fertilization and normal growth with a single egg, no more would need to be obtained. Assuming nothing further is done with the unimplanted embryos, there is nothing disrespectful going on. The demise of the unimplanted embryos would be analogous to the loss of numerous embryos wasted in the normal *in vivo* attempts to generate a child. It is estimated that over 50 percent of eggs successfully fertilized during unprotected sexual intercourse fail to implant, or do not remain implanted, in the uterine wall, and are shed soon thereafter, before a diagnosis of pregnancy could be made. Any couple attempting to conceive a child tacitly accepts such embryonic wastage as the perfectly acceptable price to be paid for the birth of a (usually) healthy child. Current procedures to initiate pregnancy with laboratory fertilization thus differ from the natural "procedure" in that what would normally be spread over four or five months *in vivo* is compressed into a single effort, using all at once a four or five months' supply of eggs.[6]

Parenthetically, we should note that the natural occurrence of embryo and fetal loss and wastage does not necessarily or automatically justify all deliberate, humanly caused destruction of fetal life. For example, the natural loss of embryos in early pregnancy cannot in itself be a warrant for deliberately aborting them or for invasively experimenting on them *in vitro,* any more than stillbirths could be a justification for newborn infanticide. There are many things that happen naturally that we ought not to do deliberately. It is curious how the same people who deny the relevance of nature as a guide for evaluating human interventions into human generation, and who deny that the term "unnatural" carries any ethical weight, will themselves appeal to "nature's way" when it suits their purposes.[7] Still, in this present matter, the closeness to natural procreation—the goal is the same, the embryonic loss is unavoidable and not desired, and the amount of loss is similar—leads me to believe that we do no more intentional or unjustified harm in the one case than in the other, and practice no disrespect.

But must we allow *in vitro* unimplanted embryos to die? Why should they not be either transferred for "adoption" into another infertile woman, or else used for investigative purposes, to seek new knowledge, say about gene action? The first option raises questions about the nature of parenthood and lineage to which I will return. But even on first glance, it would seem likely to raise a large objection from the original couple, who were seeking a child of their own and not the dissemination of their "own" biological children for prenatal adoption.

But what about experimentation on such blastocysts and early embryos? Is that compatible with the respect they deserve? This is the hard question. On balance, I would think not. Invasive and manipulative experiments involving such embryos very likely presume that they are things or mere stuff, and deny the fact of their possible viability. Certain observational and non-invasive experiments might be different. But on the whole, I would think that the respect for human embryos for which I have argued—I repeat, not their so-called right to life—would lead one to oppose most potentially interesting and useful experimentation. This is a dilemma, but one which cannot be ducked or defined away. Either we accept certain great restrictions on the permissible uses of human embryos or we deliberately decide to override—though I hope not deny—the respect due to the embryos.

I am aware that I have pointed toward a seemingly paradoxical conclusion about the treatment of the unimplanted embryos: Leave them alone, and do not create embryos for experimentation only. To let them die "naturally" would be the most respectful course, grounded on a reverence, generically, for their potential humanity, and a respect, individually, for their being the seed and offspring of a particular couple who were themselves seeking only to have a child of their own. An analysis which stressed a "right to life," rather than respect, would of course lead to different conclusions. Only an analysis of the status of the embryo which denied both its so-called "rights" *or* its worthiness of all respect would have no trouble sanctioning its use in investigative research, donation to other couples, commercial transactions, and other activities of these sorts.

VI

Many people rejoiced at the birth of Louise Brown. Some were pleased by the technical accomplishment, many were pleased that she was born apparently in good health. But most of us shared the joy of her parents, who after a long, frustrating, and fruitless period, at last had the pleasure and blessing of a child of their own. The desire to have a child of one's own is acknowledged to be a powerful and deep-seated human desire—some have called it "instinctive"—and the satisfaction of this desire, by the relief of infertility, is said to be one major goal of continuing the work with *in vitro* fertilization and embryo transfer. That this is a worthy goal few, if any, would deny.

Yet let us explore what is meant by *"to have a child of one's own."* First, what is meant by "to have"? Is the crucial meaning that of gestating and bearing? Or is it "to have" as a possession? Or is it to nourish and to rear, the child being the embodiment of one's activity as teacher and guide? Or is it rather to provide someone who descends and comes after, someone who will replace oneself in the family line or preserve the family tree by new sproutings and branchings?

More significantly, what is meant by *"one's own"*? What sense of one's own is important? A scientist might define "one's own" in terms of carrying one's own genes. Though in some sense correct, this cannot be humanly decisive. For Mr. Brown or for most of us, it would not be a matter of indifference if the sperm used to fertilize the egg were provided by an identical twin brother—whose genes would be, of course, the same as his. Rather, the humanly crucial sense of "one's own," the sense that leads most people to choose their own, rather than to adopt, is captured in such phrases as "my seed," "flesh of my flesh," "sprung from my loins." More accurately, since "one's own" is not the own of one but of *two*, the desire to have a child of "one's own" is *a couple's desire* to embody, out of the conjugal union of their separate bodies, a child who is flesh of their separate flesh made one. This archaic language may sound quaint,

but I would argue that this is precisely what is being celebrated by most people who rejoice at the birth of Louise Brown, whether they would articulate it this way or not. Mr. and Mrs. Brown, by the birth of their daughter, fulfill this aspect of their separate sexual natures and of their married life together, they acquire descendants and a new branch of their joined family tree, and the child Louise is given solid and unambiguous roots from which she has sprung and by which she will be nourished.

If this were to be the *only* use made of embryo transfer, and if providing *in this sense* "a child of one's own" were indeed the sole reason for the clinical use of the techniques, there could be no objection. Yet there will almost certainly be other uses, involving third parties, to satisfy the desire "to have" a child of "one's own" in different senses of "to have" and "one's own." I am not merely speculating about future possibilities. With the technology to effect human *in vitro* fertilization and embryo transfer comes the *immediate* possibility of egg donation (egg from donor, sperm from husband), embryo donation (egg and sperm from outside of the marriage), and foster pregnancy (host surrogate for gestation).

Nearly everyone agrees that these circumstances are morally and perhaps psychologically more complicated than the intra-marital case. Here the meaning of "one's own" is no longer so unambiguous; neither is the meaning of motherhood and the status of pregnancy. On the one hand, it is argued that embryo donation, or "prenatal adoption," would be superior to present adoption, because the woman would have the experience of pregnancy and the child would be born of the "adopting" mother, rendering the maternal tie even more close. On the other hand, the mother-child bond rooted in pregnancy and delivery is held to be of little consequence by those who would endorse the use of surrogate gestational "mothers," say for a woman whose infertility is due to uterine disease rather than ovarian disease or oviduct obstruction. Clearly, the "need" and demand for extra-marital embryo transfer are real and probably large, probably even greater than the intra-marital ones. Already, the Chairman of the

Ethics Advisory Board has testified in Congress about the need to define the responsibilities of *the donor* and the recipient "parents." Thus the new techniques will not only serve to ensure and preserve lineage, but will also serve to confound and complicate it. The principle truly at work here is not to provide married couples with a child of *their own,* but to provide anyone who wants one with a child, by whatever possible or convenient means.

"So what?" it will be said. First of all, we already practice and encourage adoption. Second, we have permitted artificial insemination—though we have, after some 40 years of this practice, yet to resolve questions of legitimacy. Third, what with the high rate of divorce and remarriage, identification of "mother," "father," and "child" are already complicated. Fourth, there is a growing rate of illegitimacy and husbandless parentages. Fifth, the use of surrogate mothers for foster pregnancy has already occurred, with the aid of artificial insemination. Finally, our age in its enlightenment is no longer so certain about the virtues of family, lineage, and heterosexuality, or even about the taboos against adultery and incest. Against this background, it will be asked, why all the fuss about some little embryos that stray from the nest?

It is not an easy question to answer. Yet, consider. We practice adoption because there are abandoned children who need a good home. We do not, and would not, encourage people deliberately to generate children for others to adopt; partly we wish to avoid baby markets, partly we think it unfair to the child deliberately to deprive him of his natural ties. Recent years have seen a rise in our concern with roots, against the rootless and increasingly homogeneous background of contemporary American life. Adopted children, in particular, are pressing for information regarding their "real parents," and some states now require that such information be made available (on that typically modern ground of "freedom of information," rather than because of the profound importance of lineage for self-identity). The practice of artificial insemination has yet to be evaluated, the secrecy in which it is practiced being an apparent concession to the dangers of

publicity. Indeed, most physicians who practice artificial insemination routinely mix in some semen from the husband, to preserve some doubt about paternity—again, a concession to the importance of lineage and legitimacy. Finally, what about the changing mores of marriage, divorce, single-parent families, and sexual behavior? Do we applaud these changes? Do we want to contribute further to the confusion of thought, identity, and practice?[8]

Properly understood, the largely universal taboos against incest, and also the prohibition against adultery, suggest that clarity about who your parents are, clarity in the lines of generation, clarity about who is whose, are the indispensable foundations of a sound family life, itself the sound foundation of civilized community. Clarity about your origins is crucial for self-identity, itself important for self-respect. It would be, in my view, deplorable public policy further to erode such fundamental beliefs, values, institutions, and practices. This means, concretely, no encouragement of embryo adoption or especially of surrogate pregnancy. While it would be perhaps foolish to try to proscribe or outlaw such practices, it would not be wise for the Federal government to foster them. The Ethics Advisory Board should carefully consider whether it should and can attempt to restrict the use of embryo transfer to the married couple from whom the embryo derives.

The case of surrogate wombs bears a further comment. While expressing no objection to the practice of foster pregnancy itself, some people object that it will be done for pay, largely because of their fear that poor women will be exploited by such a practice. But if there were nothing wrong with foster pregnancy, what would be wrong with making a living at it? Clearly, this objection harbors a *tacit* understanding that to bear another's child for pay is in some sense a degradation of oneself—in the same sense that prostitution is a degradation *primarily* because it entails the loveless surrender of one's body to serve another's lust, and *only derivatively* because the woman is paid. It is to deny the meaning and worth of one's body, to treat it as a mere incubator, divested of its human meaning. It is also to deny the mean-

ing of the bond among sexuality, love, and procreation. The buying and selling of human
flesh and the dehumanized uses of the human
body ought not to be encouraged. To be sure,
the practice of womb donation could be engaged in for love not money, as it apparently
has been in the case in Michigan. A woman
could bear her sister's child out of sisterly love.
But to the degree that one escapes in this way
from the degradation and difficulties of the *sale*
of human flesh and bodily services, and the
treating of the body as stuff (the problem of cannibalism), one approaches instead the difficulties of incest and near-incest.

VII

Objections have been raised about the deliberate technological intervention into the so-called
natural processes of human reproduction.
Some would simply oppose such interventions
as "unnatural," and therefore wrong. Others
are concerned about the consequences of these
interventions, and about their ends and limits.
Again, I think it important to explore the meaning and possible significance of such interventions, present and projected, especially as they
bear on fundamental beliefs, institutions, and
practices. To do so requires that we consider
likely future developments in the laboratory
study of human reproduction. Indeed, I shall
argue that we *must* consider such future developments in reaching a decision in the present
case.

What can we expect in the way of new modes
of reproduction, as an outgrowth of present
studies? To be sure, prediction is difficult. One
can never know with certainty what will happen, much less how soon. Yet uncertainty is not
the same as simple ignorance. Some things, indeed, seem likely. They seem likely because 1)
they are thought necessary or desirable, at least
by some researchers and their sponsors, 2) they
are probably biologically possible and technically feasible, and 3) they will be difficult to
prevent or control (especially if no one anticipates their development or sees a need to worry
about them). One of the things the citizenry,
myself included, would expect from an Ethics

Advisory Board and our policy makers generally is that they face up to reasonable projections of future accomplishments, consider
whether they are cause for social concern, and
see whether or not the principles *now* enunciated and the practices *now* established are adequate to deal with any such concerns.

I project at least the following:

1. The growth of human embryos in the
laboratory will be extended beyond the blastocyst stage. Such growth must be deemed desirable under all the arguments advanced for developmental research *up* to the blastocyst stage;
research on gene action, chromosome segregation, cellular and organic differentiation, fetus-
environment interaction, implantation, etc.,
cannot answer all its questions with the blastocyst. Such *in vitro* post-blastocyst differentiation
has apparently been achieved in the mouse, in
culture; the use of other mammals as temporary hosts for human embryos is also a possibility. How far such embryos will eventually be
perpetuated is anybody's guess, but full-term
ectogenesis cannot be excluded. Neither can
the existence of laboratories filled with many
living human embryos, growing at various
stages of development.

2. Experiments will be undertaken to alter
the cellular and genetic composition of these
embryos, at first without subsequent transfer to
a woman for gestation, perhaps later as a prelude to reproductive efforts. Again, scientific
reasons now justifying Dr. Soupart's research
already justify further embryonic manipulations, including formation of hybrids or chime-
ras (within species and between species); gene,
chromosome, and plasmid insertion, excision,
or alteration; nuclear transplantation or cloning, etc. The techniques of DNA recombination, coupled with the new skills of handling
embryos, make prospects for some precise
genetic manipulation much nearer than anyone would have guessed ten years ago. And embryological and cellular research in mammals is
making astounding progress. On the cover of a
recent issue of *Science* is a picture of a hexapar-
ental mouse, born after reaggregation of an
early embryo with cells disaggregated from
three separate embryos. (Note: That sober

journal calls this a "handmade mouse"—i.e., literally a *manu-factured* mouse—and goes on to say that it was "manufactured by genetic engineering techniques.")[9]

3. Storage and banking of living human embryos (and ova) will be undertaken, perhaps commercially. After all, commercial sperm banks are already well-established and prospering.

Space does not permit me to do more than identify a few kinds of questions that must be considered in relation to such possible coming control over human heredity and reproduction: questions about the wisdom required to engage in such practices; questions about the goals and standards that will guide our interventions; questions about changes in the concepts of being human, including embodiment, gender, love, lineage, identity, parenthood, and sexuality; questions about the responsibility of power over future generations; questions about awe, respect, humility; questions about the kind of society we will have if we follow along our present course.[10]

Though I cannot discuss these questions now, I can and must face a serious objection to considering them at all. Most people would agree that the projected possibilities raise far more serious questions than do simple fertilization of a few embryos, their growth *in vitro* to the blastocyst stage, and their possible transfer to women for gestation. Why burden the present decision with these possibilities? Future "abuses," it is often said, do not disqualify present uses (though these same people also often say that "future benefits justify present questionable uses"). Moreover, there can be no certainty that "A" will lead to "B." This thin-edge-of-the-wedge argument has been open to criticism.

But such criticism misses the point, for two reasons. *First,* critics often misunderstand the wedge argument. The wedge argument is not primarily an argument of prediction, that A *will* lead to B, say on the strength of the empirical analysis of precedent and an appraisal of the likely direction of present research. It is primarily an argument about the *logic* of justification. Do the principles of justification *now* used to justify the current research proposal already

justify *in advance* the futher developments? Consider some of these principles:

1. It is desirable to learn as much as possible about the processes of fertilization, growth, implantation, and differentiation of human embryos and about human gene expression and its control.

2. It would be desirable to acquire improved techniques for *enhancing* conception and implantation, for *preventing* conception and implantation, for the treatment of genetic and chromosomal abnormalities, etc.

3. In the end, only research using *human* embryos can answer these questions and provide these techniques.

4. There should be no censorship or limitation of scientific inquiry or research.

This logic knows no boundary at the blastocyst stage, or for that matter, at any later stage. For these principles *not* to justify future extensions of current work, some independent additional principles, limiting such justification to particular stages of development, would have to be found. Here, the task is to find such a biologically defensible distinction that could be respected as reasonable and not arbitrary, a difficult—perhaps impossible—task, given the continuity of development after fertilization.

A better case to illustrate the wedge logic is the principle offered for the embryo-transfer procedures as treatment for infertility. Will we support the use of *in vitro* fertilization and embryo transfer because it provides a "child of *one's own,*" in a strict sense of *one's own,* to a married couple? Or will we support the transfer because it is treatment of involuntary infertility, which deserves treatment in or out of marriage, hence endorsing the use of any available technical means (which would produce a healthy and normal child), including surrogate wombs, or even ectogenesis?

Second, logic aside, the opponents of the wedge argument do not counsel well. It would be simply foolish to ignore what might come next, and to fail to make the *best possible* assessment of the implications of present action (or inaction). Let me put the matter very bluntly: the Ethics Advisory Board, in the decision it must now make, may very well be helping to decide whether human beings will eventually be produced in laboratories. I say this not to shock—and I do not mean to beg the question of whether that would be desirable or not. I say this to make sure that they and we face squarely the full import and magnitude of this decision. Once the genies let the babies into the bottle, it may be impossible to get them out again.

VIII

So much, then, for the meaning of initiating and manipulating human embryos in the laboratory. These considerations still make me doubt the wisdom of proceeding with these practices, both in research and in their clinical application, notwithstanding that valuable knowledge might be had by continuing the research and identifiable suffering might be alleviated by using it to circumvent infertility. To doubt the wisdom of going ahead makes one at least a fellow-traveller of the opponents of such research, but it does not, either logically or practically, require that one join them in trying to prevent it, say by legal prohibition. Not every folly can or should be legislated against. Attempts at prohibition here would seem to be both ineffective and dangerous—ineffective because impossible to enforce, dangerous because the costs of such precedent-setting interference with scientific research might be greater than the harm it prevents. To be sure, we already have legal restrictions on experimentation with human subjects, which restrictions are manifestly not incompatible with the progress of medical science. Neither is it true that science cannot survive if it must take some direction from the law. Nor is it the case that all research, because it is research, is or should be absolutely protected. But it does not seem to me that *in vitro* fertilization and embryo transfer deserve, *at least at present,* to be treated as sufficiently dangerous for legislative interference.

But if to doubt the wisdom does not oblige one to seek to outlaw the folly, neither does a decision *to permit* require a decision *to encourage or support.* A researcher's freedom to do *in vitro* fertilization, or a woman's right to have a child with laboratory assistance, in no way implies a public (or even a private) obligation to pay for such research or treatment. A right *against* interference is not an entitlement *for assistance.*

AN AFTERWORD

This has been for me a long and difficult exposition. Many of the arguments are hard to make. It is hard to get confident people to face unpleasant prospects. It is hard to get many people to take seriously such "soft" matters as lineage, identity, respect, and self-respect when they are in tension with such "hard" matters as a cure for infertility or new methods of contraception. It is hard to talk about the meaning of sexuality and embodiment in a culture that treats sex increasingly as sport and that has trivialized the significance of gender, marriage, and procreation. It is hard to oppose Federal funding of baby-making in a society which increasingly demands that the Federal government supply all demands, and which—contrary to so much evidence of waste, incompetence, and corruption—continues to believe that only Uncle Sam can do it. And, finally, it is hard to speak about restraint in a culture that seems to venerate very little above man's own attempt to master all. Here, I am afraid, is the biggest question and the one we perhaps can no longer ask or deal with: the question about the reasonableness of the desire to become masters and possessors of nature, human nature included.

Here we approach the deepest meaning of *in vitro* fertilization. Those who have likened it to artificial insemination are only partly correct. With *in vitro* fertilization, the human embryo emerges for the first time from the natural darkness and privacy of its own mother's womb, where it is hidden away in mystery, into the bright light and utter publicity of the scientist's laboratory, where it will be treated with unswerving rationality, before the clever and shameless eye of the mind and beneath the obedient and equally clever touch of the hand. What does it mean to hold the beginning of human life before your eyes, in your hands—even for 5 days (for the meaning does not depend on duration)? Perhaps the meaning is contained in the following story:

Long ago there was a man of great intellect and great courage. He was a remarkable man, a giant, able to answer questions that no other human being could answer, willing boldly to face any challenge or problem. He was a confident man, a masterful man. He saved his city from disaster and ruled it as a father rules his children, revered by all. But something was wrong in his city. A plague had fallen on generation; infertility afflicted plants, animals, and human beings. The man confidently promised to uncover the cause of the plague and to cure the infertility. Resolutely, dauntlessly, he put his sharp mind to work to solve the problem, to bring the dark things to light. No secrets, no reticences, a full public inquiry. He raged against the representatives of caution, moderation, prudence, and piety, who urged him to curtail his inquiry; he accused them of trying to usurp his rightfully earned power, of trying to replace human and masterful control with submissive reverence. The story ends in tragedy: He solved the problem but, in making visible and public the dark and intimate details of his origins, he ruined his life, and that of his family. In the end, too late, he learns about the price of presumption, of overconfidence, of the overweening desire to master and control one's fate. In symbolic rejection of his desire to look into everything, he punishes his eyes with self-inflicted blindness.

Sophocles seems to suggest that such a man is always in principle—albeit unwittingly—a patricide, a regicide, and a practitioner of incest. We men of modern science may have something to learn from our forebear, Oedipus. It appears that Oedipus, being the kind of man an Oedipus is (the chorus calls him a paradigm of man), had no choice but to learn through suffering. Is it really true that we too have no other choice?

Notes

1. In the British procedures, several eggs are taken from each woman and fertilized, to increase the chance of success, but only one embryo is transferred for implantation. In Dr. Soupart's proposed experiments, as the embryos will be produced only for the purpose of research and not for transfer, all of them will be discarded or destroyed.
2. A perhaps justifiable exception would be the case of a universal plague on childbirth, say because of some epidemic that fatally attacks all fetuses *in utero* at age 5 months. Faced with the prospect of the end of the race, might we not condone the deliberate institution of pregnancies to provide fetuses for research, in the hope of finding a diagnosis and remedy for this catastrophic blight?
3. Peter Gwynne, "Was the Birth of Louise Brown Only a Happy Accident?" *Science Digest,* October 1978, (emphasis added).
4. For the supporting analysis of the concept of "viability," see my article, "Determining Death and Viability in Fetuses and Abortuses," prepared for the National Commission for the Protection of Human Subjects of Biomedical and Behavioral Research, published in *Appendix: Research on the Fetus,* U. S. Department of Health, Education, and Welfare, HEW Publ. No. (OS) 76-128, 1975.
5. Some people have suggested that the embryo be regarded like a vital organ, salvaged from a newly dead corpse, usable for transplantation or research, and that its donation by egg and sperm donors be governed by the Uniform Anatomical Gift Act, which legitimates pre-mortem consent for organ donation upon death. But though this acknowledges that embryos are not things, it is mistaken in treating embryos as mere organs, thereby overlooking that they are early stages of a *complete, whole* human being. The Uniform Anatomical Gift Act does not apply to, nor should it be stretched to cover, donation of gonads, gametes (male sperm or female eggs), or—especially—zygotes and embryos.
6. There is a good chance that the problem of surplus embryos may be avoidable, for purely technical reasons. Some researchers believe that the uterine receptivity to the transferred embryo might be reduced during the particular menstrual cycle in which the ova are obtained, because of the effects of the hormones given to induce superovulation. They propose that the harvested *eggs* be frozen, and then defrosted one at a time each month for fertilization, culture, and transfer, until pregnancy is achieved. By refusing to fertilize all the eggs at once—i.e., not placing all one's eggs in one uterine cycle—there will not be surplus *embryos,* but at most only surplus eggs. This change in the procedure would make the demise of unimplanted embryos *exactly* analogous to the "natural" embryonic loss in ordinary reproduction.
7. The literature on intervention in reproduction is both confused and confusing on the crucial matter of the meanings of "nature" or "the natural," and their significance for the ethical issues. It may be as much a mistake to claim that "the natural" has *no* moral force as to suggest

that the natural way is best, because natural. Though shallow and slippery thought about nature, and its relation to "good," is a likely source of these confusions, the nature of nature may itself to elusive, making it difficult for even careful thought to capture what is natural.

8. To those who point out that the bond between sexuality and procreation has already been effectively and permanently cleaved by "the pill," and that this is therefore an idle worry in the case of *in vitro* fertilization, it must be said that the pill provides only sex without babies. Now the other shoe drops: babies without sex.

9. *Science, 202:*5, October 6, 1978.

10. Some of these questions are addressed, albeit too briefly and polemically, in the latter part of my 1972 "Making Babies" article, to which the reader is referred. It has been pointed out to me by an astute colleague that the tone of the present article is less passionate and more accommo-

dating than the first, which change he regards as an ironic demonstration of the inexorable way in which we get used to, and accept, our technological nightmares. I myself share his concern. I cannot decide whether the decline of my passion is to be welcomed; that is, whether it is due to greater understanding bred of more thought and experience, or to greater callousness and the contempt of familiarity bred from *too much* thought and experience. It does seem to me now that many of the fundamental beliefs and institutions that might be challenged by laboratory growth of human embryos and by laboratory-assisted reproduction are already severely challenged in perhaps more potent and important ways. Here, too, we see the creeping effect of the aggregated powers of modernity and the corrosive power of the familiar. Adaptiveness is our glory and our curse: as Raskolnikov put it, "Man gets used to everything, the beast!"

From *Progeny, Progress, and Primrose Paths*

Samuel Govovitz

Issues involving human sexuality and reproduction are second to none in generating moral debate and in prompting indecision and anxiety. Among the issues that have been highly disputed in one way or another are questions of abortion, birth control, artificial insemination, genetic screening, pornography and censorship, adolescent sexuality, prenatal sex selection, sex-related research and therapy, *in vitro* fertilization, and sex education. Each of these topics has moral dimensions that could fill a volume.

I want to look at one aspect of the debate that centers on the use of modern technology as an aid to the fulfillment of the aspirations people have about procreation. In particular, I want to examine the kind of reasoning that the debate

inspires because much of it seems to me to be faulty. In this exploration I will focus on issues related to *in vitro* fertilization, but the arguments are plainly of more general relevance.

In vitro fertilization is the process by which Louise Brown was conceived. The first of what the journalists call test tube babies, she was born in England in 1978, despite the fact that her mother had an inoperable blockage of the fallopian tubes which prevented her from getting pregnant in the usual way. Physicians removed an egg from Mrs. Brown by means of a surgical procedure, fertilized it in a Petrie dish with sperm from Mr. Brown, nurtured the fertilized egg in the laboratory for several days, then implanted it in Mrs. Brown's uterus. The result was a normal pregnancy and birth. Louise Brown is healthy, famous, and thanks to a public relations windfall, affluent.

The process used by Drs. Edwards and Steptoe in the case of Louise Brown is complicated, however, by the fact that more than a single egg gets fertilized in the Petrie dish. The technique is just not precise enough to extract and then to fertilize a single egg. (In fact, for the most part, the process doesn't work at all, and it took more than a hundred attempts before the first successful outcome.) So after a fertilized egg is implanted in the womb of the intended mother, the question remains of what to do with the extra eggs that may have been fertilized along the way. The simple answer is to discard them since they are extra, not needed, useless. But two very different objections arise.

To those who believe that personhood begins at conception, the very notion that such entities are valueless and superfluous is distressing. They argue, on the contrary, that the process involves nothing less than callous mass murder of innocent human life, a case of multiple, ex-utero abortion. So the problem of abortion is not merely parallel to the problem of IVF after all but is a part of it.

On the other side are scientists who see great research potential in the use of those extra fertilized eggs as subjects in medical research. If there is anything wrong with discarding the extras, they argue, it is the waste of a valuable opportunity to advance the frontiers of medical knowledge. For if we are concerned to reduce the incidence of congenital illness, there can be no more promising prospect than that of nurturing embryonic life *in vitro,* subjecting it to various environmental influences, and learning thereby how fetal development goes wrong. No event is more tragic than the birth of a grievously defective child; no line of research holds more promise for reducing human tragedy. So the battle lines are drawn.

In the United States there are scientists who want to do research involving IVF and women who want to have children of their own but who, like Mrs. Brown, cannot conceive in the usual way. But there are many who hold that IVF is a procedure that should not be employed —that it is, on moral grounds, a misuse of the physician's art. The government has been in the middle. It provides the funding for most medical research and is thus the target of the scientists' appeals. It is the target of the moral objections as well, and has received 60,000 letters of opposition to the use of IVF.

Let us pursue the debate about *in vitro* fertilization by imagining a woman who desperately wants to have a child of her own, for whom IVF is the only possibility. She is deeply religious, totally committed to doing the morally right thing, aware that there is controversy about the morality of IVF, and unsure what to do. She asks her gynecologist for advice, but the physician is also unsure what to do. She and her colleagues have been asked by a number of patients to make the service available through their practice, either directly or by referral to another clinic. The patient and the physician agree to survey the literature, assess the arguments they find, and try to reach agreement about whether such technologically aided reproduction is an appropriate option. What are the discussions like that they will find?

Laced through the literature of objection to abortion, IVF therapy and research is an argument variously called the primrose path argument, the thin edge of the wedge argument, and the camel's nose in the tent argument. Its structure is familiar: Once one starts sliding down a slippery slope, things get out of control. There is no stopping; disaster awaits us. No skier thinks the argument is generally good; fortunately it is often possible to start down a slippery slope and then to stop.

Paul Ramsey—a prominent Protestant theologian and a leading critic of the use of modern technology in clinical medicine— assures us of disaster in his discussions of such matters, relying heavily, as we shall see, on arguments of this kind. He claims that such measures as artificial insemination and *in vitro* fertilization are the first steps down the primrose path, and there is, in his apocalyptic view, no slowing up, no turning back short of social disaster.[1] Whether or not that view is reasonable is an empirical question. Some processes, like nuclear chain reactions or the spreading of an epidemic, once begun are difficult or impossible to stop. Others are not. It is always an empirical question which sort of process we are dealing with in any particular instance.

I will not attempt to ski the Schilthorn— though I have seen it done—because my descent, once begun on that insanely precipitous slope, would surely end in cataclysm below. I might as well attempt to ski to safety from a plane in flight. In view of my ability, the argument against my attempting that slope is conclusive. Yet I can handle slopes that beginning skiers properly shun. It is a question of control and judgment.

Is the slippery slope argument against IVF a good one? It is not enough to show that disaster awaits if the process is not controlled. A man walking East in Omaha will drown in the Atlantic—if he does not stop. The argument must also rest on evidence about the likelihood that judgment and control will be exercised responsibly. Here Ramsey's position collapses; he describes disaster and rests his argument on the unduly pessimistic assumption that such unhappy outcomes as are possible will surely occur. But Ramsey sells us short. Collectively we have significant capacity to exercise judgment and control. We have not always done well, especially in areas like foreign policy or energy planning. But our record has been rather good in regard to medical treatment and research.

Consider the vexatious problem of abortion as a case in point. Some opponents of a liberal law have argued that once we allow the killing of fetuses, nothing can stop the slide. If we sanction abortion, they fear, even where amniocentesis reveals a defect like trisomy 21 (Down's Syndrome), we will sanction capricious infanticide as well. If we would abort a fetus on the ground that it is going to be seriously defective, why not allow infanticide on the ground that the child actually has the dreaded defect? Further, such infanticide is just a short skid away from the killing of those judged socially useless, so that if one sanctions early-term abortions even in cases of demonstrable defect, one has irretrievably opened the floodgates to the selective slaughter of anyone in social disfavor.

No such disaster has ensued. Through a process of social policy determination, the society has exercised judgment. That judgment has made a lot of people on both sides unhappy, but it is nonetheless a judgment that makes clear that we can stop a process once we have begun it. Anyone who has ever had a haircut should know that.

Many other examples illustrate our capacity to exercise judgment. Consider an experiment in language acquisition and early child development. We could learn a lot by raising some children in strict isolation from linguistic input for three or four years and then immersing them in a highly verbal environment. No one denies that would be a scientifically sound and useful experiment, but nobody proposes doing it. We will not do so because we judge that on ethical grounds it is indefensible. Andre Hellegers, the late director of the Kennedy Institute for Ethics, and Richard McCormick, a leading Catholic theologian, are right when they speak of "benefits we can never enjoy because we cannot get them without being unethical".[2] There is a difference, despite our mistakes and despite the fears of the pessimists, between what we could do and what we do. That difference is largely due to our capacity for judgment.

Note that with regard to IVF applications, we do not face any single slippery slope argument. Rather, there are several. There are arguments that clinical IVF poses a threat to marriage and the family and to mankind's self-image. There is a separate argument that IVF research will lead to experimentation of an ethically undesirable sort on late-stage fetuses. Each such consideration involves an empirical assessment of the likelihood that sound judgment will prevail as well as an assessment of the magnitude of the disaster if it does not.

It is important here to recognize that the likelihood of the subsequent exercise of judgment and restraint may largely depend on the principles that are used to justify first steps. If early-term abortion were justified by the principle that parents enjoy absolute dominion over their issue, the adoption of that principle would already have constituted a sanctioning of infanticide, and there would be no basis for stopping the slide down the slippery slope. If IVF research on embryos is justified by the principle that prenatal fetal life is of no moral importance, there will be no basis for restraint in regard to research on later-stage fetuses. So it can matter decisively how the justification of first steps is formulated.

There has been considerable speculation about the impact of clinical IVF on marriage and the family. Some of the predictions based on slippery slope arguments are dire. Such prospects as the use of surrogate mothers have been especially disturbing to some writers. (The surrogate mother is a woman who allows the implantation into her uterus of a fertilized egg from another couple, the woman in which wants to have a child of her own but without undergoing pregnancy. The surrogate mother then carries the fetus to term, waiving rights in regard to the resulting child, who is given to the genetic parents.) Hellegers and McCormick warn of such outcomes, toward which they see IVF as leading: "We see in these procedures grave assaults on marriage and the family, to say nothing of the subtle devaluation of sexual intimacy that clings to them."[3] But whereas they raise concerns and call for "a serious public discussion," Ramsey speaks of "what the manipulation of embryos will surely do to ourselves and our progeny."[4] He goes on to invoke the chilling images of a Huxleyan world so sterile that "there is no poetry."[5]

These issues are of the first importance. But it is necessary not to lose sight, in the glare of that importance, of the need to examine the evidence. What reason is there to give credence to such portents of familial disaster? Much of the case seems based on concern about the separation of reproduction from sexual intercourse. But artificial insemination, with husbands' and with donors' sperm, has been practiced widely, if not very visibly, for decades. There has been no discernible deleterious effect on marriage or the family. More important, the wide availability of inexpensive and effective birth control means that for the first time in human history, sex and reproduction have already been separated. The impact on social structure will surely be astounding; no doubt it will transcend our current understanding. So it is a wholly idle worry that IVF will separate sex and procreation.

It is worth remembering, moreover, that IVF involves hospitalization and surgery, and it is a very small percentage of the population that is in any position to benefit from it. The traditional method of conception will remain the method of choice. It is inexpensive, can be performed at home, takes little time, training, or skill, and is a great deal of fun. I do not see it in serious jeopardy.

Further, we are only beginning to document what we have known all along: that there is no substitute for early parent-child interaction.[6] As we learn more fully how the family works when it is working well, I suspect that our appreciation of it and of its special capacity for nurturing will grow. Hellegers and McCormick are right; we should take the long view and look at societal consequences, not simply at individual needs, in evaluating IVF. But I do not see the family under grave assault because of IVF. Indeed, it is often a respect for family, lineage, and the traditional parental role that prompts the request for clinical IVF in the first place.

Finally, mankind's image of what it is to be human may well involve a sense of lineage and of parenting, and that image may undergo some perturbation from the few cases in which procreation has a heavy dose of technology added. But mankind's sense of what it is to be human is threatened far more seriously on other fronts. Recent work on primate language acquisition, notwithstanding debate about its significance, has challenged the belief that we alone have the capacity for abstraction or to communicate to others a sense of self-awareness, and in the process the sharpness of the distinction between humans and the higher primates has been blunted.[7] Recent work in artificial intelligence has produced machines with awesome cognitive capacities, and the sharpness of the distinction between people and machines has also been challenged.[8] We have ample reason to reflect seriously about what we are. The prospects for IVF add little to the case.

Like the slippery slope argument, the concept of what is natural plays a frequent role in writings of those who are troubled by IVF. Ramsey, for example, writes:

> Today many are testifying to the spiritual autonomy of all natural objects and to arrogance over none; to the scheme of things in which man has his place. But there is as yet no discernible evidence that we are recovering a sense for man as a natural object, too, toward whom a like form of "natural piety" is appropriate. . . . [P]rocreation, parenthood, is certainly one of those "courses of action" natural to man, which cannot without violation be disassembled and put together again—any more than we have the wisdom or the right impiously to destroy the environ-

ment of which we are a part rather than working according to its lineaments, according to the functions we discover to be the case in the whole assemblage of natural objects.[9]

He then goes on to advocate the position that "the proper objective of medicine is to serve and care for man as a natural object, to help in all our natural 'courses of action,' to tend the garden of our creation."[10] It is time this sort of argument was laid permanently to rest. That something is natural has, by itself, absolutely no moral force.

We can distinguish three senses in which an action or process can be said to be natural:

1. It conforms to the laws of nature; the contrast, I presume, is with the impossible or with the supernatural. But *everything* we do or could do—the good and bad alike—is natural in this sense. No moral distinctions can be based on it.

2. It is free of human intervention; the contrast is with processes influenced by mankind's efforts to manipulate its environment. But *nothing* we do is natural in this sense, for our action is itself the mark of the unnatural. The practice of medicine itself is a clear example of human efforts to manipulate the playing out of events, as when we deliberately destroy "natural" life forms and terminate a "natural" process by using antibiotics to cure an infection. No moral distinctions can be based on this sense of what is natural either.

3. It conforms to some natural moral law or other code or set or principles of value; the contrast here is with what is wrong, what is a violation of principles about how one ought to act. In this interpretation the concept of what is natural has moral force, but only because it is based on some prior judgment about what is right and what is wrong—a judgment then reflected in the choice of what to call natural and artificial.

The passage from Ramsey suggests that he employs the third sense of *natural;* that he sees certain processes, such as normal procreation, as desirable; and that he extols their naturalness without thereby suggesting that medical intervention is typically a violation of nature.

The claim of naturalness is thus a moral *conclusion,* not evidence that can be offered in a

moral argument. Ramsey sees atypical reproduction as undesirable but says little about why. His invocation of the concept of the natural only obscures the point that there are morally desirable and morally undesirable actions, and we must strive to discern the difference between them on reasonable grounds, not on purported grounds of naturalness. I do not understand why this confusion about the moral significance of the concept of what is natural persists as widely and tenaciously as it does.

The most central issue in the debate about IVF, however, as in the debate about abortion, is the question of the status of the embryo. In approaching this question, we must recall the crucial distinction between facts we seek to discover and decisions we need to make. If we wish to know a fact, we seek to discover it through appropriate research. Contrast that with the question of when a young person becomes an adult. Whether a person warrants classification as an adult at thirteen, eighteen, or twenty-one is not a fact to discover through research in biology, physiology, psychology, or anything else. It is social policy, a decision of the body politic. This distinction between discoveries and decisions seems straightforward, yet sometimes the two become confused. Much discussion about death, for example, proceeds on the misconception that the criterion of death is a fact to discover. Yet the appropriate criterion of death in clinical situations is not a fact to discover; it is a social policy to make. (That is one reason why the results of such discussions are somewhat unstable, why the criterion of death is a subject of ongoing dispute; the factors that go into justifying a social policy decision are always open to review and to argument.)

What, then, of the embryo—the embryo that is implanted and the embryo that is dealt with otherwise? Inevitably there arise questions of whether or not such embryos are persons or are the bearers of rights. These are not questions of fact but instead require the setting of social policy. To say that a question is a question of policy is not to say that the answers are unconstrained. There are clear cases of life and of death; the question arises—and a policy is needed—only in cases at the margin where some physiological systems still function while others are irretrievably lost. So the range within which decision can be made is rather narrow. Similarly, the questions of what to count as a person and what to count as a bearer of rights require decision only within a circumscribed range—the cases at the margins of personhood. Such cases are of various sorts—the anencephalic newborn, the linguistically proficient primate, the embryo.

I will not rehearse the extensive debate about the personhood of embryos and fetuses, a debate fueled by intense division of sentiment about abortion. Rather, I will sketch the conclusions that seem to me to provide the most reasonable basis for judgment.

Surely the concept of a person involves in some fundamental way the capacity for sentience, for an awareness of sensations at the very least. In the normal case there is much more. There is self-awareness, capacity for reflection, a sense of others and of relationships between self and others. So the condition of sentience is very weak, a necessary condition for personhood, but far from a sufficient condition.

No one seriously contends that embryos are sentient, that they are capable of even the slightest awareness of pleasure or pain. Of course, if all goes well, they will develop into people, and it is on that potential that the case for their pesonhood largely rests. The idea of potential is tricky. We often hear encomiums to it: Individuals should have the opportunity to fulfill their potential, it is somehow grounds for disappointment when someone fails to live up to his potential, and the like. But that is careless talk, for some potentials are desirable and others are not. He who has the potential to be Sherlock Holmes has the potential to be a master criminal; she who has the manual dexterity for neurosurgery perhaps has the potential to be a leading pickpocket as well. Further, he who has the potential to be a swimmer and to be a ballet dancer must choose between them; what advances one potential interferes with the other. So aphorisms about potential do little to advance the debate. Mainly what they come to is that it is good to advance those potentials that it is good to advance.

Even though *people* should be encouraged in living up to some of their more desirable potentials, we cannot use that principle to defend a claim that *embryos* have personhood or rights since the principle is about the potentials of persons—and whether or not embryos should be accorded that status is precisely the point in question. It is not obvious that rights should accrue to an object just because it has the potential, assuming that all goes well, to become a person at some later time. Indeed, the unfertilized human egg, like the embryo, has the potential to become a person if all goes well—when all going well includes getting fertilized. And no one has argued that each unfertilized egg or each spermatozoon be accorded personhood or rights.

One does hear it said of the embryo that it has the potential to become a *particular* adult person. Its genetic identity is complete; it is already a unique individual. That does distinguish it from spermatozoa and ova in isolation (apart from the possibility of twinning), but not from identified, though unjoined, pairs of sperm and egg. That no union has yet occurred does not alter the fact that any pair of sperm and egg has the potential, if all goes well, to become a genetically specific adult person. The point of conception may be, for some, a convenient place to draw the line, but there should be no mistake about the fact that it is drawn there for convenience. That is no less "arbitrary" a choice than the choice to draw the line later, which I believe it makes better sense to do. Indeed, it is a myth that conception is itself instantaneous. Even one who seeks to avoid the problem of "drawing a line" by choosing conception as an unproblematic point is in reality selecting a temporal region within which a process takes place over time. That we did not know this fact before it was possible to monitor the process of conception at the microscopic level does not make it any the less important a fact.

At the other end of fetal development we are struck by the similarity between infants and late-stage fetuses. Indeed, not only is the late-stage fetus clearly sentient, reacting to stimuli in its environment, but in most cases it already holds a place, as a specific, though unseen, individual, in a network of human emotions and expectations. In most respects it is like a child and utterly unlike an embryo.

For my part, the onset of the capacity for sentience marks a qualitative change in fetal development. From that point forward what we do may cause it, as a present actuality, to suffer. Surely that is a morally significant factor, though not the only one. It is an empirical question of neurological development when that change occurs; it happens sometime prior to quickening but well after the embryonic stage. That we have no word for this stage in the series of events that includes conception, quickening, and birth reflects only the fact that we have not historically invested it with much significance or until recently had much understanding of the development of which it is a part. It is not necessarily less significant for that.

The later it is in its development, the more seriously we should take a fetus as a person in the making. I see no reason for, and no possibility of, holding to a clear-cut distinction between the nonperson and the person as if personhood somehow snaps into place in an instant, instead of emerging organically out of a developmental process. That emergence, I suggest, begins to have moral force with the onset of fetal sentience. In any case, I know of no persuasive arguments for the position that the most reasonable social policy is to accord the embryo the status of a person.

Leon Kass, a physician and persuasive commentator on ethical issues in medicine, has argued forcefully that the human embryo is an entity of moral significance:

> The human blastocyst, even the blastocyst *in vitro,* is not humanly nothing; it possesses a power to become what everyone will agree is a human being. . . . [T]he blastocyst is not nothing, it is *at least* potential humanity, and as such it elicits, or ought to elicit, our feelings of awe and respect. In the blastocyst, even in the zygote, we face a mysterious and awesome power. . . . *The human embryo is not mere meat; it is not just stuff; it is not a thing.* Because of its origin and because of its capacity, it commands a higher respect.[11]

I agree that the human blastocyst is not humanly nothing. So, too, however, do all the advocates of IVF. It is *precisely* the human blastocyst's potential to become a human being that makes it an object of particular research interest and that accounts for the possibility of clinical IVF. From the fact that it is not humanly nothing, no conclusion directly follows about what should or should not be done.

Of course, the force of Kass's argument is intended to rest not merely on the fact that the human blastocyst has some human status but on its mysterious and awesome power, its capacity to engender awe and respect. But it is not the *human* character of the blastocyst that accounts for its splendor. Any strand of DNA confronts us with a mysterious and awesome power; any mammalian embryo embodies an "immanent plan" that dwarfs our understanding; any acorn is, as much as anything ever is, miraculous; and even the lowly hydrogen atom, reflected on with reverent disposition, is humbling in its beauty, power, and complexity. And so are cathedrals, symphonies, great literary works, and the minds of great scientists.

Surely, one might claim, I miss the point. Human blastocysts are not uniquely grounds for awe, but they do command, as Kass puts it, a "higher respect." He is not explicit, however, in the comparison; higher than what, one wonders. The context suggests an answer: higher than the respect commanded by "mere meat," by that which is "just stuff." But two problems of interpreting the point arise. First, Kass nowhere explains what he means by *respect.* He has merely *invoked* the notion of the respect due the embryo, much as Ramsey invoked the notion of the natural. Secondly, Kass does not consider the respect due to other objects than the embryo. That omission is what gives plausibility to his argument that since human blastocysts are due respect, they ought not be the subjects of research or clinical manipulation. Kass, I am certain, would agree that human cadavers should be treated with respect; they are not mere meat, not humanly nothing, not unrelated to a network of emotional attachments and deeply felt values that constrain how we treat the bodily remains of former persons. Yet Kass does not protest the use of cadavers in medical education or the practice of transplanting organs from someone who has just died. To be sure, there is a difference between using cadavers and abusing them, and it is to this difference that the concept of respect is relevant. It is simply a mistake to assume that if an object is due respect, it is therefore wrong to make practical use of it.

Finally, Kass speaks freely of the appropriateness of experimenting on animals, including primates. But are animals not also due respect? They are sentient creatures whose development and behavior are proper grounds for awe and wonder, they participate in social communities, and in some cases their communicative capacity is far greater than we had until recently imagined. The homocentricity of Kass's position enables him to make respect sound like a barrier to use. In fact, it is a barrier only to abuse. If we can justifiably experiment on animals under some circumstances, and if we can justifiably make use of human remains, despite the fact that they are not humanly nothing, I see no reason based on the concept of respect why we cannot, respectfully, make justifiable clinical and research use of human blastocysts.

Both Kass and R. G. Edwards, in reply to Kass, have discussed the proper function of medicine and whether IVF is defensible in terms of it. There are serious issues here. Kass argues:

> Just as infertility is not a disease, so providing a child by artificial means to a woman with blocked oviducts is not treatment. . . . What is being "treated" is her desire—a perfectly normal and unobjectional desire—to bear a child.[12]

Ramsey voices a similar concern:

> The important line lies between doctoring desires . . . and seeking to correct a medical condition if it is possible to do so. . . . [M]edical practice loses its way into an entirely different human activity—manufacture . . . if it undertakes either to produce a child without curing infertility as a condition or to produce simply the desired sort of child.[13]

Edwards replies:

> A great many medical advances depend on the replacement of a deficient compound or an organ. Examples include insulin, false teeth, and spectacles: the clinical condition itself remains, but treatment modifies its expression. Patients taking advantage of these three treatments are surely receiving the correct therapeutic measures, the doctors treating the desire to be nondiabetic or to see and eat properly. . . . Exactly the same argument applies to the cure of infertility: should patients have their desired children, the treatment would have achieved its purpose.[14]

We need not rely on the idea of prosthetic devices to make Edwards's point that treatment does often leave the initial condition unaltered while responding to a patient's desire to transcend the limitations imposed by that condition. The administration of tranquilizers, sleeping pills, and analgesics are examples of medical treatments which do not correct physiological deficiencies but respond, in a sense, to a patient's desires. Edwards's defense seems adequate; treating some desires is a traditional and appropriate part of medical practice.

But the problem runs deeper, for it may not be appropriate to treat all medically treatable desires. First, there is the question of the distribution of costs, a question that has heightened impact if we consider the use of public funds to pay for medical treatment. It is one thing to provide insulin, dialysis, or dentures to a patient. But should we provide cosmetic surgery when the desire does not arise out of injury or illness but rather is simply a wish to be more youthfully attractive? Perhaps such treatment is unexceptionable if the costs are borne wholly by the patient. But other desires arising out of vanity seem less legitimate. Should surgical treatment have been available to those women who, in the 1950s, had their little toes amputated in order to fit their feet into narrower and hence, in their benighted judgment, more fashionable shoes? Or is the provision of such treatment a misuse of medical skills, a perversion of the privilege that the license to practice medicine signifies? I submit that this is the case and that the underlying reason is that the treatment of a desire for self-mutilation in the service of a whimsical vanity is not the sort of desire that legitimately warrants treatment.

Value-free medicine is not fully possible. Some judgments about which desires are properly treatable, and which not, must be made. We cannot oppose clinical IVF on the ground that it is the treatment of a desire, nor can we simply approve it on the ground, as Edwards suggests, that the treatment of desires is medically legitimate. Rather, we must face directly the question of whether the desire to have a child of one's own, when IVF is the only available means, is one of the desires that warrants medical response.

At this point our hypothetical patient and physician, if they agree with me, will conclude that there is no adequate argument against the clinical use of IVF as a response to inoperable infertility. But they may remain troubled by some of the dangers to which critics like Ramsey, Hellegers, McCormick, and Kass call our attention, despite the weaknesses in their arguments. For there remains something discomforting about the notion of raising embryos in the laboratory for use as research subjects, notwithstanding the useful knowledge that might result. And there remains something discomforting about the growing incidence of surrogate motherhood arrangements that have already begun to lead us into uncharted waters of litigation, as when the surrogate mother decides during the pregnancy to try to keep the child she had agreed to incubate for someone else. But these problems must be faced on their own, and the judgments we make in response to them should remain distinguishable from the judgments we make about more straightforward uses of IVF as a clinical therapy. We need not consider all possible uses of IVF as parts of one inseparable package any more than we need endorse an absolutist position on abortion. There is no good reason why we cannot separate justifiable from unjustifiable instances on the basis of where the best arguments lie.

Notes

1. Paul Ramsey, "Shall We 'Reproduce'?" *Journal of the American Medical Association* 220 (June 12, 1972), p. 1484.
2. Andre Hellegers and Richard McCormick, "Unanswered Questions on Test Tube Life," *America* (August 19, 1978), pp. 74–78.
3. Ibid., p. 77.
4. Ramsey, "Shall We 'Reproduce'?" p. 1485.
5. Paul Ramsey, "Manufacturing Our Offspring: Weighing the Risks," *The Hastings Center Report* 8, no. 5 (October 1979), p. 9.
6. See, for example, M. Klaus and J. Kennell, "Mothers Separated from Their Newborn Infants," *Pediatric Clinics of North America* 17 (1970), pp. 1015–37.
7. See, for example, P. Jenkins, "Ask No Questions," *The Guardian*, London (July 10, 1973), excerpted under the title "Teaching Chimpanzees to Communicate," in *Animal Rights and Human Obligations,* edited by T. Regan and P. Singer (Englewood Cliffs, N.J.: Prentice-Hall, 1976), pp. 85–92.
8. See, for example, B. G. Buchanan, "Scientific Theory Formulation by Computers," in *Computer Oriented Learning Processes,* edited by J. C. Simon (Leyden: Noordhoff, 1976).
9. Ramsey, "Shall We 'Reproduce'?" p. 1484.
10. Ibid.
11. Leon Kass, "Ethical Issues in Human *In Vitro* Fertilization, Embryo Culture and Research, and Embryo Transfer," in Ethics Advisory Board, DHEW, *Appendix, HEW Support of Research Involving Human* In Vitro *Fertilization and Embryo Transfer* (Washington, D.C.: U.S. Government Printing Office, 1979), pp. 6–8, emphases in original.
12. Leon Kass, "Babies by Means of *In Vitro* Fertilization: Unethical Experiments on the Unborn?" *New England Journal of Medicine* 285 (November 18, 1971), p. 1177.
13. Ramsey, "Shall We 'Reproduce'?" p. 1482.
14. R. G. Edwards, "Fertilization of Human Eggs *In Vitro:* Morals, Ethics and the Law," *Quarterly Review of Biology* 49 (1974), pp. 3–26.

From *Buck* v. *Bell*

Oliver Wendell Holmes

We have seen more than once that the public welfare may call upon its best citizens for their lives. It would be strange if it could not call upon those who already sap the strength of the State for these lesser sacrifices, often not felt to be such by those concerned, in order to prevent our being swamped with incompetence. It is

From O. W. Holmes, *Buck* v. *Bell* 274 U.S. 200; 47 S.Ct. 584, 71 L.Ed. 1000 (1927).

better for all the world, if instead of waiting to execute degenerate offspring for crime, or to let them starve for their imbecility, society can prevent those who are manifestly unfit from continuing their kind. The principle that sustains compulsory vaccination is broad enough to cover cutting the Fallopian tubes. (*Jacobson* v. *Massachusetts*, 197 U.S. 11, 25 S.Ct. 358,49 L.Ed. 643,3 Ann. Cas. 765). Three generations of imbeciles are enough.

From "Moral Issues in Human Genetics: Counseling or Control?"

Ruth Macklin

. . . [T]he question "valuable to what end?" is one of extraordinary complexity. For example, something obviously valuable in terms of the longest possible survival of a race (or of its best adaptation to a given climate, or of the preservation of its greatest numbers) would by no means have the same value if it were a question of developing a more powerful type. The welfare of the many and the welfare of the few are radically opposite ends.*

There is no question that genetic engineering in many forms. . . will come about. It is a general rule that whatever is scientifically feasible will be attempted. The application of these technics must, however, be examined from the point of view of ethics, individual freedom and coercion. Both the scientists directly involved and, perhaps more important, the political and social leaders of our civilization must exercise utmost caution in order to prevent genetic, evolutionary and social tragedies.**

Reprinted with permission from the author and *Dialogue,* vol. XVI, no. 3 (1977).

* Friedrich Nietzsche, *The Genealogy of Morals.*
** Kurt Hirschhorn, M.D., "Practical and Ethical Problems in Human Genetics," *Birth Defects,* Vol. VIII, No. 4 (July, 1972), pp. 29–30.

I

In the field of human genetics, the last several decades have witnessed a great increase in both theoretical knowledge and technological power. Like so many other areas in biomedical ethics, the attainment of new knowledge and the develoment of new technology has given rise to moral problems that never had to be faced before. But while the biomedical contexts are new, the moral problems are ancient. Such problems arise at the level both of the individual and society, where decisions must be made about such matters as whether compulsory genetic screening programmes constitute a violation of individual privacy; whether enforced sterilization of genetically unhealthy individuals is ever justifiable in the interest of socially desirable outcomes; whether genetic counselors are obligated to tell the truth, the whole truth, and nothing but the truth to their clients even in cases where learning the truth is likely to be harmful. Ethical dilemmas about such matters as the rights of individuals when these conflict with anticipated social benefits, the morality of withholding the truth, the acceptability of paternalistic coercion of persons "for their own good"—these age-old moral problems are found in new settings created by advances in human genetics, as is the case in other biomedical areas.

Before we can begin to answer the question "who shall make the decisions?" we must first be clear about what decisions there are to be made. Since the issues in human genetics are so complex and multilayered, I shall spend a bit of time sorting them out and try to show how the practices of genetic screening, genetic counseling, and genetic engineering, pose interconnected moral problems. In the course of this talk, I shall argue for two separate but related theses. The first is that the individual (meaning also the individual couple, where appropriate) should have final decision-making authority in matters of his or her own reproductive acts and capacities, as well as continuation or termination of pregnancy, where the reasons for these decisions refer to genetic factors. The second thesis is that attempts at government-based or scientist-directed eugenic programmes— whether aimed at positive or negative eugenics—are bound to be misguided or dangerous or both. Having asserted these theses, let me now go back and lay the groundwork. I shall try, first, to identify the chief moral issues in human genetics, showing just where and in what ways the need for decision-making arises. Then I shall have the way paved for arguing the two theses just stated.

II

As the terms imply, "genetic screening" denotes a process of detection and diagnosis of heritable conditions; "genetic counseling" refers to the activity of informing or advising those who are afflicted with such conditions or are carriers; and "genetic engineering" involves manipulation of either genetic material itself, or else the reproductive acts or capacities of persons. About each of these activities the following questions must be posed: what purposes is the practice designed to serve? who stands to benefit from the practice? what individual rights or liberties stand to be abridged?

what other values are involved in decision-making in these areas?

Beginning with genetic screening, let's look briefly at each of these activities to see where the need for decision-making arises and what sorts of decisions are involved. The range of diagnostic procedures known as genetic screening can be grouped roughly into the following five categories, of which I shall discuss the first four: (a) newborn metabolic screening; (b) chromosome screening; (c) carrier screening; (d) prenatal diagnosis; and (e) susceptibility screening.[1]

(a) The most prevalent example of newborn metabolic screening is that of the relatively simple and inexpensive test for phenylketonuria (PKU), a rare autosomal recessive in which the afflicted infant has inherited one defective gene from each parent. Those suffering from phenylketonuria lack a critical enzyme for metabolizing phenylalanine, an essential amino acid. If left untreated, PKU leads to irreversible mental retardation; when treated by introducing a synthetic diet virtually free of phenylalanine and begun shortly after birth, children with PKU do not suffer the consequence of severe retardation; but there is now some evidence that the special diet does not restore intelligence totally.[2] While PKU screening is an example of genetic screening where some treatment or cure exists for afflicted individuals, its use is not free of difficulties. For one thing, there have been significant instances of false positives—a source of difficulty because the synthetic diet can be harmful to a normal child. Moreover, a serious reproduction problem has arisen, since PKU women given birth to children who are retarded, no matter what their genotype, because of a toxic uterine environment. A different sort of problem stems from the fact that most states in the U.S. have adopted a programme of mandatory PKU screening—a practice that some believe will serve as a model for increasing numbers of medical procedures compelled by law.[3] So while PKU screening has the virtue of being a diagnostic procedure for a condition having a treatment or cure that now exists, it may, for that very reason, be an unwelcome paradigm of legally compelled medical procedures, which will make inroads into the privacy of individuals in our society.

(b) The most notorious example of chromosome screening of newborns is that of the XYY chromosomal anomaly. The extra Y chromosome is thought by some to result in an unusual degree of antisocial, aggressive behavior on the part of the so-called "super-males" who possess this abnormality. Unlike the case of PKU, there is no known "cure" or even a scientifically well-confirmed treatment programme for males who have this chromosomal abnormality, nor has it been fully ascertained that this special population is significantly different in behaviour patterns from "normal" XY males who come from similar backgrounds. But XYY screening has drawn sharp criticism for reasons other than those pertaining to theoretical and diagnostic uncertainties of this sort. Severe criticism has been leveled at a study in Boston, which has offered therapy to young boys found through screening to have the extra Y chromosome. One argument runs as follows:

> Either the researcher must withhold from the parents the information that the child being studied is XYY (which is probably immoral and perhaps also illegal), or that information must be disclosed, which will alter the way the parents feel about the child (probably for the worse). It will also render the study scientifically worthless, since for the study to demonstrate whether there are behavioral problems with the XYY male it is necessary that his upbringing be as "normal" as possible, so he can be compared with an XY boy.[4]

This argument is persuasive, especially given the circumstance that the therapy for aggressive or antisocial behaviour is, at best, uncertain, and at worst, coercive. But even if it is morally permissible or even desirable to seek to alter the deviant behaviour of XYY male children, the other points in the argument remain. The moral conflict surrounding how much and what specific information should be transmitted to whom arises directly in many cases of genetic counseling, as we shall see shortly. The problem of informing parents that they have an XYY child is wider than that raised by the Bos-

ton study. Even if no therapy were offered, there would remain the problem of adverse effects on the parents' expectations about and treatment of their sons whom they knew to possess an extra Y chromosome. While many screening programmes for XYY seem to have been dropped, controversy still rages over whether it is morally permissible to employ screening technics of this kind at all.

(c) Carrier screening is different from the two varieties just discussed in that it is aimed not at those afflicted with a genetic disease, but rather, at a carrier—one

> who is clinically well himself, but risks having a child with a disease. These programs do not involve case-finding and treatment in the conventional sense, but rather represent an attempt to identify the person at risk and to intervene in his or her reproductive life, an approach not taken by any previous screening program. [5]

The two diseases for which carriers have been screened are Tay-Sachs disease, a rare metabolic disorder that leads to blindness, paralysis and death usually before the age of four; and sickle-cell anemia, a painful and often lifeshortening disease found largely among Blacks. Tay-Sachs disease, found mostly among Jews of Eastern European descent can be diagnosed *in utero* by means of amniocentesis, so afflicted fetuses can be aborted. While the condition itself has no cure, the purpose served by screening programmes is to supply information for those parents who would choose abortion rather than bear an afflicted child who will certainly suffer and die within a very few years after birth. The purpose served by screening for sickle-cell carriers is not so clear, however. The disease cannot be detected *in utero,* so screening for carriers does not present many options. Sickle-cell anemia is autosomal recessive, which means that both parents must be carriers before it is possible to give birth to a child with the disease, and there is a one-in-four chance with each pregnancy of having an afflicted child. So parents found to be carriers can either take their chances of bearing a child who will have the disease, or choose artificial insemination with a non-carrier donor, or else seek to adopt a child. Screening programmes for sickle-cell have come under fire on the grounds that they are potentially dangerous as weapons that might be used for racist purposes by Whites against Blacks. It is difficult to see what sorts of persuasive arguments could be offered for compulsory sickle-cell screening programmes, in the absence of intra-uterine detection of diseased fetuses or else a cure for the disease. Optional screening programmes can be justified on the grounds that they enable couples to make a more informed choice about whether or not to have children; while some couples may well choose to take the one-in-four chance with each pregnancy, others will not. There seem to be no clear social benefits that accrue to mandatory programmes, and their disvalue lies largely in raising fear and suspicion about the possible repressive uses such programmes might serve.

(d)   Prenatal diagnosis as a form of genetic screening overlaps with the category of chromosomal screening discussed earlier. In one form of prenatal diagnosis, fetal cells from the amniotic fluid are cultured and subjected to chromosomal analysis. In this way, XYY males can be detected *in utero* and aborted; the moral permissibility of abortion on these grounds is another issue currently under debate. A more significant use of prenatal diagnosis is found in the case of Down's syndrome. Women over 40—or even over 35—are known to be at greatly elevated risk for having a child with Down's syndrome—the type of retardation formerly known as mongolism. Again, controversy exists over whether prenatal diagnosis ought to be routinely offered to women of any age, or particularly to those over 35. While there seem to be sound reasons for having such programmes available on a voluntary basis, there appear to be no good grounds for imposing prenatal diagnosis on women unwilling to undergo the slight physical risk or to receive genetic information about their child. There is, further, the consideration that a chromosomal analysis will turn up other genetic information, which even parents who are eager to learn about Down's syndrome may not wish to know. Here is where the moral dilemmas raised by genetic screening intersect with those of genetic counseling.

It is evident that the primary purpose for which genetic screening is now employed is for transmitting such information to prospective parents through genetic counseling, so that they can make as informed a choice as the circumstances allow. The primary and intended impact of transmitting the information obtained by screening is to reduce suffering of presently existing persons or their children. Thus the aim is to lessen the suffering of people in the present or next generation by preventing the birth of defective children, as in the case of Tay-Sachs and Down's syndrome, or by treating them at birth, like PKU children. But where there is no cure and no intrauterine detection programme, as in the case of sickle-cell anemia and Huntington's Chorea, there is some question about the purposes to which the information gained through screening may be put. We shall return to this issue later in connection with genetic engineering. But first, let us look at the overlapping yet distinct set of problems that arise in the area of genetic counseling.

III

The moral issues that arise in the practice of genetic counseling are primarily those surrounding truth and information in medicine. As noted earlier, there is the overarching issue of whether the genetic counselor's role should be as neutral and objective as possible, or whether it is sometimes permissible or even desirable to offer advice or guide the patient or couple to a decision. This issue appears to be no different, in principle, in the area of genetic counseling from that of a wide range of therapeutic situations in medicine, such as elective surgery or treatment regimens for severely defective newborns. As usual in ethical contexts, it is probably unwise to adhere dogmatically to a rigid principle like ''physicians or genetic counselors should never advise, but should always and only inform.'' While a general presumption in favour of fully autonomous decision-making by the patient or client is appropriate, sometimes that presumption may justifiably be overridden. There are cases in which a patient or couple asks directly for advice from the counselor, cases where it is evident to the counselor that the prospective parents fail to comprehend the enormity of caring for and raising a severely defective child, and still other instances where some measure of denial on the part of the parents stands in the way of their facing reality and making a rational decision. As with any other intermediate moral principle, the precept that genetic counselors should remain neutral and objective may justifiably be breached. Although some may argue that the genetic counselor's role includes some eugenic obligations, the purpose of counseling is to help the pregnant woman or prospective parents as much as possible in making an informed choice that is in accord with their own preferred values.[6] It has often been noted that many people suffer guilt, react unpredictably and often irrationally in the face of information about their role in transmitting defective genes to their offspring. A sensitive and compassionate genetic counselor, observing such situations, would be acting in accordance with a sound and widely held ethical precept in helping such parents come to a decision that is in accordance with their basic value scheme and that they can live with comfortably.

There are still other situations in genetic counseling, which pose different sorts of moral dilemmas from those just described. One such problem is whether or not it is ever permissible for a genetic counselor to withhold information from patients. In our discussion of the XYY chromosomal anomaly, we noted some difficulties that might arise if parents are apprised of the fact that their son's genetic endowment is one that has been found to correlate highly with overly aggressive behaviour and even with criminal tendencies. Other sorts of cases usually revolve around potential psychological harm to an individual or damage to a marriage likely to result from disclosure of genetic information. One physician cites the following two instances in which he believes that withholding information is justifiable.

> One example is where the genetic disorder of the child opens the possibility of nonpaternity—where the husband's genotype indicates he may not be the child's father. Disclosure of full information in this case could lead the father to question his acceptance of the child, as well as of his marital relationship.
>
> Another example would be the case of testicular feminization in which a genotypic 46, XY male develops as a female because of the failure of tissues to respond to testosterone stimulation. One might withhold this information from some parents because they would have difficulty relating to the child or would withhold it from the child herself when she is old enough to be counseled. . . . In cases in which the information can do serious psychological damage, I feel withholding it is justified.[7]

In these sorts of cases, it would seem that a rigid adherence to a moral principle that enjoins persons always to tell the truth, the whole truth, and nothing but the truth is an instance of dogmatism in ethics. Other moral principles sometimes override the precept that mandates truth-telling; or, to put it another way, the duty to tell the truth is sometimes superseded by another moral duty, when the two come into conflict. The dilemma here seems to be more of an epistemological one than an ethical one: how can we know in advance when telling the truth or disclosing full information will yield greater harm than good? How can we judge whether it is better, on the whole, for one member of a couple to be told about the infidelity of the other? Do we have an adequate basis for knowing how much and what sorts of psychological harm will be done by informing parents about their child's sexual anomaly, as in the example cited earlier? The ethical principle here seems rather clear: perform that act likely to produce least harm to everyone who stands to be affected. But one can accept this consequentialist moral position and yet still not know how to act because of the epistemological difficulties just noted. This should serve to remind us that not all the problems in moral contexts arise out of uncertainty about which ethical principle to adopt or what to do when two basic moral precepts come into conflict. In the cases just noted, it is likely that general agreement can be secured about the appropriateness of a utilitarian or consequentialist approach. Disagreement is more likely to arise over just which course of action is, in fact, likely to produce more harm, on balance. Aside from other kinds of disputes concerning what properly constitutes harm in such cases, the difficulty does seem to be more of an epistemological one than an ethical one.

The foregoing treatment of moral issues in genetic counseling has rested on the presupposition that the genetic counselor's responsibility is to the patient or client. Based on this presupposition, I have supported the general presumption that favours decision-making autonomy on the part of those being counseled. If, however, the genetic counselor were properly viewed as having an obligation to society at large or to future generations, then the presumption about autonomy might have to be overridden in some cases. In answer to the question, "To whom is the genetic counselor responsible?" one geneticist replies:

> Basically, I think that genetic counselors may be misguided if they feel that their ethical obligation is in *any way* to future generations. . . . [A]ll too often, I get the feeling that some genetic counselors are acting on the hidden assumption that they are somehow participating in that particularly Western predilection for attempting to create "ideal situations," in this instance, that of building a better gene pool through "negative eugenics." . . . The genetic counselor's obligation, I will maintain, never should extend beyond the family within his purview . . . Properly, a genetic counselor's job should not, in any way, be construed as eugenic in practice.[8]

Now, if we accept this view, that the genetic counselor has a responsibility to the family he is counseling and not to society at large or to future generations, then it is but a few small steps to the conclusion that individuals or couples should have final decision-making authority in matters of their own reproductive acts and capacities. But before such a conclusion can be reached, we must first explore the question of the feasibility or desirability of genetic engineering. Even if it is not the business of the genetic counselor to make recommendations to families on the basis of what is best for the human gene pool, it might still turn out that government-based or scientist-directed eugenic programmes could override personal decisions in these matters. So before concluding that ultimate decision-making authority ought to rest with individual persons or

couples, we must first reject any presumptions to the contrary that stem from eugenic considerations. In the remaining time I shall explore some issues in genetic engineering, with the aim of showing that government-based or scientist-directed eugenic programmes are misguided or dangerous or both.

IV

The notion of genetic engineering appears to have a narrower and a broader definition. The narrow conception refers to approaches involving laboratory manipulation of genes or cells: somatic cell alteration and germ cell alteration.[9] When this meaning is assigned to genetic engineering, the term 'eugenics' is used to refer to selection of parents or of their germ cells.[10] But sometimes the term 'genetic engineering' is used in a fully general sense, to refer to any manipulation of the reproductive acts or capacities of persons or their parts. It is this latter sense that will be used in the remainder of this account.

At least the idea behind eugenics—if not the practice itself in some form—is ancient. Positive eugenics was promoted in Plato's *Republic,* long before the science of genetics provided the theoretical basis and systematic data that today's proponents of genetic engineering have to work with. The lack of personal freedoms allowed the citizens in the *Republic* is well known to those familiar with Plato's work, and is evident in the following passage discussing regulation of unions between the sexes:

> It is for you, then, as their lawgiver, who have already selected the men, to select for association with them women who are so far as possible of the same natural capacity. . . .[A]nything like unregulated unions would be a profanation in a state whose citizens lead the good life. The Rulers will not allow such a thing. . . . [I]f we are to keep our flock at the highest pitch of excellence, there should be as many unions of the best of both sexes, and as few of the inferior, as possible, and . . . only the offspring of the better unions should be kept. . . . Moreover, young men who acquit themselves well in war and other duties, should be given, among other rewards and privileges, more liberal opportunities to sleep with a

wife, for the further purpose that, with good excuse, as many as possible of the children may be begotten of such fathers.[11]

But lest we conclude that a eugenics movement can only be promoted or gain adherents in a rigidly controlled society like Plato's *Republic* or a totalitarian regime such as Nazi Germany, let us consider the view of a 20th century Nobel Prize winning geneticist. The late Hermann Muller was an arch proponent of positive eugenics, based on his belief that the human gene pool is deteriorating. Muller argued for voluntary programmes of positive eugenics, rejecting any form of state-imposed regulations. He claimed that "democratic control . . . implies an upgrading of the people in general in both their intellectual and social faculties, together with a maintenance or, preferably, an improvement in their bodily condition."[12] Muller was one of a number of contemporary geneticists who have made gloomy prophecies about the increasing load of mutations in the human gene pool. The particular brand of positive eugenics that he advocated was a voluntary artificial insemination programme using donor semen (AID). He envisaged preserving the semen of outstanding men for future use in artificial insemination, choosing such greats as Einstein, Pasteur, Descartes, Leonardo and Lincoln as men whose child no woman would refuse to bear.[13]

Muller's method of freezing the semen of intellectual and creative men is only one of several proposals favouring some form of *positive* eugenics—a programme for improving the species, breeding a better race, or trying to prevent further deterioration by taking active countermeasures. Greater attention has been directed to the question of whether *negative* eugenics should be practiced on carriers or those afflicted with heritable diseases, in the form of enforced or encouraged abortions, sterilization, or less repressive but nonetheless coercive measures. The dilemma of choosing between preserving the individual freedom to marry and procreate as one chooses, and preventing further pollution of the gene pool would, indeed, pose an agonizing moral choice if the facts were as clear-cut as the eugenicists take them to be. There seems, however, to be enough uncertainty

about the possible and probable outcomes of any attempts at eugenics to warrant extreme caution in mounting such grandiose schemes for genetic improvement. Many scientists agree that trying to reduce the load of mutations in the human gene pool through negative eugenics would be ineffective, at best. And the arguments against positive eugenics point to a number of potentially infelicitous outcomes. There are at least five separate arguments against the feasibility or desirability of any large-scale attempt at genetic engineering for eugenic purposes—arguments which, if taken together, give strong support to my conclusion that genetic engineering with this aim is misguided or dangerous or both. A sixth argument is the religious one that creating or modifying the human species is a task not for man, but for God.[14] For those to whom this sort of argument is compelling, it may lend added strength to the other five. I shall confine my discussion to four of the five considerations that do not require belief in a supernatural deity. Each of the following arguments against a systematic effort to mount any sort of eugenics programme will be discussed in turn below:

1. We're too ignorant to do it right;

2. In any case, we are likely to alter the gene pool for ill;

3. Negative eugenics can't possibly work unless carriers are eliminated, but this would soon eliminate the entire species;

4. Some methods of genetic engineering carry grave moral risks of mishap.

The fifth argument is essentially that most—if not all—methods of genetic engineering are dehumanizing in basic ways.[15] While I think this attack contains some interesting points and raises questions of value that generally deserve important consideration, it is a gratuitous argument in this context. If the first four arguments are sound, they obviate the necessity for the fifth, since the scientific and practical objections to eugenic programmes would rule them out before the value issues need be brought into consideration. So I shall treat only the first four arguments in what follows.

(1) The claim that we are too ignorant to

do the job right has several variants, each with significant implications. The first consideration points to our general ignorance about the value of a gene to a given race to the species. As one prominent geneticist notes:

> We know only about its value to the individual carrying it and then only in instances where the effect is severe. In the light of such ignorance, it seems to me that the best procedure is to avoid all changes in the environment which are likely to change the mutation rate. . . . The quality of a gene or genotype may be determined only by the reaction of the associated phenotype in the environment in which it exists. A phenotype may be disadvantageous in some environments, essentially neutral in others, and advantageous in others. In the face of a rapidly changing and entirely new environment (new in an evolutionary sense), I do not believe that we can determine the value of specific genotypes to the species.[16]

This brand of ignorance constitutes our lack of knowledge of what to select for—a form of ignorance that some may argue is confined to the present state of development of the science of genetics. But a second variant of the "we're too ignorant" argument notes that "if we alter the gene pool, independent of environment, we are acting on the basis of present environmental criteria to select a gene pool for the future. Since the environment is changing a thousandfold times faster than our gene pool, it would be a disastrous approach.[17] But the difficulty here is not simply one of our inability to predict accurately what the future will be like. Questions of value enter in—questions that invariably resurrect the memory of attempts at positive eugenics among the Nazis. One writer asks:

> Who will be the judges and where will be the separation between good and bad? The most difficult decisions will come in defining the borderline cases. Will we breed against tallness because space requirements become more critical? Will we breed against nearsightedness because people with glasses may not make good astronauts? Will we forbid intellectually inferior individuals from procreating despite their proved ability to produce a number of superior individuals?[18]

The last variant on the "we're too ignorant" theme that we shall consider here requires us to recall Hermann Muller's proposal for positive eugenics. Muller would not be alone in including Abraham Lincoln on a list of men whose child no woman would refuse to bear. Yet there is now considerable evidence that Lincoln was afflicted with Marfan's syndrome, a heritable disease of the connective tissue that is transmitted by a dominant gene. The evidence is based on a number of factors. Lincoln's bodily characteristics and facial features—the very qualities we term "Lincolnesque"—are typical features of bone deformities common to Marfan's syndrome. The disease was first named in 1896, some thirty years after Lincoln's death. It was believed for some time that Lincoln had Marfan's disease, on the basis of physical defects he was known to have had, as well as the early death of one of his children. One sign of the disease was Lincoln's abnormally long limbs. Also, casts made of Lincoln's body in the year of his inauguration reveal that his left hand was much longer than his right hand, and his left middle finger was elongated. He is also known to have suffered from severe farsightedness, in addition to having difficulty with his eyesight that stemmed from distortions in his facial bone structure. These bodily asymmetries are common to Marfan's syndrome, as is cardiac disease. It is believed that Lincoln inherited the disease from his father's side. His father was blind in one eye, his son Robert had difficulties with his eyes, and his son Tad had a speech defect and died at the age of eighteen, probably from cardiac trouble. The likelihood that Lincoln himself suffered from Marfan's syndrome was further confirmed in 1959, when a California physician named Harold Schwartz recognized the disease in a boy of seven who was known to share an ancestor with Lincoln.[19] Since the gene for Marfan's disease is dominant, those who have it and reach child-bearing age stand a fifty percent chance of having an afflicted child.

Now consider the consequences for the gene pool if Lincoln's frozen sperm were to be disseminated widely in the population. At least until the facts became evident, the result would be exactly the opposite of what Muller intended by his proposal. And if the mistake went beyond the case of Lincoln and Marfan's syndrome, including other individuals who, despite their outstanding achievements might be afflicted with or be carriers of other little known or as yet undiagnosed genetic diseases, the results would be dysgenic in the extreme. This last consideration leads directly to the second argument against eugenics programmes to which we turn next.

(2)   This argument holds that in any event, we are likely to alter the gene pool for ill. Leaving aside the less likely incidence of this occurrence as exemplified just now in the Abraham Lincoln story, we may look at another prominent consideration noted by some geneticists.

This consideration is often referred to as "heterozygote advantage." One geneticist explains as follows:

> There is . . . good evidence that individuals who carry two different forms of the same gene, that is, are heterozygous, appear to have an advantage. This is true even if that gene in double dose, that is, in the homozygous state, produces a severe disease. For example, individuals homozygous for the gene coding for sickle-cell hemoglobin invariably develop sickle-cell anemia which is generally fatal before the reproductive years. Heterozygotes for the gene are, however, protected more than normals from the effects of the most malignant form of malaria. It has been shown that women who carry the gene in single dose have a higher fertility in malarial areas than do normals.[20]

Here again, it is not only in the cases where there is known heterozygote advantage that the likelihood exists of altering the gene pool for ill by trying to eliminate genes for heritable diseases. There are, in addition, all of the cases where heterozygote advantage may exist but is at present unknown. If one uses risk-benefit ratios or something like a utilitarian schema for deciding moral issues in biomedical contexts, the evidence seems clearly to indicate a greater risk of dysgenic consequences than a possibility of beneficial results from attempts to alter the human gene pool by means of negative eugenics. A successful effort to eliminate carriers for heritable diseases would result at the same time in eliminating heterozygote advantage, which is believed to be beneficial to the species or to sub-populations within the species. While little is known at the present stage of inquiry in

genetics about all of the particular advantages that exist, it is an inference made by many experts in the field on the basis of present data and well-confirmed genetic theory. One biologist asks us to:

> Consider the gene leading to cystic fibrosis (C.F.). Until quite recently homozygotes for this gene died in infancy. Yet the gene causing C.F. is very common among all Caucasoid populations thus far studied. . . . It is too widespread in the race to be accounted for by genetic drift. The gene is also too frequent for it to be likely to be maintained by mutation pressure. Hence, we are driven to assume heterozygote advantage.[22]

It would seem, then, that what is gained by the elimination of homozygotes may well be lost by the elimination of heterozygotes, resulting in no clear benefits and possibly some significant disadvantages in populations that suffer from genetic diseases. But the argument just given assumes that it would in fact be possible to eliminate genes for heritable diseases by preventing carriers from reproducing and thereby passing on such genes to future generations. The next argument against genetic engineering questions such a possibility.

(3)   This argument maintains, in sum, that negative eugenics can't possibly work unless carriers are eliminated as well as diseased individuals; but a successful attempt to prevent all carriers of potentially lethal genes from reproducing would effectively eliminate the entire species. The effects of negative eugenics on the general population are assessed by one geneticist as follows:

> With a few exceptions, dominant diseases are rare and interfere severely with reproductive ability. They are generally maintained in the population by new mutations. Therefore, there is either no need or essentially no need for discouraging these individuals from reproduction . . . The story is quite different for recessive conditions. . . . [A]ny attempt to decrease the gene frequency of these common genetic disorders in the population by prevention of fertility of all carriers would be doomed to failure. First, we all carry between three and eight of these genes in a single dose. Secondly, for many of these conditions, the frequency of carriers in the population is about 1 in 50 or even greater.

Prevention of fertility for even one of these disorders would stop a sizable proportion of the population from reproducing. . . .[23]

If this assessment is sound, it has significant implications for the prospects of favourably altering the human gene pool by negative eugenics. Such an argument is persuasive if the purpose of negative eugenics is viewed as that of improving the human gene pool for the sake of future generations. But if the purpose of negative eugenics is seen as improving the quality of life for those in the present and next generation, then the argument just given is beside the point. We should recall the dual purpose for which proposals for genetic engineering are put forth. The one we have been discussing here is the proposed improvement or prevention of deterioration of the gene pool for the sake of future generations of humans. The other purpose, tied to voluntary genetic screening programmes and the activity of genetic counseling, is to present options to individuals or couples that will help them avoid the birth of a defective child whose quality of life will be poor and who will most likely be a burden on both parents and society. For this latter purpose, the practice of negative eugenics through voluntary screening and sensitive genetic counseling can serve to improve the quality of life of persons in this and the next generation. But when transformed into a programme designed to control the reproductive acts or capacities of people for the sake of future generations, then the practice of negative eugenics seems to be scientifically and practically misguided. Indeed, taking this argument and the previous one together, the conclusion may be put succinctly in the words of one writer:

> Neither positive nor negative eugenics can ever significantly improve the gene pool of the population and simultaneously allow for adequate evolutionary improvement of the human race. The only useful aspect of negative eugenics is in individual counseling of specific families in order to prevent some of the births of abnormal individuals.[23]

(4) The fourth argument against genetic engineering focuses specifically on those practices involving manipulation of genetic material itself. This argument raises questions about the grave risks involved in any such manipulation, especially since mishaps that may arise are likely to be far worse than what happens when nature takes its course. One geneticist sees the prospects as follows:

> The problem of altering an individual's genes by direct chemical change of his DNA presents technically an enormously difficult task. Even if it became possible to do this, the chance of error would be high. Such an error, of course, would have the diametrically opposite effect to that desired and would be irreversible; in other words, the individual would become even more abnormal.[24]

Some observers fear the creation of hapless monsters as a result of various manipulations on genetic material. Whether or not the laboratory techniques are sufficiently refined at present to enable researchers to develop procedures for widespread use, it is likely that these techniques will be available soon enough to deserve careful reflection now. We need to ask, once again, whether the purpose served by laboratory methods of genetic engineering is helping those who are at risk for bearing defective children to prevent such occurrences, or instead, breeding a genetically improved species for the future. If such techniques are perfected and become available for use in spite of the attendant risks of mishap, they would then be offered to couples on a voluntary basis in the same way that current methods of genetic intervention are employed. Where a practice is aimed at the genetic improvement of a couple's own progeny, there are no grounds for methods that involve coercion. What is needed in such cases is counseling and education, not coercion and control.

At the outset, I said I would argue for two separate but related theses. First, the individual or couple should have final decision-making authority in matters of his or her own reproductive acts and capacities, as well as continuation or termination of pregnancy where the reasons for these decisions refer to genetic factors. Second, attempts at government-based or scientist-directed eugenic programmes are bound to be misguided or dangerous or both. The four arguments at the end were offered in support of the second thesis. If those arguments are sound, they demonstrate that there is no warrant for those in power to take final decision-making authority away from the individual where the reasons for such actions refer to eugenic considerations. Recall also our earlier conclusion that final decision-making should be left to the individual or couple in the context of genetic counseling, except in cases where the decision requires medical expertise that a patient is unlikely to have. Now if genetic screening should be practiced on a voluntary basis; and if decisions arising out of counseling should be left to the individual; and if in addition, positive and negative eugenics aimed at future generations is basically misguided; then there seems to be only one consideration remaining that might argue in favour of limiting individual rights for the sake of social benefits. That consideration points to the burden placed on society for treating and maintaining defective infants and others who might have been aborted or never even conceived by dint of state policy. Time does not permit an examination of this last issue, but is worth making a final observation in closing. If the notion of social benefit is understood largely in terms of increased financial resources that would otherwise be allocated to caring for those afflicted with heritable diseases, then something crucial is being left out of the balance between individual rights and social benefits. What is socially beneficial must be viewed not only in terms of increases in financial and other tangible resources, but also in terms of a range of freedom and autonomy that members of a society can reasonably expect to enjoy. It is important to preserve that freedom and autonomy through insuring the individual's right to decide about his or her own reproductive acts and capacities. With increased availability of voluntary genetic screening programmes and widespread education of the public, it is hard to imagine that most people will choose to burden themselves and society with defective children when other options are open to them. Even if there are some who refuse screening or abortion, society as a whole would be better off to accommodate their freely chosen reproductive acts than to impose compulsory genetic screening, abortion, or sterilization on its members.

Notes

1. Tabitha Powledge, "Genetic Screening," *Encyclopedia of Bioethics* (in press).
2. *Ibid.*
3. *Ibid.*
4. Powledge, "The XYY Man: Do Criminals Really Have Abnormal Genes?" *Science Digest*, January, 1976, p. 37.
5. Powledge, "Genetic Screening," *op. cit.*
6. A view similar to this is argued by Marc Lappé. "The Genetic Counselor: Responsible to Whom?" *The Hastings Center Report*, No. 2, September 1971.
7. Robert F. Murray, Jr., *ibid.*, p. 120.
8. Marc Lappé, *op cit.*, p. 6.
9. Bernard D. Davis. "Threat and Promise in Genetic Engineering," ed. by Preston Williams in *Ethical Issues in Biology and Medicine* (Cambridge, Mass.: Schenkman Publishing Company, 1973), pp. 17–24.
10. *Ibid.*
11. Francis MacDonald Cornford (tr.). *The Republic of Plato* (New York: Oxford Unviersity Press), pp. 157–60.
12. Hermann J. Muller, "Genetic Progress by Voluntarily Conducted Germinal Choice," ed. by Gordon Wolstenholme, in *Man and His Future* (Boston: Little, Brown and Co., 1963), p. 256.
13. Theodosius Dobzhansky, *Mankind Evolving* (New Haven: Yale University Press, 1962), p. 328.
14. Such arguments are offered by Paul Ramsey in *Fabricated Man* (New Haven: Yale University Press, 1970).
15. This argument is given by Ramsey, *op. cit.*, and also by Leon R. Kass, "Making Babies—The New Biology and the 'Old' Morality," *The Public Interest*, Vol. 26, Winter, 1972.
16. Arthur Steinberg, "The Genetic Pool. Its Evolution and Significance—'Desirable' and 'Undesirable' Genetic Traits," in C.I.O.M.S. *Recent Progress in Biology and Medicine*, pp. 83–93.
17. Hirschhorn, *op. cit.*, p. 128.
18. Hirschhorn, "Practical and Ethical Problems in Human Genetics," *Birth Defects*, Vol. VIII, July, 1972, p. 28.
19. *Ibid.*, p. 23.
20. Steinberg, *op. cit.*

21. Rene Dubos and Maya Pines, *Health and Disease* (New York: Time, Inc., 1965), pp. 123–24.

22. Hirschhorn, ''Practical and Ethical Problems in Human Genetics,'' pp. 22–23.

23. *Ibid.,* p. 25.

24. *Ibid.,* p. 27.

Genetic Screening: For Better or for Worse?

Neil A. Holtzman

Cystic fibrosis, sickle cell anemia, Tay-Sachs disease, and thalassemia are autosomal-recessive diseases that occur more frequently than once in 4,000 live births in subgroups of the American population. Tay-Sachs disease can be diagnosed by mid-trimester amniocentesis, a safe procedure.[1] Early intrauterine detection of sickle cell anemia and thalassemia by placental aspiration has been reported[2,3]; the safety and accuracy of the techniques require confirmation. In the future, diagnosis of the 16-week fetus with cystic fibrosis will also be possible.

Prenatal diagnosis could drastically reduce the incidence of these disorders, but there are two prerequisites. First, couples in whom both mates are carriers must be identified before they have any children. There is as great a chance of first births being affected as any other, and they constitute over 40% of all births in the United States,[4] with the proportion rising. Carrier identification is already possible for all of the conditions mentioned except cystic fibrosis. Second, couples at risk must terminate the pregnancy of affected fetuses. Although few couples would have a child with Tay-Sachs disease if they could avoid it, those at risk for having offspring with cystic fibrosis or sickle cell anemia, in which mental retardation and early death are not the usual outcome, might not make the same choice.[5]

In order to satisfy the two prerequisites

screening could be made compulsory and those identified as carriers compelled to avoid the birth of affected children. Although such extreme and opprobrious measures seem unlikely today, coercive pressures could be subtly exerted and carriers could be sufficiently stigmatized so that they become undesirable mates. Thus, model screening programs should be carefully scrutinized for evidence of coercion and stigmatization before they are widely adopted.

Participation has been a problem in Tay-Sachs screening. Programs directed at young married couples often attract only a small proportion of the target population. . . . Clow and Scriver describe an attempt to increase participation by screening in high schools.[6] Fortunately, they provide information that enables the reader to assess some of the effects, both beneficial and harmful.

Although the most intensive effort involved the addition of material on human genetics to the high schools' biology curriculum, coercion and peer pressure cannot be excluded. The chief medical officer of the school system was recruited to recommend testing ''in an official letter to all Jewish students . . . and a school assembly was held to discuss the benefits of testing. . . . ''[7] Whether it was education, coercion, peer pressure, a captive audience, or something else, acceptance of screening improved markedly. Whereas the earlier program, directed at newlyweds, attracted only 10.8% of the target population,[7] the authors report that 75% of the eligible students were

Reprinted by permission of the author and *Pediatrics,* vol. 59, no. 1, pp. 131–133, January 1977. Copyright American Academy of Pediatrics 1977.

screened. Thus, a far greater proportion of the at-risk population now knows whether or not they are carriers. What effect will this new knowledge have?

Let us first consider the effect on non-carriers. Ten percent of them had an improved self-image after testing. A similar percentage said they would not mate with carriers. These attitudes are not consonant with the facts: those who do not carry the Tay-Sachs gene possess, on the average, genes for three or four other "bad" diseases; there is no reason for self-image to improve. Nor is there any risk of having a child with Tay-Sachs disease in matings between a non-carrier and a carrier.

Let us turn to the carriers. All of them indicated they would want to know the results of screening in their intended spouses. Twelve percent, however, said they would "reconsider" if he or she was also a carrier. This group apparently does not understand or accept prenatal diagnosis and abortion as a means of avoiding the birth of affected infants. How many other carriers lack understanding or acceptance is unknown. Until follow-up information on the actions of carriers later in life is available the encouragement of high school screening "as the preferred program" may be premature.

Screening for carriers at a time in life when choice of mate is not imminent and when self-confidence ebbs and flows may cause additional problems. Fear of stigmatization may be the reason why one third of carriers, compared to 15% of non-carriers, did not inform their friends of the result. One half of the carriers were worried or depressed immediately after learning their status; several months later 17.7% said they were still worried. Nine percent of students identified as carriers had a diminished self-image. Although anxiety also occurs in married individuals identified as carriers, fear of stigmatization is less.[8] The significance of depression or anxiety will only be determined by comparing the subsequent experience of carriers and non-carriers identified by screening. Because of the psychological and social hazards one group of physicians advised their community against Tay-Sachs screening at any age.[9]

Before concluding that risks outweigh benefits, efforts to increase participation in screening that do not endanger the individual's freedom of choice or well-being must be considered. More education about human genetics is fundamental. Greater appreciation of the laws of inheritance might result from teaching about genetic traits of humans rather than those of peas or fruit flies. Clow and Scriver have made a notable contribution by developing in-service training for high school teachers. Further evaluation of changes in students' understanding as a result of the curriculum modification is needed.

Physicians can also educate. Indeed, people in communities involved in Tay-Sachs screening expected them to do so. Yet as the actual source of information about screening, physicians were outranked by synogogues, newspapers, radio, television, and friends.[7,10] One obstacle may be infrequent contact between physicians and young adults. Another may be physicians' preoccupation with the treatment of overt illness. But medical care administered after disease becomes manifest is a less effective way of reducing untimely death and disability than earlier intervention. As a greater number of interventions that do not depend on the presence of overt illness become available, physicians may be expected to take responsibility for them. In the case of genetic screening, the doctor-patient relationship provides a confidential channel for communication of advice and results; coercion and stigmatization might be less of a problem.

Finally, the community must be among those who decide whether screening should be undertaken. It must be presented with the objectives of screening as well as the potential pitfalls. Community input and involvement could serve to reduce the harmful effects. As no group can speak for all of its constituents, each individual should receive information about the benefits and risks before being screened and have the opportunity to refuse screening.

In the immediate future the determination of how inappropriate psychological and social attitudes that result from screening can be minimized is more important than the extension of programs whose effects are still uncertain. With the knowledge that accrues, genetic screening for better, not for worse, will result.

Notes

1. NICHD National Registry for Amniocentesis Study Group: Mid-trimester amniocentesis for prenatal diagnosis. JAMA 236:1471, 1976.
2. Kan YW, Golbus MS, Trecartin R: Prenatal diagnosis of sickle cell anemia. N Engl J Med 294:1039, 1976.
3. Alter BP, Friedman S, Hobbins JC, *et al:* Prenatal diagnosis of sickle cell anemia and alpha-G-Philadelphia. N Engl J. Med 294:1040, 1976.
4. National Center for Health Statistics: Advance Report, Final Natality Statistics, 1974. Vital Stat Rep. 1976.
5. Stomatoyannopoulos G: Problems of screening and counseling in the hemoglobinopathies. In, Motulsky AG, Lenz W (eds): Birth Defects. Amsterdam, Excerpta Medica, 1974, pp. 268–276.
6. Clow CL, Scriver CR: Knowledge and attitudes about genetic screening among high school students: The Tay-Sachs experience, *Pediatrics* 59:86, 1977.
7. Beck E., Blaichman S, Scriver CR, Clow CL: Advocacy and compliance in genetic screening, behavior of physicians and clients in a voluntary program of testing for the Tay-Sachs gene. N Engl J Med 291:1166, 1974.
8. Childs B, Gordis L, Kaback MM, Kazazian HH: Tay-Sachs screening: Social and psychological impact. Am J Hum Genet, to be published.
9. Kurh MD: Doubtful benefits of Tay-Sachs screening. N Engl J of Med 295:113, 1976.
10. Childs B, Gordis L, Kaback MM, Kazazian HH: Tay-Sachs screening: Motives for participating and knowledge of genetics and probability. Am J Hum Genet, to be published.

Genetic Diseases: Can Having Children Be Immoral?

L. M. Purdy

I. INTRODUCTION

Suppose you know that there is a fifty percent chance you have Huntington's chorea, even though you are still free of symptoms, and that if you do have it, each of your children has a fifty percent chance of having it also.

Should you now have children?

There is always some possibility that a pregnancy will result in a diseased or handicapped child. But certain persons run a higher than average risk of producing such a child. Genetic counselors are increasingly able to calculate the probability that certain problems will occur; this means that more people can find out whether they are in danger of creating unhealthy offspring *before* the birth of a child.

Reprinted with permission from *Genetics Now: Ethical Issues in Genetic Research,* edited by John Buckley, Jr. Washington, D.C.: University Press of America, 1978.

Since this kind of knowledge is available, we ought to use it wisely. I want in this paper to defend the thesis that it is wrong to reproduce when we know there is a high risk of transmitting a serious disease or defect. My argument for this claim is in three parts. The first is that we should try to provide every child with a normal opportunity for health; the second is that in the course of doing this it is not wrong to prevent possible children from existing. The third is that this duty may require us to refrain from childbearing.[1]

One methodological point must be made. I am investigating a problem in biomedical ethics: this is a philosophical enterprise. But the conclusion has practical importance since individuals do face the choice I examine. This raises a question: what relation ought the outcome of this inquiry bear to social policy?[2] It may be held that a person's reproductive life should not be interfered with. Perhaps this is a reasonable position, but it does not follow from it that it is never wrong for an individual to have children or that we should not try to determine when this is the case. All that does follow is that we may not coerce persons with regard to child-bearing. Evaluation of this last claim is a separate issue which cannot be handled here.

I want to deal with this issue concretely. The reason for this is that, otherwise, discussion is apt to be vague and inconclusive. An additional reason is that it will serve to make us appreciate the magnitude of the difficulties faced by diseased or handicapped individuals. Thus it will be helpful to consider a specific disease. For this purpose I have chosen Huntington's chorea.[3]

II. HUNTINGTON'S CHOREA: COURSE AND RISK

Let us now look at Huntington's chorea. First we will consider the course of the disease, then its inheritance pattern.

The symptoms of Huntington's chorea usually begin between the ages of thirty and fifty, but young children can also be affected. It happens this way:

> Onset is insidious. Personality changes (obstinacy, moodiness, lack of initiative) frequently antedate or accompany the involuntary choreic movements. These usually appear first in the face, neck, and arms, and are jerky, irregular, and stretching in character. Contractions of the facial muscles result in grimaces; those of the respiratory muscles, lips, and tongue lead to hesitating, explosive speech. Irregular movements of the trunk are present; the gait is shuffling and dancing. Tendon reflexes are increased . . . Some patients display a fatuous euphoria; others are spiteful, irascible, destructive, and violent. Paranoid reactions are common. Poverty of thought and impairment of attention, memory, and judgment occur. As the disease progresses, walking becomes impossible, swallowing difficult, and dementia profound. Suicide is not uncommon.[4]

The illness lasts about fifteen years, terminating in death.

Who gets Huntington's chorea? It is an autosomal dominant disease; this means it is caused by a single mutant gene located on a non-sex chromosome. It is passed from one generation to the next via affected individuals. When one has the disease, whether one has symptoms and thus knows one has it or not, there is a 50% chance that each child will have it also. If one has escaped it then there is no risk to one's children.[5]

How serious is this risk? For geneticists, a ten percent risk is high.[6] But not every high risk is unacceptable: this depends on what is at stake.

There are two separate evaluations in any judgment about a given risk. The first measures the gravity of the worst possible result; the second perceives a given risk as great or small. As for the first, in medicine as elsewhere, people may regard the same result differently:

> . . . The subjective attitude to the disease or lesion itself may be quite at variance with what informed medical opinion may regard as a realistic appraisal. Relatively minor limb defects with cosmetic overtones are examples here. On the other hand, some patients regard with equanimity genetic lesions which are of major medical importance.[7]

For devastating diseases like Huntington's chorea, this part of the judgment should be unproblematic: no one could want a loved one to suffer so.

There may be considerable disagreement, however, about whether a given probability is big or little. Individuals vary a good deal in their attitude toward this aspect of risk.[8] This suggests that it would be difficult to define the "right" attitude to a particular risk in many circumstances. Nevertheless, there are good grounds for arguing in favor of a conservative approach here. For it is reasonable to take special precautions to avoid very bad consequences, even if the risk is small. But the possible consequences here *are* very bad: a child who may inherit Huntington's chorea is a child with a much larger than average chance of being subjected to severe and prolonged suffering. Even if the child does not have the disease, it may anticipate and fear it, and anticipating an evil, as we all know, may be worse than experiencing it. In addition, if a parent loses the gamble, his child will suffer the consequences. But it is one thing to take a high risk for oneself; to submit someone else to it without his consent is another.

I think that these points indicate that the morality of procreation in situations like this demands further study. I propose to do this by looking first at the position of the possible child, then at that of the potential parent.[9]

III. REPRODUCTION: THE POSSIBLE CHILD'S POSITION

The first task in treating the problem from the child's point of view is to find a way of referring to possible future offspring without seeming to confer some sort of morally significant existence upon them. I will call children who might be born in the future but who are not now conceived "possible" children, offspring, individuals, or persons. I stipulate that this term implies nothing about their moral standing.

The second task is to decide what claims about children or possible children are relevant to the morality of childbearing in the circumstances being considered. There are, I think, two such claims. One is that we ought to provide every child with at least a normal opportunity for a good life. The other is that we do not harm possible children if we prevent them from existing. Let us consider both these matters in turn.

A. Opportunity for a Good Life

Accepting the claim that we ought to try to provide for every child a normal opportunity for a good life involves two basic problems: justification and practical application.

Justification of the claim could be derived fairly straightforwardly from either utilitarian or contractarian theories of justice, I think, although a proper discussion would be too lengthy to include here. Of prime importance in any such discussion would be the judgment that to neglect this duty would be to create unnecessary unhappiness or unfair disadvantage for some persons.

The attempt to apply the claim that we should try to provide a normal opportunity for a good life leads to a couple of difficulties. One is knowing what it requires of us. Another is defining "normal opportunity." Let us tackle the latter problem first.

Conceptions of "normal opportunity" vary among societies and also within them: *de rigueur* in some circles are private music lessons and trips to Europe, while in others providing eight years of schooling is a major sacrifice. But there is no need to consider this complication since we are here concerned only with health as a prerequisite for normal opportunity. Thus we can retreat to the more limited claim that every parent should try to ensure normal health for his child. It might be thought that even this moderate claim is unsatisfactory since in some places debilitating conditions are the norm. One could circumvent this objection by saying that parents ought to try to provide for their children health normal for that culture, even though it may be inadequate if measured by some outside standard. This conservative position would still justify efforts to avoid the birth of children at risk for Huntington's chorea and other serious genetic diseases.

But then what does this stand require of us: is sacrifice entailed by the duty to try to provide normal health for our children? The most plausible answer seems to be that as the danger of serious disability increases, the greater the sacrifice demanded of the potential parent. This means it would be more justifiable to recommend that an individual refrain from childbearing if he risks passing on spina bifida than if he risks passing on webbed feet. Working out all the details of such a schema would clearly be a difficult matter: I do not think it would be impossible to set up workable guidelines, though.

Assuming a rough theoretical framework of this sort, the next question we must ask is whether Huntington's chorea substantially impairs an individual's opportunity for a good life.

People appear to have different opinions about the plight of such persons. Optimists argue that a child born into a family afflicted with Huntington's chorea has a reasonable chance of living a satisfactory life. After all, there is a fifty percent chance it will escape the disease even if a parent has already manifested it, and a still greater chance if this is not so. Even if it does have the illness, it will probably enjoy thirty years of healthy life before symptoms appear; and, perhaps, it may not find the disease destructive. Optimists can list diseased or handicapped persons who have lived fruitful lives. They can also find individuals who seem genuinely glad to be alive. One is Rick Donohue, a sufferer from the Joseph family disease: "You know, if my mom hadn't had me, I wouldn't be here for the life I have had. So there is a good possibility I will have children."[10] Optimists therefore conclude that it would be a shame if these persons had not lived.

Pessimists concede these truths, but they take a less sanguine view of them. They think a fifty percent risk of serious disease like Huntington's chorea appallingly high. They suspect that a child born into an afflicted family is liable to spend its youth in dreadful anticipation and fear of the disease. They expect that the disease, if it appears, will be perceived as a tragic and painful end to a blighted life. They point out that Rick Donohue is still young and has not yet experienced the full horror of his sickness.

Empirical research is clearly needed to resolve this dispute: we need much more information about the psychology and life history of sufferers and potential sufferers. Until we have it we cannot know whether the optimist or the pessimist has a better case: definitive judgment must therefore be suspended. In the meantime, however, common sense suggests that the pessimist has the edge.

If some diseased persons do turn out to have a worse than average life there appears to be a case against further childbearing in afflicted families. To support this claim two more judgments are necessary, however. The first is that it is not wrong to refrain from childbearing. The second is that asking individuals to so refrain is less of a sacrifice than might be thought.[11] I will examine each of these judgments.

B. The Morality of Preventing the Birth of Possible Persons

Before going on to look at reasons why it would not be wrong to prevent the birth of pos-sible persons, let me try to clarify the picture a bit. To understand the claim it must be kept in mind that we are considering a prospective situation here, not a retrospective one: we are trying to rank the desirability of various alternative future states of affairs. One possible future state is this: a world where nobody is at risk for Huntington's chorea except as a result of random mutation. This state has been achieved by sons and daughters of persons afflicted with Huntington's chorea ceasing to reproduce. This means that an indeterminate number of children who might have been born were not born. These possible children can be divided into two categories: those who would have been miserable and those who would have lived good lives. To prevent the existence of members of the first category it was necessary to prevent the existence of all. Whether or not this is a good state of affairs depends on the morality of the means and the end. The end, preventing the existence of miserable beings, is surely good; I will argue that preventing the birth of possible persons is not intrinsically wrong. Hence this state of affairs is a morally good one.

Why then is it not in itself wrong to prevent the birth of possible persons? It is not wrong because there seems to be no reason to believe that possible individuals are either deprived or injured if they do not exist. They are not deprived because to be deprived in a morally significant sense one must be able to have experiences. But possible persons do not exist. Since they do not exist, they cannot have experiences. Another way to make this point is to say that each of us might not have been born, although most of us are glad we were. But this does not mean that it makes sense to say that we would have been deprived of something had we not been born. For if we had not been born, we would not exist, and there would be nobody to be deprived of anything. To assert the contrary is to imagine that we are looking at a world in which we do not exist. But this is not the way it would be: there would be nobody to look.

The contention that it is wrong to prevent possible persons from existing because they have a right to exist appears to be equally baseless. The most fundamental objection to this view is that there is no reason to ascribe rights to entities which do not exist. It is one thing to say that as-yet-nonexistent persons will have certain rights if and when they exist: this claim is plausible if made with an an eye toward preserving social and environmental goods.[12] But what justification could there be for the claim that nonexistent beings have a right to exist?

Even if one conceded that there was a presumption in favor of letting some nonexistent beings exist, stronger claims could surely override it.[13] For one thing, it would be unfair not to recognize the prior claim of already existing children who are not being properly cared for. One might also argue that it is simply wrong to prevent persons who might have existed from doing so. But this implies that contraception and population control are also wrong.

It is therefore reasonable to maintain that because possible persons have no right to exist, they are not injured if not created. Even if they had that right, it could rather easily be overridden by counterclaims. Hence, since possible persons are neither deprived nor injured if not conceived, it is not wrong to prevent their existence.

C. Conclusion to Part III

At the beginning of Part III I said that two claims are relevant to the morality of childbearing in the circumstances being considered. The first is that we ought to provide every child with at least a normal opportunity for a good life. The second is that we do not deprive or injure possible persons if we prevent their existence.

I suggested that the first claim could be derived from currently accepted theories of justice: a healthy body is generally necessary for happiness and it is also a prerequisite for a fair chance at a good life in our competitive world. Thus it is right to try to ensure that each child is healthy.

I argued, with regard to the second claim, that we do not deprive or injure possible persons if we fail to create them. They cannot be deprived of anything because they do not exist and hence cannot have experiences. They cannot be injured because only an entity with a right to exist could be injured if prevented from

existing: but there are no good grounds for believing that they are such entities.

From the conjunction of these two claims I conclude that it is right to try to ensure that a child is healthy even if by doing so we preclude the existence of certain possible persons. Thus it is right for individuals to prevent the birth of children at risk for Huntington's chorea by avoiding parenthood. The next question is whether is it seriously wrong *not* to avoid parenthood.

IV. REPRODUCTION: THE POTENTIAL PARENT'S SITUATION

I have so far argued that if choreics live substantially worse lives than average, then it is right for afflicted families to cease reproduction. But this conflicts with the generally recognized freedom to procreate and so it does not automatically follow that family members ought not to have children. How can we decide whether the duty to try to provide normal health for one's child should take precedence over the right to reproduce?

This is essentially the same question I asked earlier: how much must one sacrifice to try to ensure that one's offspring is healthy? In answer to this I suggested that the greater the danger of serious disability, the more justifiable considerable sacrifice is.

Now asking someone who wants a child to refrain from procreation seems to be asking for a large sacrifice. It may, in fact, appear to be too large to demand of anyone. Yet I think it can be shown that it is not as great as it initially seems.

Why do people want children? There are probably many reasons, but I suspect that the following include some of the most common. One set of reasons has to do with the gratification to be derived from a happy family life—love, companionship, watching a child grow, helping mold it into a good person, sharing its pains and triumphs. Another set of reasons centers about the parents as individuals—validation of their place within a genetically continuous family line, the conception of children as a source of immortality, being surrounded by replicas of themselves.

Are there alternative ways of satisfying these desires? Adoption or technological means provide ways to satisfy most of the desires pertaining to family life without passing on specific genetic defects. Artificial insemination by donor is already available; implantation of donor ova is likely within a few years. Still another option will exist if cloning becomes a reality. In the meantime, we might permit women to conceive and bear babies for those who do not want to do so themselves.[14] But the desire to extend the genetic line, the desire for immortality, and the desire for children that physically resemble one cannot be met by these methods.

Many individuals probably feel these latter desires strongly. This creates a genuine conflict for persons at risk for transmitting serious genetic diseases like Huntington's chorea. The situation seems especially unfair because, unlike normal people, through no fault of their own, doing something they badly want to do may greatly harm others.

But if my common sense assumption that they are in grave danger of harming others is true, then it is imperative to scrutinize their options carefully. On the one hand, they can have children: they satisfy their desires but risk eventual crippling illness and death for their offspring. On the other, they can remain childless or seek nonstandard ways of creating a family: they have some unfulfilled desires, but they avoid risking harm to their children.

I think it is clear which of these two alternatives is best. For the desires which must remain unsatisfied if they forgo normal procreation are less than admirable. To see the genetic line continued entails a sinister legacy of illness and death; the desire for immortality cannot really be satisfied by reproduction anyway; and the desire for children that physically resemble one is narcissistic and its fulfillment cannot be guaranteed even by normal reproduction. Hence the only defence of these desires is that people do in fact feel them.

Now, I am inclined to accept William James' dictum regarding desires: "Take any demand, however slight, which any creature, however weak, may make. Ought it not, for its own sole sake be satisfied? If not, prove why not."[15] Thus I judge a world where more desires are satisfied to be better than one in which fewer are. But not all desires should be regarded as legitimate, since, as James suggests, there may be good reasons why these ought to be disregarded. The fact that their fulfillment will seriously harm others is surely such a reason. And I believe that the circumstances I have described are a clear example of the sort of case where a desire must be judged illegitimate, at least until it can be shown that sufferers from serious genetic diseases like Huntington's chorea do not live considerably worse than average lives. Therefore, I think it is wrong for individuals in this predicament to reproduce.

V. CONCLUSION

Let me recapitulate. At the beginning of this paper I asked whether it is wrong for those who risk transmitting severe genetic disease like Huntington's chorea to have "blood" children. Some despair of reaching an answer to this question.[16] But I think such pessimism is not wholly warranted, and that if generally accepted would lead to much unnecessary harm. It is true that in many cases it is difficult to know what ought to be done. But this does not mean that we should throw up our hands and espouse a completely laissez-faire approach: philosophers can help by probing the central issues and trying to find guidelines for action.

Naturally there is no way to derive an answer to this kind of problem by deductive argument from self-evident premises, for it must depend on a complicated interplay of facts and moral judgments. My preliminary exploration of Huntington's chorea is of this nature. In the course of discussion I suggested that, if it is true that sufferers live substantially worse lives than do normal persons, those who might transmit it should not have children. This conclusion is supported by the judgments that we ought to try to provide for every child a normal opportunity for a good life, that possible individuals are not harmed if not conceived, and that it is sometimes less justifiable for persons to exercise their right to procreate than one might think.

I want to stress, in conclusion, that my argument is incomplete. To investigate fully even a single disease, like Huntington's chorea, empirical research on the lives of members of afflicted families is necessary. Then, after developing further the themes touched upon here, evaluation of the probable consequences of different policies on society and on future generations is needed. Until the results of a complete study are available, my argument could serve best as a reason for persons at risk for transmitting Huntington's chorea and similar diseases to put off having children. Perhaps this paper will stimulate such inquiry.

Notes

1. There are a series of cases ranging from low risk of mild disease or handicap to high risk of serious disease or handicap. It would be difficult to decide where the duty to refrain from procreation becomes compelling. My point here is that there are some clear cases.

   I'd like to thank Lawrence Davis and Sidney Siskin for their helpful comments on an earlier version of this paper.

2. This issue is one which must be faced most urgently by genetic counselors. The proper role of the genetic counselor with regard to such decisions has been the subject of much debate. The dominant view seems to be that espoused by Lytt Gardner who maintains that it is unethical for a counselor to make ethical judgments about what his clients ought to do. ("Counseling in Genetics." *Early Diagnosis of Human Genetic Defects: Scientific & Ethical Considerations,* ed. Maureen Harris, [H.E.W. Publication No. (NIH) 72-25; Fogarty Center Proceedings No. 6]; p. 192.) Typically this view is unsupported by an argument. For other views see Bentley Glass "Human Heredity and Ethical Problems" *Perspectives in Biology & Medicine,* Vol. 15 (winter '72) 237–53, esp. 242–52; Marc Lappé, "The Genetic Counselor Responsible to Whom? *Hastings Center Report,* Vol. 1, No. 2 (Sept. '71) 6–8; E. C. Fraser, "Genetic Counseling" *Am. J. of Human Genetics* 26: 636–659, 1974.

3. I have chosen Huntington's chorea because it seems to me to be one of the clearest cases of high risk serious genetic disease known to the public, despite the fact that it does not usually manifest itself until the prime of life. The latter entails two

further facts. First an individual of reproductive age may not know whether he has the disease; he therefore does not know the risk of passing on the disease. Secondly, an affected person may have a substantial number of years of healthy life before it shows itself. I do not think that this factor materially changes my case, however. Even if an individual does not in fact risk passing the disease to his children, *he cannot know that this is true.* And even thirty years of healthy life may well be seriously shadowed by anticipation and fear of the disease. Thus the fact that the disease develops late does not diminish its horror. If it could be shown that these factors could be adequately circumvented, my claim that there is a *class* of genetic disease of such severity that it would be wrong to risk passing them on would not be undermined.

   It might also be thought that Huntington's chorea is insufficiently common to merit such attention. But, depending on reproductive patterns, the disease could become a good deal more widespread. Consider the fact that in 1916 nine hundred and sixty-two cases could be traced from six seventeenth-century arrivals in America. (Gordon Rattray Taylor, *The Biological Time Bomb,* [New York, 1968], p. 176.) But more importantly, even if the disease did not spread, it would still be seriously wrong. I think, to inflict it unnecessarily on *any* members of new generations. Finally, it should be kept in mind that I am using Huntington's chorea as an example of the sort of disease we should try to eradicate. Thus the arguments presented here would be relevant to a wide range of genetic diseases.

4. *The Merck Manual,* (Rahway, N.J.: Merck, 1972). p. 1346.

5. Hymie Gordon, "Genetic Counseling," *JAMA,* Vol. 217 No. 9 (August 30, 1971), 1217.

6. Charles Smith, Susan Holloway, and Alan E. H. Emery, "Individuals at Risk in Families —Genetic Disease," *J. of Medical Genetics,* 8 (1971), 453. See also Townes in *Genetic Counseling* ed. Daniel Bergsma, *Birth Defects Original Article Series,* Vol. VL No. 1 (May 1970).

7. J. H. Pearn, "Patients' Subjective Interpretation of Risks offered in Genetic Counseling," *Journal of Medical Genetics,* 10 (1973) 131.

8. Pearn, p. 132.

9. There are many important and interesting points that might be raised with respect to future generations and present society. There is no space to deal with them here, although I strongly suspect that conclusions regarding them would support my judgment that it is wrong for those

who risk transmitting certain diseases to reproduce—for some discussion of future generations, see Gerald Leach, *The Biocrats,* (Middlesex, England: Penguin Books, 1972), p. 150; M. P. Golding, "Obligations to Future Generations," *Monist* 56 (Jan. 1972) 84-99; Gordon Rattray Taylor, *The Biological Time Bomb* (New York, 1968), esp. p. 176. For some discussions of society, see Daniel Callahan, "The Meaning and Significance of Genetic Disease: Philosophical Perspectives," *Ethical Issues in Human Genetics,* ed. Bruce Hilton et al., (New York, 1973), p. 87ff.; John Fletcher, "The Brink: The Parent-Child Bond in the Genetic Revolution," *Theological Studies* 33 (Sept. '72) 457-485; Glass (supra 2ª); Marc Lappé, "Human Genetics," Annals of the *New York Academy of Sciences,* Vol. 26 (May 18, 1973) 152-59; Marc Lappé, "Moral Obligations and the Fallacies of Genetic Control," *Theological Studies* Vol. 33, No. 3 (Sept. '72) 411-427; Martin P. Golding. "Ethical Issues in Biological Engineering," *UCLA Law Review* Vol. 15: 267 (1968) 443-479; L. C. Dunn, *Heredity and Evolution in Human Populations,* (Cambridge, Mass., 1959), p. 145; Robert S. Morison in *Ethical Issues in Human Genetics,* ed. Bruce Hilton et al., (New York, 1973), p. 208.

10. *The New York Times,* September 30, 1975, p. 1. col. 6. The Joseph family disease is similar to Huntington's chorea except that symptoms start appearing in the twenties. Rick Donohue is in his early twenties.

11. There may be a price for the individuals who refrain from having children. We will be looking at the situation from their point of view shortly.

12. This is in fact the basis for certain parental duties. An example is the maternal duty to obtain proper nutrition before and during pregnancy, for this is necessary if the child is to have normal health when it is born.

13. One might argue that as many persons as possible should exist so that they may enjoy life.

14. Some thinkers have qualms about the use of some or all of these methods. They have so far failed to show why they are immoral, although, naturally, much careful study will be required before they could be unqualifiedly recommended. See, for example, Richard Hull, "Genetic Engineering: Comment on Headings," *The Humanist,* Vol. 32 (Sept./Oct. 1972). 13.

15. *Essays in Pragmatism,* ed. A. Castell (New York, 1948), p. 73.

16. For example, see Leach, p. 138. One of the ways the dilemma described by Leach could be lessened would be if society emphasized those aspects of family life not dependent on "blood" relationships and downplayed those that are.

BIRTH DEFECTS

From "Dilemmas of 'Informed Consent' in Children"

Anthony M. Shaw and Iris A. Shaw

Numerous articles have been written about "rights" of patients. We read about "right to life" of the unborn, "right to die" of the elderly, "Bill of Rights" for the hospitalized, "Declaration of Rights" for the retarded, "right of privacy" for the pregnant and, of course, "right to medical care" for us all.

Whatever the legitimacy of these sometimes conflicting "rights" there is at present general agreement that patients have at least one legal right: that of "informed consent"—i.e., when a decision about medical treatment is made, they are entitled to a full explanation by their physicians of the nature of the proposed treatment, its risks and its limitations. Once the physician has discharged his obligation fully to inform * an adult, mentally competent patient,

Reprinted by permission of the authors and *The New England Journal of Medicine,* vol. 289, no. 17, pp. 885-890, October 25, 1973.

---

* I agree with Ingelfinger that "educate" is a better concept here than "inform."

that patient may then accept or reject the proposed treatment, or, indeed, may refuse any and all treatment, as he sees fit. But if the patient is a minor, a parental decision rejecting recommended treatment is subject to review when physicians or society disagree with that decision.

The purpose of this paper is to consider some of the moral and ethical dilemmas that may arise in the area of "informed consent" when the patient is a minor. The following case reports, all but two from my practice of pediatric surgery, raise questions about the rights and obligations of physicians, parents and society in situations in which parents decide to withhold consent for treatment of their children.

Instead of presenting a full discussion of these cases at the end of the paper, I have followed each case presentation with a comment discussing the points I wish to make, relating the issues raised by that case to those raised in some of the other cases, and posing the very hard questions that I had to ask myself in dealing with the patients and parents. At present the questions are coming along much faster than the answers.

CASE REPORTS

A. Baby A was referred to me at 22 hours of age with a diagnosis of esophageal atresia and tracheoesophageal fistula. The infant, the first-born of a professional couple in their early thirties, had obvious signs of mongolism, about which they were fully informed by the referring physician. After explaining the nature of the surgery to the distraught father, I offered him the operative consent. His pen hesitated briefly above the form and then as he signed, he muttered, "I have no choice, do I?" He didn't seem to expect an answer, and I gave him none. The esophageal anomaly was corrected in routine fashion, and the infant was discharged to a state institution for the retarded without ever being seen again by either parent.

Comment

In my opinion, this case was mishandled from the point of view of Baby A's family, in that consent was not truly informed. The answer to Mr. A's question should have been, "You *do* have a choice. You might want to consider not signing the operative consent at all." Although some of my surgical colleagues believe that there is no alternative to attempting to save the life of every infant, no matter what his potential, in my opinion, the doctrine of informed consent should, under some circumstances, include the right to withhold consent. If the parents do have the right to withhold consent for surgery in a case such as Baby A, who should take the responsibility for pointing that fact out to them—the obstetrician, the pediatrician or the surgeon?

Another question raised by this case lies in the parents' responsibility toward their baby, who has been saved by their own decision to allow surgery. Should they be obligated to provide a home for the infant? If their intention is to place the baby after operation in a state-financed institution, should the initial decision regarding medical or surgical treatment for their infant be theirs alone?

B. Baby B was referred at the age of 36 hours with duodenal obstruction and signs of Down's syndrome. His young parents had a 10-year-old daughter, and he was the son they had been trying to have for 10 years; yet, when they were approached with operative consent, they hesitated. They wanted to know beyond any doubt whether the baby had Down's syndrome. If so, they wanted time to consider whether or not to permit the surgery to be done. Within 8 hours a geneticist was able to identify cells containing 47 chromosomes in a bone-marrow sample. Over the next 3 days the infant's gastrointestinal tract was decompressed with a nasogastric tube, and he was supported with intravenous fluids while the parents consulted with their ministers, with family physicians in their home community and with our geneticists. At the end of that time the B's decided not to permit surgery. The infant died 3 days later after withdrawal of supportive therapy.

Comment

Unlike the parents of Baby A, Mr. and Mrs. B realized that they did have a choice—to consent or not to consent to the intestinal surgery. They were afforded access to a wide range of resources to help them make an informed decision. The infant's deterioration was temporarily prevented by adequate intestinal decompression and intravenous fluids.

Again, some of the same questions are raised here as with Baby A. Do the parents have the right to make the decision to allow their baby to die without surgery?

Can the parents make a reasonable decision within hours or days after the birth of a retarded or brain-damaged infant? During that time they are overwhelmed by feelings of shock, fear, guilt, horror and shame. What is the proper role of the medical staff and the hospital administration? Can parents make an intelligent decision under these circumstances, or are they simply reacting to a combination of their own instincts and fears as well as to the opinions and biases of medical staff? Rickham has described the interaction of physician and parents in such situations as follows.

> Every conscientious doctor will, of course, give as correct a prognosis and as impartial an opinion about the possible future of the child as he can, but he will not be able to be wholly impartial, and, whether he wants it or not, his opinion will influence the parents. At the end it is usually the doctor who has to decide the issue. It is not only cruel to ask the parents whether they want their child to live or die, it is dishonest, because in the vast majority of cases, the parents are consciously or unconsciously influenced by the doctor's opinion.

I believe that parents often *can* make an informed decision if, like the B's, they are afforded access to a range of resources beyond the expertise and bias of a single doctor and afforded sufficient time for contemplation of the alternatives. Once the parents have made a decision, should members of the medical staff support them in their decision regardless of their own feelings? (This support may be important to assuage recurrent feelings of guilt for months or even years after the parents' decision.)

When nutritional and fluid support was withdrawn, intestinal intubation and pain medication were provided to prevent suffering. To what extent should palliative treatment be given in a case in which definitive treatment is withheld? The lingering death of a newborn infant whose parents have denied consent for surgery can have a disastrous effect on hospital personnel, as illustrated . . . by the well publicized Johns Hopkins Hospital case, which raised a national storm of controversy. In this case, involving an infant with mongoloidism and duodenal atresia, several of the infant's physicians violently disagreed with the parent's decision not to allow surgery. The baby's lingering death (15 days) severely demoralized the nursing and house staffs. In addition, it prolonged the agony for the parents, who called daily to find out if the baby was still alive. Colleagues of mine who have continued to keep such infants on gastrointestinal decompression and intravenous fluids for weeks after the parents have decided against surgery have told me of several cases in which the parents have finally changed their minds and given the surgeon a green light! Does such a change of heart represent a more deliberative decision on the part of the parents or merely their capitulation on the basis of emotional fatigue?

After the sensationalized case in Baltimore, Johns Hopkins Hospital established a committee to work with physicians and parents who are confronted by similar problems. Do such medical-ethics committees serve as a useful resource for physicians and families, or do they, in fact, further complicate the decision-making process by multiplying the number of opinions?

Finally, should a decision to withhold surgery on an infant with Down's syndrome or other genetically determined mental-retardation states be allowed on clinical grounds only, without clear-cut chromosomal evidence?

C. I was called to the Newborn Nursery to see Baby C, whose father was a busy surgeon with 3 teen-age children. The diagnosis of imperforate anus and microcephalus were obvious. Doctor C called me after being informed of the situation by the pediatrician. "I'm not going to sign that op permit," he said. When I didn't reply, he said, "What would you do, doctor, if he were your baby?" "I wouldn't let him be operated on either," I replied. Palliative support only was provided, and the infant died 48 hours later.

Comment

Doctor C asked me bluntly what I would do were it my baby, and I gave him my answer. Was my response appropriate? In this case I simply reinforced his own decision. Suppose he had asked me for my opinion before expressing his own inclination? Should my answer in any case have simply been, "It's not my baby"— with a refusal to discuss the subject further? Should I have insisted that he take more time to think about it and discuss it further with his family and clergy, like the parents of Baby B? Is there a moral difference between withholding surgery on a baby with microcephalus and withholding surgery on a baby with Down's syndrome?

Some who think that all children with mongolism should be salvaged since many of them are trainable, would not dispute a decision to allow a baby with less potential such as microcephalic Baby C to die. Should, then, decisions about life and death be made on the basis of IQ? . . .

E. A court order *was* obtained for Baby E. . . . This infant, with Down's syndrome, intestinal obstruction and congenital heart disease, was born in her mother's car on the way to the hospital. The mother thought that the retarded infant would be impossible for her to care for and would have a destructive effect on her already shaky marriage. She therefore refused to sign permission for intestinal surgery, but a local child-welfare agency, invoking the state child-abuse statute, was able to obtain a court order directing surgery to be performed. After a complicated course and thousands of dollars worth of care, the infant was returned to the mother. The baby's continued growth and development remained markedly retarded because of her severe cardiac disease. A year and a half after the baby's birth, the mother felt more than ever that she had been done a severe injustice.

Comment

Is the crux of this case parental rights versus the child's right to life? Can the issue in this case be viewed as an extension of the basic dilemma in the abortion question? Does this case represent proper application of child-abuse legislation—i.e., does the parents' refusal to consent to surgery constitute neglect as defined in child-abuse statutes? If so, under these statutes does a physician's concurrence in a parental decision to withhold treatment constitute failure to report neglect, thereby subjecting him to possible prosecution?

Baby E's mother voluntarily took the baby home, but had she not done so, could the state have forced her to take the baby? Could the state have required her husband to contribute to the cost of medical care and to the subsequent maintenance of the infant in a foster home or institution?

If society decides that the attempt must be made to salvage every human life, then, as I have written, " . . . society *must* provide the necessary funds and facilities to meet the continuing medical and psychological needs of these unfortunate children."

F. Baby F was conceived as the result of an extramarital relation. Mrs. F had sought an abortion, which she had been denied. F was born prematurely, weighing 1600 g and in all respects normal except for the presence of esophageal atresia and tracheoesophageal fistula. Mrs. F signed the operative consent, and the surgery was performed uneventfully. Mrs. F. fears that her husband will eventually realize that the baby is not his and that her marriage may collapse as a result of this discovery.

Comment

Like those of Mrs. E, Mrs. F's reasons for not wanting her baby were primarily psychosocial. However, Mrs. F never raised the question of withholding consent for surgery even though the survival of her infant might mean destruction of her marriage. Does the presence of mental retardation or severe physical malformation justify withholding of consent for psychosocial reasons (Babies B, C, . . . , and E), whereas the absence of such conditions does not (Baby F)? If she had decided to withhold consent there is no doubt in my mind that I would have obtained a court order to operate on this baby, who appeared to be normal beyond her esophageal anomaly. Although I personally would not have objected to an abortion in this situation for the sociopsychologic reasons, I would not allow an otherwise normal baby with a correctable anomaly to perish for lack of treatment for the same reasons. Although those who believe that all life is sacred, no matter what its level of development, will severely criticize me for the apparent inconsistency of this position, I believe it to be a realistic and humane approach to a situation in which no solution is ideal.

Although my case histories thus far have dealt with the forms of mental retardation most common in my practice, similar dilemmas are encountered by other physicians in different specialties, the most obvious being in the spectrum of hydrocephalus and meningomyelocele. Neurosurgeons are still grappling unsuccessfully and inconsistently with the indications for surgery in this group, trying to fit together what is practical, what is moral, and what is humane. If neurosurgeons disagree violently over criteria for operability on infants with meningomyelocele, how can the parents of such a child decide whether to sign for consent? Who would say that they *must* sign if they don't want a child whose days will be measured by operations, clinic visits and infections? I have intentionally omitted from discussion in this paper the infant with crippling deformities and multiple anomalies who does not have rapidly lethal lesions. Infants with such lesions may survive for long periods and may require palliative procedures such as release of limb contractures, ventriculoperitoneal shunts, or colostomies to make their lives more tolerable or to simplify their management. The extent to which these measures are desirable or justifiable moves us into an even more controversial area.

I must also point out that the infants discussed in the preceding case reports represent but a small percentage of the total number of infants with mental-retardation syndromes on whom I have operated. Once the usual decision to operate has been made I, of course, apply the same efforts as I would to any other child. . . .

DISCUSSION

If an underlying philosophy can be gleaned from the vignettes presented above, I hope it is one that tries to find a solution, humane and loving, based on the circumstances of each case rather than by means of a dogmatic formula approach. ([Joseph] Fletcher has best expressed this philosophy in his book, *Situation Ethics,* and in subsequent articles.) This outlook contrasts sharply with the rigid "right-to-life" philosophy, which categorically opposes abortion, for example. My ethic holds that all rights are not absolute all the time. As Fletcher points out, ". . . all rights are imperfect and may be set aside if human *need* requires it." My ethic further considers quality of life as a value that must be balanced against a belief in the sanctity of life.

Those who believe that the sanctity of life is the overriding consideration in all cases have a relatively easy time making decisions. They say that all babies must be saved; no life may be aborted from the womb, and all attempts to salvage newborn life, whatever its quality and whatever its human and financial costs to family and society, must be made. Although many philosophies express the view that "heroic" efforts need not be made to save or prolong life, yesterday's heroic efforts are today's routine procedures. Thus, each year it becomes possible to remove yet another type of malformation from the "unsalvageable" category. All pediatric surgeons, including myself, have "triumphs"—infants who, if they had been born 25 or even five years ago, would not have been salvageable. Now with our team approaches, staged surgical technics, monitoring capabilities, ventilatory support systems and intravenous hyperalimentation and elemental diets, we can wind up with "viable" children three and four years old well below the third percentile in height and weight, propped up on a pillow, marginally tolerating an oral diet of sugar and amino acids and looking forward to another operation.

Or how about the infant whose gastrointestinal tract has been removed after volvulus and infarction? Although none of us regard the insertion of a central venous catheter as a "heroic" procedure, is it right to insert a "lifeline" to feed this baby in the light of our present technology, which can support him, tethered to an infusion pump, for a maximum of a year and some months?

Who should make these decisions? The doctors? The parents? Clergymen? A committee? As I have pointed out, I think that the parents must participate in any decision about treatment and that they must be fully informed of the consequences of consenting and of withholding consent. This is a type of informed consent that goes far beyond the traditional presentation of possible complications of surgery, length of hospitalization, cost of the operation, time lost from work, and so on.

It may be impossible for any general agreement or guidelines for making decisions on cases such as the ones presented here to emerge, but I believe we should bring these problems out into public forum because whatever the answers may be, they should not be the result of decisions made solely by the attending physicians. Or should they?

Moral and Ethical Dilemmas in the Special-Care Nursery

Raymond S. Duff, M.D., and A.G.M. Campbell, M.B., F.R.C.P. (Edin.)

Between 1940 and 1970 there was a 58 percent decrease in the infant death rate in the United States.[1] This reduction was related in part to the application of new knowledge to the care of infants. Neonatal mortality rates in hospitals having infant intensive-care units have been about ½ those reported in hospitals without such units.[2] There is now evidence that in many conditions of early infancy the long-term morbidity may also be reduced.[3] Survivors of these units may be healthy, and their parents grateful, but some infants continue to suffer from such conditions as chronic cardiopulmonary disease, short-bowel-syndrome or various manifestations of brain damage; others are severely handicapped by a myriad of congenital malformations that in previous times would have resulted in early death. Recently, both lay and professional persons have expressed increasing concern about the quality of life for these severely impaired survivors and their families.[4,5] Many pediatricians and others are distressed with the long-term results of pressing on and on to save life at all costs and in all circumstances. Eliot Slater[6] stated, "If this is one of the consequences of the sanctity-of-life ethic,

perhaps our formulation of the principle should be revised."

The experiences described in this communication document some of the grave moral and ethical dilemmas now faced by physicians and families. They indicate some of the problems in a large special-care nursery where medical technology has prolonged life and where "informed" parents influence the management decisions concerning their infants.

BACKGROUND AND METHODS

The special-care nursery of the Yale-New Haven Hospital not only serves an obstetric service for over 4000 live births annually but also acts as the principal referral center in Connecticut for infants with major problems of the newborn period. From January 1, 1970, through June 30, 1972, 1615 infants born at the Hospital were admitted, and 556 others were transferred for specialized care from community hospitals. During this interval, the average daily census was 26, with a range of 14 to 37.

For some years the unit has had a liberal policy for parental visiting, with the staff placing particular emphasis on helping parents adjust to and participate in the care of their infants with special problems. By encouraging visiting, attempting to create a relaxed atmosphere within the unit, ex-

Reprinted by permission of the authors and *The New England Journal of Medicine,* vol. 289, no. 17, pp. 890–894, October 25, 1973.

ploring carefully the special needs of the infants, and familiarizing parents with various aspects of care, it was hoped to remove much of the apprehension—indeed, fear—with which parents at first view an intensive-care nursery.[7] At any time, parents may see and handle their babies. They commonly observe or participate in most routine aspects of care and are often present when some infant is critically ill or moribund. They may attend, as they choose, the death of their own infant. Since an average of two to three deaths occur each week and many infants are critically ill for long periods, it is obvious that the concentrated, intimate social interactions between personnel, infants and parents in an emotionally charged atmosphere often make the work of the staff very difficult and demanding. However, such participation and recognition of parents' rights to information about their infant appear to be the chief foundations of "informed consent" for treatment.

Each staff member must know how to cope with many questions and problems brought up by parents, and if he or she cannot help, they must have access to those who can. These requirements can be met only when staff members work closely with each other in all the varied circumstances from simple to complex, from triumph to tragedy. Formal and informal meetings take place regularly to discuss the technical and family aspects of care. As a given problem may require, some or all of several persons (including families, nurses, social workers, physicians, chaplains and others) may convene to exchange information and reach decisions. Thus, staff and parents function more or less as a small community in which a concerted attempt is made to ensure that each member may participate in and know about the major decisions that concern him or her. However, the physician takes appropriate initiative in final decision making, so that the family will not have to bear that heavy burden alone.

For several years, the responsibilities of attending pediatrician have been assumed chiefly by ourselves, who, as a result, have become acquainted intimately with the problems of the infants, the staff, and the parents. Our almost constant availability to staff, private pediatricians and parents has resulted in the raising of more and more ethical questions about various aspects of intensive care for critically ill and congenitally deformed infants. The penetrating questions and challenges, particularly of knowledgeable parents (such as physicians, nurses, or lawyers), brought increasing doubts about the wisdom of

many of the decisions that seemed to parents to be predicated chiefly on technical considerations. Some thought their child had a right to die since he could not live well or effectively. Others thought that society should pay the costs of care that may be so destructive to the family economy. Often, too, the parents' or siblings' rights to relief from the seemingly pointless, crushing burdens were important considerations. It seemed right to yield to parent wishes in several cases as physicians have done for generations. As a result, some treatments were withheld or stopped with the knowledge that earlier death and relief from suffering would result. Such options were explored with the less knowledgeable parents to ensure that their consent for treatment of their defective children was truly informed. As Eisenberg[8] pointed out regarding the application of technology, "At long last, we are beginning to ask, not *can* it be done, but *should* it be done?" In lengthy, frank discussions, the anguish of the parents was shared, and attempts were made to support fully the reasoned choices, whether for active treatment and rehabilitation or for an early death.

To determine the extent to which death resulted from withdrawing or with-holding treatment, we examined the hospital records of all children who died from January 1, 1970, through June 30, 1972.

RESULTS

In total, there were 299 deaths; each was classified in one of two categories; deaths in Category 1 resulted from pathologic conditions in spite of the treatment given; 256 (86 per cent) were in this category. Of these, 66 per cent were the result of respiratory problems or complications associated with extreme prematurity (birth weight under 1000 g). Congenital heart disease and other anomalies accounted for an additional 22 per cent (Table 1).

Deaths in Category 2 were associated with severe impairment, usually from congenital disorders (Table 2): 43 (14 per cent) were in this group. These deaths or their timing was associated with discontinuance or withdrawl of treatment. The mean duration of life in Category 2 (Table 3) was greater than that in Category 1. This was the result of a mean life of 55 days for eight infants who became chronic cardiopulmonary cripples but for whom pro-

TABLE 1 Problems Causing Death in Category 1.

Problem	No. of Deaths	Percentage
Respiratory	108	42.2
Extreme prematurity	60	23.4
Heart disease	42	16.4
Multiple anomalies	14	5.5
Other	32	12.5
Totals	256	100.0

longed and intensive efforts were made in the hope of eventual recovery. They were infants who were dependent on oxygen, digoxin and diuretics, and most of them had been treated for the idiopathic respiratory-distress syndrome with high oxygen concentrations and positive-pressure ventilation.

Some examples of management choices in Category 2 illustrate the problems. An infant with Down's syndrome and intestinal atresia, like the much-publicized one at Johns Hopkins Hospital,[9] was not treated because his parents thought that surgery was wrong for their baby and themselves. He died seven days after birth. Another child had chronic pulmonary disease after positive-pressure ventilation with high oxygen concentrations for treatment of severe idiopathic respiratory-distress syndrome. By five months of age, he still required 40 percent oxygen to survive, and even then, he was chronically dyspneic and cyanotic. He also suffered from cor pulmonale, which was difficult to control with digoxin and diuretics. The nurses, parents and physicians considered it cruel to continue, and yet difficult to stop. All were attached to this child, whose life they had tried so hard to make worthwhile. The family had endured high expenses (the hospital bill exceeding $15,000), and the strains of the illness were believed to be threatening the marriage bonds and to be causing sibling behavioral disturbances. Oxygen supplementation was stopped, and the child died in about three hours. The family settled down and 18 months later had another baby, who was healthy.

A third child had meningomyelocele, hydrocephalus and major anomalies of every organ in the pelvis. When the parents understood the limits of medical care and rehabilitation, they believed no treatment should be given. She died at five days of age.

We have maintained contact with most families of children in Category 2. Thus far, these families appear to have experienced a normal mourning for their losses. Although some have exhibited doubts that the choices

TABLE 2 Problems Associated with Death in Category 2.

Problem	No. of Deaths	Percentage
Multiple anomalies	15	34.9
Trisomy	8	18.6
Cardiopulmonary	8	18.6
Meningomyelocele	7	16.3
Other central-nervous-system defects	3	7.0
Short-bowel syndrome	2	4.6
Totals	43	100.0

TABLE 3 Selected Comparisons of 256 Cases in Category 1 and 43 in Category 2.

Attribute	Category 1	Category 2
Mean length of life	4.8 days	7.5 days
Standard deviation	8.8	34.3
Range	1–69	1–150
Portion living for < 2 days	50.0%	12.0%

were correct, all appear to be as effective in their lives as they were before this experience. Some claim that their profoundly moving experience has provided a deeper meaning in life, and from this they believe they have become more effective people.

Members of all religious faiths and atheists were participants as parents and as staff in these experiences. There appeared to be no relation between participation and a person's religion. Repeated participation in these troubling events did not appear to reduce the worry of the staff about the awesome nature of the decisions.

DISCUSSION

That decisions are made not to treat severely defective infants may be no surprise to those familiar with special-care facilities. All laymen and professionals familiar with our nursery appeared to set some limits upon their application of treatment to extend life or to investigate a pathologic process. For example, an experienced nurse said about one child, "We lost him several weeks ago. Isn't it time to quit?" In another case, a house officer said to a physician investigating an aspect of a child's disease, "For this child, don't you think it's time to turn off your curiosity so you can turn on your kindness?" Like many others, these children eventually acquired the "right to die."

Arguments among staff members and families for and against such decisions were based on varied notions of the rights and interests of defective infants, these families, professionals and society. They were also related to varying ideas about prognosis. Regarding the infants, some contended that individuals should have a right to die in some circumstances such as anencephaly, hydranencephaly, and some severely deforming and incapacitating conditions. Such very defective individuals were considered to have little or no hope of achieving meaningful "humanhood."[10] For example, they have little or no capacity to love or be loved. They are often cared for in facilities that have been characterized as "hardly more than dying bins,"[11] an assessment with which, in our experience, knowledgeable parents (those who visited chronic-care facilities for place-

ment of their children) agreed. With institutionalized well children, social participation may be essentially nonexistent, and maternal deprivation severe; this is known to have an adverse, usually disastrous, effect upon the child.[12] The situation for the defective child is probably worse, for he is restricted socially both by his need for care and by his defects. To escape "wrongful life,"[13] a fate rated as worse than death, seemed right. In this regard, Lasagna[14] notes, "We may, as a society, scorn the civilizations that slaughtered their infants, but our present treatment of the retarded is in some ways more cruel."

Others considered allowing a child to die wrong for several reasons. The person most involved, the infant, had no voice in the decision. Prognosis was not always exact, and a few children with extensive care might live for months, and occasionally years. Some might survive and function satisfactorily. To a few persons, withholding treatment and accepting death was condemned as criminal.

Families had strong but mixed feelings about management decisions. Living with the handicapped is clearly a family affair, and families of deformed infants thought there were limits to what they could bear or should be expected to bear. Most of them wanted maximal efforts to sustain life and to rehabilitate the handicapped; in such cases, they were supported fully. However, some families, especially those having children with severe defects, feared that they and their other children would become socially enslaved, economically deprived, and permanently stigmatized, all perhaps for a lost cause. Such a state of "chronic sorrow" until death has been described by Olshansky.[15] In some cases, families considered the death of the child right both for the child and for the family. They asked if that choice could be theirs or their doctors.

As Feifel has reported,[16] physicians on the whole are reluctant to deal with the issues. Some, particularly specialists based in the medical center, gave specific reasons for this disinclination. There was a feeling that to "give up" was disloyal to the cause of the profession. Since major research, teaching and patient-care efforts were being made, professionals expected to discover, transmit and apply knowledge and skills; patients and families were supposed to co-operate fully even if they were not always grateful. Some physicians recognized that the wishes of families went against their own, but they were resolute. They commonly agreed that if they were the parents of very defective children, with-holding treatment would be most desirable for them. However, they argued that aggressive management was indicated for others. Some believed that allowing death as a management option was euthanasia and must be stopped for fear of setting a "poor ethical example" or for fear of personal prosecution or damage to their clinical departments or to the medical center as a whole. Alexander's report on Nazi Germany [17] was cited in some cases as providing justification for pressing the effort to combat disease. Some persons were concerned about the loss through death of "teaching material." They feared the training of professionals for the care of defective children in the future and the advancing of the state of the art would be compromised. Some parents who became aware of this concern thought their children should not become experimental subjects.

Practicing pediatricians, general practitioners and obstetricians were often familiar with these families and were usually sympathetic with their views. However, since they were more distant from the special-care nursery than the specialists of the medical center, their influence was often minimal. As a result, families received little support from them, and tension in community-medical relations was a recurring problem.

Infants with severe types of meningomyelocele precipitated the most controversial decisions. Several decades ago, those who survived this condition beyond a few weeks usually became hydrocephalic and retarded, in addition to being crippled and deformed. Without modern treatment, they died earlier.[18] Some may have been killed or at least not resuscitated at birth.[19] From the early 1960's, the tendency has been to treat vigorously all infants with meningomyelocele. As advocated by Zachary[20] and Shurtleff,[21] aggressive management of these children became the rule in our unit as in many others. Infants were usually referred quickly. Parents routinely signed permits for

operation though rarely had they seen their children's defects or had the nature of various management plans and their respective prognoses clearly explained to them. Some physicians believed that parents were too upset to understand the nature of the problems and the options for care. Since they believed informed consent had no meaning in these circumstances, they either ignored the parents or simply told them that the child needed an operation on the back as the first step in correcting several defects. As a result, parents often felt completely left out while the activities of care proceeded at a brisk pace.

Some physicians experienced in the care of these children and familiar with the impact of such conditions upon families had early reservations about this plan of care.[22] More recently, they were influenced by the pessimistic appraisal of vigorous management schemes in some cases.[5] Meningomyelocele, when treated vigorously, is associated with higher survival rates,[21] but the achievement of satisfactory rehabilitation is at best difficult and usually impossible for almost all who are severely affected. Knowing this, some physicians and some families[23] decide against treatment of the most severely affected. If treatment is not carried out, the child's condition will usually deteriorate from further brain damage, urinary-tract infections and orthopedic difficulties, and death can be expected much earlier. Two thirds may be dead by three months, and over 90 per cent by one year of age. However, the quality of life during that time is poor, and the strains on families are great, but not necessarily greater than with treatment.[24] Thus, both treatment and nontreatment constitute unsatisfactory dilemmas for everyone, especially for the child and his family. When maximum treatment was viewed as unacceptable by families and physicians in our unit, there was a growing tendency to seek early death as a management option, to avoid that cruel choice of gradual, often slow, but progressive deterioration of the child who was required under these circumstances in effect to kill himself. Parents and the staff then asked if his dying needed to be prolonged. If not, what were the most appropriate medical responses?

Is it possible that some physicians and some

families may join in a conspiracy to deny the right of a defective child to live or to die? Either could occur. Prolongation of the dying process by resident physicians having a vested interest in their careers has been described by Sudnow.[25] On the other hand, from the fatigue of working long and hard some physicians may give up too soon, assuming that their cause is lost. Families, similarly, may have mixed motives. They may demand death to obtain relief from the high costs and the tensions inherent in suffering, but their sense of guilt in this thought may produce the opposite demand, perhaps in violation of the sick person's rights. Thus, the challenge of deciding what course to take can be most tormenting for the family and the physician. Unquestionably, not facing the issue would appear to be the easier course, at least temporarily; no doubt many patients, families, and physicians decline to join in an effort to solve the problems. They can readily assume that what is being done is right and sufficient and ask no questions. But pretending there is no decision to be made is an arbitrary and potentially devastating decision of default. Since families and patients must live with the problems one way or another in any case, the physician's failure to face the issues may constitute a victimizing abandonment of patients and their families in times of greatest need. As Lasagna[14] pointed out, "There is no place for the physician to hide."

Can families in the shock resulting from the birth of a defective child understand what faces them? Can they give truly "informed consent" for treatment or with-holding treatment? Some of our colleagues answer no to both questions. In our opinion, if families regardless of background are heard sympathetically and at length and are given information and answers to their questions in words they understand, the problems of their children as well as the expected benefits and limits of any proposed care can be understood clearly in practically all instances. Parents *are* able to understand the implications of such things as chronic dyspnea, oxygen dependency, incontinence, paralysis, contractures, sexual handicaps and mental retardation.

Another problem concerns who decides for a child. It may be acceptable for a person to reject treatment and bring about his own death. But it is quite a different situation when others are doing this for him. We do not know how often families and their physicians will make just decisions for severely handicapped children. Clearly, this issue is central in evaluation of the process of decision making that we have described. But we also ask, if these parties cannot make such decisions justly, who can?

We recognize great variability and often much uncertainty in prognoses and in family capacities to deal with defective newborn infants. We also acknowledge that there are limits of support that society can or will give to assist handicapped persons and their families. Severely deforming conditions that are associated with little or no hope of a functional existence pose painful dilemmas for the laymen and professionals who must decide how to cope with severe handicaps. We believe the burdens of decision making must be borne by families and their professional advisers because they are most familiar with the respective situations. Since families primarily must live with and are most affected by the decisions, it therefore appears that society and the health professions should provide only general guidelines for decision making. Moreover, since variations between situations are so great, and the situations themselves so complex, it follows that much latitude in decision making should be expected and tolerated. Otherwise, the rules of society or the policies most convenient for medical technologists may become cruel masters of human beings instead of their servants. Regarding any "allocation of death"[26] policy we readily acknowledge that the extreme excesses of Hegelian "rational utility" under dictatorships must be avoided.[17] Perhaps it is less recognized that the uncontrolled application of medical technology may be detrimental to individuals and families. In this regard, our views are similar to those of Waitzkin and Stoekle.[27] Physicians may hold excessive power over decision making by limiting or controlling the information made available to patients or families. It seems appropriate that the profession be held accountable for presenting fully all management options and their expected consequences. Also, the public should be aware that professionals often face conflicts of interest that may result in decisions against individual preferences.

What are the legal implications of actions like those described in this paper? Some persons may argue that the law has been broken, and others would contend otherwise. Perhaps more than anything else, the public and professional silence on a major social taboo and some common practices has been broken further. That seems appropriate, for out of the ensuing dialogue perhaps better choices for patients and families can be made. If working out these dilemmas in ways such as those we suggest is in violation of the law, we believe the law should be changed.

Notes

1. Wegman ME: Annual summary of vital statistics—1970. *Pediatrics* 48:979–983, 1971.

2. Swyer PR: The regional organization of special care for the neonate. *Pediatr Clin North Am* 17:761–776, 1970.

3. Rawlings G, Reynold EOR, Stewart A, et al: Changing prognosis for infants of very low birth weight. *Lancet* 1:516–519, 1971.

4. Freeman E: The god committee. *New York Times Magazine*, May 21, 1972, pp. 84–90.

5. Lorber J: Results of treatment of myelomeningocele. *Dev Med Child Neurol* 13:279–303, 1971.

6. Slater E: Health service or sickness service. *Br Med J* 4:734–736, 1971.

7. Klaus MH, Kennell JH: Mothers separated from their newborn infants. *Pediatr Clin North Am* 17:1015–1037, 1970.

8. Eisenberg L: The human nature of human nature. *Science* 176:123–128. 1972.

9. Report of the Joseph P. Kennedy Foundation International Symposium on Human Rights, Retardation and Research. Washington, DC, The John F. Kennedy Center for the Performing Arts, October 16, 1971.

10. Fletcher J: Indicators of humanhood: a tentative profile of man. The Hastings Center Report Vol. 2. No. 5. Hasting-on-Hudson. New York, Institute of Society, Ethics and Life Sciences, November, 1972, pp 1–4.

11. Freeman HE, Brim OG Jr., Williams G: New dimensions of dying. *The Dying Patient.* Edited by OG Brim, Jr., New York, Russell Sage Foundation. 1970, pp. xiii–xxvi.

12. Spitz RA: Hospitalism: an inquiry into the genesis of psychiatric conditions in early childhood. *Psychoanal Study Child* 1:53–74, 1945.

13. Engelhardt HT Jr: Euthanasia and children: the injury of continued existence. *J Pediatr* 83:170–171, 1973.

14. Lasagna L: *Life, Death and the Doctor.* New York, Alfred A. Knopf, 1968.

15. Olshansky S: Chronic sorrow: a response to having a mentally defective child. *Soc Casework* 43:190–193, 1962.

16. Feifel H: Perception of death. *Ann NY Acad Sci* 164:669–677, 1969.

17. Alexander L: Medical science under dictatorship. *N Engl J Med* 241:39–47, 1949.

18. Laurence KM and Tew BJ: Natural history of spina bifida cystica and cranium bifidum cysticum: major central nervous system malformations in South Wales. Part IV. *Arch Dis Child* 46:127–138, 1971.

19. Forrest DM: Modern trends in the treatment of spina bifida: early closure in spina bifida: results and problems. *Proc R Soc Med* 60:763–767, 1967.

20. Zachary RB: Ethical and social aspects of treatment of spina bifida. *Lancet* 2:274–276, 1968.

21. Shurtleff DB: Care of the myelodysplastic patient. *Ambulatory Pediatrics.* Edited by M Green, R Haggerty. Philadelphia, WB Saunders Company, 1968, pp. 726–741.

22. Matson DD: Surgical treatment of myelomeningocele. *Pediatrics* 42:225–227, 1968.

23. Mac Keith RC: A new look at spina bifida aperta. *Dev Med Child Neurol* 13:277–278, 1971.

24. Hide DW, Williams HP, Ellis HL: The outlook for the child with a myelomeningocele for whom early surgery was considered inadvisable. *Dev Med Child Neurol* 14:304–307, 1972.

25. Sudnow D: *Passing On.* Englewood Cliffs, New Jersey, Prentice-Hall, 1967.

26. Manning B: Legal and policy issues in the allocation of death. *The Dying Patient.* Edited by OG Brim Jr. New York, Russell Sage Foundation. 1970, pp. 253–274

27. Waitzkin H, Stoeckle JD: The communication of information about illness. *Adv Psychosom Med* 8:180–215, 1972.

To Save or Let Die:
The Dilemma of Modern Medicine

Richard A. McCormick, SJ

On Feb 24, the son of Mr. and Mrs. Robert H. T. Houle died following court-ordered emergency surgery at Maine Medical Center. The child was born Feb 9, horribly deformed. His entire left side was malformed; he had no left eye, was practically without a left ear, had a deformed left hand; some of his vertebrae were not fused. Furthermore, he was afflicted with a tracheal esophageal fistula and could not be fed by mouth. Air leaked into his stomach instead of going to the lungs, and fluid from the stomach pushed up into the lungs. As Dr. Andre Hellegers recently noted, "It takes little imagination to think there were further internal deformities" (*Obstetrical and Gynecological News*, April 1974).

As the days passed, the condition of the child deteriorated. Pneumonia set in. His reflexes became impaired and because of poor circulation, severe brain damage was suspected. The tracheal esophageal fistula, the immediate threat to his survival, can be corrected with relative ease by surgery. But in view of the associated complications and deformities, the parents refused their consent to surgery on "Baby Boy Houle." Several doctors in the Maine Medical Center felt differently and took the case to court. Maine Superior Court Judge David G. Roberts ordered the surgery to be performed. He ruled: "At the moment of live birth there does exist a human being entitled to the fullest protection of the law. The most basic right enjoyed by every human being is the right to life itself."

"MEANINGFUL LIFE"

Instances like this happen frequently. In a recent issue of the *New England Journal of Medicine*,

Drs. Raymond S. Duff and A. G. M. Campbell[1] reported on 299 deaths in the special-care nursery of the Yale-New Haven Hospital between 1970 and 1972. Of these, 43 (14%) were associated with discontinuance of treatment for children with multiple anomalies, trisomy, cardiopulmonary crippling, meningomyelocele, and other central nervous system defects. After careful consideration of each of these 43 infants, parents and physicians in a group decision concluded that the prognosis for "meaningful life" was extremely poor or hopeless, and therefore rejected further treatment. The abstract of the Duff-Campbell report states: "The awesome finality of these decisions, combined with a potential for error in prognosis, made the choice agonizing for families and health professionals. Nevertheless, the issue has to be faced, for not to decide is an arbitrary and potentially devastating decision of default."

In commenting on this study in the *Washington Post* (Oct 28, 1973), Dr. Lawrence K. Pickett, chief-of-staff at the Yale-New Haven Hospital, admitted that allowing hopelessly ill patients to die "is accepted medical practice." He continued: "This is nothing new. It's just being talked about now."

It has been talked about, it is safe to say, at least since the publicity associated with the famous "Johns Hopkins Case" some three years ago. In this instance, an infant was born with Down syndrome and duodenal atresia. The blockage is reparable by relatively easy surgery. However, after consultation with spiritual advisors, the parents refused permission for this corrective surgery, and the child died by starvation in the hospital after 15 days. For to feed him by mouth in this condition would have killed him. Nearly everyone who has commented on this case has disagreed with the decision.

It must be obvious that these instances—and they are frequent—raise the most agonizing and delicate moral problems. The problem is best seen in the ambiguity of the term "hopelessly ill." This used to and still may refer to lives that cannot be saved, that are irretrievably in the dying process. It may also refer to lives that can be saved and sustained, but in a wretched, painful, or deformed condition. With regard to infants, the problem is, which infants, if any, should be allowed to die? On what grounds or according to what criteria, as determined by whom? Or again, is there a point at which a life that can be saved is not "meaningful life," as the medical community so often phrases the question? If our past experience is any hint of the future, it is safe to say that public discussion of such controversial issues will quickly collapse into slogans such as "There is no such thing as a life not worth saving" or "Who is the physician to play God?" We saw and continue to see this far too frequently in the abortion debate. We are experiencing it in the euthanasia discussion. For instance, "death with dignity" translates for many into a death that is fast, clean, painless. The trouble with slogans is that they do not aid in the discovery of truth; they co-opt this discovery and promulgate it rhetorically, often only thinly disguising a good number of questionable value judgments in the process. Slogans are not tools for analysis and enlightenment; they are weapons for ideological battle.

Thus far, the ethical discussion of these truly terrifying decisions has been less than fully satisfactory. Perhaps this is to be expected since the problems have only recently come to public attention. In a companion article to the Duff-Campbell report,[1] Dr. Anthony Shaw[3] of the Pediatric Division of the Department of Surgery, University of Virginia Medical Center, Charlottesville, speaks of solutions "based on the circumstances of each case rather than by means of a dogmatic formula approach." Are these really the only options available to us? Shaw's statement makes it appear that the ethical alternatives are narrowed to dogmatism (which imposes a formula that prescinds from circumstances) and pure concretism (which denies the possibility or usefulness of any guidelines).

ARE GUIDELINES POSSIBLE?

Such either-or extremism is understandable. It is easy for the medical profession, in its fully justified concern with the terrible concreteness of these problems and with the issue of who makes these decisions, to trend away from any substantive guidelines. As *Time* remarked in reporting these instances: "Few, if any, doctors are willing to establish guidelines for determining which babies should receive lifesaving surgery or treatment and which should not" (*Time*, March 25, 1974). On the other hand, moral theologians, in their fully justified concern to avoid total normlessness and arbitrariness wherein the right is "discovered," or really "created," only in and by brute decision, can easily be insensitive to the moral relevance of the raw experience, of the conflicting tensions and concerns provoked through direct cradleside contact with human events and persons.

But is there no middle course between sheer concretism and dogmatism? I believe there is. Dr. Franz J. Ingelfinger,[4] editor of the *New England Journal of Medicine*, in an editorial on the Duff-Campbell-Shaw articles, concluded, even if somewhat reluctantly: "Society, ethics, institutional attitudes and committees can provide the broad guidelines, but the onus of decision-making ultimately falls on the doctor in whose care the child has been put." Similarly, Frederick Carney of Southern Methodist University, Dallas, and the Kennedy Center for Bioethics stated of these cases: "What is obviously needed is the development of substantive standards to inform parents and physicians who must make such decisions" (*Washington Post*, March 20, 1974).

"Broad guidelines," "substantive standards." There is the middle course, and it is the task of a community broader than the medical community. A guideline is not a slide rule that makes the decision. It is far less than that. But it is far more than the concrete decision of the parents and physician, however seriously and conscientiously this is made. It is more like a light in a room, a light that allows the individual objects to be seen in the fullness of their context. Concretely, if there are certain infants that we agree ought to be saved in spite of illness or deformity, and if there are certain infants that we agree should be allowed to die, then there is a line to be drawn. And if there is a line to be drawn, there ought to be some criteria, even if very general, for doing this. Thus, if nearly every commentator has disagreed with the Hopkins decision, should we not be able to distill from such consensus some general wisdom that will inform and guide future decisions? I think so.

This task is not easy. Indeed, it is so harrowing that the really tempting thing is to run from it. The most sensitive, balanced, and penetrating study of the Hopkins case that I have seen is that of the University of Chicago's James Gustafson.[2] Gustafson disagreed with the decision of the Hopkins physicians to deny surgery to the mongoloid infant. In summarizing his dissent, he notes: "Why would I draw the line on a different side of mongolism than the physicians did? While reasons can be given, one must recognize that there are intuitive elements, grounded in beliefs and profound feelings, that enter into particular judgments of this sort." He goes on to criticize the assessment made of the child's intelligence as too simplistic, and he proposes a much broader perspective on the meaning of suffering than seemed to have operated in the Hopkins decision. I am in full agreement with Gustafson's reflections and conclusions. But ultimately, he does not tell us where he would draw the line or why, only where he would *not,* and why.

This is very helpful already, and perhaps it is all that can be done. Dare we take the next step, the combination and analysis of such negative judgments to extract from them the positive criterion or criteria inescapably operative in them? Or more startlingly, dare we *not* if these decisions are already being made? Gustafson is certainly right in saying that we cannot always establish perfectly rational accounts and norms for our decisions. But I believe we must never cease trying, in fear and trembling to be sure. Otherwise, we have exempted these decisions in principle from the one critique and control that protects against abuse. Exemption of this sort is the root of all exploitation whether personal or political. Briefly, if we must face the frightening task of making quality-of-life

judgments—and we must—then we must face the difficult task of building criteria for these judgments.

FACING RESPONSIBILITY

What has brought us to this position of awesome responsibility? Very simply, the sophistication of modern medicine. Contemporary resuscitation and life-sustaining devices have brought a remarkable change in the state of the question. Our duties toward the care and preservation of life have been traditionally stated in terms of the use of ordinary and extraordinary means. For the moment and for purposes of brevity, we may say that, morally speaking, ordinary means are those whose use does not entail grave hardships to the patient. Those that would involve such hardship are extraordinary. Granted the relativity of these terms and the frequent difficulty of their application, still the distinction has had an honored place in medical ethics and medical practice. Indeed, the distinction was recently reiterated by the House of Delegates of the American Medical Association in a policy statement. After disowning intentional killing (mercy killing), the AMA statement continues: "The cessation of the employment of extraordinary means to prolong the life of the body when there is irrefutable evidence that biological death is imminent is the decision of the patient and/or his immediate family. The advice and judgment of the physician should be freely available to the patient and/or his immediate family" (*JAMA* 227:728, 1974).

This distinction can take us just so far—and thus the change in the state of the question. The contemporary problem is precisely that the question no longer concerns only those for whom "biological death is imminent" in the sense of the AMA statement. Many infants who would have died a decade ago, whose "biological death was imminent," can be saved. Yesterday's failures are today's successes. Contemporary medicine with its team approaches, staged surgical techniques, monitoring capabilities, ventilatory support systems, and other methods, can keep almost anyone alive. This has tended gradually to shift the problem from the means to reverse the dying process to the quality of the life sustained and preserved. The questions, ''Is this means too hazardous or difficult to use'' and ''Does this measure only prolong the patient's dying,'' while still useful and valid, now often become ''Granted that we can easily save the life, what kind of life are we saving?'' This is a quality-of-life judgment. And we fear it. And certainly we should. But with increased power goes increased responsibility. Since we have the power, we must face the responsibility.

A RELATIVE GOOD

In the past, the Judeo-Christian tradition has attempted to walk a balanced middle path between medical vitalism (that preserves life at any cost) and medical pessimism (that kills when life seems frustrating, burdensome, ''useless''). Both of these extremes root in an identical idolatry of life—an attitude that, at least by inference, views death as an unmitigated, absolute evil, and life as the absolute good. The middle course that has structured Judeo-Christian attitudes is that life is indeed a basic and precious good, but a good to be preserved precisely as the condition of other values. It is these other values and possibilities that found the duty to preserve physical life and also dictate the limits of this duty. In other words, life is a relative good, and the duty to preserve it a limited one. These limits have always been stated in terms of the *means* required to sustain life. But if the implications of this middle position are unpacked a bit, they will allow us, perhaps, to adapt to the type of quality-of-life judgment we are now called on to make without tumbling into vitalism or a utilitarian pessimism.

A beginning can be made with a statement of Pope Pius XII[5] in an allocution to physicians delivered Nov 24, 1957. After noting that we are normally obliged to use only ordinary means to preserve life, the Pontiff stated: ''A more strict obligation would be too burdensome for most men and would render the attainment of the higher, more important good too difficult. Life, death, all temporal activities are in fact subordinated to spiritual ends.'' Here it would be helpful to ask two questions. First, what are these spiritual ends, this ''higher, more important good?'' Second, how is its attainment rendered too difficult by insisting on the use of extraordinary means to preserve life?

The first question must be answered in terms of love of God and neighbor. This sums up briefly the meaning, substance, and consummation of life from a Judeo-Christian perspective. What is or can easily be missed is that these two loves are not separable. St. John wrote: ''If any man says I love God and hates his brother, he is a liar. For he who loves not his brother, whom he sees, how can he love God whom he does not see?'' (1 John 4:20–21). This means that our love of neighbor is in some very real sense our love of God. The good our love wants to do Him and to which He enables us, can be done only for the neighbor, as Karl Rahner has so forcefully argued. It is in others that God demands to be recognized and loved. If this is true, it means that, in Judeo-Christian perspective, the meaning, substance, and consummation of life is found in human *relationships*, and the qualities of justice, respect, concern, compassion, and support that surround them.

Second, how is the attainment of this ''higher, more important (than life) good'' rendered ''too difficult'' by life-supports that are gravely burdensome? One who must support his life with disproportionate effort focuses the time, attention, energy, and resources of himself and others not precisely on relationships, but on maintaining the condition of relationships. Such concentration easily becomes overconcentration and distorts one's view of and weakens one's pursuit of the very relational goods that define our growth and flourishing. The importance of relationships gets lost in the struggle for survival. The very Judeo-Christian meaning of life is seriously jeopardized when undue and unending effort must go into its maintenance.

I believe an analysis similar to this is implied in traditional treatises on preserving life. The illustrations of grave hardship (rendering the means to preserve life extraordinary and nonobligatory) are instructive, even if they are outdated in some of their particulars. Older moralists often referred to the hardship of moving to another climate or country. As the late

Gerald Kelly, SJ,[6] noted of this instance: "They (the classical moral theologians) spoke of other inconveniences, too: e.g., of moving to another climate or another country to preserve one's life. For people whose lives were, so to speak, rooted in the land, and whose native town or village was as dear as life itself, and for whom, moreover, travel was always difficult and often dangerous—for such people, moving to another country or climate was a truly great hardship, and more than God would demand as a 'reasonable' means of preserving one's health and life."

Similarly, if the financial cost of life-preserving care was crushing, that is, if it would create grave hardships for oneself or one's family, it was considered extraordinary and non-obligatory. Or again, the grave inconvenience of living with a badly mutilated body was viewed, along with other factors (such as pain in preanesthetic days, uncertainty of success), as constituting the means extraordinary. Even now, the contemporary moralist, M. Zalba, SJ,[7] states that no one is obliged to preserve his life when the cost is "a most oppressive convalescence" (molestissima convalescentia).

THE QUALITY OF LIFE

In all of these instances—instances where the life could be saved—the discussion is couched in terms of the means necessary to preserve life. But often enough it is the kind of, the quality of the life thus saved (painful, poverty-stricken and deprived, away from home and friends, oppressive) that establishes the means as extraordinary. That type of life would be an excessive hardship for the individual. It would distort and jeopardize his grasp on the overall meaning of life. Why? Because, it can be argued, human relationships—which are the very possibility of growth in love of God and neighbor—would be so threatened, strained, or submerged that they would no longer function as the heart and meaning of the individual's life as they should. Something other than the "higher, more important good" would occupy first place. Life, the condition of other values and achievements, would usurp the place of these and become itself the ultimate value. When that happens, the value of human life has been distorted out of context.

In his Morals in Medicine, Thomas O'Donnell, SJ, hinted at an analysis similar to this. Noting that life is a relative, not an absolute good, he asks: Relative to what? His answer moves in two steps. First, he argues that life is the fundamental natural good God has given to man, "the fundamental context in which all other goods which God has given man as means to the end proposed to him, must be exercised." Second, since this is so, the relativity of the good of life consists in the effort required to preserve this fundamental context and "the potentialities of the other goods that still remain to be worked out within that context."

Can these reflections be brought to bear on the grossly malformed infant? I believe so. Obviously there is a difference between having a terribly mutilated body as the result of surgery, and having a terribly mutilated body from birth. There is also a difference between a long, painful, oppressive convalescence resulting from surgery, and a life that is from birth one long, painful, oppressive convalescence. Similarly, there is a difference between being plunged into poverty by medical expenses and being poor without ever incurring such expenses. However, is there not also a similarity? Can not these conditions, whether caused by medical intervention or not, equally absorb attention and energies to the point where the "higher, more important good" is simply too difficult to attain? It would appear so. Indeed, is this not precisely why abject poverty (and the systems that support it) is such an enormous moral challenge to us? It simply dehumanizes.

Life's potentiality for other values is dependent on two factors, those external to the individual, and the very condition of the individual. The former we can and must change to maximize individual potential. That is what social justice is all about. The latter we sometimes cannot alter. It is neither inhuman nor unchristian to say that there comes a point where an individual's condition itself represents the negation of any truly human—i.e., relational—potential. When that point is reached, is not the best treatment no treatment?

I believe that the *implications* of the traditional distinction between ordinary and extraordinary means point in this direction.

In this tradition, life is not a value to be preserved in and for itself. To maintain that would commit us to a form of medical vitalism that makes no human or Judeo-Christian sense. It is a value to be preserved precisely as a condition for other values, and therefore insofar as these other values remain attainable. Since these other values cluster around and are rooted in human relationships, it seems to follow that life is a value to be preserved only insofar as it contains some potentiality for human relationships. When in human judgment this potentiality is totally absent or would be, because of the condition of the individual, totally subordinated to the mere effort for survival, that life can be said to have achieved its potential.

HUMAN RELATIONSHIPS

If these reflections are valid, they point in the direction of a guideline that may help in decisions about sustaining the lives of grossly deformed and deprived infants. That guidelines is the potential for human relationships associated with the infant's condition. If that potential is simply nonexistent or would be utterly submerged and undeveloped in the mere struggle to survive, that life has achieved its potential. There are those who will want to continue to say that some terribly deformed infants may be allowed to die *because* no extraordinary means need be used. Fair enough. But they should realize that the term "extraordinary" has been so relativized to the condition of the patient that it is this condition that is decisive. The means is extraordinary because the infant's condition is extraordinary. And if that is so, we must face this fact head-on—and discover the substantive standard that allows us to say this of some infants, but not of others.

Here several caveats are in order. First, this guideline is not a detailed rule that preempts decisions; for relational capacity is not subject to mathematical analysis but to human judgment. However, it is the task of physicians to provide some more concrete categories or presumptive biological symptoms for this human judgment. For instance, nearly all would very likely agree that the anencephalic infant is without relational potential. On the other hand, the same cannot be said of the mongoloid infant. The task ahead is to attach relational potential to presumptive biological symptoms for the gray area between such extremes. In other words, individual decisions will remain the anguishing onus of parents in consultation with physicians.

Second, because this guideline is precisely that, mistakes will be made. Some infants will be judged in all sincerity to be devoid of any meaningful relational potential when that is actually not quite the case. This risk of error should not lead to abandonment of decisions; for that is to walk away from the human scene. Risk of error means only that we must proceed with great humility caution, and tentativeness. Concretely, it means that if err we must at times, it is better to err on the side of life—and therefore to tilt in that direction.

Third, it must be emphasized that allowing some infants to die does not imply that "some lives are valuable, others not" or that "there is such a thing as a life not worth living." Every human being, regardless of age or condition, is of incalculable worth. The point is not, therefore, whether this or that individual has value. Of course he has, or rather *is* a value. The only point is whether this undoubted value has any potential at all, in continuing physical survival, for attaining a share, even if reduced, in the "higher, more important good." This is not a question about the inherent value of the individual. It is a question about whether this wordly existence will offer such a valued individual any hope of sharing those values for which physical life is the fundamental condition. Is not the only alternative an attitude that supports mere physical life as long as possible with every means?

Fourth, this whole matter is further complicated by the fact that this decision is being made for someone else. Should not the decision on whether life is to be supported or not be left to the individual? Obviously, wherever possible. But there is nothing inherently objectionable in the fact that parents with physicians must make this decision at some point for infants. Parents must make many crucial decisions for children. The only concern is that the decision not be shaped out of the utilitarian perspectives so deeply sunk into the consciousness of the contemporary world. In a highly technological culture, an individual is always in danger of being valued for his function, what he can do, rather than for who he is.

It remains, then, only to emphasize that these decisions must be made in terms of the child's good, this alone. But that good, as fundamentally a relational good, has many dimensions, Pius XII,[5] in speaking of the duty to preserve life, noted that this duty "derives from well-ordered charity, from submission to the Creator, from social justice, as well as from devotion towards his family." All of these considerations pertain to that "higher, more important good." If that is the case with the duty to preserve life, then the decision not to preserve life must likewise take all of these into account in determining what is for the child's good.

Any discussion of this problem would be incomplete if it did not repeatedly stress that it is the pride of Judeo-Christian tradition that the weak and defenseless, the powerless and unwanted, those whose grasp on the goods of life is most fragile—that is, those whose potential is real but reduced—are cherished and protected as our neighbor in greatest need. Any application of a general guideline that forgets this is but a racism of the adult world profoundly at odds with the gospel, and eventually corrosive of the humanity of those who ought to be caring and supporting as long as that care and support has human meaning. It has meaning as long as there is hope that the infant will, in relative comfort, be able to experience our caring and love. For when this happens, both we and the child are sharing in the "greater, more important good."

Were not those who disagreed with the Hopkins decision saying, in effect, that for the infant, involved human relationships were still within reach and would not be totally submerged by survival? If that is the case, it is potential for relationships that is at the heart of these agonizing decisions.

Notes

1. Duff S, Campbell AGM: Moral and ethical dilemmas in the special-care nursery. *N Engl J Med* 289:890–894, 1973.
2. Gustafson JM: Mongolism, parental desires, and the right to life. *Perspect Biol Med* 16:529–559, 1973.
3. Shaw A: Dilemmas of "informed" consent in children. *N Engl J Med* 289:885–890, 1973.
4. Ingelfinger F: Bedside ethics for the hopeless case. *N Engl J Med* 289:914, 1973.
5. Pope Pius XII: *Acta Apostolicae Sedis.* 49:1031–1032, 1957.
6. Keily G: *Medico-Moral Problems.* St. Louis, Catholic Hospital Association of the United States and Canada, 1957, p. 132.
7. Zalba M: *Theologiae Moralis Summa.* Madrid, La Editorial Catolica, 1957, vol 2, p. 71.
8. O'Donnell T, *Morals in Medicine.* Westminster, Md, Newman Press, 1957, p. 66.

Spina Bifida

The Editors

Spina bifida is the result of faulty embryological development of the spinal cord and the vertebral column. In serious cases of spina bifida, the infant is born with a men-

Reprinted from *Teaching Medical Ethics: A Report on One Approach,* Moral Problems in Medicine Project, Department of Philosophy, Case Western Reserve University, Cleveland, 1973, pp. 29-30.

ingomyelocele (also called myelomeningocele), a protruding sac filled with cerebrospinal fluid and containing a defective spinal cord. The sac is not usually covered by anything resembling normal skin and may leak fluid. These lesions occur most commonly at the small of the back, but may be higher or lower.

As a consequence of the spinal cord deformity, the child is paralyzed below the level of the lesion. This always involves loss of bladder and bowel control and, depending on the level of the sac, paraplegia. The kidneys may also be dysfunctional. There is usually impairment of normal circulation of cerebrospinal fluid, leading to hydrocephalus—an accumulation of excess fluid in the brain which can result in mental retardation. Without this complication the child may have normal or above average intelligence.

The incidence of spina bifida with a meningomyelocele is about two per 1000 live births. The cost of years of spina bifida treatment is several hundred thousand dollars per patient. For a family with one child with spina bifida, the chances of having another damaged child are about 9%.

Treatment of these infants involves immediate closure of the defect to prevent infection and further rapid neurologic loss. A surgical shunt may be necessary to alleviate the hydrocephalus. Efforts at correcting orthopedic problems may include putting the legs in casts. Later, incontinence may be modified surgically or with devices. Even with vigorous therapy, the results are seldom very good. In a study of 323 "vigorously attended" children, British physician John Lorber found that 134 were still alive after 8 to 12 years. But most lived pitiful lives. About half had shunts draining their hydrocephalus (many of these with an IQ below 80), 40% were totally incontinent, 43% had chronic urinary infections, and only 17 of the 134 survivors could walk unaided. Although the advent of new drugs and new therapies has enabled physicians to treat these children more actively, Lorber feels that it has not improved the quality of their lives, but instead has kept alive a larger percentage of more severely handicapped retarded children. He has proposed that the worst cases not be treated, citing studies that over 90% of untreated cases are dead by their first birthday.

Dr. John Freeman, of Johns Hopkins Medical School, who has also treated many spina bifida children, is concerned about these untreated survivors, some of whom live for years, whose quality of life is worse than if they had been treated initially. Therefore, given the choice of treating or not treating, he feels that one is compelled to give maximum treatment.

Ethical and Social Aspects of Treatment of Spina Bifida

R. B. Zachary

In our society the actions of one individual towards another are not without their effect on the rest of the community. Our plans of action in the treatment of myelomeningocele and their attainment are directed in the first place to the patient, but there are also important and significant effects on the family and on the community. Although we acknowledge and accept these wider effects of our treatment, we have always thought that our primary duty is to the patient, and that the most important decision is to do what is right and best for him.

Reprinted with permission of author and publisher from *The Lancet*, 274–76, August 3, 1968.

I shall therefore consider first the question of the treatment of the patient and afterwards the important social implications of this treatment.

THE CHILD

The first and the most serious ethical problem arising in the case of a child with myelomeningocele is whether he should receive medical treatment or not. The relative merits of early operation, secondary operation, or no operation at all, can only be decided when this basic principle has been established.

When a baby is born with a serious spina

bifida (i.e., a myelomeningocele with a plaque of neural tissue exposed on the surface and with all the associated complications) there are three possible lines of thought: (1) he should be killed; (2) he should be encouraged to die, either by giving no treatment at all (e.g., no feeding) or by not treating complications (e.g., no treatment of infection by antibiotics); or (3) he should be encouraged to live.

The ethical principle that the direct and deliberate killing of a human being is wrong is widely accepted on a religious and philosophical basis, and has been the basis of medical practice since the time of Hippocrates, and even earlier. (I am talking of medical matters here, not of crime and war.) The second alternative has no better justification. To leave a child without food is to kill it as deliberately and directly as if one was cutting its throat. Even the prescribing of antibiotics for infection, such as pneumonia, must now be considered as ordinary care of patients.

Once the principle has been established that the child should be encouraged to live, we are then in a position to consider which method of management gives the child the best chance to live, and secondly, which method of treatment will reduce the handicap to a minimum.

There is a widely held but mistaken view that the purpose of early operation in myelomeningocele is to save the child's life—that if operation is undertaken the child will live, and if operation is not undertaken the child will die. Pediatric surgeons will at once recognize that this is untrue, and that it contrasts with the treatment of many other congenital abnormalities. For example, in esophageal atresia we know for certain that the child will die unless a neonatal operation is undertaken, but quite a number of patients with myelomeningocele survive without any operation at all on the back, and some die as a direct result of operation when otherwise they might have survived.

In other words, there is no necessary connection between early operation and survival. It is true that in a large series of cases treated with and without operation, the results favour surgery as far as mortality is concerned. Yet this is probably not a valid reflection of the effect of operation on survival-rates. Surgical patients are receiving active treatment from all points of view: infections are treated vigorously whether they are local infections, systemic infections, or ventriculitis, and the child will probably be getting better attention to the renal tract than those who are receiving no treatment at all. I do not think it has been proved, from a concurrent study of two large series of cases, that the mortality is less in those receiving early operation than in those who do not have early operation but, in every other respect, receive the same care and attention as the surgical series.

The question at issue is whether there are advantages of early operation which outweigh any possible extra risks that such operation might have for the life of the child.

The surgeon who operates on such a child in the neonatal period has a continuing concern for the fullest development of the child; and I think it is right to emphasize the maximum development of the child, rather than the reduction of handicaps to the minimum, for this will influence the whole attitude to the child and his future.

The doctor who accepts the responsibility for the early treatment of the child, whether he be pediatrician, or pediatric surgeon, or neurosurgeon, has a duty to see that the long-term total development of the child is always kept in mind. The treatment of the hydrocephalus is only a part of the total care of these children, and we have no hesitation in calling upon other specialists to help in those aspects of the total care of the child in which we ourselves are not competent. The amount of outside help required will vary from one centre to another, but we must be quite certain that the child's orthopedic difficulties, those of the lower limbs and the spine, his renal-tract problems, and his ophthalmic problems, are dealt with competently.

What will be the effect of this treatment on the child himself? Most of the survivors who have had a severe myelomeningocele will still remain severely handicapped—they will have considerable weakness of the lower limbs and will probably be wearing callipers. About 10% will be permanently in a wheelchair, but others may use a wheelchair for most of the time, but will be able to walk a little. Few will have normal renal tracts, either because of poor control of the bladder or because of renal-tract infection and renal damage, and there will be many with urinary diversions. In most cases the hydrocephalus will be well controlled, but even as the children approach school age it may still be necessary for revision operations on the ventriculocaval shunt.

As the child grows up, therefore, his disabilities are mainly those of the lower part of the body—his arms are normal, and his head circumference will usually be within the normal range or only slightly above, and 90% of the children will be educable. In fact it is likely that between two-thirds and three-quarters of them will have an intelligence quotient within the normal range, and from this point of view be capable of receiving normal education.

THE FAMILY

But the child is not going to develop in vacuo, he is going to be brought up in a family as part of a community, and his prospects will depend very much on his integration into the life of the family and the possibility of the community supplying any special needs.

We should consider first the effect on the family of the birth of a seriously handicapped child such as one with serious myelomeningocele. Such an event is not merely a disappointment after nine months of pregnancy, it is a shattering blow to the confidence of the parents in themselves, and one which we must understand if we are to be able to help. It is strange that in these days of equality of the sexes, there is a very common and frequent feeling among the mothers that they have failed their husbands by producing a baby who is not perfect, and there is an immediate searching back in the memory for any event in the early part of pregnancy which could have contributed to this catastrophe. Later comes the recognition on the part of each parent that this may be not entirely due to them, that perhaps the other partner is partly or mainly to blame, and I think it is very important to foresee these doubts, particularly when the parents ask whether there is an hereditary factor concerned with the deformity. If parents ask me whether it is likely that another child in the family will also have spina bifida my immediate answer is that it is most unlikely to happen. If they would like some further information on this point, I give them the figures that we have used for a long time as the basis of our advice, namely, that there is, perhaps a 5–10% chance of another child having this congenital anomaly. This is, of course, about 20–30 times the incidence in the rest of the community, and such a risk would deter some parents from having further children. However, I think it should be pointed out to them that this means that there is perhaps a 90–95% chance of a subsequent child being normal in this respect: strangely, this alternative way of expressing the same facts seems much more promising to them (indeed, compared with the odds that they get on the football pools, the prospects seem very good indeed).

Parents are entitled to have this information, but it can produce a serious rift in domestic harmony unless some further explanation is given. Very soon you will find that the wife's knowledge about her husband's ancestors is only equalled by that of the husband's knowledge of the wife's ancestors, and I think it is vital to make clear two aspects of family incidence: firstly, that there is a genetic factor which is almost certainly derived from both sides of the family and, secondly, that the genetic factor is not the only one, there must be some environmental factor which may be of great importance. The clearest way of explaining this to the parents is to tell them that it is possible for one of a pair of identical twins to have spina bifida and the other to be perfectly normal; indeed, there is some evidence to show that the incidence among twins is less than the incidence among non-twin siblings.

A most important step in integrating the handicapped child into the life of the family is the acceptance of the child back home by the parents at the earliest possible moment. In many cases the child will only have been shown to the mother for a brief moment and the father may not have seen him at all before he is sent to a special centre for treatment. This may involve a child travelling a long distance from home, and separation from the mother at this stage will do harm unless special efforts are made to prevent it. Firstly, the mere fact of the child going to a special centre for treatment should in itself give the parents some hope that the child can be helped to overcome his disability. If there is no attempt to send the child for special treatment, if the parents are told that the case is hopeless, that the baby will not survive, that he will be mentally defective, or that he will never be able to walk or go to school or earn his living, the parents are left without any hope at all and their morale drops to zero.

If, on the other hand, they are told that their child is seriously handicapped but active treatment is to be undertaken to help the child to develop himself more fully, and to reduce the handicaps to the minimum, they look forward to having the child back home to do what they can to help him. The child should not be kept in hospital any longer than is absolutely necessary, and if there are to be delays of even two or three weeks between operations it is most important that he should be allowed home. Moreover, if at all possible, the mother should be encouraged to visit the child in hospital, and to learn how to feed him and take care of him under the supervision of the sister. With this attitude of optimistic realism, with the encouragement of visiting by the mother and the early discharge of the patient, it is very seldom indeed that the child is rejected by the parents, no matter how serious his disabilities. The rejection-rate is far greater in those areas where there is no policy of active treatment, and, even if the child is not left for months in the hospital or in an institution, the family has a heavy burden of unhappiness because they have been given no hope.

Besides the anxieties which the parents have about the survival of their child, his disabilities, and their feelings of guilt, there are also other heavy burdens which they must bear. During infancy the task of the mother may not be very much greater than with a normal child, but as he grows older there is considerable extra work which the parents accept so very willingly. They find themselves tied to the household very much more than the parents of normal children, for they feel a grave responsibility which will not permit them to leave the child in the care of a baby-sitter, so that free evenings and even holidays become very difficult indeed, unless the parents get help from outside.

There is also a considerable financial burden which is sometimes overlooked. Although apparatus and special shoes may be supplied by the Health Service, the wear and tear on clothing is very much greater than with other children, as a result of the apparatus and appliances which they wear. In addition, the frequent admissions to hospital for the various operations which are going to be required mean that the parents have to spend quite a lot of money on travelling to the hospital, for which they may have to give up some of the ordinary dangerous habits such as smoking.

As the children grow the anxiety of the parents does not diminish, and they are extremely worried about the prospects of education for their children, and about their chances of being accepted by the community.

THE COMMUNITY

What are the responsibilities of the community in the care of the children with myelomeningocele? I think the health authorities in Britain are only now becoming aware of the size of this problem and of its gravity. It has taken a considerable time to obtain a clear idea of the incidence of serious spina bifida in our country, and of the survival-rates to be expected. We know that there is a considerable variation in incidence from one country to another, and even in different parts of the same country—for example, in South Wales and in the area around Liverpool the incidence is about twice as great as in some other parts of England. For the country as a whole it seems likely that a figure approaching 2 per 1000 live births is not very far off the mark. Survival-rates are even more difficult to assess, but when all cases are accepted for treatment it seems likely that at least 70% will be surviving at the end of one year, and probably between 50% and 60% will be alive at five years of age.

In the first place the health authorities should make themselves aware of the extent of the problem. It will be necessary to provide treatment centres, and we have found in this special type of neonatal surgery that there are very great advantages in operations being undertaken in special units designed for neonatal surgery, where the whole hospital is geared to the special needs of seriously ill neonates and infants. There are also many advantages in concentrating this work so that not merely 5 or 6 cases are done in the course of a year, but perhaps a minimum of 20 or 30. I think the maximum that we have had has been 170 in a year, and I think this is too many, and we have now persuaded other centres to undertake this work and we do about 120 a year at present.

An adult who sustains a spinal injury causing paraplegia has already received his education, and in many countries there are opportunities for retraining of the adult paraplegic. The child paraplegic, the child with a serious myelomeningocele, has many handicaps in his struggle to obtain even a basic education.

How can these children be fitted into the educational system of the country? In the first place, if the intelligence quotient of a child is normal, he should go to an ordinary school if at all possible. His two major problems are difficulty in walking and incontinence. Many modern schools are built on one floor and have no steps, and so children can attend them even though they spend most of their time in a wheelchair or use callipers; but if there are many steps in a school, it is quite impossible for the child to attend.

A more serious barrier to attendance at a normal school is incontinence, and it is largely for this reason that special day-schools are needed, where frequent attention can be given to the children and, most important, where the child does not feel embarrassed and become emotionally disturbed by being the only incontinent child in the class.

A small number of residential schools for the seriously handicapped are important when parents live too far away from a day-school for handicapped children, or when the child's condition needs very frequent supervision, and I think there are advantages in having such a residential school closely related to a centre for treatment.

We must also look forward to the time when they are about to leave school and consider in what way they are going to make their living. Education is even more important than for those children who have no handicap at all, and vocational training should be specially directed towards the needs of the seriously handicapped.

They will have to rely on their brains and their arms and hands to earn a living, and I think it is most important that the vocational training should not be narrow, simply learning how to undertake mechanical procedures with the hands; it should also have a wide scope, with the possibilities of developing the talents and abilities of these young people in many directions. Simple clerical and manual mechanical work is well within the capacity of most of these young people, but there must be many who are potentially great authors, artists, linguists, musicians, scientists, and philosophers, and yet they may have no opportunity to advance themselves in this way because of the lack of educational opportunities and the lack of vocational training.

It is here, I think, that the parents' associations have proved most valuable. These associations are now scattered widely throughout Great Britain, and although their aim at first was to provide moral support for the parents in the management and care of their children, it has now become clear that a major concern of the parents is education.

In helping these children the community is helping itself. If it provides adequate treatment these children will be less handicapped than they would otherwise be: if it provides adequate educational and vocational training, they will be able to earn their living. In simple economic terms the potential for a child with myelomeningocele must be very much greater than that of the old person with carcinoma of the lung or stomach. Let us be fair to children born with myelomeningocele. Let us plan their treatment so that their handicap is minimal. Let us develop their minds and bodies so as to compensate for their serious disability, and give them education and vocational training to fit them for a career.

Letters: Ethical and Social Aspects of Treatment of Spina Bifida

Sir,—I feel that the ethical justification given by Mr. Zachary for the treatment of children with severe spina bifida is shallow and cruel. It is no longer accepted that the preservation of life as such is the doctor's most important task. We now consider the patient's wellbeing and happiness to the equally at stake. It is now an accepted principle that we treat terminal patients in a way that makes for comfort rather than long survival. Surely we should apply the same sort of principles to children whose prognosis is despairingly poor? If long-term survival entails many operations, much pain and disfigurement, an inability to lead a normal life because of incontinence and paraplegia, and mental strain and distress to parents, should we always attempt it?

R. C. Sanders

This letter has been shown to Mr. Zachary, whose reply follows.—Ed. L.

Sir,—The whole point of my paper has been missed by Dr. Sanders. I would have thought that the three main premises of the argument were abundantly clear: (1) babies with spina bifida should not be killed; (2) the main purpose of all treatment is not to save the child's life, but to improve his function and reduce his handicaps to the minimum; (3) the child with spina bifida deserves that every effort should be made to improve his wellbeing and happiness. If Dr. Sanders thinks these babies should be killed he should say so. If not he should encourage efforts to enable the child to walk, to help his mental development, and to overcome the problems of incontinence.

Dr. Sanders is welcome to visit our follow-up clinic any Tuesday afternoon, when we see 40–70 patients. He will see for himself whether our outlook is "shallow and cruel" and whether

we have a real concern for "the patient's wellbeing and happiness."

R. B. Zachary

Sir,—In his well-written and beguiling paper Mr. Zachary makes out a good case for treating all babies with severe spina bifida surgically, yet Dr. Sanders describes this as "shallow and cruel," to which Mr. Zachary retorts that the alternative is to kill these babies. Clearly this is a highly emotional subject. There is, of course, a third approach—namely, to let Nature take its course. Over the years without any active intervention on my part, over 90% of the untreated babies I have seen have died before their first birthday.

Now that surgical treatment is available for such babies, the easiest way out for the doctor is to transfer the neonates to a unit where all such babies are operated upon without delay. The parents, in their confused and highly disappointed state, will gladly clutch at any offer to help, fervently hoping that the miracle of modern surgery will put the baby right. It will take time before the awful truth dawns upon them and by then it will be too late to step back. Then their only course is to put on a brave face—one that warms the heart of the surgeon in the follow-up clinic. The advent of such a severely handicapped child into a family will transform the lives of all its members—in some cases permanently and completely. That some parents gain fulfilment by dedicating their lives to the care of such children is one of the saving graces of this tragic story, but who can be sure that their lives would have been emptier with a healthy replacement?

The haste that is recommended in order to get the best surgical results often precludes careful consideration of the implications for the family as a whole if the neonate survives. Whenever possible, I try to put the argument for and against surgery to the parents as objectively as I can—a difficult task in the emotionally charged atmosphere that surrounds the

Reprinted with permission from *The Lancet*, August 24, 1968, September 9, 1968, October 12, 1968, November 2, 1968, and November 9, 1968, respectively.

birth of any baby, let alone a seriously deformed one. Some down-to-earth parents have no hesitation in letting Nature solve the problem so that they can try again, knowing that the risk of a recurrence is not very great. In such cases we offer to keep the baby in the ward indefinitely should they so wish. Others are grateful for the hope which surgery offers and here there is no problem. But it is the waverers, who can be swayed either way according to the views of the doctor interviewing them, who constitute the heart of the problem—which is most easily, though not necessarily correctly, dealt with by the unquestioning committal of the baby to surgery. One can argue that this is the baby's fundamental right, but have we forgotten that parents and their living children also have rights? Should they not also be considered and consulted?

Ian G. Wickes

Sir,—Every chronic and disabling condition in medicine necessarily presents an emotional problem to the patient's family. Except in this sense, and certainly at professional level, discussion of the management of the severe forms of spina bifida should be kept to the facts.

Dr. Wickes claims that a policy of "letting Nature take its course"—he does not define that phrase though it is highly ambiguous—achieves, if that is the word, a mortality of more than 90% of such cases in the first year of life. What is the alternative? It is difficult to compare figures without knowing the criteria on which Dr. Wickes judges that a case is only suitable for expectant treatment; but even restricting the discussion to the most severe form of the disorder, that in which without treatment anything short of complete paraplegia is unusual and the incidence of hydrocephalus 96%—namely, open thoracolumbar myelocele—we find that with adequate surgical treatment 35% survive to the age of 16 years, and that 70% of these are of normal intelligence. Moreover there is, at the time of birth, an important group among these (48%) which can be detected by clinical methods and in which immediate operation gives an even chance of preserving useful function in the legs. Similar findings have been reported by Zachary and his colleagues in Sheffield and from other centres.

We believe that it is doubt about the realities of the prognosis which causes parents (and physicians) to be "waverers." No reasonable person would advise "the unquestioning committal of the baby to surgery." Instead one can and should tell the parents of a baby born with severe spina bifida, as defined above:

1. Whether with immediate operation there is a good chance that he will achieve natural ambulation. If not, then the haste which Dr. Wickes deplores is unnecessary. More conservative methods can be used.

2. That there is a serious risk of hydrocephalus, but that this can be surgically controlled with a reasonable mortality and morbidity.

3. That orthopaedic and urological treatment will be required also, but that there is a better than even chance that, if he survives, the baby will grow up as a normally intelligent human being.

Whether these results are to be preferred to Dr. Wickes' 90% mortality within the first year (we trust that at least he encourages treatment of hydrocephalus in the survivors), is a matter for personal judgment. But parents are not interested in percentages: they want to know what we can do for their own individual children.

A. A. Fernandez-Serrats
A. N. Guthkelch
S. A. Parker

Sir,—Pediatricians cannot possibly assess the prognosis of individual cases unless they have themselves been involved in the operative treatment. By his attitude Dr. Wickes is denying neonates their right to a surgical opinion. No-one would quarrel with his expressions of dismay over handicapped survivors, but what of the many metabolic disorders and known mental defects obvious at birth? Dr. Wickes should have the courage to publish the progress of his 10% untreated survivors. They probably have brain damage which could have been spared and paralysis more extensive than it need have been. Dr. Wickes is extending the principles of social abortion into the neonatal period. This influence is unhealthy in the nurseries of maternity units.

D. F. Ellison Nash

Sir,—Dr. Wickes is by no means the only pediatrician who prefers to let Nature take its course in cases of severe thoracolumbar myelocele with paraplegia. I, for one, have not been impressed by the long-term results of surgical treatment, and after a period of treating these with immediate operation have now returned to a conservative approach to this problem. As Dr. Fernandez-Serrats and his colleagues themselves admit, 65% of surgically treated patients will be dead by the age of sixteen anyway. In the meantime, however, the care of such a child will have been an intolerable strain on the family, especially the mother. In the vast majority of cases she will forego her chances of having further normal children. As for the survivors, only two-thirds of whom are of normal intelligence, they have to find their place in society as paraplegics with incontinence, subject to repeated urinary infections and bedsores.

Mr. Ellison Nash surely exaggerates when he talks of "social abortion" in the neonatal period. The old dictum we were taught as medical students, "Thou shalt not kill; but need'st not strive officiously to keep alive," is a very different principle from that of abortion, which means the active physical destruction of a presumably healthy, normal fetus. I should like to assure Mr. Ellison Nash that spina bifida is not the only state in neonatal pediatrics in which non-interference is the kinder course of action if one considers the well-being of the family as a whole. I personally never see the problem of the untreated survivor with severe thoracolumbar myelocele, hydrocephalus, and paraplegia. Nature if left alone will always correct its own mistakes in these cases.

L. Haas

Sir,—Dr. Wickes and Dr. Haas last week probably command more support amongst pediatricians than is evident in your columns. It is comforting that a surgeon also has doubts about current approaches.

Dr. Fernandez-Serrats and his colleagues appreciate only half the problem when they suggest a detailed conference with the parents before an infant is submitted to operation. Current surgical advice insists that immediate transfer to a surgical unit is imperative. How is this compatible with the careful conference? A half-anaesthetised mother and a distraught father are in no position to make rational decisions. In any case it is doubtful whether they should be allowed to take part in a decision at this stage. Whether the results are death, or handicapped survival, they are likely to feel some guilt if the decision has been theirs.

Mr. Ellison Nash says that by selecting some children (and accepting the responsibility ourselves) we are denying infants the right to a surgical opinion. But it is not the infant who needs the opinion—it is his parents. In how many cases would it be possible to say that the parents have read and *understood* the operation consent-form which they sign? This refers to an operation "the effect and nature of which have been explained to me." All too often the referral for surgical opinion means that the infant will be swept up into the machinery of a first-rate specialist hospital which is operation-oriented. In how many cases has the consultant surgeon, before operation, fully explained the intended programme and the odds against complete normality? Has he explained about the likelihood of urinary diversion, and the prospects of education—and of life as an independent citizen? Has he waited for the question " . . . and if he survives will he have children of his own, and will they also be affected?" It is the very essence of the problem that these questions are often neither asked nor answered, and make the operation consent-form a blank cheque. It is partly because of this that some pediatricians have some doubts.

Some of us think that as well as the right to live there is also the right to die. This has been well stated for the sick and for the aged. It is well that this view should also be aired by pediatricians, who are increasingly involved both with the initial decisions and with the aftermath.

R. M. Forrester

From "Health Service or Sickness Service?"

Eliot Slater

PERINATAL RISKS

The processes of meiosis and mitosis, of spermatogenesis and oogenesis, and after them of the development of the embryo through all its stages are very delicately controlled. But they are extremely complex and have no margin for error; any error, however minor, has cumulative effects. Nevertheless, the defective embryos are progressively eliminated. Out of every 1,000 conceptuses 120 to 150 die in the first four weeks of life. Probably all of them are seriously abnormal. They cause no more disturbance in the mother than perhaps an unusually heavy menstrual bleeding. Between the end of the first four weeks and the seventh month of pregnancy there will be a further 100 to 150 miscarriages. More than half of these spontaneously aborted fetuses can be seen to be abnormal, even on superficial examination. These are nature's discards.

Of the babies who come to term some 2% are stillborn and a further 4% or so have gross defects. The save-all policy has become the rule in our obstetric and pediatric services, with results which could become grave in terms of human suffering. About three in every 1,000 babies born are affected by spina bifida, in a high proportion of cases to a moderate or severe degree. When I was a student and no treatment was known the usual course was put the little mistake of nature in a cool spot while attention was diverted to the mother. The baby died, the mother wept. But a few months later she would be entering on another pregnancy with every chance of having a normal healthy child.

Then came the time when these damaged babies were given their chance of surviving and got the same support as any other baby. Then the life span was somewhat longer, though only the very mildest cases ever reached adolescence. The most heavily handicapped babies died off rapidly, and four out of five were gone in the first year.

Nowadays pediatric surgery proceeds stage by stage to ward off all the dangers. There is operation after operation, always new adjustments having to be made as the child grows. Attention is needed because the child is spastic and paralysed and incontinent. There has to be special education to help him to adjust to the combination of defects, among which there is often superadded mental subnormality.

It appears that the proportion of spina bifida babies now having an immediate operation is rising. So too no doubt are the numbers of severely handicapped survivors; and so too the medical, educational, social, and family burdens. In the first five years of life most survivors spend an average of two years in hospital, mainly in spells of one to two weeks. Admissions are numbered in dozens, and the child is hardly out of hospital before the time is nearing for him to go back again. Special schooling can usually enable these children to walk and to get their incontinence under a socially acceptable degree of control. But if Britain were to provide special schools for every spina bifida child who is now being salvaged Leach estimated that it would have to build one with 50 places, and staff it with about 10 skilled people, each and every month for the next 15 years.

These children are now beginning to come into puberty and adolescence, when their sufferings will really begin. Only the most miserably impaired social life will be open to them; they will be equipped with normal sex drive but no normal sex function; all around them they will see the normal, the vigorous, and the healthy. Will they really be grateful to the fates, the all too human fates, but for whose intervention they would have died before their miseries began?

Perhaps the whole procedure is mistaken. If

Reprinted with permission by author and publisher from *The British Medical Journal*, 4, 734–35, December 18, 1971.

this is one of the necessary consequences of the sanctity-of-life ethic perhaps our formulation of the principle should be revised. The spina bifida baby is a mistake of nature not equipped to survive. Who suffers if he dies at birth? Certainly not the child, though if he is forced to survive he faces years of suffering. Do the parents suffer if he dies? Yes, in the disappointment of not having a baby when they had hoped for a normal little boy or girl; but in a few months they can try again. If the child survives, however, they have years of servitude, of tortured love, trying to make up to him for all his disadvantages. And society, the community? The death costs nothing; the life costs not only money but the pre-emption of precious medical, nursing, social, and educational resources.

It is sometimes said that the handicapped child has the same right as the normal child to a normal family life. But the mentally subnormal and the severely handicapped child cannot have a normal family life. The abnormal child causes emotional reactions in his parents and sibs that distort normal relationships, and these families suffer severely. . . . The true ethic is, I believe, that normal parents have a right to a normal child. It is their first duty to preserve the normality of their home, the welfare of their marriage, their mutual relationship, and their family life. They should think it wrong to inflict an abnormal sib on their other normal children, who cannot defend themselves against this trauma. Sometimes parents do reject the abnormal baby when he is born, but if so it is in the face of strong emotional pressures from everyone—doctors, nurses, and neighbours. Yet common sense and humanity are on the side of rejecton. The spina bifida baby, the mongol, the phenylketonuric are not babies so much as attempts at babyhood that misfired. If as a community we impose on our medical services the duty of keeping them alive, then through these and other State services we should bear the whole burden. It is one for specialists. We should not shuffle it off on to untrained women and men of only average ability and stability, who by their relationship with the abnormal infant are put under particular strain.

Is There a Right to Die—Quickly?

John M. Freeman

A child born with a meningomyelocele has a readily and accurately diagnosable lesion at birth. The degree of neurologic deficit is ascertainable and irreversible; the risks of hydrocephalus and mental retardation are largely predictable, as is the risk of bladder involvement and urinary incontinence. While 10 to 15 years ago few physicians were enthusiastic about treating children with meningomyeloceles, under the leadership of the English groups there has been an increasing interest in early, vigorous, and comprehensive treatment. Dr. John Lorber, one of the leading exponents of early and vigorous intervention in these

Reproduced with premission of author and publisher from J. Pediatr. 80, 904–905, 1972; copyrighted by The C. V. Mosby Company, St. Louis, Missouri.

children, has recently assessed his long-term results, with some second thoughts. After careful analysis of his data, Lorber states that not all children with meningomyeloceles should be treated. He states that depending on the level of the lesion, the presence of hydrocephalus, and other factors, certain children should be left unoperated—to die. He quotes from the few available studies of untreated meningomyeloceles to show that untreated, a large percentage (60 to 80 per cent) die within the first year of life. While some might interpret the quoted studies differently, the significant factor is that many do not die quickly, but slowly over months or years, dying of meningitis, hydrocephalus, or renal disease. However, of equal importance is the fact that many survive, and the quality of their survival after drying and infection of the spinal cord, hydrocephalus, and renal decompensation is poorer than if they had had early, vigorous—optimal—treatment.

We are thus between the Scylla of treating all children with meningomyeloceles with resultant increase in the number of survivors with severe handicapping conditions, and the Charybdis of not treating some children and permitting nature to take its often long, lingering course. There are all gradients of this latter position: One could not feed the child and allow him to starve to death; one could feed, but not treat meningitis or infection if they occur; one could close the back so that the child is aesthetically more desirable and could be cared for at home, but not treat the hydrocephalus; one could close the back and shunt the hydrocephalus, but allow the child to die later of renal disease, with or without orthopedic treatment. In short, when one decides not to treat, or to treat only partially, patients survive. It is not the patient or the problem that goes away—it is the physician who goes away from the problem, leaving the family and the patient to suffer.

One of the recent "advances" in medicine is prenatal diagnosis. By this technique, we can now detect certain genetic or metabolic diseases before birth and "allow the family to have only normal children." This is the current euphemism used for abortion on fetal indication. Physicians, to a large extent backed by society, have decided that it may not only be permissible, but laudable, to kill at 20 weeks a fetus who might die of Tay-Sachs disease at 2 years, or one with mongolism who might lead an impaired life for many years. Indeed, if there were mechanisms for the diagnosis of meningomyeloceles at 20 to 24 weeks of gestation, would we not encourage parents to request termination of pregnancy? If it is permissible to kill a fetus at 20 to 24 weeks, should it not also be permissible to kill such an infant at 40 weeks of gestation?

A discussion of killing is an anathema to most of us who are trained and dedicated to saving lives. However, physicians should admit that in deciding that some children with meningomyeloceles should not be operated upon, as Lorber has done, they are making a decision between life and death. The unoperated infant is being condemned to death, sooner or later, by less than optimal care—what might be termed passive euthanasia. The physician does not take into account the increased pain and suffering to both child and parent attendant to "letting nature take its course." If we make that decision for a given child, should we not then, as physicians, also have the opportunity to alleviate the pain and suffering by accelerating that death? This conversion from passive euthanasia to active euthanasia is not an easy one for society or for the individual physician faced with the decisions and with their consequences. Having seen children with unoperated meningomyeloceles lie around the ward for weeks or months untreated, waiting to die, one cannot help but feel that the highest form of medical ethic would have been to end the pain and suffering, rather than wishing that the patient would go away.

It is time that society and medicine stopped perpetuating the fiction that withholding treatment is ethically different from terminating life. It is time that society began to discuss mechanisms by which we can alleviate the pain and suffering for those individuals whom we cannot help.

People will ask: If we are to kill some children with meningomyeloceles, then where will we draw the line? At children with mongolism who may have a long, if impaired life? At children with muscular dystrophy who have a shorter life, but a number of normal years? At the severely retarded child? At the mildly retarded child? At the child with phocomelia, or with a congenital amputation? These are areas where I do not believe euthenasia should be considered, but which physicians and society can and should discuss. However, in those rare instances where the decision has been made to avoid "heroic" measures and to allow "nature to take its course," should society not allow physicians to alleviate the pain and suffering and help nature to take its course—quickly?

Whose Suffering?

Robert E. Cooke

In an accompanying editorial, "Is there a right to die—quickly?," Dr. John Freeman raises old issues concerning a new problem. New dilemmas are being created with the advances of science. Before meningomyeloceles could be repaired, the physician had no options. Now that a poor prognosis is no longer a certainty new dilemmas arise—who should be operated upon, when should antibiotics be given, and at what stage should the physician admit defeat in his efforts to prolong life?

The comments in this editorial are not addressed to the issue of operating or not operating, but to the handling of the case not operated upon. Dr. Freeman adequately states the case for the infant's suffering. In so doing, he adopts understandable, commonplace, yet to my mind erroneous, reasoning. He applies what may loosely be called the anthropomorphic approach to the infant, attributing to it perceptions and emotions characteristic of the mature adult. Yet the infants that Dr. Freeman says, "lie around the ward for weeks or months untreated, *waiting to die*" are not fully conscious in adult terms, not capable of abstraction, and respond only to relatively simple stimuli with relatively simple internal as well as external behavior. Quite simply, "waiting to die," is a nonexistent thought of the infant.

Dr. Freeman refers to the "suffering of society." It is an unfortunate fact that society suffers very little: So many competing pains and pleasures exist that only a small percentage of society is even aware that the unoperated hydrocephalic patient exists. One aspect of suffering may be fiscal hardship. If that is the case, all of us should suffer the tortures of the damned as billions go to the Defense Department. Only a small portion of the fiscal hardship could result if all such children were cared for for a lifetime.

The word "suffering" is often appropriate to the parents. Yet how many of us in pediatrics

have seen love and devotion, not misery, come at least occasionally to the parents of the handicapped. Surely all of us know of many cases in which even a severely handicapped child has brought great joy to a family. How much the hopelessly handicapped infant or the unoperated-upon patient decreases or augments the humanity of the doctors or the parents about him, cannot readily be measured. In an indirect way at least, he makes a contribution to our heritage—primarily personal—but occasionally public, and this qualifies him as human, according to Monod's definition. "Unwanted by both family and society" might apply as a criterion for termination of life, but let us be careful since much of the pediatrician's "heroics," such as intensive care for the 1,200 Gm. offspring of the 13-year-old unmarried girl from the ghetto, would come to an end.

Medicine is the science of care, not the science of cure, and in caring, we as physicians must suffer. Such difficult experiences are part of the fabric of medicine that bring humane people to medicine, not drive them away. Medicine would change for the worse if the physician joined too fully the new discomfort-free society.

Lest the reader consider the author a harbinger of the ethic of suffering, let us examine another aspect of Dr. Freeman's argument. If it is acceptable to kill the defective fetus by abortion before birth, why not the infant with non-correctable serious abnormalities after birth? Dr. Freeman is correct that biologically there is little difference between the fetus and infant; the birth process or viability conveys few new biological properties. In the newborn infant, the respiratory system is adequately developed and no functioning umbilical cord is necessary. But without external support, i.e., feeding, every human new born infant would die. The potential for humanity in the fetus and neonate is the same. The newborn infant directly contributes little more or benefits little more than the fetus from the heritage of our culture. Yet I cannot agree with Dr. Freeman. There is indeed a vast difference, in a large part of our society, between the fetus and the noenate. The neonate is perceived as human, giving and receiving and inspiring love. The differences are psychological, but nevertheless real in both the public and the private mind. Individuals in most societies see in the infant's face and appearance human goodness and love; yet it would be difficult for them to imagine the fetus in these terms. The public mind also views the fetus and the neonate differently. The law regards termination of the fetus' life as "abortion"—considered acceptable by many in society, and desirable by many in some circumstances. Yet infanticide is "murder." The difference in attitude toward the fetus and neonate does not exist because of the law, rather the law exists because of the attitude of the public. Whether abortion is condoned or condemned is irrevelant—the difference still exists between it and infanticide. We do not know if these differences will persist or disappear in generations to come, but the fact is that at the moment they do exist.

I can only conclude that pediatricians must accept the suffering and offer corrective measures as needed to all who have a probability of response, as long as it is impossible to predict with a high degree of precision the outcome in an individual case. Therapy without cure, if it contributes to *care*, is a necessary part of medicine in spite of the fact that the physician must sometimes suffer. Death of the unoperated patient is an unacceptable means of alleviating this suffering.

Human and Handicapped

Karen M. Metzler

In preparing these remarks, I was undecided as to whether I should use lecture form to give you my experience of society's attitudes toward handicappedness, or should continue by allowing both of us to do our questioning, searching, and experiencing out loud together. I have decided to begin by sharing my experience with you so that you can know how deeply I am willing to probe into being aware of and understanding myself, you, our encounters, and life itself.

I am a humanist—I see life, growth, and potential in every human circumstance. I also see the pain, sorrow, and grief in them. But I work towards choosing to empathize the former qualities. Such an attitude is truly me. It is real. It is no pretense. But I do know that I learned at an early age that if I wanted to be praised and accepted I had to smile. And smile I did, always, even when the pain inside wanted

This article was presented originally to an undergraduate course on Moral Problems in Medicine at Case Western Reserve University. It is published here by permission of the author.

to howl like a pack of wolves in the dark. And I smiled and people said, "Look at Karen, how she's always smiling. Boy, she's strong. She's accepted her handicap. She never complains." I wanted to be strong, to be healthy. But most of all, I wanted to be accepted by others. And it appeared to me that the rules were that in order to be accepted, I had to keep to myself any of the negative aspects of being handicapped, because society had to deny them in order for society to be free of discomfort. I am taking, now, a big risk in being honest and open about my feelings and perceptions, which means that I do not sugarcoat any which may need it for social acceptability. The risk is of being accused, by both the able-bodied and the disabled persons in society, of not having accepted being handicapped. Knowing my own life process, I believe that it was not until I was able to begin to accept myself that I was able to speak honestly not only to myself, but to others as well. When I speak out against what I perceive as injustices, though they often be unintentional, in such areas as education, employment, and even daily living, I am not complaining, but confronting. To complain means just to express undirected, immature hostility with no goal in mind except the mere release of inner tension caused by the abrasion of one's personal existence against Existence itself. But to confront means that I have as my goal the bringing about of awareness and action upon that awareness.

Let me allow you to become aware of what it is like to be me—a white, female, middle-class handicapped person. Not a black or an upper-class or a male handicapped person, but me. Though there are commonalities among persons who are handicapped, there are differences, because we are all individuals. I do not presume to say that my feelings, perceptions, and experiences are the way it is for all. I can only say that it is the way it is for me.

I think that the underlying emotion behind my total experience of being a person with a handicap is that because I am imperfect in one way, I *must* be perfect in all other ways. Admittedly, this comes from a need within me to compensate. But you, as a society and as individuals, also help to create this need, because you—as a society and as individuals—become fixated to the fact that I am different and unable to do certain things, and then generalize this fixation into a belief that I am unable to do anything at all. It is this generalization which leads you to discriminate against allowing me to do those things which I am in fact capable of doing. It would or should not be as important to me that I am unable to do certain things. After all, isn't that part of being human?

But am I human? Am I less human as a person because my body is not like that of other humans? Are my feelings, thoughts, needs, and desires different from theirs because my body is? Is the development of my potential distorted, or just in some ways delayed? It is my belief that the development of a person with a handicap should not be considered abnormal, and need not be abnormal. His or her development, just like that of any other person, has meaning and consistency within itself. For instance, when I was sixteen my emotional energies were invested in dealing with an unknown blood disorder and the impending loss of a leg. How, emotionally, could I have been at the same place it is expected that

sixteen-year-olds be, for instance in regard to social development—e.g., dating? For my situation, I was normal, but for the hypothetical or average situation, I was abnormal. But consider this. What would you think about a sixteen-year-old who had come to grips with the concept and reality of death? You would call her mature for her age or situation, would you not? But the hypothetical or average situation of a sixteen-year-old does not include the achievement of that particular developmental task. In this sense, he or she is not being "normal" but "abnormal." Why then do we make such distinctions and value judgments about the direction in which a person can deviate from the developmental norms? It is because we make comparisons of persons, rather than accepting them as they are and where they are.

However, even those individuals who are able to accept the handicapped person as he is—that is, as handicapped—are often unable to accept where the handicapped person is emotionally in dealing with his handicappedness. The individuals around him and society in general expect him to have reached the stage of acceptance, while emotionally and behaviorally they are only willing to allow him to go through the first stage—denial of the existence of his or her handicap—in his struggle towards acceptance. They often will not even let him talk about it. But there are intermediate and succeeding stages which are just as necessary and valid for the handicapped person to go through if he is ever to reach the stage of acceptance. These stages consist of such emotional reactions as anger, self-pity, and self-rejection. To allow a handicapped person to experience and express such emotions threatens other people, particularly those who are deeply involved with him or her, because their own feelings of anger, pity, and rejection may become surfaced. What people must realize, particularly if they are professionally or personally involved, is that there are ways of showing respect for a handicapped person's need to be at a certain stage without having necessarily to reinforce him or her so that he or she never grows beyond the earlier stages to that of acceptance.

Some people are able to recognize the existence of and need for this process more easily in situations involving a person who becomes handicapped after having lived as a nonhandicapped person. But a child born with a birth defect must also go through the same process. The difference is that the onset of the process is undatable. Any one of the stages may become his mode of personality, since they are occurring during his formative years, and he has not established a prior personality on which to build or with which to buffer against any permanent adoption of the emotional responses (i.e., hostility, self-rejection, denial, etc.).

And for some persons, like myself, even though we have gone through the process before, since our bodies and body-images continue to undergo repeated trauma and mutilation, the process must be gone through again each time. But people do not easily recognize this. For instance, when I told people that my leg was going to be amputated, some responded by saying that since I had gone through so much already, I should be able to handle this easily. It was as though they were saying that it was less of a trauma for me than it would be for someone else! This only complicated the guilt feelings I had later about my having to go through the less socially acceptable stages in the process of acceptance.

One element of acceptance is the ability to feel a positive regard towards oneself and to feel that others hold one in positive regard as well. One source in our society of positive regard is through the achievement of expectations and goals as set for one by himself or others. The fulfillment of these expectations or goals constitutes, in the general mind, success. But one like myself wonders if he or she has truly achieved success, when its acknowledgement is accompanied by such statements as, "For someone handicapped like yourself," or "Despite your handicaps." It makes me wonder if what I have done would be only mediocre, or less, if I were able-bodied, but because I am not, it deserves praise. To assure myself that when I succeed, I truly succeed, I set out towards goals that would be difficult for anyone, whether or not he had a handicap. I do not want the left-overs or what might only be the spoils after everyone else's victories.

In my case, goals and success centered around my mind, my intellect. But even though my mind earned me recognition and

respect, I still felt insecure about it. I had grown up from birth hearing the words, "And you should have been retarded, but you are not." Well, with such an expectation as that, even mediocrity would seem praiseworthy. But whether or not I was the genius that I thought I had to be, I did at least have enough intelligence. I felt compelled to use what I had because I was concerned about what might have happened if I had not had a mind which was capable of compensating for my imperfect body. What would have given my life value so that people would want me? I wondered often about those children who were not as lucky as myself. I am bothered when I see a documentary about a handicapped boy which ends by saying that he can be a physicist someday. What if he becomes a plumber instead? Would his success as a handicapped person be any less?

Putting myself in the place of the other person has always been something which I have tried to do. But I have never liked to be compared with another person—that was something only I could do in my perennial profession as self-criticizer. It bothered me, though I understood their good intentions, to have people always telling me about some other handicapped person they knew who was able to do this, that, or the other thing. My initial response would be that they were not really listening to me. I was not that person, but me! I was an individual, separate from the other to whom I was being compared, with a different set of problems and potentialities whether or not they were greater or less than someone else's—for in the end they were mine, and only mine. Comparisons tend to imply at an unconscious level a test of one's adequacy. And at some level within me, it made me feel inadequate. For instance, I knew that amputees could swim, but I had not always been an amputee. Instead, I had spent my life with my legs in casts, unable to go in water. If I had had the opportunity, I would have learned. And when the opportunity did arise, I did learn. Still, if I had never been able to learn to swim, knowing that it was something which amputees could in fact do, there would have been a part of me asking, "Have I failed? Am I less well-adjusted than others?"

A successful handicapped person is one who

has not only gained his own acceptance of himself, but the acceptance of himself from others as well. But from whom and how does a handicapped person gain his acceptance? His parents, who have been trained by society to react towards handicappedness with rejection, discomfort, and denial add to these feelings those of guilt and anger. They have also incorporated from society a set of expectations about their child's behavior and potential. Thus, they are given the difficult task of re-educating their emotions so that they may become compassionate and accepting facilitators of their child's development. They are often left to do this alone, unaided by professional or non-professional help and support while they are attempting to re-educate the emotions of other people in order that their child eventually be accepted as the human being he is. His parents must also supply him with what he needs to be successful in life as a handicapped person, while they themselves do not know the experience of being handicapped. Other children will see the child who is handicapped as something to be feared and ridiculed, because they are learning from unenlightened adults the same old attitudes. And because he is a handicapped child, adults will see him as someone to be pitied and babied. When he becomes a handicapped teenager or adult, people will choose to ignore his existence in order not to have to deal with their own feelings.

Relationships with people then, become the responsibility of the handicapped person, if for no other reason than that he is the only person who has the experience of dealing with such encounters where there is included an added negative element to be overcome—that is, his or her handicap. His encounters with persons who will be able to become his friends are subject to the same filteration process that all peoples' possibilities must go through, but his handicap forces some possibilities to go through a filter once more. Thus, a handicapped person can not afford to have any further obstacles to his having relationships with other people, particularly any placed before him by his personality. I, for instance, have felt pressures against being the quiet and shy person I believe myself naturally to be. Since people are most often deterred from wanting to know me

because of my first impression—that is, my disfigured body—I am forced to become the initiator. Also, oftentimes quietness on my part has led people to think that I was withdrawn and inhibited due to my handicap. The problem is that sometimes this is true and sometimes it is not. Thus, I do not have the freedom to be a quiet person in circumstances where other people might be allowed to be. Yet, I also learned that I must move with caution and not reach out to people too eagerly, for there are those people who feel uncomfortable having attention called to them in my presence. If people are staring at me, that means that they are staring at those who are with me as well.

I might also include here my feelings about the matter of staring. In our culture, people are not supposed to look directly at other people—which adds to the discomfort people have about staring. There is also the problem that the person doing the staring feels guilty about doing it and the person being stared at feels attacked. The attitude that I have tried to maintain, since I have been older, is that staring is a way of making familiar something which is unfamiliar. Such reasoning came out of my examination of my own reaction to when I see another handicapped person. I want to stare, too; but I do it out of curiosity and not attack. Still, there are those times when I feel attacked by stares and want to attack back.

But it is acceptance, not attack, which is going to bridge the gap between handicapped and non-handicapped persons. Yet, there are those individuals whose attitude, implicit if not explicit, remains one of rejection of me because I am handicapped. I strive, however, to accept even those who reject me. For I have realized that in essence I reject others when I do not accept their own rejection of me. Therefore, I do not think that it was best for people to console me by saying, "They're just small-minded people, or ignorant," etc. Such a condemning attitude is ineffective, both for me and those to whom it is directed. It unrightfully places me in a position of superiority and also makes me defensive. If I am defensive, I am walled within my own experience and feelings. And thus, I have no empathy for the person rejecting me. But if I do not allow myself to become defensive, I am open to the rejecting person's experience, and thus I am able not only to learn from him, but to help him to deal with his own feelings. Although I see him as an individual, I also see the context within which he is an individual. He is a member of a society in which handicappedness is not a universal, but a uniqueness—a stigmatized one. Knowing this, I can not condemn nor judge him, for he has not actively sought such personal attitudes. Thus when one of my peers says to me, "When I first saw you, I decided then that I did not want to get to know you. I guess this is bad and that I should not feel this way. I'm sorry." I ask him not to apologize or feel guilty, but to accept his feelings without judgment. I assure him that I do not judge or criticize his feelings. After we both have accepted his feelings, it is up to me to help him come to understand them so that in the future they need not be in the way of him and other handicapped people. For I realize that I and others like me are not seen as individuals, but as a stereotype or category. Thus, in order to gain acceptance I must compete against that stereotype. Yet, since I am seen as a stereotype, anything which I may be or do is added to that generalized image. Thus, I have always felt a responsibility to insure that I do not become a detriment to those who may come after me.

It is my hope then, that I have enabled you to feel more comfortable and willing to deal with the emotions surrounding handicappedness for both sides. It is my hope to facilitate honest acceptance and healthy support. As I discussed the handicapped person, I wanted to impress upon you the reality that although he is handicapped, he is as human as those who are not, although while he is human, he is also handicapped. The "humanness" and the "handicappedness" of the person are not separate, for they are integrated throughout his entire existence. Just as man's soul may be surrounded by his body, so is his humanness by his handicaps, whether physical or otherwise.

DEATH

A Definition of Irreversible Coma
The Ad Hoc Committee of the Harvard Medical School*

Our primary purpose is to define irreversible coma as a new criterion for death. There are two reasons why there is need for a definition: (1) Improvements in resuscitative and suppor-

Reprinted by permission of the American Medical Association from *JAMA*, vol. 205, no. 6, August 5, 1968, pp. 337–340. Copyright 1968, American Medical Association.

*The Ad Hoc Committee includes Henry K. Beecher, MD, *chairman;* Raymond D. Adams, MD; A. Clifford Barger, MD; William J. Curran, LLM, SMHyg; Derek Denny-Brown, MD; Dana L. Farnsworth, MD; Jordi Folch-Pi, MD; Everett I. Mendelsohn, PhD; John P. Merrill, MD; Joseph Murray, MD; Ralph Potter, ThD; Robert Schwab, MD; and William Sweet, MD.

tive measures have led to increased efforts to save those who are desperately injured. Sometimes these efforts have only partial success so that the result is an individual whose heart continues to beat but whose brain is irreversibly damaged. The burden is great on patients who suffer permanent loss of intellect, on their families, on the hospitals, and on those in need of hospital beds already occupied by these comatose patients. (2) Obsolete criteria for the definition of death can lead to controversy in obtaining organs for transplantation.

Irreversible coma has many causes, but *we are concerned here only with those comatose individuals who have no discernible central nervous system activity.* If the characteristics can be defined in satisfactory terms, translatable into action—and we believe this is possible—then several problems will either disappear or will become more readily soluble.

More than medical problems are present. There are moral, ethical, religious, and legal issues. Adequate definition here will prepare the way for better insight into all of these matters as well as for better law than is currently applicable.

CHARACTERISTICS OF IRREVERSIBLE COMA

An organ, brain or other, that no longer functions and has no possibility of functioning again is for all practical purposes dead. Our first problem is to determine the characteristics of a *permanently* nonfunctioning brain.

A patient in this state appears to be in deep coma. The condition can be satisfactorily diagnosed by points 1, 2, and 3 to follow. The electroencephalogram (point 4) provides confirmatory data, and when available it should be utilized. In situations where for one reason or another electroencephalographic monitoring is not available, the absence of cerebral function has to be determined by purely clinical signs, to be described, or by absence of circulation as judged by standstill of blood in the retinal vessels, or by absence of cardiac activity.

1.   *Unreceptivity and Unresponsivity.* —There is a total unawareness to externally applied stimuli and inner need and complete unresponsiveness—our definition of irreversible coma. Even the most intensely painful stimuli evoke no vocal or other response, not even a groan, withdrawal of a limb, or quickening of respiration.

2.   *No Movements or Breathing.* —Observations covering a period of at least one hour by physicians is adequate to satisfy the criteria of no spontaneous muscular movements or spontaneous respiration or response to stimuli such as pain, touch, sound, or light. After the patient is on a mechanical respirator, the total absence of spontaneous breathing may be established by turning off the respirator for three minutes

and observing whether there is any effort on the part of the subject to breathe spontaneously. (The respirator may be turned off for this time provided that at the start of the trial period the patient's carbon dioxide tension is within the normal range, and provided also that the patient had been breathing room air for at least 10 minutes prior to the trial.)

3.   *No reflexes.* —Irreversible coma with abolition of central nervous system activity is evidenced in part by the absence of elicitable reflexes. The pupil will be fixed and dilated and will not respond to a direct source of bright light. Since the establishment of a fixed, dilated pupil is clear-cut in clinical practice, there should be no uncertainty as to its presence. Ocular movement (to head turning and to irrigation of the ears with ice water) and blinking are absent. There is no evidence of postural activity (decerebrate or other). Swallowing, yawning, vocalization are in abeyance. Corneal and pharyngeal reflexes are absent.

As a rule the stretch of tendon reflexes cannot be elicited; ie, tapping the tendons of the biceps, triceps, and pronator muscles, quadriceps and gastrocnemius muscles with the reflex hammer elicits no contraction of the respective muscles. Plantar or noxious stimulation gives no response.

4.   *Flat Electroencephalogram.* —Of great confirmatory value is the flat or isoelectric EEG. We must assume that the electrodes have been properly applied, that the apparatus is functioning normally, and that the personnel in charge is competent. We consider it prudent to have one channel of the apparatus used for an electrocardiogram. This channel will monitor the ECG so that, if it appears in the electroencephalographic leads because of high resistance, it can be readily identified. It also establishes the presence of the active heart in the absence of the EEG. We recommend that another channel be used for a noncephalic lead. This will pick up space-borne or vibration-borne artifacts and identify them. The simplest form of such a monitoring noncephalic electrode has two leads over the dorsum of the hand, preferably the right hand, so the ECG will be minimal or absent. Since one of the requirements of this state is that there be no mus-

cle activity, these two dorsal hand electrodes will not be bothered by muscle artifact. The apparatus should be run at standard gains $10\mu v/mm$, $50\mu v/5$ mm. Also it should be isoelectric at double this standard gain which is $5\mu v/mm$ or $25\mu v/5$ mm. At least ten full minutes of recording are desirable, but twice that would be better.

It is also suggested that the gains at some point be opened to their full amplitude for a brief period (5 to 100 seconds) to see what is going on. Usually in an intensive care unit artifacts will dominate the picture, but these are readily identifiable. There shall be no electroencaphalographic response to noise or to pinch.

All of the above tests shall be repeated at least 24 hours later with no change.

The validity of such data as indications of irreversible cerebral damage depends on the exclusion of two conditions: hypothermia (temperature below 90 F [32.2 C]) or central nervous system depressants, such as barbiturates.

OTHER PROCEDURES

The patient's condition can be determined only by a physician. When the patient is hopelessly damaged as defined above, the family and all colleagues who have participated in major decisions concerning the patient, and all nurses involved, should be so informed. Death is to be declared and *then* the respirator turned off. The decision to do this and the responsibility for it are to be taken by the physician-in-charge, in consultation with one or more physicians who have been directly involved in the case. It is unsound and undesirable to force the family to make the decision.

LEGAL COMMENTARY

The legal system of the United States is greatly in need of the kind of analysis and recommendations for medical procedures in cases of irreversible brain damage as described. At present, the law of the United States, in all 50 states and in the federal courts, treats the question of human death as a question of fact to be decided in every case. When any doubt exists, the courts seek medical expert testimony concerning the time of death of the parcicular individual involved. However, the law makes the assumption that the medical criteria for determining death are settled and not in doubt among physicians. Furthermore, the law assumes that the traditional method among physicians for determination of death is to ascertain the absence of all vital signs. To this extent, *Black's Law Dictionary* (fourth edition, 1951) defines death as

> The cessation of life; the ceasing to exist; *defined by physicians* as a total stoppage of the circulation of the blood, and a cessation of the animal and vital functions consequent thereupon, such as respiration, pulsation, etc [italics added]

In the few modern court decisions involving a definition of death, the courts have used the concept of the total cessation of all vital signs. Two cases are worthy of examination. Both involved the issue of which one of two persons died first.

In *Thomas vs Anderson*, (96 Cal App 2d 371, 211 P 2d 478) a California District Court of Appeal in 1950 said, "In the instant case the question as to which of the two men died first was a question of fact for the determination of the trial court . . ."

The appellate court cited and quoted in full the definition of death from *Black's Law Dictionary* and concluded, ". . . death occurs precisely when life ceases and does not occur until the heart stops beating and respiration ends. Death is not a continuous event and is an event that takes place at a precise time."

The other case is *Smith vs Smith* (229 Ark, 579, 317 SW 2d 275) decided in 1958 by the Supreme Court of Arkansas. In this case the two people were husband and wife involved in an auto accident. The husband was found dead at the scene of the accident. The wife was taken to the hospital unconscious. It is alleged that she "remained in coma due to brain injury" and died at the hospital 17 days later. The petitioner in court tried to argue that the two people died simultaneously. The judge writing the opinion said the petition contained a "quite unusual and unique allegation." It was quoted as follows:

> That the said Hugh Smith and his wife, Lucy Coleman Smith, were in an automobile accident on the 19th day of April, 1957, said accident being instantly fatal to each of them at the same time, although the doctors maintained a vain hope of survival and made every effort to revive and resuscitate said Lucy Coleman Smith until May 6th, 1957, when it was finally determined by the attending physicians that their hope of resuscitation and possible restoration of human life to the said Lucy Coleman Smith was entirely vain, and
>
> That as a matter of modern medical science, your petitioner alleges and states, and will offer the Court competent proof that the said Hugh Smith, deceased, and said Lucy Coleman Smith, deceased, lost their power to will at the same instant, and that their demise as earthly human beings occurred at the same time in said automobile accident, neither of them ever regaining any consciousness whatsoever.

The court dismissed the petition as a *matter of law*. The court quoted *Black's* definition of death and concluded,

> Admittedly, this condition did not exist, and as a matter of fact, it would be too much of a strain of credulity for us to believe any evidence offered to the effect that Mrs. Smith was dead, scientifically or otherwise, unless the conditions set out in the definition existed.

Later in the opinion the court said, "Likewise, we take judicial notice that one breathing, though unconscious, is not dead."

"Judicial notice" of this definition of death means that the court did not consider that definition open to serious controversy; it considered the question as settled in responsible scientific and medical circles. The judge thus makes proof of uncontroverted facts unnecessary so as to prevent prolonging the trial with unnecessary proof and also to prevent fraud being committed upon the court by quasi "scientists" being called into court to controvert settled scientific principles at a price. Here, the Arkansas Supreme Court considered the definition of death to be a settled, scientific, biological fact. It refused to consider the plaintiff's offer of evidence that "modern medical science" might say otherwise. In simplified form, the above is the state of the law in the United States concerning the definition of death.

In this report, however, we suggest that responsible medical opinion is ready to adopt new criteria for pronouncing death to have occurred in an individual sustaining irreversible coma as a result of permanent brain damage. If this position is adopted by the medical community, it can form the basis for change in the current legal concept of death. No statutory change in the law should be necessary since the law treats this question essentially as one of fact to be determined by physicians. The only circumstance in which it would be necessary that legislation be offered in the various states to define "death" by law would be in the event that great controversy were engendered surrounding the subject and physicians were unable to agree on the new medical criteria.

It is recommended as a part of these procedures that judgment of the existence of these criteria is solely a medical issue. It is suggested that the physician in charge of the patient consult with one or more other physicians directly involved in the case before the patient is declared dead on the basis of these criteria. In this way, the responsibility is shared over a wider range of medical opinion, thus providing an important degree of protection against later questions which might be raised about the particular case. It is further suggested that the decision to declare the person dead, and then to turn off the respirator, be made by physicians not involved in any later effort to transplant organs or tissue from the deceased individual. This is advisable in order to avoid any appearance of self-interest by the physicians involved.

It should be emphasized that we recommend the patient be declared dead before any effort is made to take him off a respirator, if he is then on a respirator. This declaration should not be delayed until he has been taken off the respirator and all artificially stimulated signs have ceased. The reason for this recommendation is that in our judgment it will provide a greater degree of legal protection to those involved. Otherwise, the physicians would be turning off the respirator on a person who is, under the present strict, technical application of law, still alive.

COMMENT

Irreversible coma can have various causes: cardiac arrest; asphyxia with respiratory arrest; massive brain damage; intracranial lesions, neoplastic or vascular. It can be produced by other encephalopathic states such as the metabolic derangements associated, for example, with uremia. Respiratory failure and impaired circulation underlie all of these conditions. They result in hypoxia and ischemia of the brain.

From ancient times down to the recent past it was clear that, when the respiration and heart stopped, the brain would die in a few minutes; so the obvious criterion of no heart beat as synonymous with death was sufficiently accurate. In those times the heart was considered to be the central organ of the body; it is not surprising that its failure marked the onset of death. This is no longer valid when modern resuscitative and supportive measures are used. These improved activities can now restore "life" as judged by the ancient standards of persistent respiration and continuing heart beat. This can be the case even when there is not the remotest possibility of an individual recovering consciousness following massive brain damage. In other situations "life" can be maintained only by means of artificial respiration and electrical stimulation of the heart beat, or in temporarily by-passing the heart, or, in conjunction with these things, reducing with cold the body's oxygen requirement.

In an address, "The Prolongation of Life," (1957),[1] Pope Pius XII raised many questions; some conclusions stand out: (1) In a deeply unconscious individual vital functions may be maintained over a prolonged period only by extraordinary means. Verification of the moment of death can be determined, if at all, only by a physician. Some have suggested that the moment of death is the moment when irreparable and overwhelming brain damage occurs. Pius XII acknowledged that it is not "within the competence of the Church" to determine this. (2) It is incumbent on the physician to take all reasonable, ordinary means of restoring the spontaneous vital functions and consciousness, and to employ such extraordinary means as are available to him to this end. It is not obligatory, however, to continue to use extraordinary means indefinitely in hopeless cases. "But normally one is held to use only ordinary means—according to circumstances of persons, places, times, and cultures—that is to say, means that do not involve any grave burden for oneself or another." It is the church's view that a time comes when resuscitative efforts should stop and death be unopposed.

SUMMARY

The neurological impairment to which the terms "brain death syndrome" and "irreversible coma" have become attached indicates diffuse disease. Function is abolished at cerebral, brain-stem, and often spinal levels. This should be evident in all cases from clinical examination alone. Cerebral, cortical, and thalamic involvement are indicated by a complete absence of receptivity of all forms of sensory stimulation and a lack of response to stimuli and to inner need. The term "coma" is used to designate this state of unreceptivity and unresponsivity. But there is always coincident paralysis of brain-stem and basal ganglionic mechanisms as manifested by an abolition of all postural reflexes, including induced decerebrate postures; a complete paralysis of respiration; widely dilated, fixed pupils; paralysis of ocular movements; swallowing; phonation; face and tongue muscles. Involvement of spinal cord, which is less constant, is reflected usually in loss of tendon reflex and all flexor withdrawal or nocifensive reflexes. Of the brain-stem-spinal mechanisms which are conserved for a time, the vasomotor reflexes are the most persistent, and they are responsible in part for the paradoxical state of retained cardiovascular function, which is to some extent independent of nervous control, in the face of widespread disorder of cerebrum, brain stem, and spinal cord.

Neurological assessment gains in reliability if the aforementioned neurological signs persist over a period of time, with the additional safeguards that there is no accompanying hypothermia or evidence of drug intoxication. If either of the latter two conditions exist, interpretation of the neurological state should await the return of body temperature to normal level and elimination of the intoxicating agent.

Under any other circumstances, repeated examinations over a period of 24 hours or longer should be required in order to obtain evidence of the irreversibility of the condition.

Notes

1. Pius XII: The Prolongation of Life, *Pope Speaks* 4:393–398 (No. 4) 1958.

The Concept of Death: Tradition and Alternative

R. B. Schiffer

> If we are aware of what indicates life, which everyone may be supposed to know, though perhaps no one can say that he truly and clearly understands what constitutes it, we at once arrive at the discrimination of death. It is the cessation of the phenomena with which we are so especially familiar—the phenomena of life. [J. G. Smith, *Principles of Forensic Medicine* (London, 1821)]

Although some problems in philosophy seem to remain the same from decade to decade, the problem of defining death has proven a relatively new obstacle for the philosophy of medicine. Where once there was no problem, now discussion is widespread and disagreement the rule. One finds variability across major medical centers in encoded criteria for determining death, and variability in legislative definition across states (Kennedy 1971). This is a philosophic problem with important practical implications. It is the purpose of this paper to clarify some of the issues involved in the debate, and to provide arguments in favor of a central nervous system—oriented definition of death.

Part of the problem has to do with the distinction between the statement of a concept for a state of affairs, for an object, or for anything, and the statement of the criteria for that concept. The Ad Hoc Committee of the Harvard Medical School introduced this confusion into the debate with the opening sentence of their 1968 Report (Beecher 1968): "Our primary purpose is to define irreversible coma as a new

Reprinted with permission of the author and *The Journal of Medicine & Philosophy*, vol. 3, no. 1, 1978, pp. 24–37.

criterion for death.'' One defines a concept by giving a statement of what it is, or of what it means. Thus one might define the state of rheumatic fever by saying, ''For any patient, that patient is in a state of rheumatic fever if and only if that patient is in the state of having an autoimmune, inflammatory reaction following a Group A strep infection.'' But when one states the criteria for a given concept, one lists a family of features which can signal the presence of the conceptualized state. Thus one might list the Jones criteria, which are used to diagnose rheumatic fever: carditis, polyarthritis, chorea, etc. Wittgenstein (1958) helped us with this distinction when he characterized a criterion: ''A criterion for a given thing's being so is something that can show the thing to be so, and show by its absence that the thing is not so; it is something by which one may be justified in saying that the thing is so and by whose absence one may be justified in saying that the thing is not so.'' The point is that a definition for a given state of affairs, such as the state of death, is not the same as the criteria for the state. A concept is an idea; a criterion must be an observable. These two notions are interrelated, of course, as by a family relationship to which no single criterion is essential, but to which each contributes. And criteria, no matter how carefully selected, may err. A patient may have rheumatic fever in fact, yet not fit the criteria. We seem to believe, however, that the state of affairs is what it is, and is either present or absent without necessary regard for what the criteria say.

Perhaps because they did not fully appreciate this distinction, the Harvard Committee initiated the debate over the problem of defining death at both levels: criteria and concept. The characteristics of irreversible coma which they listed (unreceptivity and unresponsivity, no movements or breathing, no reflexes, flat EEG) clearly refer to observable features, and are meant to function as criteria. However, these are the criteria for irreversible coma, the state of having a "permanently nonfunctioning brain." When the committee stated that any patient meeting these criteria should be declared dead, they were also proposing a new concept for death itself; that it is a state of irreversible coma. Although this last point was less emphasized in their paper, it may have been the more significant. For once we agree on what death *is* as a state, we will be able to work toward a set of acceptable criteria. But it is just this agreement at the conceptual level which has proved elusive over the eight years subsequent to the committee's report.

Once the debate over the definition of death has been joined at the conceptual level, one often finds that the debaters are soon talking about life instead—personal life. This is an important point, one which lays the ground rules for the discussion. J. G. Smith, as quoted in the epigraph to this paper, appreciated this point in saying, "If we are aware of what indicates life . . . we at once arrive at the discrimination of death." Death is the *absence* for which life is the *presence*. Veatch (1975) has recently called this the "formal definition" of death, and stated it as, "Death is the irreversible loss of that which is essentially significant to the nature of man." As Veatch indicates in his formal definition, the life which is at issue is life at a high level of organization, the living "nature of man," or life as human personal life. Of course, there is also human life at other organizational levels, such as cellular or biochemical. But it is not cellular or biochemical death of which we are speaking; rather the death of the person. Therefore, it is the meaning of human personal life as a concept which is at issue in understanding the concept of death. The features essential to human personal life will show, through their absence, the concept of death.

It is just this direction which the current debate over the definition of death has taken. Veatch, in the same article, suggested the following features as those essential to personal life: the capacity to integrate bodily function, the capacity for rationality, and the capacity to experience. Dr. H. K. Beecher, the chairman of the Ad Hoc Committee, produced a different list of features, stating that a person is dead when he has lost his "personality, his conscious life, his uniqueness, his capacity for remembering, judging, reasoning, acting, enjoying, worrying, and so on" (Beecher 1970, as quoted in Veatch 1975). Fletcher has also written at some length upon this subject, and in his last article (Fletcher 1974) listed fifteen positive "indicators of humanhood," ranging from "a sense of the past" to "idiosyncrasy."

My objection is not with the thrust of these writings, but with the difficulty of choosing among them. Why is one list or one feature "better" than any other? Surely these features are compellingly important in our estimation of what goes into a human person, but the issue here is the *essence* of that person, that minimum feature(s) without which a person would not be a person. This is not a literary use of the term "essence," but a philosophical one, and philosophical arguments are required to defend the naming of any feature as a feature essential to personal life. None of the authors quoted above offers such arguments. It is the purpose of this paper to offer a central nervous system-oriented definition of death based upon the absence of a single feature from personal life, and to offer arguments to justify the choice of this feature. First, however, it may be worthwhile to examine the more traditional concept of death, that oriented to cardiac and respiratory function, to indicate some of its shortcomings.

THE CARDIORESPIRATORY CONCEPT

Despite a good deal of recent discussion, it is difficult to find a clear statement of the cardiorespiratory definition of death. It has been referred to as the "concept which focuses on the hearts and lungs" (Veatch 1975), and its essential features have been stated as "the respiratory movements and heart contractions" (Jonas 1974). The only more explicit statement of this particular death concept is that offered by Black's Law Dictionary (4th ed., 1951), defining death as "the cessation of life; the ceasing to exist; defined by physicians as a total stoppage of the circulation of the blood, and a cessation of the animal and vital functions consequent thereon, such as respiration, pulsation, etc." And this statement is at best philosophically misleading, since its first two phrases are tautologous, and its closing list of "vital functions" is capable of endless extension.

Let me suggest that the fundamental intuition concerning features essential to personal life within the cardiorespiratory-oriented death concept is that concerning the flow of vital fluids, both respiratory and circulatory. Spontaneity does not seem to be an essential feature, nor does there seem any compelling reason why artificial systems cannot provide the vital flows, as long as those flows continue. The concept statement then becomes, "X is in a state of death if and only if both respiratory and circulatory fluids have irreversibly ceased to flow." The claim here is that, although the loss of each separate fluid's flow is an essential feature of the death state, both features are required for sufficiency of the statement. The criteria of the concept seem to be understood as "cardiac pulsation" and "respiratory excursion," each of which refers to a standard set of procedures and observations in order to determine its presence or absence.

What is to be said about this concept statement? First, we should ask whether it is true. That is, would the set of features in the definiens always pick out the concept state and only that state, in any conceivable circumstance? These truth requirements are the logical requirements of necessity and sufficiency, and no empirical counterexample need be given to prove the concept statement false, but only a conceivable one. I would like to offer two paradigmatic cases which suggest that the cardiorespiratory definition of death is neither necessary nor sufficient to the concept defined.

Case A. A person X at time t_1 has the following properties at time t_2 in the operating room:

(1) Cardiorespiratory functions are provided in their entirety by extracorporeal pump and oxygenator. (2) The last closure sutures are being inserted in a massive, posterior, midline incision from occipital pole to sacrum. Through this incision the entire central nervous system has been removed in pieces, and sent to Anatomy for medical student use. No upper motor, association, or preganglionic neurons remain within X; X is completely flaccid and limp; pupils fixed and dilated; no spontaneous movement or reflex of any sort; flat EEG; no response to any stimulation.

Case B. A person X at time t_1 has the following properties at time t_2: (1) No respiratory movements discernible over a prolonged period of time by any of the usual, observational procedures. (2) No cardiac pulsations can be identified. There is no apical impulse; no radial pulse; no auscultatory evidence of vascular flow. (3) Despite properties 1 and 2, X shows clear evidence of a continuing, responsive consciousness. When addressed, X slowly rolls his eyes toward the speaker, moves his lips just perceptibly, and emits appropriate replies in a voice which seems to come from deep within. He also conveys sensation reports, concerning feelings of coldness, and of pain when his legs are tested with a pin.

Case A attempts to clarify the basic issues actually presented by an increasing number of cases which are considered candidates for a brain-oriented concept of death of some sort.[1] In these cases, the "patient" does not have the features which would justify a death pronouncement under the cardiorespiratory concept, but seems clearly to have lost most of what is fundamental to our notion of "person" or "personal life." The question is whether we can say that case A describes a living person. Of course, there will be some living cellular systems in case A as long as the cardiorespiratory support is continued, and for a while thereafter. This is not the issue. The issue is the life of the whole person. Is this a living person? Or is the person dead, leaving only some nonessential cellular systems behind? Although some would say that case A does describe a living person, a growing group of people, particularly within the medical profession, would say that it does not. This group contends that the cardiorespiratory death concept fails the logical requirement of necessity; the features it identifies (absence of cardiac and respiratory functions) do not seem necessary to the concept they define, because cases similar to A exist as counterexamples. For those who hold rigorously to the cardiorespiratory death concept in the face of examples such as A, the debate must shift to the notion of personhood, and to the features which are philosophically essential to a living person. For if cardiac and respiratory functions are not essential features of what we mean by "living person," then there is no basis for defining death as their absence. Case B is meant to suggest that these functions are, indeed, nonessential components of personhood.

Case B sounds a little fanciful, and I do not pretend to have encountered such a case in an intensive care unit, or elsewhere. It draws upon Edgar Allen Poe's fictional description of a patient mesmerized at the moment of death in "The Facts in the Case of M. Valdemar" (Poe [1846] 1944). And for the purposes of logical argument, all that is required is that the case be clearly described, and not self-contradictory in its content. There is no doubt that we *can* imagine such a case. The question is, do we want to say that this "person" is dead? The case clearly fits the cardiorespiratory concept of death, as stated above. But isn't there something about case B which makes it seem closer to our notion of personal life than the "person" described in case A? Of course, this question remains at the level of "notions" of personal life, and intuitions about what persons are. No arguments have yet been offered concerning which features of personal life may indeed be the essential features. It does seem, however, that there is something about case B which prevents us from saying that personal life is clearly absent. To this extent, the cardiorespiratory death concept fails the logical requirement of sufficiency: a state description may meet the features required by the concept, yet leave us in doubt as to whether the defined concept applies. Poe, by the way, was not sure whether to call M. Valdemar "dead" until the trance was terminated after several months and the "person" collapsed in putrefaction.

THE CNS CONCEPT

Suggestions come before arguments and make them possible. Cases A and B are intended to suggest to the reader that the traditional, cardiorespiratory death concept fails at the conceptual level; that a death concept statement using the features of absent respiratory and vascular flow is a statement neither necessary nor sufficient to the concept defined. Those who would take up this suggestion contend that a cardiorespiratory death definition omits mention of those features which are essential to personal life—features having to do with central nervous system function. Some of the candidates for this list of CNS features, such as "responsivity," "the capacity for experience and social interaction," "subjectivity," and "intelligence" have been mentioned above. The contention is that a death concept statement based upon the absence of some such list of nervous system features will avoid the difficulties posed by cases A and B: in no actual or imagined case would such a definition fail to diagnose the state of death. Still, these features of nervous system function are presented as *plausibly, reasonably,* or *intuitively* features essential to personal life. Careful arguments have not been presented, and theorists of cardiorespiratory persuasion remain free to disagree. Let me now present a definition of death based upon a central nervous system feature, and defend that definition with five arguments to show that this feature is, indeed, essential to personal life.

THE DEATH CONCEPT

I propose the following concept statement of death: A former person is in a state of death if and only if he/she has lost irreversibly the property of embodied consciousness. This statement is similar to Veatch's contention that a "man" is dead when he has irreversibly lost the "embodied capacity for experience and social interaction." There are differences. "Person" is substituted for "man" and "human life" because, although there probably are forms of human life which are not persons (zygotes, cell culture systems), we are not interested in defining their death. In addition, the proposed concept statement says nothing of "capacities," and confines itself to a single, necessary feature. Most importantly, arguments will be adduced to support this statement based upon features essential to personhood.

Before turning to the arguments, let me mention my use of the term "person." I use this term, initially, to refer to a usual human being in the fullness of his life. Of course, it is a task of this paper partially to clarify what is meant by "a usual human being in the fullness of his life." To justify the death concept stated above, it must be shown that the feature of having an embodied consciousness is an essential feature of what we mean by "person," in the sense of a usual human being in the fullness of his life. The point is that I am using "person" in a descriptive sense, to refer to a human being with a certain set of factual features, some of which are essential and some of which are contingent. I am specifically excluding moral arguments, or language about values and rights. Presumably values and rights should be accorded to entities, not arbitrarily, but in virtue of factual features which those entities possess. History, through its examples of slaves in our society and Jews in the Third Reich, teaches that this is not necessarily so. At any rate, whether there is an entailment relation between these factual features and rights or values is a question I do not address. What is required for my argument is to show that the possession of an embodied consciousness is the possession of a property which persons must have in order to be persons. Although a single feature is discussed, the following arguments begin with consciousness as a separate aspect of that feature.

1. Argument from Mind–Body Question

Is there something irreducibly psychic about conscious states, events, and features? Does a statement about such states, events, and features report something which could never fully be reported by a statement couched in terms of atoms, molecules, nerve cells, and electrical impulses? If not, it would be odd to contend that consciousness was an essential feature of the human person. One could just as easily say

that the having of a certain set of neurophysical impulses was the feature essential to personhood. If there *is* something irreducibly psychic about features of consciousness, however, *and* a human person is the sort of entity to which at least one such feature is always attributable, then the having of conscious features is an essential personal property.

To ask whether conscious phenomena are irreducibly psychic is to ask what the relationship is between conscious states, events, features, and physical states, events, features. Whatever this relationship may be in fact, all that is required for my point is to show that this relationship cannot be one of "strict identity." Strict identity is usually defined in terms of the principle of the identity of indiscernibles; that two nonsynonymous names or descriptions refer to the same thing if and only if a predicate is truly predicated of one if and only if it is also truly predicated of the other. Unless this principle applies, there are at least some properties correctly attributable to conscious phenomena, which are not correctly attributable to corresponding neurphysical phenomena. And to this extent, one is justified in claiming that there is something irreducibly psychic about the conscious phenomena.

No one would contend that a conscious event, such as the having of a pain, is intensionally, or analytically identical with some neurophysical event. Pains are nagging, sharp, constant, while neurophysical events are discussed in terms of synaptic firing, inhibition, thresholds, etc. One can very well know that he is having a pain, and yet know nothing at all about his neurophysical state. If analytic reasoning is inadequate to identify these events, most psychophysical identity theorists have concluded that such an identity will have to be de facto, if it exists at all. That is, empirical evidence will be required to support the identification. As Jaegwon Kim has pointed out (Kim 1966), however, empirical evidence could never establish the strict identity required by the principle of the identity of indiscernibles. At most, an absolutely comprehensive neurophysical explanation of all conscious states, features, and events would establish a *correlation* between the conscious and physical phenomena. Thus we might know that, whenever a person had a pain, he was at that same time in neurophysical state p. Such evidence might well support a "weaker" sort of identity, such as theoretical identity (Nagel 1965), or functional identity (Fodor 1968), but such evidence could not justify strict identity. It could never give sense to speaking of neurophysical processes as nagging, or dull. Therefore, there are some features of consciousness which are irreducibly psychic.

To say that language about human persons is the same thing as language about entities to which at least some conscious features are always attributable does not seem controversial. And it can be shown that there is at least one such feature (or at least that language must attribute such a feature) by the following examples:

That person Jerry and his motorcycle annoy me.
That person Jerry and his club foot depress me.
That person Jerry and his low back pain bore me.

A motorcycle annoys, a club foot depresses, and a back pain bores, but "Jerry and" all of these is a construction which requires a plural verb. This notion of a person as a potential subject of his possessions, physical states, and mental states seems built into the language. Therefore, there is always at least one irreducibly psychic feature attributable to any person—that of being a potential subject for mental and physical events. Thus, at least some features of consciousness are essential to what we mean by the term "person."

2. Argument from Consciousness as Locus of Personal Identity

When John Dewey wrote in 1886 (Dewey [1886] 1970) that "the soul does not write in water, but in the plastic brain and spinal cord," he was expressing no necessary truth. We can just as well imagine a metaphor of the "soul" written in the heart or lungs. It just happens to be, however, that conscious states and features have an intimate connection with the central nervous system.[2] We need not specify the exact nature of this connection is an essential feature of personhood.

Let us consider a complete description of the person of Richard Milhous Nixon, one includ-

ing the entire set of bodily features and habits, plus the entire set of mentalistic features and states which can be ascribed correctly to this person. Anyone armed with this information, plus any requisite technical skills for comparing descriptions with realities, could measure the real R. M. N. against the description and determine that he was, indeed, "this person."

If R. M. N. has recently had a heart transplant, however, he will no longer fit the exhaustive description in every detail. The heart will be different. Does this mean that he is no longer Richard Milhous Nixon? Clearly not. For persons continuously alter certain details of physical appearance (such as by having a heart transplant), and we have no trouble in identifying them as the "same persons." It would be equivalent to say that, although some features had changed, those features essential to personal identification had not changed.

What if the real R. M. N. now experiences a catastrophic automobile accident, severing both legs, both arms, and badly mutilating his face? An interviewer, using the complete description noted above, would find a number of discrepancies. He would certainly say that R. M. N. had changed significantly. But after an extensive interview, could he say that he was unable to identify this person as R. M. N. any longer? This seems doubtful. Catastrophes such as this occur all too frequently, but they do not provide problems in personal identification.

But now, what if we imagine our interviewer confronted by an "R. M. M." who has had a complete central nervous system transplantation, and who has received the CNS of George McGovern? This new subject would match the physical description fairly well, but he would have all of George McGovern's attitudes, beliefs, dispositions, and knowledge. After an exhaustive interview, could a reasonable man identify this person as R. M. N.? This seems unlikely. That is not to say that he would have an easier time identifying this person as George McGovern, which would be the case if the set of CNS functions were the same thing as the person. The example does indicate, however, that by changing the total set of CNS functions, features have been changed which seem essential to our process of identifying persons.

If the above example is compelling, it shows that at least some states and features of consciousness (attitudes, beliefs, knowledge) are essential to personal identity. Without some unspecified level of constancy in these features, we just cannot pick someone out as "the same person." And if these features are essential to the identity of a person, they are essential features of the person as well. For it is unclear what might be different between a concept statement for a particular person, and an identity statement for that same person.[3]

3. Argument that Consciousness Is Essential from the Nature of Embodiment

Persons are embodied. Leaving aside temporarily the question of whether this is necessarily so, we can ask whether there is something about the embodiment of persons which requires consciousness essentially. That is, can we even make sense of the notion, "embodied person" without adding to that notion features and states of consciousness? It is my contention that we cannot.

There is a disingenuous sense of embodiment of which we are not speaking. The still, stark embodiment of the decomposing corpse; the unmoving, objective embodiment described in case A above; this is not the sense of embodiment at issue. For in these cases personhood is in doubt. There is something about the embodiment in these cases which seems to say, "no person here." The question then becomes, what is it about the usual, embodied person which is different; which shows conscious life at work? The instructor at the blackboard writes his signature through broad, sweeping strokes of arm and shoulder movements. None of the fine musculature of the hand which customarily demonstrates this signature is involved in the act. Yet the signature writ large is of the same character as the small signature; an indelibly personal character. What does this mean? One can turn his attention away from the bodies of other persons, to experience his own body in action. Then one notices that this body in action, this hand performing its task of signature writing, absolutely cannot be understood

in the same way as other, external, physical objects. The shoulder muscles, though they have never demonstrated a signature before, yet seem to "know how" to produce the same personal signature. Previous learning, or previously reinforced neural circuitry provide no explanation, for neither has occurred. What one senses is that by its very movements, and through them, this arm has an awareness of the external world in which it is engaged. This is what these movements *mean*. Merleau-Ponty has termed this bodily awareness which is sensed through action, "praktognosia," and has stated that "the plunge into action is, from the subject's point of view, an original way of relating himself to the object, and is on the same footing as perception" (Merleau-Ponty 1962).

It is more difficult to make the same point concerning the embodiment of other persons as we encounter them in daily life. If we remove ourselves to a purely objective standpoint, it seems that we can imagine the subtly sensitive responsiveness of a loved one as just so much behavior, without conscious states and intentions underlying. The questions would remain, however, whether behavior so understood would not have a fundamentally different meaning from personal behavior as actually encountered, and whether something essential to the meaning of that personal behavior had been left out. Engelhardt (Engelhardt 1975) has recently contended that such a purely objective understanding of others' personal behavior does represent such an essentially changed understanding. Whether this point can be made convincingly or not, it still seems that there are cases, such as the example concerning signatures above, in which consciousness or awareness is right there—an essential part of the physical action—rather than as a potential ghost lurking behind.

ARGUMENTS THAT EMBODIMENT IS ESSENTIAL

The contention of this paper is that the possession of an embodied consciousness, as a single feature, is the possession of a feature essential to human persons. Although I have discussed first some arguments for considering consciousness a necessary feature, it is clear that personal consciousness cannot be considered fully apart from the embodiment which it partly is. An "inverted glimpse" of this point was provided by argument 3 above, where it was suggested that the notion of personal embodiment includes within it the notion of consciousness. If we ask now whether embodiment is a necessary feature of personhood, we find that the answer is "yes"—by the nature of consciousness. Two arguments follow.

4. Argument from Perspective

Most philosophers agree that it is possible to imagine a disembodied consciousness. The argument then runs that by this fact we have proved embodiment to be merely contingently and unnecessarily connected with consciousness. I doubt that we can imagine a disembodied consciousness at all. Or if we can, such a disembodied consciousness would be so qualitatively different from the embodied consciousness we know that the necessity of embodiment to personal consciousness would be proved instead of its contingency.

A person's every conscious act has a point of view. A sighting, a smelling, a grasping; each refers necessarily to a place from which the act occurred. This place is the place of the person's body. H. T. Engelhardt (1975) has made this point explicit: "Our place in the world is our bodies, which feel, see, hear, taste, and smell. We feel, see, hear, taste, and smell the world from a perspective which is always our body's perspective or that of some extension of our body. At any time we are always at a space, and in any space we are always in a time. And our time and space in the world are the time and space of our bodies. Experience and action, thus, are always perspectival" (p. 488).

A person's every conscious act has the perspective which his body provides. To see, hear, taste, and smell the world is the same thing as to be this body which sees, hears, tastes, and smells the world. We tell ourselves in a facile manner that we can easily imagine a perspective which is not a physical perspective, from a place at which our bodies would not be. But En-

gelhardt's description of the fundamental sameness of "personal counscious act" and "bodily conscious act" helps us to see that this is a false claim. When I imagine a point of view upon these circumstances which might exist upon the moon, it is still this eye which I imagine to do the looking, and I imagine that things would appear as they appear to this eye. I cannot do otherwise, because I do not know what it would mean to speak of a visual perspective which was not a potentially physical perspective; the perspective of this eye. Therefore, embodiment is a necessary part of what is meant by personal consciousness.

5. Argument from the Location of Mental Events

Can we even think of a mental event without thinking of that event as having a location? Would it make sense to speak of a pain, a thought, or a longing, and then to claim that it had occurred nowhere? It does not seem that this is possible.

Of course, a neurophysiologist might claim that such events are to be located in terms of CNS circuitry, so we could say that one particular event just now occurred in the temporal lobe of a certain person. This sort of locating seems odd for such events, however. Would it make sense to say that my sudden fear was located in the middle gyrus of my left temporal lobe? How could it, while the fear belongs to all of me, as a person, and not to any part? Still, it seems clear that the fear did have a location—that of my person. And this location seems to have been that entire person, from the thoughts which were interrupted to the erector pilae muscles which straightened the hairs of the forearm.

And just as clearly, it seems required that a mental event be located in terms of the person to whom it occurs. As Shaffer (1966) has put it, "It is a logically essential feature of a mental event that it occurs to a particular person, and to pick it out uniquely we must indicate *whose* mental event it was. It is senseless to say that just that mental event might have occurred, all right, but not to the person to whom it occurred" (p. 66).

The last step in this argument is to note that

this personal location could not be in terms of personal consciousness alone (which, without embodiment, would be without location) but must be in terms of an embodied consciousness. There is no other way to understand the statement, ''just this mental event occurred at just that personal location.'' Therefore, embodiment is an essential feature of what is meant by personal consciousness.

Arguments 1–5 have been designed to show that the having of an embodied consciousness is the having of a feature essential to personal life. Thus, a death definition based upon the irreversible loss of the feature of embodied consciousness, as proposed, is a definition based upon the loss of a feature essential to personal life. In this respect, this definition is superior to the traditional cardiorespiratory definition, which was based upon important, but not essential, features. Some closing observations are in order.

It may be that there are persons who are not human persons. Martians come to mind. I see no reason why the arguments and death concept would not apply equally well to them.

The arguments, especially numbers 4 and 5, make clear why we cannot treat ''brain death'' cases in a way which some have advocated—by declaring the ''person'' dead but the ''body'' alive. Such statements conjure views of a person/body dualism to replace the older mind/body dualism. This is untenable. Of course, pieces may be cultured and maintained after the death of the whole person. But the sense of ''bodily life'' here is not the sense of ''personal bodily life.''

And last, it should be pointed out that proving a feature *necessary* to personal life does not prove that feature *sufficient*. Indeed, the having of an embodied consciousness seems clearly an insufficient ground of personhood for those who maintain that persons are qualitatively different from other animal life. For we do not doubt that animals have an embodied consciousness of some kind, do we? The question then becomes whether there are some other features of human persons which we can add to the death concept in order to ''tighten'' its grasp of personal death as opposed to merely animal death. I doubt that this can be done, although

something called ''self-consciousness'' is often mentioned as setting persons apart from animals.[4] In any event, this is not required. A death concept which applies broadly to animal life, such as the above, is much more useful than one specially designed for personal life alone. After all, should we not require that man and ape be equally dead before we pronounce them so?

Notes

1. For a recent article giving full medical and pathologic details of two such cases, see Brierly et al. (1971).
2. See especially classical works by Fritzsch and Hitzig, Paul Broca, Carl Wernicke, Josef Gerstmann (1927).
3. For a similar example, see Quinton (1962).
4. Michael Tooley (1974) has recently offered such a contention.

References

BEECHER, H. K. ''A Definition of Irreversible Coma: Report of the Ad Hoc Committee of the Harvard Medical School to Examine the Definition of Brain Death.'' *Journal of the American Medical Association* 205, no. 6 (August 1968): 337–40.

BEECHER, H. K. ''The New Definition of Death: Some Opposing Views,'' Paper presented to the annual meeting of the American Association for the Advancement of Science, December 1970.

BRIERLY, J. B., et al. ''Neocortical Death after Cardiac Arrest.'' *Lancet* (September 11, 1971), pp. 560–65.

DEWEY, JOHN, ''Soul and Body.'' In *The Philosophy of the Body,* edited by Stuart Spicker, New York: Quadrangle/New York Times Book Co., 1970.

ENGELHARDT, H. T., JR. ''Bioethics and the Process of Embodiment.'' *Perspectives in Biology and Medicine* 18, no. 4 (Summer 1975): 486–500.

FLETCHER, J. F. ''Four Indicators of Humanhood: The Enquiry Matures.'' *Hastings Center Report* 4, no. 6 (December 1974): 4–7.

FODOR, JERRY. ''Materialism.'' In *Psychological Explanation.* New York: Random House, 1968.

JONAS, HANS. ''Against the Stream: Comments on the Definition and Redefinition of Death.'' In

Philosophical Essays: From Ancient Creed to Technological Man. Englewood Cliffs, N.J.: Prentice-Hall, Inc., 1974.

KENNEDY, IAN McCOLL. "The Kansas Statute on Death: An Appraisal." *New England Journal of Medicine* 285 (October 1971): 946–50.

KIM, JAEGWON. "On the Psycho-Physical Identity Theory." *American Philosophical Quarterly* 3, no. 3 (July 1966): 227–35.

MERLEAU-PONTY, M. *Phenomenology of Perception.* New York: Humanities Press, 1962.

NAGEL, THOMAS. "Physicalism." *Philosophical Review* 74, no. 3 (July 1965): 339–56.

POE, EDGAR ALLEN. "The Facts in the Case of M. Valdemar." In *Great Tales of Terror and the Supernatural,* edited by Herbert A. Wise. New York: Modern Library, Random House, 1944.

QUINTON, A. "The Soul." *Journal of Philosphy* 59 (1962): 401.

SHAFFER, JEROME. "Persons and Their Bodies." *Philosophical Review* 75 (January 1966): 59–79.

TOOLEY, MICHAEL. "Abortion and Infanticide." In *The Rights and Wrongs of Abortion.* Princeton, N.J.: Princeton University Press, 1974.

VEATCH, ROBERT M. "The Whole-Brain-oriented Concept of Death: An Outmoded Philosophical Formulation." *Journal of Thanatology* 3 (1975): 13–30.

WITTGENSTEIN, L. *Philosophical Investigations.* 2d ed. Translated by G. E. M. Anscombe. New York: Macmillan Co., 1958.

From *Epistula Morales,* "On Suicide"

Seneca (1st Century A.D.*)*

. . . life has carried some men with the greatest rapidity to the harbour, the harbour they were bound to reach even if they tarried on the way, while others it has fretted and harassed. To such a life, as you are aware, one should not always cling. For mere living is not a good, but living well. Accordingly, the wise man will live as long as he ought, not as long as he can. He will mark in what place, with whom, and how he is to conduct his existence, and what he is about to do. He always reflects concerning the quality, and

Reprinted from *Ethical Choice,* eds. R. N. Beck and J. B. Orr (New York: The Free Press, 1970), p. 54, with permission of the publisher and The Loeb Classical Library, from *Epistula Morales* Vol. II, trans. R. M. Gumere (Cambridge: Harvard University Press, 1920).

not the quantity, of his life. As soon as there are many events in his life that give him trouble and disturb his peace of mind, he sets himself free. And this privilege is his, not only when the crisis is upon him, but as soon as Fortune seems to be playing him false; then he looks about carefully and sees whether he ought, or ought not, to end his life on that account. He holds that it makes no difference to him whether his taking-off be natural or self-inflicted, whether it comes later or earlier. He does not regard it with fear, as if it were a great loss; for no man can lose very much when but a driblet remains. It is not a question of dying earlier or later, but of dying well or ill. And dying well means escape from the danger of living ill.

Duties Towards the Body in Regard to Life

Immanuel Kant

What are our powers of disposal over our life? Have we any authority of disposal over it in any shape or form? How far is it incumbent upon us to take care of it? These are questions which fall to be considered in connexion with our duties towards the body in regard to life. We must, however, by way of introduction, make the following observations. If the body were related to life not as a condition but as an accident or circumstance so that we could at will divest ourselves of it; if we could slip out of it and slip into another just as we leave one country for another, then the body would be subject to our free will and we could rightly have the disposal of it. This, however, would not imply that we could similarly dispose of our life, but only of our circumstances, of the movable goods, the furniture of life. In fact, however, our life is entirely conditioned by our body, so that we cannot

Reprinted by permission of the publisher from Immanuel Kant, *Lectures on Ethics,* trans. Louis Infield (New York: Harper & Row, 1963), pp. 147–48.

not conceive of a life not mediated by the body and we cannot make use of our freedom except through the body. It is, therefore, obvious that the body constitutes a part of ourselves. If a man destroys his body, and so his life, he does it by the use of his will, which is itself destroyed in the process. But to use the power of a free will for its own destruction is self-contradictory. If freedom is the condition of life it cannot be employed to abolish life and so to destroy and abolish itself. To use life for its own destruction, to use life for producing lifelessness, is self-contradictory. These preliminary remarks are sufficient to show that man cannot rightly have any power of disposal in regard to himself and his life, but only in regard to his circumstances. His body gives man power over his life; were he a spirit he could not destroy his life; life in the absolute has been invested by nature with indestructibility and is an end in itself; hence it follows that man cannot have the power to dispose of his life.

Suicide

Immanuel Kant

Suicide can be regarded in various lights; it might be held to be reprehensible, or permissible, or even heroic. In the first place we have the specious view that suicide can be allowed and tolerated. Its advocates argue thus. So long as he does not violate the proprietary rights of others, man is a free agent. With regard to his body there are various things he can properly do; he can have a boil lanced or a limb amputated, and disregard a scar; he is, in fact, free to

Reprinted by permission of the publisher from Immanuel Kant, *Lectures on Ethics,* trans. Louis Infield (New York: Harper & Row, 1963), pp. 148–154.

do whatever he may consider useful and advisable. If then he comes to the conclusion that the most useful and advisable thing that he can do is to put an end to his life, why should he not be entitled to do so? Why not, if he sees that he can no longer go on living and that he will be ridding himself of misfortune, torment and disgrace? To be sure he robs himself of a full life, but he escapes once and for all from calamity and misfortune. The argument sounds most plausible. But let us, leaving aside religious considerations, examine the act itself. We may treat our body as we please, provided our motives are those of self-preservation. If, for instance, his foot is a hindrance to life, a man might have it amputated. To preserve his person he has the right of disposal over his body. But in taking his life he does not preserve his person; he disposes of his person and not of its attendant circumstances; he robs himself of his person. This is contrary to the highest duty we have towards ourselves, for it annuls the condition of all other duties; it goes beyond the limits of the use of free will, for this use is possible only through the existence of the Subject.

There is another set of considerations which make suicide seem plausible. A man might find himself so placed that he can continue living only under circumstances which deprive life of all value; in which he can no longer live conformably to virtue and prudence, so that he must from noble motives put an end to his life. The advocates of this view quote in support of it the example of Cato. Cato knew that the entire Roman nation relied upon him in their resistance to Caesar, but he found that he could not prevent himself from falling into Caesar's hands. What was he to do? If he, the champion of freedom, submitted, every one would say, "If Cato himself submits, what else can we do?" If, on the other hand, he killed himself, his death might spur on the Romans to fight to the bitter end in defence of their freedom. So he killed himself. He thought that it was necessary for him to die. He thought that if he could not go on living as Cato, he could not go on living at all. It must certainly be admitted that in a case such as this, where suicide is a virtue, appearances are in its favour. But this is the only example which has given the world the opportunity of defending suicide. It is the only example of its kind and there has been no similar case since. Lucretia also killed herself, but on grounds of modesty and in a fury of vengeance. It is obviously our duty to preserve our honour, particularly in relation to the opposite sex, for whom it is a merit; but we must endeavour to save our honour only to this extent, that we ought not to surrender it for selfish and lustful purposes. To do what Lucretia did is to adopt a remedy which is not at our disposal; it would have been better had she defended her honour unto death; that would not have been suicide and would have been right; for it is no suicide to risk one's life

against one's enemies, and even to sacrifice it, in order to observe one's duties towards oneself.

No one under the sun can bind me to commit suicide; no sovereign can do so. The sovereign can call upon his subjects to fight to the death for their country, and those who fall on the field of battle are not suicides, but the victims of fate. Not only is this not suicide; but the opposite, a faint heart and fear of the death which threatens by the necessity of fate, is no true self-preservation; for he who runs away to save his own life, and leaves his comrades in the lurch, is a coward; but he who defends himself and his fellows even unto death is no suicide, but noble and high-minded; for life is not to be highly regarded for its own sake. I should endeavour to preserve my own life only so far as I am worthy to live. We must draw a distinction between the suicide and the victim of fate. A man who shortens his life by intemperance is guilty of imprudence and indirectly of his own death; but his guilt is not direct; he did not intend to kill himself; his death was not premeditated. For all our offences are either *culpa* or *dolus.* There is certainly no *dolus* here, but there is *culpa;* and we can say of such a man that he was guilty of his own death, but we cannot say of him that he is a suicide. What constitutes suicide is the intention to destroy oneself. Intemperance and excess which shorten life ought not, therefore, to be called suicide; for if we raise intemperance to the level of suicide, we lower suicide to the level of intemperance. Imprudence, which does not imply a desire to cease to live, must, therefore, be distinguished from the intention to murder oneself. Serious violations of our duty towards ourselves produce an aversion accompanied either by horror or by disgust; suicide is of the horrible kind, *crimina carnis* of the disgusting. We shrink in horror from suicide because all nature seeks its own preservation; an injured tree, a living body, an animal does so; how then could man make of his freedom, which is the acme of life and constitutes its worth, a principle for his own destruction? Nothing more terrible can be imagined; for if man were on every occasion master of his own life, he would be master of the lives of others; and being ready to sacrifice his life at any and every time rather than be captured, he could perpetrate every conceivable crime and vice. We are, therefore, horrified at the very thought of suicide; by it man sinks lower than the beasts; we look upon a suicide as carrion, whilst our sympathy goes forth to the victim of fate.

Those who advocate suicide seek to give the widest interpretation to freedom. There is something flattering in the thought that we can take our own life if we are so minded; and so we find even right-thinking persons defending suicide in this respect. There are many circumstances under which life ought to be sacrificed. If I cannot preserve my life except by violating my duties towards myself, I am bound to sacrifice my life rather than violate these duties. But suicide is in no circumstances permissible. Humanity in one's own person is something inviolable; it is a holy trust; man is master of all else, but he must not lay hands upon himself. A being who existed of his own necessity could not possibly destroy himself; a being whose existence is not necessary must regard life as the condition of everything else, and in the consciousness that life is a trust reposed in him, such a being recoils at the thought of committing a breach of his holy trust by turning his life against himself. Man can only dispose over things; beasts are things in this sense; but man is not a thing, not a beast. If he disposes over himself, he treats his value as that of a beast. He who so behaves, who has no respect for human nature and makes a thing of himself, becomes for everyone an Object of freewill. We are free to treat him as a beast, as a thing, and to use him for our sport as we do a horse or a dog, for he is no longer a human being; he has made a thing of himself, and, having himself discarded his humanity, he cannot expect that others should respect humanity in him. Yet humanity is worthy of esteem. Even when a man is a bad man, humanity in his person is worthy of esteem. Suicide is not abominable and inadmissible because life should be highly prized; were it so, we could each have our own opinion of how highly we should prize it, and the rule of prudence would often indicate suicide as the best means. But the rule of morality does not admit of it under any condition because it degrades human nature below the level of animal nature and so destroys it. Yet there is much in the world far more important than life. To observe

morality is far more important. It is better to sacrifice one's life than one's morality. To live is not a necessity; but to live honourably while life lasts is a necessity. We can at all times go on living and doing our duty towards ourselves without having to do violence to ourselves. But he who is prepared to take his own life is no longer worthy to live at all. The pragmatic ground of impulse to live is happiness. Can I then take my own life because I cannot live happily? No! It is not necessary that whilst I live I should live happily; but it is necessary that so long as I live I should live honourably. Misery gives no right to any man to take his own life, for then we should all be entitled to take our lives for lack of pleasure. All our duties towards ourselves would then be directed towards pleasure; but the fulfilment of those duties may demand that we should even sacrifice our life.

Is suicide heroic or cowardly? Sophistication, even though well meant, is not a good thing. It is not good to defend either virtue or vice by splitting hairs. Even right-thinking people declaim against suicide on wrong lines. They say that it is arrant cowardice. But instances of suicide of great heroism exist. We cannot, for example, regard the suicides of Cato and of Atticus as cowardly. Rage, passion and insanity are the most frequent causes of suicide, and that is why persons who attempt suicide and are saved from it are so terrified at their own act they they do not dare to repeat the attempt. There was a time in Roman and in Greek history when suicide was regarded as honourable, so much so that the Romans forbade their slaves to commit suicide because they did not belong to themselves but to their masters and so were regarded as things, like all other animals. The Stoics said that suicide is the sage's peaceful death; he leaves the world as he might leave a smoky room for another, because it no longer pleases him; he leaves the world, not because he is no longer happy in it, but because he disdains it. It has already been mentioned that man is greatly flattered by the idea that he is free to remove himself from this world, if he so wishes. He may not make use of this freedom, but the thought of possessing it pleases him. It seems even to have a moral aspect, for if man is capable of removing himself from the world at his own will, he need not submit to any one; he can retain his independence and tell the rudest truths to the cruellest of tyrants. Torture cannot bring him to heel, because he can leave the world at a moment's notice as a free man can leave the country, if and when he wills it. But this semblance of morality vanishes as soon as we see that man's freedom cannot subsist except on a condition which is immutable. This condition is that man may not use his freedom against himself to his own destruction, but that, on the contrary, he should allow nothing external to limit it. Freedom thus conditioned is noble. No chance or misfortune ought to make us afraid to live; we ought to go on living as long as we can do so as human beings and honourably. To bewail one's fate and misfortune is in itself dishonourable. Had Cato faced any torments which Caesar might have inflicted upon him with a resolute mind and remained steadfast, it would have been noble of him; to violate himself was not so. Those who advocate suicide and teach that there is authority for it necessarily do much harm in a republic of free men. Let us imagine a state in which men held as a general opinion that they were entitled to commit suicide, and that there was even merit and honour in so doing. How dreadful everyone would find them. For he who does not respect his life even in principle cannot be restrained from the most dreadful vices; he recks neither king nor torments.

But as soon as we examine suicide from the standpoint of religion we immediately see it in its true light. We have been placed in this world under certain conditions and for specific purposes. But a suicide opposes the purpose of his Creator; he arrives in the other world as one who has deserted his post; he must be looked upon as a rebel against God. So long as we remember the truth that it is God's intention to preserve life, we are bound to regulate our activities in conformity with it. We have no right to offer violence to our nature's powers of self-preservation and to upset the wisdom of her arrangements. This duty is upon us until the time comes when God expressly commands us to leave this life. Human beings are sentinels on earth and may not leave their posts until relieved by another beneficent hand. God is our owner; we are His property; His providence works for our good. A bondman in the care of a beneficent master deserves punishment if he opposes his master's wishes.

But suicide is not admissible and abominable because God has forbidden it; God has forbidden it because it is abominable in that it degrades man's inner worth below that of the animal creation. Moral philosophers must, therefore, first and foremost show that suicide is abominable. We find, as a rule, that those who labour for their happiness are more liable to suicide; having tasted the refinements of pleasure, and being deprived of them, they give way to grief, sorrow, and melancholy.

From "Essay on Suicide"

David Hume

One considerable advantage that arises from Philosophy consists in the sovereign antidote which it affords to superstition and false religion. All other remedies against that pestilent distemper are vain, or at least uncertain. Plain good sense and the practice of the world, which

Reprinted with permission from *Ethics and Metaethics,* ed. R. Abelson, (New York: St. Martin's Press, 1963) pp. 108–16.

alone serve most purposes of life, are here found ineffectual: History as well as daily experience furnish instances of men endowed with the strongest capacity for business and affairs, who have all their lives crouched under slavery to the grossest superstition. Even gaiety and sweetnes of temper, which infuse a balm into every other wound, afford no remedy to so virulent a poison; as we may particularly observe of the fair sex, who, though commonly possest of these rich presents of nature, feel many of their joys blasted by this importunate intruder. But when sound Philosophy has once gained possession of the mind, superstition is effectually excluded; and one may fairly affirm that her triumph over this enemy is more complete than over most of the vices and imperfections incident to human nature. Love or anger, ambition or avarice, have their root in the temper and affections, which the soundest reason is scarce ever able fully to correct; but superstition being founded on false opinion, must immediately vanish when true philosophy has inspired juster sentiments of superior powers. The contest is here more equal between the distemper and the medicine, and nothing can hinder the latter from proving effectual, but its being false and sophisticated.

It will here be superfluous to magnify the merits of philosophy by displaying the pernicious tendency of that vice of which it cures the human mind. The superstitious man, says Tully, is miserable in every scene, in every incident of life; even sleep itself, which banishes all other cares of unhappy mortals, affords to him matter of new terror; while he examines his dreams, and finds in those visions of the night prognostications of future calamities. I may add, that though death alone can put a full period to this misery, he dares not fly to this refuge, but still prolongs a miserable existence from a vain fear lest he offend his maker by using the power with which that beneficient being has endowed him. The presents of God and nature are ravished from us by this cruel enemy; and notwithstanding that one step would remove us from the regions of pain and sorrow, her menaces still chain us down to a hated being, which she herself chiefly contributes to render miserable.

'Tis observed by such as have been reduced by the calamities of life to the necessity of employing this fatal remedy, that if the unseasonable care of their friends deprive them of that species of Death which they proposed to themselves, they seldom venture upon any other, or can summon up so much resolution a second time, as to execute their purpose. So great is our horror of death that when it presents itself, under any form, besides that to which a man has endeavoured to reconcile his imagination, it acquires new terrors and overcomes his feeble courage: But when the menaces of superstition are joined to this natural timidity, no wonder it quite deprives men of all power over their lives, since even many pleasures and enjoyments, to which we are carried by a strong propensity, are torn from us by this inhuman tyrant. Let us here endeavour to restore men to their native liberty by examining all the common arguments against Suicide, and shewing that that action may be free from every imputation of guilt or blame, according to the sentiments of all the ancient philosophers.

If Suicide be criminal, it must be a transgression of our duty either to God, our neighbour, or ourselves. To prove that suicide is no transgression of our duty to God, the following considerations may perhaps suffice. In order to govern the material world, the almighty Creator has established general and immutable laws by which all bodies, from the greatest planet to the smallest particle of matter, are maintained in their proper sphere and function. To govern the animal world, he has endowed all living creatures with bodily and mental powers; with senses, passions, appetites, memory and judgment, by which they are impelled or regulated in that course of life to which they are destined. These two distinct principles of the material and animal world continually encroach upon each other, and mutually retard or forward each other's operations. The powers of men and of all other animals are restrained and directed by the nature and qualities of the surrounding bodies; and the modifications and actions of these bodies are incessantly altered by the operation of all animals. Man is stopt by rivers in his passage over the surface of the earth; and rivers, when properly directed, lend their force to the motion of machines, which serve to the use of man. But though the provinces of material and animal powers are not kept entirely separate, there results from thence no discord or disorder in the creation; on the contrary, from the mixture, union and contrast of all the various powers of inanimate bodies and living creatures, arises that surprising harmony and proportion which affords the surest argument of supreme wisdom. The providence of the Deity appears not immediately in any operation, but governs everything by those general and immutable laws, which have been established from the beginning of time. All events, in one sense, may be pronounced the action of the Almighty; they all proceed from those powers with which he has endowed his creatures. A house which falls by its own weight is not brought to ruin by his providence more than one destroyed by the hands of men; nor are the human faculties less his workmanship than the laws of motion and gravitation. When the passions play, when the judgment dictates, when the limbs obey; this is all the operation of God, and upon these animate principles, as well as upon the inanimate, has he established the government of the universe. Every event is alike important in the eyes of that infinite being, who takes in at one glance the most distant regions of space and remotest periods of time. There is no event, however important to us, which he has exempted from the general laws that govern the universe, or which he has peculiarly reserved for his own immediate action and operation. The revolution of states and empires depends upon the smallest caprice or passion of single men; and the lives of men are shortened or extended by the smallest accident of air or diet, sunshine or tempest. Nature still continues her progress and operation; and if general laws be ever broke by particular volitions of the Deity, 'tis after a manner which entirely escapes human observation. As, on the one hand, the elements and other inanimate parts of the creation carry on their action without regard to the particular interest and situation of men; so men are entrusted to their judgment and discretion, in the various shocks of matter, and may employ every faculty with which they are endowed, in order to provide for their ease, happiness, or preservation. What is the meaning then of that principle that a man, who, tired of life, and haunted by pain and misery, bravely overcomes all the natural terrors of death and makes his escape from this cruel scene; that such a man, I say, has incurred the indignation of his Creator by encroaching on the office of divine providence, and disturbing the order of the universe? Shall we assert that the Almighty has reserved to himself in any pe-

culiar manner the disposal of the lives of men, and has not submitted that event, in common with others, to the general laws by which the universe is governed? This is plainly false; the lives of men depend upon the same laws as the lives of all other elements; and these are subjected to the general laws of matter and motion. The fall of a tower, or the infusion of poison, will destroy a man equally with the meanest creature; an inundation sweeps away every thing without distinction that comes within the reach of its fury. Since therefore the lives of men are for ever dependent on the general laws of matter and motion, is a man's disposing of his life criminal, because in every case it is criminal to encroach upon these laws, or disturb their operation? But this seems absurd; all animals are entrusted to their own prudence and skill for their conduct in the world, and have full authority, as far as their power extends, to alter all the operations of nature. Without the exercise of this authority they could not subsist a moment; every action, every motion of a man, innovates on the order of some parts of matter, and diverts from their ordinary course the general laws of motion. Putting together, therefore, these conclusions, we find that human life depends upon the general laws of matter and motion, and that it is no encroachment on the office of providence to disturb or alter these general laws: Has not everyone, of consequence, the free disposal of his own life? And may he not lawfully employ that power with which nature has endowed him? In order to destroy the evidence of this conclusion, we must shew a reason why this particular case is excepted; is it because human life is of so great importance, that 'tis a presumption for human prudence to dispose of it? But the life of a man is of no greater importance to the universe than that of an oyster. And were it of ever so great importance, the order of nature has actually submitted it to human prudence, and reduced us to a necessity in every incident of determining concerning it. Were the disposal of human life so much reserved as the peculiar province of the Almightly that it were an encroachment of his right for men to dispose of their own lives; it would be equally criminal to act for the preservation of life as for its destruction. If I turn aside a stone which is falling upon my head, I disturb the course of nature, and I invade the peculiar province of the Almighty by lengthening out my life beyond the period which by the general laws of matter and motion he had assigned it.

A hair, a fly, an insect is able to destroy this mighty being whose life is of such importance. Is it an absurdity to suppose that human prudence may lawfully dispose of what depends on such insignificant causes? It would be no crime in me to divert the Nile or Danube from its course, were I able to effect such purposes. Where then is the crime of turning a few ounces of blood from their natural channel? Do you imagine that I repine at providence or curse my creation, because I go out of life, and put a period to a being, which, were it to continue, would render me miserable? Far be such sentiments from me; I am only convinced of a matter of fact, which you yourself acknowledge possible, that human life may be unhappy, and that my existence, if further prolonged, would become ineligible; but I thank providence, both for the good which I have already enjoyed, and for the power with which I am endowed of escaping the ill that threatens me. To you it belongs to repine providence, who foolishly imagine that you have no such power, and who must still prolong a hated life, though loaded with pain and sickness, with shame and poverty. Do you not teach that when any ill befalls me, though by the malice of my enemies, I ought to be resigned to providence, and that the actions of men are the operations of the Almighty as much as the actions of inanimate beings? When I fall upon my own sword, therefore, I receive my death equally from the hands of the Deity as if it had proceeded from a lion, a precipice, or a fever. The submission which you require to providence in every calamity that befalls me excludes not human skill and industry, if possibly by their means I can avoid or escape the calamity: And why may I not employ one remedy as well as another? If my life be not my own, it were criminal for me to put it in danger, as well as to dispose of it; nor could one man deserve the appellation of *hero* whom glory or friendship transports into the greatest dangers, and another merit the reproach of *wretch* or *miscreant* who puts a period to his life for like motives. There is no being which possesses any power or

faculty that it receives not from its Creator, nor is there any one which by ever so irregular an action can encroach upon the plan of his providence, or disorder the universe. Its operations are his works equally with that chain of events which it invades, and whichever principle prevails, we may for that very reason conclude it to be most favoured by him. Be it animate, or inaminate, rational, or irrational; 'tis all a case: Its power is still derived from the supreme creator, and is alike comprehended in the order of his providence. When the horror of pain prevails over the love of live; when a voluntary action anticipates the effects of blind causes; 'tis only in consequence of those powers and principles which he has implanted in his creatures. Divine providence is still inviolate and placed far beyond the reach of human injuries. 'Tis impious, says the old Roman superstition, to divert rivers from their course, or invade the prerogatives of nature. 'Tis impious, says the French superstition, to inoculate for the smallpox, or usurp the business of providence, by voluntarily producing distempers and maladies. 'Tis impious, says the modern European superstition, to put a period to our own life, and thereby rebel against our creator; and why not impious, say I, to build houses, cultivate the ground, or sail upon the ocean? In all these actions we employ our powers of mind and body to produce some innovation in the course of nature; and in none of them do we any more. They are all of them therefore equally innocent, or equally criminal. *But you are placed by providence, like a sentinel in a particular station, and when you desert it without being recalled, you are equally guilty of rebellion against your almighty sovereign, and have incurred his displeasure.* I ask, why do you conclude that providence has placed me in this station? For my part I find that I owe my birth to a long chain of causes, of which many depend upon voluntary actions of men. *But Providence guided all these causes, and nothing happens in the universe without its consent and cooperation.* If so, then neither does my death, however voluntary, happen without its consent; and whenever pain or sorrow so far overcome my patience as to make me tired of life, I may conclude that I am recalled from my station in the clearest and most express terms. 'Tis Providence surely that has placed me at this present moment in this chamber: But may I not leave it when I think proper, without being liable to the imputation of having deserted my post or station? When I shall be dead, the principles of which I am composed will still perform their part in the universe, and will be equally useful in the grand fabric, as when they composed this individual creature. The difference to the whole will be no greater than betwixt my being in a chamber and in the open air. The one change is of more importance to me than the other; but not more so to the universe.

'Tis a kind of blasphemy to imagine that any created being can disturb the order of the world or invade the business of providence! It supposes that being possesses powers and faculties which it received not from its creator, and which are not subordinate to his government and authority. A man may disturb society no doubt, and thereby incur the displeasure of the Almighty: But the government of the world is placed far beyond his reach and violence. And how does it appear that the Almighty is displeased with those actions that disturb society? By the principles which he has implanted in human nature, and which inspire us with a sentiment of remorse if we ourselves have been guilty of such actions, and with that of blame and disapprobation, if we ever observe them in others. Let us now examine, according to the method proposed, whether Suicide be of this kind of actions, and be a breach of our duty to our *neighbour* and to *society*.

A man who retires from life does no harm to society: He only ceases to do good; which, if it is an injury, is of the lowest kind. All our obligations to do good to society seem to imply something reciprocal. I receive the benefits of society and therefore ought to promote its interests, but when I withdraw myself altogether from society, can I be bound any longer? But, allowing that our obligations to do good were perpetual, they have certainly some bounds; I am not obliged to do a small good to society at the expense of a great harm to myself; why then should I prolong a miserable existence, because of some frivolous advantage which the public may perhaps receive from me? If upon account of age and infirmities I may lawfully resign any office, and employ my time altogether in fencing against these calamities, and alleviating as

much as possible the miseries of my future life: Why may I not cut short these miseries at once by an action which is no more prejudicial to society? But suppose that it is no longer in my power to promote the interest of society; suppose that I am a burthen to it; suppose that my life hinders some person from being much more useful to society. In such cases my resignation of life must not only be innocent but laudable. And most people who lie under any temptation to abandon existence are in some such situation; those who have health, or power, or authority, have commonly better reason to be in humour with the world.

A man is engaged in a conspiracy for the public interest; is seized upon suspicion; is threatened with the rack; and knows from his own weakness that the secret will be extorted from him: Could such a one consult the public interest better than by putting a quick period to a miserable life? This was the case of the famous and brave Strozi of Florence. Again, suppose a malefactor is justly condemned to a shameful death; can any reason be imagined why he may not anticipate his punishment, and save himself all the anguish of thinking on its dreadful approaches? He invades the business of providence no more than the magistrate did, who ordered his execution; and his voluntary death is equally advantageous to society by ridding it of a pernicious member.

That suicide may often be consistent with interest and with our duty to ourselves, no one can question who allows that age, sickness, or misfortune may render life a burthen, and make it worse even than annihilation. I believe that no man ever threw away life while it was worth keeping. For such is our natural horror of death that small motives will never be able to reconcile us to it; and though perhaps the situation of a man's health or fortune did not seem to require this remedy, we may at least be assured that any one who, without apparent reason, has had recourse to it, was curst with such an incurable depravity or gloominess of temper as must poison all enjoyment, and render him equally miserable as if he had been loaded with the most grievous misfortunes. If suicide be supposed a crime 'tis only cowardice can impel us to it. If it be no crime, both prudence and courage should engage us to rid ourselves at once of existence, when it becomes a burthen. 'Tis the only way that we can then be useful to society, by setting an example, which, if imitated, would preserve to everyone his chance for happiness in life and would effectually free him from all danger or misery.

Suicide and the Right to Die

George E. Murphy

At least one recent court case has upheld a patient's right to freedom from unwanted intervention in the process of dying. Medical societies across the country are publicly supporting carefully considered decisions to limit intervention in terminal illness. Excesses of therapeutic zeal, bred of a burgeoning life-support technology, are giving way to a more careful consideration of the patient's humanity. At the same time, euthanasia receives little public support. The deliberate induction of death is foreign to the spirit of medicine. But we are once again becoming aware of the mortally ill individual's right to die with dignity.

Physicians know full well they cannot prevent death. They can only postpone it. Where death is imminent—and every clinician knows that judgment is fugitive at times—the questions are when and how, not whether. Suicide, or the theat of it, raises the question of *whether*, in the sense that death is not otherwise near. Symposia, panel discussions, and debates have been held on the question of the individual's right to suicide. But the assertion of such a "right" leaves out of consideration what is known about those who have taken their lives. So-called "rational" suicide is a rarity. Only a few persons who commit suicide are suffering from a terminal illness (and may perhaps be excluded from the discussion that follows). The descriptive facts are that most persons who commit suicide are suffering from clinically recognizable psychiatric illnesses often carry-

ing an excellent prognosis; that the majority have sought help from physicians for their symptoms; and that few have received the indicated treatment. To say that this person is exercising a right is to mock him in his frustration at failing to find the understanding and the technical skill he sought.

To be sure, there are those who condemn any effort to interfere with an individual's behavior against his wishes. But their grounds are philosophical, not clinical, and foreign to our concerns as physicians. Others, in the hope of de-stigmatizing suicide, would establish "thanatoria" to facilitate, regulate, and sanitize the act. This idea seems to be the intellectual toy of frustrated would-be suicide preventers. There is much to be frustrated about. Our ability to predict suicide is still crude. Our ability to prevent suicide is at best unproven. The loss of federal support for research in these vital areas coincides with an unprecedented rise in suicide among the young. But suicide is not a topic on which to take the position: "If you can't beat them, join them!"

From our knowledge of the natural history of the psychiatric disorders underlying the suicidal urge, we can confidently predict recovery from that urge in the great majority of cases, when other symptoms of depression lift. The desire to terminate one's life is usually transient. The "right" to suicide is a "right" desired only temporarily. Every physician should feel the obligation to support the desire for life, which will return even in a patient who cannot believe that such a change can occur. To cooperate in the patient's hopelessness violates an important responsibility of the physician.

From "The Right to Suicide: A Psychiatrist's View"

Jerome A. Motto

To speak as a psychiatrist may suggest to some that psychiatrists have a certain way of looking at things. This would be a misconception, though a common one. I know of no professional group with more diverse approaches to those matters concerning it than the American psychiatric community. All physicians, however, including psychiatrists, share a tradition of commitment to both the preservation and the quality of human life. With this one reservation, I speak as a psychiatrist strictly in the singular sense.

The emergence of thoughts or impulses to bring an end to life is a phenomenon observed in persons experiencing severe pain, whether that pain stems from physical or emotional sources. Thus physicians, to whom persons are inclined to turn for relief from suffering, frequently encounter suicidal ideas and impulses in their patients. Those who look and listen do, at least.

From a psychiatric point of view, the question as to whether a person has the right to cope with the pain in his world by killing himself can be answered without hesitation. He does have that right. With a few geographical exceptions the same can be said from the legal and social point of view as well. It is only when philosophical or theological questions are raised that one can find room for argument about the right to suicide, as only in these areas can restrictions on behavior be institutionalized without requiring social or legal support.

The problem we struggle with is not whether the individual *has* the right to suicide; rather, we face a twofold dilemma stemming from the fact that he does have it. Firstly, what is the extent to which the exercise of that right should be subject to limitations? Secondly, when the right

Reprinted with permission of author and publisher from *Life-Threatening Behavior,* 2. No. 3 (Fall 1972), 183–88. Copyright 1972 by Behavioral Publications, Inc., 72 Fifth Ave., New York, N.Y. 10011.

is exercised, how can we eliminate the social stigma now attached to it?

LIMITATIONS ON THE INDIVIDUAL'S RIGHT TO SUICIDE

Putting limitations on rights is certainly not a new idea, since essentially every right we exercise has its specified restrictions. It is generally taken for granted that certain limitations must be observed. In spite of this, it is inevitable that some will take the position that unless the right is unconditional it is not "really" granted.

I use two psychological criteria as grounds for limiting a person's exercise of his right to suicide: (*a*) the act must be based on a realistic assessment of his life situation, and (*b*) the degree of ambivalence regarding the act must be minimal. Both of these criteria clearly raise a host of new questions.

Realistic Assessment of Life Situation

What is reality? Who determines whether a realistic assessment has been made? Every person's perception is reality to *him,* and the degree of pain experienced by one can never be fully appreciated by another, no matter how empathic he is. Differences in capacity to *tolerate* pain add still another crucial yet unmeasurable element.

As formidable as this sounds, the psychiatrist is obliged to accept this task as his primary day-to-day professional responsibility, whether or not the issue of suicide is involved. With an acute awareness of how emotions can—like lenses—distort perceptions which in turn shape one's thoughts and actions, and with experience in understanding and dealing with this underlying substrate of emotion, he is constantly working with his patients on the process of differentiating between what is realistic and what is distorted. The former must be dealt with on a rational level; the latter must be explored and modified till the distortion is reduced at least to the point where it is not of handicapping severity. He is aware of the nature and extent of his own tendency of distort ("Physician, heal thyself"), and realizes that the entire issue is one of degree. Yet he must use his own perception of reality as a standard, shortcomings notwithstanding, realizing full well how much information must be carefully considered in view of the frailty of the human perceptual and reality-testing apparatus.

Some persons have a view of reality so different from mine that I do not hesitate to interfere with their right to suicide. Others' perceptions are so like mine that I cannot intercede. The big problem is that large group in between.

In the final analysis, then, when a decision has to be made, what a psychiatrist calls "realistic" is whatever looks realistic to *him*. At the moment of truth, that is all any person can offer. This inherent human limitation in itself is a reality that accounts for a great deal of inevitable chaos in the world; it is an article of faith that not to make such an effort would create even greater chaos. On a day-to-day operational level, one contemporary behavioral scientist expressed it this way: "No doubt the daily business of helping troubled individuals, including suicides, gives little time for the massive contemplative and investigative efforts which alone can lead to surer knowledge. And the helpers are not thereby to be disparaged. They cannot wait for the best answers conceivable. They must do only the best they can *now*."

Thus if I am working with a person in psychotherapy, one limitation I would put on his right to suicide would be that his assessment of his life situation be realistic as *I* see it.

A related concept is that of "rational suicide," which has enjoyed a certain vogue since at least the seventeenth century, when the "Rationalist Era" saw sharp inroads being made into the domination of the church in determining ethical and social values. According to one contemporary philosopher, "the degree of rationality of the [suicidal] act would depend on the degree of rationality of the philosophy which was guiding the person's deliberations." Rationality is defined as a means of problem solving, using "methods such as logical,

mathematical, or experimental procedures which have gained men's confidence as reliable tools for guiding instrumental actions." The rationality of one's philosophy is determined by the degree to which it is free of mysticism. Further, "A person who is considering how to act in an intensely conflicting situation cannot be regarded as making the most rational decision, unless he has been as critical as possible of the philosophy that is guiding his decision. If the philosophy is institutionalized as a political ideology or a religious creed, he must think critically about the institution in order to acquire maximum rationality of judgment. This principle is clear enough, even if in practice it is enormously difficult to fulfill."

The idea of "rational suicide" is a related yet distinctly different issue from the "realistic assessment of one's life situation" referred to above. Making this assessment involves assembling and understanding all the facts clearly, while the idea of a "rational suicide" can only be entertained after this assessment is done and the question is "what to do" in the light of those facts.

The role of the psychiatrist and the thinking of the rationalist tend to merge, at one point, however. In the process of marshaling all the facts and exploring their meaning to the person, the psychiatrist must ensure that the patient does indeed critically examine not only his perception of reality but his own philosophy. This often entails making that philosophy explicit for the first time (without ever using the term "philosophy"), and clarifying how it has influenced his living experience. The implication is clear that modification of the person's view of his world, with corresponding changes in behavior, may lead to a more satisfying life.

The rationalist concedes that where one's philosophy is simply an "intellectual channeling of emotional forces," rational guidelines have severe limitations, since intense emotional conflicts cut off rational guidance. These circumstances would characterize "irrational" grounds for suicide and would identify those persons whose suicide should be prevented.

The argument for "rational suicide" tends to apply principally to two sets of circumstances; altruistic self-sacrifice for what is perceived as a noble cause; and the severe, advanced physical illness with no new therapeutic agents anticipated in the foreseeable future. This does not help us very much because these circumstances generate relatively little real controversy among behavioral scientists. The former situations are not usually recognized till after the act, and the latter at present are receiving a great deal of well-deserved attention from the point of view of anticipating (and sometimes hastening) the foreseeable demise in comfort and dignity.

Our most difficult problem is more with the person whose pain is emotional in origin and whose physical health is good, or at most constitutes a minor impairment. For these persons, the discussion above regarding "rational" and "irrational" distinctions seems rather alien to the clinical situation. This is primarily due to the rationalist's emphasis on intellectual processes, when it is so clear (at least to the psychiatrist) that it is feelings of worthiness of love, of relatedness, of belonging, that have the strongest stabilizing influence on the suicidal person.

I rarely hear a patient say, "I've never looked at it that way," yet no response is more frequently encountered than, "Yes, I understand, but I don't feel any differently." It is after a continuing therapeutic effort during which feelings of acceptance and worthiness are generated that emotional pain is reduced and suicidal manifestations become less intense. Either exploring the philosophy by which one lives or carefully assessing the realities of one's life can provide an excellent means of accomplishing this, but it is rarely the influence of the philosophy or the perception of the realities per se that brings it about. Rather, it is through the influence of the therapeutic relationship that the modified philosophy or perception develops, and can then be applied to the person's life situation.

Manifestations of Ambivalence

The second criterion to be used as the basis for limiting a person's exercise of his right to suicide is minimal ambivalence about ending his life. I make the assumption that if a person has no ambivalence about suicide he will not be in my office, nor write to me about it, nor call me on the telephone. I interpret, rightly or

wrongly, a person's calling my attention to his suicidal impulses as a request to intercede that I cannot ignore.

At times this call will inevitably be misread, and my assumption will lead me astray. However, such an error on my part can be corrected at a later time; meanwhile, I must be prepared to take responsibility for having prolonged what may be a truly unendurable existence. If the error is made in the other direction, no opportunity for correction may be possible.

This same principle regarding ambivalence applies to a suicide prevention center, minister, social agency, or a hospital emergency room. The response of the helping agency may be far from fulfilling the needs of the person involved, but in my view, the ambivalence expressed is a clear indication for it to limit the exercise of his right to suicide. . . .

It seems inevitable to me that we must eventually establish procedures for the voluntary cessation of life, with the time, place, and manner largely controlled by the person concerned. It will necessarily involve a series of deliberate steps providing assurance that appropriate criteria are met, such as those proposed above, as we now observe specific criteria when a life is terminated by abortion or by capital punishment.

The critical word is "control." I would anticipate a decrease in the actual number of suicides when this procedure is established, due to the psychological power of this issue. If I know something is available to me and will remain available till I am moved to seize it, the chances of my seizing it now are thereby much reduced. It is only by holding off that I maintain the option of changing my mind. During this period of delay the opportunity for therapeutic effort—and the therapy of time itself—may be used to advantage.

Finally, we have to make sure we are not speaking only to the strong. It is too easy to formulate a way of dealing with a troublesome problem in such a manner, that if the person in question could approach it as we suggest, he would not be a person who would have the problem in the first place.

When we discuss—in the abstract—the right to suicide, we tend to gloss over the intricacies of words like "freedom," "quality of life," "choice," or even "help," to say nothing of "rational" and "realistic." Each of these concepts deserves a full inquiry in itself, though in practice we use them on the tacit assumption that general agreement exists as to their meaning.

Therefore it is we who, in trying to be of service to someone else, have the task of determining what is rational for us, and what our perception of reality is. And we must recognize that in the final analysis it will be not only the suicidal person but we who have exercised a choice, by doing what we do to resolve our feelings about this difficult human problem.

The Definition of Euthanasia

Tom L. Beauchamp
and Arnold I. Davidson

Although debate about the moral justifiability of euthanasia has increased in recent years, no sustained attention has been devoted to the development of an adequate definition of euthanasia. Since significantly different moral and legal sanctions will be implied by the classification of an act as euthanasia, abortion, suicide, or murder, the development of an adequate definition will have important practical consequences. The way we classify actions is indicative of the way we think about them, and in the present case such classifications have immediate relevance for medicine, ethics, and law.

We attempt in this paper to provide both a nonprescriptive definition of euthanasia (one which dictates no moral conclusions) and one which is not subject to refutation by counterexample. All other definitions in the literature on euthanasia, we shall argue, are open to fatal counterexamples. We begin by examining a representative sample of these definitions and their difficulties (Sec. I). Next we propose and argue for a definition containing logically necessary and sufficient conditions (Sec. II). Finally, we consider and rebut possible objections and counterexamples to our definition (Sec. III).

I

One common definition of euthanasia is the following offered by Marvin Kohl: (1) "the

Reprinted with permission from the authors and *The Journal of Medicine & Philosophy*, Vol. 4, No. 3, 1979, pp. 294–312.

painless inducement of a quick death" (1974, p. 94). This definition is virtually identical with the one given in the *Oxford English Dictionary*[1] and is widely relied upon in writings on euthanasia. Unfortunately, numerous counterexamples can be adduced against this definition, because neither painlessness nor quickness is a necessary condition of euthanasia. Consider the following case. Smith sneaks up behind an innocent but disliked member of his department and injects a painless and quick-acting lethal agent into his bloodstream. This is murder simpliciter, not euthanasia. Similarly, Smith could quickly and painlessly induce his own death by accidently walking under a load of falling bricks, yet none would say euthanasia had occurred. In his quest for simplicity, Kohl has proposed a definition which is overly simplistic. It omits all the subtle aspects of our notion of euthanasia.

A more satisfactory approximation to the correct definition of euthanasia includes the elements of suffering or disease. Three representative definitions including this element are the following: (2) "a mode or act of inducing or permitting death painlessly as a relief from suffering" (Kohl and Kurtz 1975); (3) "an act or practice of painlessly putting to death persons suffering from incurable conditions or diseases [*Webster's International Dictionary*]";[2] (4) "administering . . . an easy painless death to one who is suffering from an incurable and perhaps agonizing ailment" (Healy 1956).

Although these writers correctly recognize the indispensable role played by the notion of suffering in any adequate definition, their formulations remain deficient. Definitions 3 and 4—as well as 1—give no consideration at all to the reasons an administering agent has for causing the death of a second human being. On these definitions, if we were to kill a person suffering from an incurable disease because we stood to gain financially from his demise, then we would have committed an act of euthanasia. But again, if our motive is primarily one of self-interest, the case is one of murder simpliciter, not euthanasia. Furthermore, definitions 1–4 all stipulate that the death must be painless. Although consideration relating to the pain caused by the death are relevant, as we shall show, *painlessness* of death is not a necessary condition of euthanasia. Suppose someone is suffering from intractable pain and there are two means by which to cause death. One of these means is painless but requires days to work, while the second is (minimally) painful but works significantly more quickly. If the painful means were to be used on the patient, the act would not be disqualified as euthanasia simply because the person died a less than painless death. Other considerations, such as the length of time required for death to take place, might militate against selection of a completely painless death, and yet the act would still be one of euthanasia.

Although other features of the above definitions are also inadequate, as will become clear in Section II, the counterexamples already adduced seem to us to provide sufficient reason for rejecting these basic definitions as deficient. Accordingly, we pass on to other proposed definitions.

In an attempt to deal with the role of motives in the definition of euthanasia, Baruch Brody has proposed a definition which requires beneficence: (5) "an act of euthanasia is one in which one person . . . (*A*) kills another person (*B*) for the benefit of the second person, who actually does benefit from being killed" (1975, p. 218). Unlike the previous definitions, this one gives no role to suffering and seems deficient for this reason, among others. While Brody is to be commended for giving a role to the reason why A kills B, his condition of a beneficent reason is too vague. For reasons later to be explained (see condition 3*a* of our

definition in Sec. II), the beneficent reason for which A kills B must be a very specific one (relating to the cessation of B's actual or future predicted condition), and B need not *actually* benefit from A's action in order for that action to be one of euthanasia since the *intention* to benefit B is sufficient, if the person actually dies.[3] But even more importantly, Brody's formulation is too broad, for it fails to recognize that many instances of benefit have no connection with proper use of the term "euthanasia," as the following hypothetical cases illustrate. Suppose it is known that after death all human beings are guaranteed a supernatural life of eternal bliss. It could plausibly be claimed that, if this assumption were true, all human beings would actually benefit from being killed, since they would receive the unmitigated benefits of eternal bliss in contrast to the infrequent and shortlived benefits of life before death. According to Brody's definition (granted this assumption), if we decided to kill the entire human race because we wanted everyone to benefit from this state of eternal bliss, and they did actually benefit, then the deaths of anyone and everyone whom we killed would be instances of euthanasia. A less fanciful case is the following. A perfectly healthy man, B, has been given a choice by a dictatorial government of either ending his own life or having his family killed by governmental agents. Knowing that he will become a national hero by sacrificing himself (and wanting this above all else), B asks his friend A to assist him, and A complies. Both cases satisfy Brody's conditions, but to classify such deaths as euthanasia is nothing less than a reductio ad absurdum of Brody's definition.

On the other hand, Brody does display a useful insight in claiming that a necessary condition of euthanasia is that one person, A, kills another person, B. Some such condition is necessary to distinguish euthanasia from (unassisted) suicide. Unfortunately, the word "kill" is not acceptable and requires reformulation in terms of "causing death," for reasons later to be indicated.

The final definition we shall consider is Glanville Williams's. He says that euthanasia is (6) "either an assisted suicide or a killing by another for humanitarian reasons and by merciful means, generally with the consent of the person killed, in which case it is referred to specifically as voluntary euthanasia'' (1966, p. 43). Since we are concerned with comprehensive definitions of euthanasia which cover both voluntary and involuntary cases, we can safely disregard Williams's last clause.

Williams's definition contains three elements. First euthanasia must be either an assisted suicide or a killing. ''Assisted suicide'' is an improvement over Brody's simple killing condition, but Williams too fails to realize that there are theoretical reasons for preferring the language of ''*causing* the death of another person'' (see condition 1 below). Second, Williams stipulates that the killing must be done for humanitarian reasons. Like Brody's condition of a beneficent reason, Williams's humanitarian reason is too vague to be helpful. But more importantly, according to Williams's definition the condition of the person who dies plays no role in our concept of euthanasia, and this latitude is clearly inadequate. If a doctor kills a defective newborn out of sympathy for the poverty-ridden parents who will suffer by raising the child, he has no more performed an act of euthanasia than Robin Hood would have by killing the rich and evil sheriff of Nottingham in order to distribute the wealth to the starving poor. Third, Williams says that the killing must be done by a merciful means. The mercifulness of the means is no doubt related to Kohl's conditions of painlessness and quickness. But, as we have shown above, neither painlessness nor quickness is a necessary condition of euthanasia. Although there are limitations on the kind of means which can be used, the notion of a merciful means is too porous to be a satisfactory characterization of these limitations. For these reasons, Williams's definition is open to the same type of counterexamples as those definitions already considered.

We have now criticized the best available sources known to us which discuss the definition of euthanasia—with the exception of a recent paper by Philippa Foot, which will be considered below in Section III. Rather than considering other definitions, which are generally more inadequate,[4] we proceed to our own definition, in the form of five conditions which we take to be individually necessary and jointly

sufficient for a death to be an instance of euthanasia.

II

Before we actually construct an alternative to those definitions rejected in Section I, a methodological consideration requires attention. It is clear in the case of many actions that they are correctly classifiable as acts of euthanasia. Other actions, however, are less clearly instances of euthanasia; and still others are borderline cases between euthanasia and, for example, suicide. Any satisfactory definition of euthanasia must be able to account for the clear cases. But, just as important, if one is supplied with a definition which contains theoretical power, one might be called upon to *revise* one's (intuitive) judgments concerning less clear or borderline cases in such a way that the revised judgments cohere with the definition.

We believe that the definition for which we shall now argue adequately accounts for all clear cases, though some actions which have commonly been denominated euthanasia— such as the overused Nazi examples—would not be euthanasia on our definition. In Section III we shall adduce some hard cases and borderline cases about which we have either unclear or conflicting judgments. When examples such as these are presented, a comprehensive theory ought to prevail over vague intuitive judgments. We believe that our definition strikes a stable balance between intuition and theory and that, better than any other definition known to us, it matches what Rawls has called our ''judgments in reflective equilibrium.''[5]

Two unargued presuppositions are made throughout our analysis. First, it is a well-known fact about the etymology of the term ''euthanasia'' that it derives from the Greek for ''good death'' or perhaps ''easy death.'' We think it would be impossible to explicate the meaning of euthanasia without reference to such notions, which for many years have been associated with ideas such as death with dignity, death with a minimum of suffering, assisted death where there are humanitarian reasons, etc. One of our goals is to refine and give precise content to the broad notion of a ''good death.'' On the other hand, our analysis would be unacceptable if it resulted in a commitment to the proposition that all acts of euthanasia are good. Despite the explicit appeals we make to the notion of a good death, we remain neutral on the question whether euthanasia is either bad or good. Our appeals to ''good death'' are appeals only to standard associations with that term which have emerged in the euthanasia literature. (As we explain in Sec. IV, it is paradoxical but conceptually possible in our descriptive sense of ''good death'' that a ''good death'' [euthanasia] is not a good death.)

Second, there are two distinctions which are commonly observed in the literature on euthanasia, and we assume that any definition which could not accommodate these distinctions is incorrect. These distinctions are between (*a*) voluntary and involuntary euthanasia and (*b*) active and passive euthanasia. This presupposition is important for at least two reasons. Whether there is a viable conceptual distinction between active and passive euthanasia is a matter of considerable contemporary controversy. We take no position on this issue, our only concern being that whatever the standing of this distinction, no definition of euthanasia would be correct if it appealed to the distinction between active and passive means of death and then allowed only cases of active or only cases of passive dying to be properly in the extension of the term ''euthanasia.'' Also, some writers have been led by their moral views on euthanasia to declare that ''letting die'' or passive euthanasia should not be considered euthanasia. We take no such moral position, it being our assumption that no fair or objective definition can be reached if one bends the definition to one's moral preferences while ignoring distinctions basic to present understandings of the concept. On these questions of standard contemporary usage, including recent modifications, we accept the following account (from *The New Columbia Encyclopedia*) as definitive:''*euthanasia,* either painlessly putting to death or failing to prevent death from natural causes in cases of terminal illness. The term formerly referred only to the act of painlessly putting incurably ill persons to death. However, technological advances in the field of medicine, which have

made it possible to prolong the life of patients who have no hope of recovery, have led to the use of the term *negative euthanasia,* i.e., the withdrawal of extraordinary means used to preserve life. Accordingly, the term *positive euthanasia* has come to refer to actions that actively cause death.'' Armed with these two presuppositions, we turn now to defense of our five-condition definition.

Intending Death and Causing Death

In each of the definitions previously considered in Section I it is implicit, though not explicitly acknowledged, that the death of the person euthanatized is *intended* by at least one other person. Intentionality is important to the definition of euthanasia since, on a definition such as Kohl's, an *accidental* death could be an instance of euthanasia. But must the intention be that of *killing* the second person, as Brody suggests? Like ''murder,'' ''killing'' is often used in an evaluative or value-laden sense, as entailing a wrongful taking of life, and it would be unfortunate if this sense were incorporated into the definition. Moreover, *if* there is a viable distinction between killing and letting die, then most instances of euthanasia would probably be instances of letting die and not of killing. For these reasons it would seem better to eliminate the language of killing and to replace it with more neutral language, along the lines of ''causing the death of. . . .'' Accordingly, one logically necessary condition of euthanasia would seem to be the following:

> 1. A's death is intended by at least one other human being, B, where B is either the cause of death or a causally relevant feature of the event resulting in death (whether by action or by omission).

This condition asserts that the death of a human being, A, is an instance of euthanasia only if intended by and caused by another person.[6] It is preferable to use the language of causation, rather than that of assisted suicide (Williams), since suicide entails that the dead person played a role in killing himself. But even in paradigm cases of euthanasia it is not *necessary* that the euthanasia person killed himself, though it is conceptually *possible* that he killed himself. (That is, it is possible, but not necessary, that euthanasia is also suicide, as long as the suicide involves a second human being as a causally relevant feature of the event resulting in death.)

Suffering and Evidence of Suffering

According to Williams, as well as others who write on euthanasia, an act of euthanasia must employ a *merciful* means. It is hard to understand such language except as meaning "merciful in the alleviation of suffering." The whole point of performing euthanasia would seem to be the alleviation of suffering (actual or future predicted) or, in the case of neurologically impoverished vegetables, to end their irreversibly comatose state. It is only *because* there exists the intention to relieve the suffering or to terminate the coma that it is considered a merciful action. However, one reason we would not consider all actions which are intended to alleviate suffering instances of euthanasia is that some might be based on ignorance or on insufficient evidence. Mere guesswork about the suffering of another, for example, would be too insubstantial to justify calling an action resulting in that person's death "euthanasia." We would require good evidence that there exists an acutely suffering individual. For all these reasons, we suggest a second condition of euthanasia as follows. The death of a human being A is an instance of euthanasia only if:

2. There is either sufficient current evidence for B to believe that A is acutely suffering or irreversibly comatose, or there is sufficient current evidence related to A's present condition such that one or more known causal laws supports B's belief that A will be in a condition of acute suffering or irreversible comatoseness.

The concept of suffering is notoriously difficult to analyze, yet its importance for discussions of euthanasia and other topics in medical ethics is undeniable. Although no detailed conceptual analysis will be provided here, we intend the notion to cover at least the following kinds of acute suffering: (*a*) conscious pain, (*b*) mental anguish, (*c*) serious self-burdensomeness. While the first two sorts of suffering will

be readily accepted by most persons, the third is more problematic. We regard this third kind of suffering as necessary to our analysis, since there are many states of human existence where there is no conscious pain or mental anguish and yet the person is severely suffering as a result of his condition. Examples would include spinal transsections, and tetraplegia after fracture of the cervical vertebrae (involving total paralysis from the neck down). One of the premiere films of the British Euthanasia Society deals with a patient of this description—a dedicated artist irreversibly paralyzed from the neck down. It is made clear that further existence is to him an unacceptable burden. He is unwilling to live without the capacity for artistic practice, which cannot be provided (even though life can be made relatively painless for him). There is an almost embarrassing lack of precision in the term "acute suffering" as it appears in condition 2, but we doubt that it can be improved by any substitute.

Also, predictability based on known causal laws is required in this formulation because it may be the case that although A is not presently suffering or irreversibly comatose, B has sufficient current evidence that, on the basis of known causal laws, A will be in a condition of acute suffering or irreversible comatoseness. This well-grounded, predicted suffering of A would play the same role for B as his belief in A's present suffering and thus must be included in the above condition.

Reasons for Death and the Means to Death

The notion that there must be a beneficient motive or a humanitarian reason in cases of euthanasia is one we previously encountered, and it is recurrent in the literature on euthanasia. While it is surely false that any beneficent reason is sufficient for euthanasia, it seems reasonable to require that the primary reason be to relieve another's actual or predicted future suffering or irreversible comatoseness. Any other primary reason would seem inconsistent with the intent to produce a "good death." If A is acutely suffering and B kills A for A's money, this *may* in fact produce a desirable death for A, but it hardly seems a case of euthanasia precisely because B's motives are inconsistent with our understanding of an act of euthanasia. More precisely, the notion of "causing death" requires further analysis in terms of the reasons the agent has for causing death. Clearly not any reason will do. The concept of euthanasia only admits a certain set of reasons which form a set *because* they are connected with cessation of suffering or irreversible comatoseness. Any other reason might be present and play a minor role, but it seems necessary that the primary reason be the cessation of suffering. And a corollary would seem to be that the causal means to the person's death must not produce any more suffering than would be produced for that person if a second person were not to intervene. If *more* suffering were produced by the intervention than would be produced by nonintervention, this again does not seem to be an instance of a "good death." For these reasons, we suggest a two-part third condition as follows. The death of a human being, A, is an instance of euthanasia only if:

3. (*a*) B's primary reason for intending A's death is cessation of A's (actual or predicted future) suffering or irreversible comatoseness, where B does not intend A's death for a different primary reason, though there may be other relevant reasons; and (*b*) there is sufficient current evidence for either A or B that the causal means to A's death will not produce any more suffering than would be produced for A if B were not to intervene.

Painlessness

We have previously considered proposals which require that an act of euthanasia be *painless* as well as *merciful,* and we have seen that these proposals require amendment. The general theoretical reason which forces this amendment is that a person might choose a more painful means of inducing death if it would hasten death, or if there were some similar overriding reasons for not choosing the least painless means. Such an overriding reason could actually require an act that involved more suffering than is strictly necessary without ceasing to be a genuine instance of euthanasia. However, if there is sufficient evidence that the means to death involves more total suffering in life than would be produced if death were not caused by

B (and not merely a "more painful means" than is necessary for death), then A's death would be worse with B's intervention than without it. If such a means were still chosen, the resulting death being *worse* than it would otherwise have been, then it is analytically true that A's death would not be a "good death." For all these reasons, we suggest a fourth condition of euthanasia as follows. The death of a human being A is an instance of euthanasia only if:

4. The causal means to the event of A's death are chosen by A or B to be as painless as possible, unless either A or B has an overriding reason for a more painful causal means, where the reason for choosing the later causal means does conflict with the evidence in 3*b*.

Nonfetal Humanity

Finally, a simple qualification of the above conditions is necessary. According to all the definitions of euthanasia considered in the previous section, it would not be possible to distinguish many abortions from acts of euthanasia. "The painless inducement of a quick death," for example, can be administered to fetuses as well as the acutely ill. If there were such a category as "fetal euthanasia" which paralleled "pediatric euthanasia," these definitions and other similar ones might be judged faultless. But we do sharply distinguish between abortion and euthanasia, and it would seem important to perpetuate the distinction in a formal definition. Also, we do on occasion euphemistically use the language of euthanasia in reference to animals, yet this extended usage seems to be a derivative one. In order to confine euthanasia to the human domain, we have always required that the death of A be a *human* death. However, we still need the following fifth condition. The death of human being A is an instance of euthanasia only if A is a nonfetal organism.

In summary, we have argued in this section that the death of a human being, A, is an instance of euthanasia if and only if (1) A's death is intended by at least one other human being, B, where B is either the cause of death or a causally relevant feature of the event resulting in death (whether by action or by omission); (2)

there is either sufficient current evidence for B to believe that A is acutely suffering or irreversibly comatose, or there is sufficient current evidence related to A's present condition such that one or more known causal laws supports B's belief that A will be in a condition of acute suffering or irreversible comatoseness; (3) (*a*) B's primary reason for intending A's death is cessation of A's (actual or predicted future) suffering or irreversible comatoseness, where B does not intend A's death for a different primary reason, though there may be other relevant reasons, and (*b*) there is sufficient current evidence for either A or B that causal means to A's death will not produce any more suffering than would be produced for A if B were not to intervene; (4) the causal means to the event of A's death are chosen by A or B to be as painless as possible, unless either A or B has an overriding reason for a more painful causal means, where the reason for choosing the latter causal means does not conflict with the evidence in 3*b*; (5) A is a nonfetal organism.

III

In this final section several objections to the above definition of euthanasia are considered, and each objection is rebutted. The three objections to be considered are the following: (1) the definition is too broad; (2) the definition is too narrow; and (3) the definition does not adequately handle borderline and similarly difficult cases.

1. Is the Definition Too Broad?

Definitions are too broad when they allow instances into the term's extension which are not in fact members of that class of instances which constitutes the normal extension of the term. That is, a definition is too broad when it allows an instance *Y* into the class *X* of the term's extension which is not a member of that class. It might be thought that our definition suffers from this defect because cases such as the following can be constructed. A person, B, pulls the plug on his brother A, who is acutely suffering. His motives are primarily to relieve A's suffering, and his action satisfies all our conditions (1–5). However, it is also the case

that A is not a terminal case, would have recovered fully (after prolonged agony), and does not want to die. Many would feel inclined to say that in this case B murdered his brother and that it is not a case of euthanasia. If so, the definition seems too broad.

We do not think, however, that this example is a genuine counterexample to our definition. The first thing to notice about the sorts of euthanasia cases which are commonly referred to as mercy killings is that under virtually all existent laws they are also homicides. There is no conceptual exclusion of murder, legally defined, when employing the notion of euthanasia, though there may be some question whether murder in the moral sense (wrongful killing from immoral motives) could be a case of euthanasia. Second, whether or not this case or any similar case is one of murder, we think it *is* one of euthanasia. The notion of "good death" as determined by the word "euthanasia" does not exclude a painful and even an unjust death, except as limited by condition 3*b*. It also does not exclude a "wrongful death" in the sense that someone with good motives might take the life of another when the life of the other ought not to have been taken. Perhaps the most difficult kind of case would be the following: B is a hospital attendant who has good reason, based on orders from A's doctor, to unplug A's respirator. When competent, A signed a living will granting the hospital permission to cease artificial respiration whenever A reached the present level of degeneration. However, A's doctor fails to inform the hospital attendant, B, that A's one-hundreth birthday is tomorrow and that A's only remaining wish in life was to reach 100. This case may involve murder and negligence in the legal sense, but it still seems to us a case of euthanasia, precisely because of B's good evidence, justified beliefs, and appropriate intention to produce a good death for A—and despite the wrongfully produced death for A. When B's evidence, beliefs, and intentions conform to our conditions 1–4 (and when 5 is met as well), this satisfaction of the conditions is solely sufficient for the classification of the act as one of euthanasia—independent of A's actual condition. (This sufficiency condition is further justified in our reply to objection 2 below.)

It is tempting to say that cases of this sort involve the *intent* to perform euthanasia or are cases of attempted euthanasia, not euthanasia itself, just as one can attempt murder without murdering. But in our euthanasia case A is dead, and his death cannot be understood as a mere attempt to allow him to die; B would be attempting euthanasia only if he tried but failed. Also, to say that he failed for reasons of ignorance would produce intolerable counterexamples. For example, consider a case where a man's aged grandfather, a physician, slips into irreversible coma. Involuntary euthanasia is performed. After he is buried, an authentic but heretofore undisclosed and completely unanticipated will is discovered. It contains a provision which forbids termination of his life while he is in a coma. We would surely not, in retrospect, say that euthanasia was *not* performed. The dead person's wishes perhaps make a moral difference in any judgment of what ought to have been done; but we cannot see that these wishes make a conceptual difference in regard to what was done. And if one is still inclined to say that there is a conceptual difference, it should be noticed that similar but even more problematic cases can be constructed, such as the following: (1) there is a bona fide legal will, though it is never discovered; (2) the dead person feared and did not want to have artificial respiration ceased while comatose, though he neglected to communicate this conviction; and (3) the dead person would have denied permission if he had (counterfactually) thought about it, but he just never got around to thinking about it.

Another objection is advanced in a most interesting recent article by Philippa Foot, who dismisses as too broad any definition of the sort we have defended in this paper. She argues that no definition is acceptable which includes under its instances persons who are comatose, such as Karen Quinlan. Her general theoretical reason is that the concept of euthanasia should apply only in cases where there is the intent to benefit an individual by relieving him from *suffering*. Her most direct argument for this claim seems to be the following: "Given the importance of the question, For whose sake are we acting? it is good to have a definition of euthanasia which brings under this heading only cases of opting for death for the sake of the one who dies. Perhaps what is most important is to say either that euthanasia is to be for the good of the subject or at least that death is to be no evil to him, thus refusing to talk Hitler's language. However, in this paper it is the first condition that will be understood . . ." (1977, p. 86). This argument seems to us to beg the question. We would not deny that the death should be a "good death" for the person who dies, as that term has been used throughout our paper. The problem is to determine what counts as a good death. Foot insists—without argument, so far as we can determine—that there can be a good death for a person only if that person is actually suffering. But why is this the only possible instance of a good death? Two common reasons in favor of euthanasia are the preservation of human dignity and the fulfillment of the express wishes of the patient. It is well known that patients in Quinlan's condition suffer a continuous decline in human functioning that can only be described as progressive loss of integrating capacities. It does not seem unreasonable to say that these persons are benefited by euthanasia, even though they are not relieved of suffering.

Foot confronts us with a false dilemma: Either you benefit such persons by the alleviation of suffering or you do not benefit them. What she overlooks is the possibility of a benefit which is not an alleviation of suffering. Yet if Foot were correct on this point, unacceptable consequences would follow. Suppose that Karen Quinlan had completed a legally supported "living will" which directed that in the event condition X should cause progressive degeneration no measures should be taken to preserve her life. Moreover, Quinlan could have specifically requested that even if she were not conscious, and therefore not suffering, she would still want to be allowed to die. One of the reasons for making such a request could be the (correct) belief that a person in these circumstances would be benefited by the observance of her directive. However, on Foot's argument such a person could not be benefited and therefore could not be an act of euthanasia, despite the living will on the basis of which the action is performed. Indeed, Foot's analysis would make one function of the living will unintelligible, since it is designed to authorize euthanasia even when a person is irreversibly comatose. Foot seems herself committed to this conclusion by another of her arguments. She argues that life itself is not to be considered a good, but that only "life coming up to some standard of normality" should be considered a good life (1977, p. 95). One who anticipates a comatose condition for himself and who considers it well below the threshold of an acceptable state of normality, and for this reason requests noncontinuance when the threshhold is reached, is benefited and not deprived by having his wish carried out.

Finally, in regard to the charge that our definition is too broad, some writers seem to feel quite strongly that an act of ending someone's life cannot be euthanasia unless the person is suffering either from a terminal illness or a mortal injury. We think this claim has strong intuitive appeal yet is without conceptual foundation. We previously mentioned the British Euthanasia Society film involving a patient with paralysis from the neck down. This person is seriously injured, but the injury is not a mortal one and he suffers no illness whatsoever. Cases of this sort can be multiplied indefinitely. Virtually all pediatric euthanasia cases are relevantly similar, since common operations usually can be performed to save the life of the infant who is neither mortally injured nor terminally ill. To say that all such cases are not cases of euthanasia simply because there are no conditions of terminal illness or mortal injury would be stipulative and would involve a substantial change in our ordinary use of the term.

It might also be thought that the inclusion of the notion of predicted suffering based on known causal laws makes our definition too broad. Suppose a degenerative disease exists which does not cause suffering until ten or twenty years after its initial onset. It might be claimed that an act would not really be one of euthanasia if it were committed at the time of onset of the disease, since it could be predicted that suffering would not have taken place until many years after the time the act was actually performed. However, diseases satisfying the above description, such as Huntington's Chorea, do exist, and we do want to accept examples such as this one as an instance of euthanasia. Any attempt to introduce temporal limitations into the prediction of suffering and the time of death seems to us to create insoluble problems. How *much* time would have to elapse between the act and the (predicted) suffering in order for that act to be no longer correctly classified as one of euthanasia? Any answer to this question specifying a determinate amount of time would be purely stipulative. If a causal law allowed one to predict that B would be acutely suffering or irreversibly comatose ten minutes from now, then an act which met our five conditions would clearly be one of euthanasia. We can find no justification for differentiating, in principle, between such a case and one in which the predicted suffering would not take place for ten years. In both cases it is the fact that suffering will occur which is decisive. It is not a matter of remoteness or proximity in the future.

2. Is the Definition Too Narrow?

Definitions are too narrow when they exclude instances in the term's extension which are in fact members of that class of instances which constitutes the normal extension of the term. That is, a definition is too narrow when it excludes an instance Y from the class X of the term's extension when Y is a member of that class. It might be thought that our definition is too narrow because it excludes cases such as the following. R. M. Hare adduces an interesting case of a driver in a petrol lorry which, after overturning, leaves the driver trapped inside and certain to be roasted to death (1975, p. 45). The driver requests that he be clubbed over the head with a bat in order that he not roast to death. Should the request be honored, Hare takes it to be an instance of euthanasia, and so do we. Suppose, however, that a case somewhat different from Hare's is considered in which B's clubbing of A actually produces more suffering for A than would be produced if he were not to intervene, and B knows before beginning that his action will produce more suffering. Still B is only complying with A's request. On our grounds it would seem that this is not an instance of euthanasia, and yet if one agrees, in the case of Hare's original example, that it is an instance of euthanasia, as we do, we would seem to be arbitrarily excluding such a case of (voluntary) euthanasia merely on grounds of the means employed to end the driver's life.

We think however, that this variation on Hare's case is *not* a case of euthanasia. In these circumstances B may be morally innocent for clubbing A over the head, since A requested it. Here we pass no judgment. However, since B knowingly chooses a means involving more suffering, then despite any commendable intentions he may have, we think this is not a case of euthanasia. By choosing a means which involves more suffering for A, B has created a worse death for A than would have been produced had he not intervened. For this reason, A's death cannot be said to be a "good death." Our root assumption here is that if the total volume of suffering is knowingly increased rather than decreased, then the person's death cannot be a *good death* in any acceptable sense of that term. Without some condition of this sort, unacceptable counterexamples would emerge involving torture and other excruciating means of producing death. However, it is to be noted that our condition 3*b* requires only that B have sufficient evidence that his intervention will not produce more suffering. It does not require that suffering cannot *unknowingly* be increased rather than decreased. As we have argued in our response to the objection that our definition is too broad, B's evidence, beliefs, and intentions do make a decisive difference to whether his action is a case of euthanasia. If B believes that his action will produce less suffering, on the basis of good evidence which he has to this effect, then it does not cease to become an act of euthanasia merely because the actual outcome involves a greater volume of suffering as the result of B's intervention.

In all these cases it is important to separate *moral* acceptability and unacceptability (since B may be morally innocent) from *conceptual* acceptability and unacceptability. We are, of course, exclusively concerned with the latter.

3. Is the Definition Too Vague?

Definitions are unacceptably general, vague, and therefore unhelpful when they cannot precisely place certain cases either within or outside the term's extension. That is to say, a definition is too vague when it does not precisely place an instance, Y, either within or outside of the class X of the term's extension. It might be argued that our definition is like this because cases such as the following can be constructed. A recovering patient, A, who is suffering acutely from painful tubes entering his nose and throat snatches them out in an effort to kill himself. A doctor sympathetic to A's discomfort, B, watches intently and decides not to prolong A's suffering by reinserting the tubes, though he could have done so easily and painlessly. This case seems to satisfy our conditions, since B (by omission) is a causally relevant feature of the event resulting in death; yet it seems to be a case of suicide, not of enthanasia. At least, so it can be argued, this case is not clearly one of euthanasia, and our definition does nothing to help us decide whether this and similar cases are ones of euthanasia or suicide. For this reason our definition seems unacceptably vague.

Although the charge of vagueness is correct, it is not a valid criticism of our definition. In cases such as the above, what is vague is whether or not B is in fact a causally relevant feature of the event resulting in death. If B is causally relevant (and all the other conditions are met) then the action is one of euthanasia. If B is not causally relevant, then the action is suicide and not euthansia. It is the vagueness which surrounds the notion of causal relevance that creates problems, leaving us uncertain how to classify individual cases. But this criticism is not a criticism of our definition; rather, it is a call for an analysis of the concept of causal relevance, especially as it is connected to that of causal responsibility. This latter clarification, although necessary and important, is beyond the scope of the present paper.

It is important to notice that the problem of B's causal role is a common and perplexing problem in the literature on euthanasia. It is left unclear or is arbitrarily decided in much of this literature which instances of physician responsibility do and which do not count as causally relevant features of an event in such a way that the event is one of euthanasia. For example, we think it is an arbitrary stipulation on the part of both Pope Pius XII and the AMA to exclude cases of letting die from the class of euthanasia acts.[7] As mentioned at the beginning of Section II, there is a commonly observed distinction between active and passive euthanasia. This distinction indicates that although "letting die" euthanasia may be distinguished by its passivity from active euthanasia, it is nevertheless a subclass of euthanasia acts. If one accepts this distinction, then there is no reason to disqualify letting die as euthanasia. On the other hand, if one rejects this distinction, then the only plausible principle by which to decide if an act is an instance of euthanasia seems to be some principle which explicates causal relevance. The notion of causal relevance plays this central role here because of its intimate connection with the notion of causal responsibility. If A is causally responsible for the death of B, then it is of no conceptual significance (even though it may be of moral importance) whether A's responsibility is active or passive; in either case he is still causally responsible. If one accepts some such principle, then those cases of death which include a second human being as a causally relevant feature are instances of euthanasia, while any cases of death which do not include a second causally relevant human being are not. This principle determines which cases of letting die are euthanasia cases and which are not. In addition, those cases of patient refusal of life-saving therapeutic procedures which satisfy our last four conditions and also include a second causally relevant human being are also instances of euthanasia on our definition.[8]

Consider now a case which *does not satisfy our conditions* yet which also *seems* to be a euthanasia case. A husband and wife are both nearing deaths which will involve lengthy suffering. They decide they want to die together before the onslaught of the worst phases of their illnesses. They do everything they can to make each other comfortable, and then she administers to herself, and he to himself, a fatal overdose. This is not a case of euthanasia by our definition, even if it is a good death, because neither of these individuals is a *causal* factor in the death of the other. Suppose, however, that only this one detail of the circumstances is altered: they feed the pills to each other rather

than self-feeding them. This would be a case of (double) euthanasia by our definition, since now each is a causal factor in the death of the other. Yet this is such a small and morally irrelevant change in the circumstances that it seems arbitrary to segregate one way of dying as euthanasia and the other as noneuthanasia. Moreover, an infinite string of similar cases which builds on a change in *morally irrelevant* causal intervention can be constructed, and this change will determine whether the case is one of euthanasia or not.

While this objection can be recast to make an interesting point, it is misguided as a criticism of our definition. It is a benefit, and not a detriment, of our definition that it preserves the distinction between unassisted suicide and the form of euthanasia which Williams categorizes as assisted suicide. There is conceptual distinction, inherent in the way we think about such actions, which it is desirable to keep as clear as possible, between the killing of oneself alone and the killing of oneself with the assistance of another. It is this distinction which Williams seeks to preserve with his notion of assisted suicide. Our causal formulation is, we think, as precise as one can be in the attempt to keep clear the difference between our concepts of suicide and euthanasia. It is precisely the causal agency which makes a difference wherever there is a difference.

IV

In conclusion, a methodological point underlying the analysis throughout this paper must be considered.

We have attempted to provide a descriptive definition of euthanasia which dictates no moral conclusions. Unlike a concept such as murder, euthanasia includes no inherently evaluative component. "Murder" entails *wrongful* killing, and therefore possesses both prescriptive and descriptive force; but "euthanasia" is not analogous. Some may claim that, because of its derivation from the Greek for "good death," "euthanasia," like "murder" must be inherently evaluative. But such a claim rests on the mistaken belief that, in this context, "good death" is an evaluative term. That "good death" does not here function as an evaluative term can be proved in the following way: If "euthanasia" is synonymous with "good death," then they are intersubstitutable *salva sensu* in referentially transparent and opaque contexts. Yet it is not a contradiction to say, "an act of euthanasia is immoral." Given the condition of synonymy, it must therefore not be a contradiction to say, "a good death is immoral." If "good death" were an evaluative term, both the former and later phrases would be contradictions, which they are not. We do not believe that it is conceptually required that all instances of euthanasia are either right or morally good. We are therefore using "good death," throughout our paper, criteriologically and not prescriptively. That is, we are using "good death" in accordance with the five conditions or criteria which we have argued determine the extension of the term, without in any way implying that a good death is (morally) good. As we have emphasized, we wish to provide a nonprescriptive definition of euthanasia, and we have accordingly sharply distinguished the descriptive meaning of the term from its prescriptive meaning. Since we have only been concerned with the former, the seeming paradox that a good death might not be good is really no paradox at all. Normative questions about euthanasia are entirely independent of the problem of the correct definition.

Notes

1. Quoted in Bok and Behnke 1975, p. 1.
2. Ibid.
3. On this point, see esp. Sec. III below. Perhaps Brody means to say that if B does not actually benefit from A's action, then the action is not justified. But this is a moral, and not a conceptual, point. In addition, one should not underestimate the epistemological problems inherent in Brody's definition. What type of evidence would be necessary to conclude that someone has *actually benefited* from being killed?
4. Other proposed definitions of euthanasia include the following (1–3 are from the collection of definitions found in Gorovitz et al. [1972]): (1) the intentional putting to death by artificial means of persons with incurable or painful disease (*Stedman's Medical Dictionary*); (2) the deliberate easing into death of a patient suffering from a painful and fatal disease (Joseph Fletcher); (3) the termination of human life by painless means for the purpose of ending severe physical suffering (Euthanasia Society of America); (4) the deliberate killing by a physician or other party of a person suffering from a painful and terminal illness (Cantor 1973). Our discussion in Sec. I and our discussion to follow in Secs. II and III should make clear the reasons for the deficiencies in all these definitions.
5. John Rawls (1971), pp. 19–21, 48–51. "Reflective equilibrium" is Rawl's term for that state of affairs in which our principles and judgments coincide, and which is arrived at by revising judgments to conform to principle and altering principles to account for judgments.
6. We use the language of "a second human being B" in order to distinguish human agency from nonhuman agency. It is possible that the cause of death, and even the *intended* cause of death, could be an animal's action (or robot's, or extraterrestrial's etc.). William's language of "assisted suicide" is especially regrettable in this connection. An example is the following: C, the owner of a pet rattlesnake which acts only on his owner's command, desires a good death. He therefore orders the rattlesnake to bite him, and dies as a result of the bite. This is clearly assisted suicide, even though the assistance is nonhuman; yet it is not an act of euthanasia. Still we do not wish to pass judgment on all of those actions intended by a nonhuman which result in another's death. Some of these actions may in fact qualify as euthanasia. Also, we have not attempted to distinguish between direct intent and implied intent. Whether or not it makes sense to claim that someone intended to do *X* even though he sincerely disavows any such intention, is a question the answer to which depends in part upon one's views on the epistemological status of first-person utterances. Such questions are beyond the scope of this paper.
7. James Rachels (1975) has uncovered some important elements of arbitrariness in the AMA's position.
8. Several patient refusal cases which illustrate this point are conveniently summarized and analyzed in Bryn (1975).

References

Bok, Sissela, and Behnke, John A., eds. *The Dilemmas of Euthanasia.* Garden City, N.Y.: Anchor/Doubleday, 1975.

BRODY, BARUCH. "Voluntary Euthanasia and the Law." In *Beneficient Euthanasia,* edited by Marvin Kohl. Buffalo, N.Y.: Prometheus Books, 1975.

BYRN, ROBERT M. "Compulsory Lifesaving Treatment for the Competent Adult." *Fordham Law Review* 44 (1975): 1–36.

CANTOR, N. "A Patient's Decision to Decline Lifesaving Medical Treatment: Bodily Integrity versus the Preservation of Life." *Rutgers Law Review* 26, no. 2 (Winter 1973): 228–64.

FOOT, PHILLIPA. "Euthanasia." *Philosophy and Public Affairs* 6, no. 2 (Winter 1977): 85–112.

GOROVITZ, S., et al. *Teaching Medical Ethics.* Cleveland: Case Western Reserve Press, 1972.

HARE, R. M. "Euthanasia." *Philosophic Exchange* 6, no. 2 (Summer 1975): 43–52.

HEALY, EDWIN F., S.J. *Medical Ethics.* Chicago: Loyola University Press, 1956.

KOHL, MARVIN. *The Morality of Killing.* New York: Humanities Press, 1974.

KOHL, MARVIN, and KURTZ, PAUL. "A Plea for Beneficient Euthanasia." In *Beneficient Euthanasia,* edited by Marvin Kohl. Buffalo, N.Y.: Prometheus Books, 1975.

RACHELS, JAMES. "Active and Passive Euthanasia." *New England Journal of Medicine* 292 (January 9, 1975): 78–80.

RAWLS, JOHN. *A Theory of Justice.* Cambridge, Mass.: Harvard University Press, 1971.

WILLIAMS, GLANVILLE. "Suicide." In *The Encyclopedia of Philosophy,* edited by Paul Edwards. Vol. 3. New York: Macmillan/Collier, 1966.

From "Euthanasia Legislation: Some Non-Religious Objections"

Yale Kamisar

A book by Glanville Williams, *The Sanctity of Life and the Criminal Law,* once again brought to the fore the controversial topic of euthanasia, more popularly known as "mercy-killing." In keeping with the trend of the euthanasia movement over the past generation, Williams concentrates his efforts for reform on the *voluntary* type of euthanasia, for example the cancer victim begging for death, as opposed to the *involuntary* variety—that is, the case of the congenital idiot, the permanently insane or the senile. . . .

As an ultimate philosophical proposition, the case for voluntary euthanasia is strong. Whatever may be said for and against suicide generally, the appeal of death is immeasurably greater when it is sought not for a poor reason or just any reason, but for "good cause," so to speak; when it is invoked not on behalf of a "socially useful" person, but on behalf of, for example, the pain-racked "hopelessly in-

Reprinted with permission from *Euthanasia and the Right to Die,* ed. A. B. Downing (New York: Humanities Press; London: Peter Owen Ltd., 1970) pp. 85–133.

curable" cancer victim. If a person is *in fact* (1) presently incurable, (2) beyond the aid of any respite which may come along in his life expectancy, suffering (3) intolerable and (4) unmitigable pain and of a (5) fixed and (6) rational desire to die, I would hate to have to argue that the hand of death should be stayed. But abstract propositions and carefully formed hypotheticals are one thing; specific proposals designed to cover everyday situations are something else again.

In essence, Williams's specific proposal is that death be authorized for a person in the above situation "by giving the medical practitioner a wide discretion and trusting to his good sense."[2] This, I submit, raises too great a risk of abuse and mistake to warrant a change in the existing law. That a proposal entails risk of mistake is hardly a conclusive reason against it. But neither is it irrelevant. Under any euthanasia programme the consequences of mistake, of course, are always fatal. As I shall endeavour to show, the incidence of mistake of one kind or another is likely to be quite appreciable. If this indeed be the case, unless the need for the authorized conduct is compelling enough to override it, I take it the risk of mistake *is* a conclusive reason against such authorization. I submit, too, that the possible radiations from the proposed legislation—for example, involuntary euthanasia of idiots and imbeciles (the typical ''mercy-killings'' reported by the press)—and the emergence of the legal precedent that there are lives not ''worth living,'' give additional cause for reflection.

I see the issue, then, as the need for voluntary euthanasia versus (1) the incidence of mistake and abuse; and (2) the danger that legal machinery initially designed to kill those who are a nuisance to themselves may some day engulf those who are a nuisance to others.

The ''freedom to choose a merciful death by euthanasia'' may well be regarded as a special area of civil liberties. This is definitely a part of Professor Williams's approach:

> If the law were to remove its ban on euthanasia, the effect would merely be to leave this subject to the individual conscience. This proposal would . . . be easy to defend, as restoring personal liberty in a field in which men differ on the question of conscience. . . . On a question like this there is surely everything to be said for the liberty of the individual.[3]

I am perfectly willing to accept civil liberties as the battlefield, but issues of ''liberty'' and ''freedom'' mean little until we begin to pin down *whose* ''liberty'' and ''freedom'' and for *what* need and at *what* price. Williams champions the ''personal liberty'' of the dying to die painlessly. I am more concerned about the life and liberty of those who would needlessly be killed in the process or who would irrationally choose to partake of the process. Williams's price on behalf of those who are *in fact* ''hopeless incurables'' and *in fact* of a fixed and rational desire to die is the sacrifice of (1) some few, who, though they know it not, because their physicians know it not, need not and should not die; (2) others, probably not so few, who, though they go through the motions of ''volunteering,'' are casualties of strain, pain or narcotics to such an extent that they really

know not what they do. My price on behalf of those who, despite appearances to the contrary, have some relatively normal and reasonably useful life left in them, or who are incapable of making the choice, is the lingering on for awhile of those who, if you will, *in fact* have no desire and no reason to linger on. . . .

Under current proposals to establish legal machinery, elaborate or otherwise, for the administration of a quick and easy death, it is not enough that those authorized to pass on the question decide that the patient, in effect, is ''better off dead.'' The patient must concur in this opinion. Much of the appeal in the current proposal lies in this so-called ''voluntary'' attribute.

But is the adult patient really in a position to concur? Is he truly able to make euthanasia a ''voluntary'' act? . . .

By hypothesis, voluntary euthanasia is not to be resorted to until narcotics have long since been administered and the patient has developed a tolerance to them. *When,* then, does the patient make the choice? While heavily drugged? Or is narcotic relief to be withdrawn for the time of decision? But if heavy dosage no longer deadens pain, indeed, no longer makes it bearable, how overwhelming is it when whatever relief narcotics offer is taken away too?

''Hypersensitivity to pain after analgesia has worn off is nearly always noted.''[4] Moreover, ''the mental side-effects of narcotics, unfortunately for anyone wishing to suspend them temporarily without unduly tormenting the patient, appear to outlast the analgesic effect'' and ''by many hours.''[5] The situation is further complicated by the fact that ''a person in terminal stages of cancer who had been given morphine steadily for a matter of weeks would certainly be dependent upon it physically and would probably be addicted to it and react with the addict's responses.''[6]

The narcotics problem aside, Dr. Benjamin Miller, who probably has personally experienced more pain than any other commentator on the euthanasia scene, observes:

> Anyone who has been severely ill knows how distorted his judgment became during the worst moments of the illness. Pain and the toxic effect of

disease, or the violent reaction to certain surgical procedures may change our capacity for rational and courageous thought.[7]

Undoubtedly, some euthanasia candidates will have their lucid moments. How they are to be distinguished from fellow-sufferers who do not, or how these instances are to be distinguished from others when the patient is exercising an irrational judgment, is not an easy matter. . . .

Assuming, for purposes of argument, that the occasion when a euthanasia candidate possesses a sufficiently clear mind can be ascertained and that a request for euthanasia is then made, there remain other problems. The mind of the pain-racked may occasionally be clear, but is it not also likely to be uncertain and variable? . . .

The concept of "voluntary" in voluntary euthanasia would have a great deal more substance to it if, as is the case with voluntary admission statutes for the mentally ill, the patient retained the right to reverse the process within a specified number of days after he gives written notice of his desire to do so—but unfortunately this cannot be. The choice here, of course, is an irrevocable one. . . .

If consent is given at a time when the patient's condition has so degenerated that he has become a fit candidate for euthanasia, when, if ever, will it be "clear and incontrovertible"? Is the suggested alternative of consent in advance a satisfactory solution? Can such a consent be deemed an informed one? Is this much different from holding a man to a prior statement of intent that if such and such an employment opportunity would present itself he would accept it, or if such and such a young woman were to come along he would marry her? Need one marshal authority for the proposition that many an "iffy" inclination is disregarded when the actual facts are at hand?

Professor Williams states that where a pre-pain desire for "ultimate euthanasia" is "reaffirmed" under pain, "there is the best possible proof of full consent." Perhaps. But what if it is alternately renounced and reaffirmed under pain? What if it is neither affirmed or renounced? What if it is only renounced? Will a physician be free to go ahead on the ground that the prior desire was "rational," but the present desire "irrational"? Under Williams's plan, will not the physician frequently "be walking in the margin of the law"—just as he is now? Do we really accomplish much more under this proposal than to put the euthanasia principle on the books?

Even if the patient's choice could be said to be "clear and incontrovertible," do not other difficulties remain? Is this the kind of choice, assuming that it can be made in a fixed and rational manner, that we want to offer a gravely ill person? Will we not sweep up, in the process, some who are not really tired of life, but think others are tired of them; some who do not really want to die, but who feel they should not live on, because to do so when there looms the legal alternative of euthanasia is to do a selfish or a cowardly act? Will not some feel an obligation to have themselves "eliminated" in order that funds allocated for their terminal care might be better used by their families or, financial worries aside, in order to relieve their families of the emotional strain involved?

It would not be surprising for the gravely ill person to seek to inquire of those close to him whether he should avail himself of the legal alternative of euthanasia. Certainly, he is likely to wonder about their attitude in the matter. It is quite possible, is it not, that he will not exactly be gratified by any inclination on their part— however noble their motives may be in fact—that he resort to the new procedure? At this stage, the patient-family relationship may well be a good deal less than it ought to be.

And what of the relatives? If their views will not always influence the patient, will they not at least influence the attending physician? Will a physician assume the risks to his reputation, if not his pocketbook, by administering the *coup de grâce* over the objection—however irrational— of a close relative. Do not the relatives, then, also have a "choice"? Is not the decision on their part to do nothing and say nothing *itself* a "choice"? In many families there will be some, will there not, who will consider a stand against euthanasia the only proof of love, devotion and gratitude for past events? What of the stress and strife if close relatives differ over the desirability of euthanatizing the patient?

At such a time, members of the family are

not likely to be in the best state of mind, either, to make this kind of decision. Financial stress and conscious or unconscious competition for the family's estate aside,

> the chronic illness and persistent pain in terminal carcinoma may place strong and excessive stresses upon the family's emotional ties with the patient. The family members who have strong emotional attachment to start with are most likely to take the patient's fears, pains and fate personally. Panic often strikes them. Whatever guilt feelings they may have toward the patient emerge to plague them.
>
> If the patient is maintained at home, many frustrations and physical demands may be imposed on the family by the advanced illness. There may develop extreme weakness, incontinence and bad odors. The pressure of caring for the individual under these circumstances is likely to arouse a resentment and, in turn, guilt feelings on the part of those who have to do the nursing. . . .[8]

Putting aside the problem of whether the good sense of the general practitioner warrants dispensing with other personnel, there still remain the problems posed by *any* voluntary euthanasia programme: the aforementioned considerable pressures on the patient and his family. Are these the kind of pressures we want to inflict on any person, let alone a very sick person? Are these the kind of pressures we want to impose on any family, let alone an emotionally shattered family? And if so, why are they not also proper considerations for the crippled, the paralyzed, the quadruple amputee, the iron-lung occupant and their families? . . . One cannot help but think of how fallible the *average* general practitioner must be, how fallible the *young doctor just starting practice* must be—and this, of course, is all that some small communities have in the way of medical care—how fallible the *worst* practitioner, young or old, must be. If the range of skill and judgment among licensed physicians approaches the wide gap between the very best and the very worst members of the bar—and I have no reason to think it does not—then the minimally competent physician is hardly the man to be given the responsibility for ending another's life.[9] Yet, under Williams's proposal at least, the marginal

physician, as well as his more distinguished brethren, would have legal authorization to make just such decisions. Under Williams's proposal, euthanatizing a patient or two would all be part of the routine day's work.

Perhaps it is not amiss to add as a final note, that no less a euthanasiast than Dr. C. Killick Millard had such little faith in the average general practitioner that as regards the *mere administering of the coup de grâce*, he observed:

> In order to prevent any likelihood of bungling, it would be very necessary that only medical practitioners who had been specially licensed to euthanize (after acquiring special knowledge and skill) should be allowed to administer euthanasia. Quite possibly, the work would largely be left in the hands of the official euthanizors who would have to be appointed specially for each area.[10]

True, the percentage of correct diagnosis is particularly high in cancer. The short answer, however, is that euthanasiasts most emphatically do not propose to restrict mercy-killing to cancer cases. Dr Millard has maintained that "there are very many diseases besides cancer which tend to kill 'by inches', and where death, when it does at last come to the rescue, is brought about by pain and exhaustion".[11] Furthermore, even if mercy-killings were to be limited to cancer, however relatively accurate the diagnosis in these cases, here, too, "incurability of a disease is never more than an estimate based upon experience, and how fallacious experience may be in medicine only those who have a great deal of experience fully realize.". . .[12]

Faulty diagnosis is only one ground for error. Even if the diagnosis is correct, a second ground for error lies in the possibility that some measure of relief, if not a full cure, may come to the fore within the life expectancy of the patient. Since Glanville Williams does not deign this objection to euthanasia worth more than a passing reference, it is necessary to turn elsewhere to ascertain how it has been met. One answer is: "It must be little comfort to a man slowly coming apart from multiple sclerosis to think that fifteen years from now, death might not be his only hope."[13]

To state the problem this way is of course, to

avoid it entirely. How do we know that fifteen *days* or fifteen *hours* from now, "death might not be [the incurable's] only hope"?

A second answer is: "No cure for cancer which might be found 'tomorrow' would be of any value to a man or woman 'so far advanced in cancerous toxemia as to be an applicant for euthanasia.'"[14]

As I shall endeavour to show, this approach is a good deal easier to formulate than it is to apply. For one thing, it presumes that we know to-day *what* cures will be found tomorrow. For another, it overlooks that if such cases can be said to exist, the patient is likely to be *so far* advanced in cancerous toxemia as to be no longer capable of understanding the step he is taking and hence *beyond* the stage when euthanasia ought to be administered.

Thirty-six years ago, Dr Haven Emerson, then President of the American Public Health Association, made the point that "no one can say today what will be incurable tomorrow. No one can predict what disease will be fatal or permanently incurable until medicine becomes stationary and sterile." Dr Emerson went so far as to say that "to be at all accurate we must drop altogether the term "incurables" and substitute for it some such term as 'chronic illness.'"[15]

At that time Dr Emerson did not have to go back more than a decade to document his contention. Before Banting and Best's insulin discovery, many a diabetic had been doomed. Before the Whipple-Minot-Murphy liver treatment made it a relatively minor malady, many a pernicious anaemia sufferer had been branded "hopeless." Before the uses of sulphanilomide were disclosed, a patient with widespread streptococcal blood-poisoning was a condemned man.

Today, we may take even that most resolute disease, cancer, and we need look back no further than the last two decades of research in this field to document the same contention. True, many types of cancer still run their course virtually unhampered by man's arduous efforts to inhibit them. But the number of cancers coming under some control is ever increasing. With medicine attacking on so many fronts with so many weapons, who would bet a man's life on when and how the next type of cancer will yield, if only just a bit? Of course, we would not be betting much of a life. For even in those areas where gains have been registered, the life is not "saved," death is only postponed. In a sense this is the case with every 'cure' for every ailment. But it may be urged that, after all, there is a great deal of difference between the typical "cure" which achieves an indefinite postponement, more or less, and the cancer respite which results in only a brief intermission, so to speak, of rarely more than six months or a year. Is this really long enough to warrant all the bother?

Well, how long *is* long enough? In many recent cases of cancer respite, the patient, though experiencing only temporary relief, underwent sufficient improvement to retake his place in society. Six or twelve or eighteen months is long enough to do most of the things which socially justify our existence, is it not? Long enough for a nurse to care for more patients, a teacher to impart learning to more classes, a judge to write a great opinion, a novelist to write a stimulating book, a scientist to make an important discovery and, after all, for a factory-hand to put the wheels on another year's Cadillac. . . .

A relevant question, then, is what is the need for euthanasia which leads us to tolerate the mistakes, the very fatal mistakes, which will inevitably occur? What is the compelling force which requires us to tinker with deeply entrenched and almost universal precepts of criminal law?

Let us first examine the qualitive need for euthanasia.

Proponents of euthanasia like to a present for consideration the case of the surgical operation, particularly a highly dangerous one: risk of death is substantial, perhaps even more probable than not; in addition, there is always the risk that the doctors have misjudged the situation and that no operation was needed at all. Yet it is not unlawful to perform the operation.

The short answer is the witticism that whatever the incidence of death in connection with different types of operations, "no doubt, it is in all cases below 100 per cent, which is the incidence rate for euthanasia."[16] But this may not be the full answer. There are occasions where the law permits action involving about a 100 per cent incident of death—for example, self-defence. There may well be other instances where the law should condone such action—for example, the "necessity" cases illustrated by the overcrowded lifeboat, the starving survivors of a shipwreck and—perhaps best of all—by Professor Lon Fuller's penetrating and fascinating tale of the trapped cave explorers.

In all these situations, death for some may well be excused, if not justified, yet the prospect that some deaths will be unnecessary is a real one. He who kills in self-defence may have misjudged the facts. They who throw passengers overboard to lighten the load may no sooner do so than see "masts and sails of rescue . . . emerge out of the fog."[17] But no human being will ever find himself in a situation where he knows for an absolute certainty that one or several must die that he or others may live. "Modern legal systems . . . do not require divine knowledge of human beings."[18]

Reasonable mistakes, then, may be tolerated if, as in the above circumstances and as in the case of the surgical operation, these mistakes are the inevitable by-products of efforts to save one or more human lives.

The need the euthanasiast advances, however, is a good deal less compelling. It is only to ease pain. . . .

That of those who do suffer and must necessarily suffer the requisite pain, many *really* desire death, I have considerable doubt. Further, that of those who may desire death at a given moment, many have a fixed and rational desire for death, I likewise have considerable doubt. Finally, taking those who may have such a desire, again I must register a strong note of scepticism that many cannot do the job themselves. It is not that I condone suicide. It is simply that I find it easier to prefer a *laissez-faire* approach in such matters over an approach aided and sanctioned by the state.

The need is only one variable. The incidence of mistake is another. Can it not be said that although the need is not very great it is great enough to outweigh the few mistakes which are likely to occur? I think not. The incidence of error may be small in euthanasia, but as I have

endeavoured to show, and as Professor Williams has not taken pains to deny, under our present state of knowledge appreciable error is inevitable.

Even if the need for voluntary euthanasia could be said to outweigh the risk of mistake, this is not the end of the matter. That "all that can be expected of any moral agent is that he should do his best on the facts as they appear to him"[19] may be true as far as it goes, but it would seem that where the consequence of error is so irreparable it is not too much to expect of society that there be *a good deal more than one moral agent* "to do his best on the facts as they appear to him."

Notes

1. Williams, p. 278. This seems to be the position taken by Bertrand Russell in reviewing Williams's book: 'The central theme of the book is the conflict in the criminal law between the divergent systems of ethics which may be called respectively utilitarian and taboo morality. . . . Utilitarian morality in the wide sense in which I am using the word, judges actions by their effects. . . . In taboo morality . . . forbidden actions are sin, and they do not cease to be so when their consequences are such as we should all welcome.' (*Stanford Law Review,* 10 [1958], 382) I trust Russell would agree, should he read this article, that the issue is not quite so simple. At any rate, I trust he would agree that I stay within the system of utilitarian ethics.

2. Id., p. 302.

3. Id., pp. 304, 309.

4. Goodman and Gilman, *The Pharmacological Basis of Therapeutics* (2nd edn, 1955), p. 235. To the same effect is Seevers and Pfeiffer, 'A study of the Analgesia, Subjective Depression and Euphoria Produced by Morphine, Heroin, Dilaudid and Codeine in the Normal Human Subject', *Journal of Pharmacological and Experimental Therapy,* 56 (1936), 166, 182, 187.

5. Sharpe, 'Medication as a Threat to Testamentary Capacity', *N. Carolina Law Review,* 35 (1957), 380, 392, and medical authorities cited therein. In the case of ACTH or cortisone therapy, the situation is complicated by the fact that 'a frequent pattern of recovery' from psychoses induced by such therapy is 'by the occurrence of

lucid intervals of increasing frequency and duration, punctuated by relapses in psychotic behavior'. (Clark *et al.,* 'Further Observations on Mental Disturbances Associated with Cortisone and ACTH Therapy', *New England Journal of Medicine,* 249 [1953], 178, 183)

6. Sharpe, op. cit., 384. Goodman and Gilman observe that while 'different individuals require varying periods of time before the repeated administration of morphine results in tolerance . . . as a rule . . . after about two or three weeks of continued use of the same dose of alkaloid the usual depressant effects fail to appear', whereupon 'phenomenally large doses may be taken'. (Op. cit. [*n.* 24 above]. p. 234) For a discussion of 'the nature of addiction', see Maurer and Vogel, *Narcotics and Narcotic Addiction* (1954), pp. 20-31.

7. 'Why I Oppose Mercy Killings', *Woman's Home Companion* (June 1950), pp. 38, 103.

8. Zarling, 'Psychological Aspects of Pain in Terminal Malignancies', *Management of Pain in Cancer* (Schiffrin edn, 1956), pp. 211-12.

9. As to how bad the bad physician can be, see generally, even with a grain of salt, Belli, *Modern Trials,* 3 (1954), §§ 327-53. See also Regan, *Doctor and Patient and the Law* (3rd edn, 1956), pp. 17-40.

10. 'The Case for Euthanasia', *Fortnightly Review,* 136 (1931), 701-717. Under his proposed safeguards (two independent doctors, followed by a 'medical referee') Dr. Millard viewed error in diagnosis as a non-deterrable 'remote possibility'. (Ibid.)

11. Op. cit., 702.

12. Frohman, 'Vexing Problems in Forensic Medicine: A Physician's View' *N.Y.U. Law Review* 31 (1956), 1215, 1216. Dr Frohman added: 'We practice our art with the tools and information yielded by laboratory and research scientists, but an ill patient is not subject to experimental control, nor are his reactions always predictable. A good physician employs his scientific tools whenever they are useful, but many are the times when intuition, change, and faith are his most successful techniques.'

13. Pro & Con: Shall We Legalize ''Mercy Killing''?', *Reader's Digest* (Nov. 1938), pp. 94, 96.

14. James, 'Euthanasia—Right or Wrong?', *Survey Graphic* (May 1948), pp. 241, 243; Wolbarst, 'The Doctor Looks at Euthanasia', *Medical Record,* 149 (1939), 354, 355.

15. Emerson, 'Who Is Incurable? A Query and a Reply', *New York Times* (Oct. 22, 1933), § 8, p. 5 col. I.

16. Rudd, 'Euthanasia', *Journal of Clinical & Experimental Psychopathology,* 14 (1953), I, 4.

17. Cardozo, 'What Medicine Can Do for Law', *Law and Literature* (1931), p. 113.

18. Hall, *General Principles of Criminal Law* (1947), p. 399. Cardozo, on the other hand, seems to say that without such certainty it is wrong for those in a 'necessity' situation to escape their plight by sacrificing any life. (Loc. cit. [*n.* 20 above]) On this point, as on the whole question of 'necessity', his reasoning, it is submitted, is paled by the careful, intensive analyses found in Hall, op. cit., pp. 377-426, and Williams, *Criminal Law: The General Part* (Wm Stevens, 1953; 2nd edn, 1961), pp. 737-44. See also Cahn, *The Moral Decision* (1955). Although he takes the position that in the Holmes' situation, 'if none sacrifice themselves of free will to spare the others—they must all wait and die together', Cahn rejects Cardozo's view as one which 'seems to deny that we can ever reach enough certainty as to our factual beliefs to be morally justified in the action we take'. (Ibid., pp. 70-71)

Section 3.02 of the *Model Penal Code* (Tent, Draft No. 8, 1958) provides (unless the legislature has otherwise spoken) that certain 'necessity' killings shall be deemed justifiable so long as the actor was not 'reckless or negligent in bringing about the situation requiring a choice of evils or in appraising the necessity for his conduct'. The section only applies to a situation where 'the evil sought to be avoided by such conduct is greater than that sought to be prevented by the law', e.g. killing one that several may live. The defence would not be available, e.g. 'to one who acted to save himself at the expense of another, as by seizing a raft when men are shipwrecked'. (Ibid., *Comment* Section 3.02. p. 8) For 'in all ordinary circumstances lives in being must be assumed . . . to be of equal value, equally deserving of the law'. (Ibid.)

19. Williams, p. 283.

"Mercy-Killing" Legislation —
A Rejoinder

Glanville Williams

I welcome Professor Kamisar's reply[1] to my argument for voluntary euthanasia, because it is on the whole a careful, scholarly work, keeping to knowable facts and accepted human values. It is, therefore, the sort of reply that can be rationally considered and dealt with.[2] In this short rejoinder I shall accept most of Professor Kamisar's valuable footnotes, and merely submit that they do not bear out his conclusion.

The argument in favour of voluntary euthanasia in the terminal stages of painful diseases is quite a simple one, and is an application of two values that are widely recognised. The first value is the prevention of cruelty. Much as men differ in their ethical assessments, all agree that cruelty is an evil—the only difference of opinion residing in what is meant by cruelty. Those who plead for the legalization of euthanasia think that it is cruel to allow a human being to linger for months in the last stages of agony, weakness and decay; and to refuse him his demand for merciful release. There is also a second cruelty involved—not perhaps quite so compelling, but still worth consideration: the agony of the relatives in seeing their loved one in his desperate plight. Opponents of euthanasia are apt to take a cynical view of the desires of relatives, and this may sometimes be justified. But it cannot be denied that a wife who has to nurse her husband through the last stages of some terrible disease may herself be so deeply affected by the experience that her health is ruined, either mentally or physically. Whether the situation can be eased for such a person by voluntary euthanasia I do not know; probably it depends very much on the individuals concerned, which is as much as to say that no solution in terms of a general regulatory law can be satisfactory. The conclusion should be in favour of individual discretion.

Reprinted with permission from the author and *Minnesota Law Review*, vol. 43:1, November 1958.

The second value involved is that of liberty. The criminal law should not be invoked to repress conduct unless this is demonstrably necessary on social grounds. What social interest is there in preventing the sufferer from choosing to accelerate his death by a few months? What positive value does his life still possess for society, that he is to be retained in it by the terrors of the criminal law?

And, of course, the liberty involved is that of the doctor as well as that of the patient. It is the doctor's responsibility to do all he can to prolong worth-while life, or, in the last resort, to ease his patient's passage. If the doctor honestly and sincerely believes that the best service he can perform for his suffering patient is to accede to his request for euthanasia, it is a grave thing that the law should forbid him to do so.

This is the short and simple case for voluntary euthanasia, and, as Kamisar admits, it cannot be attacked directly on utilitarian grounds. Such an attack can only be by finding possible evils of an indirect nature. These evils, in the view of Professor Kamisar, are (1) the difficulty of ascertaining consent, and arising out of that the danger of abuse; (2) the risk of an incorrect diagnosis; (3) the risk of administering euthanasia to a person who could later have been cured by developments in medical knowledge; (4) the "wedge" argument.

Before considering these matters, one preliminary comment may be made. In some parts of his Article Kamisar hints at recognition of the fact that a practice of mercy-killing exists among the most reputable of medical practitioners. Some of the evidence for this will be found in my book.[3] In the first debate in the House of Lords, Lord Dawson admitted the fact, and claimed that it did away with the need for legislation. In other words, the attitude of conservatives is this: let medical men do mercy-killing, but let it continue to be called murder, and be treated as such if the legal machinery is by some unlucky mischance made to work; let us, in other words, take no steps to translate the new morality into the concepts of the law. I find this attitude equally incomprehensible in a doctor, as Lord Dawson was, and in a lawyer, as Professor Kamisar is. Still more baffling does it become when Professor Kamisar seems to claim as a virtue of the system that the jury can give a merciful acquittal in breach of their oaths.[4] The result is that the law frightens some doctors from interposing, while not frightening others—though subjecting the braver group to the risk of prosecution and possible loss of liberty and livelihood. Apparently, in Kamisar's view, it is a good thing if the law is broken in a proper case, because that relieves suffering, but also a good thing that the law is there as a threat in order to prevent too much mercy being administered; thus, whichever result the law has is perfectly right and proper. It is hard to understand on what moral principle this type of ethical ambivalence is to be maintained. If Kamisar does approve of doctors administering euthanasia in some clear cases, and of juries acquitting them if they are prosecuted for murder, how does he maintain that it is an insuperable objection to euthanasia that diagnosis may be wrong and medical knowledge subsequently extended?

However, the references to merciful acquittals disappear after the first few pages of the Article, and thenceforward the argument develops as a straight attack on euthanasia. So although at the beginning Kamisar says that he would hate to have to argue against mercy-killing in a clear case, in fact he does proceed to argue against it with some zest.

In my book I reported that there were some people who opposed the Euthanasia Bill as it stood, because it brought a ridiculous number of formalities into the sickroom, and pointed out, without any kind of verbal elaboration, that these same people did not say that they would have supported the measure without the safeguards. I am puzzled by Professor Kamisar's description of these sentences of mine as "more than bitter comments."[5] Like his references to my "ire," my "neat boxing" and "gingerly parrying," it seems to be justified by considerations of literary style. However, if the challenge is made, a sharper edge can be given

to the criticism of this opposition than I incorporated in my book.

The point at issue is this. Opponents of voluntary euthanasia say that it must either be subject to ridiculous and intolerable formalities, or else be dangerously free from formalities. Kamisar accepts this line of argument, and seems prepared himself to ride both horses at once. He thinks that they present an ordinary logical dilemma, saying that arguments made in antithesis may each be valid. Perhaps I can best explain the fallacy in this opinion, as I see it, by a parable.

In the State of Ruritania many people live a life of poverty and misery. They would be glad to emigrate to happier lands, but the law of Ruritania bans all emigration. The reason for this law is that the authorities are afraid that if it were relaxed there would be too many people seeking to emigrate, and the population would be decimated.

A member of the Ruritanian Senate, whom we will call Senator White, wants to see some change in this law, but he is aware of the power of traditional opinion, and so seeks to word his proposal in a modest way. According to his proposal, every person, before being allowed to emigrate, must fill up a questionnaire in which he states his income, his prospects and so on; he must satisfy the authorities that he is living at near-starvation level, and there is to be an Official Referee to investigate that his answers are true.

Senator Black, a member of the Government Party, opposes the proposal on the ground that it is intolerable that a free Ruritanian citizen should be asked to write out these humiliating details of his life, and particularly that he should be subject to the investigation of an Official Referee.

Now it will be evident that this objection of Senator Black may be a reasonable and proper one *if* the Senator is prepared to go further than the proposal and say that citizens who so wish should be entitled to emigrate without formality. But if he uses his objections to formality in order to support the existing ban on emigration, one can only say that he must be muddle-headed, or self-deceptive, or hypocritical. It may be an interesting exercise to decide which of these three adjectives fit him, but one of them must do so. For any unbiased mind can perceive that it is better to be allowed to emigrate on condition of form-filling than not to be allowed to emigrate at all.

I should be sorry to have to apply any of the three adjectives to Professor Kamisar, who has conducted the debate on a level which protects him from them. But, although it may be my shortcoming, I cannot see any relevant difference between the assumed position of Senator Black on emigration and the argument of Kamisar on euthanasia. Substitute painful and fatal illness for poverty, and euthanasia for emigration, and the parallel would appear to be exact.

I agree with Kamisar and the critics in thinking that the procedure of the Euthanasia Bill was over-elaborate, and that it would probably fail to operate in many cases for this reason. But this is no argument for rejecting the measure, if it is the most that public opinion will accept.

Let me now turn to the proposal for voluntary euthanasia permitted without formality, as I have put it forward in my book.

Kamisar's first objection, under the heading of "The Choice," is that there can be no such thing as truly voluntary euthanasia in painful and killing diseases. He seeks to impale the advocates of euthanasia on an old dilemma. Either the victim is not yet suffering pain, in which case his consent is merely an uninformed and anticipatory one—and he cannot bind himself by contract to be killed in the future—or he is crazed by pain and stupified by drugs, in which case he is not of sound mind. I have dealt with this problem in my book; Kamisar has quoted generously from it, and I leave the reader to decide. As I understand Kamisar's position, he does not really persist in the objection. With the laconic "Perhaps," he seems to grant me, though unwillingly, that there are cases where one can be sure of the patient's consent. But having thus abandoned his own point, he then goes off to a different horror, that the patient may give his consent only in order to relieve his relatives of the trouble of looking after him.

On this new issue, I will return Kamisar the compliment and say: "Perhaps." We are certainly in an area where no solution is going to make things quite easy and happy for everybody, and all sorts of embarrassments may be conjectured. But these embarrassments are not avoided by keeping to the present law: we suffer from them already. If a patient, suffering pain in a terminal illness, wishes for euthanasia partly because of this pain and partly because he sees his beloved ones breaking under the strain of caring for him, I do not see how this decision on his part, agonizing though it may be, is necessarily a matter of discredit either to the patient himself or to his relatives. The fact is that, whether we are considering the patient or his relatives, there are limits to human endurance.

The author's next objection rests on the possibility of mistaken diagnosis. There are many reasons why this risk cannot be accurately measured, one of them being that we cannot be certain how much use would actually be made of proposed euthanasia legislation. At one place in his Article the author seems to doubt whether the law would do much good anyway, because we don't know it will be used. ("Whether or not the general practitioner will accept the responsibility Williams would confer on him is itself a problem of major proportions."[6]) But later, the Article seeks to extract the maximum of alarm out of the situation by assuming that the power will be used by all and sundry—young practitioners just starting in practice, and established practitioners who are minimally competent.[7] In this connection, the author enters in some detail into examples of mistaken diagnosis for cancer and other diseases. I agree with him that, before deciding on euthanasia in any particular case, the risk of mistaken diagnosis would have to be considered.[8] Everything that is said in the Article would, therefore, be most relevant when the two doctors whom I propose in my suggested measure come to consult on the question of euthanasia; and the possibility of mistake might most forcefully be brought before the patient himself. But have these medical questions any real relevance to the legal discussion?

Kamisar, I take it, notwithstanding his wide reading in medical literature, is by training a lawyer. He has consulted much medical opinion in order to find arguments against changing the law. I ought not to object to this, since I have consulted the same opinion for the opposite purpose. But what we may well ask ourselves is this: is it not a trifle bizarre that we should be doing it at all? Our profession is the law, not medicine; how does it come about that lawyers have to examine medical literature to assess the advantages and disadvantages of a medical practice?

If the import of this question is not immediately clear, let me return to my imaginary State of Ruritania. Many years ago, in Ruritania as elsewhere, surgical operations were attended with great risk. Pasteur had not made his discoveries, and surgeons killed as often as they cured. In this state of things, the legislature of Ruritania passed a law declaring all surgical operations to be unlawful in principle, but providing that each specific type of operation might be legalized by a statute specially passed for the purpose. The result is that, in Ruritania, as expert medical opinion sees the possibility of some new medical advance, a pressure group has to be formed in order to obtain legislative approval for it. Since there is little public interest in these technical questions, and since, moreover, surgical operations are thought in general to be inimical to the established religion, the pressure group has to work for many years before it gets a hearing. When at last a proposal for legalization is seriously mooted, the lawyers and politicians get to work upon it, considering what possible dangers are inherent in the new operation. Lawyers and politicians are careful people, and they are perhaps more prone to see the dangers than the advantages in a new departure. Naturally they find allies among some of the more timid or traditional or less knowledgeable members of the medical profession, as well as among the priesthood and the faithful. Thus it is small wonder that whereas appendicectomy has been practised in civilised countries since the beginning of the present century, a proposal to legalize it has still not passed the legislative assembly of Ruritania.

It must be confessed that on this particular matter the legal prohibition has not been an unmixed evil for the Ruritanians. During the great popularity of the appendix operation in much of the civilised world during the twenties and thirties of this century, large numbers of these organs were removed without adequate cause, and the citizens of Ruritania have been spared this inconvenience. On the other hand, many citizens of that country have died of appendicitis, who would have been saved if they had lived elsewhere. And whereas in other countries the medical profession has now learned enough to be able to perform this operation with wisdom and restraint, in Ruritania it is still not being performed at all. Moreover, the law has destroyed scientific inventiveness in that country in the forbidden fields.

Now, in the United States and England we have no such absurd general law on the subject of surgical operations as they have in Ruritania. In principle, medical men are left free to exercise their best judgment, and the result has been a brilliant advance in knowledge and technique. But there are just two—or possibly three—operations which are subject to the Ruritanian principle. These are abortion,[9] euthanasia, and possibly sterilization of convenience. In these fields we, too, must have pressure groups, with lawyers and politicians warning us of the possibility of inexpert practitioners and mistaken diagnosis, and canvassing medical opinion on the risk of an operation not yielding the expected results in terms of human happiness and the health of the body politic. In these fields we, too, are forbidden to experiment to see if the foretold dangers actually come to pass. Instead of that, we are required to make a social judgment on the probabilities of good and evil before the medical profession is allowed to start on its empirical tests.

This anomaly is perhaps more obvious with abortion than it is with euthanasia. Indeed, I am prepared for ridicule when I describe euthanasia as a medical operation. Regarded as surgery it is unique, since its object is not to save or prolong life but the reverse. But euthanasia has another object which it shares with many surgical operations—the saving of pain. And it is now widely recognised, as Lord Dawson said in the debate in the House of Lords, that the saving of pain is a legitimate aim of medical practice. The question whether euthanasia will effect a net saving of pain and distress is, perhaps, one that can be only finally answered by trying it. But it is obscurantist to forbid the experiment on the ground that until it is performed we cannot certainly know its results. Such an attitude, in any other field of medical endeavor, would have inhibited progress.

The argument based on mistaken diagnosis leads into the argument based on the possibility of dramatic medical discoveries. Of course, a new medical discovery which gives the opportunity of remission or cure will almost at once put an end to mercy-killings in the particular group of cases for which the discovery is made. On the other hand, the discovery cannot affect patients who have already died from their disease. The argument based on mistaken diagnosis is therefore concerned only with those patients who have been mercifully killed just before the discovery becomes available for use. The argument is that such persons may turn out to have been "mercy-killed" unnecessarily, because if the physician had waited a bit longer they would have been cured. Because of this risk for this tiny fraction of the total number of patients, patients who are dying in pain must be left to do so, year after year, against their entreaty to have it ended.

Just how real is the risk? When a new medical discovery is claimed, some time commonly elapses before it becomes tested sufficiently to justify large-scale production of the drug, or training in the techniques involved. This is a warning period when euthanasia in the particular class of the case would probably be halted anyway. Thus it is quite probable that when the new discovery becomes available, the euthanasia process would not in fact show any mistakes in this regard.

Kamisar says that in my book I "did not deign this objection to euthanasia more than a passing reference." I still do not think it is worth any more than that.

The author advances the familiar but hardly convincing argument that the quantitative need for euthanasia is not large. As one reason for this argument, he suggests that not many patients would wish to benefit from euthanasia, even if it were allowed. I am not impressed by the argument. It may be true, but it is irrelevant. So long as there are *any* persons dying in weakness and grief who are refused their re-

quest for a speeding of their end, the argument for legalizing euthanasia remains. Next, the Article suggests that there is no great need for euthanasia because of the advances made with pain-killing drugs. Kamisar has made so many quotations from my book that I cannot complain that he has not made more, but there is one relevant point that he does not mention. In my book, recognising that medical science does manage to save many dying patients from the extreme of physical pain, I pointed out that it often fails to save them from an artificial, twilight existence, with nausea, giddiness, and extreme restlessness, as well as the long hours of consciousness of a hopeless condition. A dear friend of mine, who died of cancer of the bowel, spent his last months in just this state, under the influence of morphine, which deadened pain, but vomiting incessantly, day in and day out. The question that we have to face is whether the unintelligent brutality of such an existence is to be imposed on one who wishes to end it.

The Article then makes a suggestion which, for once, really is a new one in this rather jaded debate. The suggestion appears to be that if a man really wants to die he can do the job himself.[10] Whether the author seriously intends this as advice to patients I cannot discover, because he adds that he does not condone suicide, but that he prefers a *laissez-faire* approach. Whatever meaning may be attached to the author's remarks on this subject, I must say with deep respect that I find them lacking in sympathy and imagination, as well as inconsistent with the rest of his approach. A patient may often be unable to kill himself when he has reached the last and terrible stage of the disease. To be certain of committing suicide, he must act in advance; and he must not take advice, because then he might be prevented. So this suggestion multiplies the risks of false diagnosis on which the author lays such stress. Besides, has he not considered what a messy affair the ordinary suicide is, and what a shock it is for the relatives to find the body? The advantage that the author sees in suicide is that it is not "an approach aided and sanctioned by the state." This is another example of his ambivalence, his failure to make up his mind on the moral issue. But it is also a mistake, for under my legislative proposal the state would not aid and sanction euthanasia. It would merely remove the threat of punishment from euthanasia, which is an altogether different thing. My proposal is, in fact, an example of that same *laissez-faire* approach which the author himself adopts when he contemplates suicide as a solution.

The last part of the Article is devoted to the ancient "wedge" argument which I have already examined in my book. It is the trump card of the traditionalist, because no proposal for reform, however strong the arguments in favour, is immune from the wedge objection. In fact, the stronger the arguments in favour of a reform, the more likely it is that the traditionalist will take the wedge objection—it is then the only one he has. C. M. Cornford put the argument in its proper place when he said that the wedge objection means this, that you should not act justly today, for fear that you may be asked to act still more justly tomorrow.

We heard a great deal of this type of argument in England in the nineteenth century, when it was used to resist almost every social and economic change. In the present century we have had less of it, but (if I may claim the hospitality of these columns to say so) it seems still to be accorded an exaggerated importance in American thought. When lecturing on the law of torts in an American university a few years ago, I suggested that just as compulsory liability insurance for automobiles had spread practically through the civilised world, so we should in time see the law of tort superseded in this field by a system of state insurance for traffic accidents, administered independently of proof of fault. The suggestion was immediately met by one student with a horrified reference to "creeping socialism." That is the standard objection made by many people to any proposal for a new department of state activity. The implication is that you must resist every proposal, however admirable in itself, because otherwise you will never be able to draw the line. On the particular question of socialism, the fear is belied by the experience of a number of countries which have extended state control of the economy without going the whole way to socialistic state regimentation.

Kamisar's particular bogey, the racial laws of Nazi Germany, is an effective one in the democratic countries. Any reference to the Nazis is a powerful weapon to prevent change in the traditional taboo on sterilization as well as euthanasia. The case of sterilization is particularly interesting on this; I dealt with it at length in my book, though Kamisar does not mention its bearing on the argument. When proposals are made for promoting voluntary sterilization on eugenic and other grounds, they are immediately condemned by most people as the thin end of a wedge leading to involuntary sterilization; and then they point to the practices of the Nazis. Yet a more persuasive argument pointing in the other direction can easily be found. Several American states have sterilization laws, which for the most part were originally drafted in very wide terms, to cover desexualisation as well as sterilization, and authorizing involuntary as well as voluntary operations. This legislation goes back long before the Nazis; the earliest statute was in Indiana in 1907. What has been its practical effect? In several states it has hardly been used. A few have used it, but in practice they have progressively restricted it until now it is virtually confined to voluntary sterilization. This is so, at least, in North Carolina, as Mrs. Woodside's study strikingly shows. In my book I summed up the position as follows:

> The American experience is of great interest because it shows how remote from reality in a democratic community is the fear—frequently voiced by Americans themselves—that voluntary sterilization may be the 'thin end of the wedge,' leading to a large-scale violation of human rights as happened in Nazi Germany. In fact, the American experience is the precise opposite—starting with compulsory sterilization, administrative practice has come to put the operation on a voluntary footing.

But it is insufficient to answer the "wedge" objection in general terms; we must consider the particular fears to which it gives rise. Kamisar professes to fear certain other measures that the Euthanasia societies may bring up if their present measure is conceded to them. Surely, these other measures, if any, will be debated on their merits? Does he seriously fear that anyone in the United States is going to propose the extermination of people of a minority race or religion? Let us put aside such ridiculous fancies and discuss practical politics.

The author is quite right in thinking that a body of opinion would favour the legalization of the involuntary euthanasia of hopelessly defective infants, and some day a proposal of this kind may be put forward. The proposal would have distinct limits, just as the proposal for voluntary euthanasia of incurable sufferers has limits. I do not think that any responsible body of opinion would now propose the euthanasia of insane adults, for the perfectly clear reason that any such practice would greatly increase the sense of insecurity felt by the borderline insane and by the large number of insane persons who have sufficient understanding on this particular matter.

Kamisar expresses distress at a concluding remark in my book in which I advert to the possibility of old people becoming an overwhelming burden on mankind. I share his feeling that there are profoundly disturbing possibilities here; and if I had been merely a propagandist, intent upon securing agreement for a specific measure of law reform, I should have done wisely to have omitted all reference to this subject. Since, however, I am merely an academic writer, trying to bring such intelligence as I have to bear on moral and social issues, I deemed the topic too important and threatening to leave without a word. I think I have made it clear, in the passages cited, that I am not for one moment proposing any euthanasia of the aged in present society; such an idea would shock me as much as it shocks Kamisar and would shock everybody else. Still, the fact that we may one day have to face is that medical science is more successful in preserving the body than in preserving the mind. It is not impossible that, in the foreseeable future, medical men will be able to preserve the mindless body until the age, say, of 1000, while the mind itself will have lasted only a tenth of that time. What will mankind do then? It is hardly possible to imagine that we shall establish huge hospital-mausolea where the aged are kept in a kind of living death. Even if it is desired to do this, the cost of the undertaking may make it impossible.

This is not an immediately practical problem, and we need not yet face it. The problem of maintaining persons afflicted with senile dementia is well within our economic resources as the matter stands at present. Perhaps some barrier will be found to medical advance which will prevent the problem becoming more acute. Perhaps, as time goes on, and as the alternatives become more clearly realised, men will become more resigned to human control over the mode of termination of life. Or the solution may be that after the individual has reached a certain age, or a certain degree of decay, medical science will hold its hand, and allow him to be carried off by natural causes.[11] But what if these natural causes are themselves painful? Would it not be better kindness to substitute human agency?

In general, it is enough to say that we do not have to know the solutions to these problems. The only doubtful moral question on which we have to make an immediate decision in relation to involuntary euthanasia is whether we owe a moral duty to terminate the life of an insane person who is suffering from a painful and incurable disease. Such a person is left unprovided for under the legislative proposal formulated in my book. The objection to any system of involuntary euthanasia of the insane is that it may cause a sense of insecurity. It is because I think that the risk of this fear is a serious one that a proposal for the reform of the law must leave the insane out.

Notes

1. Kamisar, *Some Non-Religious Views Against Proposed "Mercy-Killing" Legislation,* 42 Minn. L. Rev. 969 (1958).

2. Professor Kamisar professes to deal with the issue from a utilitarian point of view and generally does so. But he lapses when he says that "the need the euthanasiast advances. . .is a good deal less compelling (than the need to save life). It is only to ease pain." Kamisar, *supra* note 1, at 1008. This is, of course, on Benthamite principles, an inadmissible remark.

3. The Sanctity of Life and the Criminal Law 334–39 (1957).

4. Kamisar, *supra* note 1, 971–72.

5. *Id.* at 982.
6. *Id.* at 984.
7. *Id.* at 996.
8. The author is misleading on my reference to capital punishment, which I did not mention in connection with the occurrence of mistakes. See Kamisar, *supra* note 1, at 1005. I merely pointed out the inconsistency of the theological position which admits capital punishment and war as exceptions from the Sixth Commandment although not expressed therein, and says that they are not "murder," while maintaining that a killing done with a man's consent and for his benefit as an act of mercy is "murder." Whatever moral distinction may be found between these rules, they cannot by any feat of ingenuity be deduced from the text of the Commandment.
9. Lawful everywhere on certain health grounds, but not on socio-medical grounds (the overburdened mother), eugenic grounds, ethical grounds (rape, incest, etc.), or social and libertarian grounds (the unwanted child).
10. Kamisar, *Some Non-Religious Views Against Proposed "Mercy-Killing" Legislation,* 42 MINN. L. REV. 969, 1011 (1958).
11. An interesting pronouncement, on which there would probably be a wide measure of agreement, was made recently by Pope Pius XII before an international audience of physicians. The Pope said that reanimation techniques were moral, but made it clear that when life was ebbing hopelessly, physicians might abandon further efforts to stave off death, or relatives might ask them to desist "in order to permit the patient, already virtually dead, to pass on in peace." On the time of death, the Pope said that "Considerations of a general nature permit the belief that human life continues as long as the vital functions—as distinct from the simple life of organs—manifest themselves spontaneously or even with the help of artificial proceedings." By implication, this asserts that a person may be regarded as dead when all that is left is "the simple life of organs." The Pope cited the tenet of Roman Catholic doctrine that death occurs at the moment of "complete and definitive separation of body and soul." In practice, he added, the terms "body" and "separation" lack precision. He explained that establishing the exact instant of death in controversial cases was the task not of the Church but of the physician. N.Y. Times, November 25, 1957, p. 1, col. 3.

From "Apologia for Suicide"

Mary Rose Barrington

The root cause of the widespread aversion to suicide is almost certainly death itself rather than dislike of the means by which death is brought about. The leaf turns a mindless face to the sun for one summer before falling for ever into the mud; death, however it comes to pass, rubs our clever faces in the same mud, where we too join the leaves. The inconceivability of this transformation in status is partly shot through with an indirect illumination, due to the death of others. Yet bereavement is not death. Here to mourn, we are still here, and the imagination boggles at the notion that things could ever be otherwise. Not only does the imagination boggle, as to some extent it must, but the mind unfortunately averts. The averted mind acknowledges, in a theoretical way, that death does indeed happen to people here and there and now and then, but to some extent the attitude to death resembles the attitude of the heavy smoker to lung cancer; he reckons that if he is lucky it will not happen to *him,* at least not yet, and perhaps not ever. This confused sort of faith in the immortality of the body must underlie many a triumphal call from the hospital ward or theatre, that the patient's life has been saved—and he will therefore die next week instead of this week, and in rather greater discomfort. People who insist that life must always be better than death often sound as if

Reprinted with permission from *Euthanasia and the Right to Die,* ed. A. B. Downing (New York: Humanities Press; London: Peter Owen Ltd., 1970) pp. 152–70.

they are choosing eternal life in contrast to eternal death, when the fact is that they have no choice in the matter; it is death now, or death later. Once this fact is fully grasped it is possible for the question to arise as to whether death now would not be preferable.

Opponents of suicide will sometimes throw dust in the eyes of the uncommitted by asking at some point why one should ever choose to go on living if one once questions the value of life; for as we all know, adversity is usually round the corner, if not at our heels. Here, it seems to me, a special case must be made out for people suffering from the sort of adversity with which the proponents of euthanasia are concerned: namely, an apparently irremediable state of physical debility that makes life unbearable to the sufferer. Some adversities come and go; in the words of the Anglo-Saxon poet reviewing all the disasters known to Norse mythology, "That passed away, so may this." Some things that do not pass away include inoperable cancers in the region of the throat that choke their victims slowly to death. Not only do they not pass away, but like many extremely unpleasant conditions they cannot be alleviated by pain-killing drugs. Pain itself can be controlled, provided the doctor in charge is prepared to put the relief of pain before the prolongation of life; but analgesics will not help a patient to live with total incontinence, reduced to the status of a helpless baby after a life of independent adulthood. And for the person who manages to avoid these grave afflictions there remains the spectre of senile decay, a physical and mental crumbling into a travesty of the normal person. Could anything be more reasonable than for a person faced with these living deaths to weigh up the pros and cons of living out his life until his heart finally fails, and going instead to meet death half-way?

It is true, of course, that, all things being equal, people do want to go on living. If we are enjoying life, there seems no obvious reason to stop doing so and be mourned by our families and forgotten by our friends. If we are not enjoying it, then it seems a miserable end to die in a trough of depression, and better to wait for things to become more favourable. Most people, moreover, have a moral obligation to continue living, owed to their parents while they are still alive, their children while they are dependent, and their spouses all the time. Trained professional workers may even feel that they have a duty to society to continue giving their services. Whatever the grounds, it is both natural and reasonable that without some special cause nobody ever wants to die *yet*. But must these truisms be taken to embody the whole truth about the attitude of thinking people to life and death? A psychiatrist has been quoted as saying: "I don't think you can consider anyone normal who tries to take his own life."[1] The abnormality of the suicide is taken for granted, and the possibility that he might have been doing something sensible (for him) is not presented to the mind for even momentary consideration. It might as well be argued that no one can be considered normal who does not want to procreate as many children as possible, and this was no doubt urged by the wise men of yesterday; today the tune is very different, and in this essay we are concerned with what they may be singing tomorrow. . . .

It may be worth pausing here to consider whether the words, "natural end," in the sense usually ascribed to the term, have much bearing on reality. Very little is "natural" about our present-day existence, and least natural of all is the prolonged period of dying that is suffered by so many incurable patients solicitously kept alive to be killed by their disease. The sufferings of animals (other than man) are heart-rending enough, but a dying process spread over weeks, months or years seems to be one form of suffering that animals are normally spared. When severe illness strikes them they tend to stop eating, sleep and die. The whole weight of Western society forces attention on the natural right to live, but throws a blanket of silence over the natural right to die. If I seem to be suggesting that in a civilized society suicide ought to be considered a quite proper way for a well-brought-up person to end his life (unless he has the good luck to die suddenly and without warning), that is indeed the tenor of my argument; if it is received with astonishment and incredulity, the reader is referred to the reception of recommendations made earlier in the century that birth control should be practiced and encouraged. The idea is no more extraordinary, and would be equally calculated to diminish the sum total of suffering among humankind. . . .

. . . It is frequently said that hard-hearted people would be encouraged to make their elderly relatives feel that they had outlived their welcome and ought to remove themselves, even if they happened to be enjoying life. No one can say categorically that nothing of the sort would happen, but the sensibility of even hard-hearted people to the possible consequences of their own unkindness seems just as likely. A relation who had stood down from life in a spirit of magnanimity and family affection would, after an inevitable period of heart-searching and self-recrimination, leave behind a pleasant memory; a victim of callous treatment hanging like an accusing albatross around the neck of the living would suggest another and rather ugly story. Needless to say, whoever was responsible would not in any event be the sort of person to show consideration to an aged person in decline.

Whether or not some undesirable fringe results would stem from a free acceptance of suicide in our society, the problem of three or four contemporaneous generations peopling a world that hitherto has had to support only two or three is with us here and now, and will be neither generated nor exacerbated by a fresh attitude to life and death. The disabled, aged parent, loved or unloved, abnegating or demanding, is placed in one of the tragic dilemmas inherent in human existence, and one that becomes more acute as standards of living rise. One more in the mud-hut is not a problem in the same way as one more in a small, overcrowded urban dwelling; and the British temperament demands a privacy incompatible with the more sociable Mediterranean custom of packing a grandmother and an aunt or two in the attic. Mere existence presents a mild problem; disabled existence presents a chronic problem. The old person may have no talent for being a patient, and the young one may find it intolerable to be a nurse. A physical decline threatens to be accompanied by an inevitable decline in the quality of important human relationships—human relationships, it is worth repeating, not superhuman ones. Given superhuman love, patience, fortitude and all other sweet-natured qualities in a plenitude not normally present in ordinary people, there would be no problem. But the problem is there, and voluntary termination of life offers a possible solution that may be better than none at all. The young have been urged from time immemorial to have valiant hearts, to lay down their lives for their loved ones when their lives have hardly started; it may be that in time to come the disabled aged will be glad to live in a society that approves an honourable death met willingly, perhaps in the company of another "old soldier" of the same generation, and with justifiable pride. Death taken in one's own time, and with a sense of purpose, may in fact be far more bearable than the process of waiting to be arbitrarily extinguished.[2] A patient near the end of his life who arranged his death so as, for example, to permit an immediate transfer of a vital organ to a younger person, might well feel that he was converting his death into a creative act instead of waiting passively to be suppressed.

A lot of kindly people may feel that this is lacking in respect for the honourable estate of old age; but to insist on the obligation of old people to live through a period of decline and helplessness seems to me to be lacking in a feeling for the demands of human *self*-respect. They may reply that this shows a false notion of what constitutes self-respect, and that great spiritual qualities may be brought out by dependence and infirmity, and the response to such a state. It is tempting in a world dominated by suffering to find all misery purposeful, and indeed in some situations the "cross-to-bear" and the willing bearer may feel that they are contributing a poignant note to some cosmic symphony that is richer for their patience and self-sacrifice. Since we are talking of options and not of compulsions, people who felt like this would no doubt continue to play their chosen parts; but what a truly ruthless thing to impose those parts on people who feel that they are meaningless and discordant, and better written out.

What should be clear is that with so many men and so many opinions there is no room here for rules of life, or ready-made solutions by formula, least of all by the blanket injunction that, rather than allow any of these questions to be faced, life must be lived out to the bitter end, in sickness and in health, for better or for worse, until death brings release. It is true that the embargo on suicide relieves the ailing dependent of a choice, and some would no doubt be glad of the relief, having no mind for self-sacrifice. But in order to protect the mildly disabled from the burden of choice, the severely sick and suffering patient who urgently wants to die is subjected to the same compulsion to live. The willingness of many people to accept this sheltering of the stronger at the expense of the crying needs of the incomparably weaker may be because the slightly ailing are more visible and therefore make a more immediate claim on sympathy. Everyone knows aged and dependent people who might find themselves morally bound to consider the advisability of continuing to live if an option were truly available; the seriously afflicted lie hidden behind hospital windows, or secluded from sight on the upper floors of private houses. *They* are threatened not with delicate moral considerations, but with the harder realities of pain, disease and degeneration. Not only are they largely invisible, but their guardians are much given to the issuing of soothing reports about, for example, the hundred thousand or more patients who die of cancer every year, reports in which words like "happiness" and "dignity" are used liberally, and words like "pain" and "humiliation" tactfully suppressed. Let us not be misled by the reassuring face so often assumed by doctors who would have us believe that terminal suffering is just a bad fairy tale put out by alarmist bogey-men. One can only hope that the pathetic human wrecks who lie vomiting and gasping their lives out are as sanguine and cheerful about their lamentable condition as the smiling doctor who on their behalf assures us that no one (including the members of the Euthanasia Society) really wants euthanasia.

That voluntary euthanasia is in fact assisted suicide is no doubt clear to most people, but curiously enough many who would support the moral right of an incurably sick person to commit suicide will oppose his having the right to seek assistance from doctors if he is to effect his wish. The argument has so far been concentrated upon the person who clearly sees the writing on the wall (perhaps because he has a doctor who is prepared to decipher it) and has

the moral courage, whether or not encouraged by a sympathetic society, to anticipate the dying period. Further, this hypothetical person has access to the means of suicide and knows how to make use of those means. How he has acquired the means and the knowledge is obscure, but a determined person will make sure that he is equipped with both as a standby for the future. Yet the average patient desperately in need of help to cut short his suffering could well be a person unaccustomed to holding his own against authority, enfeebled by illness, dependent on pain-killing drugs, having no access to the means of suicide and not knowing how to make use of the means even if they were available; an entirely helpless person, in no way in a position to compass his own death. To acknowledge the right of a person to end his own life to avoid a period of suffering is a mere sham unless the right for him to call on expert assistance is also acknowledged. . . .

Hostile sections of the medical profession will continue to assert that it is their business to cure and not to kill, and that in any case a patient who is in a miserable state from having his body invaded with cancers (or whatever) is in no state to make a decision about life and death. A patient who is in so pitiable a condition that he says he wishes to die is *ipso facto* not in a fit condition to make a reliable statement about his wishes. Arguments of this ilk seem at times to pass from black comedy to black farce. With the same sort of metaphysical reasoning it will be maintained that a patient who requested, and was given, euthanasia on Monday evening might, had he lived until Tuesday morning, have changed his mind. It has even been suggested that patients would, if voluntary euthanasia were available for incurable patients, feel themselves reluctantly obliged to ask for it to spare the nursing staff. And, as was remarked earlier, although laying down one's life in battle is generally considered praiseworthy, to lay down your life to spare yourself pointless suffering, to release medical staff so that they can tend people who would have some chance of living enjoyable lives given greater attention and assistance, to release your family and friends from anxiety and anguish, *these* motives are considered shocking. More accurately, a mere contemplation of these motives shocks the conditioned mind so severely that no rational comment can fight its way through to the surface; it is forced back by the death taboo.

Here again it must be made clear that what is needed is the fostering of a new attitude to death that should ultimately grow from within, and not be imposed from without upon people psychologically unable to rethink their ingrained views. The suffering and dying patients of today have been brought up to feel that it is natural and inevitable, and even some sort of a duty, to live out their terminal period, and it would do them no service to try to persuade them into adopting an attitude that to most of them would seem oppressive, as aimed against them rather than for their benefit. If people have an ineradicable instinct, or fundamental conviction, that binds them to cling to life when their body is anticipating death by falling into a state of irrevocable decay, they clearly must be given treatment and encouragement consistent with their emotional and spiritual needs, and kindness *for them* will consist of assurances that not only is their suffering a matter of the greatest concern, but that so also is their continued existence. It is future generations, faced perhaps with a lifespan of eighty or ninety years, of which nearly half will have to be dependent on the earning power of the other half, who will have to decide how much of their useful, active life is to be devoted to supporting themselves through a terminal period *"sans everything,"* prolonged into a dreaded ordeal by ever-increasing medical skill directed to the preservation of life. It may well be that, as in the case of family planning, economic reality will open up a spring, the waters of which will filter down to deeper levels, and that then the new way of death will take root. The opponents of euthanasia conjure up a favourite vision of a nightmare future in which anxious patients will be obsessed with the fear that their relatives and doctors may make surreptitious plans to kill them; the anxiety of the twenty-first century patient may, on the contrary, be that they are neglecting to make such plans.

Notes

1. Reported in *The Observer* (June 26, 1967).

2. It will be noted that reference is made here in all cases to the aged. In a longer exposition I would argue that very different considerations apply to the young disabled who have not yet enjoyed a full lifespan, and who should be given far greater public assistance to enable them to enjoy life as best they can.

From "The Adolescent Patient's Decision to Die"

John E. Schowalter, Julian B. Ferholt, and Nancy M. Mann

Those who are treating a severely ill patient who decides to die are faced with an agonizing dilemma. The problem is magnified when life can be sustained for a significant period if the patient accepts dependence on a drug, a pro-

Reprinted with permission from *Pediatrics* 51:1, 97–103. January 1973. Copyright 1973, American Academy of Pediatrics.

cedure, or a machine. A patient may, however, refuse further transfusions, another course of a cytotoxic drug, further cancer surgery or radiation, an organ transplant, renal dialysis or an artificial organ or pacemaker. New techniques to prolong life make this problem increasingly common in situations where death is not imminent, but the quality of life is greatly impaired. In pediatrics the problem of a patient's decision to die is complicated even more by special developmental ethical, legal, and family considerations. . . . The basic question to be faced is should a physician always oppose a patient's request to end his life and, if not, under what conditions should he respect or even support a patient in his decision to die? These are situations of conflict between our commitment to relieve suffering and our commitment to prolong life. Sometimes it is evident to everyone that death is imminent, the suffering severe, and that efforts to prolong life will only prolong suffering, while at other times it is clear that the wish to die is irrationally out of proportion to the suffering. There is also, however, a very difficult middle ground. Especially in these cases patients may disagree with their parents, patient and family may disagree with the medical staff, various members of the medical staff may disagree with each other.

On the Adolescent Ward of Yale-New Haven Hospital, the authors recently helped to treat an adolescent who chose to die. This paper is an outcome of our considerations prior to and following her death.

Case Report

Karen was a 16-year-old Catholic girl, the second oldest of seven siblings. She was first hospitalized in September 1968, after a three-week course of nephrotic syndrome. She did not respond to medical management. A renal biopsy in April 1969 revealed "chronic, active glomerulonephritis," and by spring of 1970 a rapid decrease in renal function prompted the decision to plan for dialysis and transplantation. A bilateral nephrectomy was performed in August 1970, and Karen received a transplant of her father's kidney the following month. The transplant functioned quite well initially, but several months later proteinuria became increasingly severe, and suddenly in March 1971 the kidney completely ceased to function. Prior to surgery and following the transplant's failure, thrice-weekly hemodialysis was performed. Karen tolerated dialysis poorly, routinely having chills, nausea, vomiting, severe headaches, and weakness.

In April 1970 and prior to transplantation, a child psychiatrist (J.F.) was asked to evaluate the family. Karen was found to have reactive depression, but this was considered appropriate. The father responded to his daughter's illness by immersing

himself in his profession. The mother evidenced a suspiciousness of Karen's medical management that contained circumferential speech, loosening of thought associations, and an inappropriate lability of affect. Referral of the mother for psychiatric outpatient treatment was recommended but never accomplished.

The child psychiatrist was again consulted in July 1970. Karen and her parents met regularly with the social worker (N.M.) and the child psychiatrist (J.F.) prior to and after the transplant. The family did well psychologically during the immediate posttransplant period, but as Karen's new kidney failed, she became moderately depressed and the parents became increasingly distraught. Marital difficulties developed as the family could not deal directly with their disappointment at the transplant failing. The marital problems lessened with open discussion of the parents' feelings about the possible failure of the transplant.

In early April 1971, after it was clear that the kidney would never function, Karen and her parents expressed the wish to stop medical treatment and let "nature take its course." The medical staff was upset and they could not agree on the proper course of action. The social worker and psychiatrist attempted to have the girl and her family explore their decision in the hope that with further understanding of the decision, they would reject it. Most other staff members conveyed to the family that such wishes were unheard of and unacceptable, and that a decision to stop treatment could never be an alternative. The family did decide to continue dialysis, medication, and diet therapy. Karen's renal incapacity returned to pretransplant levels and she returned to a socially isolated life, diet restriction, chronic discomfort, and fatigue.

On May 10, Karen was hospitalized following ten days of high fever. Three days later the transplant was removed. Its pathology resembled that of the original kidneys, and the possibility of a similar reaction forming in subsequent transplants was established.

On May 21, the arteriovenous shunt placed in Karen's arm for hemodialysis was found to be infected, and part of the vein wall was excised and the shunt revised. During this portion of the hospitalization, Karen and the parents grudgingly went along with the medical recommendations, but they continued to ponder the possibility of stopping treatment. The child psychiatrist was out of town from the end of April, and the social worker was now counseling Karen as well as her parents. On May 24, the shunt clotted closed. Karen, with her parents' agreement, refused shunt revision and any further dialysis.

Those connected with Karen's treatment were stunned by frustration and anger. They felt that the decision was immoral and unsound medically. The idea of a 16-year-old patient deciding her own fate was anathema. Karen had occasionally spoken to her parish priest. Following her decision she stopped seeing him but continued talking with the hospital chaplain. She came to the personal conclusion that there was no such place as hell and even if there was not a heaven, nothingness would be far better than the suffering which would continue if she lived. On May 26, the child psychiatry consultant for the ward (J.S.), who was familiar with the situation from the time of the transplant, was asked to evaluate the girl. He found no evidence of psychotic thinking and was convinced that Karen had carefully thought out her decision and had grasped its implications.

The child psychiatrist and the attending ward physician (who happened to be a nephrologist) decided independently that Karen's decison was made as rationally as any such decision could be. They believed the staff had little choice but to comply with her request, making her dying as comfortable as possible and providing the opportunity through daily counseling for her to change her mind at any time. At first no other staff member agreed with this decision. Nurses, house officers, and consultants spent sleepless nights; faces were haggard, tempers short, and the ward morale, which usually ran high, was undermined. Almost daily staff meetings were held to discuss the policy toward Karen. Alternative suggestions ranged from having the courts take custody of the child and force treatment to demanding the parents take the girl home to die so as not to taint the hospital or staff with the voluntary death. Some staff members felt they were being forced to act as accomplices to what they believed was a suicide. Much anger was expressed at the parents for participating in Karen's decision ("It's on their heads not ours"), and many voiced a belief that if the parents gave Karen back to "Medicine" that all would be well.

The attitude of the ward staff changed, however, as the bleak medical alternatives were discussed in the ward meetings and when Karen's appetite and spirits improved after she made her decision. By May 30, when a nurse from the dialysis unit visited Karen and upset her by insisting that she return to dialysis, a majority of the staff agreed

with the family that this strident approach was undesirable, and the nurse was asked not to visit. Those that knew Karen the best found it easier to acquiesce to her decision than those, especially the house officers, who recently came onto the floor. This reaction was consistent with a previous finding that those who directly witness a dying patient's suffering are less eager than more remote physicians to prolong the life of the child in extremis.

Karen died on June 2, with both parents at her bedside. The relative speed and peacefulness of her dying were unusual for a uremic death. Shortly prior to her death she thanked the staff for what she said she knew had been a hard time for them and she told her parents she hoped they would be happy. We later learned that before her death she had written a will and picked a burial spot near her home and near her favorite horseback riding trail. In the final days she supported her parents as they faltered in their decision; she told her father, "Daddy, I will be happy there (in the ground) if there is no machine and they don't work on me any more." Six months later the family is proceeding through a quite normal grief sequence with a minimum of psychiatric (J.F.) and pastoral assistance.

It is clear in this case that issues of morality are entangled for the staff with feelings of omnipotence, impotence, control, and altruism. For the family also the motivations are complex and multidetermined. However, it is not our intent to discuss this case further but to use it to illustrate the dilemma facing those who care for an ill child who chooses to die. We will present a brief review of the literature and a summary of our approach to these difficult problems.

DEVELOPMENTAL CONSIDERATIONS

Although Freud stated that probably no one can ever fully comprehend his own death, a crucial consideration in evaluating a patient's wish to die is whether or not he can understand the concept of death. The school of Piagetian psychology suggests that the grasping of the possibilities and limitations of one's self in relation to a finite future develop within the stage of formal operations, occurring during adolescence. Other psychologists as well as pediatric clinicians concur. So, it is generally agreed that by age 14 or 15 most adolescents can understand the meaning of death.

It is rare for children who have not yet reached adolescence to decide to die. When this does occur, it is likely that the child does not comprehend the meaning of death, and the real meaning of his wish must be investigated and responded to. When an adolescent decides to die, his understanding of death's meaning and permanence must also be assessed.

On the one hand it must be kept in mind that the cognitive understanding of death can exist without the emotional maturity necessary to make final decisions regarding one's own life. On the other hand, older adolescents, like our patient, can appreciate their suffering and fatigue and can comprehend when it is likely that life will never offer any more than continued disability, doubt, and suffering.

PSYCHOLOGICAL REACTIONS OF STAFF

A patient's wish for death forces staff members to confront their personal mortality and sometimes a latent self-destructive wish. This experience can be very uncomfortable, and some people must react with denial. Studies have shown that physicians and medical students are often individuals with especially strong feelings about death and with strong wishes to avoid facing death. Our society reinforces the tendency to deny death and condemn suicide. Suicide is punished by everything from life insurance nonpayment to the threat of criminal prosecution and from incarceration in a mental hospital to religious damnation. In addition, for a physician the choosing of death by a patient represents defeat and a rebuff of his role as healer.

So if, as Kasper suggests, the physician considers his own fears about death, puts them as intellectual questions and tries to answer them for other people, a patient's decision to die can threaten the physician on both personal and professional grounds.

McKegney and Lange reported on four adults in dialysis who chose to die. These authors stress the importance of the staff recognizing the possibility of a patient wishing to die and aiding the patient to bring forth and discuss this wish before it becomes crystallized into a firm conviction. In these reported cases the dialysis staff members continued to operate on the assumption that life was always preferable to death. When the patients did not share this value judgment, the staff became angry, accusing them of not living up to their part of the bargain. This staff reaction, which we also noted, is understandable, especially since dialysis staff seem to especially demand that patients do well in return for devoted care.

As a result of these psychological stresses, staff often react with anger, irritability, or depression which may trigger an attempt to seek a rapid conclusion of events without proper exploration. A staff member may deny the obvious fact that a patient wishes to die and even transmit to the family that such thoughts are not acceptable. On the other hand, he may avoid strong feelings by a too easy compliance with the wishes of the patient. If unnoticed, these psychological reactions may interfere with the professional's ability to determine and serve the best interests of his patient.

PSYCHOLOGICAL REACTIONS OF PATIENTS WITH CHRONIC RENAL DISEASE

Patients with chronic renal disease are the best studied group in terms of their reacting to a very uncomfortable, usually fatal disorder. Suicidal behavior has been one focus of this literature. In the study of one group of 14 patients, the fear of living the unsatisfactory life of the chronically ill and handicapped seemed almost as intolerable as the fear of imminent death; while in another study of 25 patients, the main concern was not in dying or living as much as "that it would be decided one way or the other quickly." Other studies emphasize the patient's concern about the quality of his life. Abram *et al.,* in a questionnaire study including 127 centers and involving 3,478 renal dialysis patients, found that if suicides were considered as those patients who died suddenly by their own hand as well as those who died following voluntary withdrawal from the program or following refusal to adhere to the treatment regimen, that the suicide rate was 400 times that of the general population. If only outright suicides and deaths following withdrawal from treatment were included, this "suicide" rate was 100 times that in the general population. Although the accuracy of the percentages from such a questionnaire study is suspect, the fact that many patients with chronic renal disease do choose death over prolonged dying does seem substantiated.

Although most reports of reactions of patients with chronic kidney disease have been in adults, cases of nonpsychotic children on dialysis who exhibited self-destructive behavior, including trying to remove their shunt, have been reported and discussed. Reinhart's experience in Pittsburgh led him to the extreme position of seriously questioning the value of chronic dialysis or renal transplantation for children at all at this time.

Many reports question the quality of life on chronic dialysis for some patients and their families. Perhaps this is an area where in our enthusiasm for a new procedure we frequently underestimate the psychological suffering of patients. In our opinion, psychological services to these patients are essential, and indications for the procedure must include psychosocial factors. No matter how useful it is to have the statistics of other patients' experiences with a disease, every evaluation must consider the patient's specific handicaps in relation to the personal values of each family, the developmental stage of each patient, and the services in the community available to support and improve the quality of the patient's life.

MORAL AND LEGAL CONSIDERATIONS

. . . Honoring a child's wish to die can be viewed as committing a homicide, abetting a suicide, or administering euthanasia, depending on the circumstances and one's philosophy. Euthanasia is commonly understood to only mean actively causing a patient's death rather than passively allowing it to occur, and suicide is commonly understood to mean taking one's own life rather than allowing death to occur by "natural" causes. Fletcher, however, categorizes euthanasia as voluntary (depending on the patient's knowledge and wishes) and as active

or passive (depending on whether death is hastened by action or inaction). Karen's death would be considered passive, voluntary euthanasia. That is, the physicians chose to honor an informed rational choice to die by inaction based on the judgment that the child accurately perceived her own best interests.

Most physicians' ethics oppose actively causing death. In Williams' questionnaire study of 333 members of the Association of Professors of Medicine and the Association of American Physicians, 87% voted in favor of passive euthanasia and 80% have practiced it, while 85% of the physicians opposed active euthanasia. In a study of 418 physicians in Seattle, 59% favored passive euthanasia (after having obtained a signed request from relatives), and 31% favored active euthanasia. Morison and Kass have recently debated whether or not it is correct to distinguish ethically between intent and means. Intent in all euthanasia is the same, but the means differ. . . .

Passive, voluntary and even active, nonvoluntary euthanasia are occasionally performed in the terminally ill child or the monstrously deformed newborn. Voluntary euthanasia in a child who is chronically but not terminally ill is rare but may become increasingly common with the increasing number of patients' lives being sustained by artificial and often uncomfortable and expensive means. Karen, for example, was not terminal at the time of the decision, because dialysis could have prolonged her life for a considerable period of time.

Those against legalized euthanasia emphasize its possible misuses and associate it with totalitarian eugenics. They stress that approval of euthanasia would contradict the physician's commitment to heal and undermine the confidence of all patients in their physicians. The possibility of a mistaken diagnosis or of a cure being discovered during the patient's prolonged dying are also cited as objections to the practice of euthanasia. Religious opposition to all forms of euthanasia rests on belief in the divine nature of suffering or the exclusive right of God to determine the time of death. . . .

Those who accept limited euthanasia try to define guidelines. Catholic moral theology makes the useful distinction between ordinary and extraordinary means of actions. Pope Pius XII stated that "it is not obligatory for physicians to use extraordinary means to prolong life indefinitely in hopeless cases." Gerald Kelly, the Catholic Theologian, wrote that "extraordinary means of preserving life are all medicines, treatments and operations which cannot be obtained or used without excessive expense, pain, or other inconvenience for the patient or for others or which, if used, would not offer reasonable hope of benefit to the patient." Gustafson points out one difficulty with the definition of "extraordinary"; the same procedure may be ordinary for one patient but extraordinary for another, depending on the extent of the problems the patient has.

A second difficulty in using the ordinary-extraordinary distinction as a guideline is the interpretation of the word hopeless. An assessment of hopelessness includes the patient's nearness to death and the amount of his suffering, as well as the physician's attitudes toward physical suffering, psychological suffering, and the relative importance of quality to quantity of life. Gustafson warns that in assessing the quality of life no single quality can be allowed to be considered determinative. We need to encompass the variety, complexity, and interplay of the qualities we value. Major considerations might include self-determination, happiness, satisfaction in fulfilling even limited goals, and providing occasion for meaningful experiences for others, both distressing and joyful. . . .

DISCUSSION AND CONCLUSION

We believe there are instances when a physician should honor an adolescent patient's wish to die. Until the courts, hospitals, and medical societies take a stand on the issue of passive, voluntary euthanasia, the decision is left to the physician. Many considerations must be brought to bear on each case, and the use of a team of consulting specialists, including colleagues in pediatrics, psychiatry, theology, and the law is optimal. Whether the ultimate responsibility for the decision to allow passive euthanasia should rest with the responsible physician or be diffused onto a small team is a question that warrants much further debate.

As when approaching any dying patient, it is wise to arrive unencumbered with formulas for the occasion, since it will not be covered by rote. It must first be determined whether or not the child has made his decision in a rational and informed manner. Such a decision cannot be obtained in the presence of definable mental illness or persuading outside pressures. The child's cognitive ability to understand death must also be assessed. This ability would be unusual before age 14 or 15. From the physician's personal point of view, he will undoubtedly be influenced by the amount of the child's suffering, the likelihood of improvement in the quality of life now judged unsatisfactory, the closeness of death, the extent of his participation in "causing" the death, as well as his philosophy regarding the dignity of life and the importance of quality as well as length of life.

The purpose of this paper is to draw attention to the dilemma of the medical team and the individual physician who are caring for an adolescent who chooses to die. We have outlined the general areas which we think must be considered in each case. Perhaps uniform criteria to weigh these considerations are not sensible at this time, but a body of medical literature on individual cases would be helpful by providing precedents which could be studied and debated. Karen's case was the stimulant for this paper, and the need for further thought in this area remains our most compelling conclusion.

Autonomy for Burned Patients When Survival Is Unprecedented

Sharon H. Imbus, R.N., M.Sc. and
Bruce E. Zawacki, M.D.

No burn is certainly fatal until the patient dies; the most severely burned patient may speak of hope with his last breath. Unable to prophesy, and unwilling to strip the patient of any hope he may cherish, we therefore prefer to diagnose burns as "fatal" or "hopeless" only in retrospect. Every year, however, several patients are admitted to our burn center with injuries so severe that survival is not only unexpected but, to our knowledge, unprecedented. Although difficult to face, the problems that these patients present must be anticipated and not simply ignored.

The surgical literature gives little attention to these patients except for brief phrases allowing an occasional glimpse into a particular surgeon's philosophy.[1-3] The literature on death and dying, voluminous since Kubler-Ross's work,[4] offers rich background but says little about the unique situation of our patients, who, after their injury, often have only a few hours of mental clarity in which to respond to their predicament. Several recent articles about withholding intensive care seem to ignore or incompletely answer the problem of obtaining the patient's informed consent. In some of these discussions, the authors simply assign to the physician what we believe to be the patient's ultimate right to decide whether he will or will not receive a particular form of therapy.[5-7] One suggests, perhaps unconstitutionally, that "certain competent patients" may be excluded from such decision making "when, in the physician's judgment, the patient will probably be unable to cope with it psychologically."[8] Still others, who recognize patient primacy in such decision making, offer no practical suggestion how it is best honored in practice.[9]

Reprinted with permission from the authors and *The New England Journal of Medicine*, vol. 297, no. 6, pp. 309–311, August 11, 1977.

Our approach, developed empirically over several years, is based on our conviction that the decision to begin or to withhold maximal therapeutic effort is more of an ethical than a medical judgment. The physician and his colleagues on the burn-care team present to the patient the appropriate medical and statistical facts together with authoritative medical opinion about the available therapeutic alternatives and their consequences. Thus informed, the patient may give or withhold his consent to receive a particular form of therapy, but it is his own decision based on his value system, and it is arrived at before communication and competence are seriously impaired by intubation or altered states of consciousness.

DEFINITIONS AND METHODS

The patient whose management this paper addresses is characterized by some combination of massive burns, severe smoke inhalation or advanced age. Such a patient's condition is designated by "1" on the Bull Mortality Probability Chart[10] and "0" in the National Burn Information Exchange Survival Analysis Diagrams,[11] both indicating nonsurvival from the indexes of age and percentage of body-surface area burned. Furthermore, our staff members cannot, from their own experiences, our burn-unit statistics, or references from the literature, recall survival in a similar patient.

To allow the patient maximal clarity of thought in decision making, several points must be communicated to the paramedic teams in the field and to local hospitals who transfer burned patients to our burn center immediately after injury: no administration of morphine or other narcotics before arrival; prompt fluid resuscitation; oxygen administration in treatment of possible carbon monoxide intoxication; avoidance of tracheostomy or endotracheal-tube insertion unless absolutely necessary to preserve the airway and maintain ventilation; and rapid transportation to the burn center.

Upon admission of a patient for whom survival seems in doubt, the burn center's most experienced physician is consulted, day or night, to evaluate the patient. His assessment, combined with a social and family history, is presented to all involved team members. Standard works are rechecked to determine if there has ever been a precedent for survival.

When the diagnosis is confirmed, the physician and other team members enter the room. Family members are not invited into the room to ensure that the decision of the patient is specifically his own. In an attempt to establish a relation with the patient, the attending physician or resident under his guidance tries to assume the role of a compassionate friend who is willing to listen. Hands are often held, and an effort is made to look deeply into the patient's eyes to perceive the unspoken questions that may lie there. Nonverbal cues are watched for closely. The presence of the burn team serves to witness and validate the patient's desires and requests, gives consensus to the gravity of the situation and supports the physician member of the team in this delicate, painful task.

At times, when the question of impending death does not spontaneously arise, suggestions such as "You are seriously ill", "You are sicker than you have ever been" or "Your life is in immediate danger" may be made, always in a caring, gentle way.

Some patients will not respond because of coma or mental incompetency. In those circumstances, the burn team and the family confer, again in a compassionate, concerned relation. All attempts are made to determine and do what the patient would be most likely to want if he were able to communicate.

A few patients will hear but not listen because of a need to deny their predicament. In general, such denials, if persistent, are considered an expression of a strong desire to live, and the patients are treated accordingly with maximal therapeutic effort.

A large majority of patients, however, understand the gravity of their situation and make further inquiries. The very frequent question— "Am I going to die?"—is answered truthfully by the statement, "We cannot predict the future. We can only say that, to our knowledge, no one in the past of your age and with your size of burn has ever survived this injury, either with or without maximal treatment." At this point, those who interpret this diagnosis of a burn without precedent of survival as an indication to avoid heroic measures typically become quite peaceful. Regularly, they then try to live their lives completely and fully to the end, saying things that they must say to those important to them, making proper plans, reparations and apologies and, in general, obtaining what Kavanaugh refers to as "permission to die."[12] These patients receive only ordinary medical measures and sufficient amounts of pain medication to assure comfort after their choice is made explicit. Fluid resuscitation is discontinued, they are admitted to a private room, and visiting hours become unlimited. An experienced nurse and, frequently, a chaplain are in constant attendance, using their expertise to comfort and sustain the patient and his family, chiefly by their continued presence and willingness to listen.

The patients who understand that survival is unprecedented in their case but, nevertheless, choose a maximal therapeutic effort are admitted to the burn intensive-care unit. Fluid resuscitation is continued, and full treatment measures are instituted, as with any other patient in the unit. As with those who choose only ordinary care, however, they may change their minds at any time; their decision is reviewed with them on a daily basis.

In general, when patients are mentally incompetent on admission because of head injury or inhalation injury or some other injury and may reasonably be expected to remain so indefinitely, the socially designated next of kin or other relatives are allowed to speak for the patient.[13] With children who are legally incompetent because of age, however, we have for the past five years been unwilling to declare any burn as being without precedent of survival, chiefly because mortality rates for very large burns in pediatric patients appear to be improving more rapidly than can be reported.

After interviewing the patient or his family, the physician is responsible for recording the salient points and decision in the patient's chart. Accurate documentation serves to clarify communication with other team members and avoids legal ambiguity.

"Postvention," described by Shneidman as "those activities which serve to reduce the aftereffects of a traumatic event in the lives of survivors,"[14] is now being evolved on our unit. Nurses are learning how to help survivors comfort each other and, together with the chaplain and social worker, are arranging for safe transportation of the bereaved to their homes, counseling families on the difficult matters of explaining death to children and explaining such points as legal necessity of an unwanted autopsy. Our hospital chaplain is available to conduct the funeral services if the family does not have its own pastor. He gets in touch with the families on the first anniversary of their loved one's death to answer any unfinished questions that may have been bothering them. The social worker also offers her continuing services to the bereaved.

RESULTS

During 1975 and 1976 there were 748 dispositions from our burn center, excluding readmissions, transfers and nonthermal injuries. Of these patients 126 died—18 children and 108 adults. Of the adults who died, 24, or 22 per cent, were diagnosed on admission as having injury without precedent of survival. Twenty-one of these patients or their families chose nonheroic or ordinary medical care. Only three chose full treatment measures, and their desires were fulfilled.

The following case histories illustrate our approach.

Cases 1 and 2. Two sisters, 68 and 70 years of age, and their husbands were searching for a schizophrenic daughter who had disappeared after her discharge from a psychiatric hospital. While their car waited for a stoplight, a nearby construction machine hit a gasoline line. The spraying gas exploded, leveling a city block and igniting the car.

The sisters arrived in our burn center two hours later. The younger sister had 91 per cent full-thickness, 92 per cent total-body burn, with moderate smoke inhalation; the older had 94.5 per cent full-thickness, 95.5 per cent total-body burn, with severe smoke inhalation. The burn team agreed that survival was unprecedented in both cases. Both women were alert and interviewed separately.

The younger sister asked about death directly, looking intently into the physician's eyes. When he answered, she replied matter-of-factly, "Well, I never dreamed that life would end like this, but since we all have to go sometime, I'd like to go quietly and comfortably. I don't know what to do about my daughter . . . "

After she was made comfortable, the nurse obtained a description of the missing daughter and possible whereabouts. The social worker alerted the police to look for her, and telephoned relatives, informing them of the accident as gently as could be conveyed by telephone. The husbands were located at another burn unit. An attempt was made to arrange a final spousal conversation, but both husbands were intubated.

Meanwhile, the older sister doubted whether her injuries were as serious as reported. "I feel so good, wouldn't I be hurting horribly if I were going to die?" The effect of full-thickness burns on nerve endings was explained. The physician reiterated that we wished to do what she thought was best for her. She hedged, "What did my sister say? I'll go along with her decision." Since the patient seemed unsure of her decision, she was offered full therapy in the room with her sister. She then refused the therapy adamantly but denied that she was dying.

The sisters' beds were placed next to each other so that they could see and touch each other easily. They discussed funeral arrangements and then joked, in the next breath, about the damage done to their hair. The hospital chaplain prayed with them. By active listening, he was able to convey to the older that her husband was not to blame for the accident as she had thought. "It's good to go out not cursing him after all our years together," she said. The younger sister died several hours later after her sister lapsed into a coma; the older died the next day. The daughter was not located.

Case 3. A 58-year-old man was cleaning his kitchen with an aerosol when the fumes were ignited by the stove pilot. He arrived at the hospital one hour later with a 97 per cent full-thickness burn, severe smoke inhalation and corneal abrasions. The team consensus that survival was unprecedented was unanimous. When the physicians talked with him, the man replied that he preferred his wife and her mother-in-law to decide for him. His wife and her mother, stunned and horrified by the accident, refused. Further conversation with the patient revealed that he wished to live by any and all means "until God is ready for me." In the burn intensive-care unit he required a tracheostomy and respirator. He continued to communicate, although imperfectly, by "writing" letters in the air. Despite an armamentarium of intensive nursing care, a cardiac-output monitor, silver nitrate dressings, Swan-Ganz catheter, and intravenous dopamine, he died three days later in septic shock.

DISCUSSION

Unlike diseases such as uncontrolled cancer, the prognosis of burns without precedent of survival is evident almost immediately at the time of admission, because the extent and severity of burn are easily recognized and rapidly quantifiable, and mortality statistics are more detailed and complete than for most other pathologic processes. Although such severe burns are rapid and even violent in onset, the patient is usually alert and mentally competent on admission and may remain so for hours to a day after the burn—longer if aggressive fluid resuscitation is given. There is no way to predict the length of this lucid interval for a particular patient, but certainly there is little time for the patient to gain a gradual awareness of his condition or for the burn team suddenly to acquire insight into the ethical issues involved.

The California Natural Death Act requires a 14-day waiting period after a "terminal" condition is diagnosed and the appropriate document is signed and witnessed before a person's wish for nonheroic measures is legally binding. It is not applicable to these patients because death almost always occurs before the waiting period has lapsed. The lack of specific legal guidelines, however, does not negate the desirability of a planned and efficient approach.

The approach described above evolved slowly and unevenly through experience, interdisciplinary conferences and informal debate. Although medical factors were always involved, the final issues invariably proved to be primarily ethical and could be stated approximately by the question, "Which is better for this patient, maximal therapy or ordinary care, and upon whose value system should the judgment be based?"

As pointed out by Kubler-Ross, when a patient is severely ill, he is often treated like a person with no right to an opinion.[4] Yet it is the patient's life and rights that are at stake. Statistics may describe past experience with a given type of injury receiving maximal therapy or ordinary care; physicians may cite such an experience and are experts in carrying out programs of maximal therapy or ordinary care, but only the patient may choose between them because only he has the right to consent to one or the other.

Just as Lincoln stated that "No man is good enough to govern another man without that other's consent,"[15] so no physician is so skilled that he may treat another without the other's consent.[16] If asked, the physician may offer his opinion about the choice, but it will be merely his personal, inexpert opinion about whether it is better to accept death or fight to make history as the first survivor in such an injury.

Bioethicists Joseph Fletcher and Paul Ramsey, as interpreted by Robb,[17] urge that *agape* or unselfish love for the patient and regard for his full stature as a person should be the criterion upon which we base our answers to bioethical questions such as those posed above. When dealing with an alert, competent patient, we need not struggle against distractions and prejudice to imagine what the patient wants; we need only to ask. Who is more likely to be totally and lovingly concerned with the patient's best interest than the patient himself? Whenever in the past we as care-givers tried to decide these matters for the patient, issues such as what was best for the morale of the nursing service, or for the solvency of the hospital, constantly clouded our judgment. It is for this reason that we oppose decision making by select committees convened "[to] explore what the best interest of the patient and his relatives require . . ." without necessarily asking or respecting the opinions of either.[5]

It took many months before we could shed a "we-know-best" defense and actually ask the patient what he wanted on admission when he was most competent to decide. Our approach seems obvious and right to us now; the first few times were agonizing. Our words seemed clumsy and awkward. If we had acted individually, without colleague support, the plan would probably have reverted rapidly to denial, or even worse, to a paternalistic decision making for the patient. Our patients and their families were able to see the human concern behind our first faltering phrases. Their warmth, gratitude and peace confirmed what we later read: that what we say to the patient, the exact words, matters less than how we say it in an atmosphere of honesty, caring and constant human presence.[18]

Weisman wrote, "The pervasive dread in dying seems not only to be the extinction of consciousness, but the fear that the death we die will not be our own. This is the singular distinction between death as a property of life and being put to death."[19] We believe that on our burn unit, death for these patients has become a property of life. It would be hypocritical to imply that all life-and-death decision making or all "decisions not to resuscitate" are now straightforward and anxiety-free on our burn service. Many patients admitted with head injuries or inhalation injuries are confused or unconscious on admission and never regain competency. Initially competent patients with small but measurable chances of survival still tend to have complications and to become incompetent before we learn what they would want us to do in the event that continued therapy became more a prolongation of death than a prolongation of life. Turning to the family for decision making when death seems imminent for an incompetent patient is rarely satisfactory; guilt-ridden families often find it very difficult to be objective and unselfish in their decision making. The more voiceless and vulnerable the patient, the more easily we have found ourselves slipping into a paternalistic role, using terms such as "hopeless," which we realize now are so obviously prejudicial (literally, judging before the fact). Yet our experience continues to convince us that "truth is the greatest kindness." It seems inevitable that more and earlier communication with the patient will prove to be the most honest and compassionate answer to many of the remaining problems of ethical decision making in the intensive-care unit.

Notes

1. Jackson DM: The psychological effects of burns. Burns 1:70–74, 1974.

2. Muir IFK, Barclay TL: Burns and Their Treatment. Second edition. Chicago, Year Book Medical Publishers. 1974, p 110.

3. Stone HH: The composite burn solution, Contemporary Burn Management. Edited by HC Polk Jr, HH Stone, Boston, Little, Brown, 1971, p. 96.

4. Kubler-Ross E: On Death and Dying. New York, Macmillan, 1969.

5. Critical Care Committee of the Massachusetts General Hospital: Optimum care for hopelessly ill patients. N Engl J Med 295:362–364, 1976.

6. Tagge GF, Adler D, Bryan-Brown CW, et al: Relationship of therapy to prognosis in critically ill patients. Crit Care Med 2:61–63, 1974

7. Skillman JJ: Intensive Care. Boston, Little, Brown, 1975, p 21

8. Rabkin MT, Gillerman G, Rice NR: Orders not to resuscitate. N Engl J Med 295:364–366, 1976

9. Cassem NH: Confronting the decision to let death come. Crit Care Med 2:113–117, 1974

10. Bull JP: Revised analysis of mortality due to burns. Lancet 2:1133–1134, 1971

11. Feller I, Archembeault C: Nursing the Burned Patient. Ann Arbor, Institute for Burn Medicine, 1973, p 10

12. Kavanaugh RE: Facing Death. Los Angeles, Nash, 1972, p 67

13. Brody H: Ethical Decisions in Medicine. Boston, Little, Brown, 1976 p 98

14. Shneidman E: Death of Man. New York, NY Times Book Company, 1973, p 33

15. Lincoln Abraham. In Peoria, Illinois during Lincoln-Douglas debate on Oct. 16, 1854. Quoted in Bartlett J: Familiar Quotations. Boston, Little, Brown, 1968, p 635a

16. Ramsey P: The Patient as Person. New Haven, Yale University Press, 1970, p 7

17. Robb JW: The Joseph Fletcher/Paul Ramsey debate in bioethics and the Christian ethical tradition. Religion in Life (in press)

18. Feifel H: Attitudes toward death in some normal and mentally ill populations. The Meaning of Death. Edited by H Feifel. New York, McGraw-Hill, 1959, p 124

19. Weisman AD: On Dying and Denying: A psychiatric study of terminality. New York, Behavioral Publications, 1972

Letters:
Autonomy for Severely Burned Patients

To the Editor: I was struck by the sensitivity and concern for patients expressed in the recent paper by Imbus and Zawacki (N Engl J Med 297:308–311, 1977). The tone of the article was so warm and the sentiments so obviously genuine that I read it repeatedly.

The authors state that when a patient enters their burn unit with an injury so severe that survival is unprecedented, the patient is allowed to decide whether the team should go all out or remain supportive. It is obvious that major barriers had to be overcome to allow a highly motivated team to be able to accept a patient's wish not to have vigorous care.

Physicians are highly trained to do the involved technical tasks of patient care. Regrettably, we are poorly trained in knowing when to let go or permit a dreadfully ill patient to die. Invariably, when an elderly patient, severely injured, comes to the hospital, a struggle begins. Do we go "all out" despite overwhelming evidence that the outcome will be death, or do we support, comfort and attend? Experience teaches that we do what we know best—calculate fluid losses, caloric needs and surface areas denuded. It is extremely difficult to "stand by."

The refreshing paper by Imbus and Zawacki has a cleansing effect. It points out that there is an alternative to knee-jerk intervention. Patient autonomy in the face of devastating injury is helpful to patient, family and health-care providers. There are obvious carryover implications into hematology-oncology, pulmonary disease and renal medicine. We all need to remember that there is an alternative to all-out efforts.

Beyond the work of the authors lies another, more formidable hurdle. They state that in the unconscious patient, despite age or extent of injury, full efforts are applied. Furthermore, they continue that "issues such as what was best for the morale of the nursing service, or the sol-

Reprinted with permission from *The New England Journal of Medicine,* vol. 297, no. 21, November 24, 1977, pp. 1182–1183.

vency of the hospital . . . clouded our judgment." Their honesty is disarming. However, full-fledged efforts to save a 75-year-old man with 80 per cent full-thickness burns, including face and hands, seem to beg for an answer to the question: Why? If such a patient lived for three weeks, the cost would probably be nearly $10,000. Survival is extremely doubtful—hence enormous investment and ultimate loss. In the near future we who provide care to critically ill persons will have to face these issues head on. The cost in dollars is staggering. The toll in human terms is likewise impressive. The struggle to save an unsalvageable patient drains nurses, doctors, family and friends of emotional resources, thus diminishing our collective ability to "give" to others. Soon, we will have to consider the likelihood of survival, age of the patient and the cost in dollars and human resources when we make our decision to intervene.

David S. Pratt, M.D.
Veterans Administration Hospital
Denver, CO 80220

To the Editor: The quality of professional caring for the fatally ill and dying patient has certainly been the subject of much examination and debate in the past decade. The article by Imbus and Zawacki offers compassionate operational guidelines for the care of the fatally burned patient, but I do not think that the issue of human, or patient, autonomy is relevantly examined. In effect, what the authors state has become an acceptable approach to certain patients entering their unit is frankly, but compassionately, to offer to them an analysis of their predicament (that there is little expectation of recovery), and then the information that the best available treatment, an intensive-care regimen, is not capable of changing the expectation of nonrecovery but would impose additional burdens and interference with what little is left of life. Thus, the patient is not offered an alternative form of possible treatment, but rather is informed that there is no effective treatment, although one noneffective treatment may be excessively burdensome. The observation that 88 per cent of the patients elect not to choose the intensive form of treatment does not seem much of a surprise. The issue does not pose much conflict between the patients and the medical staff, and thus the medical group is not really supporting autonomous, or independent responsible, decision making. No conflicts in the values of the staff and patients are involved.

Since there were many other deaths of patients in the unit, who apparently were treated with the intensive-care regimen, but who, by inference, were not offered a choice of their management (since the diagnosis of "burned beyond precedence for recovery" was not made), the question arises whether true autonomy, defined as patient-centered responsible decision making, was contemplated. A person who refused intensive care when the possibility (large or slight) of recovery was present, and who therefore bore responsibly the consequences of his decision, would probably be more worthily defined as acting autonomously. The staff would support a patient's decision even if that decision conflicted with the staff's wishes.

Therefore, a major medical ethical dilemma is raised. Why offer at all a treatment form that is not considered by the medical team to have benefit? Not offering the treatment would not be the equivalent of abandoning the patient, if continued compassionate palliative care were instituted and continued. And, on the other hand, if a treatment form is potentially or marginally beneficial, is that not the time to explain options carefully to a patient, and permit a lucid and responsible decision to reject or accept the treatment to be made?

MELVIN J. KRANT, M.D.
University of Massachusetts Medical Center
Worcester, MA 01605

To the Editor: I read with dismay the article by Imbus and Zawacki. I agree that patients with terminal illness should be allowed to die without heroic measures, but it seems that the decision should be made spontaneously by them and without even the faintest possibility of psychologic coercion. There is a great difference between a patient's request to be allowed to die and the physician's raising the issue as described in the article. Even the caveat that "We cannot predict the future . . . no one in the past of your age and . . . size of burn has ever survived" is unfair. For example, until quite recently, we knew unequivocally that four minutes or so of oxygen deprivation because of drowning led to irreversible brain damage. Now, we are aware of the diving reflex and the possibility of return of function after considerably longer periods of anoxia.

Another point that has bearing on this discussion is that clinical therapy in part evolves out of "heroic" measures (witness the development of renal transplantation as an effective therapeutic modality). These two considerations—namely, our ultimate ignorance about the curability or reversibility of any pathologic process and the need to push back the frontiers of our medical ignorance—seem to mandate a strong attempt to cure, provided needless pain and suffering are avoided. This effort is, I think, even more important with a burn, which is an acute insult to a patient who may have been in good general health. This situation is quite different from that of a terminally ill victim of carcinoma with extensive metastasis.

There are, of course, problems involved in a heroic approach to burn therapy in apparently hopeless cases. It requires that the physician be skilled and innovative and capable of thinking of new approaches, rather than a mere technician. However, if all the diseases that were once thought incurable had been treated by allowing the afflicted patient to "die with dignity," those diseases would still be incurable. Even aside from this consideration, however, I have a great concern that we are at the beginning of a new trend. Instead of a patient asking to be treated in a minimal manner, the physician now raises the question and in effect asks the patient if he (the physician) can be allowed to treat him thus. From there it is a simple step not even to bother to ask the patient's permission. This, I am sure, is not an idle concern, in the light of the authors' assertion that when the patients are unresponsive, "all attempts are made to determine and do what the patient would be most likely to want if he were able to communicate.''

STANLEY COHEN, M.D.
University of Connecticut Health Center
Farmington, CT 06032

The above letters were referred to the authors of the article in question, who offer the following reply:

To the Editor: We and the other members of our burn team appreciate these thought-provoking responses to our approach to caring for burned patients when survival is unprecedented.

Dr. Pratt's letter was kind. The interpersonal warmth that we try to achieve is difficult to express in prose; we are encouraged that he was able to sense its presence. We recognize his concern about struggling against all odds at great expense. However, those who choose all that medical technology has to offer are the ones who ''without . . . coercion'' join us in pushing back ''the frontiers of our medical ignorance.'' The challenge then is even more exciting because the patient and we are working toward the same goal.

The next two letters demonstrate different possible attitudes to maximal medical therapy. Dr. Krant believes that offering maximal care is fraudulent when survival is unprecedented. Dr. Cohen thinks that offering less than maximal efforts denies medical progress. We acknowledge the dilemma and do not dispute either perspective. It is an individual decision: the patient's.

SHARON H. IMBUS, R.N., M.Sc.
BRUCE E. ZAWACKI, M.D.
University of Southern California
Medical Center
Los Angeles, CA 90033

Chapter 5

HEALTH POLICY

INTRODUCTION

In many areas of human enterprise, differences among people are easy to accept. But when differences become so great that some people are unable to meet their basic needs whereas others lead rich and easy lives, it is difficult to maintain that we live in a just world. For a society to be just, it is necessary that its benefits and burdens be fairly distributed. Individual health status is not evenly distributed in the United States. Some differences are attributable to chance, age, and other factors beyond human control; others are due to personal lifestyles. But many differences in health status are attributable to social factors. Poverty is highly correlated with illness and other health problems, and poverty is primarily a creation of society. Environmental pollutants that cause cancer or birth defects are social products. Some people are exposed to these risks more than others. For example, inner-city working-class people suffer from more diseases than their suburban counterparts. Poor elderly people eat less nutritious diets and live in more poorly heated homes than younger or wealthier people. The wealthiest fifth of the world's population lives twenty-two years longer on the average than the poorest fifth.[1]

Because inequalities in health are partly caused by general social inequalities, we could argue that a just health care system should tend to equalize as well as maximize the distribution of good health. Instead, the health care system reflects and hence aggravates existing social inequalities. We thus confront questions of justice with regard to health care delivery: Is it unjust that some people get better care than others because of differences in geographic location or ability to pay? How just is it for society to invest in health care as compared to other important social programs, such as income maintenance? What principles of justice should govern access to health care? Can we simultaneously provide equal access to health care facilities and maintain high-quality care for everyone?

Before discussing the issue of justice in health care, we need to see clearly how the issue arises in this context. We need to step back and bring into focus our views on justice in society generally. Justice has three main areas of application: distribution of benefits and burdens (distributive justice), punishment (retributive justice), and the orderly process of relations between the government and individuals, such as due process of law, the right to a speedy trial, and so forth (procedural justice). The discussions in this chapter apply to distributive justice.

DISTRIBUTIVE JUSTICE

The terms *just* and *unjust* can be used to describe social arrangements, sets of laws, formal or informal social practices, acts of institutions, and attitudes and actions of individuals. The terms are not identified with any single social arrangement or type of action. Depending on circumstances, a wide variety of social rules or individual actions might be counted as just or unjust. To say that the rules of a society are just is to claim by implication that its members should follow those rules. Appropriate responses to just actions of individuals include cooperation and praise. Injustice, on the other hand, is grounds for noncooperation, resistance, and condemnation.

Although *just* is sometimes used as a general term of approval, a more specific conception is sought when we talk of distributive justice. For example, to say that the general inadequacy of nursing homes in the United States is unjust is to say that elderly people have a *right* to better treatment, that it is *unfair* to neglect them, and that their treatment fails to show full *respect* for them. The claim of injustice is a stronger one than if we were simply to say that it would be *better* if they received more care. Moreover, a society using much of its health services for the care of a privileged segment of the population distributes health care unjustly, even though it may provide more health care overall than under more equitable arrangements. Justice differs from the maximization of benefits overall. To appeal to justice is to use a special sort of argument; injustice is a special sort of wrong.

Basic to various conceptions of distributive

justice are such notions as the harmony and balance of human affairs, dignity of human beings, merit, personal liberty, participation in decision making, equality, fairness, and give-and-take. A complete conception of justice will combine several of these notions. Disagreement rests on which is the root conception and which are the branches. The philosophical treatments of justice in this chapter highlight different elements, attempt to characterize these elements exactly, and distinguish justice from other moral concepts.

William Frankena places *equality* in the distribution of goods at the root of his account of justice. A just society begins with the assumption of equality among people and treats everyone equally except as unequal treatment is required by important considerations. Frankena calls these ''justicizing'' considerations to distinguish the narrower reasoning about justice from more general ''justifying'' reasons.

Frankena's first task is to characterize differences between people justifying or justicizing different treatment. For example, a heart attack clearly justicizes different treatment than a broken leg. Frankena makes a list of qualities that are generally taken to justicize different treatment by society—capacity, need, merit, keeping agreements, and avoiding injury, interference, and impoverishment. Frankena's next task is to say what these justicizing differences have in common. He argues that differences in treatment are justified only if they further equality of happiness in the long run. He concludes that a just state makes a minimum standard contribution to each person supplemented by the same relative contribution to the good life of each. By appealing to the equal happiness of each rather than to overall happiness, Frankena distinguishes justice from utilitarian approaches to happiness. The equal happiness of each as a condition of a just society, Frankena believes, is rooted in human dignity.

John Rawls represents the inexact ordinary conception of justice by means of a more exact conception suited to moral theory. He calls this process the formation of an ''analytic construction'' of justice. In so doing, he works at a higher level of abstraction than Frankena.

Rawls mentions no particular goods, liberties, or human qualities to which standards of justice apply. Instead, he offers a framework into which, he argues, any complete theory of justice must fit.

For Rawls, justice and fairness are related concepts, the former applying to major social institutions and societies as a whole. These concepts, he suggests, have in common the idea of *reciprocity*. Reciprocity, however, is not simply give-and-take; it is equal and mutual decision making in which each person has a voice and vote to express personal interests. In his view, justice is generated by conflicts of interests among individuals at a grass-roots level. His notion contrasts with Frankena's and some classical notions of justice. The latter see justice as governing goods generated by society as a whole or handed down by a central executive. Rawls's conception also differs from utilitarianism. Justice is concerned with the well-being of each, not the aggregate happiness of all. Moreover, the utilitarian conception of good counts all the good consequences of an institution in its favor regardless of how the good is produced. In contrast, Rawls claims that happiness produced unjustly should not be counted in favor of an institution or practice.

The image underlying Rawls's conception of justice is that of a group of individuals gathered together to negotiate the ground rules of a society they intend to establish. He imagines those present as being consciously self-interested but kept by a "veil of ignorance" from knowing exactly what position, advantages, and disadvantages each will occupy in this society. The group will need to agree on some principles of justice in order to ensure that each participant's interests will not be ignored, no matter what his or her position in the new society is.

Rawls argues that two basic principles of justice would be generated by reciprocal self-interest in such negotiations. The first principle is one of equal liberty: Each shall have maximum liberty compatible with a like liberty for all. Liberty is a formula to cover as much as possible—the use of goods, access to positions and procedures, and expression of personal tastes and opinions. The second principle asserts that differences in what is distributed to people are justifiable only if it can be reasonably expected that such differences will work out for the benefit of all—and then only if the privileges and offices in question are open to all.

Kai Nielsen defends what he considers to be a "radical egalitarian" concept of justice, strong enough, he believes, to require a socialist organization of society to support it. He claims that human beings should be treated equally with respect to certain characteristics, that is, those that constitute "things that all people should have." However, he does not mean that all people should receive the same goods and burdens or the same amount of them. Rather, he believes that people should be treated with equal *respect* in regard to these and that equal respect sometimes requires different treatment. Nielsen's first principle of egalitarian justice is much like Rawls's in urging maximum and equal basic liberty, but he disagrees with Rawls on the second principle of justice. The view of Rawls he criticizes is one that Rawls expressed in his work *A Theory of Justice*. This is Rawls's "difference principle," stating that social and economic inequalities should be arranged to give the greatest benefit to the least advantaged. Since Rawls's later position is more egalitarian than his earlier one, Nielsen would also criticize the position stated here. Nielsen argues that the difference principle is consistent with an unjust state of affairs. Specifically, it is consistent with welfare capitalism, under which a few are permitted great economic benefits in order to foster investment in institutions giving basic support to the worst off. Nielsen believes that this practice inevitably undermines the equality of respect necessary to justice, because equal respect is impossible where gross inequalities exist in economics and status.

It is not clear that Nielsen's equality of respect is all that it appears to be. In his discussion of specific allocations of scarce resources, he defends decisions based on differences in people's social contribution—a practice Gene Outka, James J. Childress, and others argue is inegalitarian. Nielsen could reply that in any socially stratified society like ours, judgments of social *contribution* inevitably reduce to judgments of relative social *status* but that in the framework of an egalitarian society, these judgments can be made fairly and objectively.

RIGHTS AND JUSTICE IN HEALTH CARE

Two questions dominate this section: What principles of justice should guide the delivery of health care? And to what aspects of health care can people justly claim access? Some of the discussion here is conducted in terms of the *right* to health care. To say ''People have a right to health care'' is to say more than ''Health care should be distributed justly,'' but most of the arguments about the right to health care are conducted in terms of principles of justice.

Three conceptions of health care dominate discussions on the right to health care. (1) For some, such as Daniel Callahan and Outka, health care is a system for treating disease and illness. Outka focuses even more narrowly on acute care for unexpected health problems. (2) For others, such as Laurence B. Mc-Cullough, health care refers to the wide range of measures that support good health, such as clean water, adequate diet, heat in the winter, and so on. (3) A third important conception of health care given little attention by these writers is the provision of care, comfort, and protection for those suffering from disease. Such services are good in themselves and constitute a major *humanitarian* function of health care. We can argue that people are entitled to such things as palliative terminal care, aspirin for minor headaches, and considerate attention while recovering from diseases independent of the long-term health impact of these activities.

Callahan, recognizing that it is difficult to define health, offers an explanation. He rejects the widely accepted World Health Organization definition of health—a ''state of complete physical, mental, and social well-being''—as too ambitious to be useful for a practical understanding. It also wrongly tends to make ''medicine the keystone in the search for human happiness.'' He believes that a more limited concept of health should be used: freedom from disease and illness. At least we have wide agreement on what counts as an illness and can obtain a rough idea of where and how it occurs.

Callahan argues that even if we can say what health is, we still have a basic problem of what weight we should place on freedom from illness in our thinking about justice. What other concerns would we be justified in sacrificing, if we had to, in order to maintain health? Callahan does not answer this question; instead, he gives us reasons why it is hard to make such judgments. He believes that the commitment to economic growth and technological progress in the United States impedes our ability to make judgments about justice in health care. The need for growth makes it difficult for us to distinguish our *needs* from our *desires,* and our technological optimism makes it hard to accept the limitations of medicine as a means to solving problems. Callahan believes we have a choice between two ways to conduct the debate over justice in health care. We can continue simply to struggle *politically* with each other for medical resources, and claim, for example, that our wants are needs in order to dominate the polemic; or we can move toward a *philosophical* consensus on what we *should* seek in the name of health.

Callahan assumes that health care should be distributed according to need. But not everyone agrees with him. One of the most extreme attacks on this assumption is mounted by Robert M. Sade. He denies that patients have a right to health care. According to his conception of justice, all rights rest with the *providers* of care (who seem to him all to be physicians). Sade argues that physicians should make the decisions about health care distribution because their skills are in effect their *property.* The right to use one's property without interference from others is, according to Sade, the most universal and basic freedom. Appealing to John Locke, he argues that free use of property is necessary to protect one's right to life, since one's income and possessions are necessary for survival. A just allocation of health care thus depends on the freedom of physicians to decide how to use their skills. Although Sade's language is quaint and his position unsympathetic to patients, his views are deeply held by many in the United States.

Laurence B. McCullough turns Sade's Lockean principles to the defense of the consumer. He takes greater care than Sade to explain what Locke means by a ''right'' and why Locke's concept of *natural rights* is important to the debate. McCullough emphasizes that the debate should be conducted on the basis of *reasons.* Since our discussion is about what we *should* accept in our society, not about what we *do* accept, we need a source of reasons more basic than society's approval or disapproval. Natural rights are more basic because they derive from the concept of what a human being is. Like Sade, McCullough believes that a right to life is the most basic right and that health care (in the broad sense) is necessary to life, so that a just allocation of health care is one that maintains human life. For McCullough, this means three things: a right to equal access to existing health care services, a right to basic health services adequate for survival, and (less important) enough health care to enhance health. The first two are needed to maintain humanity according to our minimal and basic concept of it; the last is needed to realize our full humanity.

McCullough rejects Sade's position by pointing out that the physician's relation to medical skills is not like Locke's conception of owning property. Locke only defends the free use of property that one acquires from nature by means of one's own personal efforts; but medical skills are socially produced and gained partly through public support. Thus, McCullough argues, medical skills belong to the public as well as to physicians.

McCullough recognizes that natural rights may conflict, as when the rights of providers to allocate their work freely conflict with the rights of patients to equal access to care. But, he argues, the key to resolving the conflict lies in the basic appeal of both principles to the right to life. Health care needed for life is more important than a large income for physicians; income necessary to keep physicians alive is more important than services for the enhancement of health.

However, we should not assume that a principle based on need is the only one that might govern the consumption of health services. Gene Outka sensitively explores five plausible principles of justice in health policy. He rejects three of them—merit, social contribution, and financial power—and favors two—need, and treating similar cases similarly.

Yet, need is Outka's main candidate for a reasonable principle of justice in helath care. It is easy to see that need should be a *necessary* con-

dition for receiving health care. Unneeded health care is a burden to both provider and recipient. But whether need is a *sufficient* condition for receiving health care is a more difficult question. Outka effectively rules out the main candidates for additonal necessary conditions by eliminating merit, social contribution, and financial power. More positively, he argues that our lack of control over health and our commitment to show equal respect to persons favor distribution according to need.

Outka's fifth principle, "treating similar cases similarly," is the empty form of the principle of justice. Why then does he include it? He is concerned that even if we allocate health care according to need, we still may not have enough to go around. In this case, he would prefer that additional principles of justice avoid the rejected principles and introduce something fairer, such as limiting care to certain categories of disease.

Amy Gutmann also accepts something like need as the principle of justice in health care. "Equal access" to health care is her key concept; it links access to health care with health status, that is, need. She sees this as a "one class" system of care distinuished from two or more classes based on the ability to pay. She sees equal access to health care, like access to similar services such as police protection, as a necessary condition of equal opportunity in general. She also argues that physical pain deserves a response whatever the ability to pay and that equality in health care is important to our cultural concept of self-respect.

Gutmann considers the problem of establishing a minimal level of care to which we would all be entitled. She believes that the question cannot be answered in advance by philosophical principles alone; instead, a consensus must be found by democratic processes. However, she sees a problem here. It has been our practice to establish a basic level of services for those in need and at the same time to permit the free practice of health care according to desire and ability to pay. Gutmann asks what we should do if the latter practice impinges on our ability to provide equal access to basic services? This is indeed a problem. Many critics of health care have pointed out that our focus on acute care and highly technological services interferes with our ability to address more basic and chronic health services. For example, the approximate annual bill for coronary artery bypass surgery in 1981 was $2 billion, while many of our nursing homes languished in disrepair. A more vivid example is the story of a group of physicians working at a public hospital who build a clinic across the street and refer patients with more profitable illnesses and better ability to pay to their own practices. A consequence of this practice is that the public hospital is less able to support its services. Gutmann is inclined to think that a free market in health care is inconsistent with meeting basic needs justly, but she thinks it politically imprudent to support limitations on markets in health care in the United States at the present time.

Dan E. Beauchamp draws out this fundamental conflict between two conceptions of justice in health care. He groups such principles as merit, social contribution, ability to pay, and freedom of property under the heading of "market justice." He pits this principle against a form of social justice he calls "public health justice." He attacks market justice not so much from arguments of justice but from those based on overall public good. Beauchamp sees health care as one of the common human goods not well supported by market economics. A common good is one that nearly everyone values, that requires collective support and understanding, and that is affected by the welfare of others. For example, all of us are affected by unclean water, and if my neighbor has an infectious disease, I too am in danger. Beauchamp sees health care under market justice as neglecting chronic care and preventive measures while focusing on highly technological acute care. Moreover, market justice tends to involve "victim-blaming"—holding individuals responsible for health problems beyond their control. He treats public health justice as a "counter-ethic" to market justice; much of it is defined by negating market justice, and since public health justice is as yet unrealized, it is harder to define. It involves our broadest definition of health care—prevention of illness, control of pollution, collective actions for health, and fair share of burdens for health problems.

The debate between market justice and public health justice is an important one. Justice is a distributive concept and applies to all. There should thus be justice for both providers and patients. Moreover, production and consumption are related. The goods and services that people consume are normally the same goods and services that others produce. So, a just system of production must be coordinated with a just system of consumption. Market justice is particularly inappropriate in health care, since as some economists point out, health care is distinguished by provider-induced demand; that is, many health services are decided upon largely by providers. Public health justice better expresses justice for consumers but does not very clearly address fairness for providers. We need a principle of justice that reconciles fairness for producers with fairness for consumers.

None of the articles looks at this problem of overall balance very closely. But we find principles of justice relating production and consumption expressed in a simple way in discussions of responsibility for health and in merit conceptions of justice in health care delivery. These conceptions of reciprocity are expressed by the common formula, "rights depend on responsibilities." Thus, three discussions of responsibility for health care are included here.

RESPONSIBILITY FOR HEALTH CARE

Attention has focused in recent years on individual efforts to maintain health. People recognize that personal habits like smoking and heavy drinking present serious health risks. Health professionals sometimes express anger toward smokers, alcoholics, and drug addicts, feel such patients are wasting their time, and express the judgment that such people should not receive health care at all, especially at public expense. This reaction is extreme but raises a serious question of justice. How much self-care do fairness and reciprocity require of individuals as compared to care from others?

To answer this question we need to understand something about the *causation* of illness. What makes us sick? What makes us healthy? Fate and luck are good traditional answers. More common modern answers are biological factors, social factors, and individual behavior. In explaining a heart attack, therefore, some emphasize the patient's genetic predisposition to heart disease; others focus on the patient's stressful work; and others look into the patient's exercise and dietary habits. Each type of explanation suggests a different approach to treatment. The biologist thinks of medication, the social theorist would change our working and living conditions, and the individualist would urge us to lead healthier lives. These choices therefore have *political* dimensions. Technology, social change, and education must compete for our energy and resources. Each view also characterizes a different relationship between production of health care and consumption. The biological model places a heavy responsibility for health on the professions; the social model affects work and production broadly; and individualism focuses on the consumer.

Robert M. Veatch canvasses these and other common positions on responsibility for health and concludes that there is no one type of cause of health problems. Like Outka, he is disinclined to use personal responsibility as a criterion for access to health care because it is too harsh a sanction for self-abuse and neglect. But since the multicausal model recognizes a role for individual conduct, he accepts that other kinds of sanctions, such as insurance rates, taxes, regulations, and the like, could be used to modify health-risking behavior.

Veatch points out that many who talk about responsibility for health are not primarily interested in it. They are ready, for example, to support health risks taken by firefighters who voluntarily risk their lives. They are actually worried about *culpability* for bad health. Veatch believes that there exists a question of justice about who should shoulder the health costs of conduct that "is not socially ennobling." He believes that some of these costs should be placed on individuals responsible for them. For example, there would be nothing wrong in establishing a cigarette tax earmarked for treating cancer. He only demands that such measures be taken with regard to truly voluntary conduct.

Daniel I. Wikler pursues in some detail the question of government measures to encourage healthy lifestyles, first considering what the goals of such intervention might be. He thinks that education as well as mild sanctions are justifiable where they would benefit people, even though some claim this would be paternalistic. He looks less favorably on arguments appealing to the costs to others of self-inflicted health problems. He thinks it is unclear that they really impose burdens on others. (The classic case is of the smoker who dies young and relieves us of his or her Social Security payments.) Even if such behavior is voluntary, people are not responsible for the fact that their acts place burdens on others; and disincentives, such as an alcohol health tax, would be paid by both abusers and nonabusers alike. Nevertheless, he claims that the abuser wishing to escape sanctions is in a double bind: Insofar as such acts are *voluntary,* the abuser can be blamed for placing burdens on others; insofar as such acts are *involuntary,* intervention cannot be charged with paternalism.

Wikler considers what might be the proper means of encouraging healthy behavior; he supports education as nonmanipulative and is willing to accept some incentives and taxes. He emphasizes, however, that focus on lifestyle can become moralistic and distract us from some of our most important health problems, such as environmental ones.

Henry Sigerist, writing in the 1930s, takes these considerations of justice as reciprocity in a more collective direction. He claims that the chief cause of disease is poverty. Failure to provide jobs for those who want to work, food for the hungry, and so on constitutes culpable behavior by society as a collective whole. The major faults that create health risks lie not with individuals but with society. If society cannot provide the means to be healthy it should at least provide treatment for disease, and thus, Sigerist argues, we have a right to health care.

Indeed, the arguments about the causation of health and disease are not as neutral as they may at first seem. Although our individual decisions affect our health, these decisions must be understood in the context of constraints created by society. The risks of driving a car—a voluntary act—are profoundly affected by automobile safety, speed limits, and highway construction. If I choose to jog to improve my health, I do so along city streets not of my making. Changing my lifestyle does little to protect me from environmental carcinogens or nuclear war. One could argue that in certain social contexts it is *unfair* to focus on individual behavior when the bulk of controllable health problems have social sources. The appropriate individual response to health problems may therefore be to support political action to find collective solutions.

REGULATION OF RESEARCH

Our beliefs about ethics and justice, insofar as they are widely shared and adhered to in conduct, constitute a system of regulation of conduct. Distributive justice, because it applies to everyone broadly, regulates our exchanges well only when we have a common sense of fair distribution. But there are areas of conduct where either we are unsure of how to apply principles of justice or some of us are likely to act in conflict with widely held conceptions of justice. In such cases, it may be necessary to undertake more active forms of regulation in order both to provide a forum in which a consensus on doubtful areas can be found and to restrict activities in conflict with the consensus. The ethical conduct of human experimentation has proved in the past decades to be just such an area. We include in this collection two case studies of ethical problems in human experimentation.

The article by Elinor Langer confirms that some medical researchers are willing to conduct work that according to the consensus is unethical. When they injected live cancer cells into elderly institutionalized patients, researchers did not tell patients about it because they believed, no doubt rightly, that had the patients known they would have refused to consent. Yet this is a case of invalid reasoning. That patients would have refused had they known is a reason for *not* giving them injections of live cancer cells. It is also a reason that patients be at least fully informed so that they can decide whether or not to serve as experimental subjects.

The Willowbrook case, about which we include several discussions, is more controversial. Like the cancer cell case, experiments were conducted on an institutionalized population, and a particularly vulnerable one—mentally retarded children. The Willowbrook studies involved giving children hepatitis under controlled conditions and then studying the blood chemistry of the disease. The studies were not intended as a possible course of therapy for the children and so constituted *nontherapeutic* research. Nontherapeutic research clearly involves using people for purposes remote from their interests. Lest experimenters use people simply as a means to an end, it is important that voluntary and informed *consent* be obtained from subjects. Consent is called for partly in the interests of justice. The requirement of consent protects powerless and disadvantaged people from being exploited by bearing more than their share of research risks. Young children, although they cannot consent for themselves, are usually allowed to participate in nontherapeutic research through the proxy consent of their parents, but only when the research needs to be conducted on children, when it may benefit children as a class, and when it is of low risk.

The experimenters claimed that they obtained parental consent only after thorough discussion and that the children were better off as a result of their participation. They were cared for in a special unit which protected them from diseases on other hospital units, where they would have contracted hepatitis anyway. In a close study of the case, Paul Ramsey challenges and explores some of these arguments. He claims that the children were exploited: Parents were under pressure because their children could obtain early admission to Willowbrook only if they participated in the study, and the study appeared beneficial only in the context of the wretched conditions at Willowbrook.

Research on human subjects does not exhaust the possibilities of experimental harm to human beings. Research on recombinant DNA, which makes uncertain and conceivably dangerous changes in organisms, has led to much public discussion about the regulation of research. Carl Cohen argues that the usual general objections to recombinant DNA research either employ unsound principles, or if sound, are inapplicable to the subject. His arguments are interesting in the light of the debate over responsibility for health. Like risky individual conduct, recombinant DNA research may damage health and place burdens on the public. Are the two areas of concern similar and therefore subject to the same principles of justice, or are they sufficiently different to require separate consideration? One consideration in favor of recombinant DNA research over individual unhealthy lifestyles is that this new technology could prove extremely beneficial. A consideration against recombinant DNA as compared with unhealthy lifestyles is that the research could conceivably result in a biological nightmare, an outcome not possible from unhealthy lifestyles.

Since both debate and examples of abuse have occurred with regard to human experimentation and recombinant DNA research, both have come to be regulated in an active way. A system of review has been established in all institutions receiving federal research funds to assess protocols for experiments concerning their risk–benefit ratio and the adequacy of their provisions for obtaining informed consent. These "human subjects" committees or "institutional review boards" discuss proposals and make suggestions to researchers about how to make studies safer and how to obtain more adequate consent. Studies may not be conducted on human beings unless they are approved by these committees. A system of "biosafety" committees has been established to ensure that recombinant DNA research is conducted safely according to federal standards. Discussion in such committees permits us to continue to study issues in ethics and to arrive at a better understanding of them.

ALTRUISM, MARKETS, AND MEDICAL RESOURCES

Scarcity forces unwelcome decisions that may lead to care for some and suffering or dying for others. The ideal resolution of such problems is to eliminate scarcity. For example, decisions about access to kidney dialysis were so painful that the government undertook to support the treatment of end-stage renal disease; now, dialysis is plentiful, although costly to provide for all who need it. But scarcity cannot always be

eliminated, and the newest treatments are inevitably scarce.

Scarce health care resources raise three different kinds of problems:

1. Because overall national resources are limited, to what extent should there be investment in health care as opposed to housing, recreation, transportation, and the like? For example, is it unjust that in 1982 we spent about $2.6 billion going to the movies and about $180 billion on armaments while millions around the world starved, languished in nursing homes, slept under bridges, and so on?

2. Within the aggregate of health care expenditures there must be allocation of scarce resources. Paul Freund raises some of these questions. Should health care capital and labor be directed to research and technological advance, or should it be directed to distribution of known benefits? Is there too much spent on acute and critical care and not enough on labor-intensive health care, such as nursing, rehabilitation, hospices, and the like?

3. Suppose that we have followed accepted principles of justice in allocating care and still have more individuals in need than we can care for. Whom should we select for scarce life-saving treatment? Outka claims that we should find some new principle of justice of the form "treat similar cases similarly." James F. Childress disagrees. He believes that justice must be to some degree "blind." The differences and similarities among us to be assessed by justice should be limited; otherwise, we lose our ability to be just. We become lost in detail, and our objectivity fades as we eventually characterize ourselves uniquely.

Instead, Childress argues that we should use *randomness* or a similar principle, such as first-come-first-serve, to make the next selection. He believes that even if we were entirely self-interested, few would be so certain of their value, once the details were investigated, to pit themselves in a contest of social worth for a place on a kidney machine. A gamble is fairer for all.

In making judgments based on scarcity, it is important that we avoid seeing shortages where there are none and moving too quickly to selection of individual patients. Recent public attention to the higher dollar *costs* of health care has led many to misperceive the problem of scarcity. We could mean any of four different things by the worry that "health care costs too much," and none of these concerns clearly requires that we become very selective about who receives care:

1. "We cannot afford so much health care because justice requires we spend money for other things." Before we can assess the justice of this claim, we need to know what else we need the money for. We also need to consider whether real shifts in labor and capital are necessary. There are thousands of registered nurses not now working in health care who would do so if pay and working conditions were appropriate to their tasks; physicians have begun to worry about a coming *excess* of physicians; and millions of people are now unemployed and willing to work. Fiscal restrictions do not translate into scarcity of resources.

2. "We are being overcharged for health care." It is true that some excess salaries and profits are made in health care. But the solution to this problem is not to limit *access* by patients; instead, we should limit excess income and profits.

3. "Health care is not *worth* what we pay for it." Where procedures are unnecessary or inefficacious, they should be eliminated even if they are cheap.

4. "There are cheaper ways to deliver health care." This may be true, but the major system under consideration in 1982 for delivering health care more cheaply is a system of competition among health maintenance organizations. Far from returning money to consumers, widespread use of large business organizations in health care would make care increasingly bureaucratic, and savings would be returned to investors as profits rather than to consumers.

The *appearance* of scarcity inspired by the fiscal crisis in health care is a prime motive for the inquiry into individual responsibility for health. Health professionals express anger toward such things as the abuse of emergency departments for minor complaints and the repetitive treatment of alcoholic derelicts. Yet, ascertaining individual responsibility for health care addresses *none* of these cost considerations. A sense of justice requires understanding limitations of resources on a broad scale and not blaming individuals for worldwide problems affecting us all.

Most crucially, the dollar costs of an enterprise measure little that is relevant to issues of justice. When dollar costs are incurred, money is always payed *to* someone. Thus the *costs* of health care are also *benefits*.[2] The more we spend on health care, the more providers earn. Thus, dollar measures of costs are meaningless until we know who is paying, who is receiving, and how the exchange affects the welfare of all involved. We need to employ principles of justice in health care that coordinate the whole picture of justice for consumers and providers. *How* we make these allocation decisions will affect both the manner of their production and their pattern of distribution.

Richard Titmuss compares the systems of blood distribution in the United States and Britain. Characterizing the U.S. system as a *market* system and the British system as a *donorship* system, his studies show that the British system is preferable in terms of cost, quality, and efficiency. This conclusion is surprising because many assume that market systems are superior to altruistic systems in these areas, even if self-interested actions appear less moral than altruistic ones.

Exchanges of blood can be viewed as a microcosmic model for the health care system as a whole. Blood is also a symbol of human unity and the hopes and fears invested in health care. Blood is transferable, so that it is possible to improve the existing distribution of health by transferring blood from the healthy to the unhealthy. Unlike kidneys, blood is regenerated by the donor, so that it represents renewable altruism rather than outright human sacrifice.

Titmuss's argument is that the market system poisons the well of altruism. If others are selling their blood, the donor enjoys less pleasure in giving blood. In this way the market system reduces our liberty to act altruistically. Blood for money tends to drive out blood for love, and turns out to be poorer quality blood as well. A self-interested hepatitis carrier is more likely to sell blood for money than to donate it from altruism. The market system also fortifies inequalities in health: The wealthy buy blood from the poor, who risk their health for limited monetary gain. In contrast, Titmuss sees the donor system as economically sound because blood is sought only to meet health needs and not to make profits.

Critics of socialized health care sometimes see it as a coercive system, but the British system of blood donorship under socialism indicates that health care might be provided in a noncoercive fashion by government. Society can rely on those motivated to provide health care to work where needed, instead of having to draft health personnel into public service. But if Titmuss and Gutmann are right, this is so only if there is no coexisting system of health care for profit.

Titmuss's views invite vigorous disagreement, as indicated by the letter by A. J. Culyer. Critics like Culyer challenge Titmuss's facts and interpretations. Blood distribution in Britain may not be all he says it is, and observed altruism in Britain may result from a cultural unity not possible in the United States. Moreover, the highly organized British National Health Service may make more efficient use of blood and use it in different ways than the more variegated U.S. system.

Is the health care system in the United States unjust? Unequal access, the hegemony of technology over treatment, the power of professionals and investors, the inadequacy of care for the elderly and those with chronic illnesses, and neglect of the "care" functions of health care lead many to judge that it is. These features of health care grow out of the normal social relations of production and consumption in the United States. Does injustice in health care indicate that economic relations in the United States (and the world) as a whole are unjust, or is health care a special case? If it is a special case, is it possible to reform health care in isolation and protect it from the mechanics of market justice in the United States at large? And if it is not a special case, how do issues of justice in health care help us to understand and assess the problems of injustice in the United States and the world as a whole?

Titmuss's discussion of altruism as a means of distributing resources suggests a second look at the concept of justice. Justice, as presented here, is for the most part rooted in self-interest. Is altruism part of the concept of justice, or does it stand outside justice and introduce social virtues of another kind? Or is recognizing the equality and dignity of human beings precisely to take an altruistic stance? If it is true that justice simply balances competing individual interests, the failure of an institution to meet the demands of justice is not the failure to meet an ideal. It is, rather, a failure to meet the minimum standards necessary to justify associations among human beings.

Andrew L. Jameton

Notes

1. Ruth Leger Sivard, *World Military and Social Expenditures 1981* (Leesburg, Va: World Priorities, Inc., 1981), p. 5.
2. The University of California, San Francisco, health sciences center general catalog states, "USCF is one of the largest employers in San Francisco and attracts many millions of dollars to the city and state each year. As a result, UCSF is one of the city and state's most important economic resources."

SOCIAL JUSTICE

From "The Concept of Social Justice"

William K. Frankena

PRELIMINARIES

I propose to take social justice, not as a property of individuals and their actions, but as a predicate of societies—particularly such societies as are called nations—and of their acts and institutions. The terms "justice" and "injustice" may also refer to the actions of individuals, but our concern is with their social application—with justice and injustice writ large, to use Plato's phrase—that is, with their manifestation by a society in its dealings with its individual members and subsocieties.

Although social justice will be considered as a property or virtue of national societies, it is not simply a property or virtue of such a society in its *formal*, or legal aspect—what is called the state. That is political justice, a part of social justice. But society does not consist merely of the law or the state: it has also a more *informal* aspect, comprised of its cultural institutions, conventions, moral rules, and moral sanctions. In order for a society to be fully just, it must be just in its informal as well as in its formal aspect.

Niebuhr and many other theologians usually associate justice with love. They assert, on the one hand, that justice is a function or political application of the law of love, and, on the other, that love is the fulfillment of justice. Now, it is true that in a society of love all of the demands of justice would be fulfilled. But, to use medieval terminology, they would be fulfilled *eminently*, not *formally*—that is, they would be overfulfilled rather than literally fulfilled. Such a society would not be called unjust, of course, but it would hardly be correct to describe it as just. It seems more accurate to contrast love and justice than to link them, even

the theologians referred to like to say there is a "tension" between them. I shall, therefore, here adopt the view that social justice cannot be defined in terms of love. This view is represented by Emil Brunner.[1]

> The sphere in which there are just claims, rights, debits and credits, and in which justice is therefore the supreme principle, and the sphere in which the gift of love is supreme, where there are no deserts, where love, without acknowledging any claim, gives all—these two spheres lie as far apart as heaven from hell. . . . If ever we are to get clear a conception of the nature of justice, we must also get a clear idea of it as differentiated from and contrasted with love.

That is a bit strong, as theological pronouncements sometimes are, but it is on the right track. Also it implies what is the last of my preliminary points: that social justice is not the only feature of an ideal society. Societies can be loving, efficient, prosperous, or good, as well as just, but they may well be just without being notably benevolent, efficient, prosperous, or good. Our problem is to define the concept of a just society, not that of an ideal society.

AN ANCIENT FORMULA FOR JUSTICE

To define the concept of social justice we must answer two questions which it is important to distinguish from one another. First, what are the criteria or principles of social justice? In other words, what features make or render a society just or unjust? Second, what are we doing or saying when we say of a society that it is just or unjust? Let us begin with the former. As is stated in an ancient formula, a society is just if it renders to it various members what is due them. But what is it that is due them? To reply that that is due them which is justly theirs or to which they have a right, is to add nothing. For we must still determine what it is that is their due or their right. To specify that their due or their right is what is accorded to them by the laws of the state may, speaking legally, suffice. The laws of the state, however, may be themselves unjust, and if so, it follows that social justice cannot consist wholly in their observance. Since social justice includes moral as well as legal justice, one might say that a society is just if its laws and actions conform to its moral standards. But even the prevailing moral principles of a society may be unjust or oppressive.

It may be said that a man's due or right is that which is his by virtue not merely of the law or of prevailing moral rules, but of valid moral principles, and that a society is just if it accords its members what it is required to accord them by valid moral principles. According to this view, social justice consists in the apportionment of goods and evils, rewards and punishments, jobs and privileges, in accordance with moral standards which can be shown to be valid. In other words, social justice is any system of distribution and retribution which is governed by valid moral principles. This view, if true, still leaves unsolved the very difficult question of which moral principles are valid, but at least simplifies matters by telling us that the answer to this question will provide the definition of justice. The concept of justice, it says, involves no special problems; all we have to do is to find out what is right.

This view is indeed plausible, for what could be more obvious than that a society is just if it treats its members as it ought to? And yet can justice be so simply equated with acting rightly? It does not seem to me that it can. Not all rights act—for example, acts of benevolence, mercy, or returning good for evil—can be properly described as just. Nor are all wrong acts unjust. As R. B. Brandt points out, incest may be wrong but the terms "just" and "unjust" simply do not apply.[2] Not all moral principles are "principles of justice" even if they are valid— for example, the principles J. S. Mill calls generosity and beneficence are not. Justice, then, is acting in accordance with the principles

of justice; it is not simply acting in accordance with valid moral principles.

This point may be emphasized in another way. Whether justice can be defined as a process of distributing and retributing in accordance with valid moral principles seems to depend on which moral principles turn out to be valid. Suppose the so-called principle of utility is understood, as some utilitarians seem to understand it, to mean that the right course of action is simply that which produces the greatest quantitative balance of something good (say, pleasure) over something evil (say, pain) regardless of how this quantity is distributed. Suppose, furthermore, that this principle of utility turns out to be the only valid principle of morality. Then distributing and retributing in accordance with valid moral principles will not coincide with what is called justice, though it may yield what is called beneficence. Justice is not simply the greatest possible balance of pleasure over pain or of good over evil. Justice has to do, not so much with the quantity of good or evil, as with the manner in which it is distributed. Two courses of action may produce the same relative quantities of good and evil, yet one course may be just and the other unjust because of the ways in which they apportion these quantities.

Therefore, unless we depart from our ordinary understanding of the term "justice," social justice cannot be defined merely by saying that a society is just which acts, distributes, and so on, in accordance with valid moral principles. If this is correct, however, then right-making characteristics or justifying considerations must be distinguished from just-making or justicizing considerations. Just-making considerations are only one species of right-making considerations. And, theoretically at least, a consideration of one kind may overrule a consideration of the other. In particular, a just-making consideration may be overruled by a right-making one which is not included under justice. As Portia says to Shylock,

. . . earthly power doth then show likest God's
When mercy seasons justice.

Furthermore, an inequality may sometimes be justified by its utility; the action or policy that promotes the inequality would then be right—but it might not be, strictly speaking, just.

It is true, as Brandt has pointed out,[3] that in such a case we should not call the action or policy unjust—that we hesitate to speak of something as unjust if we cannot also correctly speak of it as wrong. And this seems to imply that justice can be defined in terms of right-dealing after all. The answer may perhaps lie in an interesting passage in Mill. He writes that in order to save a life, "it may not only be allowable, but a duty" to do something which is contrary to the principles of justice—for example, "to steal or take by force the necessary food or medicine, or to kidnap and compel to officiate the only qualified medical practitioner." He continues:[4]

> In such cases, as we do not call anything justice which is not a virtue, we usually say, not that justice must give way to some other moral principle, but that what is just in ordinary cases is, by reason of that other principle, not just in the particular case. By this useful accommodation of language, the character of indefeasibility attributed to justice is kept up, and we are saved from the necessity of maintaining that there can be laudable injustice.

The point is that "just" and "unjust" seem to play a double role. On the one hand, they refer to certain sorts of right-making considerations as against others; on the other hand, they have much the same force as do the more general terms "right" and "wrong," so much so that one can hardly conjoin "just" and "wrong," or "right" and "unjust." It is the first of these roles which is especially important in defining the criteria of social justice, and which is neglected by the view we have been discussing. . . .

EQUALITY AND JUSTICE

Justice, whether social or not, seems to have at its center the notion of an allotment of something to persons—duties, goods, offices, opportunities, penalties, punishments, privileges, roles, status, and so on. Moreover, at least in the case of distributive justice, it seems

centrally to involve the notion of *comparative* allotment. In the paradigm case, two things, A and B, are being allotted to two individuals, C and D, A to C and B to D. Whether justice is done depends on how A's being given to C compares with B's being given to D. In this sense Aristotle was right in saying that justice involves a proportion in which A is to B as C is to D. It is a requirement both of reason and of common thinking about justice that similar cases be treated similarly. This means that if C and D are similar, then A and B must be similar. But, if this is so, then it would appear that justice also demands that if C and D are dissimilar, then A and B must be dissimilar. That is to say, justice is comparative.

Actually, of course, justice does not require that all similarities and dissimilarities be respected in this way. We do not regard it as unjust to treat similar blocks of wood dissimilarly or dissimilar ones similarly: we are concerned only about human beings (and possibly animals). Even in the case of human beings, however, justice does not call for similar treatment of every similarity or for dissimilar treatment of every dissimilarity. We do not think it is necessarily unjust, even if other things are equal, to deal similarly with people of different colors or dissimilarly with people of the same color. In fact, the historical quest for social justice has consisted largely of attempts to eliminate certain dissimilarities as bases for difference of treatment and certain similarities as bases for sameness of treatment. That is, it seems to be part of the concept of justice that not all similarities justify (or justicize) similar treatment or all differences different treatment. The point of the quest for social justice has not been merely that similarities and differences in people have too often been arbitrarily ignored; it has been mainly that the wrong similarities and differences have been taken as a basis for action. Similarities and differences should form the basis for action if it is to be just, but not all of them are relevant. The question is "Which of them are just- or unjust-making? Which of them are relevant? And is there a relation between them?"

It is important to remember that not all morally justifying considerations are just-making or justicizing. "Relevant" considerations in matters of justice cannot therefore be identified with "moral" ones, as D. D. Raphael does.[5] And it will not do to say, as Brandt does, that justice consists in treating people equally except as unequal treatment is justified by *moral* considerations of substantial weight in the circumstances.[6] If I am right, this description should be revised: justice is treating persons equally, except as unequal treatment is required by *just-making* considerations (i.e., by principles of *justice*, not merely *moral* principles) of substantial weight in the circumstances. With this emendation, the description seems to me to be correct, both in theory and as a reflection of the ordinary notion of justice. The only question then is whether there are any principles of *justice* which overrule the principle of equality, what they are, and whether they are such as to render the principle of equality otiose or not.

So far treating people equally has been equated with treating them similarly or in the same way. But suppose that society is allotting musical instruments to *C* and *D,* and that *C* prefers a banjo and *D* a guitar. If society gives *C* a banjo and *D* a guitar it is treating them *differently* yet *equally*. If justice is equal treatment of all men, then it is treatment which is equal in this sense and not simply identical. Surely neither morality nor justice, however stuffy and universalizing they may be in the eyes of Nietzsche and the existentialists, can require such monotony as identical treatment would involve. It is hard to believe that even the most egalitarian theory of justice calls for complete uniformity and not merely for substantial equality. I shall, therefore, speak in terms of equality, except when it does not matter or when it is necessary to speak in terms of similarity of treatment.

What considerations, and especially what similarities and dissimilarities in people, are just- (or unjust-) making? It is agreed that justice prescribes equals to equals and unequals to unequals, but what are the relevant respects in which people must be equal or unequal for treatment of them to be just or unjust? I have anticipated an at least partially egalitarian answer to this question, but the classical reply of Plato, Aristotle, and their many followers was different. According to them, social justice does

not involve any kind of equal allotment to all men. Justice is not linked with any quality in which men are all necessarily similar or which they all share by virtue of being men. It is tied to some property which men may or may not have, and which, in fact, they have in varying amounts or degrees or not at all. Justice simply is the appointment of what is to be apportioned in accordance with the amount or degree in which the recipients possess some required feature—personal ability, desert, merit, rank, or wealth.

This position has lately been maintained by Sir David Ross and, inconsistently, I think, by Brunner.[7] According to W. B. Gallie, it is characteristic of "liberal" as against "socialist" morality.[8] It is, however, not necessarily inegalitarian in substance; how inegalitarian it turns out to be depends on how unequal it finds men to be in the respect which it takes as basic. If it found them to be equal in this respect it would in practice have to be egalitarian, but, of course, it would not be taking equality of treatment for all men, or indeed any pair of men, as a basic requirement of justice. In this respect it may represent the classical concept of social justice, but as Gallie and Vlastos have pointed out,[9] it hardly does justice to the modern concept in which, as Mill's list[10] shows, equality of treatment (not merely the equal treatment of equals, but the equal treatment of all human beings as such) is one of the basic principles of justice. It is, however, true, as Gallie, Vlastos, and Mill recognize, that the modern concept of social justice is complex and includes a meritarian as well as an egalitarian element. It recognizes the demand to respect differences between persons as well as the demand to respect personality as such.[11]

Views which accept the principle of equality as a basic and at least *prima facie* requirement of justice may, of course, take less complex forms. It might be held, for example, that justice calls for a strict equality in the treatment of *C* and *D*, no matter who *C* and *D* are, and that no inequality is ever justified. Or it might be maintained that, although inequalities are sometimes justified and right, they are never just. Every departure from complete equality would then be regarded as beyond the pale of justice, though not beyond that of the morally right or obligatory. Such theories are possible and have an apparent simplicity, but they limit the usual scope of justice. Not every departure from equality is ordinarily regarded as a departure from justice, let alone from morality. For one thing, such departures are allowed on the ground of differences in ability, merit, or desert. Certain other departures from a direct or simple equality, called for by differences in need, or involved in carrying out agreements, convenants, contracts, and promises, are also recognized as just, and not merely as justified or right.

Much more reasonable, as well as closer to ordinary thinking, is the conception of social justice as the equal treatment of all persons, except as inequality is required by relevant—that is, just-making—considerations or principles. This is the view which I accepted as an emendation of Brandt's. It takes equality of treatment to be a basic *prima facie* requirement of justice, but allows that it may on occasion be overruled by other principles of justice (or by some other kind of moral principle). This view, however, is not necessarily very egalitarian. It does hold that all men are to be treated equally and that inequalities must be justified. But it also allows that inequalities may be justified, and everything depends on the ease and the kinds of considerations by which they may be justified. In fact, it tells us very little until it gives us answers to the following questions: What is meant by equal or similar treatment? What considerations are relevant to the justification of inequalities or dissimilarities? Are there any respects in which men are actually to be treated equally or similarly, or is this requirement always overruled by other considerations? Are there not always differences in personality, need, desert, merit, which completely nullify the *prima facie* rule of equality?

OTHER PRINCIPLES OF JUSTICE AND THEIR RELATION TO EQUALITY

The concept of social justice which prevails in our culture has now been partly defined. According to this concept, a society is without justice insofar as it is without rules (statutes or precedents, written or unwritten rules, legal and moral rules); it must, in both its formal and informal aspects, treat similar cases similarly. It must also treat human beings equally, or it must show why—a requirement which governs its rules as well as its acts and institutions. That is, the primary similarity to be respected is that which all men, as such, have. But a just society must also respect some though not all differences. In particular it must respect differences in capacities and needs, and in contribution, desert, or merit. Such differences may often make it just to treat people unequally in certain respects, thus at least qualifying the *prima facie* requirements of equality. But many other differences—for example, differences in blood and color—are not just-making. The recognition of capacity and need and the recognition of contribution and desert are not, however, the only principles of justice which may qualify the principle of equality. There is also the principle that agreements should be kept.

Are there any other principles of social justice besides the principle of equality, that of recognizing capacity and need, and that of keeping agreements? I have argued that the principle of beneficence or utility is not a principle of justice, though it is a moral principle. That is, a society is not unjust if it is not by its own direct action bringing about the greatest possible balance of good over evil. It is still, however, an old and familiar view (which I accept) that it is unjust for society or the state to injure a citizen, to withhold a good from him, or to interfere with his liberty (except to prevent him from committing a crime, to punish him for committing one, or to procure the money and other means of carrying out its just functions), and that this is unjust even if society or the state deals similarly with all its citizens. It seems to me also that a society is unjust if, by its actions, laws, and mores, it unnecessarily impoverishes the lives of its members materially, aesthetically, or otherwise, by holding them to a level below that which some members at least might well attain by their own efforts. If such views are correct, we must add to the principles of social justice those of non-injury, non-interference, and non-impoverishment.

These additions make it harder to discover what it is, if anything, that relates these principles of justice. It has sometimes been argued, however, that they are linked in that they all involve and ultimately depend on a recognition of the equality or equal intrinsic value of every human personality—or at least that they do so insofar as they are principles of justice. If this could be established, the area of justice could then be described as the area of moral reasoning in which the final appeal is to the ideal of the equality of all men. There is much to be said for this suggestion. Raphael, for instance, has very plausibly contended that differences in treatment on grounds of special need may be construed as attempts to restore inequalities due to natural or extraneous causes.[12] This would account for the justice of giving special attention to people—for example, those who are disabled or mentally backward—who are, for no fault of their own, at a disadvantage with respect to others.

More generally, it seems as if much, if not all, of the justice of recognizing differences in capacity, need, and so on, might be accounted for in terms of the ideal of equality, as follows. One of the chief considerations which not only justifies but also establishes as *just* differences in the treatment of human beings is the fact that the good life (not in the sense of the morally good life but in the sense, roughly, of the happy life) and its conditions are not the same for all, due to their differences in needs and potentialities. I am inclined to think that it is this fact, rather than that of differences in ability, merit, and the like, which primarily justifies differences in the handling of individuals. It is what justifies, for example, giving C a banjo, D a guitar, and E a skindiving outfit. Although C, D, and E are treated differently, they are not dealt with unequally, since their differing needs and capacities so far as these relate to the good life are equally considered and equally well cared for. The ideal of equality itself may require certain differences of treatment, including for example, differences in education and training. The principle involved in this claim is independent of the principle of recognizing differences in merit, but also of the principle of utility. For the differences in treatment involved are not justified simply by arguing that they are conducive to the general good life (though they may also be justified in this

way), but by arguing that they are required for the good lives of the individuals concerned. It is not as if one must first look to see how the general good is best subserved and only then can tell what treatment of individuals is just. Justice entails the presence of equal *prima facie* rights prior to any consideration of *general* utility.

Yet inequalities and differences in treatment are often said to be justified by their general utility. I do not deny this, but I do doubt that they can be shown to be *just* merely by an appeal to general utility. They can, however, often be shown to be just by an argument which is easily confused with that from the principle of utility: that initial inequalities in the distribution of offices, rewards, and so on, are required for the promotion of equality in the long run. In fact, much of what still needs to be done consists not so much of building up the biggest possible balance of welfare over illfare as in promoting the conditions for its equal distribution. It therefore seems plausible that much, if not all, of the justification of differences of function, as well as the recognition of ability, contribution, merit, and need—at least insofar as these may be denominated "just"—is based on such an indirect appeal to the ideal of equality. It also seems plausible that the introduction of incentives into economic and social systems, the redistribution of wealth through progressive taxation, and the reformation of the law may be *justicized*, if at all, only by such a line of argument, even if they may also be *justified* on other grounds.

If the duty to keep faith is assumed to be a requirement of justice, can it be justified in terms of the principle of equality? It does seem as if the practice of keeping promises and fulfilling contracts may be at least partly justified—and justicized—by such an indirect appeal to the promotion of equality. But perhaps the breaking of a promise can also be called unjust on the ground that it entails a direct violation of equality. The man who makes a promise and then breaks it, presumably for his own interest, is not only violating a useful practice but also favoring his good life over that of the others involved in the practice—in short, he is not treating persons as equals.

Retributive justice—for example, punishment—must also be considered. Aristotle and others have brought it under the principle of equality between the offender and the injured which had been disturbed. It might also be contended that, having violated the principle of equality, the criminal may justly be regarded as having forfeited his claim to a good life on equal terms with others, and even his claim not to be pained. Critics of the retributive theory of punishment might prefer to argue that punishment is made just, and perhaps also obligatory, by the fact that it tends to promote the most equality in the long run by preventing people from infringing on the claims of others. This is a non-utilitarian line of reasoning which looks not to the past, but to the future—not to future welfare, but to future equality.

There is, then, a good deal to be said for the suggestion that the principles of justice are distinguished from other principles of morality by being governed by the ideal of equality. Certainly the *prima facie* duty of treating people as equals is not rendered otiose because it so often permits inequalities of one sort or another. Nevertheless, G. F. Hourani may not be wholly right when he says that justice is equality "evident or disguised."[13] The claims of special desert may remain at least partially recalcitrant to such an interpretation. But even if Raphael's conclusion that the unequal treatment called for by special desert is a "real deviation from equality,"[14] is false, there still remain the principles of non-injury, non-interference, and non-punishment. Although the rule that a just society must provide a certain minimum level of welfare for everyone may be construed as an offshoot of the rule of equality, violations of these negative principles are unjust but do not necessarily entail any inequality of treatment, direct or indirect. If a ruler were to boil his subjects in oil, jumping in afterward himself, it would be an injustice, but there would be no inequality of treatment.

It might be argued that the injustice involved depends on an inequality after all because the ruler did not permit his subjects to participate in the decision to commit national suicide. And perhaps it might be further argued that whenever society or the state injures, interferes, or impoverishes unjustly, the injustice consists in the fact that it does not provide the individuals victimized an equal share in the process of decision-making. Then, excepting possibly the principle of recognizing desert, the principles of justice might all be claimed to rest, directly or indirectly, on the ideal of equality. I should myself welcome this conclusion, but it seems that a so-called primitive society might be so bound by tradition that although all its members had a substantially equal voice in all decisions its rules might nevertheless be unnecessarily restrictive or injurious, and therefore unjust.

If not all of these principles can be subsumed under equality, it might be argued that the recalcitrant ones should not be regarded as principles of justice, however valid they may be as moral principles. This strikes me as a rather drastic bit of conceptual legislation. Though such a departure from our ordinary understanding of social justice may be desirable in the interests of neatness, and not objectionable in principle, I am inclined to think that there is a less radical alternative.

BASIC THEORY OF JUSTICE

What we need at this point is a plausible line of thought that will explain both the role of equality in the concept of justice and those principles of justice which are not derivable from the ideal of equality. With the rule of non-interference with liberty particularly in mind, H. L. A. Hart has maintained that the sphere of justice and rights coincide not with that of equality, but with that in which the final appeal is to the claim of equal liberty for all.[15] Using a more positive conception of liberty, Raphael contends similarly that the essential points of justice and liberty are the same. The claims of desert and equality are both subsumed under the one concept of justice, he thinks, because both are concerned with protecting the interests of the individual, and so their concern is basically that of liberty.[16] Following a somewhat different line of thought, S. M. Brown argues that justice requires of society only that it provide institutions protecting the moral interests, persons, and estates of its members.[17] By restating what I take to be a familiar position, I shall not so much question as supplement these conclusions. In doing so I propose to argue that the principles of the family of justice, insofar as they go beyond the requirements of equality, direct or indirect, go beyond them only because they express a certain limited concern for the good lives of individual persons as such.

In opposition to the classical meritarian view of social justice, I accepted as part of my own view the principle that all men are to be treated as equals, not because they are equal in any respect but simply because they are human. They are human because they have emotions and desires, and are able to think, and hence are capable of enjoying a good life in a sense in which other animals are not. They are human because their lives may be "significant" in the manner which William James made so graphic in his essays "On a Certain Blindness in Human Beings" and "What Makes a Life Significant?":

> Whenever a process of life communicates an eagerness to him who lives it, there the life becomes genuinely significant. Sometimes the eagerness is more knit up with the motor activities, sometimes with the perceptions, sometimes with the imagination, sometimes with reflective thought. But, wherever it is found . . . there *is* importance in the only real and positive sense in which importance ever anywhere can be.[18]

By the good life is meant not so much the morally good life as the happy or satisfactory life. As I see it, it is the fact that all men are similarly capable of enjoying a good life in this sense that justifies the *prima facie* requirement that they be treated as equals. To quote James again, "The practical consequence of such a philosophy [as is expressed in the passage just cited] is the well-known democratic respect for the sacredness of individuality. . . ."[19] It seems plausible to claim, however, that this insight (which Royce calls "moral" and James "religious") into the "sacredness" of human beings justifies not only their equal treatment but also a real, even if limited, concern for the goodness of their lives. It justifies treating them

not only as equals but also, at least in certain ways, as ends.

A just society, then, is one which respects the good lives of its members and respect them equally. A just society must therefore promote equality; it may ignore certain differences and similarities but must consider others; and it must avoid unnecessary injury, interference, or impoverishment—all without reference to beneficence or general utility. The demand for equality is built into the very concept of justice. The just society, then, must consider and protect the good life of each man equally with that of any other, no matter how different these men may be, and so it must allow them equal consideration, equal opportunity, and equality before the law. The equal concern for the good lives of its members also requires society to treat them differently, for no matter how much one believes in a common human nature, individual needs and capacities differ, and what constitutes the good life for one individual may not do so for another. It is the society's very concern for the good lives of its members that determines which differences and which similarities it must respect (and which are relevant to justice). A society need not respect those differences which have only an *ad hoc* bearing or none at all, on the good lives of their possessors—for example, color of skin. But it must respect differences like preferring one religion to another, which do have a bearing on the individual good life.

None of this implies that society may impose or presuppose any fixed conception of the good life. As James says, "The pretension to dogmatize about [this] is the root of most human injustices and cruelties. . . ."[20] Nor does it mean that society must seek to make the life of one man as good as that of any other, for men may well be so different that the best life of which one is capable is not as good as that of which another is capable. The good lives open to men may not be equally good—even if they are called incommensurable they may still not be equally good. Nevertheless, they must be equally respected and protected. That is why I reject Rashdall's formula for justice, that "every man's good [is] to count as equal to the *like good* of every other man,"[21] for this suggests that two people are to be treated as equals only if they are capable of equally good lives. It is more accurate, in my opinion, to say that the just society must insofar as possible make *the same relative contribution* to the good life of every individual—except, of course, in cases of reward and punishment, and provided that a certain minimum standard has been achieved by all. This is what I understand as the recognition of equal intrinsic value of individual human beings.

But the regard which the just society must have for the good lives of its members involves more than equal treatment. If I am right, it does not involve direct action on the part of society to promote the good life of its members, whether this be conceived of as pleasure, happiness, self-realization, or some indefinable quality. Such direct action is beneficence, not justice. Nevertheless, a just society must be concerned for the goodness of its members' lives, and not merely for their equality, though in a more limited way than beneficence implies. A just society must protect each member from being injured or interfered with by others, and it must not, by omission or commission, itself inflict evil upon any of them, deprive them of goods which they might otherwise gain by their own efforts, or restrict their liberty—except so far as is necessary for their protection or the achievement of equality. Although we are speaking of the *just* society, and not of the *good* society, its concern with the goodness of the lives of its members need not be considered merely negative and protective. It seems reasonable to assign to the just society a more positive interest (though one which falls short of beneficence) by saying that it must, so far as possible, provide equally the conditions under which its members can by their own efforts (alone or in voluntary associations) achieve the best lives of which they are capable. This means that the society must at least maintain some minimum standard of living, education, and security for all its members.

Social justice then does not, as Ross thinks, consist *simply* in the apportionment of happiness or good life in accordance with the recipient's degree of moral goodness. In fact, society must for the most part allow virtue to be its own reward, else it is not virtue.[22] In the poem, "Easter," Arthur Clough complains that the world

> . . . visits still
> With equalest apportionment-of ill
> Both good and bad alike, and brings to one same dust
> The just and the unjust.

Society, however, must be wary of taking on the whole enterprise of cosmic or poetic justice.[23] It must honor first of all the so-called intrinsic dignity of man, which is not the same as his moral worth. Still, it is difficult to deny that the recognition of differences in desert, merit, and service, in the form of reward and punishment and unequal apportionment, is one of the principles of social justice. It remains, therefore, to see how this principle—insofar as it is a requirement of justice and not merely of utility—can be provided for by our basic theory. It has already been suggested that recognition of this principle is required for the promotion of equality in the long run. It seems to be required also for protection, one of the duties of a just society. Punishments have often been plausibly justicized on this ground, but so may rewards and privileges of various kinds. The good life of one member of society is not independent of what other members do or do not do. Certain forms of reward may in themselves show respect for individual freedom and goodness of life, by protecting one member against the acts or failures to act on the part of others, or by guaranteeing that individual talents shall not be lost or squandered.

More might be said on this point, but it is clear that a recognition of desert, contribution, or merit can be justicized without appealing either to an ultimate principle of retribution or to the principle of beneficence. This theory of social justice lies between those of the classical liberals and those of the more extreme welfare theorists. The one group includes too little under justice, the other too much. Both tend to equate just-making or justicizing considerations with right-making or justifying ones, but classical liberals greatly restrict the range of *justified* social action while the welfare theorists unduly extend that of *justicized* social action. I hold that justice includes a more positive concern for equality and goodness of life than the classical liberals allow, and that the area of right social action may extend even further in a welfare direction. I am not so much concerned to deny the conclusions the welfare theorists draw about what society and the state may or should do—I mean to leave this an open question—as to argue that they cannot plausibly defend them all as requirements of justice.

A just society is, strictly speaking, not simply a loving one. It must in its actions and institutions fulfil certain formal requirements dictated by reason rather than love; it must be rule-governed in the sense that similars are treated similarly and dissimilars dissimilarly. But only certain similarities and differences are relevant: those relating to the good life, merit, and so on. To a considerable extent, the recognition of these differences and similarities is required by the very ideal of equality, which is part of the concept of justice. But there are other principles of justice as well. Social justice is the equal (though not always similar) treatment of all persons, at least in the long run. This equal treatment must be qualified in the light of certain principles: the recognition of contribution and desert, the keeping of agreements, non-injury, non-interference, non-impoverishment, protection, and perhaps the provision and improvement of opportunity. These principles seem to go beyond the requirements of equality, even in the long run—but, insofar as they are principles of justice, they may be roughly unified under a conception of social justice as involving a somewhat vaguely defined but still limited concern for the goodness of people's lives, as well as for their equality. This double concern is often referred to as respect for the intrinsic dignity or value of the human individual. This is not the position of the extreme egalitarian but it is essentially egalitarian in spirit; in any case it is not the position of the meritarian, although it does seek to accommodate his principles.

Notes

1. *Justice and the Social Order* (London: Lutterworth Press, 1945), pp. 104, 114.

2. *Ethical Theory* (Englewood Cliffs, N.J.: Prentice-Hall, Inc., 1959), p. 409. Cf. also J. Hospers, *Human Conduct* (New York: Harcourt, Brace and World, Inc., 1961), pp. 416f.

3. *Op. cit.*, pp. 409f. But cf Hospers, *op. cit.*, pp. 417, 421f; G. Vlastos, "Justice," *Revue internationale de philosophie*, 41 (1937), p. 17.

4. All references to Mill are to *Utilitarianism*. Ch. V. Here see, e.g., Oskar Piest's ed. (New York: Liberal Arts Press, 1949), pp. 68f.

5. "Equality and Equity," *Philosophy*, XXI (1946), p. 5.

6. *Op. cit.*, p. 410.

7. W. D. Ross, *The Right and the Good* (Oxford: The Clarendon Press, 1930), pp. 26f.; Brunner, *op. cit.*, pp. 29ff.

8. "Liberal Morality and Socialist Morality," *Philosophy, Politics and Society*, ed. Peter Laslett (Oxford: Basil Blackwell, 1956), p. 123.

9. Gallie, *op. cit.*, pp. 122, 129; Vlastos, *op. cit.*, p. 9.

10. I.e., his list of what he calls "the various modes of action and arrangements of human affairs which are classed, by universal or widely spread opinion, as just or as unjust." Cf. *Utilitarianism*, Ch. V, pp. 47ff.—Ed.

11. This complexity may, perhaps have the following justification. The formal rule of reason which we took to be central to justice, insofar as it is comparative, has two parts: to treat similars similarly and to treat dissimilars dissimilarly. The egalitarian principle may be regarded as a way of specifying the first part, and the meritarian as a way of specifying the second.

12. *Op. cit.*, p. 9.

13. *Ethical Value* (Ann Arbor: University of Michigan Press, 1955), p. 86.

14. *Op. cit.*, p. 10.

15. "Are There Any Natural Rights?" *Philosophical Reivew*, LXIV (1955), pp. 177ff.

16. *Moral Judgment* (London: Allen & Unwin Ltd., 1955), pp. 67, 94.

17. "Inalienable Rights," *Philosophical Review*, LXIV (1955), pp. 192–211.

18. *Talks to Teachers on Psychology, and to Students on Some of Life's Ideals* (New York: Holt, Rinehart and Winston, Inc., 1899), pp. 264f.

19. *Ibid.*, pp. vi.

20. *Ibid.*, p. 265.

21. H. Rashdall, *The Theory of Good and Evil* (London: Oxford University Press, 1907); 1 p. 240.

22. Cf. Rashdall, *op. cit.*, pp. 256ff.

23. Cf. Hospers, *op. cit.*, pp. 462ff.

From "Justice as Reciprocity"

John Rawls

I

It might seem at first sight that the concepts of justice and fairness are the same, and that there is no reason to distinguish between them. To be sure, there may be occasions in ordinary speech when the phrases expressing these notions are not readily interchangeable, but it may appear that this is a matter of style and not a sign of important conceptual differences. I think that this impression is mistaken, yet there is, at the same time, some foundation for it. Justice and fairness are, indeed, different concepts, but they share a fundamental element in common, which I shall call the concept of reciprocity. They represent this concept as applied to two distinct cases: very roughly, justice to a practice in which there is no option whether to engage in it or not, and one must play; fairness to a practice in which there is such an option, and one may decline the invitation. In this paper I shall present an analytic construction of the concept of justice from this point of view, and I shall refer to this analysis as the analysis of justice as reciprocity.

Throughout I consider justice as a virtue of social institutions only, or of what I have called practices.[1] Justice as a virtue of particular actions or of persons comes in at but one place, where I discuss the prima facie duty of fair play. Further, the concept of justice is to be understood in its customary way as representing but one of the many virtues of social institutions; for these institutions may be antiquated, inefficient, or degrading, or any number of other things, without being unjust. Justice is not to be confused with an all-inclusive vision of a good society, or thought of as identical with the concept of right. It is only one part of any such conception, and it is but one species of right. I shall focus attention, then, on the usual sense of justice in which it means essentially the

Reprinted with permission of the author. Originally published version in *Utilitarianism: Text and Commentary* ed. S. Gorovitz (Indianapolis: Bobbs-Merrill, 1971) pp. 242–68.

elimination of arbitrary distinctions and the establishment within the structure of a practice of a proper share, balance, or equilibrium between competing claims. The principles of justice serve to specify the application of "arbitrary" and "proper," and they do this by formulating restrictions as to how practices may define positions and offices, and assign thereto powers and liabilities, rights and duties. While the definition of the sense of justice is sufficient to distinguish justice as a virtue of institutions from other such virtues as efficiency and humanity, it does not provide a complete conception of justice. For this the associated principles are needed. The major problem in the analysis of the concept of justice is how these principles are derived and connected with this moral concept, and what is their logical basis; and further, what principles, if any, have a special place and may properly be called the principles of justice? The argument is designed to lay the groundwork for answering these questions. . . .

II

The conception of justice which I want to consider has two principles associated with it. Both of them, and so the conception itself, are extremely familiar; and, indeed, this is as it should be, since one would hope eventually to make a case for regarding them as the principles of justice. It is unlikely that novel principles could be candidates for this position. It may be possible, however, by using the concept of reciprocity as a framework, to assemble these principles against a different background and to look at them in a new way. I shall now state them and then provide a brief commentary to clarify their meaning.

First, each person participating in a practice, or affected by it, has an equal right to the most extensive liberty compatible with a like liberty for all; and second, inequalities are arbitrary unless it is reasonable to expect that they will work out to everyone's advantage, and provided that the positions and offices to which they attach, or from which they may be gained, are open to all. These principles express justice as a complex of three ideas: liberty, equality, and reward for services contributing to the common good. . . .[2]

A word about the term "person." This expression is to be construed variously depending on the circumstances. On some occasions it will mean human individuals, but in others it may refer to nations, provinces, business firms, churches, teams, and so on. The principles of justice apply to conflicting claims made by persons of all of these separate kinds. There is, perhaps, a certain logical priority to the case of human individuals: it may be possible to analyze the actions of so-called artificial persons as logical constructions of the actions of human persons, and it is plausible to maintain that the worth of institutions is derived solely from the benefits they bring to human individuals. Nevertheless an analysis of justice should not begin by making either of these assumptions, or by restricting itself to the case of human persons; and it can gain considerably from not doing so. As I shall use the term "person," then, it will be ambiguous in the manner indicated.

The first principle holds, of course, only if other things are equal: that is, while there must always be a justification for departing from the initial position of equal liberty (liberty being defined by reference to the pattern of rights and duties, powers and liabilities, established by a practice), and the burden of proof is placed on him who would depart from it, nevertheless, there can be, and often there is, a justification for doing so. Now, that similar particular cases, as defined by a practice, should be treated similarly as they arise, is part of the very concept of a practice; in accordance with the analysis of justice as regularity, it is involved in the notion of an activity in accordance with rules, and expresses the concept of equality in one of its forms: that is, equality as the impartial and equitable administration and application of the rules whatever they are, which define a practice. The first principle expresses the concept of equality in another form, namely, as applied to the definition and initial specification of the structure of practices themselves. It holds, for example, that there is a presumption against the distinctions and classifications made by legal systems and other practices to the extent that they infringe on the original and equal liberty of the persons participating in them, or affected by them. The second principle defines how this presumption may be rebutted.

It might be argued at this point that justice requires only that there be an equal liberty. If, however, a more extensive liberty were possible for all without loss or conflict, then it would be irrational to settle upon a lesser liberty. There is no reason for circumscribing rights unless their exercise would be incompatible, or would render the practice defining them less effective. Where such a limitation of liberty seems to have occurred, there must be some special explanation. It may have arisen from a mistake or misapprehension; or perhaps it persists from a time past when it had a rational basis, but does so no longer. Otherwise, such a limitation would be inexplicable; the acceptance of it would conflict with the premise that the persons engaged in the practice want the things which a more extensive liberty would make possible. Therefore no serious distortion of the concept of justice is likely to follow from associating with it a principle requiring the greatest equal liberty. This association is necessary once it is supposed, as I shall suppose, that the persons engaged in the practices to which the principles of justice apply are rational.

The second principle defines what sorts of inequalities are permissible; it specifies how the presumption laid down by the first principle may be put aside. Now by inequalities it is best to understand not any differences between offices and positions, but differences in the benefits and burdens attached to them either directly or indirectly, such as prestige and wealth, or liability to taxation and compulsory services. Players in a game do not protest against there being different positions, such as that of batter, pitcher, catcher, and the like, nor to there being various privileges and powers specified by the rules. Nor do citizens of a country object to there being the different offices of government such as that of president, senator, governor, judge, and so on, each with its special rights and duties. It is not differences of this kind that are normally thought of as inequalities, but differences in the resulting distribution established by a practice, or made possible by it, of the things men strive to attain or to avoid. Thus they may complain about the pattern of honors and rewards set up by a practice (e.g., the privileges and salaries of government officials) or they may object to the distribution of power and wealth which results from the various ways in which men avail themselves of the opportunities allowed by it (e.g., the concentration of wealth which may develop in a free price system allowing large entrepreneurial or speculative gains).

It should be noted that the second principle holds an inequality is allowed only if there is a reason to believe that the practice with the inequality, or resulting in it, will work for the advantage of *every* person engaging in it. Here it is important to stress that every person must gain from the inequality. Since the principle applies to practices, it implies then that the representative man in every office or position defined by a practice, when he views it as a going concern, must find it reasonable to prefer his condition and prospects with the inequality to what they would be under the practice without it. The principles exclude, therefore, the justification of inequalities on the grounds that the disadvantages of those in one position are outweighed by the greater advantages of those in another position. This rather simple restriction is the main modification I wish to make in the utilitarian principle as usually understood. When coupled with the notion of a practice, it is a restriction of consequence, and one which some utilitarians, notably Hume and Mill, have used in their discussions of justice without realizing apparently its significance, or at least without calling attention to it.[3]

Further, it is also necessary that the various offices to which special benefits or burdens attach are open to all. It may be, for example, to the common advantage, as just defined, to attach special benefits to certain offices. Perhaps by doing so the requisite talent can be attracted to them and encouraged to give its best efforts. But any offices having special benefits must be won in a fair competition in which contestants are judged on their merits. If some offices were not open, those excluded would normally be justified in feeling unjustly treated, even if they benefited from the greater efforts of those who were allowed to compete for them. Moreover, they would be justified in their complaint not only because they were excluded from certain external emoluments of office, but because they were barred from attaining the great intrinsic goods which the skillful and devoted exercise of some offices represents, and so they would be deprived, from the start, of one of the leading ways to achieve a full human life.

Now if one can assume that offices are open, it is necessary only to consider the design and structure of practices themselves and how they jointly, as a system, work together. It will be a mistake to focus attention on the varying relative positions of particular persons, who may be known to us by their proper names, and to require that each such change, as a once and for all transaction viewed in isolation, must be in itself just. It is the practice, or the system of practices, which is to be judged, and judged from a general point of view: unless one is prepared to criticize it from the standpoint of a representative man holding some particular office, one has no complaint against it. Thus, as one watches players in a game and is moved by the changing fortunes of the teams one may be downcast by the final outcome; one may say to oneself that the losing team deserved to win on the basis of its skill, endurance, and pluck under adverse circumstances. But it will not follow from this that one thinks the game itself, as defined by its rules, is unfair. Again, as one observes the course of a free price system over time one witnesses the rise of one particular group of firms and the decline of another. Some entrepreneurs make profits, others have to take losses; and these profits and losses are not always correlated with their foresight and ability, or with their efforts to turn out worthwhile products. The fate of entrepreneurs is often the outcome of chance, or determined by changes in tastes and demand which no one could have foreseen; it is not always, by any means, founded on their deserts. But it does not follow from this that such an economic system is unjust. That the relative positions of particular entrepreneurs should be determined in this way is a consequence of the rules of the capitalist game. If one wishes to challenge it, one must do so, not from the changing relative positions of this or that entrepreneur, in this or that particular turn of fortune, but from the standpoint of the representative entrepreneur and his legitimate expectations in the system as a working institution, also, of course, keeping in mind the relation of this institution to the other practices of society.

Nothing is more natural than for those who suffer from the particular changes taking place in accordance with a practice to resent it as unjust, especially when there is no obvious correlation between these changes and ordinary conceptions of merit. This is as natural as that those who gain from inequities should overlook them, and even in time come to regard them as their due. Yet since the principles apply to the form and structure of practices as such, and not to particular transactions, the conception of justice they express requires one to appraise a practice from a general point of view, and thus from that of a representative man holding the various offices and positions defined by it. One is required to take a reasonably long view, and to ascertain how the practice will work out when regarded as a continuing system. At a later point I shall argue that unless persons are prepared to take up this standpoint in their social criticism, agreement on questions of justice is hardly possible; and that once they are prepared to do so, an argument can be given for taking these principles as the principles of justice.

III

Given these principles one might try to derive them from a priori principles of reason, or claim that they were known by intuition. These are familiar enough steps and, at least in the case of the first principle, might be made with some success. Of all principles of justice that of equality in its several forms is undoubtedly the one most susceptible to a priori argument. But it is obvious that the second principle, while certainly a common one, cannot be claimed as acceptable on these grounds. Indeed, to many persons it will surely seem overly restrictive; to others it may seem too weak. Some will want to

hold that there are cases where it is just to balance the gains of some against the losses of others, and that the principle as stated contains an exaggerated bias in the direction of equality; while there are bound to be those to whom it will seem an insufficient basis upon which to found an account of justice. These opinions are certainly of considerable force, and it is only by a study of the background of the principle and by an examination of its intended applications that one can hope to establish its merits. In any case, a priori and intuitive arguments, made at this point, are unconvincing. They are not likely to lead to an understanding of the basis of the principles of justice, not at least as principles of justice: for what one wants to know is the way in which these principles complete the sense of justice, and why they are associated with this moral concept, and not with some other. I wish, therefore, to look at the principles in a different way; I want to bring out how they are generated by imposing the constraints of having a morality upon persons who confront one another on those occasions when questions of justice arise.

In order to do this, it seems simplest to present a conjectural account of the derivation of these principles as follows. Imagine a society of persons amongst whom a certain system of practices is already well established. Now suppose that by and large they are mutually self-interested; their allegiance to their established practices is normally founded on the prospect of their own advantage. One need not, and indeed ought not, to assume that, in all senses of the term "person," the persons in this society are mutually self-interested. If this characterization holds when the line of division is the family, it is nevertheless likely to be true that members of families are bound by ties of sentiment and affection and willingly acknowledge duties in contradiction to self-interest. Mutual self-interestedness in the relations between families, nations, churches, and the like, is commonly associated with loyalty and devotion on the part of individual members. If this were not so the conflicts between these forms of association would not be pursued with such intensity and would not have such tragic consequences. If Hobbes' description of relations between persons seems unreal as applied to human individuals, it is often true enough of the relations between artificial persons; and these relations may assume their Hobbesian character largely in consequence of that element which that description professedly leaves out, the loyalty and devotion of individuals. Therefore, one can form a more realistic conception of this society if one thinks of it as consisting of mutually self-interested families, or some other association. Taking the term "person" widely from the start prepares one for doing this. It is not necessary to suppose, however, that these persons are mutually self-interested under all circumstances, but only in the usual situations in which they participate in their common practices concerning which the question of justice aprises.

Now suppose further that these persons are rational: they know their own interests more or less accurately; they realize that the several ends they pursue may conflict with each other, and they are able to decide what level of attainment of one they are willing to sacrifice for a given level of attainment of another; they are capable of tracing out the likely consequences of adopting one practice rather than another, and of adhering to a course of action once they have decided upon it; they can resist present temptations and the enticements of immediate gain; and the bare knowledge or perception of the difference between their condition and that of others is not, within certain limits and in itself, a source of great dissatisfaction. Only the very last point adds anything to the standard definition of rationality as it appears say in the theory of price; and there is no need to question the propriety of this definition given the purposes for which it is customarily used. But the notion of rationality, if it is to play a part in the analysis of justice should allow, I think, that a rational man will resent or will be dejected by differences of condition between himself and others only where there is an accompanying explanation: that is, if they are thought to derive from injustice, or from some other fault of institutions, or to be the consequence of letting chance work itself out for no useful common purpose. At any rate, I shall include this trait of character in the notion of rationality for the purpose of analyzing the concept of justice. The legitimacy of doing so will, I think, become clear as the analysis proceeds. So if these per-

sons strike us as unpleasantly egoistic in their relations with one another, they are at least free in some degree from the fault of envy.[4]

Finally, assume that these persons have roughly similar needs, interests, and capacities, or needs, interests, and capacities in various ways complementary, so that fruitful cooperation amongst them is possible; and suppose that they are sufficiently equal in power and the instruments thereof to guarantee that in normal circumstances none is able to dominate the others. This condition (as well as the other conditions) may seem excessively vague; but in view of the conception of justice to which the arguments leads, there seems to be no reason for making it more exact at this point.[5]

Since these persons are conceived as engaging in their common practices, which are already established, there is no question of our supposing them to come together to deliberate as to how they will set up these practices for the first time. Yet we can imagine that from time to time they discuss with one another whether any of them has a legitimate complaint against their established institutions. This is only natural in any normal society. Now suppose that they have settled on doing this in the following way. They first try to arrive at the principles by which complaints and so practices themselves are to be judged. That is, they do not begin by complaining; they begin instead by establishing the criteria by which a complaint is to be counted legitimate. Their procedure for this is to let each person propose the principles upon which he wishes his complaints to be tried with the understanding that, if acknowledged, the complaints of others will be similarly tried; and moreover, that no complaints will be heard at all until everyone is roughly of one mind as to how complaints are to be judged. Thus while each person has a chance to propose the standards he wishes, these standards must prove acceptable to the others before his charges can be given a hearing. They all understand further that the principles proposed and acknowledged on this occasion are binding on future occasions. So each will be wary of proposing a principle which would give him a peculiar advantage in his present circumstances, supposing it to be accepted (which is, perhaps, in most cases unlikely). Each person knows that he will be bound by it in future circumstances the peculiarities of which cannot be known, and which might well be such that the principle is then to his disadvantage. The basic idea in this procedure is that everyone should be required to make in advance a firm commitment to acknowledge certain principles as applying to his own case and such that others also may reasonably be expected to acknowledge them; and that no one be given the opportunity to tailor the canons of a legitimate complaint to fit his own special conditions, and then to discard them when they no longer suit his purpose.[6] Hence each person will propose principles of a general kind which will, to a large degree, gain their sense from the various applications to be made of them, the particular circumstances of these applications being as yet unknown. These principles will express the conditions in accordance with which each person is the least unwilling to have his interests limited in the design of practices, given the competing interests of the others, on the supposition that the interests of others will be limited likewise. The restrictions which would so arise might be thought of as those a person would keep in mind if he were designing a practice in which his enemy were to assign him his place.

The elements of this conjectural account can be divided into two main parts so that each part has a definite significance. Thus the character and respective situations of the parties, that is, their rationality and mutual self-interestedness, and their being of roughly similar needs, interests and capacities, and their having needs, interests and capacities in various ways complementary, so that fruitful forms of cooperation are possible, can be taken to represent the typical circumstances in which questions of justice arise. For questions of justice are involved when conflicting claims are made upon the design of a practice and where it is taken for granted that each person will insist, so far as possible, on what he considers his rights. It is typical of cases of justice to involve persons who are pressing on one another their claims, between which a fair balance or equilibrium must be found. So much is expressed by the sense of the concept.

On the other hand, the procedure whereby principles are proposed and acknowledged can

be taken to represent the constraints of having a morality; it is these constraints which require rational and mutually self-interested persons to act reasonably, in this case, to acknowledge familiar principles of justice. (The condition that the parties be sufficiently equal in power and the instruments thereof to guarantee that in normal circumstances none is able to dominate the others is to make the adoption of such a procedure seem more realistic; but the argument is not affected if we do without this condition, and imagine that the procedure is simply laid down.) Once the procedure is adopted and carried through each person is committed to acknowledge principles as impartially applying to his own conduct and claims as well as to another's, and he is committed moreover to principles which may constitute a constraint, or limitation, upon the pursuit of his own interests. Now a person's having a morality is analogous to having made a firm commitment in advance to acknowledge principles having these consequences for one's own conduct. A man whose moral judgments always coincided with his interests could be suspected of having no morality at all. There are, of course, other aspects to having a morality: the acknowledgment of moral principles must not only show itself in accepting a reference to them as reasons for limiting one's claims, but also in acknowledging the burden of providing a special explanation, or excuse, when one acts contrary to them, or else in showing shame and remorse (although not on purpose!), and (sincerely) indicating a desire to make amends, and so on. These aspects of having a morality and, more particularly, the place of moral feelings such as shame and remorse cannot be considered here. For the present it is sufficient to remark that the procedure of the conjectural account expresses an essential aspect of having a morality: namely, the acknowledgment of principles as impartially applying to one's own claims as well as to others, and the consequent constraint upon the pursuit of one's own interests.[7]

The two parts into which the foregoing account may be divided are intended, then, to represent the kinds of circumstances in which questions of justice arise (as expressed by the sense of the concept of justice) and the constraints which having a morality would impose upon persons so situated. By imposing these constraints on persons in the occasions of justice one can see how certain principles are generated, and one understands why these principles, and not others, come to be associated with the concept of justice; for given all the conditions as described in the conjectural account, it would be natural if the two principles of justice were to be jointly acknowledged. Since there is no way for anyone to win special advantages for himself, each would consider it reasonable to acknowledge equality as in initial principle. There is, however, no reason why they should regard this position as final. If there are inequalities which satisfy the conditions of the second principle, the immediate gain which equality would allow can be considered as intelligently invested in view of its future return. If, as is quite likely, these inequalities work as incentives to draw out better efforts, the members of this society may look upon them as concessions to human nature: they, like us, may think that people ideally should want to serve one another. But as they are mutually self-interested, their acceptance of these inequalities is merely the acceptance of the relations in which they actually stand, and a recognition of the motives which lead them to engage in their common practices. Being themselves self-interested, they have no title to complain of one another. And so provided the conditions of the principle are met, there is no reason why they should not allow such inequalities. Indeed, it would be short-sighted of them not to do so, and could result, in most cases, only from their being dejected by the bare knowledge, or perception, that others are better situated. Each person will, however, insist on an advantage to himself, and so on a common advantage, for none is willing to sacrifice anything for the others.[8]

These remarks are not offered as a rigorous proof that persons conceived and situated as the conjectural account supposes, and required to adopt the procedure described, would settle on the two principles of justice stated and commented upon in section 2. For this a much more elaborate and formal argument would have to be given. I shall not undertake a proof in this sense. In a weaker sense, however, the argument may be considered a proof, or as a sketch of a proof, although there still remain certain details to be filled in, and various alternatives to be ruled out. These I shall take up in later lectures. For the moment the essential point is simply that the proposition I seek to establish is a necessary one, or better, it is a kind of theorem: namely, that when mutually self-interested and rational persons confront one another in the typical circumstances of justice, and when they are required by a procedure expressing the constraints of having a morality to jointly acknowledge principles by which their claims on the design of their common practices are to be judged, they will settle upon these two principles as restrictions governing the assignment of rights and duties, and thereby accept them as limiting their rights against one another. It is this theorem which accounts for these principles as principles of justice, and explains how they come to be associated with this moral concept. Moreover it is analogous to theorems about human conduct in other branches of social thought. That is, a simplified situation is described in which rational persons, pursuing certain ends and related to one another in a definite way, are required to act, subject to certain limitations. Then, given this situation, it is shown that they will act in a certain manner. The failure so to act would only mean that one or more of the conditions did not obtain. The proposition we are interested in is not, then, an empirical hypothesis. This is, of course, as it should be; for this proposition is to play a part in an analysis of the concept of justice. Its point is to bring out how the principles associated with the concept derive from its sense, and to show the basis for saying that the principles of justice may be regarded as those principles which arise when the constraints of having a morality are imposed upon persons in typical circumstances of justice.

Notes

1. I use the word ''practice'' throughout as a sort of technical term meaning any form of activity specified by a system of rules which defines offices and roles, rights and duties, penalties and

defenses, and so on, and which gives the activity its structure. As examples one may think of games and rituals, trials and parliaments, markets and systems of property.

2. These principles are, of course, well known in one form or another. They are commonly appealed to in daily life to support judgments regarding social arrangements and they appear in many analyses of justice even where the writers differ widely on other matters. Thus if the principle of equal liberty is commonly associated with Kant (see *The Philosophy of Law*, W. Hastie, trans. [Edinburgh, 1887], pp. 561), it can also be found in works so different as J. S. Mills' *On Liberty* (1859) and Herbert Spencer's *Justice* (pt. IV of *Principles of Ethics*) (London, 1891). Recently H. L. A. Hart has argued for something like it in his paper "Are There Any Natural Rights?" *Philosophical Review*, 64 (1955), 175–191. The injustice of inequalities which are not won in return for a contribution to the common advantage is, of course, a frequent topic in political writings of all sorts. If the conception of justice developed here is distinctive at all, it is only in selecting these two principles in this form; but for another similar analysis, see W. D. Lamont, *The Principles of Moral Judgment*; (Oxford: Clarendon Press, 1946), ch. V. Moreover, the essential elements could, I think, be found in St. Thomas Aquinas and other medieval writers, even though they failed to draw out the implicit equalitarianism of their premises. See Ewart Lewis, *Medieval Political Ideas* (London: Routledge and Paul, 1954), vol. I, the introduction to ch. IV, especially pp. 220f. Obviously the important thing is not simply the announcement of these principles, but their interpretation and application, and the way they related to one's conception of justice as a whole.

3. It might seem as if J. S. Mill, in paragraph 36 of chapter V of *Utilitarianism,* expressed the utilitarian principle in this form, but in the remaining two paragraphs of the chapter, and elsewhere in the essay, he would appear not to grasp the significance of the change. Hume often emphasizes that every man must benefit. For example, in discussing the utility of general rules, he holds that they are requisite to the "well-being" of every individual; from a stable system of property "every individual person must find himself a gainer in balancing the account. . . ." "Every member of society is sensible of this interest; everyone expresses this sense to his fellows along with the resolution he has taken of squaring his actions by it, on the condition that others will do the same." (*A Treatise of Human Nature*, bk. III, pt. II, sect. II, par 22.) Since in the discussion of the

common good, I draw upon another aspect of Hume's account of justice, the logical importance of general rules, the conception of justice which I set out is perhaps closer to Hume's view than to any other.

4. There is no need to discuss here this addition to the usual conception of rationality. The reason for it will become clear as the argument proceeds, for it is analogous to, and is connected with, the modification of the utilitarian principle which the argument as a whole is designed to explain and to justify. In the same way that the satisfaction of interests, the representative claims of which violate the principles of justice, is not a reason for having a practice, unfounded envy, within limits, need not be taken into account. One could, of course, have another reason for this addition, namely, to see what conception of justice results when it is made. This alone would not be without interest.

5. In this description of the situation of the persons, I have drawn on Hume's account of the circumstances in which justice arises, see *A Treatise of Human Nature*, bk. III, pt. II, sec. II, and *An Enquiry Concerning the Principles of Morals*, sec. III, pt. I. It is, in particular, the scarcity of good things and the lack of mutual benevolence that leads to conflicting claims, and which gives rise to the "cautious, jealous virtue of justice," a phrase from the *Enquiry*, ibid., par. 3.

6. Thus everyone is, so far as possible, prevented from acting on the kind of advice which Aristotle summarizes in the *Rhetoric*, k. I, ch. 15. There he describes a number of ways in which a man may argue his case, and which are, he observes, especially characteristic of forensic oratory. For example, if the written law tells against his case, a man must appeal to the universal law and insist on its greater equity and justice; he must argue that the juror's oath "I will give my verdict according to my honest opinion" means that one will not simply follow the letter of the unwritten law. On the other hand, if the law supports his case, he must argue that not to apply the law is as bad as to have no laws at all, or that less harm comes from an occasional mistake than from the growing habit of disobedience; and he must contend that the juror's oath is not meant to make the judges give a verdict contrary to law, but to save them from the guilt of perjury if they do not understand what the law really means. Such tactics are, of course, common in arguments of all kinds; the notion of a considered judgment, and Adam Smith's and Hume's idea of an impartial spectator, is in part derived from the conception of a person so placed that he has no incentive to make these manoeuvers.

7. The idea that accepting a principle as a moral principle implies that one generally acts on it, failing a special explanation, has been stressed by R. M. Hare, *The Language of Morals* (Oxford: The University Press, 1952). His formulation of it needs to be modified, however, along the lines suggested by P. L. Gardiner, "On Assenting to a Moral Principle," *Proceedings on the Aristotelian Society*, n.s. 55 (1955), 23–44. See also C. K. Grant, "Akrasia and the Criteria of Assent to Practical Principles," *Mind* 65 (1956), 400–407,

where the complexity of the criteria for assent is discussed. That having a morality at all involves acknowledging and acting on principles which may be contrary to one's self-interest is mentioned below, see section 5.

8. A similar argument is given by F. Y. Edgeworth in "The Pure Theory of Taxation." *Economic Journal* 7 (1897). Reprinted in *Classics in the Theory of Public Finance*, ed. Musgrave and Peacock (New York: St. Martin's, 1958), pp. 120f.

From "Radical Egalitarian Justice: Justice as Equality"

Kai Nielsen

Let me say first crudely and oversimply what I want to do. I want to explicate and defend an egalitarian conception of justice both in production and in distribution that is even more egalitarian than John Rawls's conception of justice. In the course of arguing for this I shall argue that such a conception of justice requires, if it is to be anything other than an ideal which turns no machinery, a socialist organization of society. I am well aware that there are a host of very diverse objections that will immediately spring to mind. I shall try to make tolerably clear what I am claiming and why I want to claim it and I shall try to go some way toward at least considering, and, I hope, in some degree meeting, some of the most salient of these objections.

I shall first give four formulations of such a radical egalitarian conception of justice, formulations which, if there is anything like a concept of social justice, capture something of it, though it is more likely that such a way of putting things is not very helpful and what we have here are four conceptualizations of social justice which together articulate what the Left takes

social justice to be. I shall follow that with a statement of what I take to be the two most fundamental principles of radical egalitarian justice.

I

Four Conceptions of Radical Egalitarian Justice

1. Justice in society as a whole ought to be understood as requiring that each person be treated with equal respect irrespective of desert and that each person be entitled to self-respect irrespective of desert.[1]

2. Justice in society as a whole ought to be understood as requiring that each person be so treated such that we approach, as close as we can, to a condition where everyone will be equal in satisfaction and in such distress as is necessary for achieving our commonly accepted ends.[2]

3. Justice in society as a whole ought to be understood as a complete equality of the overall level of benefits and burdens of each member of that society.[3]

4. Justice in society as a whole ought to be understood as a structuring of the institutions of society so that each person can, to the fullest extent compatible with all other people doing likewise, satisfy her/his genuine needs.

Reprinted (with deletions) by permission of the author and *Social Theory and Practice*, vol. 5, no. 2, 1979.

These conceptualizations are, of course, vague and in various ways indeterminate. What counts as 'genuine needs', 'fullest extent', 'complete equality of overall level of benefits', 'as close as we can', 'equal respect' and the like? Much depends on how these notions function and in what kind of a theory they are placed. However, I will not pursue these matters here. I take it, however, that these conceptualizations will help us locate social justice on the conceptual and moral map.

The stress and intent of these egalitarian understandings of the concept of social justice is on the equal treatment of all people in various crucial respects. The emphasis is in attaining social justice, some central equality of condition for everyone. Some egalitarians stress some prized condition such as self-respect or a good life; others, more mundanely, but at least as crucially, stress an overall equal sharing of the various good things and bad things of the society. And such talk of needs postulates a common condition of life that is to be the common property of everyone.

When egalitarians speak of equality they should be understood as asserting that everyone is to be treated equally in certain respects, namely, that there are certain conditions of life that should be theirs. What they should be understood as saying is that all human beings are to be treated equally in respects F_1, F_2, $F_3 \ldots$, F_n, where the predicate variable will range over the conditions of life which are thought to be things that all people should have. This is to say that each person has an equal right to them, but it is not to say, or to give to understand, that each person is to have identical or uniform amounts of them. Talking about identical or uniform amounts has no clear sense for respect, self-respect, satisfaction of needs, or attaining the best life of which a person is capable. The equality of condition to be coherently sought is that they all have F_1, F_2, $F_3 \ldots$, F_n. Not that they must all have them equally, since for some F's this does not even make sense. Everyone has a right to respect and to an equal respect in that none can be treated as second-class people, but this does not mean that in treating them with respect you treat them in an identical way. In treating with equal respect a baby, a young person, or an enfeebled old man

out of his mind on his death-bed, we do not treat them equally, that is, identically or uniformly, but with some kind of not very clearly defined proportional equality.[4] (It is difficult to say what we mean here but we know how to work with the notion.) Similarly, in treating an Andaman Islander and a Bostonian with respect, we do not treat them identically, for what counts as treating someone with respect will not always be the same.

I want now to turn to a statement and elucidation of my egalitarian principles of justice. They are principles of just distribution, and it is important to recognize at the outset that they do not follow from any of my specifications of the concept of social justice. Someone might accept one of those specifications and reject my principles, and someone might accept my principles and reject any or all of those specifications or indeed believe that there is no coherent concept of social justice at all and believe that there are only different conceptualizations of justice that different theorists with different aims propound. But there is, I believe, an elective affinity between my principles and the egalitarian understanding of what the concept specified above involves. I think that if one does take justice in this egalitarian way one will find it reasonable to accept my principles.

I state my principles in a way parallel to Rawl's for ease of comparison. I will briefly compare them with his principles and show why I think an egalitarian or someone committed to Dworkin's underlying belief about the moral equality of persons, as both Rawls and I are, should opt for something closer to my principles than to Rawls's.[5]

Principles of Egalitarian Justice

1. Each person is to have an equal right to the most extensive total system of equal basic liberties and opportunities (including equal opportunities for meaningful work, for self-determination and political participation) compatible with a similar treatment of all. (This principle gives expression to a commitment to attain and/or sustain equal moral autonomy and equal self-respect.)

2. After provisions are made for common social (community) values, for capital overhead to preserve the society's productive capacity and

allowances are made for differing unmanipulated needs and preferences, the income and wealth (the common stock of means) is to be so divided that each person will have a right to an equal share. The necessary burdens requisite to enhance wellbeing are also to be equally shared, subject, of course, to limitations by differing abilities and differing situations (natural environment, not class position).

Principles of Justice as Fairness

1. Each person is to have an equal right to the most extensive total system of equal basic liberties compatible with a similar system of liberty for all.

2. Social and economic inequalities are to be arranged so that they are both: (a) to the greatest benefit of the least advantaged, consistent with the just savings principle, and (b) attached to offices and positions open to all under conditions of fair equality of opportunity.[6]

I shall start with a comparison of Rawls's principles and my own, setting out a brief criticism of Rawls's principles as I go along. (I shall be brief here as I have given that criticism at greater length elsewhere.)[7] We both, as a glance at our respective first principles of justice makes clear, have an equal liberty principle, though I do not claim the strict priority for mine over my second principle that Rawls does for his. Over the statement of the equal liberty principle, there is no serious difference between us; and I am plainly indebted to Rawls here. The advantage of my principle is that it makes more explicit what is involved in such a commitment to equal liberty than does Rawls's principle. They both give expression to the importance of moral autonomy and to the equality of self-respect, and they both acknowledge the underlying importance of a commitment to a social order where there is an equal concern and respect for all persons. This must show itself in seeing humankind as a community in which we view ourselves as "a republic of equals." This, at the very least, requires an acceptance of each other's moral autonomy and indeed equal moral autonomy. There can be no popes or dictators, no bosses and bossed; any authority that obtains must be rooted in at least some form of hypothetical consent. ("What one would choose if one were . . .''). The crucial thing about my first principle is its insistence that in a through-and-through just society we must all, if we are not children, mentally defective or senile, be in a position to control the design of our own lives and we must in our collective decisions have the right to an equal say. (The devices for doing this, of course, are numerous and the difficulties in its implementation are staggering. It is here that demanding, concrete socio-political-economic thinking is essential.)

The sharp differences between Rawls and myself come over our second principles of justice. My claim is that, given our mutual commitment to equal self-respect and equal moral autonomy, in conditions of moderate scarcity (conditions similar to those in most of North America, Japan, and much of Europe) equal self-respect and equal moral autonomy require something like my second principle for their attainability. There are circumstances where Rawls's second principle is satisfiable where equal liberty and equal self-respect are not obtainable. In short, I shall argue, his first and second principles clash. Rawls would respond, of course, that, given the lexical priority of the first principle over the second, this just couldn't obtain. But he, on his interpretation of the second principle, allows inequalities which undermine any effective application of the equal liberty principle.

Rawls would argue against a radical egalitarianism such as my own by claiming that "an equal division of all primary goods is irrational in view of the possibility of bettering everyone's circumstances by accepting certain inequalities."[8] The difference principle tells us that if the worst off will be better off—better off in monetary terms—they should accept the inequality. Justice and rationality conspire to require it. The rub, however, is in Rawls's understanding of 'better off' or 'improving the position' of the worst off. He cashes these notions in purely monetary terms. This prompts the response that either this is too narrow a notion of being 'better off' or of 'improving your position', or we are not justified in believing that rational agents, who have a tolerably adequate conception of fairness, will always give first priority to being 'better off' or 'improving their position'. They might very well, in conditions of moderate scarcity, recognize other things to be of greater value. Concerning these alternatives, it is well to remark, as Wittgenstein might, "Say what you will, it still doesn't alter the substance of the matter." Either 'being better off' is being construed too narrowly by Rawls or it does not always have first priority in deliberations about what is desirable. Indeed Rawls's own notion of the good of self-respect provides us with a jarring conception of what can, in circumstances such as ours, be a conflicting assessment of what is most desirable. Self-respect is for Rawls the most important primary good and it is something which is to be shared equally. In situations of moderate scarcity (relative abundance), we cannot, in Rawls's system, trade off a lesser self-respect for more of the other primary goods. But the disparities in power, authority, and autonomy that obtain, even in welfare state capitalism, and are not only allowed but justified by the difference principle, undermine, for the worst off, and indeed for many others as well, their self-respect. Certainly it does not make for a climate of equal self-respect.

Rawls recognizes this as an "unwelcome complication" and tries to show that self-respect need not be undermined or even diminished by the disparities in power and authority allowable in his system by the difference principle. But he concedes that if they did so undermine self-respect the difference principle should be altered.[9] He argues that a well-ordered society, in which his difference principle is in operation, would not be a society in which these inequalities in power, authority and the ability to direct your own life, would, for the worst off, and the strata which are near relatives to them, be particularly visible, hence their self-respect would not be diminished.[10] There would be, as Rawls puts it, a "plurality of associations in a well-ordered society, with their own secure internal life. . . ."[11] The more disadvantaged strata will have their various peer groups in which they will find positions that they regard as relevant to their aspirations. There various associations, Rawls remarks, will "tend to divide into . . . many noncomparing groups," where "the discrepancies between these divisions" will not attract "the kind of attention which unsettles the lives of those less well-placed."[12] This itself is a tendentious sociological description of life in contemporary class societies. It is in particular very innocent about the nature of work in those societies. Such a view of things could hardly withstand reflection on the facts about work in the twentieth century brought out, for example, in Harry Braverman's *Labor and Monopoly Capital*.

However, even if that were not so and even if Rawl's account here is in some way "telling it like it is," it still reflects an incredible elitism and paternalism. People are to be kept in ignorance and are to moderate their own aspirations and to accept their station and its duties with their respective roles—roles which often will not bear comparing, if self-respect is to be retained. However, they can, if they are so deceived, retain self-respect and society will not be destabilized by their agitation. They will not make comparisons and will unreflectively accept their social roles. Here we not only have elitism and paternalism, we have the ghost of aristocratic justice. Rawls's 'realism' here has driven him into what in effect, though I am sure not in intention, is a crass apology for the bourgeois order.

However, Rawls does not retreat here for he sees it as the only acceptable way in which self-respect can be preserved. The equality of self-respect must be preserved or achieved in this way, for we cannot rationally go for a levelling of wealth and status—an alternative way of achieving equal self-resect—because it would be irrational to undermine the incentive value of those limited inequalities of wealth which will produce more goods for all including the worst off. But that appeal, even if the motivational hypothesis behind it is true, begs the question. Some would say—and there are conflicting elements in Rawls's theory which would support them—"Better a greater equality in self-respect than more goods." Even if—indeed particularly if—that claim is made by the worst off in conditions of moderate scarcity (relative abundance), that claim, as far as anything Rawls has shown, is not irrational, or even less rational, than his worst off chaps sticking with the difference principle. (Even with the links stressed by Rawls between self-respect and liberty and given the priority of liberty, this is also what he should say. Indeed, given Rawls's and Dworkin's own deeply embedded belief that there should be equal respect and concern across persons, it would seem here that the response, "Better a greater equality in self-respect than more goods" would be, morally speaking, more appropriate, though, for reasons that Bertolt Brecht has made unforgettable, we must never forget that we are, in making such a claim, talking about conditions of relative abundance.)

Rawls might counter that he was not talking about our societies but, operating from within his ideal theory, about an 'ideal type' called a well-ordered society, where, by definition, there would not be such disparities in authority and power and effective control over one's life. But he also claims that his account is meant (a) to be applicable in the real world and (b) even there to some forms of capitalism. But my point was that his difference principle sanctions inequalities that are harmful to the sense of self-respect of people in the worse off strata of any capitalist society, actual or realistically possible. They simply, if they are being rational, must accept as justified, disparities in power, wealth, and authority which are harmful to them. Indeed these disparities attack their self-respect through undermining their moral autonomy; in such social conditions, men do not have effective control over their own lives. Thus his difference principle, in a way my second more egalitarian principle is not, is in conflict with his principle and, given Rawls's doctrine of the priority of liberty, should be abandoned.

Rawls tries to square his two principles and provide moral and conceptual space for both liberty and socio-economic inequalities by distinguishing between liberty and the *worth* of liberty. Norman Daniels, in an impressive series of both internal and external criticisms, has, I believe, demolished that defense.[13] So I shall be brief and stick with the simplest and most direct points. Even allowing the coherence and nonarbitrariness of the distinction, it will not help to say that the socio-economic disparities affect the *worth* of liberty but not liberty itself, for a liberty that cannot be exercised is of no value; and, indeed, it is in reality no liberty at all. What is the sense of having something, even assuming it makes sense to say here that you have it, which you cannot exercise? A 'liberty'

that we cannot effectively exercise, particularly because of some powerful *external* contraints, is hardly a liberty. Certainly it is of little value. If I have a right to vote but am never allowed to vote, I certainly do not have much of a right. Moreover, a rational contractor, or indeed any thoroughly rational person not bamboozled by ideology, would judge it rational to choose an equal *worth* of liberty, if he judged it rational to choose equal basic liberties. To will the end is to will the necessary means to the end. It is hardly reasonable to opt for equal liberty and then opt for a difference principle which accepts an unequal worth of liberty which, in turn, makes the equal liberty principle inoperable, that is, which makes it impossible for people actually to achieve equal liberty.

I want now to return to Rawls's arguments that equal self-respect in class societies can be achieved when inequalities remain invisible or at least invisible to those who are on the deprived side of the inequality. This hardly accords with Rawls's insistence that the principles of justice are "principles that rational persons with true general beliefs would acknowledge in the original position."[14] As Keat and Miller aptly remark, "a theory is not acceptable if the stability of a society based upon it depends upon the members of that society not knowing its principles and the way in which it is organized."[15] There is, they continue, something morally distressing—they actually say abhorrent—about a theory of justice relying on "the worse-off members of society continuing not to compare their position with that of the better off. This narrowing of reference groups, and the concomitant lowering of expectations, is something which should be a main object of criticism for any theory of justice which claims, as Rawls's does, to be 'democratic' and 'egalitarian'."[16]

My above arguments—as well as the arguments of Keat and Miller and Daniels—should push Rawls, if they are near their mark, in a more egalitarian direction. Specifically, they should require either an abandonment or an extensive modification of his second principle. If the preservation of self-respect is regarded as a conception at the heart of any theory of social justice and is taken, as Rawls would take it, to be directly relevant to questions about the just distribution of primary goods, then it seems that we would be forced to adopt more egalitarian principles of just distribution than Rawls adopts.

2

However, to go in a more egalitarian direction, is not, of course, necessarily to accept my principles. There are no doubt other alternatives. I shall now directly examine my egalitarian principles, starting with an elucidation of my own second principle and then proceeding to a consideration of some of the criticisms that would naturally be made of it.

What is now at issue is my second principle.

> After provisions are made for common social (community) values, for capital overhead to preserve the society's productive capacity and allowances are made for differing unmanipulated needs and preferences, the income and wealth (the common stock of means) is to be so divided that each person will have a right to an equal share. The necessary burdens requisite to enhance well being are also to be equally shared, subject, of course, to limitations by differing abilities and different situations (natural environment, not class position).

A central intent of this principle is to try to reduce inequalities in primary or basic social goods and goods that are the source of or ground for distinctions that give one person power or control over another. All status distinctions should be viewed with suspicion. Everyone should be treated equally as moral persons and, in spite of what will often be rather different moral conduct, everyone should be viewed as having equal moral worth.

The second principle is meant as a tool for attaining a state of affairs where there are no considerable differences in life prospects between different groups of people because some have a far greater income, power, authority, or privilege than others. My second principle tries to distribute the benefits and burdens so that they are, as far as is compatible with people having different abilities, equally shared. It does not say that all wealth should be divided equally,

like equally dividing up a pie. Unlike such pie dividing, part of the social product must be used for things that are of collective value, for example, hospitals, schools, roads, clean air, recreation facilities, and the like. And part of it must be used to protect future generations. Another part must be used to preserve the society's productive capacity so that there will be a continuous and adequate supply of goods to be divided. However, all of us—especially those of us who live in an economically authoritarianly controlled capitalist society primarily geared to production for profit and capital accumulation and only secondarily to meeting needs—must be aware of becoming captivated or entrapped by productivism. We need democratically controlled decisions about what is to be produced, who is to produce it and how much is to be produced. The underlying rationale must be to meet (as fully as possible, as equally as possible, and while allowing for different needs) the needs of all the people. Care must be taken, particularly in the period of transition out of a capitalist society, that the needs referred to are needs people would acknowledge if they were fully aware of the various hidden persuaders operating on them. And the satisfaction of a given person's needs must, as far as possible, be compatible with other people being able to similarly so satisfy their needs.

A similar attitude should be taken toward preferences. People at different ages, in different climates, with different needs and preferences will, in certain respects, need different treatment. However, they all must start with a baseline in which their basic needs are met—needs that they will have in common. (Again what exactly they are and how this is to be ascertained is something which needs careful examination.)

Rawls's notion of primary goods captures something of what they are. What more is required will be a matter of dispute and will vary culturally and historically. However, there is enough of a core here to give us a basis for consensus; and, given an egalitarian understanding of the concept of social justice, there will be a tendency to expand what counts as basic needs. Beyond that, the differing preferences and needs should, as far as possible, be equally satisfied, though what is involved in the rider "as far as possible" is not altogether evident. But it is only fair to give them all a voice. No compossible need should be denied satisfaction where the person with the need wants it satisfied and is well-informed and would continue to want it satisfied even after rational deliberation. Furthermore, giving all people a voice has other worthwhile features. It is evident enough that people are different. These differences are sometimes the source of conflict. Attaching the importance to them that some people do, can, in certain circumstances, be ethnocentric and chauvinistic. But it is also true that these differences are often the source of human enrichment. Both fairness and human flourishing are served by the stress on giving equal play to the satisfaction of all desires that are compossible.

So my second principle of justice is not the same as a principle which directs that a pie be equally divided, though it is like it in its underlying intent, namely, that fairness starts with a presumption of equality and only modifies a strict equal division of whatever is to be divided in order to remain faithful to the underlying intent of equal treatment. For example, both children aren't given skates; one is given skates, which is what she wants, and the other is given snowshoes, which is what she wants. Thus both, by being in a way treated differently, are treated with equal concern for the satisfaction of their preferences. Treating people like this catches a central part of our most elemental sense of what fair treatment comes to.

It should also be noted that my second principle says that each person, subject to the above qualifications, has a right to an equal share. But this does not mean that all or even most people will exercise that right or will feel that they should do so. This is generally true of rights. I have a right to run for office and to make a submission to a federal regulatory agency concerning the running of the CBC. But I have yet even to dream of exercising either of those rights, though I would be very aggrieved if they were taken away, and, in not exercising them, I have done nothing untoward. People, if they are rational, will exercise their rights to shares in primary goods, since having them is necessary to achieving anything else they want, but they will not necessarily demand equal shares and they will surely be very unlikely to demand equal shares of all the goods of the world. People's wants and needs are simply too different for that. I have, or rather should have, an equal right to have fish pudding or a share in the world's stock of bubble gum. *Ceteris paribus,* I have an equal right to as much of either as anyone else, but, not wanting or liking either, I will not demand my equal share.

When needs are at issue something even stronger should be said. If I need a blood transfusion, I have, *ceteris paribus,* an equal right to blood as anyone else. But I must actually need it before I have a right to an equal share or, indeed, to any blood plasma at all. Moreover, people who need blood have an equal right to the amount they require, compatible with others who are also in need having the same treatment; but, before they can have blood at all, they must need it. My wanting it does not give me a right to any of the common stock, let alone an equal share. And, even for the people actually getting the blood, a fair share would probably not be an equal share. Their needs here would probably be too different.

How does justice as equality work where it is impossible to give equal shares? Consider the equal right to have a blood transfusion. Suppose at a given time two people in a remote community both need an immediate transfusion to survive, and suppose it is impossible to give them both a transfusion at that time. There is no way of getting blood of the requisite type and there is no way of dividing up the available plasma and giving them each half or something like that. In order to live, each person needs the whole supply. There can be no equal division here. Still are not some distributions just and others unjust? If there are no relevant differences between the people needing the plasma, the only just thing to do is to follow some procedure like flipping a coin. But there almost always are relevant differences and then we are in a somewhat different ball game.

It might be thought that, even more generally in such a situation, the radical egalitarian should say: "In such a situation a coin should be tossed,'' but suppose the two people involved were quite similar in all relevant respects except that A had been a frequent donor of blood and B had never given blood. There is certainly a temptation to bring in desert and say that A is entitled to it and B is not. A had done his fair share in a cooperative situation and B had not, so it is only fair that A gets it. (We think of justice not only as equality but also as reciprocity.) Since 'ought' implies 'can', and since we cannot divide the blood equally, it does not violate my second principle or the conception of justice as equality to so distribute the plasma.

I would not say that to do so is unjust, but also, given my reservations about the whole category of desert, I would hesitate to say that justice requires it. But the central thing to see here is that such a distribution according to desert does not violate my second principle or run counter to justice as equality.

Suppose the individuals involved were A^1 and B^1. They are alike in all relevant respects except that A^1 is a young woman who has three children and who would soon be back in good health after the transfusion, and that B^1 is a woman ninety years of age, severely mentally enfeebled, without dependents and who would most probably die within the year anyway. It seems to me that the right thing to do under the circumstances is to give the plasma to A^1. Again it does not violate my second principle for an equal division is rationally impossible. But it is not correct to say A^1 deserves it more than B^1 or even, in a straightforward way, needs it more. However, we can relevantly say, because of the children and people who would be affected by the children, that more needs would be satisfied if A^1 gets it than B^1. This is bringing in utilitarian reasoning here, but, whatever we would generally say about utilitarianism as a complete moral theory, it seems to me perfectly appropriate to use such reasoning here. We could also say—and notice the role universalizability and role reversal play here—that, after all, B^1 had lived her life to the full, was now quite incapable of having the experiences and satisfactions that we normally can be expected to prize and indeed will soon not have any experiences at all, while A^1, by contrast, has much

of the fullness of her life before her. Fairness here, since we have to make such a horrible choice, would seem to require that we give the plasma to A^1 or, if 'fairness' is not the correct notion here, a certain conception of rightness seems to dictate that, everything considered, that is the right thing to do.

Let me briefly consider a final pair A^2 and B^2. Again they are alike in very respect except that A^2 is the community's only doctor while B^2 is an unemployable hopeless drunk. Both are firm bachelors and they are both middle-aged. B^2 is not likely to change his ways or A^2 to abandon what is a competently and conscientiously done practice. Here it seems to me we again quite rightly appeal to social utility—to the overall good of the community—and give the plasma to A^2. Even if, since after all he is the only doctor, A^2 makes the decision himself in his favour, it is still a decision that can be impartially sustained. Again my second principle has not been violated since an equal division is impossible.

I think that all three of those cases—most particularly the last two with their utilitarian rationale—might be resisted because of the feeling that they, after all, violate not my second principle, but, more generally, justice as equality in not giving equal treatment to persons. B, B^1 and B^2 are simply treated as expendable in a utilitarian calculation. They are treated merely as means.

This response seems to me to be mistaken. B, B^1 and B^2 are not being ignored. If the roles were reversed and they had the features of the A they are paired with, then they would get the plasma. They are not being treated differently as *individuals*. We start from a baseline of equality. If there were none of these differences between them, and if there were no other relevant differences, there would be no grounds to choose between them. We could not, from a moral point of view, simply favor A because he was A. Just as human beings, as moral persons or persons who can become capable of moral agency, we do not distinguish between them. We must treat them equally. In the limiting case, where they are only spatiotemporally distinct, this commitment to equality of treatment is seen most clearly. Morality turns into favoritism and privilege when this commitment is broken or ignored. *Within* morality there is no bypassing it; that is fixed by the very language-game of morality (by what the concept is, if you don't like that idiom).

Notes

1. David Miller, "Democracy and Social Justice," *British Journal of Political Science* 8 (1977) 1–19.
2. Ted Honderich, *Three Essays on Political Violence* (Oxford, England: Basil Blackwell Ltd., 1976), pp. 37–44.
3. Christopher Ake, "Justice as Equality," *Philosophy and Public Affairs* 5, no. 1 (Fall, 1975): 69–89.
4. Sidney Hook, *Revelation, Reform and Social Justice,* (Oxford, England: Basil Blackwell Ltd., 1975) pp. 269–287.
5. Ronald Dworking, *Taking Rights Seriously,* (Cambridge, MA: Harvard University Press, 1977) pp. 150–83; Kai Nielsen, "Class and Justice," in *Justice and Economic Distribution,* ed. John Arthur and William Shaw (Englewood Cliffs, New Jersey: Prentice-Hall, Inc. 1978), pp. 225–245.
6. These are, of course, Rawls's principles of justice. See John Rawls, *A Theory of Justice,* (Cambridge, MA: Harvard University Press, 1971) p. 302.
7. Kai Nielsen "Class and Justice" in *Justice and Economic Distribution,* "On the Very Possibility of a Classless Society," *Political Theory,* 6, No. 2 (1978): 191–208 and "The Priority of Liberty Examined," *The Indian Political Science Review,* 11, no. 1 (1977): 48–59.
8. Rawls, *Theory of Justice,* p. 546.
9. Ibid.
10. Ibid., p. 535.
11. Ibid., p. 536.
12. Ibid., pp. 536–7.
13. Norman Daniels, "Equal Liberty and Unequal Worth of Liberty," *Reading Rawls,* ed. Norman Daniels (New York, NY: Basic Books Inc., 1975), pp. 253–81.
14. Rawls, *Theory of Justice,* p. 547.
15. Russell Keat and David Miller, "Understanding Justice," *Political Theory,* 2, No. 1 (1974): 24.
16. Ibid.

RIGHTS AND JUSTICE IN HEALTH CARE

From "Health and Society: Some Ethical Imperatives"

Daniel Callahan

A new "right to health care" has been affirmed, but what it means and just what solutions are possible when there is a scarcity of resources are yet to be determined. Medical technology offers a more efficient and productive medicine. But are productivity and efficiency the only goals of medicine? Are there not, in any case, other areas where the need for better technologies is no less imperative—hous-

Reprinted by permission of the author and *Daedalus,* Journal of the American Academy of Arts and Sciences, Winter 1977, Boston, MA.

ing, agriculture, transportation? Some basic moral choices will have to be made; all of them will not be possible. Power and limitation of power, uses and abuses, promises and dangers: that has been the story of modern technology, and a story not yet fully unfolded.

A logical place to begin an examination of the moral choices at stake is with the concept of "health" itself. From there it will be possible to move to the special problems posed by technology, not only in medicine but in the culture more generally. Finally, a direct examination of the increasingly vexing questions of rights and obligations and of decision-making processes can be confronted.

THE CONCEPT OF "HEALTH"

Like most other very general concepts—"peace," "truth," "justice," "freedom"—that of "health" poses enormous difficulties of definition. We all know experientially and intuitively what it means to be sick: we hurt, and, to a greater or lesser extent, we cannot function well. That the pain or misery we feel can lead in many cases to death—either socially, by disability or impairment, or literally—only increases the burden; a reminder that we are mortal. Yet even when we attempt to grasp the notion of "health" by looking at what are normally taken to be its opposites—illness, pain, death—complications immediately arise. People can adapt to illness, learn to put up with their "dis-ease," and to cope with the fact that their body is performing in something less than an optimal way. Moreover, as the sociologists of medicine have taught us, people respond to and interpret illness in very different ways; what is considered sick in one culture or group may be considered health in another. Nevertheless, most people in most places have a rough idea of what they mean by "ill"; a recognizable area of human experience is evoked by the term, even if the borderlines can be exceedingly fuzzy.

To move from a definition of "sickness" to one for "health" is, however, not so easy. The term connotes bodily integrity, the absence of pain and infirmity, the state of a well-functioning and thus unremarkable organism. In a curious way, like "goodness," it can seem bland, if only because the alternative states of human affairs are so marked by drama and suffering. However bland the concept, the reality it invokes is regarded as eminently desirable. When one is in "good health" it is not even noticed; when one is not, it is desperately desired.

Whatever the conceptual problems posed by a philosophical attempt to define "health," and they are very real, the attempt to define the term for ethical or policy purposes brings forth even greater ones. Oddly enough, for all the debates about "health," few attempts have ever been made to give the term some substance; it seems to be taken for granted that everyone knows what is being talked about. The most notable, and undoubtedly still the most influential, definition of health was that of the World Health Organzation (WHO) in the late forties: ". . . a state of complete physical, mental, and social well-being and not merely the absence of disease or infirmity." The historical origin of that definition was the conviction of the organizers of the WHO that the security of future world peace would lie in the improvement of health, both physical and mental. That no reputable historian of the origins of the Second World War would trace it to bad health is probably beside the point. The great strides made by medicine during the war no doubt encouraged the development of this strain of utopian thinking, and it continues up to the present time.

It is dangerous definition, and it desperately needs replacement by something more modest. Its emphasis on "complete physical, mental, and social well-being" puts both medicine and society in the untenable position of being required to attain unattainable goals. There is no reason whatever to think that medicine can, for instance, make more than a modest contribution to "complete . . . social well-being," which involves (among others) political, cultural, and economic factors. Health may be, most of the time, a necessary condition for well-being, but it is not a sufficient condition. By even suggesting that medicine can succeed in such a goal—which is tantamount to making medicine the keystone in the search for human happiness—there is posited for it an impossible and illusory task.

The consequences of this definition, or at least of the ambitious spirit which it represents, can be seen all around us. Health so defined can encompass every human state. This bottomless conceptual pit makes it impossible in any practical way to specify the limits of the health enterprise, that is, to distinguish what is a political, or ethical, or cultural problem from what is a "health" problem. It has even permeated our everyday speech: how many of us designate any political or cultural movement or any person we do not like as "sick"? The ground is thus laid for a limitless economic burden on society. If anything and everything from the state of the prisons, the schools, and the economy to the anxieties invoked by life can be called a "health problem," there is no end to the resources that can be expended in the name of medicine to cope with those unpleasantries.

The difficulty legislators have had in trying to determine who, under what circumstances, and with what "medical" conditions should qualify for governmental assistance is direct testimony to the depth of the confusion. Far from clarifying our notions of human health, and thus our systems of care and distribution, the WHO definition has only made matters worse. Our society cannot continue to work with a concept of "health" that is infinite in its scope, and, at the same time, try to carry on a sensible discussion of the "right to health" or the "right to health care." A narrow, limited concept of "health" would make it possible to have a rational discussion of "rights": a vague and woolly one does not.

NEEDS, DESIRES, AND TECHNOLOGY

Nothing accounts for the strides and successes of modern medicine so much as the combination of basic biomedial research with ingenious technological application. And nothing accounts for the rising cost of medical care and the exasperation many feel at the gap between the cost of that care and the meager gain in general health so much as that same combination. Perhaps it is beside the point that costs keep rising: medicine is big business, providing profits, jobs, and social diversion; its practice can thus become an end in itself, quite apart from whether it results in significantly improved health. This has happened with other technologies, and there is no reason to think that medicine should prove the exception. That possibility aside, the place of technology in medicine—and the place of technology more generally in contemporary life—provides the most significant obstacle to the development of a reasonable and limited concept of "health."

How much health do people need? How much and what kind of sickness should be combatted? These are exceedingly difficult ques-

tions to answer, in great part, as I noted above, because of the enormous variation among individuals and groups in their tolerance for, and interpretation of, illness. Nonetheless, attempts have been made to find some reasonably objective standards for defining "illness," because without a working definition, there is no way to determine the nation's health needs. These efforts have, on the whole, taken the form of trying to establish a cost in dollars for various illnesses, both in terms of lost wages and in terms of the cost to the economy from illness and disease. Complementary to these calculations are those that employ cost-benefit techniques to determine the net economic gain resulting from investment in research and delivery systems sufficient significantly to reduce the incidence and impact of various diseases. Parallel attempts are made on social grounds: these ordinarily point to the disparities in the incidence of various diseases and disabilities among different groups and classes of people that indicate, not surprisingly, that the downtrodden (whether because of race, age, poverty, or geographic location) bear a disproportionate and thus inequitable burden of poor health.

The advantage of attempts to determine national health needs is that they allow in principle a considerable degree of quantification; reasonably accurate comparisons can be made between alternative health-policy strategies. In practice, however, the objectivity of their figures are frequently more illusory than real. Statistics can only be developed by making a number of arbitrary assumptions, some quantitative, others entailing value judgments. While it may be possible, for instance, to calculate in a rough way the economic cost to society of arthritis, it is by no means as easy to calculate the psychological cost to the afflicted individuals or their families. While unhappiness (even if those afflicted are economically "productive") ought surely to have a place in any full equation, it does not readily lend itself to calculation. In making comparisons between the full costs of different diseases (economic and psychological), is it possible, say, to find any very reasonable way to compare arthritis and hemophilia? Because of the far greater incidence of the former, one might say that the total sum of suffering is greater, but the impact of the latter (not to mention the cost) is probably far greater in terms of individual suffering.

In short, the more involved one becomes in making calculations and comparisons, the more problematic the venture. It is very well to argue that money invested in preventive medicine would, in the long run, produce more health per dollar than any other investment; that may or may not be true. But even if it is true, it could only be acted upon by systematically ignoring the presently ill. They would have to be deprived of help as allocations were shifted away from them to those who would benefit in times to come. The argument can only rest on the highly problematic premise that the value of averting future suffering is greater than the value of relieving present pain.

I am not trying to argue here that techniques for determining health needs should be abandoned. They at least reveal some interesting and suggestive figures, speculations, and projections providing those responsible for making policy decisions with something to work on, and something in this case is better than nothing. But they do evade the most difficult problem: that of determining the positive moral weight to be given to the pursuit of health in a society and the negative moral weight to be given to illness and disease. Just what is good about "health" anyway, and just what is evil about illness, disease, and death? These are nasty questions to ask, because if put too bluntly they imply a callousness to a major source of human misery and an indifference to the destructive effect of illness. But if they are not asked, it will be impossible to reach some decision regarding the limits to be placed on the quest for health and the priority to be given to societal health needs within those limits.

Two social realities are, at present, bedeviling that necessary task. The first is the almost total breakdown of the ethical distinction between "need" and "desire" in our culture. The second, closely related to the first, is the continuing utopian lure of technology, a lure whose net effect is to thwart any attempt to place limits on medical aspiration.

I would define "need" as the minimal requirements for a satisfactory life, and "desire" as those things human beings want and demand as requirements for what they would consider an optimal life. Working with that kind of distinction, it ought to be possible for societies to find ways of providing for minimal needs. Once that is accomplished, if there is a surplus, they can then set about improving the "quality of life," that is, trying to provide people with some of the things they would like to have beyond their requirements for survival. But this simple model breaks down immediately in Western technological societies. First, through habit and the requirements of the economic order, what people think they "need" for a minimally satisfactory life is set at an extremely high level. What a poor society might consider optimal (plentiful meat, spacious dwellings, refrigerators, and television sets, for instance), Western technological societies consider imperative. That many people, both in and out of government, could seriously contemplate going to war as a means of combating a fuel crisis which somewhat lowered our standard of living (but posed no possible threat to survival) is as good an indicator as any of the terms in which "need" is defined, at least in the United States.

Second, technological societies are committed to economic growth. Despite occasional discussions of a "steady-state society," most people still believe that a society which does not continue to grow economically is doomed. The key to continuous growth is the stimulation of production through increasing consumption; and the key to increasing consumption is the stimulation of desire. People must be induced to want more and more. Hence, to bring matters full circle, "needs" and "desires" become one—the satisfactory life and the optimal life turn out to be one and the same life; the satisfactory life is defined as one in which the optimal life can be, and must be, provided. Unless the individual pursues what he desires, and not just what he needs, the economy cannot continue to give him even what he needs. Desire becomes king.

The import of this process for medicine may not be so immediately apparent as it is, say, in the case of the environment. Whatever the weaknesses of the environmental movement, it has probably succeeded at least in convincing people that there must be a limit to our utilizing and exploiting natural resources. The globe is a finite resource; therefore we cannot have everything we desire.

No comparable wisdom is yet apparent in medicine. On the contrary, technological optimism is a vital as ever. It rests on two assumptions: One is that, technologically, something can be done about any medical condition. The "something" may not be much in many cases—perhaps only painkillers, when medicine can do nothing further—but that in itself is taken to be sufficient evidence that even in the most difficult cases medicine is not totally devoid of technological resources. The other is that all physical and mental ills are potentially subject to cure, control, or amelioration. This is a guiding heuristic proposition of biomedical research, fueled by the remarkable, almost unimaginable progress medicine has in fact made in recent decades and, negatively, by the fact that there is no conceivable way to disprove it. Since there is no way of disproving that proposition, a systematic optimum can remain enthroned. There is "hope against hope," if not for this generation then for the next, or the next after that, *ad infinitum.* (The equivalent argument applied to the environment is to say, yes, the resources of the earth are limited, but the ingenuity of technology in finding substitutes and in learning how to recycle resources counteracts the limitations, and is therefore tantamount to having unlimited resources.)

Against that systematic biomedical optimism (which has been no small element in the sharp increases in the funds demanded for biomedical research in recent decades), a curbing of aspiration and desire is now in order. Two strategies, not mutually incompatible, might be tried to achieve it. The first is to allow every person, whether patient, physician, researcher, or special-interest group, to press his case as far as he can. It can be stated in terms either of need or desire (it hardly matters which). The case made, a resolution is then achieved through the political process: the public through its representatives decides to which plea(s) it will respond and to what extent. The allocation of medical resources is left to public decision; public opinion will fight out the

conflicting moral and value judgments. To do so, it is not necessary for the public to have uniform theoretical ideas about that nature of health, the limits to health, or the relationship of health to other human goods (education, housing, national defense, etc.) On the contrary, desire can continue to dictate, knowing no theoretical limits at all. Conflicts will be resolved by brokerage politics, pragmatic judgments, and the trading off of relative values.

The trouble is that there is no real reason, other than lack of political power, for people to curb their desires about what they would like medicine to deliver to fulfull their notions of the optimal life. It is a system bound, therefore, to breed injustice, since some groups will have more power than others, if only by virtue of the larger pool of sick people they represent; and the individual will ineluctably ask of medicine more ("complete social well-being") than it can reasonably be expected to provide.

The other strategy (which still lacks a program) centers its attention more directly on philosophical and ethical questions. It would ask just what human beings *should* seek in the name of health and what they should avoid in the name of forestalling sickness and death. It would try to distinguish between what people need (while also trying to establish a reasonable notion of what "need" is) and what they desire. It would emphasize not just the contributions medicine could make with ample research funds, but also the limits to medicine's role in securing human happiness and security. It would encourage answering some fundamental questions about the goals of medicine, assuming that what people desire from medicine is not necessarily what they need. Medicine would be in less trouble today had it long ago promoted such an inquiry. But neither the profession nor the public (for it shares the blame) was willing to face these questions, for they are questions that threaten individualism, easy ethical relativism, and that systematic optimism which has been the stock-in-trade of medical research and technology. And that is so even if the answers might end up supporting the present system.

From "Medical Care as a Right: A Refutation"

Robert M. Sade

The current debate on health care in the United States is of the first order of importance to the health professions, and of no less importance to the political future of the nation, for precedents are now being set that will be applied to the rest of American society in the future. In the enormous volume of verbiage that has poured forth, certain fundamental issues have been so often misrepresented that they have now become commonly accepted fallacies. This paper will be concerned with the most important of these misconceptions, that health care is a right, as well as a brief consideration of some of its corollary fallacies.

RIGHTS—MORALITY AND POLITICS

The concept of rights has its roots in the moral nature of man and its practical expression in the political system that he creates. Both morality and politics must be discussed before the relation between political rights and health care can be appreciated.

A "right" defines a freedom of action. For instance, a right to a material object is the uncoerced choice of the use to which that object will be put; a right to a specific action, such as free speech, is the freedom to engage in that activity without forceful repression. The moral foundation of the rights of man begins with the fact that he is a living creature: he has the right to his own life. All other rights are corollaries of this primary one; without the right to life, there can be no others, and the concept of rights itself becomes meaningless.

The freedom to live, however, does not automatically ensure life. For man, a specific course of action is required to sustain his life, a course of action that must be guided by reason and reality and has as its goal the creation or ac-

Reprinted with permission from the author and *The New England Journal of Medicine*, vol. 285, no. 23, pp. 1288–1292, December 2, 1971.

quisition of material values, such as food and clothing, and intellectual values, such as self-esteem and integrity. His moral system is the means by which he is able to select the values that will support his life and achieve his happiness.

Man must maintain a rather delicate homeostasis in a highly demanding and threatening environment, but has at his disposal a unique and efficient mechanism for dealing with it: his mind. His mind is able to perceive, to identify percepts, to integrate them into concepts, and to use those concepts in choosing actions suitable to the maintenance of his life. The rational function of mind is volitional, however; a man must *choose* to think, to be aware, to evaluate, to make conscious decisions. The extent to which he is able to achieve his goals will be directly proportional to his commitment to reason in seeking them.

The right to life implies three corollaries: the right to select the values that one deems necessary to sustain one's own life; the right to exercise one's own judgment of the best course of action to achieve the chosen values; and the right to dispose of those values, once gained, in any way one chooses, without coercion by other men. The denial of any one of these corollaries severely compromises or destroys the right to life itself. A man who is not allowed to choose his own goals, is prevented from setting his own course in achieving those goals and is not free to dispose of the values he has earned is no less than a slave to those who usurp those rights. The right to private property, therefore, is essential and indispensable to maintaining free men in a free society.

Thus, it is the nature of man as a living, thinking being that determines his rights—his "natural rights." The concept of natural rights was slow in dawning on human civilization. The first political expression of that concept had its beginnings in 17th and 18th century England through such exponents as John

Locke and Edmund Burke, but came to its brilliant debut as a form of government after the American Revolution. Under the leadership of such men as Thomas Paine and Thomas Jefferson, the concept of man as a being sovereign unto himself, rather than a subdivision of the sovereignty of a king, emperor or state, was incorporated into the formal structure of government for the first time. Protection of the lives and property of individual citizens was the salient characteristic of the Constitution of 1787. Ayn Rand has pointed out that the principle of protection of the individual against the coercive force of government made the United States the first moral society in history.

In a free society, man exercises his right to sustain his own life by producing economic values in the form of goods and services that he is, or should be, free to exchange with other men who are similarly free to trade with him or not. The economic values produced, however, are not given as gifts by nature, but exist only by virtue of the thought and effort of individual men. Goods and services are thus owned as a consequence of the right to sustain life by one's own physical and mental effort.

If the chain of natural rights is interrupted, and the right to a loaf of bread, for example, is proclaimed as primary (avoiding the necessity of earning it), every man owns a loaf of bread, regardless of who produced it. Since ownership is the power of disposal,[1] every man may take his loaf from the baker and dispose of it as he wishes with or without the baker's permission. Another element has thus been introduced into the relation between men: the use of force. It is crucial to observe who has initiated the use of force: it is the man who demands unearned bread as a right, not the man who produced it. At the level of an unstructured society it is clear who is moral and who immoral. The man who acted rationally by producing food to support his own life is moral. The man who expropriated the bread by force is immoral.

To protect this basic right to provide for the support of one's own life, men band together for their mutual protection and form governments. This is the only proper function of government: to provide for the defense of individuals against those who would take their lives or property by force. The state is the repository for retaliatory force in a just society wherein the only actions prohibited to individuals are those of physical harm or the threat of physical harm to other men. The closest that man has ever come to achieving this ideal of government was in this country after its War of Independence.

When a government ignores the progression of natural rights arising from the right to life, and agrees with a man, a group of men, or even a majority of its citizens, that every man has a right to a loaf of bread, it must protect that right by the passage of laws ensuring that everyone gets his loaf—in the process depriving the baker of the freedom to dispose of his own product. If the baker disobeys the law, asserting the priority of his right to support himself by his own rational disposition of the fruits of his mental and physical labor, he will be taken to court by force or threat of force where he will have more property forcibly taken from him (by fine) or have his liberty taken away (by incarceration). Now the initiator of violence is the government itself. The degree to which a government exercises its monopoly on the retaliatory use of force by asserting a claim to the lives and property of its citizens is the degree to which it has eroded its own legitimacy. It is a frequently overlooked fact that behind every law is a policeman's gun or soldier's bayonet. When that gun and bayonet are used to initiate violence, to take property or to restrict liberty by force, there are no longer any rights, for the lives of the citizens belong to the state. In a just society with a moral government, it is clear that the only "right" to the bread belongs to the baker, and that a claim by any other man to that right is unjustified and can be enforced only by violence or the threat of violence.

RIGHTS—POLITICS AND MEDICINE

The concept of medical care as the patient's right is immoral because it denies the most fundamental of all rights, that of a man to his own life and the freedom of action to support it. Medical care is neither a right nor a privilege: it is a service that is provided by doctors and others to people who wish to purchase it. It is the provision of this service that a doctor depends upon for his livelihood, and is his means of supporting his own life. If the right to health care belongs to the patient, he starts out owning the services of a doctor without the necessity of either earning them or receiving them as a gift from the only man who has the right to give them: the doctor himself. In the narrative above substitute "doctor" for "baker" and "medical service" for "bread." American medicine is now at the point in the story where the state has proclaimed the nonexistent "right" to medical care as a fact of public policy, and has begun to pass the laws to enforce it. The doctor finds himself less and less his own master and more and more controlled by forces outside of his own judgment. . . .

Any doctor who is forced by law to join a group or a hospital he does not choose, or is prevented by law from prescribing a drug he thinks is best for his patient, or is compelled by law to make any decision he would not otherwise have made, is being forced to act against his own mind, which means forced to act against his own life. He is also being forced to violate his most fundamental professional commitment, that of using his own best judgment at all times for the greatest benefit of his patient. It is remarkable that this principle has never been identified by a public voice in the medical profession, and that the vast majority of doctors in this country are being led down the path to civil servitude, never knowing that their feelings of uneasy foreboding have a profoundly moral origin, and never recognizing that the main issues at stake are not those being formulated in Washington, but are their own honor, integrity and freedom, and their own survival as sovereign human beings.

SOME COROLLARIES

The basic fallacy that health care is a right has led to several corollary fallacies, among them the following:

That health is primarily a community or social rather than an individual concern.[2] A simple calculation from American mortality statistics[3] quickly corrects that false concept: 67 per cent of deaths in 1967 were due to diseases known to be caused or exacerbated by alcohol, tobacco smoking or overeating, or were due to accidents. Each of those factors is either largely or wholly correctable by individual action. Although no statistics are available, it is likely that morbidity, with the exception of common respiratory infections, has a relation like that of mortality to personal habits and excesses.

That state medicine has worked better in other countries than free enterprise has worked here. There is no evidence to support that contention, other than anecdotal testimonials and the spurious citation of infant mortality and longevity statistics. There is, on the other hand, a good deal of evidence to the contrary.[4,5]

That the provision of medical care somehow lies outside the laws of supply and demand, and that government-controlled health care will be free care. In fact, no service or commodity lies outside the economic laws. Regarding health care, market demand, individual want, and medical need are entirely different things, and have a very complex relation with the cost and the total supply of available care, as recently discussed and clarified by Jeffers et al.[6] They point out that " 'health is purchaseable', meaning that somebody has to pay for it, individually or collectively, at the expense of foregoing the current or future consumption of other things." The question is whether the decision of how to allocate the consumer's dollar should belong to the consumer or to the state. It has already been shown that the choice of how a doctor's services should be rendered belongs only to the doctor: in the same way the choice of whether to buy a doctor's service rather than some other commodity or service belongs to the consumer as a logical consequence of the right to his own life.

That opposition to national health legislation is tantamount to opposition to progress in health care. Progress is made by the free interaction of free minds developing new ideas in an atmosphere conducive to experimentation and trial. If group practice really is better than solo, we will find out because the success of groups will result in more groups (which has, in fact, been happening); if prepaid comprehensive care really is the best form of practice, it will succeed and the health industry will swell with new Kaiser-Permanente plans. But let one of these or any other form of practice become the law, and the system is in a straight jacket that will stifle progress. Progress requires freedom of action, and that is precisely what national health legislation aims at restricting.

That doctors should help design the legislation for a national health system, since they must live with and within whatever legislation is enacted. To accept this concept is to concede to the opposition its philosophic premises, and thus to lose the battle. The means by which nonproducers and hangers-on throughout history have been able to expropriate material and intellectual values from the producers has been identified only relatively recently: the saction of the victim.[7] Historically, few people have lost their freedom and their rights without some degree of complicity in the plunder. If the American medical profession accepts the concept of health care as the right of the patient, it will have earned the Kennedy-Griffiths bill by default. The alternative for any health professional is to withhold his sanction and make clear who is being victimized. Any physician can say to those who would shackle his judgment and control his profession: I do not recognize your right to my life and my mind, which belong to me and me alone; I will not participate in any legislated solution to any health problem.

In the face of the raw power that lies behind government programs, nonparticipation is the only way in which personal values can be maintained. And it is only with the attainment of the highest of those values—integrity, honesty and self-esteem—that the physician can achieve his most important professional value, the absolute priority of the welfare of his patients.

The preceding discussion should not be interpreted as proposing that there are no problems in the delivery of medical care. Problems such as high cost, few doctors, low quantity of available care in economically depressed areas may be real, but it is naïve to believe that governmental solutions through coercive legislation can be anything but shortsighted and formulated on the basis of political expediency. The only long-range plan that can hope to provide for the day after tomorrow is a "nonsystem"—that is, a system that proscribes the imposition by force (legislation) of any one group's conception of the best forms of medical care. We must identify our problems and seek to solve them by experimentation and trial in an atmosphere of freedom from compulsion. Our sanction of anything less will mean the loss of our personal values, the death of our profession, and a heavy blow to political liberty.

Notes

1. Rand A: Man's rights, Capitalism: The unknown ideal. New York, New American Library, Inc. 1967, pp. 320–329.
2. Millis JS: Wisdom? Health? Can society guarantee them? N Engl J Med 283:260–261, 1970.
3. Department of Health, Education, and Welfare, Public Health Service: Vital Statistics of the United States 1967. Vol II, Mortality. Part A. Washington, DC, Government Printing Office, 1969, p. 1–7.
4. Financing Medical Care: An appraisal of foreign programs. Edited by H Shoeck. Caldwell, Idaho, Caxton Printers, Inc. 1962.
5. Lynch MJ, Raphael SS: Medicine and the State. Springfield, Illinois, Charles C Thomas, 1963.
6. Jeffers JR, Bognanno MF, Bartlett JC: On the demand versus need for medical services and the concept of "shortage." Am J Publ Health 61:46–63, 1971.
7. Rand A: Atlas Shrugged. New York, Random House, 1957, p 1066.

The Right to Health Care

Laurence B. McCullough

"Health care is in a state of crisis", is a refrain become all too common in recent years. One of the many responses to this "crisis" has been a concern and even a demand for the right to health care. It is thought that everyone, regardless of their ability to pay or their geographical circumstances is entitled to adequate health care. The temptation of many is to extend this initial claim to a right to quality health care. That is, what is sought is not merely health maintenance but the kind of medical care and services ministered to the well-to-do. The rhetoric of such language is to expose what is taken to be an unjust or unfair state of affairs: people are being deprived of that which they are entitled to claim for themselves.

What is perceived to be unjust is the present strucure of health care. It is such that possibilities for human life are frequently diminished or even eliminated. What I propose to do here is to reflect on talk about a right to health care as a way of exposing this injustice. I shall frame my reflections in terms of natural rights since this concept of rights is best suited to analyzing what is involved in this talk of a right to health care.

Historically, rights have been spoken of in three ways, determined by their origin: whether in God, in man, or in nature. Divine rights are known by revelation and are thought to be conferred upon men by the will of God. Quite clearly, then, for any divine right, God could have refrained from granting it. Consider for example, the older notion of the divine right of kings. We can just as easily think in terms of a divine right of self-government. The one is just as plausible as the other. There is no necessity, therefore, that one should obtain and the other not. Divine rights are contingent and, because they could have failed to obtain, they cannot serve as those constraints on a moral or political order by which we determine the justice of that order.

Reprinted with permission from the author and *Ethics in Science & Medicine,* vol. 6, pp. 1–9. Copyright 1979, Pergamon Press, Ltd.

Man-made rights—the conferred, societal, or civil rights—are those rights men agree to respect for one another. Like divine rights, they also could fail to obtain: men could, quite simply, disagree on whether or not to create or respect this or that right. Men might, for example, decide to dispense with the legal right of due process under law or the right to vote. Man-made rights, therefore, cannot serve as a basis for providing a fundamental critique of a moral or political order as talk of a right to health is meant to do. Instead, man-made rights reflect and give expression to such orders.

Natural rights differ from both divine and man-made rights in that these rights could not fail to obtain. They obtain—that is, men possess them—no matter what the circumstances of a particular moral or political order. They can, therefore, serve as fundamental, moral constraints by which the justice of a political order is to be judged.

In my judgement, claims of a right to health care are best analyzed in terms of natural rights, because only such an analysis displays adequately the critique that such claims are meant to advance, *viz.,* that the present structure of medicine and health care appears to be unjust and that this structure must be changed in accordance with fundamental (in the sense of unavoidable) constraints placed upon *any* just social order. By contrast, talk of a right to health care, as either a divine or man-made right, is not adequate, as a logical matter, to the thrust of current discussion of the future of medicine and health care. There is, therefore, good reason to cast talk of a right to health care in terms of a natural right.

RIGHTS: SOME PRELIMINARY OBSERVATIONS

Claiming rights, of whatever sort, is a powerful moral and political move—thus, it is one frequently made. This is so despite the present-day discomfort with rights talk on the part of some philosophers.[1] When someone says that he has a right to something, he does so, in part, to arrest our attention. Rights talk signals that what is at issue is not taken by the claimant(s) to be some private matter that others can ignore but is, instead, something that has a claim on someone. The point of announcing something as a right is to express to others an interest in something one might not have, retain, or acquire in the absence of recognition of that right. So, for example, if I were to claim as a right a certain freedom of expression, this freedom is announced as something that I *ought* to enjoy, and not merely as something that I happen to enjoy or would like to enjoy. I am, so I claim in my right, entitled to freedom of expression and others are, therefore, bound to acknowledge that freedom.

Moreover, when a right is claimed, it is announced to someone, including society at large, governments, and other individuals. Rights and rights talk have, then, a *public* character. First, rights are not private, else they would be empty. That is, if there can be no one morally bound to me by obligation regarding my right, then I would have no such right. Second, rights are not idiosyncratic. Instead, they are general, even universal: anyone similarly situated can and ought to enjoy the same rights. Finally, if one is to succeed in claiming something as a right, one must be prepared to adduce reasons in support of this claim, i.e. to display the grounds of the right.

Any talk of a right to health care as a natural right, then, must be preceded by some consideration of the grounding of natural rights. This I propose to do in two parts. First, I shall consider the main themes of Locke's theory of natural rights. His account of natural rights is useful here in that it is especially revealing of the logic of natural rights and of claims made in terms of them. Second, I shall propose a revision of Locke's theory. This revised theory of natural rights will then serve as the basis for discussion of talk of the right to health care. This discussion will focus on (a) the different senses of the right to health care, and (b) the moral constraints that these different senses of the right place upon us.

LOCKE ON NATURAL RIGHTS

Locke argued that man possesses certain basic rights independently of—that is, logically and morally prior to—any political order. Indeed, natural rights constitute the fundamental moral order to which any political order must conform, if it is to be just. Locke used "natural rights" to designate the rights man possesses in this state, the state of nature.

In the state of nature, men are free and equal. In this state, freedom and equality obtain with respect to preservation. Preservation means freedom from harm in those conditions necessary to realize freedom and equality in the community and, subsequently, in the political order, *viz.*, life, health, liberty, and possessions (one's body and one's property). Men, then, are entitled, under the law of nature, to those things required for their preservation "and such other things as Nature affords for their Subsistence."[2] Because these conditions have been met, men can realize their nature as free and equal creatures living the life of reason, i.e., living in accord with the law of nature.

Although its metaphysical origin is in God's will, natural law can be known by man without the aid of revelation.[3] It can be known by reason alone. Hence, all rational creatures must assent to it. To refuse to assent to it is to abandon the very ground of rationality and, hence, of moral judgement. With this is lost, as well, the means to assess and defend on moral grounds any political order. In short, denial of the law of nature entails the abandonment of any rational, common basis for moral, civil, or political order.[4]

Reason, Locke maintains, discovers and does not invent or create the law of nature. "Positive laws of Commonwealths", on the other hand, *are* created by men.[5] The law of nature, therefore, enjoys logical and, hence, moral, priority over man's laws.

. . . yet it is certain there is such a law, and that too, as intelligible and plain to a rational Creature, and a Studier of that Law, as the positive Laws of Commonwealths, nay possibly plainer; As much as Reason is easier to be understood, than the Phansies and intricate Contrivances of Men, following contrary and hidden interest put into Words: For so truly are a great part of the Municipal Laws of Countries, which are only so far right, as they are founded on the Law of Nature, by which they are to be regulated and interpreted.[6]

Since the Law of Nature does not follow from the "phansies and contrivances of men" but from the requirements of reason, it is not "contrary and hidden", i.e. contingent, but is, instead, clear and necessary.

Employing the law of nature, men can know with certainty that necessarily they are equal and free. These elements in man's nature are tempered by and realized in preservation. Whatever is entailed by preservation as its immediate necessary conditions is a natural right for Locke. These rights, in turn, *imply* (the relation is contingent) other rights. The natural right to liberty, for example, implies a right to self-government or the possibility of justifying the breaking of the compact of trust with governors in the political order. Hence, political self-determination is derivative of a natural right.

Locke maintained that man is a creature possessed of reason. What reason knows clearly—by the "light of nature"—is what is necessary. Among the things known in this way is the law of nature. And what we know when we reason according to the law of nature is something about the very nature, or essence, of man. In particular, we know that to *be* a man includes certain inalienable rights. Such rights can, therefore, never be justifiably ignored. Hence, they serve as fundamental constraints on any moral, social, or political order.

NATURAL RIGHTS: A REVISED THEORY

From the above, it should be clear that a natural right is an entitlement one possesses principally by virtue of being a certain kind of thing, *viz.,* a human being: a natural right is grounded in our nature. Natural rights are best understood, therefore, as meta-physical, as well as moral claims. They are claims about what it is to be, what is included in being, a human being. Though metaphysical, natural rights are not

wholly so. They do have serious pragmatic implications bearing on what one can will to do: they possess a profound moral dimension. That is, claims of natural rights are meant to determine the wills of others *always* to regard us in certain specified manners, e.g. as entitled to possession of property that is the product of our own labors. To fail to satisfy such a right, i.e. to fail to treat the claimant as the kind of being that he is clearly would be irrational. Hence the origin of the compelling character of natural rights: failure to acknowledge them is a patent absurdity. Natural rights, therefore, always have a claim on us insofar as we are rational social beings. The difficult issue at this point is to determine the nature of this claim.

In discussing rights it is commonplace to distinguish absosolute from *prima facie* rights. That is, rights may be construed such that their *exercise* is without limit or constraint: that exercise is never to be denied. This is the way Locke seems at times to have understood natural rights: their exercise must be respected no matter what other rights or duties conflict with the duties created by natural rights. On the other hand, rights may be construed in more limited terms. It may be held that, where significant duties and/or rights conflict with the duty generated by a right, the claimant of that right has no absolute purchase on what he claims. So, for example, the right to own property—which Locke treated as a natural right—may be, and in practice is, restricted in scope, despite Locke's apparent views to the contrary. One has the right to possess property up to that point where other rights must give way, e.g. another's right to property or even to life. In this way natural rights are but *prima facie* in their exercise. Natural rights, like all *prima facie* rights, are difficult to implement.

There is an important sense, however, in which natural rights are absolute.

Those who have spoken of human rights as universal and inalienable have not intended to assert that the actual exercise of those rights on a given substantive human right may properly be denied or overridden if the force of other morally relevant considerations is stronger in a given situation. What we can *never* do is rule out a human right as a morally relevant consideration.[7]

Thus, natural rights, as was said at the beginning of this section, must always be *acknowledged:* they shall always enjoy a central place in moral reasoning and discourse. As a moral matter, one ought never to fail to consider obligations originating in natural rights when one seeks to determine the morally proper course of action. This is the nature of their claim upon us.

Natural rights, then, may not be absolute constraints on action. For example, I may not have an absolute duty to give my life to save another, say by hurling myself on the proverbial live handgrenade. Nor is it clear that I am morally constrained to refrain from killing another to save a life: I may be justified in killing someone who is trying to murder another. At the same time, though, I am *not* morally free to ignore altogether others' rights to life in trying to determine the proper course of action. There are two points to emphasize here; (a) that those obliged to another because of his natural rights are not bound absolutely to fulfill those duties, since more compelling obligations may bind them;[8] but (b) that natural rights must always be included in moral discourse as fundamental constraints upon it.

Some considerations concerning the conditions under which rights obtain or fail to obtain are in order next. It has been maintained that only beings of a certain sort have rights. After all, a right is a claim to something. A claim to something, though, entails a choice of that something and someone's ability to realize that choice. Making choices, it seems, is the activity only of a being that can be aware of what it chooses as distinct from itself. Also, the realization of choices entails the capacity to form action in accordance with what is chosen, i.e. to act in a reasoned manner. In short, only rational, self-conscious, and free beings have rights. As Professor Engelhardt has put it, only *persons* have rights. Non-persons, including some human beings, he says, have no rights.[9]

I take issue with his conclusion, for it is not adequate to the character of natural rights. Those entitlements that derive from our nature as human beings must always be recognized *since such conditions do not affect our nature.* Infants, children, the mentally retarded, the senile, and

the comatose, for example, do not fail—simply as a result of being in such conditions—to possess those natural rights also belonging to a fully competent and rational adult. The senile or retarded, for example, are not non-human, though their capacity to realize that nature may be diminished. Therefore, natural rights can always be claimed, on behalf of others or for oneself. In particular, if some human being (distinguished as a genus from persons, one of the species of human, the other being non-persons) cannot claim his natural rights, one must acknowledge his entitlements nonetheless and claim them as rights for him, since he cannot fail to possess them and we cannot fail to claim them for him. A natural right, then, is a right that obtains for any being in virtue of its being of its kind; a human being with the *capacity* or potential for, if not always the actuality of, rational, self-conscious, free life is entitled to those special freedoms appropriate to that essence. Here, the language of essence enters into our consideration of natural rights. An examination of the different senses of essence reveals dimensions of natural rights which Locke overlooked, and which come to play a central role in understanding the right to health care.

Let me explain what I mean here in terms of a tradition that predates Locke. Following Aristotle, I maintain that essence includes the form of the thing (and sometimes matter). Form, for the present purposes, can be understood as that principle by which it is the kind of thing that it is. This is of course, the formal cause of the thing. Second, the form is the principle toward the realization of which the thing tends. It is the principle of what it is to *become* or *enjoy* the fullness of being that kind. This tending is the final cause. By the formal cause I exist as a man. By the final cause I strive to realize in my life history the fullness of human life.

Natural rights, if we follow Locke are to be understood as those rights included in man's nature by entailment: natural rights are the necessary conditions for man's essence. But what Locke failed to appreciate is that natural rights take on one of two emphases or aspects, according to the two aspects of essence. The first concerns those conditions for humanity *qua* formal cause. The second concerns those conditions that permit not merely the existence of humanity but its fulfilment or full realization in each of us: the necessary conditions for humanity *qua* final cause.

This revision of Locke's theory and the revision of the sense in which natural rights are absolute are important for understanding the various senses of the right to health care.

THE RIGHT TO HEALTH CARE AS A NATURAL RIGHT

A right to health care, I said at the outset, is claimed in order to call attention to a state of affairs perceived to be unjust. The remedy for this injustice is to extend our awareness of the full scope of rights talk and to arrange the world accordingly. What is gained by the former is a recognition that all men have a certain entitlement to health care, independent of their socio-politico-economic status. What is gained by the latter is justice. At issue is the guarantee of comprehensive health services for everyone irrespective of income or geographic location. Failure of the socio-political order to recognize and to secure the exercise of this right would be judged unjust. The logic of this argument is the logic of natural rights.

Before explaining how that is, we must get clear as to what we mean by "health care" and "a right to health care". First, health care usually means *medical* care. But this is not an adequate rendering, since it is also meant to include requirements for good health like nutrition and clean water. (The latter seems already to be recognized as a fundamental right.) I shall not attempt to give a full definition here. Indeed, the concept of health care seems so open-textured as to defy final definition. In what follows, I shall use the term in a broad sense, not in the restricted sense of medical care (though I shall use its medical aspect as my paradigm).

Second, if "health care" is ambiguous, then the term "right to health care" cannot be unequivocal either. There are at least two ways of understanding it. The first sense of the term is that in which "right to health care" means equality of (access to) health care, irrespective of any considerations other than the fact that

one is a human being subject to losses of health. Consideration of merit or capacity to pay, etc. are to be put aside. This sense emphasizes that no one should be deprived of available health care and services. Each is equally entitled to health care resources already available.

The second sense is more penetrating. It suggests that health care of a variety not now available to all ought to be. The second sense of the right to health care can itself be taken in two ways. The first is what I want to call its negative aspect: what is claimed are those conditions of health necessary for survival as a human being. Hence, preventive medicine, cure of (curable) life-threatening ailments (like acute appendicitis), proper nutrition, etc. can be claimed as the right of all men, because in their absence we would not exist at all. The positive aspect of the right to health care is considerably more ambitious in scope than the negative sense. Under this rubric are claimed those facets of health care that *enhance* human life and do not simply or exclusively permit or maintain human life. It is not clear to me what exactly is to be included here. The revisionary emphasis of this aspect of talk of a right to health care is, in spite of the vagueness concerning the scope of the claim, a prominent feature in contemporary talk of a right to health care. The two major senses of a right to health care require separate analysis.

The first sense of the right to health care has been analyzed recently by Professor Outka. He begins by pointing out that we are all equal with respect to "being randomly susceptible to (health) crises".[10] That is, the loss of health and the occurrence of disease are by and large not a matter of will but are "acts of God". It makes no sense, then, to treat individuals or classes of individuals as unequal regarding their vulnerability. In particular, "health crises seem non-meritarian because they occur so often for reasons beyond our control or power to predict".[11]

Clearly, though, it is not true of all losses of health that they are non-meritarian. We do know, for example, that smoking is causally linked with the occurrence of various cancers. Outka, though, is aware of this obvious point. "People suffer in varying ratios the effects of their natural and undeserved vulnerabilities, the irresponsibility and brutality of others and their own desires and weaknesses".[12] Outka goes on, though, to discount this qualification of his position on pragmatic grounds.

> In some final reckoning then dessert considerations seem not irrelevant to many health crises. The practical applicability of this admission, however, in the instance of health care delivery, appears limited. . . . Would it be feasible to allocate additional tax monies from taxes on alcohol and tobacco to the man with leukemia before [allocating them to] the overweight man suffering a heart attack on the ground of difference of dessert? At the point of emergency care at least, it seems impracticable for the doctor to discriminate between these cases, to make meritarian judgments at the points of catastrophe. And the number of persons who are in need of medical treatment for reasons utterly beyond their control remains a datum with tenacious relevance.[13]

Surely it is true that we persistently fall prey to the villainies of man and the "fate" of nature. But we also fall prey to our own folly and pernicious lack of self-regard. With respect to the villainies of man against man, it may well be impracticable, even unjust, to discriminate among losses of health. In such cases, the villainy of man may be taken as equivalent to the vicissitudes of nature, the so-called acts of God: we are all equally likely to fall prey to misfortune, whether at the hands of our fellows or of nature. But, unlike Outka, I do want to separate those losses of health whose causes *are* within "our control and power to predict" and consequently, to prevent, from those that are not. It is not at all clear to me that a person who has contracted lung cancer after fifteen or twenty years of smoking is like the five-year-old stricken with acute appendicitis. They are, indeed, not alike. Of the cancer-ridden man we can say, reasonably, that the outcome of his habit was predictable. In some measure, therefore, he was responsible for the results of a habit whose dangers have been well-known for some time. It would be unreasonable, even nonsensical, to say the same of the small child with appendicitis. His affliction is fortuitous.

Now, admittedly, the distinction between deserved and undeserved losses of health may be hard to draw exactly. But the absence of a sharp distinction does not entail the absence of the distinction altogether, as Outka would have it. Hence, those who can for good reasons be said to deserve their losses of health will be excluded from the set of those who have a right to health care *on the basis of the right to equality.* With regard to those cases, then, where losses of health are within our control, a natural right of equality does not apply. Otherwise one can speak in terms of a natural right to equal treatment for losses of health.

The sense of a right to health care just outlined is understood as depending on another right, that to equal treatment. By contrast, the right to health care in the second of our two senses is understood directly as a natural right and not as depending on one. That is, it is claimed that the right to health care is an ingredient in what it is to be a human being. The analysis here differs for each of the two aspects of this sense of the right to health care.

The first aspect is the negative one: a right to health care cast in terms of necessary conditions for one's very survival as human. At issue here is the denial of those conditions. It will help at this point to recall Locke's views on the natural right to health. For Locke, what is entailed by preservation can be claimed as a natural right and it is unjustifiable to take away what tends to the preservation of health. Hence, without at least minimal health care, preservation of health and life itself would be impossible. Any health care delivery system that fails to provide such care to all men would, therefore, be unjust and must be altered according to the conditions necessary for survival as human. It would appear, then, that the negative sense of the right to health care falls within the scope of natural rights. More exactly, the analysis turns on taking the natural right to health care as entailed by man's essence *qua* formal cause.

The requirements for taking the positive sense of the right to health care as a natural right are different. Recall that under this rubric are claimed those aspects of health care that enhance life and do not merely maintain or preserve it. Thus, the necessary conditions for the realization of the fullness of human life (essence *qua* final cause) may also be claimed in a right to health care: in the absence of these conditions, we would be deprived of that to which we are entitled to become, by virtue of being the kinds of things we are. Claims of a right to sophisticated medical treatment, e.g. corrective surgery for physical defects, can be analyzed in this way.

The analysis so far has proceeded by displaying the nature of the different restraints that claims regarding a right to health care place upon us. What this analysis shows is that these claims are not homogeneous and that care should, consequently, be taken in distinguishing which sense (or senses) is (are) appropriate in particular cases. One, should, therefore, not expect public policy formed in response to claims to a right to health care to be woven all of a single fabric. In whatever sense the right to health care is taken, however, it is, in its exercise, a *prima facie* and not an absolute right. This important point is apparent upon consideration of conflicts of the duties generated by the right to health care and other rights and/or duties of health practitioners.

In an interesting article, "Medical Care as a Right: A Refutation", Dr Robert Sade takes up this issue. His argument is illustrative in the way it raises problems concerning conflicting exercise of rights. He fails, however, to understand the roots of his own position adequately and so skews his argument badly. Putting that argument back on the right track will help here, by bringing into focus what is at issue in the conflicts of the right to health care with other rights, in particular, conflicts with the rights of health care practitioners.

Dr Sade points to two kinds of conflicts which may defeat the right to health care. The first is a conflict with the natural right of any man to his property, what Locke called the right to Possessions. The second is a conflict with the natural right of freedom. On the first of these two points, as I shall show, Dr Sade's position fails. On the second, his argument can be taken to illuminate a point that should not be ignored by anyone advocating the right to health care (in any of its senses).

Dr Sade's first claim is that a physician's knowledge and skills are within the scope of the natural right to property. He argues as follows:

In a free society, man exercises his right to sustain his own life by producing economic values in the form of goods and services that he is, or should be free to exchange with other men who are similarly free to trade with him or not. The economic values produced, however, are not given as gifts by nature, but exist only by virtue of the thought and effort of individual men. Goods and services are thus owned as a consequence of the right to sustain life by one's own physical and mental effort. . . . Medical care is neither a right nor a privilege: it is a service that is provided by doctors and others to people who wish to purchase it.[14]

In this claim, however, Dr Sade is incorrect. In answering his argument, I shall depend on Locke, as Dr Sade himself has done in an explicit way.[15]

According to Locke, possessions to which man is entitled as a natural right are the product of *his own individual* labor "mixed with" the material of nature.[16] Dr Sade captures this point in the phrase: "the thought and individual effort of individual men". But the thought and effort of the individual practitioner is not produced by him *alone* and nature. On the contrary, it is reasonable to argue that the knowledge and skills of the contemporary practitioner are, without exception, made possible only by virtue of the enormous investment that society has made in the form of expenditures, facilities, and institutions for medical education, research, and care. Hence, it is the individual's labor, *only as mediated by society* and not as that individual's labor alone, that produces the "property" of medical knowledge and skills rendered in service to patients. If this analysis is correct, then it clearly follows that the practitioner has no *natural* right to his services as property. At most, he has a civil right to them.

The more significant sort of conflict that could be generated in the wake of a claim to health care would be with the freedom and not the property of the practitioner.

American medicine is now at the point in the story where the state has proclaimed the nonexistent "right" to medical care as a fact of public policy, and has begun to pass laws to enforce it. The doctor finds himself less his own master and more and more controlled by forces outside his own judgment.[17]

This passage shows that Sade is aware of this

kind of conflict in his consideration of what he terms the "outrages" of Senator Kennedy's proposed legislation.[18] Some of these are serious violations of the natural right to freedom and not to property. An interesting example of this is the bill's provision of forcing health care personnel to locate and practice in specified areas. This situation, if it came to pass, would result in a conflict of the right to health care with the right to freedom. In whatever way the right to health care is understood, it must eventually give way before the demands of freedom, because freedom itself is one of the natural rights, if any is.[19] This conflict is more difficult to resolve. The resolution should turn on which of the two rights in conflict are primary. As a natural right, health care is necessary to preservation of life. Without freedom, it seems, we would be no better off. Similarly, the denial of either or both diminishes the prospects for a full life. Here we encounter an invincible difficulty accompanying natural rights theory: balancing competing claims of natural rights in the simultaneous implementation of them.

The dual emphasis of natural rights has special application at this point. Clearly, a natural right in its aspect as a necessary condition for existing as a human being is logically prior to its aspect as an entitlement to an enhanced or fuller life. Hence, the moral status or authority of the former is greater than the latter. *Ceteris paribus,* the claims of natural rights to an enhanced human life must give way before the claims of natural rights to exist as a human being. Thus, for example, if one claims a natural right to health care in the negative aspect of the second sense and if making good this claim would, say, halve the average income of physicians, then it is morally justifiable, indeed imperative, to provide that health care, since at even half their average wage physicians could exist, quite comfortably, as human beings.

THE RIGHT TO HEALTH CARE AND PUBLIC POLICY

This brings us to the following conclusions. There is adequate reason for analyzing the right to health care in terms of natural rights. The right to health care, on this interpretation, has a number of senses, each with its own special character and limits. Inescapably, it would seem, serious conflicts will arise as we seek to realize any right to health care, if we focus on the *exercise* of rights. We are left, then, with the view that as a natural right the right to health care is *prima facie vis-á-vis* its exercise. It is nevertheless a fundamental moral constraint. As a natural right the right to health care could never be ignored as a factor in the formulation of public policy, *pace* Dr Sade, for natural rights compel our attention and require us to form our *reasons* for acting in accord with their conditions. This brings us full circle, to the issue outlined at the beginning of this paper: the alleged injustice of the present structure of the health care system.

As a result of the foregoing, we can now see that the moral constraints placed on us by claims to a right to health care will vary according to the senses of that right. These constraints will be of two kinds. The more authoritative constraint is that generated by the right to health care in its sense of a natural right derivative of man's essence *qua* formal cause. Included here are both the first sense of the right to health care, based on a right to equal treatment, and negative aspect of the second sense of the right to health care, both of which derive from man's essence *qua* formal cause. A less authoritative, but nevertheless persistent constraint is that generated by the right to health care as a natural right derivative of man's essence *qua* formal cause. The positive aspect of the second sense of the right to health care is included here.

The task, then, in addressing claims to a right to health care is, first, to determine in which of its senses the right is claimed. This, in turn, permits us to determine the place such claims are to be given among the fundamental constraints that bound our moral lives and the public policies regarding health care still to be established. The final step will be to come to grips with these different constraints and to negotiate a coherent response to claims to a right to health care within the inescapable limits that this and other natural rights together place

upon us as moral agents. Following these prescriptions should advance us toward the goal of
implementing this increasingly important
right.

Notes

1. See, for example, Ruth Macklin. Moral Concerns and Appeals to Rights and Duties.
   Hastings Center Report **6**, 31–38. 1976.
2. John Locke, *Two Treatises of Government,* with introduction and notes by Peter Laslett, Mentor
   Books, New York, second treatise, para. 25.
   1965.
3. See *ibid.,* Laslett's introduction, p. 104.
4. For a good discussion of this point, see Leo
   Strauss. *Natural Right and History,* University of
   Chicago Press, Chicago, p. 229, 1974.
5. John Locke, *op. cit.,* second treatise, para. 12.
6. *Ibid.*
7. W. T. Blackstone. Equality and human rights.
   The Monist **52,** 627–628. 1968, his emphasis.
8. See Richard B. Brandt. *Ethical Theory,* Prentice-
   Hall, Inc., Englewood Cliffs, N.J., p. 444,
   1959.
9. H. T. Engelhardt, Jr. The ontology of abortion.
   Ethics **84,** 217–234, 1974.
10. Gene Outka. Social justice and equal access to
    health care. *J. Religious Ethics* **2,** 11, 1974.
11. *Ibid.*
12. *Ibid.,* 17.
13. *Ibid.,* emphasis added.
14. Robert M. Sade, Medical care as a right: a
    refutation. *New England J. Med.* **285,** 1289,
    1971.
15. *Ibid.,* 1288.
16. John Locke, *op. cit.,* second treatise, para. 25ff.
    especially para. 27.
17. Robert M. Sade, *op. cit.,* 1289.
18. *Ibid.,* 1289–1290.
19. H. L. A. Hart, Are there any natural rights?
    Philosoph. Rev. **64,** 175–191, 1955.

Social Justice and Equal Access to Health Care[1]

Gene Outka

I want to consider the following question. Is it
possible to understand and to justify morally a
societal goal which increasing numbers of
people, including Americans, accept as normative? The goal is: the assurance of comprehensive health services for every person irrespective of income or geographic location.
Indeed, the goal now has almost the status of a
platitude. Currently in the United States politicians in various camps give it at least verbal
endorsement (see, e.g., Nixon, 1972:1; Kennedy, 1972:234–252). I do not propose to examine the possible sociological determinants in
this emergent consensus. I hope to show that
whatever these determinants are, one may offer
a plausible case in defense of the goal on rea-

Reprinted with permission from the author and *Journal
of Religious Ethics,* Vol. 2, No. 1, 1974, pp. 11–29.

sonable grounds. To demonstrate why appeals
to the goal get so successfully under our skins, I
shall have recourse to a set of conceptions of
social justice. Some of the standard conceptions, found in a number of writings on justice,
will do (these writings include Bedau, 1971;
Hospers, 1961:416–468; Lucas, 1972; Perelman, 1963; Rescher, 1966; Ryan, 1916; Vlastos, 1962). By reflecting on them it seems to me
a prima facie case can be established, namely,
that every person in the entire resident population should have equal access to health care
delivery.

The case is prima facie only. I wish to set
aside as far as possible a related question which
comes readily enough to mind. In the world of
"suboptimal alternatives," with the constraints for example which impinge on the

government as it makes decisions about resource allocation, what is one to say? What criteria should be employed? Paul Ramsey, in *The Patient as Person* (1970:240), thinks that the large question of how to choose between medical and other societal priorities is "almost, if not altogether, incorrigible to moral reasoning." Whether it is or not is a matter which must be ignored for the present. One may simply observe in passing that choices are unavoidable nonetheless, as Ramsey acknowledges, even where the government allows them to be made by default, so that in some instances they are determined largely by which private pressure groups prove to be dominant. In any event, there is virtue in taking up one complicated question at a time and we need to get the thrust of the case for equal access before us. It is enough to observe now that Americans attach an obviously high priority to organized health care. National health expenditures for the fiscal year 1972 were $83.4 billion (Hicks, 1973:52). Even if such an enormous sum is not entirely adequate, we may still ask: how are we to justify spending whatever we do in accordance as far as possible with the goal of equal access? The answer I propose involves distinguishing various conceptions of social justice and trying to show which of these apply or fail to apply to health care considerations. Only toward the end of the paper will some institutional implications be given more than passing attention, and then in a strictly programmatic way.

Another sort of query should be noted as we begin. What stake does someone in religious ethics have in this discussion? For the reasonable case envisaged is offered after all in the public forum. If the issue is how to justify morally the societal goal which seems so obvious to so many, whether or not they are religious believers, does the religious ethicist then simply participate qua citizen? Here I think we should be wary of simplifying formulae. Why for example should a Jew or a Christian not welcome wide support for a societal goal which he or she can affirm and reaffirm, or reflect only on instances where such support is not forthcoming? If a number of ethical schemes, both religious and humanist, converge in their acceptance of the goal of equal access to health

care, so be it. Secularists can join forces with believers, at least at some levels or points, without implying there must be unanimity on every moral issue. Yet it also seems too simple if one claims to wear only the citizen's hat when making the case in question. At least I should admit that a commitment to the basic normative principle which in Christian writings is often called *agape* may influence the account to follow in ways large and small (see Outka, 1972). For example, someone with such a commitment will quite naturally take a special interest in appeals to the generic characteristics all persons share rather than the idiosyncratic attainments which distinguish persons from one another, and in the playing down of desert considerations. As I shall try to show, such appeals are centrally relevant to the case for equal access. And they are nicely in line with the normative pressures agapeic considerations typically exert.

One issue of theoretical importance in religious ethics also emerges in connection with this last point. The approach in this paper may throw a little indirect light on the traditional question, especially prominent in Christian ethics, of how love and justice are related. To distinguish different conceptions of social justice will put us in a better position, I think, to recognize that often it is ambiguous to ask about "*the* relation." There may be different relations to different conceptions. For the conceptions themselves may sometimes produce discordant indications, or turn out to be incommensurable, or reflect, when different ones are seized upon, rival moral points of view. I shall note several of these relations as we proceed.

Which then among the standard conceptions of social justice appear to be particularly relevant or irrelevant? Let us consider the following five:

I. To each according to his merit or desert.

II. To each according to his societal contribution.

III. To each according to his contribution in satisfying whatever is freely desired by others in the open marketplace of supply and demand.

IV. To each according to his needs.

V. Similar treatment for similar cases.

In general I shall argue the first three of these are less relevant because of certain distinctive features which health crises possess. I shall focus on crises here not because I think preventive care is unimportant (the opposite is true), but because the crisis situation shows most clearly the special significance we attach to medical treatment as an institutionalized activity or social practice, and the basic purpose we suppose it to have.

I

To each according to his merit or desert. Meritarian conceptions, above all perhaps, are grading ones: advantages are allocated in accordance with amounts of energy expended or kinds of results achieved. What is judged is particular conduct which distinguishes persons from one another and not only the fact that all the parties are human beings. Sometimes a competitive aspect looms large.

In certain contexts it is illuminating to distinguish between efforts and achievements. In the case of efforts one characteristically focuses on the individual: rewards are based on the pains one takes. Some have supposed, for example, that entry into the kingdom of heaven is linked more directly to energy displayed and fidelity shown than to successful results attained.

To assess achievements is to weigh actual performance and productive contributions. The academic prize is awarded to the student with the highest grade-point average, regardless of the amount of midnight oil he or she burned in preparing for the examinations. Sometimes we may exclaim, "it's just not fair," when person X writes a brilliant paper with little effort while we are forced to devote more time with less impressive results. But then our complaint may be directed against differences in innate ability and talent which no expenditure of effort altogether removes.

After the difference between effort and achievement, and related distinctions, have been acknowledged, what should be stressed I think is the general importance of meritarian or desert criteria in the thinking of most people

about justice. These criteria may serve to illuminate a number of disputes about the justice of various practices and institutional arrangements in our society. It may help to explain, for instance, the resentment among the working class against the welfare system. However wrongheaded or self-deceptive the resentment often is, particularly when directed toward those who want to work but for various reasons beyond their control cannot, at its better moments it involves in effect an appeal to desert considerations. "Something for nothing" is repudiated as unjust; benefits should be proportional (or at least related) to costs; those who can make an effort should do so, whatever the degree of their training or significance of their contribution to society; and so on. So, too, persons deserve to have what they have labored for; unless they infringe on the works of others their efforts achievements are justly theirs.

Occasionally the appeal to desert extends to a wholesale rejection of other considerations as grounds for just claims. The most conspicuous target is need. Consider this statement by Ayn Rand.

> A morality that holds *need* as a claim, holds emptiness—nonexistence—as its standard of value; it rewards an absence, a defect: weakness, inability, incompetence, suffering, disease, disaster, the lack, the fault, the flaw—the *zero*.
>
> Who provides the account to pay these claims? Those who are cursed for being non-zeros, each to the extent of his distance from that ideal. Since all values are the product of virtues, the degree of your virtue is used as the measure of your penalty; the degree of your faults is used as the measure of your gain. Your code declares that the rational man must sacrifice himself to the irrational man, the independent man to parasites, the honest man to the dishonest, the man of justice to the unjust, the productive man to thieving loafers, the man of integrity to compromising knaves, the man of self-esteem to sniveling neurotics. Do you wonder at the meanness of soul in those you see around you? The man who achieves these virtues will not accept your moral code; the man who accepts your moral code will not achieve these virtues. (1957–958)

I have noted elsewhere (1972:89–90; 165–167) that *agape*, while it characteristically plays down, need not formally disallow attention to considerations falling under merit or desert; for in the case of merit as well as need it may be possible, the quotation above notwithstanding, to reason solely from egalitarian premises. A major reason such attention is warranted concerns what was called there the differential exercise of an equal liberty. That is, one may fittingly revere another's moral capacities and thus the efforts he makes as well as the ends he seeks. Such reverence may lead one to weigh expenditure of energy and specific achievements. I would simply hold now (1) that the idea of justice is not exhaustively characterized by the notion of desert, even if one agrees that the latter plays an important role; and (2) that the notion of desert is especially ill-suited to play an important role in the determination of policies which should govern a system of health care.

Why is it so ill-suited? Here we encounter some of the distinctive features which it seems to me health crises possess. Let me put it in this way. Health crises seem non-meritarian because they occur so often for reasons beyond our control or power to predict. They frequently fall without discrimination on the (according-to-merit) just and unjust, i.e., the virtuous and the wicked, the industrious and the slothful alike.

While we may believe that virtues and vices cannot depend upon natural contingencies, we are bound to admit, it seems, that many health crises do. It makes sense therefore to say that we are equal in being randomly susceptible to these crises. Even those who ascribe a prominent role to desert acknowledge that justice has also properly to do with pleas of "But I could not help it" (Lucas, 1972:321). One seeks to distinguish such cases from those acknowledged to be praiseworthy or blameworthy. Then it seems unfair as well as unkind to discriminate among those who suffer health crises on the basis of their personal deserts. For it would be odd to maintain that a newborn child deserves his hemophilia or the tumor afflicting her spine.

These considerations help to explain why the following rough distinction is often made. Bernard Williams, for example, in his discussion of "equality in unequal circumstances," identifies two different sorts of inequality, inequality of merit and inequality of need, and two corresponding goods, those earned by effort and those demanded by need (1971:126–137). Medical treatment in the event of illness is located under the umbrella of need. He concludes: "Leaving aside preventive medicine, the proper ground of distribution of medical care is ill health: this is a necessary truth" (1971:127). An irrational state of affairs is held to obtain if those whose needs are the same are treated unequally, when needs are the ground of the treatment. One might put the point this way. When people are equal in the relevant respects—in this case when their needs are the same and occur in a context of random, undeserved susceptibility—that by itself is a good reason for treating them equally (see also Nagel, 1973:354).

In many societies, however, a second necessary condition for the receipt of medical treatment exists de facto: the possession of money. This is not the place to consider the general question of when inequalities in wealth may be regarded as just. It is enough to note that one can plausibly appeal to all of the conceptions of justice we are embarked in sorting out. A person may be thought to be entitled to a higher income when he works more, contributes more, risks more, and not simply when he needs more. We may think it fair that the industrious should have more money than the slothful and the surgeon more than the tobacanist. The difficulty comes in the misfit between the reasons for differential incomes and the reasons for receiving medical treatment. The former may include a pluralistic set of claims in which different notions of justice must be meshed. The latter are more monistically focused on needs, and the other notions not accorded a similar relevance. Yet money may nonetheless remain as a causally necessary condition for receiving medical treatment. It may be the power to secure what one needs. The senses in which health crises are distinctive may then be insufficiently determinative for the policies which govern the actual availability of treatment. The nearly automatic links between income, prestige, and the receipt of comparatively higher quality medical treatment should then be subjected to critical scrutiny. For unequal treatment of the rich ill and the poor ill is unjust if, again, needs rather than differential income constitute the ground of such treatment.

Suppose one agrees that it is important to recognize the misfit between the reasons for differential incomes and the reasons for receiving medical treatment, and that therefore income as such should not govern the actual availability of treatment. One may still ask whether the case so far relies excessively on "pure" instances where desert considerations are admittedly out of place. That there are such pure instances, tumors afflicting the spine, hemophilia, and so on, is not denied. Yet it is an exaggeration if we go on and regard all health crises as utterly unconnected with desert. Note for example that Williams leaves aside preventive medicine. And if in a cool hour we examine the statistics, we find that a vast number of deaths occur each year due to causes not always beyond our control, e.g., automobile accidents, drugs, alcohol, tobacco, obesity, and so on. In some final reckoning it seems that many persons (though crucially, not all) have an effect on, and arguably a responsibility for, their own medical needs. Consider the following bidders for emergency care: (1) a person with a heart attack who is seriously overweight; (2) a football hero who has suffered a concussion; (3) a man with lung cancer who has smoked cigarettes for forty years; (4) a 60 year old man who has always taken excellent care of himself and is suddenly stricken with leukemia; (5) a three year old girl who has swallowed poison left out carelessly by her parents; (6) a 14 year old boy who has been beaten without provocation by a gang and suffers brain damage and recurrent attacks of uncontrollable terror; (7) a college student who has slashed his wrists (and not for the first time) from a psychological need for attention; (8) a woman raised in the ghetto who is found unconscious due to an overdose of heroin.

These cases help to show why the whole subject of medical treatment is so crucial and so perplexing. They attest to some melancholy elements in human experience. People suffer in varying ratios the effects of their natural and undeserved vulnerabilities, the irresponsibility and brutality of others, and their own desires

and weaknesses. In some final reckoning then desert considerations seem not irrelevant to many health crises. The practical applicability of this admission, however, in the instance of health care delivery, appears limited. We may agree that it underscores the importance of preventive health care by stressing the influence we sometimes have over our medical needs. But if we try to foster such care by increasing the penalties for neglect, we normally confine ourselves to calculations about incentives. At the risk of being denounced in some quarters as censorious and puritannical, perhaps we should for example levy far higher taxes on alcohol and tobacco and pump the dollars directly into health care programs rather than (say) into highway building. Yet these steps would by no means lead necessarily to a demand that we correlate in some strict way a demonstrated effort to be temperate with the receipt of privileged medical treatment as a reward. Would it be feasible to allocate the additional tax monies to the man with leukemia before the overweight man suffering a heart attack on the ground of a difference in desert? At the point of emergency care at least, it seems impracticable for the doctor to discriminate between these cases, to make meritarian judgments at the point of catastrophe. And the number of persons who are in need of medical treatment for reasons utterly beyond their control remains a datum with tenacious relevance. There are those who suffer the ravages of a tornado, are handicapped by a genetic defect, beaten without provocation, etc. A commitment to the basic purpose of medical care and to the institutions for achieving it involves the recognition of this persistent state of affairs.

II

To each according to his societal contribution. This conception gives moral primacy to notions such as the public interest, the common good, the welfare of the community, or the greatest good of the greatest number. Here one judges the social consequences of particular conduct. The formula can be construed in at least two ways (Rescher, 1966:79–80). It may refer to the interest of the social group considered collectively, where the group has some independent life all its own. The group's welfare is the decisive criterion for determining what constitutes any member's proper share. Or the common good may refer only to an aggregation of distinct individuals and considered distributively.

Either version accords such a primacy to what is socially advantageous as to be unacceptable not only to defenders of need, but also, it would seem, of desert. For the criteria of effort and achievement are often conceived along rather individualistic lines. The pains an agent takes or the results he brings about deserve recompense, whether or not the public interest is directly served. No automatic harmony then is necessarily assumed between his just share as individually earned and his proper share from the vantage point of the common good. Moreover, the test of social advantage *simpliciter* obviously threatens the agapeic concern with some minimal consideration due each person which is never to be disregarded for the sake of long-range social benefits. No one should be considered as *merely* a means or instrument.

The relevance of the canon of social productiveness to health crises may accordingly also be challenged. Indeed, such crises may cut against it in that they occur more frequently to those whose comparative contribution to the general welfare is less, e.g., the aged, the disabled, children.

Consider for example Paul Ramsey's persuasive critique of social and economic criteria for the allocation of a single scarce medical resource. He begins by recounting the imponderables which faced the widely-discussed "public committee" at the Swedish Hospital in Seattle when it deliberated in the early 1960's. The sparse resource in this case was the kidney machine. The committee was charged with the responsibility of selecting among patients suffering chronic renal failure those who were to receive dialysis. Its criteria were broadly social and economic. Considerations weighed included age, sex, marital status, number of dependents, income, net worth, educational background, occupation, past performance and future potential. The application of such criteria proved to be exceedingly problematic. Should someone with six children always have

priority over an artist or composer? Were those who arranged matters so that their families would not burden society to be penalized in effect for being provident? And so on. Two critics of the committee found "a disturbing picture of the bourgeoisie sparing the bourgeoisie" and observed that "the Pacific Northwest is no place for a Henry David Thoreau with bad kidneys" (quoted in Ramsey, 1970:248).

The mistake, Ramsey believes, is to introduce criteria of social worthiness in the first place. In those situations of choice where not all can be saved and yet all need not die, "the equal right of every human being to live, and not relative personal or social worth, should be the ruling principle" (1970:256). The principle leads to a criterion of "random choice among equals" expressed by a lottery scheme or a practice of "first-come, first-served." Several reasons stand behind Ramsey's defense of the criterion of random choice. First, a religious belief in the equality of persons before God leads intelligibly to a refusal to choose between those who are dying in any way other than random patient selection. Otherwise their equal value as human beings is threatened. Second, a moral primacy is ascribed to survival over other (perhaps superior) interests persons may have, in that it is the condition of everything else. "... Life is a value incommensurate with all others, and so not negotiable by bartering one man's worth against another's" (1970:256). Third, the entire enterprise of estimating a person's social worth is viewed with final skepticism. "... We have no way of knowing how really and truly to estimate a man's societal worth or his worth to others or to himself in unfocused social situations in the ordinary lives of men in their communities" (1970:256). This statement, incidentally, appears to allow something other than randomness in *focused* social situations; when, say, a President or Prime Minister and the owner of the local bar rush for the last place in the bomb shelter, and the knowledge of the former can save many lives. In any event, I have been concerned with a restricted point to which Ramsey's discussion brings illustrative support. The canon of social productiveness is notoriously difficult to apply as a workable criterion for distributing medical services to those who need them.

One may go further. A system of health care delivery which treats people on the basis of the medical care required may often go against (at least narrowly conceived) calculations of societal advantage. For example, the health care needs of people tend to rise during that period of their lives, signaled by retirement, when their incomes and social productivity are declining. More generally:

> Some 40 to 50 per cent of the American people—the aged, children, the dependent poor, and those with some significant chronic disability are in categories requiring relatively large amounts of medical care but with inadequate resources to purchase such care. (Somers, 1971a:20)

If one agrees, for whatever reasons, with the agapeic judgment that each person should be regarded as irreducibly valuable, then one cannot succumb to a social productiveness criterion of human worth. Interests are to be equally considered even when people have ceased to be, or are not yet, or perhaps never will be, public assets.

III

To each according to his contribution in satisfying whatever is freely desired by others in the open marketplace of supply and demand. Here we have a test which, though similar to the preceding one, concentrates on what is desired de facto by certain segments of the community rather than the community as a whole, and on the relative scarcity of the service rendered. It is tantamount to the canon of supply and demand as espoused by various laissez-faire theoreticians (cf. Rescher, 1966:80–81). Rewards should be given to those who by virtue of special skill, prescience, risk-taking, and the like discern what is desired and are able to take the requisite steps to bring satisfaction. A surgeon, it may be argued, contributes more than a nurse because of the greater training and skill required, burdens borne, and effective care provided, and should be compensated accordingly. So too perhaps a star quarterback on a pro-football team should be remunerated even more highly because of the rare athletic prowess needed, hazards involved, and widespread demand to watch him play.

This formula does not then call for the weighing of the value of various contributions, and tends to conflate needs and wants under a notion of desires. It also assumes that a prominent part is assigned to consumer free-choice. The consumer should be at liberty to express his preferences, and to select from a variety of competing goods and services. Those who resist many changes currently proposed in the organization and financing of health care delivery in the U.S.A.—such as national health insurance—often do so by appealing to some variant of this formula.

Yet it seems health crises are often of overriding importance when they occur. They appear therefore not satisfactorily accommodated to the context of a free marketplace where consumers may freely choose among alternative goods and services.

To clarify what is at stake in the above contention, let us examine an opposing case. Robert M. Sade, M.D., published an article in *The New England Journal of Medicine* entitled "Medical Care as a Right: A Refutation" (1971). He attacks programs of national health insurance in the name of a person's right to select one's own values, determine how they may be realized, and dispose of them if one chooses without coercion from other men. The values in question are construed as economic ones in the context of supply and demand. So we read:

> In a free society, man exercises his right to sustain his own life by producing economic values in the form of goods and services that he is, or should be, free to exchange with other men who are similarly free to trade with him or not. The economic values produced, however, are not given as gifts by nature, but exist only by virtue of the thought and effort of individual men. Goods and services are thus owned as a consequence of the right to sustain life by one's own physical and mental effort. (1971:1289)

Sade compares the situation of the physician to that of the baker. The one who produces a loaf of bread should as owner have the power to dispose of his own product. It is immoral simply to expropriate the bread without the baker's permission. Similarly, "medical care is neither a right nor a privilege: it is a service that is provided by doctors and others to people who wish to purchase it" (1971:1289). Any coercive regulation of professional practices by the society at large is held to be analogous to taking the bread from the baker without his consent. Such regulation violates the freedom of the physician over his own services and will lead inevitably to provider-apathy.

The analogy surely misleads. To assume that doctors autonomously produce goods and services in a fashion closely akin to a baker is grossly oversimplified. The baker may himself rely on the agricultural produce of others, yet there is a crucial difference in the degree of dependence. Modern physicians depend on the achievements of medical technology and the entire scientific base underlying it, all of which is made possible by a host of persons whose salaries are often notably less. Moreover, the amount of taxpayer support for medical research and education is too enormous to make any such unqualified case for provider-autonomy plausible.

However conceptually clouded Sade's article may be, its stress on a free exchange of goods and services reflects one historically influential rationale for much American medical practice. And he applies it not only to physicians but also to patients or "consumers."

> The question is whether the decision of how to allocate the consumer's dollar should belong to the consumer or to the state. It has already been shown that the choice of how a doctor's services should be rendered belongs only to the doctor: in the same way the choice of whether to buy a doctor's service rather than some other commodity or service belongs to the consumer as a logical consequence of the right to his own life. (1971:1291)

This account is misguided, I think, because it ignores the overriding importance which is so often attached to health crises. When lumps appear on someone's neck, it usually makes little sense to talk of choosing whether to buy a doctor's service rather than a color television set.

References to just trade-offs suddenly seem out of place. No compensation suffices, since the penalties may differ so much.

There is even a further restriction on consumer choice. One's knowledge in these circumstances is comparatively so limited. The physician makes most of the decisions: about diagnosis, treatment, hospitalization, number of return visits, and so on. In brief:

> The consumer knows very little about the medical services he is buying—probably less than about any other service he purchases. . . . While [he] can still play a role in policing the market; that role is much more limited in the field of health care than in almost any other area of private economic activity. (Schultze, 1972:214–215)

For much of the way, then, an appeal to supply and demand and consumer choice is not quite fitting. It neglects the issue of the value of various contributions. And it fails to allow for the recognition that medical treatments may be overridingly desired. In contexts of catastrophe at any rate, when life itself is threatened, most persons (other than those who are apathetic or seek to escape from the terrifying prospects) cannot take medical care to be merely one option among others.

IV

To each according to his needs. The concept of needs is sometimes taken to apply to an entire range of interests which concern a person's "psycho-physical existence" (Outka, 1972: esp. 264–265). On this wide usage, to attribute a need to someone is to say that the person lacks what is thought to conduce to his or her "welfare"—understood in both a physiological sense (e.g., for food, drink, shelter, and health) and a psychological one (e.g., for continuous human affection and support).

Yet even in the case of such a wide usage, what the person lacks is typically assumed to be basic. Attention is restricted to recurrent considerations rather than to every possible individual whim or frivolous pursuit. So one is not surprised to meet with the contention that a preferable rendering of this formula would be:

"to each according to his essential needs" (Perelman, 1963:22). This contention seems to me well taken. It implies, for one thing, that basic needs are distinguishable from felt needs or wants. For the latter may encompass expressions of personal preference unrelated to considerations of survival or subsistance in the society at large.

Essential needs are also typically assumed to be given rather than acquired. They are not constituted by any action for which the person is responsible by virtue of his or her distinctively greater effort. It is almost as if the designation "innocent" may be linked illuminatingly to need, as retribution, punishment, and so on, are to desert, and in complex ways, to freedom. Thus essential needs are likewise distinguishable from deserts. Where needs are unequal, one thinks of them as fortuitously distributed; as part, perhaps, of a kind of "natural lottery" (see Rawls, 1971:e.g., 104). So very often the advantages of health and the burdens of illness, for example, strike one as arbitrary effects of the lottery. It seems wrong to say that a newborn child deserves as a reward all of his faculties when he has done nothing in particular which distinguishes him from another newborn who comes into the world deprived of one or more of them. Similarly, though crudely, many religious believers do not look on natural events as personal deserts. They are not inclined to pronounce sentences such as, "That evil person with incurable cancer got what he deserved." They are disposed instead to search for some distinction between what they may call the conditions of finitude on the one hand and sin and moral evil on the other. If the distinction is "ultimately" invalid, in this life it seems inscrutably so. Here and now it may be usefully drawn. Inequalities in the need for medical treatment are taken, it appears, to reflect the conditions of finitude more than anything else.

One can even go on to argue that among our basic or essential needs, the case of medical treatment is conspicuous in the following sense. While food and shelter are not matters about which we are at liberty to please ourselves, they are at least predictable. We can plan, for instance, to store up food and fuel for the winter. It may be held that responsibility increases

along with the power to predict. If so, then many health crises seem peculiarly random and uncontrollable. Cancer, given the present state of knowledge at any rate, is a contingent disaster, whereas hunger is a steady threat. Who will need serious medical care, and when, is then perhaps a classic example of uncertainty.

Finally, and more theoretically, it is often observed that a need-conception of justice comes closest to charity or *agape* (e.g., Perelman, 1963:23). I think there are indeed crucial overlaps (see Outka, 1972:91–92, 309–312). To cite several of them: the equal consideration *agape* enjoins has to do in the first instance with those generic endowments which people share, the characteristics of a person qua human existent. Needs, as we have seen, likewise concern those things essential to the life and welfare of men considered simply as men (see also Honoré, 1968). They are not based on particular conduct alone, on those idiosyncratic attainments which contribute to someone's being such-and-such a kind of person. Yet a certain sort of inequality is recognized, for needs differ in divergent circumstances and so treatments must if benefits are to be equalized. *Agape* too allows for a distinction between equal consideration and identical treatment. The aim of equalizing benefits is implied by the injunction to consider the interests of each party equally. This may require differential treatments of differing interests.

Overlaps such as these will doubtless strike some as so extensive that it may be asked whether *agape* and a need-conception of justice are virtually equivalent. I think not. One contrast was pointed out before. The differential treatment enjoined by *agape* is more complex and goes deeper. In the case of *agape,* attention may be appropriately given to varying *efforts* as well as to unequal *needs*. More generally one may say that agapeic considerations extend to all of the psychological nuances and contextual details of individual persons and their circumstances. Imaginative concern is enjoined for concrete human beings: for what someone is uniquely, for what he or she—as a matter of personal history and distinctive identity—wants, feels, thinks, celebrates, and endures. The attempt to establish and enhance mutual affection between individual persons is taken likewise to be fitting. Conceptions of social justice, including "to each according to his essential needs," tend to be more restrictive; they call attention to considerations which obtain for a number of pesons, to impersonally specified criteria for assessing collective policies and practices. *Agape* involves more, even if one supposes never less.

Other differences could be noted. What is important now however is the recognition that, in matters of health care in particular, *agape* and a need-conception of justice are conjoined in a number of relevant respects. At least this is so for those who think that, again, justice has properly to do with pleas of "But I could not help it." It seeks to distinguish such cases from those acknowledged to be praiseworthy or blameworthy. The formula "to each according to his needs" is one cogent way of identifying the moral relevance of these pleas. To ignore them may be thought to be unfair as well as unkind when they arise from the deprivation of some essential need. The move to confine the notion of justice wholly to desert considerations is thereby resisted as well. Hence we may say that sometimes "questions of social justice arise just because people are unequal in ways they can do very little to change and . . . only by attending to these inequalities can one be said to be giving their interests equal consideration" (Benn, 1971:164).

V

Similar treatment for similar cases. This conception is perhaps the most familiar of all. Certainly it is the most formal and inclusive one. It is frequently taken as an elementary appeal to consistency and linked to the universalizability test. One should not make an arbitrary exception on one's own behalf, but rather should apply impartially whatever standards one accepts. The conception can be fruitfully applied to health care questions and I shall assume its relevance. Yet as literally interpreted, it is necessary but not sufficient. For rightly or not, it is often held to be as compatible with no positive treatment whatever as with active promotion of others peoples' interests, as long as all

are equally and impartially included. Its exponents sometimes assume such active promotion without demonstrating clearly how this is built into the conception itself. Moreover, it may obscure a distinction which we have seen agapists and others make: between equal consideration and identical treatment. Needs may differ and so treatments must, if benefits are to be equalized.

I have placed this conception at the end of the list partly because it moves us, despite its formality, toward practice. Let me suggest briefly how it does so. Suppose first of all one agrees with the case so far offered. Suppose, that is, it has been shown convincingly that a need-conception of justice applies with greater relevance than the earlier three when one reflects about the basic purpose of medical care. To treat one class of people differently from another because of income or geographic location should therefore be ruled out, because such reasons are irrelevant. (The irrelevance is conceptual, rather than always, unfortunately, causal.) In short, all persons should have equal access, "as needed, without financial, geographic, or other barriers, to the whole spectrum of health services" (Somers and Somers, 1972a:122).

Suppose however, secondly, that the goal of equal access collides on some occasions with the realities of finite medical resources and needs which prove to be insatiable. That such collisions occur in fact it would be idle to deny. And it is here that the practical bearing of the formula of similar treatment for similar cases should be noticed. Let us recall Williams' conclusion: "the proper ground of distribution of medical care is ill health: this is a necessary truth." While I agree with the essentials of his argument—for all the reasons above—I would prefer, for practical purposes, a slightly more modest formulation. Illness is the proper ground for the *receipt* of medical care. However, the *distribution* of medical care in less-than-optimal circumstances requires us to face the collisions. I would argue that in such circumstances the formula of similar treatment for similar cases may be construed so as to guide actual choices in the way most compatible with the goal of equal access. The formula's allowance of no positive treatment whatever may justify exclusion of entire classes of cases from a priority list. Yet it forbids doing so for irrelevant or arbitrary reasons. So (1) if we accept the case for equal access, but (2) if we simply cannot, physically cannot, treat all who are in need, it seems more just to discriminate by virtue of categories of illness, for example, rather than between the rich ill and poor ill. All persons with a certain rare, non-communicable disease would not receive priority, let us say, where the costs were inordinate, the prospects for rehabilitation remote, and for the sake of equalized benefits to many more. Or with Ramsey we may urge a policy of random patient selection when one must decide between claimants for a medical treatment unavailable to all. Or we may acknowledge that any notion of "comprehensive benefits" to which persons should have equal access is subject to practical restrictions which will vary from society to society depending on resources at a given time. Even in a country as affluent as the United States there will surely always be items excluded, e.g., perhaps over-the-counter drugs, some teenage orthodontia, cosmetic surgery, and the like (Somers and Somers, 1972b:182). Here too the formula of similar treatment for similar cases may serve to modify the application of a need-conception of justice in order to address the insatiability-problem and limit frivolous use. In all of the foregoing instances of restriction, however, the relevant feature remains the illness, discomfort, etc. itself. The goal of equal access then retains its prima facie authoritativeness. It is imperfectly realized rather than disregarded.

VI

These latter comments lead on to the question of institutional implications. I cannot aim here of course for the specificity rightly sought by policy-makers. My endeavor has been conceptual elucidation. While the ethicist needs to be apprised about the facts, he or she does not, qua ethicist, don the mantle of the policy-expert. In any case, only rarely does anyone do both things equally well. Yet cross-fertilization is extremely desirable. For experts should not be isolated from the wider assumptions their

recommendations may reflect. I shall merely list some of the topics which would have to be discussed at length if we were to get clear about the implications. Examples will be limited to the current situation in the United States.

Anyone who accepts the case for equal access will naturally be concerned about de facto disparities in the availability of medical treatment. Let us consider two relevant indictments of current American practice. They appear in the writings not only of those who attack indiscriminately a system seen to be governed only by the appetite for profit and power, but also of those who denounce in less sweeping terms and espouse more cautiously reformist positions. The first shortcoming has to do with the maldistribution of supply. Per capita ratios of physicians to populations served vary, sometimes notoriously, between affluent suburbs and rural and inner city areas. This problem is exacerbated by the distressing data concerning the greater health needs of the poor. Chronic disease, frequency and duration of hospitalization, psychiatric disorders, infant death rates, etc.—these occur in significantly larger proportions to lower income members of American society (Appel, 1970; Hubbard, 1970). A further complication is that "the distribution of health insurance coverage is badly skewed. Practically all the rich have insurance. But among the poor, about two-thirds have none. As a result, among people aged 25 to 64 who die, some 45 to 50 per cent have neither hospital nor surgical coverage" (Somers, 1971a:46). This last point connects with a second shortcoming frequently cited. Even those who are otherwise economically independent may be shattered by the high cost of a "catastrophic illness" (see some eloquent examples in Kennedy, 1972).

Proposals for institutional reforms designed to overcome such disparities are bound to be taken seriously by any defender of equal access. What he or she will be disposed to press for, of course, is the removal of any double standard or "two class" system of care. The viable procedures for bringing this about are not obvious, and comparisons with certain other societies (for relevant alternative models) are drawn now with perhaps less confidence (see Anderson, 1973). One set of commonly discussed proposals includes (1) incentive subsidies to physicians, hospitals, and medical centers to provide services in regions of poverty (to overcome in part the unwillingness—to which no unique culpability need be ascribed—of many providers and their spouses to work and live in grim surroundings); (2) licensure controls to avoid comparatively excessive concentrations of physicians in regions of affluence; (3) a period of time (say, two years) in an undeserved area as a requirement for licensing; (4) redistribution facilities which allow for population shifts.

A second set of proposals is linked with health insurance itself. While I cannot venture into the intricacies of medical economics or comment on the various bills for national health insurance presently inundating Congress, it may be instructive to take brief note of one proposal in which, once more, the defender of equal access is bound to take an interest (even if he or she finally rejects it on certain practical grounds). The precise details of the proposal are unimportant for our purposes (for one much-discussed version, see Feldstein, 1971). Consider this crude sketch. Each citizen is (in effect) issued a card by the government. Whenever "legitimate" medical expenses (however determined for a given society) exceed, say 10 per cent of his or her annual taxable income, the card may be presented so that additional costs incurred will be paid for out of general tax revenues. The reasons urged on behalf of this sort of arrangement include the following. In the case of medical care there is warrant for proportionately equalizing what is spend from anyone's total taxable income. This warrant reflects the conditions, discussed earlier, of the natural lottery. Insofar as the advantages of health and the burdens of illness are random and undeserved, we may find it in our common interest to share risks. A fixed percentage of income attests to the misfit, also mentioned previously, between the reasons for differential total income and the reasons for receiving medical treatment. If money remains a causally necessary condition for receiving medical treatment, then a way must be found to place it in the hands of those who need it. The card is one such means. It is designed effectively to equalize purchasing power. In this way it seems

to accord nicely with the goal of equal access. On the other side, the requirement of initial out-of-pocket expenses—sufficiently large in comparison to average family expenditures on health care—is designed to discourage frivolous use and foster awareness that medical care is a benefit not to be simply taken as a matter of course. It also safeguards against an excessively large tax burden while providing universal protection against the often disastrous costs of serious illnesses. Whether 10 per cent is too great a chunk for the very poor to pay, and whether by itself the proposal will feed price inflation and neglect of preventive medicine are questions which would have to be answered.

Another kind of possible institutional reform will also greatly interest the defender of equal access. This has to do with the "design of health care systems" or "care settings." The prevalent setting in American society has always been "fee-for-service." It is left up to each person to obtain the requisite care and to pay for it as he or she goes along. Because costs for medical treatment have accelerated at such an alarming rate, and because the sheer diffusion of energy and effort so characteristic of American medical practice leaves more and more people dissatisfied, alternatives to fee-for-service have been considered of late with unprecedented seriousness. The alternative care setting most widely discussed is prepaid practice, and specifically the "health maintenance organization" (HMO). Here one finds "an organized system of care which accepts the responsibility to provide or otherwise assure comprehensive care to a defined population for a fixed periodic payment per person or per family . . ." (Somers, 1972b:v). The best-known HMO is the Kaiser-Permanente Medical Care Program (see also Garfield, 1971). Does the HMO serve to realize the goal of equal access more fully? One line of argument in its favor is this. It is plausible to think that equal access will be fostered by the more economical care setting. HMO's are held to be less costly per capita in at least two respects: hospitalization rates are much below the national average; and less often noted, physician manpower is as well. To be sure, one should be sensitive to the corruptions in each type of setting. While fee-for-service has resulted in a suspiciously high number of surgeries (twice as many per capita in the United States as in Great Britain), the HMO physician may more frequently permit the patient's needs to be overridden by the organization's pressure to economize. It may also be more difficult in an HMO setting to provide for close personal relations between a particular physician and a particular patient (something commended, of course, on all sides). After such corruptions are allowed for, the data seem encouraging to such an extent that a defender of equal access will certainly support the repeal of any law which limits the development of prepaid practice, to approve of "front-aid" subsidies for HMO's to increase their number overall and achieve a more equitable distribution throughout the country, and so on. At a minimum, each care setting should be available in every region. If we assume a common freedom to choose between them, each may help to guard against the peculiar temptations to which the other is exposed.

To assess in any serious way proposals for institutional reform such as the above is beyond the scope of this paper. We would eventually be led, for example, into the question of whether it is consistent for the rich to pay more than the poor for the same treatment when, again, needs rather than income constitute the ground of the treatment (Ward, 1973), and from there into the tangled subject of the "ethics of redistribution" in general (see, e.g., Benn and Peters, 1965:155–178; de Jouvenal, 1952). Other complex issues deserve to be considered as well, e.g., the criteria for allocation of limited resources,[2] and how conceptions of justice apply to the providers of health care.[3]

Those committed to self-conscious moral and religious reflection about subjects in medicine have concentrated, perhaps unduly, on issues about care of individual patients (as death approaches, for instance). These issues plainly warrant the most careful consideration. One would like to see in addition, however, more attention paid to social questions in medical ethics. To attend to them is not necessarily to leave behind all of the matters which reach deeply into the human condition. Any detailed case for institutional reforms, for example, will be enriched if the proponent asks soberly whether certain conflicts and certain perplex-

ities allow for more than partial improvements and provisional resolutions. Can public and private interests ever be made fully to coincide by legislative and administrative means? Will the commitment of a physician to an individual patient and the commitment of the legislator to the "common good" ever be harmonized in every case? Our anxiety may be too intractable. Our fear of illness and of dying may be so pronounced and immediate that we will seize the nearly automatic connections between privilege, wealth, and power if we can. We will do everything possible to have our kidney machines even if the charts make it clear that many more would benefit from mandatory immunization at a fraction of the cost. And our capacity for taking in rival points of view may be too limited. Once we have witnessed tangible suffering, we cannot just return with ease to public policies aimed at statistical patients. Those who believe that justice is the pre-eminent virtue of institutions and that a case can be convincingly made on behalf of justice for equal access to health care would do well to ponder such conflicts and perplexities. Our reforms might then seem, to ourselves and to others, less abstract and jargon-filled in formulation and less sanguine and piecemeal in substance. They would reflect a greater awareness of what we have to confront.

Notes

1. Much of the research for this paper was done during the Fall Term, 1972–73, when I was on leave in Washington, D.C. I am very grateful for the two appointments which made this leave possible: as Service Fellow, Office of Special Projects, Health Services and Mental Health Administration, Department of Health, Education, and Welfare; and as Visiting Scholar, Kennedy Center for Bioethics, Georgetown University.

2. The issue of priorities is at least threefold: (1) between improved medical care and other social needs, e.g., to restrain auto accidents and pollution; (2) between different sorts of medical treatments for different illnesses, e.g., prevention vs. crisis intervention and exotic treatments; (3) between persons all of whom need a single scarce resource and not all can have it, e.g., Ramsey's

discussion of how to decide among those who are to receive dialysis. Moreover, (1) can be subdivided between (a) improved medical care and other social needs which affect health directly, e.g., drug addiction, auto accidents, and pollution; (b) improved medical care and other social needs which serve the overall aim of community-survival, e.g., a common defense. In the case of (2), one would like to see far more careful discussion of some general criteria which might be employed, e.g., numbers affected, degree of contagion, prospects for rehabilitation, and so on.

3. What sorts of appeals to justice might be cogently made to warrant, for instance, the differentially high income physicians receive? Here are three possibilities: (1) the greater skill and responsibility involved should be rewarded proportionately, i.e., one should attend to considerations of *desert;* (2) there should be *compensation* for the money invested for education and facilities in order to restore circumstances of approximate equality (this argument, while a common one in medical circles, would need to consider that medical education is received in part at public expense and that the modern physician is the highest paid

professional in the country); (3) the difference should benefit the least advantaged more than an alternative arrangement where disparities are less. We prefer a society where the medical profession flourishes and everyone has a longer life expectancy to one where everyone is poverty-striken with a shorter life expectancy ("splendidly equalized destitution"). Yet how are we to ascertain the minimum degree of differential income required for the least advantaged members of the society to be better off?

Discussions of "justice and the interests of providers" are, I think, badly needed. Physicians in the United States have suffered a decline in prestige for various reasons, e.g., the way many used Medicare to support and increase their own incomes. Yet one should endeavor to assess their interests fairly. A concern for professional autonomy is clearly important, though one may ask whether adequate attention has been paid to the distinction between the imposition of cost-controls from outside and interference with professional medical judgments. One may affirm the former, it seems, and still reject—energetically— the latter.

For and Against Equal Access to Health Care

Amy Gutmann

There is a fairly widespread consensus among empirical analysts that access to health care in this country has become more equal in the last quarter century. Agreement tends to end here; debate follows as to whether this trend will or should persist. But before debating these questions, we ought to have a clear idea of what equal access to health care means. Since equality of access to health care cannot be defined in a morally neutral way, we must choose a definition that is morally loaded with a set of values (Daniels, 1981b). The definition offered here is by no means the only possible one. It has,

Reprinted with permission from the author and Milbank Memorial Fund Quarterly/Health and Society, vol. 59, no. 4, 1981, pp. 542–560.

however, the advantage not only of clarity but also of having embedded within it strong and commonly accepted liberal egalitarian values. The debate is better focused upon arguments for and against a strong *principle* of equal access than disputes over definitions, which tend to hide fundamental value disagreements instead of making them explicit.

An equal access principle, clearly stated and understood, can serve at best as an ideal toward which a society committed to equality of opportunity and equal respect for persons can strive. It does not provide a blueprint for social change, but only a moral standard by which to judge marginal changes in our present institutions of health care.

My purpose here is not only to evaluate the strongest criticisms that are addressed to the principle, ranging from libertarian arguments for more market freedom to arguments supporting a more egalitarian principle of health care. I also propose to examine the sorts of theoretical and practical problems that arise when one tries to defend an egalitarian principle directed at a particular set of institutions within an otherwise inegalitarian society. Since it is extremely unlikely that such a society will be transformed all at once into an egalitarian one, there ought to be room within political and philosophical argument for reasoned consideration and advocacy of "partial" distributive justice, i.e., of principles that are directed only to a particular set of social institutions and whose implementation is not likely to create complete justice even within those institutions.

THE PRINCIPLE DEFINED

A principle of equal access to health care demands that every person who shares the same type and degree of health need must be given an equally effective chance of receiving appropriate treatment of equal quality so long as that treatment is available to anyone. Stated in this way, the equal access principle does not establish whether a society must provide any particular medical treatment or heath care benefit to its needy members. I shall suggest later that the level and type of provision can vary within certain reasonable boundaries according to the priorities determined by legitimate democratic procedures. The principle requires that if anyone within a society has an opportunity to receive a service or good that satisfies a health need, then everyone who shares the same type and degree of health need must be given an equally effective chance of receiving that service or good.

Since this is a principle of equal *access,* it does not guarantee equal *results,* although it probably would move our society in that direction. Discriminations in health care are permitted if they are based upon type or degree of health need, willingness of informed adults to be treated, and choices of lifestyle among the population. The equal access principle con-

strains the distribution of opportunities to receive health care to an egalitarian standard, but it does not determine the total level of health care available or the effects of that care (provided the care is of equal quality) upon the health of the population. Of course, even if equality in health care were defined according to an "equal health" principle (Veatch, 1976), one would still have to admit that a just health care system could not come close to producing an equally healthy population, given the unequal distribution of illness among people and our present medical knowledge.

PRACTICAL IMPLICATIONS

Since the equal access principle requires equality of effective opportunity to receive care, not merely equality of formal legal access, it does not permit discriminations based upon those characteristics of people that we can reasonably assume they did not freely choose. Such characteristics include sex, race, genetic endowment, wealth, and, often, place of residence. Even in an ideal society, equally needy persons will not use the same amount of quality of health care. Their preferences and their knowledge will differ as will the skills of the providers who treat them.

A One-Class System

The most striking result of applying the equal access principle in the United States would be the creation of a one-class system of health care. Services and goods that meet health care needs would be equally available to everyone who was equally needy. As a disincentive to overuse, only small fees for service could be charged for health care, provided that charges did not prove a barrier to entry to the poorest people who were needy. A one-class system need not, of course, be a uniform system. Diversity among medical and health care services would be permissible, indeed even desirable (Starr, 1975), so long as the diversity did not create differential access along nonconsensual lines such as wealth, race, sex, or geographical location.

Equal access also places limits upon the market freedoms of some individuals, especially, but not exclusively, the richest members of society. The principle does not permit the purchase of health care to which other similarly needy people do not have effective access. The extent to which freedom of the rich must be restricted will depend upon the level of public provision for health care and the degree of income inequality. As the level of health care guaranteed to the poor decreases and the degree of income inequality increases, the equal access standard demands greater restrictions upon the market freedom of the rich. Where income and wealth are very unevenly distributed, and where the level of publicly guaranteed access is very low, the rich can use the market to buy access to health care goods unavailable to the poor, thereby undermining the effective equality of opportunity required by an equal access principle.

The restriction upon market freedoms to purchase health care under these circumstances creates a certain discomforting irony: the equal access principle permits (or is at least agnostic with respect to) the free market satisfaction of preferences for nonessential consumer goods. Thus, the rigorous implementation of equal access to health care would prevent rich people from spending their extra income for preferred medical services, if those services were not equally accessible to the poor. It would not prevent their using those same resources to purchase satisfactions in other areas—a Porsche or any other luxurious consumer good. In discussing additional problems created by an attempt to implement a principle of equal access to health care in an otherwise inegalitarian society, I return later to consider whether advocates of equal access can avoid this irony.

Hard Cases

As with all principles, hard cases exist for the equal access principle. Without dwelling upon these cases, it is worth considering how the principle might deal with two hard but fairly common cases: therapeutic experimentation in medicine, and alternative treatments of different quality.

Each year in the United States, many potentially successful therapies are tested. Since their

value has not been proved, there may be good reason to limit their use to an appropriate sample of sick experimental subjects. The equal access principle would insist that experimenters choose these subjects at random from a population of relevantly sick consenting adults. A randomized clinical trial could be advertised by public notice, and individuals who are interested might be registered and enrolled on a lottery basis. The only requirement for enrollment would be the health conditions and personal characteristics necessary for proper scientific testing.

How does one apply the principle of equal access when alternative treatments are each functionally adequate but aesthetically or socially quite disparate? Take the hypothetical case of a societal commitment to adequate dentition among adults. Replacement of carious or mobile teeth with dentures may preserve dental function at relatively minor cost. On the other hand, full mouth reconstruction, involving periodontal and endodontal treatment and capping of affected teeth, may be only marginally more effective but substantially more satisfying. The added costs for the preferred treatment are not inconsiderable. The principle would seem to demand that at equal states of dental need there be equal access to the preferred treatment. It is unclear, however, whether the satisfaction of subjective desire is equivalent to fulfillment of objective need.

In cases of alternative treatments, proponents of equal access could turn to another argument for providing access to the same treatments for all. A society that publicly provides the minimal acceptable treatment freely to all, and also permits a private market in more expensive treatments, may result in a two-class system of care. The best providers will service the richest clientele, at the risk of inadequate treatment for the poorest. Approval of a private market in alternative treatments would rest upon the empirical hypothesis that, if the publicly funded level of adequate treatment were high enough, few people would choose to short-circuit the public (i.e., equal access) sector; the small additional free market sector would not threaten to lower the quality of services universally available.

Most cases, like the one of dentistry, are difficult to decide merely on principle. Proponents of equal access must take into account the consequences of alternative policies. But empirical knowledge alone will not decide these issues, and arguments for or against a particular policy can be entertained in a more systematic way once one exposes the values that underlie support for an equal access principle. One can then judge to what extent alternative policies satisfy these values.

SUPPORTING VALUES

Advocates of equal access to health care must demonstrate why health care is different from other consumer goods, unless they are willing to support the more radical principle of equal distribution of all goods. Norman Daniels (1981a) provides one foundation for distinguishing between health care and other goods. He establishes a category of health care needs whose satisfaction provides an important condition for future opportunity. Like police protection and education, some kinds of health care goods are necessary for pursuing most other goods in life. Any theory of justice committed to equalizing opportunity ought to treat health care as a good deserving of special distributive treatment. Equal access to health care provides a necessary, although certainly not a sufficient, condition for equal opportunity in general.

A precept of egalitarian justice that physical pains of a sufficient degree be treated similarly, regardless of who experiences them, establishes another reason for singling out certain kinds of health care as special goods (Gutmann, 1980). Some health conditions cause great pain but are not linked to a serious curtailment of opportunity. The two values are, however, mutually compatible.

A theory of justice that gives priority to the value of equal respect among people might also be used to support a principle of equal access to health care. John Rawls (1971:440), for example, argues that without self-respect "nothing may seem worth doing, or if some things have value for us, we lack the will to strive for them. . . . Therefore the parties in the original

position would wish to avoid at almost any cost the social conditions that undermine self-respect.''

Conditions of Self-Respect

It is not easy to determine what social conditions support or undermine self-respect. One might plausibly assume that equalizing opportunity and treating similar pains similarly would be the most essential supports for equal respect within a health care system. And so, in most cases, the value of equal respect provides additional support for equal access to the same health care goods that are warranted by the values of equal opportunity and relief from pain. But at least some kinds of health care treatment not essential to equalizing opportunity or bringing equal relief from pain may be necessary to equalize respect within a society. It is conceivable that much longer waiting time, in physicians' offices or for admission to hospitals, may not affect the long-term health prospects of the poor or of blacks. But such discriminations in waiting times for an essential good probably do adversely affect the self-respect of those who systematically stand at the end of the queue.

Some of the conditions necessary for equal respect are socially relative; we must arrive at a standard of equal respect appropriate to our particular society. Universal suffrage has long been a condition for equal respect; the case for it is independent of the anticipated results of equalizing political power by granting every person one vote. More recently, equal access to health care has similarly become a condition for equal respect in our society. Most of us do not base our self-respect on the way we are treated on airplanes, even though the flight attendants regularly give preferential treatment to those traveling first class. This contrast with suffrage and health care treatment (and education and police protection) no doubt is related to the fact that these goods are much more essential to our security and opportunities in life than is airplane travel. But it is still worth considering that unequal treatment in health care, as in education, may be understood as a sign of unequal respect even where there are no discernible adverse effects on the health or education of those receiving less favored treatment. Even where a dual health care system will not produce inferior medical results for the less privileged, the value of equal respect militates against the perpetuation of such a system in our society.

CHALLENGES

Equality of opportunity, equal efforts to relieve pain, and equal respect are the three central values providing the foundation of support for a principle of equal access to health care. Any theory of justice that gives primacy to these values (as do many liberal and egalitarian theories) will lend prima facie support to a health care system structured along equal access lines.

We are not in a position to consider alternative values and empirical claims that would lead someone to challenge, or reject, a principle of equal access to health care. These challenges also enable us to elaborate further the moral and political implications of the principle.

Proponents of the Market

The most radical and vocal opposition comes from those who support a pure free market principle in heath care. A foundation of support for the free market principle is the idea that the relative importance of satisfying different human desires is a purely subjective matter: we can distinguish between one person's desire for good medical care and another person's desire for a good Beaujolais only by the price they are willing to pay for each. If no goods are special because there is no way of ranking desires except by individual processes of choice, then what better way than the unconstrained market to allow us to decide among the smorgasbord of goods society has to offer (Fried, 1979; Nozick, 1974; Sade, 1971)?

Health care goods and services are likely to be more equally allocated through the market if income and wealth are more equally distributed. Several defenders of the market as a means of allocating goods and services also support a moderate degree of income redistribution on grounds of its diminishing marginal utility, or because they believe that every person has a right to a "basic minimum" (Friedman, 1962; Fried, 1978). Neither rationale for redistribution takes us very far toward a principle of equal access to health care. If one retains the basic assumption that human preferences are totally subjective, then the market remains the best way to order human priorities. Only the market appropriately decentralizes decision-making and eliminates all nonconsensual exchanges of goods and services (Fried, 1978: 124–26).

Although a minimum income floor under all individuals increases *access* to most goods and services, even at a higher level than that supported by Friedman and others, a guaranteed income will be inadequate to sustain the costs of a catastrophic illness. An exceptionally high guaranteed minimum might result in almost universal insurance coverage at a fairly high level. Supporters of free market allocation do not, however, press for a very high minimum for at least two reasons. They fear its effects on incentives, and they cannot justify a high guaranteed income without admitting that there are many expensive goods that are essential to all persons, and are not just mere consumer preferences.

The first reason for opposing an exceptionally high minimum is probably a good one. A principle approaching equality of income and wealth is likely to have serious disincentive effects on productive work and investment. There are also better reasons for treating health care as a special good, a good that society has an obligation to provide equally to all its members, than there are for equally distributing most consumer goods.

A significant step beyond the pure free market principle is a position that preserves the role of the market in allocating different "packages" of health care according to consumer preferences, but concedes a role for government in supplying every adult with a "voucher" of a certain monetary value redeemable exclusively for health care goods and services. Proponents of health vouchers must assume that there is something special about health care to justify government in taxing its citizens to provide universally for these goods, and not all others. But if health care is a more important good, because it preserves life and expands opportunity, then what is the rationale for effectively limiting the demand a sick but poor person can make upon the health care system? Why should access to health care be dependent upon income or wealth at all?

Opponents of equal access generally imply that more than minimal access will unjustly curtail the freedom of citizens as taxpayers, as consumers, and as providers of health care. Let us consider separately the arguments with regard to the many citizens who are taxpayers and consumers, and the few citizens who are providers of health care.

The Charge of Paternalism

Charles Fried (1976:31) has argued that equal access to health care is a particularly intrusive form of paternalism toward citizens. He claims further that "apart from a rather general commitment to equality and, indeed, to state control of the allocation and distribution of resources, to insist on the right to health care, where that right means a right to equal access, is an anomaly. For as long as our society considers that inequalities of wealth and income are morally acceptable, . . . it is anomalous to carve out a sector like health care and say that *there* equality must reign."

Would an equal access system necessarily be intrusive or paternalistic in its operation? A national health care system simply cannot be said to take away the income entitlement of citizens, since citizens are not entitled to their gross incomes. We can determine our income entitlements only after we deduct from our gross income the amount we owe the state to support the rights of others. To the extent that the rationale of an equal access principle is redistributive, those individuals who otherwise could not afford certain health care services will experience an expansion of their freedom (if we assume an adequate level of social provision). Of course, part of the justification of a national health care system is that it would also guarantee health care coverage to people who could afford adequate health care but who would not be prudent enough to save or to invest in in-

surance. Even if we accept the common definition of paternalistic actions as those that restrict an individual's liberty so as to further his or her interest, we still have to assess the assertion that this (partial) rationale for an equal access system entails a restriction of individual liberty. Unlike a law banning the sale of cigarettes or forcing people to wear seat belts, the institution of a national health care system forces no one to use it. If a majority of citizens decide that they want to be taxed in order to ensure health care for themselves, the resulting legislation could not be considered paternalistic: "Legislation requiring contributions to some cooperative scheme (such as medical care) . . . is not necessarily paternalistic, so long as its purpose is to give effect to the desires of a democratic majority, rather than simply to coerce a minority who do not want the benefits of the legislation" (Thompson, 1980:247). It is significant in this regard that for the past twenty years the Michigan survey of registered voters has found a consistent and solid majority supporting government measures designed to ensure universal access of medical care.

The charge of paternalism levied against an equal access system is therefore dubious because it is extremely difficult, if not impossible, to isolate the self-protectionist rationale from the redistributive and the democratic rationales. Those who object to a national health care system on the grounds that it is coercing some people for their own good forget that such a system still could be justified as a means to avoid the threat to a one-class system that exempting the rich would create. To condemn such a system as paternalistic would commit us to criticizing all legislation in which a democratic majority decides to protect itself against the wishes of a minority when exemption from the resulting policy would undermine it. Other critics wrongly assume that people have an entitlement to the cash equivalent of the medical care to which society grants them a right. People do not have such an entitlement because taxpayers have a right to demand that their tax dollars are spent to satisfy health needs, not to buy luxuries. Indeed, our duty to pay taxes is dependent upon the fact that certain needs of other people must be given priority over our own desires for more commodious living.

Other Restrictions

Nonetheless, two restrictions upon consumer freedom are entailed in an equal access system. One is the restriction imposed by the taxation necessary to provide all citizens, but especially the poorest, with access to health care goods. This restriction does not raise unique or particularly troublesome moral problems so long as one believes that the freedom to retain one's gross income is not an absolute right and that the resulting redistribution of income to the health care sector increases the life chances and thereby the effective freedom of many citizens.

But there is a second restriction of consumer market freedom sanctioned by the equal access principle: the limitation upon freedom to buy health care goods above the level publicly provided. Aside from reasserting the primary values of equality, there is at least one plausible argument for such a restriction. Without restricting the free market in extra health care goods, a society risks having its best medical practitioners drained into the private market sector, thereby decreasing the quality of medical care received by the majority of citizens confined to the publicly funded sector. The lower the level of public provision of health care and the less elastic the supply of physicians, the more problematic (from the perspective of the values underlying equal access) will be an additional market sector in health care.

Without an additional market sector, would the freedom of physicians and other providers to practice wherever and for whomever they choose be unduly restricted? The extent of such restrictions will also vary with the level of public provision and with the diversity of the health care system. Public funds already are crucial to providing many physicians with basic income (through Medicare and Medicaid fees), research opportunities through the National Institutes of Health (NIH), and many with hospitals and other institutions in which to practice (through the provisions of the Hill-Burton act). In place of the time and resources now directed to privately purchased add-ons, an equal access system would redirect providers toward meeting previously unserved needs. These types of redirections of supply and redistributions of demand are commonly accepted in other professions that are oriented toward satisfying an important public interest. The legal and teaching professions are analogous in this regard. The equal access principle, strictly interpreted, however, adds another restriction, a limitation upon private practice that supplies health care goods not equally accessible to the entire population of relevantly needy persons. This restriction upon the freedom of providers does not have an analogue in the present practice of law or of education, although the arguments for equal access to the goods of these professions might be similar. And so, one's assessment of the strength of the case for such a restriction is likely to have implications beyond the health care system.

It is hard to see why one ought to prevent people, rich or poor, from spending money upon health care goods while permitting them to spend money on consumer goods that are clearly not essential, and perhaps even detrimental to health. One reason might be the possible systemic effect, mentioned above, that such additional expenditures would deprive the less advantaged of the best physicians. The freedom of providers as well as consumers would have to be restricted in order to curtail this effect. But beyond this empirically contingent argument for restricting any market in health care goods that are not equally accessible to all, the strict limitations upon market freedom in "extra" health care goods are hard to accept if one believes that medical services are at least as worthy items of expense as other consumer goods. One could argue that physicians ought to be free to meet the demand for additional medical goods, especially when that demand is a substitute for demand for less important goods.

This criticism illuminates a more general problem of attempting to equalize access to any good in an otherwise inegalitarian society. The more unequal the distribution of income and wealth within our society, the more likely that the freedom of consumers and providers to buy and sell health care outside the publicly funded sector will result in inequalities that cannot properly be regarded merely as the product of differences in consumer preferences. Therefore, in an inegalitarian society, we must live with a moral tension between granting providers the freedom to leave the publicly funded sector and achieving more equality in the satisfaction of health care needs.

A principle of equal access to health care applied within an otherwise egalitarian society might give little or no reason to restrict the freedom of providers or consumers. One argument often voiced against a publicly funded system that permits a marginal free-market sector is that the government is a less efficient provider of goods than are private parties. But the equal access principle does not require that the government directly provide medical services through, for example, a national health service. Government need only be a regulator of the use and distribution of essential health-care goods and services. This is a role that most people concede to government for many other purposes deemed essential to the welfare of all individuals.

Government regulation may, of course, be more expensive and hence less efficient than government provision of health care services of similar extent and quality. The tradeoff here would be between the additional market choice facilitated by government regulation of private providers and the decreased public cost of government provision. Despite utilitarian claims to the contrary, no simple moral calculus exists that would enable an impartial spectator to determine where the balance of advantage lies. Philosophers ought to cede to a fairly constituted democratic majority the right to decide this issue. What constitutes a fair process of democratic decision-making is an important question of procedural justice that lies beyond the scope of this paper.

Liability for Voluntary Risks?

Another important criticism of the equal access principle cuts across advocacy of the free market and government regulation of health care. Supporters of both views might consistently ask whether it is fair to provide the same level of access for all people, including those who voluntarily adopt bad health habits, and who quite knowingly and willingly take greater-than-average risks with their lives and health. Even if it might be unjust not to provide health care for those people once the need arises, why would it not be fair to force those who choose to drink, smoke, rock climb, and skydive also to bear a greater burden of their ensuing medical costs than that borne by people who deliberately avoid these risky pursuits? An equal access principle seems to neglect the distinction between voluntary and nonvoluntary health risks in its eagerness to ensure that all people have an equal opportunity to receive appropriate health care.

Gerald Dworkin (1979) extensively and convincingly argues that it would not be unfair to force individuals to be financially liable for voluntarily undertaken health risks, but only under certain conditional assumptions. These include our ability 1) to determine the relative causal role of voluntary versus nonvoluntary factors in the genesis of illness; 2) to differentiate between purely voluntary behavior and what is nonvoluntary or compulsive; and 3) to distinguish between genetic and nongenetic predispositions to illness. For example, to satisfy the first condition one would have to determine the relative causal role of smoking and environmental pollution in the genesis of lung cancer; to fulfill the second, one must know when smoking (or drinking or obesity) is voluntary and when it is compulsive behavior; and to satisfy the third condition, one must distinguish among those who smoke and get cancer, and those who smoke and do not. In addition, so long as there are no good institutional mechanisms for monitoring certain risky activities or for differentiating between moderate and immoderate users of unhealthy substances, qualifying the equal access principle to take account of voluntary health risks is likely to create more unfairness rather than less. Finally, given great inequalities in income distribution, the poor will be less able to bear the consequences of their risky behavior than will the rich, creating a situation of unfairness at least as serious as the unfairness of equally distributing the burdens of health care costs between those who voluntarily impose risks upon themselves and those who do not. With respect to the health hazards of overeating and obesity, for example, the rich have recourse to expensive programs of weight control unavailable to the poor. Since we have such scanty knowledge of situations when sickness can be attributable to voluntary health risks, criticisms of the equal access principle from this perspective have more weight in principle than they do in practice.

Equal Access to All Health Goods

All criticisms considered so far are directed at the equal access principle from a perspective suggesting that government involvement and public funding of health care would be too great and the role of the market too small in an equal access system. Now let us consider a powerful criticism of the principle for including too little, rather than too much, in the public sector. The criticism can be posed in the form of a challenge: if one crucial reason for supporting a principle of equal access is that health goods are much more essential than many other goods because they provide a basis for equalizing opportunity and relieving substantial pain, then why not require a government to provide equal access to *all* those health goods that would move a society further in the direction of equalizing opportunity and relieving pain for the physically and mentally ill? Without pretending that our society could ever arrive at a condition of absolute equality of health (or therefore strict equality of opportunity), proponents of this principle could still argue that we should move as far as possible in that direction.

In a society in which no tradeoffs had to be made between health care and other goods, equal access to *all* health goods might be the most acceptable principle of equity in health care (Veatch, 1976:127–153). Of course, we do not live in such a society. Given the advanced state of our medical and health care technology, and the prevalence of chronic degenerative diseases and mental disorders in our population, a requirement that society provide access to every known health care good would place an enormous drain upon social resources (Somers, 1971).

Costliness per se is not the main issue. The problem with the principle of equal access to all health goods is that it demands an absolute tradeoff between satisfaction of health care needs and other needs and desires. The simplest argument against this principle is that other needs, such as education, police protec-

tion, and legal aid, will be sacrificed to health care, if the principle is enforced. But this argument is too simple. A proponent of equal access to all health goods could consistently establish some priority principle among these goods, all of which satisfy needs derived in large part from a principle of equal opportunity. The weightier counterargument is that, above some less-than-maximum level in the provision of opportunity goods, it seems reasonable for people to value what, for want of a better term, one might call "quality of life" goods: cultural, recreational, noninstrumental educational goods, and even consumer amenities. A society that maximized the satisfaction of needs before it even began to provide access to "quality of life" goods would be a dismal society indeed. Most people do not want to devote their entire lives to being maximally secure and healthy. Why, then, should a society devote all of its resources to satisfying human *needs?*

Democracy and Equal Access

We need to find some principle or procedure by which to draw a line at an appropriate level of access to health care short of what is socially and technologically possible, but greater than what an unconstrained market would afford to most people, particularly to the least advantaged. I suspect that no philosophical argument can provide us with a cogent principle by which we can draw a line within the enormous group of goods that can improve health or extend the life prospects of individuals.

This problem of determining a proper level of guaranteed social satisfaction of need is not unique to health care. Something similar can be said about police protection or education in our society. Philosophers can provide reasons why police protection and education are rightly considered basic collective needs and why they should be given priority over individual consumer preferences. But no plausible philosophical principle can tell us what level of police protection or how much education a society ought to provide on an egalitarian basis.

The principle of equal access to health care establishes a criterion of distribution for whatever level of health care a society provides for any of its members. And further philosophical argument might establish some criteria by which to judge when the publicly funded level of health care was so low as to be unfair to the least advantaged, or so high as to create undue restrictions upon the ability of most people to live interesting and fulfilling lives. The remaining question of establishing a precise level of priorities among health care and other goods (at the "margin") is appropriately left to democratic decision-making. The advantage of the democratic process in determining the precise level of health care provision is that citizens have an equal and collective voice in determining a decision that, according to the equal access principle, ought to be mutually binding. Citizens not only reap the benefits; they also share the burdens of the decision to expand or limit access to health care.

There is yet another advantage to this procedural method of establishing a fair level of health care provision. If the democratic decision will be binding upon all citizens, as the equal access principle assumes it must be, then one might expect the most advantaged citizens to exercise more political pressure to increase access to health care and hence increase the opportunity of the least advantaged above the level that they could afford in a free market system, or in a system where the rich were not included within the publicly funded health care sector. One finds some evidence to support this hypothesis in comparing the relative immunity from budget cutbacks of the program under universal entitlement of Medicare compared with the income-related Medicaid program. Of course, if costliness to the taxpayer is one's only concern, this added political pressure for health care expenditures is a liability rather than a strength of a one-class system. But from the perspective of equal access, the cost of a two-class system, one privately and one publicly funded, is an inequitable distribution of quantity and quality of care according to wealth, not need. The added nonproductive costs required merely to keep the two classes apart are seldom taken into account. And from the perspective of those supporters of an equal access principle who also want to increase the total level of health care provision, the two-class system threatens to work in the opposite direction, siphoning off the pressure of citizens who have a disproportionate share of political influence. A democratic decision, the results of which are constrained by the principle of equal access, will give a relatively accurate reading of what most people believe to be an adequate level of health care protection. The major disadvantage of the equal access constraint is that the decision of the majority or its representatives binds everyone, even those people who want more than the socially mandated level of health care.

Given the great economic inequalities of our society, it is politically impossible for advocates of equal access to fulfill their task. No democratic legislator could possibly succeed in winning support for a proposal that restricted market freedom as extensively as a strict interpretation of the equal access principle requires. And it probably would be a mistake to insist upon strict philosophical standards: one thereby risks throwing the possibility of greater access to health care for the poor out with the insistence upon curtailing access for the rich.

CONCLUSION

I began by arguing that a principle of equal access to health care was at best an ideal toward which our society might strive. I shall end by qualifying that statement. A sufficiently high level of public provision of health care for all citizens and a sufficiently elastic supply of health care would significantly reduce the threat to universal provision of quality health care of a private market in extra health care goods, just as a very high level of police protection and education reduces the inequalities of opportunity resulting from purchase of private bodyguards or of private school education by the rich.

In the best of all imaginable worlds of egalitarian justice, the equal access principle would be sufficiently supported by other egalitarian social and economic institutions that a market in health care would complement rather than undercut the goals of equal respect and opportunity.* In our society, the best that we can

* Editors' Note: At the author's request, the remainder of this paragraph has been substituted for the final sentence of the article as originally published.

reasonably hope to achieve is a more universal and higher level of health care coupled with a greater supply of qualified primary care physicians and paramedics. These measures alone will not satisfy the equal access principle, but they would move us a long way towards fulfilling those ideals that inform support for equal access. It is politically infeasible as well as morally problematic to fulfill the equal access principle by restricting the market in health care goods above the guaranteed social minimum. Recognition of the limits of partial distributive justice thus requires that we be prepared to live with moral deficiencies within a system of health care as long as we live within a fundamentally inegalitarian society. Given the effects of economic and political inequalities upon the distribution of health care in the United States, our best alternative is to strive for imperfection.

References

DANIELS, N. 1981a. Health-Care Needs and Distributive Justice. *Philosophy and Public Affairs* 10:146–179.

———. 1981b. Equity of Access to Health Care: Some Conceptual and Ethical Issues. Paper delivered to *The President's Commission for the Study of Ethical Issues in Medicine and Biomedical and Behavioral Research,* March 13, Washington, D.C.

DWORKIN, G. 1979. Responsibility and Health Risks. Paper delivered to the *Institute of Society, Ethics and the Life Sciences,* Hastings-on-Hudson, New York, October.

FRIED, C. 1976. Equality and Rights in Medical Care. *Hasting Center Report* 6:30–32.

———. 1977. Difficulties in the Economic Analysis of Rights. In Dworkin, G., Bermant, G., Brown, P.G., eds., *Markets and Morals,* 175–195. Washington, D.C.: Hemisphere.

———. 1978. *Right and Wrong.* Cambridge, Mass.: Harvard University Press.

———. 1979. Health Care, Cost Containment, Liberty. Paper delivered to the *Institute of Society, Ethics and the Life Sciences,* Hastings-on-Hudson, New York, October.

FRIEDMAN, M. 1962. *Capitalism and Freedom.* Chicago: Chicago University Press.

GUTMANN, A. 1980. *Liberal Equality.* New York: Cambridge University Press.

NOZICK, R. 1974. *Anarchy, State and Utopia.* New York: Basic Books.

RAWLS, J. 1971. *A Theory of Justice.* Cambridge, Mass.: Harvard University Press.

SADE, R.N. 1971. Medical Care as a Right: A Refutation. *New England Journal of Medicine* 285:1288–1292.

SOMERS, A.R. 1971. *Health Care in Transition: Directions for the Future.* Chicago: Hospital Research and Educational Trust.

STARR, P. 1975. A National Health Program: Organizing Diversity. *The Hastings Center Report* 5:11–13.

THOMPSON, D.F. 1980. Paternalism in Medicine, Law and Public Policy. In Callahan, D., and Bok, S., eds., *Ethics Teaching in Higher Education,* 245–275. New York: Plenum.

VEATCH, R.M. 1976. What Is a "Just" Health Care Delivery? In Veatch, R. M. and Branson, R., eds., *Ethics and Health Policy,* 127–153. Cambridge, Mass.: Ballinger.

From "Public Health as Social Justice"

Dan E. Beauchamp

Anthony Downs[1] has observed that our most intractable public problems have two significant characteristics. First, they occur to a relative minority of our population (even though that minority may number millions of people). Second, they result in significant part from arrangements that are providing substantial benefits or advantages to a majority or to a powerful minority of citizens. Thus solving or minimizing these problems requires painful losses, the restructuring of society and the acceptance of new burdens by the most powerful and the most numerous on behalf of the least powerful or the least numerous. As Downs notes, this bleak reality has resulted in recent years in cycles of public attention to such problems as poverty, racial discrimination, poor housing, unemployment or the abandonment of the aged; however, this attention and interest rapidly wane when it becomes clear that solving these problems requires painful costs that the dominant interests in society are unwilling to pay. Our public ethics do not seem to fit our public problems.

It is not sufficiently appreciated that these same bleak realities plague attempts to protect the public's health. Automobile-related injury and death; tobacco, alcohol and other drug damage; the perils of the workplace; environmental pollution; the inequitable and ineffective distribution of medical care services; the hazards of biomedicine—all of these threats inflict death and disability on a minority of our society at any given time. Further, minimizing or even significantly reducing the death and disability from these perils entails that the majority or powerful minorities accept new burdens or relinquish existing privileges that they presently enjoy. Typically, these new

Abridged and reprinted, with permission of the author and the Blue Cross Association, from *Inquiry*, Vol. XIII, No. 1 (March 1976), pp. 3-14. © 1976 Blue Cross Association. All rights reserved.

burdens or restrictions involve more stringent controls over these and other hazards of the world.

This somber reality suggests that our fundamental attention in public health policy and prevention should not be directed toward a search for new technology, but rather toward breaking existing ethical and political barriers to minimizing death and disability. This is not to say that technology will never again help avoid painful social and political adjustments.[2] Nonetheless, only the technological Pollyannas will ignore the mounting evidence that the critical barriers to protecting the public against death and disability are not the barriers to technological progress—indeed the evidence is that it is often technology itself that is our own worst enemy. The critical barrier to dramatic reductions in death and disability is a social ethic that unfairly protects the most numerous or the most powerful from the burdens of prevention.

This is the issue of justice. In the broadest sense, justice means that each person in society ought to receive his due and that the burdens and benefits of society should be fairly and equitably distributed.[3] But what criteria should be followed in allocating burdens and benefits: Merit, equality or need?[4] What end or goal in life should receive our highest priority: Life, liberty or the pursuit of happiness? The answer to these questions can be found in our prevailing theories or models of justice. These models of justice, roughly speaking, form the foundation of our politics and public policy in general, and our health policy (including our prevention policy) specifically. Here I am speaking of politics not as partisan politics but rather the more ancient and venerable meaning of the political as the search for the common good and the just society.

These models of justice furnish a symbolic framework or blueprint with which to think about and react to the problems of the public, providing the basic rules to classify and categorize problems of society as to whether they necessitate public and collective protection, or whether individual responsibility should prevail. These models function as a sort of map or guide to the common world of members of society, making visible some conditions in society as public issues and concerns, and hiding, obscuring or concealing other conditions that might otherwise emerge as public issues or problems were a different map or model of justice in hand.

In the case of health, these models of justice form the basis for thinking about and reacting to the problems of disability and premature death in society. Thus, if public health policy requires that the majority or a powerful minority accept their fair share of the burdens of protecting a relative minority threatened with death or disability, we need to ask if our prevailing model of justice contemplates and legitimates such sacrifices.

MARKET-JUSTICE

The dominant model of justice in the American experience has been market-justice.[5] Under the norms of market-justice people are entitled only to those valued ends such as status, income, happiness, etc., that they have acquired by fair rules of entitlement, e.g., by their own individual efforts, actions or abilities. Market-justice emphasizes individual responsibility, minimal collective action and freedom from collective obligations except to respect other persons's fundamental rights.

While we have as a society compromised pure market-justice in many ways to protect the public's health, we are far from recognizing the principle that death and disability are collective problems and that all persons are entitled to health protection. Society does not recognize a general obligation to protect the individual against disease and injury. While society does prohibit individuals from causing direct harm to others, and has in many instances regulated clear public health hazards, the norm of market-justice is still dominant and the primary duty to avert disease and injury still

rests with the individual. The individual is ultimately alone in his or her struggle against death.

Barriers to Protection

This individual isolation creates a powerful barrier to the goal of protecting all human life by magnifying the power of death, granting to death an almost supernatural reality.[6] Death has throughout history presented a basic problem to humankind,[7] but even in an advanced society with enormous biomedical technology, the individualism of market-justice tends to retain and exaggerate pessimistic and fatalistic attitudes toward death and injury. This fatalism leads to a sense of powerlessness, to the acceptance of risk as an essential element of life, to resignation in the face of calamity, and to a weakening of collective impulses to confront the problems of premature death and disability.

Perhaps the most direct way in which market-justice undermines our resolve to preserve and protect human life lies in the primary freedom this ethic extends to all individuals and groups to act with minimal obligations to protect the common good.[8] Despite the fact that this rule of self-interest predictably fails to protect adequately the safety of our workplaces, our modes of transportation, the physical environment, the commodities we consume, or the equitable and effective distribution of medical care, these failures have resulted so far in only half-hearted attempts at regulation and control. This response is explained in large part by the powerful sway market-justice holds over our imagination, granting fundamental freedom to all individuals to be left alone—even if the "individuals" in question are giant producer groups with enormous capacities to create great public harm through sheer inadvertence. Efforts for truly effective controls over these perils must constantly struggle against a prevailing ethical paradigm that defines as threats to fundamental freedoms attempts to assure that all groups—even powerful producer groups—accept their fair share of the burdens of prevention.

Market-justice is also the source of another

major barrier to public health measures to minimize death and disability—the category of voluntary behavior. Market-justice forces a basic distinction between the harm caused by a factory polluting the atmosphere and the harm caused by the cigarette or alcohol industries, because in the latter case those that are harmed are perceived as engaged in "voluntary" behavior.[9] It is the radical individualism inherent in the market model that encourages attention to the individual's behavior and inattention to the social preconditions of that behavior. In the case of smoking, these preconditions include a powerful cigarette industry and accompanying social and cultural forces encouraging the practice of smoking. These social forces include norms sanctioning smoking as well as all forms of media, advertising, literature, movies, folklore, etc. Since the smoker is free in some ultimate sense to not smoke, the norms of market-justice force the conclusion that the individual voluntarily "chooses" to smoke; and we are prevented from taking strong collective action against the powerful structures encouraging this so-called voluntary behavior.

Yet another way in which the market ethic obstructs the possibilities for minimizing death and disability, and alibis the need for structural change, is through explanations for death and disability that "blame the victim."[10] Victim-blaming misdefines structural and collective problems of the entire society as individual problems, seeing these problems as caused by the behavioral failures or deficiencies of the victims. These behavioral explanations for public problems tend to protect the larger society and powerful interests from the burdens of collective action, and instead encourage attempts to change the "faulty" behavior of victims.

Market-justice is perhaps the major cause for our over-investment and over-confidence in curative medical services. It is not obvious that the rise of medical science and the physician, taken alone, should become fundamental obstacles to collective action to prevent death and injury. But the prejudice found in market-justice against collective action perverts these scientific advances into an unrealistic hope for "technological shortcuts"[11] to painful social change. Moreover, the great emphasis placed on individual achievement in market-justice has further diverted attention and interest away from primary prevention and collective action by dramatizing the role of the solitary physician-scientist, picturing him as our primary weapon and first line of defense against the threat of death and injury.

The prestige of medical care encouraged by market-justice prevents large-scale research to determine whether, in fact, our medical care technology actually brings about the result desired—a significant reduction in the damage and losses suffered from disease and injury. The model conceals questions about our pervasive use of drugs, our intense specialization, and our seemingly boundless commitment to biomedical technology. Instead, the market model of justice encourages us to see problems as due primarily to the failure of individual doctors and the quality of their care, rather than to recognize the possibility of failure from the structure of medical care itself.[12] Consequently, we seek to remedy problems by trying to change individual doctors through appeals to their ethical sensibilities, or by reshaping their education, or by creating new financial incentives. . . .

Public Health Measures

I have saved for last an important class of health policies—public health measures to protect the environment, the workplace, or the commodities we purchase and consume. Are these not signs that the American society is willing to accept collective action in the face of clear public health hazards?

I do not wish to minimize the importance of these advances to protect the public in many domains. But these separate reforms, taken alone, should be cautiously received. This is because each reform effort is perceived as an isolated exception to the norm of market-justice; the norm itself still stands. Consequently, the predictable career of such measures is to see enthusiasm for enforcement peak and wane. These public health measures are clear signs of hope. But as long as these actions are seen as merely minor exceptions to the rule of individual responsibility, the goals of public health will remain beyond our reach. What is required is for the public to see that protecting the public's health takes us beyond the norms of market-justice categorically, and necessitates a completely new health ethic.

I return to my original point: Market-justice is the primary roadblock to dramatic reductions in preventable injury and death. More than this, market-justice is a pervasive ideology protecting the most powerful or the most numerous from the burdens of collective action. If this be true, the central goal of public health should be ethical in nature: The challenging of market-justice as fatally deficient in protecting the health of the public. Further, public health should advocate a "counter-ethic" for protecting the public's health, one articulated in a different tradition of justice and one designed to give the highest priority to minimizing death and disability and to the protection of all human life against the hazards of this world . . . .

Ideally . . . the public health ethic[13] is not simply an alternative to the market ethic for health—it is a fundamental critique of that ethic as it unjustly protects powerful interests from the burdens of prevention and as that ethic serves to legitimate a mindless and extravagant faith in the efficacy of medical care. In other words, the public health ethic is a *counter-ethic* to market-justice and the ethics of individualism as these are applied to the health problems of the public.

This view of public health is admittedly not widely accepted. Indeed, in recent times the mission of public health has been viewed by many as limited to that minority of health problems that cannot be solved by the market provision of medical care services and that necessitate organized community action.[14] It is interesting to speculate why many in the public health profession have come to accept this narrow view of public health—a view that is obviously influenced and shaped by the market model as it attempts to limit the burdens placed on powerful groups.[15]

Nonetheless, the broader view of public health set out here is logically and ethically justified if one accepts the vision of public health as being the protection of all human life. The central task of public health, then, is to complete its unfinished revolution: The elaboration of a health ethic adequate to protect and preserve all human life. This new ethic has several key implications which are referred to here as "principles"[16]: 1) Controlling the hazards of this world, 2) to prevent death and disability, 3) through organized collective action, 4) shared equally by all except where unequal burdens result in increased protection of everyone's health and especially potential victims of death and disability.

These ethical principles are not new to public health. To the contrary, making the ethical foundations of public health visible only serves to highlight the social justice influences as work behind pre-existing principles.

Controlling the Hazards

A key principle of the public health ethic is the focus on the identification and control of the hazards of this world rather than a focus on the behavioral defects of those individuals damaged by these hazards. Against this principle it is often argued that today the causes of death and disability are multiple and frequently behavioral in origin.[17] Further, since it is usually only a minority of the public that fails to protect itself against most known hazards, additional controls over these perilous sources would not seem to be effective or just. We should look instead for the behavioral origins of most public health problems,[18] asking why some people expose themselves to known hazards or perils, or act in an unsafe or careless manner.

Public health should—at least ideally—be suspicious of behavioral paradigms for viewing public health problems since they tend to "blame the victim" and unfairly protect majorities and powerful interests from the burdens of prevention.[19] It is clear that behavioral models of public health problems are rooted in the tradition of market-justice, where the emphasis is upon individual ability and capacity, and individual success and failure.

Public health, ideally, should not be concerned with explaining the successes and failures of differing individuals (dispositional explanations)[20] in controlling the hazards of this world. Rather these failures should be seen as signs of still weak and ineffective controls or limits over those conditions, commodities, services, products or practices that are either hazardous for the health and safety of members of the public, or that are vital to protect the public's health.

Prevention

Like the other principles of public health, prevention is a logical consequence of the ethical goal of minimizing the numbers of persons suffering death and disability. The only known way to minimize these adverse events is to prevent the occurrence of damaging exchanges or exposures in the first place, or to seek to minimize damage when exposures cannot be controlled.

Prevention, then, is that set of priority rules for restructuring existing market rules in order to maximally protect the public. These rules seek to create policies and obligations to replace the norm of market-justice, where the latter permits specific conditions, commodities, services, products, activities or practices to pose a direct threat or hazard to the health and safety of members of the public, or where the market norm fails to allocate effectively and equitably those services (such as medical care) that are necessary to attend to disease at hand.

Thus, the familiar public health options: [21]

1. Creating rules to minimize exposure of the public to hazards (kinetic, chemical, ionizing, biological, etc.) so as to reduce the rates of hazardous exchanges.

2. Creating rules to strengthen the public against damage in the event damaging exchanges occur anyway, where such techniques (fluoridation, seat-belts, immunization) are feasible.

3. Creating rules to organize treatment resources in the community so as to minimize damage that does occur since we can rarely prevent all damage.

Collective Action

Another principle of the public health ethic is that the control of hazards cannot be achieved through voluntary mechanisms but must be undertaken by governmental or non-governmental agencies through planned, organized and collective action that is obligatory or non-voluntary in nature. This is for two reasons.

The first is because market or voluntary action is typically inadequate for providing what are called public goods. [22] Public goods are those public policies (national defense, police and fire protection, or the protection of all persons against preventable death and disability) that are universal in their impacts and effects, affecting everyone equally. These kinds of goods cannot easily be withheld from those individuals in the community who choose not to support these services (this is typically called the "free rider" problem). Also, individual holdouts might plausibly reason that their small contribution might not prevent the public good from being offered.

The second reason why self-regarding individuals might refuse to voluntarily pay the costs of such public goods as public health policies is because these policies frequently require burdens that self-interest or self-protection might see as too stringent. For example, the minimization of rates of alcoholism in a community clearly seems to require norms or controls over the substance of alcohol that limit the use of this substance to levels that are far below what would be safe for individual drinkers. [23]

With these temptations for individual non-compliance, justice demands assurance that all persons share equally the costs of collective action through obligatory and sanctioned social and public policy.

Fair-Sharing of the Burdens

A final principle of the public health ethic is that all persons are equally responsible for sharing the burdens—as well as the benefits—of protection against death and disability, except where unequal burdens result in greater protection for every person and especially potential victims of death and disability. [24] In practice this means that policies to control the hazards of a given substance, service or commodity fall unequally (but still fairly) on those involved in the production, provision or consumption of the service, commodity or substance. The clear implication of this principle is that the automotive industry, the tobacco industry, the coal industry and the medical care industry—to mention only a few key groups—have an unequal responsibility to bear the costs of reducing death and disability since their actions have far greater impact than those of individual citizens.

DOING JUSTICE: BUILDING A NEW PUBLIC HEALTH

I have attempted to show the broad implications of a public health commitment to protect and preserve human life, setting out tentatively the logical consequences of that commitment in the form of some general principles. We need, however, to go beyond these broad principles and ask more specifically: What implications does this model have for doing public health and the public health profession?

The central implication of the view set out here is that doing public health should not be narrowly conceived as an instrumental or technical activity. Public health should be a way of doing justice, a way of asserting the value and priority of all human life. The primary aim of all public health activity should be the elaboration and adoption of a new ethical model or paradigm for protecting the public's health. This new ethical paradigm will necessitate a heightened consciousness of the manifold forces threatening human life, and will require thinking about and reacting to the problems of disability and premature death as primarily collective problems of the entire society.

These new definitions would reveal the collective and structural aspects of what are termed voluntary risks, challenging attempts to narrowly and persuasively limit public attention to the behavior of the smoker or the drinker, and exposing pervasive myths that "blame the victim."[25] These collective definitions and descriptions would focus attention on the industry behind these activities, asking whether powerful producer groups and supporting cultural and social norms are not primary factors encouraging individuals to accept unreasonable risks to life and limb, and whether these groups or norms constitute aggressive collective structures threatening human life.

A case in point: Under the present definition of the situation, alcoholism is mostly defined in individual terms, mainly in terms of the at-

tributes of those persons who are "unable" to control their drinking. But I have shown elsewhere that this argument is both conceptually and empirically erroneous. Alcohol problems are collective problems that require more adequate controls over this important hazard.[26]

This is not to say that there are no important issues of liberty and freedom in these areas. It is rather to say that viewing the use of, for example, alcohol or cigarettes by millions of American adults as "voluntary" behavior, and somehow fundamentally different from other public health hazards, impoverishes the public health approach, tending (as Terris has suggested)[27] to divorce the behavior of the individual from its social base.

In building these collective redefinitions of health problems, however, public health must take care to do more than merely shed light on specific public health problems. The central problems remain the injustice of a market ethic that unfairly protects majorities and powerful interests from their fair share of the burdens of prevention, and of convincing the public that the task of protecting the public's health lies categorically beyond the norms of market-justice. This means that the function of each different redefinition of a specific problem must be to raise the common and recurrent issue of justice by exposing the aggressive and powerful structures implicated in all instances of preventable death and disability, and further to point to the necessity for collective measures to confront and resist these structures.

I also believe that the realism inherent in the public health ethic dictates that the foundation of all public health policy should be primarily (but not exclusively) national in locus. I simply disagree with the current tendency, rooted in misguided pluralism and market metaphors, to build from the bottom up. This current drift will, in my opinion, simply provide the medical care industry and its acolytes (to cite only one powerful group) with the tools necessary to further elaborate and extend its hegemony. Confronting organizations, interests, ideologies and alliances that are national and even international in scope with such limited resources seems hopelessly sentimental. We must always remember that the forces opposed to full protection of the public's health are fundamental and powerful, deeply rooted in our national character. We are unlikely to successfully oppose these forces with appeals or strategies more appropriate for an earlier and more provincial time.

Finally, the public health movement must cease being defensive about the wisdom or the necessity of collective action. One of the most interesting aspects of market-justice—and particularly its ideological thrusts—is that it makes collective or governmental activity seem unwise if not dangerous. Such rhetoric predictably ignores the influence of private power over the health and safety of every individual. Public health need not be oblivious to the very real concerns about a proliferating bureaucracy in the emergent welfare state. In point of fact, however, the preventive thrust of public health transcends the notion of the welfare or service state and its most recent variant, the human services society. Much as the ideals of service and welfare are improvements over the simple working of market-justice, the service society frequently functions to spread the costs of public problems among the entire public while permitting the interests, industries, or professions who might remedy or prevent many of these problems to operate with expanding power and autonomy.

CONCLUSION

The central thesis of this article is that public health is ultimately and essentially an ethical enterprise committed to the notion that all persons are entitled to protection against the hazards of this world and to the minimization of death and disability in society. I have tried to make the implications of this ethical vision manifest, especially as the public health ethic challenges and confronts the norms of market-justice.

I do not see these goals of public health as hopelessly unrealistic nor destructive of fundamental liberties. Public health may be an "alien ethic in a strange land."[26] Yet, if anything, the public health ethic is more faithful to the traditions of Judeao-Christian ethics than is market-justice.

The image of public health that I have drawn here does raise legitimate questions about what it is to be a professional, and legitimate questions about reasonable limits to restrictions on human liberty. These questions must be addressed more thoroughly than I have done here. Nonetheless, we must never pass over the chaos of preventable disease and disability in our society by simply celebrating the benefits of our prosperity and abundance, or our technological advances. What are these benefits worth if they have been purchased at the price of human lives?

Notes

1. Downs, A. "The Issue-Attention Cycle and the Political Economy of Improving Our Environment," revised version of the Royer Lectures presented at the University of California at Berkeley, April 13–14, 1970.
2. Etzioni, A. and Remp, R. "Technological 'Shortcuts' to Social Change," *Science* 175:31–38 (1972).
3. Jonsen, A. R. and Hellegers, A. E. "Conceptual Foundations for an Ethics of Medical Care," in: Tancredi, L. R. (ed.) *Ethics of Health Care* (Washington, D.C.: National Academy of Sciences, 1974).
4. Outka, E. "Social Justice and Equal Access to Health Care," *The Journal of Religious Ethics* 2:11–32 (1974).
5. Some might object strenuously to the marriage of the two terms "market" and "justice." One theory of the market holds that it is a blind hand that rewards without regard to merit or individual effort. For this point of view, see: Friedman, M. *Capitalism and Freedom* (Chicago: University of Chicago Press, 1962); and Hayek, F. *The Constitution of Liberty* (Chicago: University of Chicago Press, 1960). But Irving Kristol, in his "When Virtue Loses All Her Loveliness," [*The Public Interest* 21:3–15 (1970)], argues that this is a minority view: most accept the marriage of the market ideal and the merits of individual effort and performance. I agree with this point of view—which is to say I see the dominant model of justice in America as a merger of the notions of meritarian and market norms.
6. Marcuse, H. "The Ideology of Death," in: Feifel, H. *The Meaning of Death* (New York: McGraw-Hill, 1959).
7. Illich, I. "The Political Uses of Natural Death," *Hastings Center Studies* 2:3–20 (1974).

8. For excellent discussions of the notion of market "externalities," see: Hardin, G. *Exploring New Ethics for Survival* (Baltimore, Md.: Penguin Books, 1972); Mishan, E. *The Costs of Economic Growth* (New York: Praeger, 1967); and Kapp, W. *Social Costs of Business Enterprise,* 2d ed. (New York: Asia Publishing House, 1964).

9. Brotman, R. and Suffet, F. "The Concept of Prevention and Its Limitations," *The Annals of the American Academy of Political and Social Science* 417:53-65 (1975).

10. Ryan, W. *Blaming the Victim* (New York: Vintage Books, 1971). See Barry, P. "Individual Versus Community Orientation in the Prevention of Injuries," *Preventive Medicine* 4:45-56 (1975), for an excellent discussion of "victim-blaming" in the field of injury-control. Also, see Beauchamp, D. "Alcoholism As Blaming the Alcoholic," *The International Journal of Addictions* 11 (1) (1976); and "The Alcohol Alibi: Blaming Alcoholics," *Society* 12:12-17 (1975), for discussion of the process of victim-blaming in the area of alcoholism policy.

11. Etzioni and Remp, *op cit.*

12. Freidson, E. *Professional Dominance* (Chicago: Aldine, 1971).

13. By the "public health ethic" I mean several things: The assignment of the highest priority to the preservation of human life, the assurance that this protection is extended maximally (consistent with maintaining basic political liberties: See Rawls, *op. cit.,* and note 33), that no person or group should be arbitrarily excluded, and finally that all persons ought accept these burdens of preserving life as just.

14. Two examples of this point: A standard text in health administration, John Hanlon's *Public Health Administration and Practice* (St. Louis, Missouri: C. V. Mosby, 1974), does reference very broad definitions of public health but quickly settles down to discussing public health in terms of those various programs designed to deal with market failures or inadequacies. Nowhere does Hanlon seem to view the concept of public health as an ethical concept standing as a fundamental critique of the existing measures to protect human life. Second, a recent proposed policy statement on prevention for adoption by the American Public Health Association (*The Nation's Health,* October 1975), does give a very high priority to prevention but contains within it a major concession to the norm of market-justice—the category of voluntary or self-imposed risks and the treatment of this category as distinctively different from other public health hazards.

15. Beauchamp, D. "Public Health: Alien Ethic in a Strange Land?" *American Journal of Public Health* 65:1338-1339 (December 1975).

16. I hasten to add that I am not arguing that there are exactly four principles of the public health ethic. Actually, the four offered here can be easily collapsed to two—controls over the hazards of this world and the fair sharing of the burdens of these controls. However, the reason for expanding these two key principles is to draw out the character of the public health ethic as a counter-ethic or counter-paradigm to the market model, and to demonstrate that the public health ethic focuses on different aspects of the world, asserts different priorities and imposes different obligations than the market ethic.

17. Brotman and Suffet, *op. cit.*

18. Sade, R. "Medical Care As A Right: A Refutation," *The New England Journal of Medicine* 285:1288-1292 (1971).

19. Ryan, *op. cit.* See also: Terris, M. "A Social Policy for Health," *American Journal of Public Health* 58: 5-12 (1968).

20. See Brown, R. *Explanation in Social Science* (Chicago: Aldine, 1963) for an excellent discussion of the limitations of dispositional explanations in social science. Also, see Beauchamp, D. "Alcoholism as Blaming the Alcoholic," *op. cit.,* for a further discussion of the pitfalls of dispositional explanations in the specific area of alcohol policy.

21. For excellent discussions of the strategies of public health, see: Haddon, W., Jr. "Energy Damage and the Ten Countermeasure Strategies," *The Journal of Trauma* 13:321-331 (1973); Haddon, W., Jr. "The Changing Approach to the Epidemiology, Prevention, and Amelioration of Trauma," *American Journal of Public Health* 58:1431-1438 (1968); and Terris, M. "Breaking the Barriers to Prevention," paper presented to the Annual Health Conference, New York Academy of Medicine, April 26, 1974.

22. Olson, M. *The Logic of Collective Action* (Cambridge: Harvard University Press, 1965).

23. Beauchamp, D. "Federal Alcohol Policy: Captive to an Industry and a Myth," *Christian Century* 92:788—791 (1975).

24. This principle is similar to Rawls' "difference principle." See Rawls, *op. cit.*

25. Destroying these "myths" could be a major task of public health activity. See Ryan, *op. cit.,* for the best discussion of "victim-blaming" myths. See Beauchamp, "The Alcohol Alibi," *op. cit.,* for a foray against the "myth" of alcoholism. I am using myth here in the specific sense: The

confusion and false definitions that arise when we discuss a *public* problem and an individual idiom. For a good discussion of the concept of myths in general, see Ryle, G. *The Concept of*

Mind (New York: Barnes and Noble, 1949).
26. Beauchamp, ''The Alcohol Alibi,'' *op. cit.*
27. Terris, ''A Social Policy For Health,'' *op. cit.*
28. Terris, ''A Social Policy For Heath,'' *op. cit.*

RESPONSIBILITY FOR HEALTH CARE

From "Socialized Medicine"

Henry E. Sigerist

In a report published last year by the American Foundation, a professor of medicine in a grade A medical school in the Middle West, member of the Association of American Physicians, wrote: ''I do not believe that a patient is entitled to free medical service any more than he is entitled to free housing, free clothing, and free feeding.'' In other words: if a society is unable to provide work for all its members, it is perfectly normal for the unemployed to be evicted from his home and to run around naked, sick, and starving. Such a view is not only barbaric but it is utterly foolish. Nobody seriously believes that any group of unemployed American workers would sit down quietly and wait for death to relieve them. They would kick before they starved, and any government that shared the professor's view would be overthrown at the first major economic crisis.

If our professor's statement represented the general view of American society, there would be no reason for discussing our present system of medical care. Medical service then would be a commodity sold on the market to whoever could afford to purchase it. American society, however, like any other civilized society, feels differently in the matter. It has come to realize that a highly specialized modern industrial nation cannot function normally if its members are sick and that it is a wasteful burden to carry a large number of sick and half sick people. The propertied class, moreover, knows very well that a diseased working class is a menace to its own health. Tuberculosis to-day is largely con-

fined to the low income groups, but venereal diseases have not yet learned to respect class barriers.

Most people agree that it is in the interest of society to fight disease and to provide medical care for the whole population regardless of the economic status of the individual. This is, to begin with, a purely practical and utilitarian consideration. Our attitude, however, is also influenced by humanitarian motives. After all, some of the humanitarian ideals of the nineteenth century are still alive. Every society has many thousands of perfectly useless members, mostly feeble-minded and mentally diseased people who will never be able to work and will never contribute anything to society. And yet we do not destroy them. We consider them unfortunate fellow citizens. We feed them, nurse them, try to provide tolerable living conditions for them, hoping that science, some day, will give us sufficient data to allow us to reduce their number.

There are people to-day—their number is increasing—who think that man has a right to health. The chief cause of disease is poverty. If we are unable to provide work for everybody and to guarantee a decent standard of living to every individual willing to work, whatever his intelligence may be, we are collectively responsible for the chief cause of disease. The least we can do is to make provisions for the protection and restoration of the people's health. They have an undeniable right to such provisions.

Once we accept the principle that medical care must be available to all, we must examine whether the people actually receive the services they need, under the present system. There are still doctors who pretend quite ingenuously that there is not one man in the United States who could not get medical care in case of illness if he took the trouble to ask for it. They point out proudly that our hospitals have charity wards and that the medical profession, conscious of its humanitarian traditions, has always been ready to help the poor without remuneration.

Nobody will deny the good will and idealism of the medical profession. It has made desperate efforts to remain a liberal profession and has refused steadily but in vain to be dragged into business, into a competitive world that is ruled by iron economic necessities. The doctors are not responsible for the fact that the social and economic structure of society has changed. They did the best they could and kept to the job under increasingly adverse conditions. Their good will and idealism are still wanted, more than ever before; not for charity services, however, but to enable them to face the present conditions with an open mind and courageously, and to cooperate in their readjustment.

Long before the depression, it was felt that medicine had infinitely more to give than the people actually received. At the height of prosperity, in 1928, the Committee on the Costs of Medical Care was appointed to survey conditions. Whoever looked around without prejudice saw people, many people, who had not sufficient medical care. We all knew families whose budget was wrecked by a sudden illness, and we all had friends who hesitated to enter a hospital or to undergo certain treatments because they could not afford them. The many reports of the Committee on the Costs of Medical Care gave us facts and figures for what we vaguely knew, and demonstrated unmistakably that large sections of our population lacked adequate medical care.

If any doubts are left, they will be dispelled by the results of the National Health Survey that was undertaken by the United States Public Health Service as a W.P.A. project. From preliminary reports we already know that the lower a family's income is, the higher is the incidence of disease and the smaller the volume of medical care received. We know that hundreds of thousands of cases of illness are needless and could have been prevented, that

many thousands of people die prematurely; and we also know that one-third of the population of this wealthy country is not only ill-fed, ill-housed, and ill-clothed, but also ill-cared for in sickness.

The facts that have become known as a result of the various surveys are so overwhelming that even the American Medical Association could not ignore them and had to admit recently that ''a varying number of people may at times be insufficiently supplied with medical service.''

The present conditions are not only most depressing and harmful to society but also unnecessary and stupid in a country that has such splendid medical equipment. No country in the world has a better standard of physicians, public health officers, nurses, and social workers; no country has better hospital or laboratory facilities. It is almost a miracle how the United States in less than half a century caught up with European medicine and surpassed it in many respects. Accumulated wealth and the wisdom of a group of medical leaders made it possible. And yet, one-third of the population has no medical service or not enough, and great possibilities of preventive medicine have not even been considered yet.

The cause of this maladjustment is easy to guess. Medical service, as a result of the progress of medicine, has become increasingly expensive. A hundred years ago a man with an indefinite pain in his belly went to see a doctor who asked a few questions, palpated the abdomen, and prescribed a laxative. The procedure did not cost much. Most people could afford the fee, or if they were totally indigent they were given the advice free of charge. In most such cases, the patient recovered as he probably would have done without consulting a doctor. In some cases, however, a tumor possibly developed from which the patient died.

The same type of patient consulting a doctor to-day has a series of X-ray pictures and a number of laboratory tests made which may lead to the early recognition of a disease at a time when successful treatment is still possible. It is obvious, however, that such an examination, not to mention the treatment, costs money, more than most people can afford to pay at the time.

In other words, it is not only difficult for the

indigent to secure for himself adequate medical care, but for all families of moderate income, all those whose income does not exceed $3,000 or even more. This, however means more than three quarters of the entire population. The fee-for-service system may have worked—I doubt if it ever did—as long as medicine had little to give. Today it is impossible to protect the people's health effectively under any such system because there is too wide a gap between the scientific status of medicine and the economic status of the population. Therefore, if we think that the people's health is a major concern of society, we must necessarily devise some other system.

Voluntary Risks to Health: The Ethical Issues

Robert M. Veatch

In an earlier era, one's health was thought to be determined by the gods or by fate. The individual had little responsibility for personal health. In terms of the personal responsibility for health and disease, the modern medical model has required little change in this view. One of the primary elements of the medical model was the belief that people were exempt from responsibility for their condition.[1] If one had good health in old age, from the vantage point of the belief system of the medical model, one would say he had been blessed with good health. Disease was the result of mysterious, uncontrollable microorganisms or the random process of genetic fate.

A few years ago we developed a case study[2] involving a purely hypothetical proposal that smokers should be required to pay for the costs of their extra health care required over and above that of nonsmokers. The scheme involved taxing tobacco at a rate calculated to add to the nation's budget an amount equal to the marginal health cost of smoking.

Recently a number of proposals have been put forth that imply that individuals are in some sense personally responsible for the state of their health. The town of Alexandria, Va, refuses to hire smokers as fire fighters, in part because smokers increase the cost of health and disability insurance (*The New York Times,* Dec. 18, 1977, p. 28). Oral Roberts University insists that students meet weight requirements to attend school. Claiming that the school was concerned about the whole person, the school dean said that the school was just as concerned about the students' physical growth as their intellectual and spititual growth (*The New York Times,* Oct. 9, 1977, p. 77). Behaviors as highly diverse as smoking, skiing, playing professional football, compulsive eating, omitting exercise, exposing oneself excessively to the sun, skipping needed immunizations, automobile racing, and mountain climbing all can be viewed as having a substantial voluntary component. Health care needed as a result of any voluntary behavior might generate very different claims on a health care system from care conceptualized as growing out of some other causal nexus. Keith Reemtsma, MD, chairman of the Department of Surgery at Columbia University's College of Physicians and Surgeons, has called for "a more rational approach to improving national health," involving "a reward/punishment system based on individual choices." Persons who smoked cigarettes, drank whiskey, drove cars, and owned guns would be taxed for the medical consequences of their choices (*The New York Times,* Oct. 14, 1976, p. 37). That individuals should be personally responsible for their health is a new theme, implying a new model for health care and perhaps for funding of health care.[3-6]

Reprinted by permission of the author and the American Medical Association from *JAMA,* vol. 243, no. 1, January 4, 1980, pp. 50–55. Copyright 1980, American Medical Association.

Some data correlating life-style to health status are being generated. They seem to support the conceptual shift toward a model that sees the individual as more personally responsible for his health status. The data of Belloc and Breslow[7-9] make those of us who lead the slovenly life-style very uncomfortable. As Morison[3] has pointed out, John Wesley and his puritan brothers of the covenant may not have been far from wrong after all. Belloc and Breslow identify seven empirical correlates of good health: eating moderately, eating regularly, eating breakfast, no cigarette smoking, moderate or no use of alcohol, at least moderate exercise, and seven to eight hours of sleep nightly. They all seem to be well within human control, far less mysterious than the viruses and genes that exceed the comprehension of the average citizen. The authors found that the average physical health of persons aged 70 years who reported all of the preceding good health practices was about the same as persons aged 35 to 44 years who reported fewer than three.

We have just begun to realize the policy implications and the ethical impact of the conceptual shift that begins viewing health status as, in part, a result of voluntary risk taking in personal behavior and life-style choices. If individuals are responsible to some degree for their health and their need for health resources, why should they not also be responsible for the costs involved? If national health insurance is on the horizon, it will be even more questionable that individuals should have such health care paid for out of the same money pool generated by society to pay for other kinds of health care. Even with existing insurance plans, is it equitable that all persons contributing to the insurance money pool pay the extra costs of those who voluntarily run the risk of increasing their need for medical services?

The most obvious policy proposals—banning from the health care system risky behaviors and persons who have medical needs resulting from such risks—turns out to be the least plausible.[10-11] For one thing, it is going to be extremely difficult to establish precisely the cause of the lung tumor at the time the patient is standing at the hospital door. Those who have carcinoma of the lung possibly from smoking or from unknown causes should not be excluded.

Even if the voluntary component of the cause could be determined, it is unlikely that our society could or would choose to implement a policy of barring the doors. While we have demonstrated a capacity to risk statistical lives or to risk the lives of citizens with certain socioeconomic characteristics, it is unlikely that we would be prepared to follow an overall policy of refusing medical service to those who voluntarily brought on their own conditions. We fought a similar battle over social security and concluded that—in part for reasons of the stress placed on family members and on society as a whole—individuals would not be permitted to take the risk of staying outside the social security system.

A number of policy options are more plausible. Additional health fees on health-risk behavior calculated to reimburse the health care system would redistribute the burden of the cost of such care to those who have chosen to engage in it. Separating health insurance pools for persons who engage in health-risk behavior and requiring them to pay out of pocket the marginal cost of their health care is another alternative. In some cases the economic cost is not the critical factor; it may be scarce personnel or equipment. Some behaviors might have to be banned to free the best neurosurgeons or orthopedic specialists for those who need their services for reasons other than for injuries suffered from the motorcycle accident or skiing tumble. Of course, all of these policy options require not only judgments about whether these behaviors are truly voluntary, but also ethical judgments about the rights and responsibilities of the individual and the other, more social components of the society.

There are several ethical principles that could lead us to be concerned about these apparently voluntary behaviors and even lead us to justify decisions to change our social policy about paying for or providing health care needed as a result of such behavior. The most obvious, the most traditional, medical ethical basis for concern is that the welfare of the individual is at stake. The Hippocratic tradition is committed to having the physician do what he thinks will benefit the patient. If one were developing an insurance policy or a mode of approaching the individual patient for private practice, paternalistic concern about the medical welfare of the patient might lead to a conclusion that, for the good of the patient, this behavior ought to be prevented or deferred. The paternalistic Hippocratic ethic, however, is suspect in circles outside the medical profession and is even coming under attack from within the physician community itself.[12] The Hippocratic ethic leaves no room for the principle of self-determination—a principle at the core of liberal Western thought. The freedom of choice to smoke, ski, and even race automobiles may well justify avoiding more coercive policies regarding these behaviors—assuming that it is the individual's own welfare that is at stake. The hyperindividualistic ethics of Hippocratism also leaves no room for concern for the welfare of others or the distribution of burdens with the society. A totally different rationale for concern is being put forward, however. Some, such as Tom Beauchamp,[13] have argued that we have a right to be concerned about such behaviors because of their social costs. He leaves unanswered the question of why it would be considered fair or just to regulate these voluntary behaviors when and only when their total social costs exceed the total social benefits of the behavior. This is a question we must explore.

Clearly, the argument is a complex one requiring many empirical, conceptual, and ethical judgments. Those judgments will have to be made regardless of whether we decide to continue the present policy or adopt one of the proposed alternatives. At this point, we need a thorough statement of the kinds of questions that must be addressed and the types of judgments that must be made.

ARE HEALTH RISKS VOLUNTARY?

The first question, addressed to those advocating policy shifts based on the notion that persons are in some sense responsible for their own health, melds the conceptual and empirical issues. Are health risks voluntary? Several models are competing for the conceptual attention of those working in the field.

The Voluntary Model. The model that considers the individual as personally responsible for his health has a great deal going for it. The empirical correlations of life-style choices with health status are impressive. The view of humans as personally responsible for their destiny is attractive to those of us within modern Western society. Its appeal extends beyond the view of the human as subject to the forces of fate and even the medical model, which as late as the 1950s saw disease as an attack on the individual coming from outside the person and outside his control.

The Medical Model. Of course, that it is attractive cannot justify opting for the voluntarist model if it flies in the face of the empirical reality. The theory of external and uncontrollable causation is central to the medical model.[14] It is still probably the case that organic causal chains almost totally outside human control account now and then for a disease. But the medical model has been under such an onslaught of reality testing in the last decade that it can hardly provide a credible alternative to the voluntarist model. Even for those conditions that undeniably have an organic causal component, the luxury of human innocence is no longer a plausible defense against human accountability. The more we learn about disease and health and their causal chains, the more we have the possibility of intervening to change those chains of causation. Since the days of the movement for public health, sanitation, and control of contagion, there has been a rational basis for human responsibility. Even for those conditions that do not yet lend themselves to such direct voluntary control, the chronic diseases and even genetic diseases, there exists the possibility of purposeful, rational decisions that have an indirect impact on the risk. Choices can be made to minimize our exposure to potential carcinogens and risk factors for cardiovascular disease. Parents now have a variety of potential choices to minimize genetic disease risk and even eliminate it in certain cases. We may not be far from the day when we can say that all health problems can be viewed as someone's fault—if not our own fault for poor sanitary practices and life-style choices, then the fault of our parents for avoiding carrier status diagnosis, amniocentesis, and selective abortion; the fault of industries that pollute our environment; or the fault of the National Institutes of Health for failing to make the scientific breakthroughs to understand the causal chain so that we could intervene. Although there remains a streak of plausibility in the medical model as an account of disease and health, it is fading rapidly and may soon remain only as a fossil-like trace in our model of health.

The Psychological Model. While the medical model seems to offer at best a limited counter to the policy options rooted in the voluntarist model, other theories of determinism may be more plausible. Any policy to control health care services that are viewed as necessitated by voluntary choices to risk one's health is based on the judgment that the behavior is indeed voluntary. The primary argument countering policies to tax or control smoking to be fair in distributing the burdens for treating smokers' health problems is that the smoker is not really responsible for his medical problems. The argument is not normally based on organic or genetic theories of determinism, but on more psychological theories. The smoker's personality and even the initial pattern of smoking are developed at such an early point in life that they could be viewed as beyond voluntary control. If the smoker's behavior is the result of toilet training rather than rational decision making, then to blame the smoker for the toilet training seems odd.

Many of the other presumably voluntary risks to health might also be seen as psychologically determined and therefore not truly voluntary. Compulsive eating, the sedentary lifestyle, and the choice of a high-stress life pattern may all be psychologically determined.

Football playing is a medically risky behavior. For the professional, the choice seems to be made consciously and voluntarily. But the choice to participate in high school and even grade school competitive leagues may not really be the voluntary choice of the student. Then, if reward systems are generated from these early choices, certainly college level football could be the result. The continuum from partially nonvoluntary choices of the youngster to the career choice of professional athlete may have a heavy psychological overlay after all.

If so-called voluntary health risks are really psychologically determined, then the ethical

and policy implications collapse. But it must seriously be questioned whether the model of psychological determinism is a much more plausible monocausal explanation of these behaviors than the medical model. Choosing to be a professional football player, or even to continue smoking, simply cannot be viewed as determined and beyond personal choice because of demonstrated irresistible psychological forces. The fact that so many people have stopped smoking or drinking or even playing professional sports reveals that such choices are fundamentally different from monocausally determined behaviors. Although state of mind may be a component in all disease, it seems that an attempt to will away pneumonia or a carcinoma of the pancreas is much less likely to be decisively influential than using the will to control the behaviors that are now being grouped as voluntary.

The Social Structural Model. Perhaps the most plausible competition to the voluntarist model comes not from a theory of organic or even psychological determinism, but from a social structural model. The correlations of disease, mortality, and even so-called voluntary health-risk behavior with socioeconomic class are impressive. Recent data from Great Britain and from the Medicaid system in the United States[15] reveal that these correlations persist even with elaborate schemes that attempt to make health care more equitably available to all social classes. In Great Britain, for instance, it has recently been revealed that differences in death rates by social class continue, with inequalities essentially undiminished, since the advent of the National Health Service. Continuing to press the voluntarist model of personal responsibility for health risk in the face of a social structural model of the patterns of health and disease could be nothing more than blaming the victim,[16-19] avoiding the reality of the true causes of disease, and escaping proper social responsibility for changing the underlying social inequalities of the society and its modes of production.

This is a powerful counter to the voluntarist thesis. Even if it is shown that health and disease are governed by behaviors and risk factors subject to human control, it does not follow that the individual should bear the sole or even primary responsibility for bringing about the changes necessary to produce better health. If it is the case that for virtually every disease, those who are the poorest, those who are in the lowest socioeconomic classes, are at the greatest risk,[20-22] then there is a piously evasive quality to proposals that insist on individuals changing their life-styles to improve their positions and their health potential. The smoker may not be forced into his behavior so much by toilet training as by the social forces of the workplace or the society. The professional football player may be forced into that role by the work alternatives available to him, especially if he is a victim of racial, economic, and educational inequities.

If one had to make a forced choice between the voluntarist model and the social structural model, the choice would be difficult. The knowledge that some socially deprived persons have pulled themselves up by their bootstraps is cited as evidence for the voluntarist model, but the overwhelming power of the social system to hold most individuals in their social place cannot be ignored.

A Multicausal Model and Its Implications. The only reasonable alternative is to adopt a multicausal model, one that has a place for organic, psychological, and social theories of causation, as well as voluntarist elements, in an account of the cause of a disease or health pattern. One of the great conceptual issues confronting persons working in this area will be whether it is logically or psychologically possible to maintain simultaneously voluntarist and deterministic theories. In other areas of competing causal theories, such as theories of crime, drug addiction, and occupational achievement, we have not been very successful in maintaining the two types of explanation simultaneously. I am not convinced that it is impossible. A theory of criminal behavior that simultaneously lets the individual view criminal behavior as voluntary while the society views it as socially or psychologically determined has provocative and attractive implications. In the end it may be no more illogical or implausible than a reductionistic, monocausal theory.

The problem parallels one of the classic problems of philosophy and theology: How is it that there can be freedom of the will while at the same time the world is orderly and predictable? In more theological language, how can humans be free to choose good and evil while at the same time affirming that they are dependent on divine grace and that there is a transcendent order to the world? The tension is apparent in the Biblical authors, the Pelagian controversy of the fourth century, Arminius's struggle with the Calvinists, and contemporary secular arguments over free will. The conclusion that freedom of choice is a pseudo-problem, that it is compatible with predictability in the social order, may be the most plausible of the alternative, seemingly paradoxical answers.

The same conclusions may be reached regarding voluntary health risks. It would be a serious problem if a voluntarist theory led to abandoning any sense of social structural responsibility for health patterns. On the other hand, it seems clear that there are disease and health differentials even within socioeconomic classes and that some element of voluntary choice of life-style remains that leads to illness, even for the elite of the capitalist society and even for the members of the classless society. The voluntarist model seems at least to apply to differentials in behavior within socioeconomic classes or within groups similarly situated. Admitting the possibility of a theory of causation that includes a voluntary element may so distract the society from attention to the social and economic components in the causal nexus that the move would become counterproductive. On the other hand, important values are affirmed in the view that the human is in some sense responsible for his own medical destiny, that he is not merely the receptacle for external forces. These values are important in countering the trend toward the professionalization of medical decisions and the reduction of the individual to a passive object to be manipulated. They are so important that some risk may well be necessary. This is one of the core problems in any discussion of the ethics of the voluntary health-risk perspective. One of the most difficult research questions posed by the voluntary health-risk theme is teasing out the implications of the theme for a theory of the causation of health patterns.

RESPONSIBILITY AND CULPABILITY

Even in cases where we conclude that the voluntarist model may be relevant—where voluntary choices are at least a minor component of the pattern of health—it is still unclear what to make of the voluntarist conclusion. If we say that a person is responsible for his health, it still does not follow that the person is culpable for the harm that comes from voluntary choices. It may be that society still would want to bear the burden of providing health care needed to patch up a person who has voluntarily taken a health risk.

To take an extreme example, a member of a community may choose to become a professional fire fighter. Certainly this is a health-risking choice. Presumably it could be a relatively voluntary one. Still it does not follow that the person is culpable for the harms done to his health. Responsible, yes, but culpable, no.

To decide in favor of any policy incorporating the so-called presumption that health risks are voluntary, it will be necessary to decide not only that the risk is voluntary, but also that it is not worthy of public subsidy. Fire fighting, an occupation undertaken in the public interest, probably would be worthy of subsidy. It seems that very few such activities, however, are so evaluated. Professional automobile racing, for instance, hardly seems socially ennobling, even if it does provide entertainment and diversion. A more plausible course would be requiring auto racers to purchase a license for a fee equal to their predicted extra health costs.

But what about the health risks of casual automobile driving for business or personal reasons? There are currently marginal health costs that are not built into the insurance system, eg, risks from automobile exhaust pollution, from stress, and from the discouraging of exercise. It seems as though, in principle, there would be nothing wrong with recovering the economic part of those costs, if it could be done. A health tax on gasoline, for instance, might be sensible as a progressive way of funding a national health service. The evidence for the direct causal links and the exact costs will be hard, probably impossible, to discover. That

difficulty, however, may not be decisive, provided there is general agreement that there are some costs, that the behavior is not socially ennobling, and that the funds are obtained more or less equitably in any case. It would certainly be no worse than some other luxury tax.

THE ARGUMENTS FROM JUSTICE

The core of the argument over policies deriving from the voluntary health-risks thesis is the argument over what is fair or just. Regardless of whether individuals have a general right to health care, or whether justice in general requires the social provision of health services, it seems as though what justice requires for a risk voluntarily assumed is quite different from what it might require in the most usual medical need.

Two responses have been offered to the problem of justice in providing health care for medical needs resulting from voluntarily assumed risks. One by Dan Beauchamp[19, 23] and others resolves the problem by attacking the category of voluntary risk. He implies that so-called voluntary behaviors are, in reality, the result of social and cultural forces. Since voluntary behavior is a null set, the special implications of meritorious or blameworthy behavior for a theory of justice are of no importance. Beauchamp begins forcefully with a somewhat egalitarian theory of social justice, which leads to a moral right to health for all citizens. There is no need to amend that theory to account for fairness of the claims of citizens who bring on their need for health care through their voluntary choices, because there are no voluntary choices.

It seems reasonable to concede to Dan Beauchamp that the medical model has been overly individualistic, that socioeconomic and cultural forces play a much greater role in the causal nexus of health problems than is normally assumed. Indeed, they probably play the dominant role. But the total elimination of voluntarism from our understanding of human behavior is quite implausible. Injuries to the socioeconomic elite while mountain climbing or waterskiing are not reasonably seen as primarily the result of social structural determinism. If there remains a residuum of the voluntary theory, then one of justice for health care will have to take that into account.

A second approach is that of Tom Beauchamp,[13] who goes further than Dan Beauchamp. He attacks the principle of justice itself. Dan Beauchamp seems to hold that justice or fairness requires us to distribute resources according to need. Since needs are not the result of voluntary choices, a subsidiary consideration of whether the need results from foolish, voluntary behavior is unnecessary. Tom Beauchamp, on the other hand, rejects the idea that needs per se have a claim on us as a society. He seems to accept the idea that at least occasionally behaviors may be voluntary. He questions whether need alone provides a plausible basis for deciding what is fair in cases where the individual has voluntarily risked his health and is subsequently in need of medical services. He offers a utilitarian alternative, claiming that the crucial dimension is the total social costs of the behaviors. He argues:

> Hazardous personal behaviors should be restricted if, and only if: (1) the behavior creates risks of harm to persons other than those who engage in such activities, and (2) a cost-benefit analysis reveals that the social investment in controlling such behaviors would produce a net increase in social utility, rather than a net decrease.

The implication is that any social advantage to the society that can come from controlling these behaviors would justify intervention, regardless of how the benefits and burdens of the policy are distributed.

A totally independent, nonpaternalistic argument is based much more in the principle of justice. This approach examines not only the impact of disease, but also questions of fairness. It is asked, is it fair that society as a whole should bear the burden of providing medical care needed only because of voluntarily taken risks to one's health? From this point of view, even if the net benefit of letting the behavior continue exceeded the benefits of prohibiting it, the behavior justifiably might be prohibited, or at least controlled, on nonpaternalistic grounds. Consider the case, for instance, where the benefits accrue overwhelmingly to persons who do engage in the behavior and the costs to those who do not. If the need for medical care is the result of the voluntary choice to engage in the behavior, then those arguing from the standpoint of equity or fairness might conclude that the behavior should still be controlled even though it produces a net benefit in aggregate.

Both Beauchamps downplay a secondary dimension of the argument over the principle of justice. Even those who accept the egalitarian formula ought to concede that all an individual is entitled to is an equal opportunity for a chance to be as healthy, insofar as possible, as other people.[24] Since those who are voluntarily risking their health (assuming for the moment that the behavior really is voluntary) do have an opportunity to be healthy, it is not the egalitarian dimensions of the principle of justice that are relevant to the voluntary health-risks question. It is the question of what is just treatment of those who have had opportunity and have not taken advantage of it. The question is one of what to do with persons who have not made use of their chance. Even the most egalitarian theories of justice— of which I consider myself to be a proponent— must at times deal with the secondary question of what to do in cases where individuals voluntarily have chosen to use their opportunities unequally. Unless there is no such thing as voluntary health-risk behavior, as Dan Beauchamp implies, this must remain a problem for the more egalitarian theories of justice.

In principle I see nothing wrong with the conclusion, which even an egalitarian would hold, that those who have not used fairly their opportunities receive inequalities of outcome. I emphasize that this is an argument in principle. It would not apply to persons who are truly not equal in their opportunity because of their social or psychological conditions. It would not apply to those who are forced into their health-risky behavior because of social oppression or stress in the mode of production.

From this application of a subsidiary component of the principle of justice, I reach the conclusion that it is fair, that it is just, if persons in need of health services resulting from true, voluntary risks are treated differently from those in need of the same services for other reasons. In fact, it would be unfair if the two groups were treated equally.

For most cases this would justify only the funding of the needed health care separately in cases where the need results from voluntary behavior. In extreme circumstances, however, where the resources needed are scarce and cannot be supplemented with more funds (eg, when it is the skill that is scarce), then actual prohibition of the behavior may be the only plausible option, if one is arguing from this kind of principle of justice.

This essentially egalitarian principle, which says that like cases should be treated alike, leaves us with one final problem under the rubric of justice. If all voluntary risks ought to be treated alike, what do we make of the fact that only certain of the behaviors are monitorable? Is it unfair to place a health tax on smoking, automobile racing, skiing at organized resorts with ski lifts, and other organized activities that one can monitor, while letting slip by failing to exercise, climbing, mountain skiing on the hill on one's farm, and other behaviors that cannot be monitored? In a sense it may be. The problem is perhaps like the unfairness of being able to treat the respiratory problems of pneumonia, but not those of trisomy E syndrome or other incurable diseases. There may be some essential unfairness in life. This may appear in the inequities of policy proposals to control or tax monitorable behavior, but not behavior that cannot be monitored. Actually some ingenuity may generate ways to tax what seems untaxable —taxing gasoline for the health risks of automobiles, taxing mountain climbing equipment (assuming it is not an ennobling activity), or creating special insurance pools for persons who eat a bad diet. The devices probably would be crude and not necessarily in exact proportion to the risks involved. Some people engaged in equally risky behaviors probably would not be treated equally. That may be a necessary implication of the crudeness of any public policy mechanism. Whether the inequities of not being able to treat equally people taking comparable risks constitute such a serious problem that it would be better to abandon entirely the principle of equality of opportunity for health is

the policy question that will have to be resolved.

COST-SAVING HEALTH-RISK BEHAVIORS

Another argument is mounted against the application of the principle of equity to voluntarily health-risking behaviors. What ought to be done with behaviors that are health risky, but that end up either not costing society or actually saving society's scarce resources? This question will separate clearly those who argue for intervention on paternalistic grounds from those who argue on utilitarian grounds or on the basis of the principle of justice. What ought to be done about a behavior that would risk a person's health, but risk it in such a way that he would die rapidly and cheaply at about retirement age? If the concern is from the unfair burden that these behaviors generate on the rest of society, and, if the society is required to bear the costs and to use scarce resources, then a health-risk behavior that did not involve such social costs would surely be exempt from any social policy oriented to controlling such unfair behavior. In fact, if social utility were the only concern, then this particular type of risky behavior ought to be encouraged. Since our social policy is one that ought to incorporate many ethical concerns, it seems unlikely that we would want to encourage these behaviors even if such encouragement were cost-effective. This, indeed, shows the weakness of approaches that focus only on aggregate costs and benefits.

REVULSION AGAINST THE RATIONAL, CALCULATING LIFE

There is one final, last-ditch argument against adoption of a health policy that incorporates an equitable handling of voluntary health risks. Some would argue that, although the behavior might be voluntary and supplying health care to meet the resulting needs unfair to the rest of the society, the alternative would be even worse. Such a policy might require the conversion of many decisions in life from spontaneous expressions based on long tradition and life-style patterns to cold, rational, calculating decisions based on health and economic elements.

It is not clear to me that that would be the result. Placing a health fee on a package of cigarettes or on a ski-lift ticket may not make those decisions any more rational calculations than they are now. The current warning on tobacco has not had much of an impact. Even if rational decision making were the outcome, however, I am not sure that it would be wrong to elevate such health-risking decisions to a level of consciousness in which one had to think about what one was doing. At least it seems that as a side effect of a policy that would permit health resources to be paid for and used more equitably, this would not be an overwhelming or decisive counterargument.

CONCLUSION

The health policy decisions that must be made in an era in which a multicausal theory is the only plausible one are going to be much harder than the ones made in the simpler era of the medical model—but then, those were harder than some of the ones that had to be made in the era where health was in the hands of the gods. Several serious questions remain to be answered. These are both empirical and normative. They may constitute a research agenda for pursuing the question of ethics and health policy for an era when some risks to health may be seen, at least by some people, as voluntary.

Notes

1. Parsons T: *The Social System,* New York, The Free Press, 1951, p. 437.
2. Steinfels P, Veatch RM: Who should pay for smokers' medical care? *Hastings Cent Rep* 4:8–10, 1974.
3. Morison RS: Rights and responsibilities: Redressing the uneasy balance. *Hastings Cent Rep.* 4:1–4, 1974.
4. Vayda E: Keeping people well: A new approach to medicine. *Hum Nature* 1:64–71, 1978.
5. Somers AR, Hayden MC: Rights and respon-

sibilities in prevention. *Health Educ* 9:37–39, 1978.
6. Kass L: Regarding the end of medicine and the pursuit of health. *Public Interest* 40:11–42, 1975.
7. Belloc NB, Breslow L: Relationship of physical status health and health practices. *Prev Med:* 1:409–421, 1972.
8. Belloc, NB: Relationship of health practices and mortality. *Prev Med:* 2:67–81, 1973.
9. Breslow L: Prospects for improving health through reducing risk factors. *Prev Med:* 7:449–458, 1978.
10. Wikler D: Coercive measures in health promotion: Can they be justified? *Health Educ Monogr* 6: 223–241, 1978.
11. Wikler D: Persuasion and coercion for health: Ethical issues in government efforts to change life-styles. *Milbank Mem Fund Q* 56:303–338, 1978.
12. Veatch RM: The Hippocratic ethic: Consequentialism, individualism and paternalism, in Smith DH, Bernstein LM (eds): *No Rush to Judgment: Essays on Medical Ethics.* Bloomington, Ind., The Poynter Center, Indiana University, 1976, pp 238–264.
13. Beauchamp T: The regulation of hazards and hazardous behaviors. *Health Educ Monogr* 6:242–257, 1978.
14. Veatch RM: The medical model: Its nature and problems. *Hastings Cent Rep* 1:59–76, 1973.
15. Morris JN: Social inequalities undiminished. *Lancet* 1:87–90, 1979.
16. Ryan, W: *Blaming the Victim.* New York, Vintage Books, 1971.
17. Crawford R: Sickness as sin. *Health Policy Advisory Center Bull* 80: 10–16, 1978.
18. Crawford R: You are dangerous to your health. *Social Policy* 8:11–20, 1978.
19. Beauchamp, DE: Public health as social justice. *Inquiry* 13:3–14, 1976.
20. Syme L, Berkman L: Social class, susceptibility and sickness. *Am J Epidemiol* 104:1–8, 1976.
21. Conover, PW: Social class and chronic illness. *Int J Health Serv* 3:357–368, 1973.
22. *Health of the Disadvantaged: Chart Book,* publication (HRA) 77–628. Hyattsville, Md, US Dept of Health, Education and Welfare, Public Health Service, Health Resources Administration, 1977.
23. Beauchamp DE: Alcoholism as blaming the alcoholic. *Int J Addict* 11:41–52, 1976.
24. Veatch RM: What is a 'just' health care delivery? in Branson R, Veatch RM (eds.): *Ethics and Health Policy.* Cambridge, Mass, Ballinger Publishing Co. 1976, pp 127–153.

Persuasion and Coercion for Health

Daniel I. Wikler

What should be the government's role in promoting the kinds of personal behavior that lead to long life and good health? Smoking, overeating, and lack of exercise increase one's chances of suffering illness later in life, as do many other habits. The role played by life-style is so important that, as stated by Fuchs (1974): "The greatest current potential for improving the health of the American people is to be found in what they do and don't do for themselves." But the public has shown little spontaneous interest in reforming. If the government uses the means at its disposal to remedy the situation, it may be faced with problems of an ethical nature. Education, exhortation, and other relatively mild measures may not prove effective in inducing self-destructive people to change their behavior. Attention might turn instead to other means, which, though possibly more effective, might also be intrusive or otherwise distasteful. In this essay, I seek to identify the moral principles underlying a reasoned judgment on whether stronger methods might justifiably be used, and, if so, what limits ought to be observed.

BACKGROUND TO GOVERNMENT INVOLVEMENT IN LIFE-STYLE REFORM

This inquiry occurs at a time when the government is widening its scope of involvement in life-style reform. Major prospective health policy documents of both the United States (Department of Health Education and Welfare, 1975) and Canadian governments (documented by Lalonde, 1974) have announced a change of orientation in this direction. Behind this shift is a host of factors, one of which is the pattern of disease in which an increasing share of ill health is attributed to chronic illnesses and accidental injuries that are aggravated by living habits. This development

Reprinted with permission from the author and the Milbank Memorial Fund Quarterly/*Health and Society,* 56: 3, 1978.

has caused increased interest in preventive behavioral change, and has been abetted by the current wave of "therapeutic nihilism," an attitude that questions medical intervention and is more friendly to health efforts that begin and end at home.

That life-style reform should be undertaken by the *government,* rather than by private individuals or associations, is part of the general emergence of the government as health-care provider. Encouragement of healthful living may also have a budgetary motive. Government officials may find that life-style reform is one of the most cost-effective ways of delivering health, especially if more effective change-inducing techniques are developed.[1] Indeed, the present cost-containment crisis may propel life-style reform to a central place in health planning before the necessary scientific and policy thinking has taken place.

Further pressure on the government to take strong steps to change unhealthy life-styles might come from those who live prudently. All taxpayers have a stake in keeping federal health costs down, but moderate persons may particularly view others' self-destructive life-styles as a kind of financial aggression against them. They may be expected to intensify their protest in the event of a national health insurance plan or national health service.

Involvement of the government in legislating healthful patterns of living is not wholly new; there have been public health and labor laws for a long time. Still, with the increased motivation for government action in life-style reform, it is time to reflect on the kinds of interventions the public wants and should have to accept. Various sorts of behavior change measures need to be examined to see if they might be used to induce healthier living. But that is not enough; goals must also be identified and subjected to ethical examination.[2]

The discussion below will examine a small number possible goals of government life-style reform, and follow with a survey of the principal kinds of steps now contemplated. The approach will be to devote attention to those behavior change measures that are likely to be unpleasant and unwelcome. Since most techniques now used or contemplated for future use do not have such properties, there is little need to justify or focus on them. The reader should also note that each possible policy goal will be discussed in isolation from others. Although in actuality most government programs would probably be expected to serve several purposes at once, and some might be justified by the aggregate but not by one end alone, it is best for our purposes to consider one goal at a time so as to determine the contribution of each. Finally, my analysis should be understood as independent of certain political currents with which my views might be associated. There is some danger that attention to health-related personal behavior will distract the government and public from examining other sources of illness, such as unsafe working conditions, environmental health hazards, and even social and commercial determinants of the injurious behavior. Further, undue stress upon the individual's role in the cause of illness could lead to a "blame-the-victim" mentality, which could be used as a pretext for failing to make curative services available. Although these matters are essentially external to the issue of reform of unhealthy living habits, they pose ethical questions of equal or greater moral gravity.

GOALS OF HEALTH BEHAVIOR REFORM

I propose to discuss three possible goals of health behavior reform with regard to their appropriateness as goals of government programs and the problems arising in their pursuit. The first goal can be simply stated: health should be valued for its own sake. Americans are likely to be healthier if they can be induced to adopt healthier habits, and this may be reason enough to try to get them to do so. The second goal is the fair distribution of the burdens caused by illness. Those who become ill because of unhealthy life-styles may require the financial support of the more prudent, as well as the sharing of what may be scarce medical facilities. If this is seen as unfair to those who do not make

themselves sick, life-style reform measures will also be seen as accomplishing distributive justice. The third goal is the maintenance and improvement of the general welfare, for the nation's health conditions have their effects on the economy, allocation of resources, and even national security.

Health as a Goal in Itself: Beneficence and Paternalism

Much of the present concern for the reform of unhealthy life-styles stems from concern over the health of those who live dangerously. Only a misanthrope would quarrel with this goal. There are several steps that might immediately be justified: the government could make the effects of unhealthy living habits known to those who practice them, and sponsor research to discover more of these facts. The chief concern over such efforts might be that the government would begin its urgings before the facts in question had been firmly established, thus endorsing living habits that might be useless or detrimental to good health.

Considerably more debate, however, would arise over a decision to use stronger methods. For example, a case in point might be a government "fat tax," which would require citizens to be weighed and taxed if overweight. The surcharges thus derived would be held in trust, to be refunded with interest if and when the taxpayers brought their weight down.[3] This pressure would, under the circumstances, be a bond imposed by the government upon its citizens, and thus can be fairly considered as coercive.

The two signal properties of this policy would be its aim of improving the welfare of obese taxpayers, and its presumed unwelcome imposition on personal freedom. (Certain individual taxpayers, of course, might welcome such an imposition, but this is not the ordinary response to penalties.) The first property might be called "beneficence," and it is generally a virtue. But the second property becomes paternalism;[4] and its status as a virtue is very much in doubt. "Paternalism" is a loaded word, almost automatically a term of reprobation. But many paternalistic policies, especially when more neutrally described, attract support and even admiration. It may be useful to consider what is bad and what is good about paternalistic practices, so that we might decide whether in this case the good outweighs the bad. For detailed discussions of paternalism in the abstract, see Feinberg (1973), Dworkin (1971), Bayles (1974), and Hodson (1977).

What is good about some paternalistic interventions is that people are helped, or saved from harm. Citizens who have to pay a fat tax, for example, may lose weight, become more attractive, and live longer. In the eyes of many, these possible advantages are more than offset by the chief fault of paternalism, its denying persons the chance to make their own choices concerning matters that affect them. Self-direction, in turn, is valued because people usually believe themselves to be the best judges of what is good for them, and because the choosing is considered a good in itself. These beliefs are codified in our ordinary morality in the form of a moral right to noninterference so long as one does not adversely affect the interests of others. This right is supposed to shield an individual's "self-regarding" actions from intervention by others, even when those acts are not socially approved ones and even when they promise to be unwise.

At the same time, the case for paternalistic intervention on at least some occasions seems compelling. There may be circumstances in which we lose, temporarily or permanently, our capacity for competent self-direction, and thereby inflict harm upon ourselves that serves little purpose. Like Ulysses approaching the Sirens, we may hope that others would then protect us from ourselves. This sort of consideration supports our imposed guardianship of children and of the mentally retarded. Although these persons often resent our paternalistic control, we reason that we are doing what they would want us to do were their autonomy not compromised. Paternalism would be a benefit under the sort of social insurance policy that a reasonable person would opt for if considered in a moment of lucidity and competence (Dworkin, 1971).

Does this rationale for paternalism support governmental coercion of competent adults to assure the adoption of healthy habits of living? It might seem to, at first sight. Although these adults may be generally competent, their decision-making abilities can be compromised in specific areas. Individuals may be ignorant of the consequences of their acts; they may be under the sway of social or commercial manipulation and suggestion; they may be afflicted by severe psychological stress or compulsion; or be under external constraint. If any of these conditions hold, the behavior of adults may fail to express their settled will. Those of us who disavow any intention of interfering with free and voluntary risk-taking may see cause to intervene when a person's behavior is not under his or her control. . . .

Indeed, the dangers involved in disregarding individual's personal values and in falsely branding their behavior involuntary are closely linked. In the absence of independent criteria for decision-making disability, the paternalist may try to determine disability by seeing whether the individual is rational, *i.e.*, whether he or she competently pursues what is valuable. An absence of rationality may be reason to suspect the presence of involuntariness and hence grounds for paternalism. The problem, however, is that this test for rationality—whether the chosen means are appropriate for the individual's personal ends—is not fully adequate. Factors that deprive an individual of autonomy—such as compulsion or constraint—not only affect a person's ability to calculate means to ends but also induce ends that are in some sense foreign. Advertisements, for example, may instill desires to consume certain substances whose pleasures would ordinarily be considered trifling. Similarly, ignorance may induce people to value a certain experience because they believe it will lead to their attainment of other ends. Alcoholics, for example, may value intoxication because they think it will enhance their social acceptance. The paternalist on the lookout for non-autonomous, self-destructive behavior will be interested not only in irrational means but also uncharacteristic, unreasonable values.

The difficulty for the paternalist at this point is plain. The desire to interfere only with involuntary risk-taking leads to designating individuals for intervention whose behavior proceeds from externally-instilled values. Pluralism commits the paternalist to use the persons' own values in determining whether a health-related practice is harmful. What is needed is some way of determining individuals' "true" personal values; but if these cannot be read off from their behavior, how can they be known?

In certain individual cases, a person's characteristic preferences can be determined from wishes expressed before losing autonomy, as was Ulysses' desire to be tied to the mast. But this sort of data is hardly likely to be available to government health planners. The problem would be at least partially solved if we could identify a set of goods that is basic and appealing, and that nearly all rational persons value. Such universal valuation would justify a presumption of involuntariness should an individual's behavior put these goods in jeopardy. On what grounds would we include an item on this list? Simple popularity would suffice: if almost everyone likes something, such approval probably stems from a common human nature, shared by even those not professing to like that thing. Hence we may suspect, that, if unconstrained, they would like it also. Alternatively, there may be experiences or qualities that, while not particularly appealing in themselves, are preconditions to attaining a wide variety of goods that people idiosyncratically value. Relief from pain is an example of the first sort of good; normal-or-better intelligence is an instance of the latter.

The crucial question for health planners is whether *health* is one of these primary goods. Considered alone, it certainly is: it is valued for its own sake; and it is a means to almost all ends. Indeed, it is a necessary good. No matter how eccentric a person's values and tastes are, no matter what kinds of activities are pleasurable, it is impossible to engage in them unless alive. Most activities a person is likely to enjoy, in fact, require not only life but good health. Unless one believes in an afterlife, the rational person must rate death as an incomparable calamity, for it means the loss of everything.

But the significance of health as a primary good should not be overestimated. The health planner may attempt to argue for coercive reform of health-destructive behavior with a line of reasoning that recalls Pascal's wager.[5] Since death, which precludes all good experience, must receive an enormously negative

valuation, contemplated action that involves risk of death will also receive a substantial negative value after the good and bad consequences have been considered. And this will hold true even if the risk is small, since even low probability multiplied by a very large quantity yields a large quantity. Hence anyone who risks death by living dangerously must, on this view, be acting irrationally. This would be grounds for suspecting that the life-threatening practices were less than wholly voluntary and thus created a need for protection. Further, this case would not require the paternalistic intervenor to turn away from pluralistic ideals, for the unhealthy habits would be faulted not on the basis of deviance from paternalistic values, but on the apparent lapse in the agent's ability to understand the logic of the acts.

This argument, or something like it, may lied behind the willingness of some to endorse paternalistic regulation of the life-styles of apparently competent adults. It is, however, invalid. Its premises may sometimes be true, and so too may its conclusion, but the one does not follow from the other. Any number of considerations can suffice to show this. For example, time factors are ignored. An act performed at age 25 that risks death at age 50 does not threaten every valued activity. It simply threatens the continuation of those activities past the age of 50. The argument also overlooks an interplay between the possible courses of action: if every action that carries some risk of death or crippling illness is avoided, the enjoyment of life decreases. This makes continued life less likely to be worth the price of giving up favorite unhealthy habits.[6] Indeed, although it may be true that death would deny one of all chances for valued experiences, the experiences that make up some people's lives have little value. The less value a person places on continued life, the more rational it is to engage in activities that may brighten it up, even if they involve the risk of ending it. Craig Claiborne (1976), food editor of *The New York Times,* gives ebullient testimony to this possibility in the conclusion of his "In Defense of Eating Rich Food":

I love hamburgers and chili con carne and hot dogs. And foie gras and sauternes and those small birds known as ortolans. I love banquettes of quail eggs with hollandaise sauce and clambakes with lobsters dipped into so much butter it dribbles down the chin. I like cheesecake and crepes filled with cream sauces and strawberries with crème fraiche . . .

And if I am abbreviating my stay on this earth for an hour or so, I say only that I have no desire to be a Methuselah, a hundred or more years old and still alive, grace be to something that plugs into an electric outlet.

The assumption that one who is endangering one's health must be acting irrationally and involuntarily is not infrequently made by those who advocate forceful intervention in suicide attempts; and perhaps some regard unhealthy life-styles as a sort of slow suicide. The more reasonable view, even in cases of imminent suicide, seems rather to be that *some* unhealthy or self-destructive acts are less-than-fully voluntary but that others are not. Claiborne's diet certainly seems to be voluntary, and suggests that the case for paternalistic intervention in life-style cannot be made on grounds of logic alone. It remains true, however, that much of the behavior that leads to chronic illness and accidental injury is not fully under the control of the persons so acting. My thesis is merely that, first, this involuntariness must be shown (along with much else) if paternalistic intervention is to be justified; and, second, this can only be determined by case-by-case empirical study. Those who advocate coercive measures to reform life-styles, whose motives are purely beneficent, and who wish to avoid paternalism except where justified, might find such study worth undertaking.

Any such study is likely to reveal that different practitioners of a given self-destructive habit act form different causes. Perhaps one obese person overeats because of an oral fixation over which he has no control, or in a Pavlovian response to enticing television food advertisements. The diminished voluntariness of these actions lends support to paternalistic intervention. Claiborne has clearly thought matters through and decided in favor of a shorter though gastronomically happier life; to pressure him into changing so that he may live longer would be a clear imposition of values and

would lack the justification provided in the other person's case.

The trouble for a government policy of life-style reform is that a given intervention is more likely to be tailored to practices and habits than to people. Although we may someday have a fat tax to combat obesity, it would be surprising indeed to find one that imposed charges only on those whose obesity was due to involuntary factors. It would be difficult to reach agreement on what constituted diminished voluntariness; harder still to measure it; and perhaps administratively impractical to make the necessary exceptions and adjustments. We may feel, after examining the merits of the cases, that intervention is justified in the compulsive eater's life-style but not in the case of Claiborne. If the intervention takes the form of a tax on obesity *per se*, we face a choice: Do we owe it to those like Claiborne *not* to enforce alien values more than we owe it to compulsive overeaters to protect them from self-destruction? The general right of epicures to answer to their own values, a presumptive right conferred by the pluralistic ethic spoken of earlier, might count for more than the need of compulsive overeaters to have health imposed on them, since the first violates a right and the second merely confers a benefit. But the situation is more complex than this. The compulsive overeater's life is at stake, and this may be of greater concern (everything else being equal) than the epicure's pleasures. Then, too, the epicure is receiving a compensating benefit in the form of longer life, even if this is not a welcome exchange. And there may be many more compulsive overeaters than there are people like Claiborne. On the other hand, the positive causal link between tax and health for either is indirect and tenuous, while the negative relation between tax and gastronomic pleasure is relatively more substantial. (For a fuller discussion of this type of trade-off, see Bayles [1974].) Perhaps the firmest conclusion one may draw from all this is that a thoroughly reasoned moral rationale for a given kind of intervention can be very difficult to carry out.

Paternalism: Problems in Practice. Even if we accept the social insurance rationale for paternalism in the abstract, then, there are theoretical reasons to question its applicability to the problem of living habits that are injurious to health. It is still possible that in some instances these doubts can be laid to rest. We may have some noncircular way of determining when self-destructive behavior is involuntary; we may have knowledge of what preferences people would have were their behavior not constrained; and there may be no way to restore their autonomy. While at least a *prima facie* case for paternalistic intervention would exist under such circumstances, I think it is important to note several practical problems that could arise in any attempt to design and carry out a policy of coercive lifestyle reform.

First, there is the distinct possibility that the government that takes over decision-making power from partially-incompetent individuals may prove even less adept at securing their interests than they would have been if left alone. Paucity of scientific data may lead to misidentification of risk factors. The primitive state of the art in health promotion and mass-scale behavior modification may render interventions ineffective or even counterproductive. And the usual run of political and administrative tempests that affect all public policy may result in the misapplication of such knowledge as is available in these fields. These factors call for recognizing a limitation on the social insurance rationale for paternalism. If rational persons doubt that the authorities who would be guiding their affairs during periods of their incompetence would themselves be particularly competent, they are unlikely to license interventions except when there is a high probability of favorable cost-benefit trade-off. This yields the strongest support for those interventions that prevent very serious injuries, and in which the danger posed is imminent (Feinberg, 1973).

These reflections count against a rationale for government involvement in vigorous health promotion efforts, as recently voiced by the Secretary of Health, Education, and Welfare (1975) and found elsewhere (McKeown and Lowe, 1974). Their statements that smoking and similar habits are "slow suicide" and should be treated as such make a false analogy, precisely because suicide often involves certain imminent dangers of the most serious sort in

situations in which there cannot be time to determine whether the act is voluntary. This is just the sort of case that the social insurance policy here described would cover; but this would not extend to the self-destruction that takes 30 years to accomplish.

Second, there is some possibility that what would be advertised as concern for the individual's welfare (as that person defines it) would turn out to be simple legal moralism, *i.e.,* an attempt to impose the society's or authorities' moral prescriptions upon those not following them. In Knowles's call for life-style reform (1976) the language is suggestive:

> The next major advances in the health of the American people will result from the assumption of individual responsibility for one's own health. This will require a change in lifestyle for the majority of Americans. The cost of sloth, gluttony, alcoholic overuse, reckless driving, sexual intemperance, and smoking is now a national, not an individual responsibility.[7]

All save the last of these practices are explicit *vices;* indeed, the first two—sloth and gluttony—use their traditional names. The intrusion of non-medical vaues is evidenced by the fact that of all the living habits that affect health adversely, only those that are sins (with smoking excepted) are mentioned as targets for change. Skiing and football produce injuries as surely as sloth produces heart disease; and the decision to postpone childbearing until the thirties increases susceptibility to certain cancers in women (Medawar, 1977). If it is the unhealthiness of "sinful" living habits that motivates the paternalist toward reform, then ought not other acts also be targeted on occasions when persons exhibit lack of self-direction? The fact that other practices are not ordinarily pointed out in this regard provides no *argument* against paternalistic life-style reform. But those who favor pressuring the slothful to engage in physical exercise might ask themselves if they also favor pressure on habits which, though unhealthy, are not otherwise despised. If enthusiasm for paternalistic intervention slackens in these latter cases, it may be a signal for reexamination of the motives.

A third problem is that the involuntariness of some self-destructive behavior may make paternalistic reform efforts ineffective. To the extent that the unhealthy behavior is not under the control of the individual, we cannot expect the kind of financial threat involved in a "fat tax" to exert much influence. Paradoxically, the very conditions under which paternalistic intervention seems most justified are those in which many of the methods available are least likely to succeed. The result of intervention under these circumstances may be a failure to change the life-threatening behavior, and a needless (and inexcusable) addition to the individual's woes through the unpleasantness of the intervention itself. A more appropriate target for government intervention might be the commercial and/or social forces that cause or support the life-threatening behavior.

Although the discussion above has focused on the problems attendant to a paternalistic argument for coercive health promotion programs, I have implicitly outlined a positive case for such interventions as well. A campaign to reform unhealthy habits of living will be justified, in my view, so long as it does not run afoul of the problems I have mentioned. It may indeed be possible to design such a program. The relative weight of the case against paternalistic intervention can be lessened, in any case, by making adjustments for the proportion of intervention, benefit, and intrusion. Health-promotion programs that are only very mildly coercive, such as moderate increases in cigarette taxes, require very little justification; noncoercive measures such as health education require none at all. And the case for more intrusive measures would be stronger if greater and more certain benefits could be promised. Moreover, even if the paternalistic rationale for coercive reform of health-related behavior fails completely, there may be other rationales to justify the intrusion. It is to these other sorts of arguments that I now turn.

Fair Distribution of Burdens

The problem of health-related behavior is sometimes seen as a straight-forward question of collective social preference:

> The individual must realize that a perpetuation of the present system of high cost, after-the-fact medicine will only result in higher costs and

greater frustration . . . This is his primary critical choice: to change his personal bad habits or stop complaining. He can either remain the problem or become the solution to it; Beneficent Government cannot—indeed, should not—do it for him or to him. (Knowles, 1977)

A good deal of the controversy is due, however, not to any one person's distaste for having to choose between bad habits and high costs, but rather some people's distaste for having to accept both high costs and someone *else's* bad habits. In the view of these persons, those who indulge in self-destructive practices and present their medical bills to the public are free riders in an economy kept going by the willingness of others to stay fit and sober. Those who hold themselves back from reckless living may care little about beneficence. When they call for curbs on the expensive health practices of others, they want the government to act as their agent primarily out of concern for their interests.

The demand for protection from the costs of calamities other people bring upon themselves involves an appeal to fairness and justice. Both the prudent person and the person with unhealthy habits, it is thought, are capable of safe and healthy living; why should the prudent have to pay for neighbors who decide to take risks? Neighbors are certainly not permitted to set fire to their houses if there is danger of its spreading. With the increasing economic and social connectedness of society, the use of coercion to discourage the unhealthy practices of others may receive the same justification. As the boundary between private and public becomes less distinct, and decisions of the most personal sort come to have marked adverse effects upon others, the state's protective function may be thought to give it jurisdiction over any health-related aspect of living.

This sort of argument presupposes a certain theory of justice; and one who wishes to take issue with the rationale for coercive intervention in health-related behavior might join the debate at the level of theory. Since this debate would be carried out at a quite general level, with only incidental reference to health practices, I will accept the argument's premise (if only for argument's sake) and comment only upon its applicability to the problem of self-destructive behavior. A number of considerations lead to the conclusion that the fairness argument as a justification of coercive intervention, despite initial appearances, is anything but straightforward. Underlying this argument is an empirical premise that may well prove untrue of at least some unhealthy habits: that those who take chances with their health *do* place a significant financial burden upon society. It is not enough to point to the costs of medical care for lung cancer and other diseases brought on by individual behavior. As Hellegers (1978) points out, one must also determine what the individual would have died of had he not engaged in the harmful practice, and subtract the cost of the care which that condition requires. There is no obvious reason to suppose that the diseases brought on by self-destructive behavior are costlier to treat than those that arise from "natural causes."

Skepticism over the burden placed on society by smokers and other risk-takers is doubly reinforced by consideration of the nonmedical costs and benefits that may be involved. It may turn out, for all we know prior to investigation, that smoking tends to cause few problems during a person's productive years and then to kill the individual before the need to provide years of social security and pension payments. From this perspective, the truly burdensome individual may be the unreasonably fit senior citizen who lives on for 30 years after retirement, contributing to the bankruptcy of the social security system, and using up savings that would have reverted to the public purse via inheritance taxes had an immoderate life-style brought an early death. Taken at face value, the fairness argument would require taxes and other disincentives on *non*-smoking and other healthful personal practices which in the end would sap the resources of the healthy person's fellow citizens. Only detailed empirical inquiry can show which of these practices would be slated for discouragement were the argument from fairness accepted; but the fact that we would find penalties on healthful behavior wholly unpalatable may weaken our acceptance of the argument itself.

A second doubt concerning the claim that the burdens of unhealthy behavior are unfairly distributed also involves an unstated premise. The risk taker, according to the fairness argument, should have to suffer not only the illness that may result from the behavior but also the loss of freedom attendant to the coercive measures used in the attempt to change the behavior. What, exactly, is the cause cited by those complaining of the financial burdens placed upon society by the self-destructive? It is not simply the burden of caring and paying for care of these persons when they become sick. Many classes of persons impose such costs on the public besides the self-destructive. For example, diabetics, and others with hereditary dispositions to contract diseases, incur unusual and heavy expenses, and these are routinely paid by others. Why are these costs not resisted as well?

One answer is that there *is* resistance to these other costs, which partly explains why we do not yet have a national health insurance system. But even those willing to pay for the costs of caring for diabetics, or the medical expenses of the poor, may still bridle when faced by the needs of those who have compromised their own health. Is there a rationale for resisting the latter kinds of costs while accepting the former? One possible reason to distinguish the costs of the person with a genetic disease from those of the person with a life-style-induced disease is simply that one can be prevented and the other cannot. Health behavior change measures provide an efficient way of reducing the overall financial burden of health care that society must shoulder, and this might be put forward as the reason why self-destructive persons may have their presumptive rights compromised while others with special medical expenses need not.

But this is not the argument we seek. The medical costs incurred by diseases caused by unhealthy life-styles may be preventable, if our behavior-modifying methods are effective; but this fact shows only that there is a utilitarian opportunity for reducing costs and saving health-care dollars. It does *not* show that this opportunity makes it right to burden those who lead unhealthy lives with governmental intrusion. If costs must be reduced, perhaps they should be reduced some other way (*e.g.,* by lessening the quality of care provided for all); or perhaps costs should not be lowered and those feeling burdened should be made to tolerate the expense. The fact that money could be saved by intruding into the choice of life-styles of the self-destructive does not *itself* show that it would be particularly fair to do so.

If intrusion is to be justified on the grounds that unhealthy life-styles impose unfair financial burdens on others, then, something must be added to the argument. That extra element, it seems, is *fault*. Instead of the *avoidability* of the ilnesses and their expenses, we point to the *responsibility* for them, which we may believe falls upon those who contract them. This responsibility, it might be supposed, makes it unfair to force others to pay the bills and makes it fair for others to take steps to prevent the behaviors that might lead to the illness, even at the cost of some of the responsible person's privacy and liberty.

The argument thus depends crucially on the premise that the person who engages in an unhealthy life-style is responsible for the costs of caring for the illness that it produces. "Responsible" has many senses, and this premise needs to be stated unambiguously. Since responsibility was brought into the argument in hopes of contrasting life-style-related diseases from others, it seems to involve the notions of choice and voluntariness. If the chronic diseases resulting from life-style were not the result of voluntary choices, then there could be no assignment of responsibility in the sense in which the term is being used. This would be the case, for example, if a person contracted lung cancer from breathing the smog in the atmosphere rather than from smoking. But what if it should turn out that even a person's smoking habit were the result of forces beyond the smoker's control? If the habit is involuntary, so is the illness; and the smoker in this instance is no more to be held liable for imposing the costs of treatment than would, say, the diabetic. Since much self-destructive behavior is the result of suggestion, constraint, compulsion, and other factors, the applicability of the fairness argument is limited.

Even if the behavior leading to illness is wholly voluntary, there is not necessarily any justification for intervention *by the state*. The only parties with rights to reform life-styles on these grounds are those who are actually being burdened by the costs involved. A wealthy man who retained his own medical facilities would not justifiably be a target of any of these interventions, and a member of a prepaid health plan would be liable to intervention primarily from others in his payments pool. He would then, of course, have the option of resigning and continuing his self-destructive ways; or he might seek out an insurance scheme designed for those who wish to take chances but who also want to limit their losses. These insured parties would join forces precisely to pool risks and remove reasons for refraining from unhealthy practices; preventive coercion would thus be out of the question. Measures undertaken by the government and applied indiscriminately to all who indulge in a given habit may thus be unfair to some (unless other justification is provided). The administrative inconvenience of restricting these interventions to the appropriate parties might make full justice on this issue too impractical to achieve.

This objection may lose force should there be a national health insurance program in which membership would be mandatory. Indeed, it might be argued that existing federal support of medical education, research, and service answers this objection now. But this only establishes another ground for disputing the responsibility of the self-destructive individual for the costs of his medical care. To state this objection, two classes of acts must be distinguished: the acts constituting the life-style that causes the disease and creates the need for care; and the acts of imposing financial shackles upon an unwilling public. Unless the acts in the first group are voluntary, the argument for imposing behavior change does not get off the ground. Even if voluntary, those acts in the second class might not be. Destructive acts affect others only because others are in financial relationships with the individual that cause the medical costs to be distributed among them. If the financial arrangement is mandatory, then the individual may not have *chosen* that his acts should have these effects on others. The situation will have been this: an individual is

compelled by law to enter into financial relationships with certain others as a part of an insurance scheme; the arrangement causes the
individual's acts to have effects on others that
the others object to; and so they claim the right
to coerce the individual into desisting from
those acts. It seems difficult to assign to this individual responsiblity for the distribution of
financial burdens. He or she may (or may not)
be responsible for getting sick, but not for having the sickness affect others adversely.

This objection has certain inherent limitations in its scope. It applies only to individuals
who are brought into a mandatory insurance
scheme against their wishes. Those who join the
scheme gladly may perhaps be assigned responsibility for the effect they have on others once
they are in it; and certainly many who will be
covered in such a plan will be glad of it. Further,
the burden imposed under such a plan does not
occur until persons who have made themselves
sick request treatment and present the bill to the
public. Only if treatment is mandatory and all
financing of care taken over by the public can
the imposition of burden be said to be wholly involuntary.

In any case, certain adjustments could be
made in a national health insurance plan or service that would disarm this objection. Two such
changes are obvious: the plan could be made
voluntary, rather than mandatory; and/or the
public could simply accept the burdens imposed by unhealthy life-styles and refrain from
attempts to modify them. The first of these may
be impractical for economic reasons (in part
because the plan would fill up with those in
greatest need, escalating costs), and the second
only ignores the problem for which it is supposed to be a solution.

There is, however, a response that would
seem to have more chance of success: allowing
those with unhealthy habits to pay their own
way. Users of cigarettes and alcohol, for example, could be made to pay an excise tax, the
proceeds of which would cover the costs of treatment for lung cancer and other resulting illnesses. Unfortunately, these costs would also
be paid by users who are not abusers: those who
drink only socially would be forced to pay for
the excesses of alcoholics. Alternatively, only
those contracting the illnesses involved could

be charged; but it would be difficult to distinguish illnesses resulting from an immoderate
life-style from those due to genetic or environmental causes. The best solution might be to
identify persons taking risks (by tests for heavy
smoking, alcohol abuse, or dangerous inactiv-
ity) and charge higher insurance premiums
accordingly. This method could be used only if
tests for these behaviors were developed that
were non-intrusive and administratively manageable.[8] The point would be to have those
choosing self-destructive life-styles assume the
true costs of their habits. I defer to economists
for devising the best means to this end.[9]

This kind of policy has its good and bad
points. Chief among the favorable ones is that it
allows a maximum retention of liberty in a
situation in which liberty carries a price. Under
such a policy, those who wished to continue
their self-destructive ways without pressure
could continue to do so, provided that they absorbed the true costs of their practices
themselves. Should they not wish to shoulder
these costs, they could submit to the efforts of
the government to induce changes in their behavior. If the rationale for coercive reform is
the burden the unhealthy life-styles impose on
others, this option seems to meet its goals; and it
does so in a way that does not require loss of
liberty and immunity from intrusions. Indeed,
committed immoderates might have reason to
welcome the imposition of these costs. Although their expenses would be greater, they
would thereby remove at one stroke the most effective device held by others to justify meddling
with their "chosen" life-styles (Detmer, 1976).

The negative side of this proposal stems
from the fact that under its terms the only way
to retain one's liberty is to pay for it. This, of
course, offers very different opportunities to
rich and poor. This inequality can be assessed
in very different ways. From one perspective,
the advantage money brings to rich people under this scheme is the freedom to ruin their own
health. Although the freedom may be valued
intrinsically (*i.e.*, for itself, not as a means to
some other end), the resulting illness cannot;
perhaps the poor, who are denied freedom but
given a better chance for health are coming off
best in the transaction. From another perspective, however, it seems that such a plan simply

adds to the degradation already attending to being poor. Only the poor would be forced to submit to loss of privacy, loss of freedom from pressure, and regulation aimed at behavior change. Such liberties are what make up full citizenship, and one might hold that they ought not to be made contingent on one's ability to purchase them.[10]

The premise that illnesses caused by unhealthy habits impose financial burdens on society, then, does not automatically give cause for adopting strong measures to change the self-destructive behavior. Still, it *may* do so, if the underlying theory of justice is correct and if its application can skirt the problems mentioned here. Besides, justification for such programs may be derived from other considerations.

Indeed, there is one respect in which the combined force of the paternalistic rationale and the fairness argument is greater than the sum of its parts. The central difficulty for the fairness argument, mentioned above, is that much of the self-destructive behavior that burdens the public is not really the fault of the individual; various forces, internal and external, may conspire to produce such behavior independently of the person's will. Conversely, a problem for the paternalist is that much of the harm from which the individual would be "protected" may be the result of free, voluntary choices, and hence beyond the paternalist's purview. The best reason to be skeptical of the first rationale, then, is doubt over the *presence* of voluntariness; the best reason to doubt the second concerns the *absence* of voluntariness. Whatever weighs against the one will count for the other.

The self-destructive individual, then, is caught in a theoretical double-bind: whether the behavior is voluntary or not, there will be at least *prime facie* grounds for coercive intervention. The same holds true for partial voluntariness and involuntariness. This consideration is of considerable importance for those wanting to justify coercive reform of health-related behavior. It reduces the significance of the notion of voluntariness in the pro-intervention arguments, and so serves to lessen concern over the intractable problems of defining the notion adequately, and detecting and measuring its occurrence. . . .

MEANS OF HEALTH BEHAVIOR REFORM

Two questions arise in considering the ethics of government attempts to bring about healthier ways of living. The first question is: Should coercion, intrusion, and deprivation be used as methods for inducing change? The other question is: How do we decide whether a given health promotion program is coercive, intrusive, or inflicts deprivations? These questions are independent of each other. Two parties who agreed on the degree of coerciveness that might be justifiably employed in a given situation might still assess a proposed policy differently in this regard, and hence reach different conclusions on whether the policy should be put into effect.

Disagreement over the degree of coerciveness of health behavior change programs is to be expected, not least because of the vagueness of the notion of coercion itself. Some of the most difficult problems addressed in the philosophical literature (Nozick, 1969; Held, 1972; Bayles, 1972; and Pennock, 1972) arise in the present context: What is the difference between persuasion and manipulation? Can offers and incentives be coercive, or is coerciveness a property only of threats? And can one party be said to have coerced another even if the latter manages to accomplish that which the first party tried to prevent?

The answers to these and similar queries will affect the evaluation of various kinds of health promotion measures.

Health Education

Health education seems harmless. Education generally provides information and this generally increases our power, since it enhances the likelihood that our decisions will accomplish our ends. For the most part, there is no inherent ethical problem with such programs, and they do not stand in need of moral justification. Still, there are certain problems with some health education programs, and these should be mentioned.

Health education *could* be intrusive. Few could object to making information available to those who seek it out. But if "providing information" were taken to mean making sure that the public attained a high level of awareness of the message, the program might require an objectionably high level of exposure. This is primarily an esthetic issue, and is unlikely to cause concern.

Can education be coercive? Information can be used as a tool for one party to get another to do its bidding, just as threats can. But the method is different: Instead of changing the prospective consequences of available actions, which is what a threat does, education alerts one to the previously unrecognized consequences of one's acts. Educators who hope to increase healthful behavior will disseminate only information that points in that direction; they cannot be expected to point out that, in addition to causing deterioration of the liver, alcohol helps certain people feel relaxed in social settings. It is difficult to know whether to regard this selective informing as manipulative. Theoretically, at least, people are free to seek out the other side on their own. Such measures acquire more definite coercive coloration when they are combined with suppression of the other side; "control over the means of persuasion" is another option open to reformers.[11]

The main threat of coerciveness in health education programs, in my opinion, lies in the possibility that such programs may turn from providing information to manipulating attitude and motivation. Education, in the sense of providing information, is a means of inducing belief and knowledge. A review of the literature indicates, however, that when health education programs are evaluated, they are not judged successful or unsuccessful in proportion to their success in *inducing belief.* Rather, evaluators look at *behavior change,* the actions which, they hope, would stem from these beliefs. If education programs are to be evaluated favorably, health educators may be led to take a wider view of their role (Rosenstock 1960). This would include attempts to motivate the public to adopt healthy habits, and this might have to be supplied by covert appeals to other interests ("smokers are unpopular," and so on). Suggestion and manipulation may replace information as the tools used by the health educators to accomplish their purpose. (American Public Health Association, 1975;

Haefner and Kirscht, 1970; and Milio, 1976). Indeed, health education may call for actual and deliberate *mis*information: directives may imply or even state that the scientific evidence in favor of a given health practice is unequivocal even when it is not (a problem noted by Lalonde, 1974).

A fine line has been crossed in these endeavors. Manipulation and suggestion go well beyond providing information to enhance rational decision making. These measures bypass rational decision-making faculties and thereby inflict a loss of personal control. Thus, health education, except when restricted to information, requires some justification. The possible deleterious effects are so small that the justification required may be slight; but the requirement is there. Ethical concerns for this kind of practice may become more pressing as the educational techniques used to induce behavior change become more effective.[12]

Incentives, Subsidies, and Taxes

Incentive measures range from pleasantly noncoercive efforts such as offering to pay citizens if they will live prudently, to coercive measures such as threatening to fine them if they do not. Various noncoercive measures designed to facilitate healthful life-styles might include: providing jogging paths and subsidizing tennis balls. Threats might include making all forms of transportation other than bicycling difficult, and making inconvenient the purchase of food containing saturated fats.

Generally speaking, justification is required only for coercive measures, not for incentives. However, the distinction is not as clear as it first appears. Suppose, for exampe, that the government wants to induce the obese to lose weight, and that a mandatory national health insurance plan is about to go into effect. The government's plan threatens the obese with higher premiums unless they lose their excess weight. Before the plan is instituted, however, someone objects that the extra charges planned for eager eaters make the program coercive. No adequate justification is found. Instead of calling off the program, however, some subtle changes are made. The insurance scheme is announced with higher premiums than had been originally planned. No extra charges are imposed on anyone; instead, discounts are offered to all those who avoid overweight. Instead of coercion, the plan now uses positive incentives; and this does not require the kind of justification needed for the former plan. Hence the new program is allowed to go into effect.

The effect of the rate structure in the two plans is, of course, identical: The obese would pay the higher rate, the slender the lower one. It seems that the distinction between coercion and incentive is merely semantic. But this is the wrong conclusion. There is a real difference, upon which much ethical evaluation must rest; the problem is in stating what the difference amounts to. A partial answer is that a given measure cannot be judged coercive or noncoercive without referring to a background standard from which the measure's effects diverge favorably or unfavorably. Ultimately, I believe, the judgment required for the obesity measure would require us to decide what a fair rate would have been for the insurance; any charges above that fair rate would be coercive, and any below, incentive. (For an account of this complex subject, see Nozick, 1969). The rate the government plans to charge as the standard premium might not be the fair rate; and this shows that one cannot judge the coerciveness of a fee structure merely by checking it for surcharges.

Even if we are able to sort the coercive from the incentive measures, however, we may have reason to hesitate before allowing the government unlimited use of incentives. A government in a position to make offers may not necessarily coerce those it makes the offers to, but is relatively more likely to get its way; in this sense its power increases. Increased government power over life-styles would seem generally to require some justification. In particular, there is inevitably some danger that, given the present scientific uncertainty over the effects of many habits, practices might be encouraged that would contribute nothing to health or even be dangerous. A further problem with financial incentives is that if they are to affect the behavior of the rich they must be sizable; and this may redistribute wealth in a direction considered unjust on other grounds.

The imposition of financial penalties as a means of inducing behavior raises questions that have been touched on above. The chief issue, of course, is the deprivation this method inflicts. Even where justifiably applied to induce behavior change, no *more* deprivation ought to be used than is necessary; but there are administrative difficulties in trying to obey this limitation. Different persons respond to different amounts of deprivation—again, the rich man will absorb costs that would deter the poor one. A disincentive set higher than that needed to induce behavior change would be unfair; a rate set too low would be ineffective. The amount of deprivation inflicted ought, then, to be tailored to the individual's wealth and psychology. This may well be administratively impossible, and injustice would result to the degree that these differences were ignored.

Regulative Measures

The coercive measures discussed above concentrate on applying influence on individuals so that their behavior will change. A different way of effecting a reform is to deprive self-destructive individuals of the means needed to engage in their unhealthy habits. Prohibition of the sale of cigarettes would discourage smoking at least as effectively as exhortations not to smoke or insurance surcharges for habitual tobacco use. Yet, these regulative measures are surely as coercive, although they do not involve direct interaction with the individuals affected. They are merely one more way of intervening in an individual's decision to engage in habits that may cause illness. As such, they are clearly in need of the same or stronger justification as those involving threats, despite the argument that these measures are taken only to combat an unhealthy *environment,* and thus cannot be counted as coercing the persons who have unhealthy ways of living (Terris, 1968). For a discussion of this indirect form of paternalism, see Dworkin (1971). What distinguishes these "environmental" causes of illness from, say, carcinogens in the water supply, is the active connivance of the victims. "Shielding" the "victims" from these external forces must involve making them behave in a way they do not choose. This puts regulative measures in the same category as those applied directly to the self-destructive individuals.

CONCLUSIONS

I have been concerned with clarifying what sorts of justification must be given for certain kinds of government involvement in the reform of unhealthy ways of living. It is apparent that more is needed than a simple desire on the part of the government to promote health and/or reduce costs. When the measures taken are intrusive, coercive, manipulative, and/or inflict deprivations—in short, when they are of the sort many might be expected to dislike—the moral justification required may be quite complex. The principles that would be used in making a case for these interventions may have limited scope and require numerous exceptions and qualifications; it is unlikely that they can be expressed as simple slogans such as "individuals must be responsible for their own health" or "society can no longer afford self-destructiveness."

My goal has been to specify the kind of justification that would have to be provided for any coercive life-style reform measure. I have not attempted to reach a judgment of right or wrong. Either of these judgments would be foolhardy, if only in view of the diversity of health-promotion measures that have been and will be contemplated. Yet it might be appropriate to recall a few negative and positive points on life-style reform.

Inherent in the subject matter is a danger that reform efforts, however rationalized and advertised, may become "moralistic," in being an imposition of the particular preferences and values of one (powerful) group upon another. Workers in medicine and related fields may naturally focus on the medical effects of everyday habits and practices, but others may not. From this perspective, trying to induce the public to change its style of living would represent an enormous expansion of the medical domain, a "medicalization of life." The parochial viewpoint of the health advocate can reach absurd limits. A recent presidential address to a prominent professional health organization, for example, came close to calling for abolition of alcohol simply on the grounds that the rate of cirrhosis of the liver had increased by 6 per 100,000 over the last 40 years. In this instance, health is being imposed upon

us as a goal from above; perhaps medicine would serve us best if it acted to remove the dangers from the pursuit of other goals.

When the motivation behind life-style reform is concern for taxpayers rather than for self-destructive individuals, problems of a different kind are posed. Insistence that individuals are "responsible" for their own health may stem from a conflation of two different phenomena: an individual's life-style playing a causal role in producing illness, and that individual being at fault and accountable for his or her life-style and illness. The former may be undeniable, but the latter may be very difficult to prove. Unless difficulties in this sort of view are acknowledged, attention may be diverted from the various external causes of dangerous health-related behavior, resulting in a lessening of willingness to aid the person whose own behavior has resulted in illness.

On the positve side, two points made earlier bear repetition. First, although I have emphasized the difficulties in justifying coercive measures to induce life-style change, I have done so in the course of outlining the sort of case that might be made in support. It is entirely possible that such measures might be fair and desirable; at least, this is consistent with the principles I have claimed are relevant to deciding the issue. Second, few of the steps called for in either the professional or lay literature have been very coercive or intrusive in nature. Little of what I have said goes against any of these. Indeed, one hopes that these measures will be funded and used to the extent they are effective. An increase in the number and scope of such research, education, and incentive programs may be the best result of the current attention to the role of life-style in maintaining health. This would serve two goals over which there cannot be serious dispute: enabling people to be as healthy as they want to be, given the costs involved; and reducing overall medical need so as to make room in the health care system for all who still require care.

Notes

1. Though there is much dispute over the effectiveness of many health-promotion measures,

efficient techniques may be developed in step with the progress of behavioral medicine generally. See Ubell (1972), Pomerleau, Bass, and Crown, (1975), and Haggerty (1977).

2. I am not attempting to determine what the actual goals of the government are in intervening in life-style; indeed, it may make little sense to speak of specific goals at all. (See MacCallum (1966). The rationale for legislation as voiced by the legislature may have the purpose of establishing the legal basis for the legislation rather than that of exhibiting the legislators' goals in passing the measures or of identifying the need to which the measure was a response. For example, a bill requiring motorcyclists to wear helmets might be accepted by the public on paternalistic grounds, but the personal motivation of the legislators may have been harassment of the cyclists. And the measure might be upheld in court as a legitimate attempt to prevent the public from being saddled with the cost of caring for injured cyclists who could not afford to pay for medical care.

   My inquiry into the goals of a proposed health policy has the sole purpose of determining whether the goals of the policy and the means to it are legitimate. Thus, if it is decided that such a helmet law is unwarranted, even on the paternalistic grounds which seem most applicable, it will not concern us that the law could be cleared through the courts by nimble use of the possibility of the cyclists becoming public charges. This is not to denigrate thee use of such methods in the practice of legislation and legal challenge; but these pursuits are different from those undertaken here.

3. This measure was concocted for the present essay, but it shares its important features with others which have been actually proposed.

4. "Coercive beneficence" is not a fully correct definition of paternalism; but I will not attempt to give adequate definition here (see Gert and Culver, 1976). The term itself is unnecessarily sex-linked; "Parentalism" carries the same meaning without this feature. However, "paternalism" is a standard term in philosophical writing, and a change from it invites confusion.

5. The agnostic should adopt the habits which would foster his own belief in God. If he does and God exists, he will receive the infinite rewards of paradise; if he does and God does not exist, he was only wasting the efforts of conversion and prayer. If he does not try to believe in God, and religion is true, he suffers the infinitely bad fate of hell; whereas if God does not exist he has

merely saved some inconvenience. Conversion is the rational choice even if the agnostic estimates the chances of God's existing as very remote, since even a very small probability yields a large index when multiplied against an infinite quantity.

6. Readers of the previous footnote might note that a similar difficulty attends Pascal's wager. If the agnostic took steps to foster belief in every diety for which the chance of existing was greater than zero, the inconvenience suffered would be considerable, after all. Yet such would be required by the logic of the wager.

7. Elsewhere, however, Dr. Knowles emphasizes that "he who hates sin, hates humanity" (Knowles, 1977). Knowles's argument in the latter essay is primarily nonpaternalistic.

8. It may be that the only way to separate smokers and drinkers taking risks from those not taking risks is to wait until illness develops or fails to develop. Perhaps smokers could save their tax seals and cash them in for refunds if they reach 65 without developing lung cancer!

9. The reader may sense a paradox by this point. Taxes on unhealthy habits would avoid inequities involved in life-style reform measures, such as taxes on unhealthy habits. And it is true that some of the steps that might be taken to permit those with unhygienic life-styles to assume the costs incurred might resemble those that could be used to induce them to give the habits up. Despite this, and despite the fact that the two kinds of programs might even have the same effects, I believe that they can and ought to be distinguished. The imposition of a fat tax has a behavior change as its goal. It is this goal that made it a topic for discussion in this paper. It would not be imposed to cover the costs of diseases stemming from unhealthy life-styles—indeed, as the reader will recall, the funds obtained through the tax were to be kept in trust and returned later if and when the behavior changed. In contrast, the taxes being mentioned as part of a "pay-as-you-go" plan would not be imposed as a means to changing behavior. Such a proposal would constitute one way of financing health costs, a topic I am not addressing in the present paper. These taxes would, of course, tend to discourage the behavior in question; but this (welcome) effect would not be their purpose nor provide their rationale (more precisely, *need* not be their purpose). Any program, of course, can serve mulitple needs simultaneously. The "pay-as-you-go" tax would succeed as a program even if no behavior change occurred, and the behavior-modifying tax would succeed if

behavior did change even if no funds were raised. In any case, surcharges and taxes would be but a few methods among many that might be used to induce behavior change; while they could consititute the whole of a policy aimed to impose costs upon those incurring them.

10. It might be possible to devise charges that would be assessed proportionately to income, so that the "bite" experienced by rich and poor would be about the same. This has not been the pattern in the past: all pay the same tax on a pack of cigarettes. In any case, this adjustment is in no way mandated by the fairness argument. The purpose of the charges would be to permit self-destructive individuals to "pay their own way" and hence remain free to indulge in favored habits. Reducing the amounts charged to low-income persons fails to realize that end; the costs of medical treatment for the poor are not any lower than for the rich. Indeed, being poor may increase the likelihood that the costs of treatment would have to be borne by the public. This suggests a scheme in which charges are assessed *inversely* proportional to income.

11. Though this most clearly recalls the banning of liquor and cigarette advertising from the air-

waves, I do not believe that the suppression of information was generally involved. The advertisements did not stress the delivery of information. The quoted phrase is Michael Walzer's (1978).

12. See Ubell (1972). It might be objected that the kind of manipulation I am speaking of is practiced continuously by commercial advertisers, and that no justification is provided by or demanded from them. It certainly is true that these techniques are used, but this does not show that there is not a need for justification when they are used in the course of a government health promotion campaign. The fact that the commercials are tolerated may indicate not that the manipulative techniques are themselves unobjectionable, but rather that private interests enjoy First Amendment freedom from regulation in their attempts to communicate with the public. The rationale for this freedom—if it exists—may not apply to government communications. The government *per se* is not an entity with interests which must be protected by rights in society; and the same holds true (officially, at least) of health education advocates, when agents of the government.

REGULATION OF RESEARCH

From "Viral Hepatitis: New Light on an Old Disease"

Saul Krugman and Joan P. Giles

Our studies on the natural history and prevention of viral hepatitis have been in progress since 1956. During the past 14 years we have collected and stored more than 25,000 serum specimens from more than 700 patients who were exposed to hepatitis in an institution where the disease has been highly endemic. Serial samples of serum were obtained before exposure, during the incubation period, and for many months and years after infection. This hepatitis serum bank has been a valuable source of materials for the study of the natural history of infectious hepatitis and serum hepatitis.

The discovery of Australia antigen by Blumberg and associates has opened a new chapter in hepatitis research. The association of this serum antigen with viral hepatitis has been confirmed by many investigators. The specific association with serum hepatitis has been demonstrated by Prince and by Giles and associates. The availability of a simple agar-gel precipitin test and a quantitative complement fixation test for the detection of Australia or hepatitis-associated antigen (HAA) and antibody (anti-HAA) represents an important technological advance. The use of these procedures for the re-evaluation of the specimens in our hepatitis serum bank has enabled us to shed new light on an old disease.

Background for Willowbrook Hepatitis Studies. The Willowbrook State School is an institution for mentally retarded children located in Staten Island, N.Y. The nature of endemic hepatitis, first recognized in Willowbrook in 1949, has been described in detail in previous reports. Subsequently, the constant admission of many susceptible children in a population which increased to more than 5,000 patients by 1960 provided fertile soil for a continuing endemic situation. In the absence of an effective, specific prophylactic agent, it has been impossible to prevent the spread of this infection. As indicated in a previous report,* "under the chronic circumstance of multiple and repeated natural exposure, it has been shown that most newly admitted children become infected within the first 6 to 12 months of residence in the institution." Studies reported in 1967 revealed evidence of two distinctive immunological types of viral hepatitis, MS-1 which resembled infectious hepatitis (IH) and MS-2 which resembled serum hepatitis (SH).

The most important source of serum specimens was children whose hepatitis infection followed artificial exposure to the Willowbrook strains of virus which have been prevalent in the institution. The decision to conduct these studies was reached after consideration of many factors.

It was inevitable that susceptible children would become infected in the institution. Hepatitis was especially mild in the 3- to 10-year age group at Willowbrook. These studies would be carried out in a special unit with optimum isolation facilities to protect the children from other infectious diseases such as shigellosis, and parasitic and respiratory infections which are prevalent in the institution. It should be emphasized that the artificial induction of hepatitis implies a "therapeutic" effect because of the immunity which is conferred.

The study groups have included only children whose parents gave written consent. Our method of obtaining informed consent has changed progressively since 1956. At that time

* Krugman S. Giles JP, Hammond J: Infectious hepatitis: Evidence for two distinctive clinical, epidemiological, and immunological types of infection. *JAMA* 200:365–73, 1967.

Reprinted from *Journal of the American Medical Association* 212:6, 1019–21, May 11, 1970. Copyright 1970, American Medical Association.

TABLE 2   Incidence of Hepatitis-Associated Antigen (HAA) in Patients at the
Willowbrook State School From 1965 to 1970

Group	Description	Age Yr.	Time in Institution	No. Tested	HAA-Positive No.	%
1.	Retarded adult men, all types, 1965 *	19–36	>6 yr	150	23	15.3
2.	Retarded adult male monogoloids, 1970	19–36	>6 yr	86	16	18.6
3.	Retarded children, all types, 1968–1969	<5	0–7 mo	130	13	10.0
4.	Retarded children, all types, 1968–1969 †	<10	0–5 yr	210	58	32.8
5.	Retarded children, congenital rubella, 1970	<10	0–7 yr	45	11	24.4

* Of 150 adults in group 1, 17 had Down's syndrome and 133 had other causes of mental retardation. The HAA was detected in 3 of 17 (18%) of those with Down's syndrome and in 20 of 133 (15%) of other retarded adults. Sixteen HAA-positive patients were retested in 1969; 14 were still abnormal.

† Of 210 children in group 4, 44 had Down's syndrome; 43% were HAA-positive. Of the remaining 166 mentally retarded children, 24.4% were HAA-positive.

the information was conveyed to individual parents by letter or personal interview. More recently, we have used the group technique of obtaining consent. The following procedure has been employed: First, a psychiatric social worker discusses the project with parents during a preliminary interview. Those who are interested are invited to attend a group session at the institution to discuss the project in greater detail. These sessions are conducted by the staff responsible for the program, including the physician, supervising nurse, staff attendants, and psychiatric social workers. Meetings have been frequently attended by outside physicians who have expressed interest. Parents in groups of six to eight are given a tour of the facilities. The purposes, potential benefits, and potential hazards of the program are discussed with them, and they are encouraged to ask questions. Thus, all parents can hear the response to questions posed by the more articulate members of the group. After leaving this briefing session parents have an opportunity to talk with their private physicians who may call the unit for more information. Approximately two weeks after the visit, the psychiatric social worker contacts the parents for their decision. If the decision is in the affirmative, the consent is signed but parents are informed that signed consent may be withdrawn any time before the beginning of the program. It has been clear that the group method has enabled us to obtain more thorough informed consent. Children who are wards of the state or children without parents have never been included in our studies.

Since 1956 the hepatitis studies have been reviewed and sanctioned by various local, state, and federal agencies. These studies have been reviewed and approved by the New York University and Willowbrook State School committees on human experimentation since their formation in February 1967. Prior to this date the functions of the present University Committee on Human Experimentation were performed by the Executive Faculty of the School of Medicine for studies of this type. The initial proposal in 1956 was reviewed and approved by the following groups: Executive Faculty, New York University School of Medicine, New York State Department of Mental Hygiene, New York State Department of Health, and Armed Forces Epidemiological Board. It is of interest that the guidelines which were adopted for the hepatitis studies at its inception in 1956 conformed to the World Medical Association's Draft Code of Ethics on Human Experimentation which was presented to its general assembly in September 1961, five years later.

Letters: Experiments at the Willowbrook State School

SIR.—You have referred to the work of Krugman and his colleagues at the Willowbrook State School in three editorials. In the first article the work was cited as a notable study of hepatitis and a model for this type of investigation. No comment was made on the rightness of attempting to infect mentally retarded children with hepatitis for experimental purposes, in an institution where the disease was already endemic.

The second editorial again did not remark on the ethics of the study, but the third sounded a note of doubt as to the justification for extending these experiments. The reason given was that some children might have been made more susceptible to serious hepatitis as the result of the administration of previously heated icterogenic material.

I believe that not only this last experiment, but the whole of Krugman's study, is quite unjustifiable, whatever the aims, and however academically or therapeutically important are the results. I am amazed that the work was published and that it has been actively supported editorially by the *Journal of the American Medical Association* and by Ingelfinger in the 1967–68 *Year Book of Medicine*. To my knowledge only the *British Journal of Hospital Medicine* has clearly stated the ethical position on these experiments and shown that it was indefensible to give potentially dangerous infected material to children, particularly those who were mentally retarded, with or without parental consent, when no benefit to the child could conceivably result.

Krugman and Giles have continued to publish the results of their study, and in a recent paper go to some length to describe their method of obtaining parental consent and list a number of influential medical boards and committees that have approved the study. They point out again that, in their opinion, their work conforms to the World Medical Association Draft Code of Ethics on Human Experimentation. They also say that hepatitis is still highly endemic in the school.

Letters reprinted from *The Lancet,* April 10, May 8, and July 10, 1971.

This attempted defence is irrelevant to the central issue. Is it right to perform an experiment on a normal or mentally retarded child when no benefit can result to that individual? I think that the answer is no, and that the question of parental consent is irrelevant. In my view the studies of Krugman serve only to show that there is a serious loophole in the Draft Code, which under General Principles and Definitions puts the onus of consent for experimentation on children on the parent or guardian. It is this section that is quoted by Krugman. I would class his work as "experiments conducted solely for the acquisition of knowledge," under which heading the code states that "Persons retained in mental hospital or hospitals for mental defectives should not be used for human experiment." Krugman may believe that his experiments were for the benefit of his patients, meaning the individual patients used in the study. If this is his belief he has a difficult case to defend. The duty of a pediatrician in a situation such as exists at Willowbrook State School is to attempt to improve that situation, not to turn it to his advantage for experimental purposes, however lofty the aims.

Every new reference to the work of Krugman and Giles adds to its apparent ethical respectability, and in my view such references should stop, or at least be heavily qualified. The editorial attitude of *The Lancet* to the work should be reviewed and openly stated. The issue is too important to be ignored.

If Krugman and Giles are keen to continue their experiments I suggest that they invite the parents of the children involved to participate. I wonder what the response would be.

Stephen Goldby

SIR.—Dr. Stephen Goldby's critical comments (April 10, p. 749) about our Willowbrook studies and our motives for conducting them were published without extending us the courtesy of replying in the same issue of *The Lancet.* Your acceptance of his criticisms without benefit of our response implies a blackout of all comment related to our studies. This decision is unfortunate because our recent studies on active and passive immunisation for the prevention of viral hepatitis, type B, have clearly demonstrated a "therapeutic effect" for the children involved. These studies have provided us with the first indication and hope that it may be possible to control hepatitis in this institution. If this aim can be achieved, it will benefit not only the children, but also their families and the employees who care for them in the school. It is unnecessary to point out the additional benefit to the world-wide populations which have been plagued by an insoluble hepatitis problem for many generations.

Dr. Joan Giles and I have been actively engaged in studies aimed to solve two infectious-disease problems in the Willowbrook State School—measles and viral hepatitis. These studies were investigated in this institution because they represented major health problems for the 5000 or more mentally retarded children who were residents. Uninformed critics have assumed or implied that we came to Willowbrook to "conduct experiments on mentally retarded children."

The results of our Willowbrook studies with the experimental live attenuated measles vaccine developed by Enders and his colleagues are well documented in the medical literature. As early as 1960 we demonstrated the protective effect of this vaccine during the course of an epidemic. Prior to licensure of the vaccine in 1963 epidemics occurred at two-year intervals in this institution. During the 1960 epidemic there were more than 600 cases of measles and 60 deaths. In the wake of our ongoing measles vaccine programme, measles has been eradicated as a disease in the Willowbrook State School. We have not had a single case of measles since 1963. In this regard the children at the Willowbrook State School have been more fortunate than unimmunised children in Oxford, England, other areas in Great Britain, as well as certain groups of children in the United States and other parts of the world.

The background of our hepatitis studies at Willowbrook has been described in detail in various publications. Viral hepatitis is so prevalent that newly admitted susceptible children become infected within 6 to 12 months after entry in the institution. These children are a

source of infection for the personnel who care for them and for their families if they visit with them. We were convinced that the solution of the hepatitis problem in this institution was dependent on the acquisition of new knowledge leading to the development of an effective immunising agent. The achievements with smallpox, diphtheria, poliomyelitis, and more recently measles represent dramatic illustrations of this approach.

It is well known that viral hepatitis in children is milder and more benign than the same disease in adults. Experience has revealed that hepatitis in institutionalised, mentally retarded children is also mild, in contrast with measles, which is a more severe disease when it occurs in institutional epidemics involving the mentally retarded. Our proposal to expose a small number of newly admitted children to the Willowbrook strains of hepatitis virus was justified in our opinion for the following reasons: (1) they were bound to be exposed to the same strains under the natural conditions existing in the institution; (2) they would be admitted to a special, well-equipped, and well-staffed unit where they would be isolated from exposure to other infectious diseases which were prevalent in the institution—namely, shigellosis, parasitic infections, and respiratory infections—thus, their exposure in the hepatitis unit would be associated with less risk than the type of institutional exposure where multiple infections could occur; (3) they were likely to have a subclinical infection followed by immunity to the particular hepatitis virus; and (4) only children with parents who gave informed consent would included.

The statement by Dr. Goldby accusing us of conducting experiments exclusively for the acquisition of knowledge with no benefit for the children cannot be supported by the true facts.

Saul Krugman

SIR.—I am astonished at the unquestioning way in which *The Lancet* has accepted the intemperate position taken by Dr. Stephen Goldby (April 10, p. 749) concerning the experimental studies of Krugman and Giles on hepatitis at the Willowbrook State School. These investigators have repeatedly explained—for over a decade—that natural hepatitis infection occurs sooner or later in virtually 100% of the patients admitted to Willowbrook, and that it is better for the patient to have a known, timed, controlled infection than an untimed, uncontrolled one. Moreover, the wisdom and human justification of these studies have been repeatedly and carefully examined and verified by a number of very distinguished, able individuals who are respected leaders in the making of such decisions.

The real issue is: Is it not proper and ethical to carry out experiments in children, which would apparently incur no greater risk than the children were likely to run by nature, in which the children generally receive better medical care when artificially infected than if they had been naturally infected, and in which the parents as well as the physician feel that a significant contribution to the future well-being of similar children is likely to result from the studies? It is true, to be sure, that the W.M.A. code says, "Children in institutions and not under the care of relatives should not be the subjects of human experiments." But this unqualified *obiter dictum* may represent merely the well-known inability of committees to think a problem through. However, it has been thought through by Sir Austin Bradford Hill, who has pointed out the unfortunate effects for these very children that would have resulted, were such a code to have been applied over the years.

Geoffrey Edsall

Children in Institutions

Paul Ramsey

Even if one granted the right of parents to consent for their children to be used in medical investigations having unknown present and future risks to them and promising future possible benefits only for others, it would still be possible to argue that children in institutions and not directly and continuously under the care of parents or relatives should *never* be so used. If we are not persuaded that *because they are children* children cannot consent (nor should anyone else consent in their behalf) to experiments primarily for the accumulation of knowledge, we at least should be convinced that such experiments ought not to be performed upon children in orphanages, reformatories, or homes for the retarded *because they are a captive population.*

In discussions of the consent-requirement more attention has been paid to the question of whether and under what possible circumstances adult prisoners can validly consent to research trials than to the question of whether

Reprinted with permission of author and publisher from Paul Ramsey, *The Patient as a Person* (New Haven: Yale University Press, 1970), pp. 40–58.

and under what possible circumstances there can be valid consent for children who cannot consent at all. Some authors seem to find it easier to include children by proxy, reducing consent to a merely formal requirement which can be met by someone else other than the real subject, than to include prisoners who may be under duress (but who, to suppose the worst, do themselves conditionally consent). In an otherwise excellent article, Professor John Fletcher of Virginia Theological Seminary, for example, comes closest to ever saying "never" in ethics when he is discussing the use of prisoners, while accepting as standard the substitution of the consent of an incompetent's legal representative.[1] This anomaly or contrast in the literature of medical ethis is worth pondering.

The usual reasons offered for not accepting prisoner volunteers are only cautionary, even if very severe, warnings. It is not impossible in local situations to overcome them so as to secure from prisoners a reasonably free as well as an adequately informed consent. It is duress that has to be avoided—the duress to give a particular consent because of too great hope of parole.

This should not be an automatic "payment." Even a pattern of always weighing heavily the consent of prisoners in considering them for parole has to be avoided. Still it is not impossible to arrange things so that a man in prison may freely volunteer to become a joint adventurer in an experiment for the sake of the knowledge and good to come, and not for the sake of the reward. It is not impossible to protect his will from duress to cooperate in such medical undertakings. To do this, some would require in the case of prisoners the complete exclusion of any possibility of reward, or of earlier parole. This seems unfairly severe on prisoners. No one who has read the noble words of Nathan Leopold concerning the purposefulness of his own and other prisoners' participation in the malaria experiments in the Illinois State Prison during World War II can deny that prisoners *may* be as free in volunteering as persons in normal life.

If the consent of prisoners to medical experimentation is not inherently or always necessarily invalid, there may still be decisive objection to the general practice of using them. This was the most persuasive argument made by Professor David Danube in the Ciba Symposium in morally forbidding the use of prisoners as donors of organs for transplantation. Daube allowed that the pressure upon familial donors may be greater than that placed upon prisoners, but "the pressure in one's family or circle belongs to the normal burden and dignity of social existence"; this is "a pressure consonant with the dignity and responsibility of free life." This we deny to prisoners. Lord Kilbrandon made something of the same point (appealing to what philosophers call *fairness*-considerations) when he said that "when we put a man in prison we deprive him of a large number of his consents, therefore it is perhaps distasteful to confer upon him a consent which is not for his benefit but for our own." In any case, from these considerations, Professor Daube drew a strict conclusion: "No person under any restraint whatsoever should be allowed to give consent"; "a person under restraint cannot be presumed to consent."[2] These statements—as we shall see in a moment—are applicable as well to children in institutions.

But the reasons so far cited that lend support to this sweeping conclusion are not adequate, unless imprisonment means that a man has been altogether drummed out of the human community. Since it does not, one might argue for quite the opposite conclusion. It can be contended that since we have deprived a prisoner of a large number of his consents, we should yield to his consent to do good if it is an understanding, voluntary consent. It can be contended that there are dignity and responsibilities consonant with prison life, and that under proper precautions participation in medical experimentation may be among them.

Interwoven with these considerations, however, was another that was more convincing. As Professor Daube put it: "Not all prison authorities throughout the world deserve the fullest trust"; ". . . it would be fatal to lower standards in an indirect manner, however laudable the purposes"; "I have no doubt that 99 out of 100 prisoners would have done this freely, but I wouldn't take the chance on the 100th."[3]

Dr. T. E. Starzl, and the other transplant surgeons at the University of Colorado, had used prisoner donors. He remained convinced of the *voluntariness* of their action. The program was announced in a low key, by a simple notice on the bulletin board of the prison. No pay or pardon or reduction of length of servitude was offered, and none was given. The incidence of enlistment was low. Many of those who volunteered had only a few weeks or months left to serve. These facts support the view that the prisoners' actions were volitional. They also lead us to question again whether the opportunity to make this consent should be withheld from prisoners if it is an opportunity to be presented to anyone. Still, Dr. Starzl was persuaded by Professor Daube for the reason stated above, and the practice was discontinued. Dr. Starzl summarized the argument very well indeed: "The use of penal volunteers, however equitably handled in a local situation, would inevitably lead to abuse if accepted as a reasonable precedent and applied broadly."[4]

This asks and gives one answer to the question: Which rule of medical practice or institutional practice, if widely adopted, can be foreseen to lead on the whole to the violation of men and to their self-violation, even if this need not be the case in each instance? Where, for example, the payment of money for blood tissue is practiced, and prisoners are not excluded from this payment, one does not have to travel far even in this enlightened land to hear rumors that local or state politicians have a concession or a kickback on the prisoner blood supply! That is wrong and was predictable, even if payment, and payment to prisoners, is not wrong in each instance.

To return to the question of investigations involving children in institutions as subjects in trials having no relation to their care, we can now say that even if this would not be (as I have argued) inherently or always necessarily wrong, still the use of captive populations in children, however equitably and safely handled in a local situation, would inevitably lead to abuse if accepted as a reasonable precedent and applied broadly. A rule of practice prohibiting the use of children in institutions simply as experimental subjects in the accumulation of knowledge for the benefit of others should govern the institutions set up to care for them. Some philosophers would call this a rule-utilitarian-rule. It is rather a rule of fidelity, expressing in a specific practice mankind's minimum loyalty to children.

The Kefauver-Harris amendments to the Federal Food, Drug, and Cosmetic Act passed in 1962 do not so rule; and the use of captive populations of children in pharmacological investigations is a practice that is not only widespread but predictably abused in this country. The bill that went before Congress for vote contained no provision for patient or subject consent. Senator Jacob Javits proposed to amend the bill to require that in investigations of a new drug the patients or subjects be "appropriately advised that such drug had not been determined to be safe in use for human beings." The outcome of debate in the House and Senate was to make subject consent mandatory while lodging the certification of this in the investigators, not in the Food and Drug Administration. The provision finally enacted introduced proxy consent and two exceptions to the procuring of consent. As finally adopted the provision requires:

... that experts using such drugs for investigational purposes certify to such manufacturer or sponsor that they will inform any human beings to whom such drugs, or any controls used in connection therewith, are being administered, or their representatives, that such drugs are being used for investigational purposes and will obtain the consent of such human beings or their representatives, except [1] where they deem it not feasible or, [2] in their professional judgment, contrary to the best interests of such human beings.[5]

The first interpretative ruling by the FDA concerning this consent requirement was not issued until August 30, 1966. Meantime, a number of investigators had thought that "not feasible" allowed them to dispense with consent if this inconvenienced the research design. In short, the provision was thought to have enacted the supremacy of *another* duty of medical experimenters, namely, to ensure that the quality of the research design is such as to secure the scientific results being sought.

The 1966 interpretative ruling, however, limited the intention of this stipulation to care for the patients or subjects consenting to drug investigations. It adopted the distinction in the Helsinki Declaration between research primarily for the accumulation of knowledge and research in therapeutic situations. No exception to the requirement of consent of the subject or his representative was allowed in the first instance. The two exceptions applied only to research having patient care primarily in view. Finally, the meaning of these exceptions was determined largely by reference to the debates in the House and Senate in 1962. "Not feasible" meant patients in coma or patients otherwise incapable of consenting whose legal representative was unavailable in an emergency. "Contrary to the best interests of such human beings" was meant to permit beneficial investigations on, for example, cancer patients without upsetting such a patient's well-being when in a physician's discretion the patient does not know he has cancer.

This interpretative ruling concerning the meaning of these exceptions is dangerous if it is taken to sanction unrelated experimentation on the seriously ill or the dying without the patient's prior participatory consent. But the main thing to be said is that these stipulations are largely irrelevant to drug research. The interpretation of the "exceptions" followed the debate in Congress; but that debate about seriously ill and dying patients was also largely irrelevant to the majority of drug research. Therefore, even after these interpretations were issued, it could fairly be said of the FDA "exceptions": "Better loopholes may be invented, but this seems a good start."[6] However, seriously ill or dying patients may need an insufficiently tested drug. Then medical ethics would require that the efficacy of the new drug be predictable with some confidence; it must be more likely to work than an established remedy. But we may allow that in the course of new-drug investigations there may be cases in which, all other therapies having failed or estimated to be likely to prove less beneficial than the new drug, a patient's consent can be constructively implied as the basis of Good Samaritan emergency treatment.

Ordinarily, however, drug research is more deliberate and preplanned. What is needed are human beings willing to consent to take the drugs or to serve as anonymous controls. What is needed is an easily controlled population. The legal representative of children in institutions would ordinarily be available, if he is to be vested with the power of consent for them but not in their medical behalf. The children themselves are ordinarily under no necessity to have the drug used without delay. Reference to the use of drugs in emergencies among the specifications of a law governing investigations in drugs is exceedingly likely to come to mean that anything that delays the solution of medical problems is unethical. The research consequences are likely to become overriding. This may happen if investigators are tempted to transfer the exceptions to the consent requirement in cases of beneficial (emergency) research to the bulk of drug research, which is nonbeneficial, and which should proceed only with the understanding of the subject. The crux, therefore, is the admission that a subject's consent can be satisfied by *his representative*.[7] This opens the door to the use of children in institutions for experimental purposes and not for drug testing that is incidental to the course of their medical care.

In 1958 and 1959 the *New England Journal of Medicine* reported a series of experiments performed upon patients and new admittees to the Willowbrook State School, a home for retarded children in Staten Island, New York.[8] These experiments were described as "an attempt to control the high prevalence of infectious hepatitis in an institution for mentally defective patients." The experiments were said to be justified because, under conditions of an existing controlled outbreak of hepatitis in the institution, "knowledge obtained from a series of suitable studies could well lead to its control." In actuality, the experiments were designed to duplicate and confirm the efficacy of gamma globulin in immunization against hepatitis, to develop and improve or improve upon that inoculum, and to learn more about infectious hepatitis in general.

The experiments were justified—doubtless, after a great deal of soul searching—for the following reasons: there was a smoldering epidemic throughout the institution and "it was apparent that most of the patients at Willowbrook were naturally exposed to hepatitis virus"; infectious hepatitis is a much milder disease in children; the strain at Willowbrook was especially mild; only the strain or strains of the virus already disseminated at Willowbrook were used: and only those small and incompetent patients whose parents gave consent were used.

The patient population at Willowbrook was 4478, growing at a rate of one patient a day over a three-year span, or from 10 to 15 new admissions per week. In the first trial the existing population was divided into two groups: one group served as uninoculated controls, and the other group was inoculated with 0.01 ml. of gamma globulin per pound of body weight. Then for a second trial new admittees and those left uninoculated before were again divided: one group served as uninoculated controls and the other was inoculated with 0.06 ml. of gamma globulin per pound of body weight. This proved that Stokes et al. had correctly demonstrated that the larger amount would give significant immunity for up to seven or eight months.[9]

Serious ethical questions may be raised about the trials so far described. No mention is made of any attempt to enlist the adult personnel of the institution, numbering nearly 1,000 including nearly 600 attendants on ward duty, and new additions to the staff, in these studies whose excusing reason was that almost everyone was "naturally" exposed to the Willowbrook virus. Nothing requires that major research into the natural history of hepatitis be first undertaken in children. Experiments have been carried out in the military and with prisoners as subjects. There have been fatalities from the experiments; but surely in all these cases the consent of the volunteers was as valid or better than the proxy consent of these children's "representatives." There would have been no question of the understanding consent that might have been given by the adult personnel at Willowbrook, if significant benefits were expected from studying that virus.

Second, nothing is said that would warrant withholding an inoculation of some degree of known efficacy from part of the population, or for withholding in the first trial less than the full amount of gamma globulin that had served to immunize in previous tests, except the need to test, confirm, and improve the inoculum. That, of course, was a desirable goal; but it does not seem possible to warrant withholding gamma globulin for the reason that is often said to justify controlled trials, namely, that one procedure is *as likely* to succeed as the other.

Third, nothing is said about attempts to control or defeat the low-grade epidemic at Willowbrook by more ordinary, if more costly and less experimental, procedures. Nor is anything said about admitting no more patients until this goal had been accomplished. This was not a massive urban hospital whose teeming population would have to be turned out into the streets, with resulting dangers to themselves and to public health, in order to sanitize the place. Instead, between 200 and 250 patients were housed in each of 18 buildings over approximately 400 acres in a semirural setting of fields, woods, and well-kept spacious lawns. Clearly it would have been possible to secure other accommodation for new admissions away from the infection, while eradicating the infection at Willowbrook building by building. This might have cost money, and it would certainly have required astute detective work to discover the source of the infection. The doctors determined that the new patients likely were not carrying the infection upon admission, and that it did not arise from the procedures and routine inoc-

ulations given them at the time of admission. Why not go further in the search for the source of the epidemic? If this had been an orphanage for normal children or a floor of private patients, instead of a school for mentally defective children, one wonders whether the doctors would so readily have accepted the hepatitis as a "natural" occurrence and even as an opportunity for study.

The next step was to attempt to induce "passive-active immunity" by feeding the virus to patients already protected by gamma globulin. In this attempt to improve the inoculum, permission was obtained from the parents of children from 5 to 10 years of age newly admitted to Willowbrook, who were then isolated from contact with the rest of the institution. All were inoculated with gamma globulin and then divided into two groups: one served as controls while the other group of new patients were fed the Willowbrook virus, obtained from feces, in doses having 50 percent infectivity, i.e., in concentrations estimated to produce hepatitis with jaundice in half the subjects tested. Then twice the 50 percent infectivity was tried. This proved, among other things, that hepatitis has an "alimentary-tract phase" in which it can be transmitted from one person to another while still "inapparent" in the first person. This, doubtless, is exceedingly important information in learning how to control epidemics of infectious hepatitis. The second of the two articles mentioned above describes studies of the incubation period of the virus and of whether pooled serum remained infectious when aged and frozen. Still the small, mentally defective patients who were deliberately fed infectious hepatitis are described as having suffered mildly in most cases: "The liver became enlarged in the majority, occasionally a week or two before the onset of jaundice. Vomiting and anorexia usually lasted only a few days. Most of the children gained weight during the course of hepatitis."

That mild description of what happened to the children who were fed hepatitis (and who continued to be introduced into the unaltered environment of Willowbrook) is itself alarming, since it is now definitely known that cirrhosis of the liver results from infectious hepatitis more frequently than from excessive consumption of alcohol! Now, or in 1958 and 1959, no one knows what may be other serious consequences of contracting infectious hepatitis. Understanding human volunteers were then and are now needed in the study of this disease, although a South American monkey has now successfully been give a form of hepatitis, and can henceforth serve as our ally in its conquest. But not children who cannot consent knowingly. If Peace Corps workers are regularly given gamma globulin before going abroad as a guard against their contracting hepatitis, and are inoculated at intervals thereafter, it seems that this is the least we should do for mentally defective children before they "go abroad" to Willowbrook or other institutions set up for their care.

Discussion pro and con of the Willowbrook experiments that have come to my attention serve only to reinforce the ethical objections that can be raised against what was done simply from a careful analysis of the original articles reporting the research design and findings. In an address at the 1968 Ross Conference on Pediatric Research, Dr. Saul Krugman raised the question, Should vaccine trials be carried out in adult volunteers before subjecting children to similar tests?[10] He answered this question in the negative. The reason adduced was simply that "a vaccine virus trial may be a more hazardous procedure for adults than for children." Medical researchers, of course, are required to minimize the hazards, but not by moving from consenting to unconsenting subjects. This apology clearly shows that adults and children have become interchangeable in face of the overriding importance of obtaining the research goal. This means that the special moral claims of children for care and protection are forgotten, and especially the claims of children who are most weak and vulnerable. (Krugman's reference to the measles vaccine trials is not to the point.)

The *Medical Tribune* explains that the 16-bed isolation unit set up at Willowbrook served "to protect the study subjects from Willowbrook's other endemic diseases—such as shigellosis, measles, rubella and respiratory and parasitic infections—while exposing them to hepatitis."[11] This presumably compensated for the infection they were given. It is not convincingly shown that the children could by no means,

however costly, have been protected from the epidemic of hepatitis. The statement that Willowbrook "had endemic infectious hepatitis and a sufficiently open population so that the disease could never be quieted by exhausting the supply of susceptibles" is at best enigmatic.

Oddly, physicians defending the propriety of the Willowbrook hepatitis project soon begin talking like poorly instructed "natural lawyers"! Dr. Louis Lasagna and Dr. Geoffrey Edsall, for example, find these experiments unobjectionable—both, for the reason stated by Edsall: "the children would apparently incur no greater risk than they were likely to run by nature." In any case, Edsall's examples of parents consenting with a son 17 years of age for him to go to war, and society's agreement with minors that they can drive cars and hurt themselves were entirely beside the point. Dr. David D. Rutstein adheres to a stricter standard in regard to research on infectious hepatitis: "It is not ethical to use human subjects for the growth of a virus for any purpose."[12]

The latter sweeping verdict may depend on knowledge of the effects of viruses on chromasomal difficulties, mongolism, etc., that was not available to the Willowbrook group when their researches were begun thirteen years ago. If so, this is a telling point against appeal to "no discernible risks" as the sole standard applicable to the use of children in medical experimentation. That would lend support to the proposition that we always know that there are unknown and undiscerned risks in the case of an invasion of the fortress of the body—which then can be consented to by an adult in behalf of a child only if it is in the child's behalf medically.

When asked what she told the parents of the subject-children at Willowbrook, Dr. Joan Giles replied, "I explain that there is no vaccine against infectious hepatitis. . . . I also tell them that we can modify the disease with gamma globulin but we can't provide lasting immunity without letting them get the disease."[13] Obviously vaccines giving "lasting immunity" are not the only kinds of vaccine to be used in caring for patients.

Doubtless the studies at Willowbrook resulted in improvement in the vaccine, to the benefit of present and future patients. In September 1966, "a routine program of GG [gamma globulin] administration to every new patient at Willowbrook" was begun. This cut the incidence of icteric hepatitis 80 to 85 percent. Then follows a significant statement in the *Medical Tribune* article: "A similar reduction in the icteric form of the disease has been accomplished among the employees, who began getting routine GG earlier in the study."[14] Not only did the research team (so far as these reports show) fail to consider and adopt the alternative that new admittees to the staff be asked to become volunteers for an investigation that might improve the vaccine against the strand of infectious hepatitis to which they as well as the children were exposed. Instead, the staff was routinely protected earlier than the inmates were! And, as we have seen, there was evidence from the beginning that gamma globulin provided at least some protection. A "modification" of the disease was still an inoculum, even if this provided no lasting immunization and had to be repeated. It is axiomatic to medical ethics that a known remedy or protection—even if not perfect or even if the best exact administration of it has not been proved—should not be withheld from individual patients. It seems to a layman that from the beginning various trials at immunization of all new admittees might have been made, and controlled observation made of their different degrees of effectiveness against "nature" at Willowbrook. This would doubtless have been a longer way round, namely, the "anecdotal" method of investigative treatment that comes off second best in comparison with controlled trials. Yet this seems to be the alternative dictated by our received medical ethics, and the only one expressive of minimal care of the primary patients themselves.

Finally, except for one episode the obtaining of parental consent (on the premise that this is ethically valid) seems to have been very well handled. Wards of the state were not used, though by law the administrator at Willowbrook could have signed consent for them. Only new admittees whose parents were available were entered by proxy consent into the project. Explanation was made to groups of these parents, and they were given time to think about it and consult with their own family phy-

sicians. Then late in 1964 Willowbrook was closed to all new admissions because of overcrowding. What then happened can most impartially be described in the words of an article defending the Willowbrook project on medical and ethical grounds:

> Parents who applied for their children to get in were sent a form letter over Dr. Hammond's signature saying that there was no space for new admissions and that their name was being put on a waiting list.
>
> But the hepatitis program, occupying its own space in the institution, continued to admit new patients as each new study group began. "Where do you find new admissions except by canvassing the people who have applied for admission?" Dr. Hammond asked.
>
> So a new batch of form letters went out, saying that there were a few vacancies in the hepatitis research unit if the parents cared to consider volunteering their child for that.
>
> In some instances the second form letter apparently was received as closely as a week after the first letter arrived.[15]

Granting—as I do not—the validity of parental consent to research upon children not in their behalf medically, what sort of consent was that? Surely, the duress upon these parents with children so defective as to require institutionalization was far greater than the duress on prisoners given tobacco or paid or promised parole for their cooperation! I grant that the timing of these events was inadvertent. Since, however, ethics is a matter of criticizing institutions and not only of exculpating or making culprits of individual men, the inadvertence does not matter. This is the strongest possible argument for saying that even if parents have the right to consent to submit the children who are directly and continuously in their care to nonbeneficial medical experimentation, this should not be the rule of practice governing institutions set up for their care.

Such use of captive populations of children for purely experimental purposes ought to be made legally impossible. My view is that this should be stopped by legal acknowledgement of the moral invalidity of parental or legal proxy consent for the child to procedures having no relation to a child's own diagnosis or treatment.

If this is not done, canons of loyalty require that the rule of practice (by law, or otherwise) be that children in institutions and not directly under the care of parents or relatives should *never* be used in medical investigations having present pain or discomfort and unknown present and future risks to them, and promising future possible benefits only for others.

In 1967, after a study of twenty-one New York City municipal hospitals, State Senator Seymour R. Thaler proposed an amendment to the New York State Civil Rights bill that would apply sweepingly to all medical research and to all research involving children as subjects. Some of the provisions of his amendment could be applied more narrowly to captive populations of children. Senator Thaler would require the "voluntary informed written consent of adult patients used in medical experiment and would prohibit research on children unless authorized by a 'court of competent jurisdiction.' " His bill stipulated that the court may authorize a medical experiment or other medical research upon a minor when such experiment or research is related to the minor's physical or mental ailment and upon a finding by the court that the best interests of the minor would thereby be served. It was the provision placing all research upon children under courts of competent jurisdiction that caused the furor. Dr. Saul Krugman, chairman of pediatrics at New York University, called the bill "a disaster—a real disaster," if passed.[16]

The version of this bill introduced by Senators Thaler and Lent in 1969 does not entirely invalidate parental consent. This, however, is set within the context of the creation of a state board on human research charged with responsibility to formulate rules and regulations and to require the establishment of institutional and regional screening committees. The bill provides that "no person shall be used in human research without his or his parent's, guardian's or legal representative's prior written informed consent, but the board may make such exceptions as it may prescribe where the proposed subject is incompetent to give such consent . . ."[17]

The objection to this legislation can be only the resistance of researchers to the development of public policy in this regard, by law and through regulatory agencies. There are more regulations governing animal experimentation than govern human experimentation; more laws regulating the interstate transportation of bodies than regulate the interstate transportation of dying patients (who may be eligible organ donors when they are pronounced dead); a great mass of case law having to do with medical negligence in cases of treatment but little that deals with investigations primarily for the accumulation of knowledge. This situation is not likely long to endure.

For this reason, let us look briefly at another attempt to draft appropriate legislation—this time not by a state senator but by Frank P. Grad, Adjunct Professor of Legislation and Associate Director of the Legislative Drafting Research Fund at Columbia University Law School. In a paper before a conference sponsored by the New York Academy of Sciences, Professor Grad stated the principle that runs throughout our legal and moral tradition. "The rationale," he wrote, "which allows parents or guardians to consent on behalf of their children or wards in the therapeutic situation are not clearly applicable to the non-therapeutic one. . . . There is no clear reason why a parent should be given the power to consent to expose his child to a risk, where taking the risk is not clearly in the child's interest or for his benefit. Nor is there any reason why a lawyer-guardian sitting in his downtown office ought to be free to expose his incompetent ward in a state hospital to hazards which he has neither chosen, nor which he has the competency to choose, for himself. Consent on behalf of minors and incompetents has, therefore, been rather closely circumscribed."[18]

But in the model legislation accompanying his paper, Professor Grad suggested the unqualified enactment of this principle only in the case of incompetents other than children as such. "Valid consent for an incompetent to become a subject may be given by his legal guardian," the draft legislation reads, "only if the human experimentation or research bears directly upon such incompetent's disability." That statement might have been repeated with regard to subjects judged incompetent for reasons of age. Instead, the draft reads: "Valid consent for a person under the age of eighteen years may be given by his parent or legal guardian only if there is no reason to believe that the human experimentation or research will result in physical or psychological injury or harm."

In other words, these legislative proposals would bring under public scrutiny both the parental consents obtained and the physiologically describable acts to be used in medical research. Neither would actually rule out the power of the consent of parents to enter their children into nontherapeutic medical trials. I suggest that—short of prohibiting the latter—our legislation would still need to go further than these proposals. Parental responsibility is necessarily weakened when children are institutionalized, when they are no longer directly, daily, and continuously under our care.

If we are going to count on parental and familial consent as sufficient protection of child-life, this should be only when parents are constantly placed on their mettle in the daily life of the home. If we than fail our children, this may be, as Professor Daube said, among the normal burdens, hazards, and dignity of a child's daily life. But surely we have the wisdom to know that even ordinary parental care must slacken when children are away in institutions; this is even more true when parents grievously need to place a child in an institution in order to provide at all for his care.

If, then, we are not going to invalidate the consents of parents and relatives except in the case of investigations proximately or remotely related to a child's own treatment, there can be no valid argument against doing exactly this in the limited case of children in orphanages, reformatories, or homes for the retarded. The legal representatives of such children—even if parents—should be able to make decisions only in the stated medical interests of the children themselves if they are part of a captive population. To require a showing that this in fact is what is being done would be a proper additional arrangement guaranteeing that institutions for the care of children exist in fact only to care for them according to the canons of the highest loyalty, and not for the accumulation of knowledge having no stated benefit to these children them-

selves. Then parents and medical experimentation in general in the case of children might be moved to come up to the standards of our institutions.

Notes

1. Fletcher, "Human Experimentation," pp. 620-49. The author "agrees with those who would put the sharpest restrictions upon the use of prisoner populations in medical research, since by virtue of their imprisonment they cannot be truly said to possess and active capacity to consent. . . . [Those who have suffered] the loss of public liberty through imprisonment, should not then be made to go through the charade of seeming to possess what has been temporarily removed" ibid., p. 636. I suggest that a child, by virtue of his childhood, cannot be truly said to possess all active capacity to consent; and that it is a dangerous charade for anyone to go through the motions of consenting for him when this is not truly done *in his behalf medically.* Particularly in regard to children in institutions, to say "never" to the consents of their legal representatives when these are not even ostensibly in the children's behalf medically would not be "to remove oneself from historical possibility" (*ibid.,* p. 636, n. 46). It would rather be to place upon ourselves the moral requirement that other historical possibilities for the accumulation of knowledge be looked for or designed.

2. Wolstenholme and O'Connor, *Ethics in Medical Progress,* pp. 198, 204, 205, 197, 204.

3. Ibid., pp. 198, 204.

4. Ibid., pp. 75-77.

5. Federal Food, Drug, and Cosmetic Act, Section 505 (i).

6. Oscar D. Ratnoff and Marian F. Ratnoff, "Ethical Responsibility in Clinical Investigation," *Perspectives in Biology and Medicine,* Autumn 1967, p. 89.

7. By contrast, the statement on "Clinical Investigations Using Human Beings as Subject" issued by the U.S. Public Health Service severely limits the consent of such human beings' legal representatives. "No subject may participate in an investigative procedure," it says, "unless (a) He is mentally competent and has sufficient mental and communicative capacity to understand his choice to participate; and (b)

He is 21 years of age or more, except that if the individual be less than 21, he may participate in a procedure intended and designed to protect or improve his personal health or otherwise for his personal benefit or advantage if the informed written consent of his parents or legal guardian be obtained as well as the written consent of the subject himself if he be mature enough to appreciate the nature of the procedure and the risks involved" (Department of Health, Education and Welfare, Bureau of Medical Services Circular No. 38, June 23, 1966).

8. Robert Ward, Saul Krugman, Joan P. Giles, A. Milton Jacobs, and Oscar Bodansky, "Infectious Hepatitis: Studies of Its Natural History and Prevention," *New England Journal of Medicine* 258, no. 9 (February 27, 1958): 407-16; Saul Krugman, Robert Ward, Joan P. Giles, Oscar Bodansky, and A. Milton Jacobs, "Infectious Hepatitis: Detection of the Virus during the Incubation Period and in Clinically Inapparent Infection," *New England Journal of Medicine* 261, no. 15 (October 8, 1959): 729-34. The following account and unannotated quotations are taken from these articles.

9. J. Stokes, Jr., et al., "Infectious Hepatitis: Length of Protection by Immune Serum Globulin (Gamma Globulin) during Epidemics," *Journal of the American Medical Association* 147 (1951): 714-19. Since the half-life of gamma globulin is three weeks, no one knows exactly why it immunizes for so long a period. The "highly significant protection against hepatitis obtained by the use of gamma globulin," however, had been confirmed as early as 1945 (see Edward B. Grossman, Sloan G. Stewart, and Joseph Stokes, "Post-Transfusion Hepatitis in Battle Casualties," *Journal of the American Medical Association* 129 no. 15 [December 8, 1945]: 991-94). The inoculation *withheld* in the Willowbrook experiments had, therefore, proved valuable.

10. Saul Krugman, "Reflections on Pediatric Clinical Investigations," in *Problems of Drug Evaluation in Infants and Children,* Report of the Fifty-eighth Ross Conference on Pediatric Research, Dorado Beach, Puerto Rico, May 5-7, 1968 (Columbus: Ross Laboratories), pp. 41-42.

11. "Studies with Children Backed on Medical, Ethical Grounds," *Medical Tribune and Medical News* 8, no. 19 (February 20, 1967): 1, 23.

12. *Daedalus.* Spring 1969, pp. 471-72, 529. See also pp. 458, 470-72. Since it is the proper business of an ethicist to uphold the proposition that only

retrogression in civility can result from bad moral reasoning and the use of inept examples, however innocent, it is fair to point out the startling comparison between Edsall's "argument" and the statement of Dr. Karl Brandt, plenipotentiary in charge of all medical activities in the Nazi Reich: "Do you think that one can obtain any worth-while, fundamental results without a definite toll of lives? The same goes for technological development. You cannot build a great bridge, a gigantic building—you cannot establish a speed record without deaths!" (quoted by Leo Alexander, "War Crimes: Their Social-Psychological Aspects," *American Journal of Psychiatry* 105, no. 3 [September 1948]: 172). Casualties to progress, or injuries accepted in setting speed limits, are morally quite different from death or maiming or even only risks, or unknown risks, directly and deliberately imposed upon an unconsenting human being.

13. *Medical Tribune,* February 20, 1967, p. 23.

14. *Medical Tribune,* February 20, 1967, p. 23.

15. *Medical Tribune,* February 20, 1967, p. 23.

16. *New York Times,* January 20, 1967. Krugman was one of the physicians who conducted the Willowbrook experiments.

17. An Act To Amend the Education Law, in Relation to the Regulation of Research on Human Subjects. In Senate, 1969-70 Regular Session, Cal. No. 1865, 4652-A. February 14, 1969.

18. Frank P. Grad, "Regulation of Clinical Research by the State," Conference on New Dimensions in Legal and Ethical Concepts for Human Research, New York Academy of Sciences, New York City, May 19-21, 1969. Professor Grad resolved the alleged problem of drawing the line between therapeutic and nontherapeutic research by imagining a patient to ask: " '*Doctor, are you doing this for me, or am I doing this for you?*' If the physician can truthfully answer that he is doing it for the patient, then it is clearly therapeutic research. If, on the contrary, the subject is undergoing a particular procedure not for his own benefit but for that of the researcher in the pursuit of a scientific goal, then the procedure is non-therapeutic." The thesis of this chapter is that since the child patient cannot ask that question, what he is doing for the researcher is simply being done to him, while what is done to him by way of treatment or investigational treatment, with legitimate parental or guardian consent or by his implied consent, has the patient as an end in view.

When May Research Be Stopped?

Carl Cohen

The uses and possible misuses of recombinant DNA are so threatening, some believe, that research into that technology should now be stopped. But reasons good enough to justify prohibition of research in this sphere must, in fairness, apply equally to other spheres, if threats of similar gravity arise there.

I ask, therefore: What are the alternative principles that, if adopted, might reasonably justify prohibition of research in a given sphere? Which of these alternative principles should be rejected, and which accepted in some form or part? And to the extent that any one of these principles is acceptable, what bearing does it have upon continued research with recombinant DNA?

My answers to these questions rest upon two fundamental propositions, very generally agreed upon. First: freedom of inquiry is a value of such profound importance that it must not be abridged without the most compelling reasons. This proposition, true generally, carries great weight in a society holding liberty as a paramount ideal; it carries extraordinary weight in universities and research institutions committed explicitly to the enlargement of knowledge. Second: some research undertakings should properly be restricted. Everyone may not agree upon particular cases, but it will be agreed that a rational commitment to freedom of inquiry does not protect every research enterprise in every circumstance.

The task is to characterize the enterprises and circumstances in which prohibition may prove defensible or even obligatory.

ALTERNATIVE PRINCIPLES OF PROHIBITION

To justify prohibition, some would present a practical syllogism in this form: Major

Reprinted by permission of the author and *The New England Journal of Medicine,* vol. 296, pp. 1203–1210, May 26, 1977.

premise: research having certain identifiable features (p,q,r. . . .) may (or must) be stopped. Minor premise: this research (in recombinant DNA, or in nuclear fission, or. . .) has precisely those features. Hence, this research may (or must) be stopped. My first objective is to formulate alternative, plausible major premises of such syllogisms.

Principles of prohibition must pertain either to the product or to the process of the research in question. The line between the two may be hard to draw, but under one or the other can be listed all the general principles that seem remotely tenable.

Set A: By-product (#1-#3)

(1) Research should not be permitted when it aims at (or is likely to result in) the discovery of knowledge that is wrong for human beings to possess.

(2) Research should not be permitted when it aims at (or is likely to result in) the discovery of knowledge that is not wise to place in human hands.

(2a) When there is any probability that the knowledge developed will be used with very injurious consequences.

(2b) When there is moderate probability that the knowledge developed will be used with very injurious consequences.

(2c) When there is high probability that the knowledge developed will be used with very injurious consequences.

(3) Research should not be permitted when it aims specifically at the development or perfection of instruments for killing or injuring human beings.

Set B: By-process (#4-#6)

(4) Research should not be permitted when it is not conducted openly, for all to examine the ongoing process and results.

(5) Research should not be permitted when its continuation is unfair, either to the subjects of the experimentation or to those otherwise involved in

the research. Research is unfair when, through coercion or deceit, or in some other way, the rights of those involved are not respected.

(6) Research should not be permitted when its conduct (as distinct from its product) presents risks so great as clearly to outweigh the benefits reasonably anticipated. Risks here must be understood to include all hazards that that process of inquiry entails, of which there are two large categories: risks of "misfire" (i.e., achieving results different from and more dangerous than those sought) and risks of "accident" (i.e., unforeseen mishap during the process).

(6a) When the risks are essentially to persons involved in the research:

(6a1) the subjects of experimentation;

(6a2) the researchers and their associates.

(6b) Where the risks are essentially to others than those involved in the research.

These exhaust the alternative principles that are at all reasonable, or arguably tenable, for the prohibition of research. Phrasing (and the degree of specificity) may vary, but every plausible candidate, I contend, will fall under one or another of the six kinds distinguished.

As an illustration: Robert Sinsheimer, professor of biophysics at the California Institute of Technology and an acute critic of recombinant DNA research, has suggested some possible answers to the question, "For what specific purposes might we wish to limit inquiry?" He proposes, or at least entertains, several candidates.[1]

(a) To preserve human dignity. "We should not do experiments that involuntarily make of man a means rather than an end."[1] But, of course, human subjects in medical experiments are means. Sinsheimer surely intends to emphasize, with Kant, that one must not treat human beings as means only, but also as ends—for which reason research committees do rigorously insist that their participation be truly voluntary and informed. This is but a more elaborate statement of principle (5), above, demanding fairness.

(b) To avoid "involuntary physical or biological hazard."[1] Sinsheimer recognizes, of course, that one cannot avoid all such hazards. He wants us all to be very sensitive to the level of danger. This is but another formulation, less precise, of principle (6), above, addressing the balance of risk and benefit.

(c) Cost. "[One] asks if the primary consequences of the inquiry, that is, the knowledge to be gained, is worth the expenditures of talent, time and resources."[1] But refusing to support research is one thing, prohibiting it is another. When the research enterprise involves heavy expense, one is right to insist that the worth of the knowledge to be gained be very carefully estimated. Protecting free inquiry does not entail irrationality in the expenditure of resources. And it is true that institutional refusal to fund a research project often has the effect of blocking that project in that context. Many research activities, however (work with recombinant DNA technology being one important example), do not require very large investments of institutional or governmental funds. Although one may conclude, therefore, that for some projects the object does not justify the expenditure, it is essential to see that cost cannot serve as grounds for prohibition. Some research is simply not worth doing, but reasons for not troubling to do certain things ourselves must not be taken as reasons for keeping other persons from doing them.

Some principles, very different from those stated above, are procedural, requiring special machinery for the approval of research protocols in certain areas. Approval (some say) must be given by the appropriate bodies, with appropriate memberhship, deliberating with appropriate care. Others say that the decision to permit research of certain kinds may be made only by some larger community (city or state) through some democratic voting procedure. Such regulation, although awkward, is being tried in some quarters. But, even when feasible and fitting, those procedural requirements are not germane here. One seeks to discover reasons that may serve to deny approval. Whatever the decision-making machinery, the individual users of that machinery need grounds for concluding yea or nay. These grounds—not the system of their application—are what I am concerned with here.

Finally, I note that the six alternative principles are not mutually exclusive; one could rationally hold (say) both (3) [on killing], and some variant of (6) [risks over benefits]. They may overlap, relying upon the same feature of a given inquiry—for example, what is objectionable under (4) [openness] may also be objectionable under (5) [unfairness].

It remains to determine which (if any) of these principles should be adopted, and which (if any) apply to the sphere of recombinant DNA research, and to indentify the restrictions (if any) that properly follow there-from.

THE SIX PRINCIPLES RECONSIDERED

What follows is a critical appraisal of the six alternative principles listed above. The conclusions reached unavoidably rely upon some personal judgments, but are put forward for general agreement.

Principles Based upon the Product of Research (#1-#3)

(1) "Research should not be permitted when it aims at (or likely to result in) the discovery of knowledge that is wrong for human beings to possess."

This principle should be rejected utterly. There is no body of knowledge, or item of knowledge, that is intrinsically wrong to possess. The conviction that there are forbidden precincts, that there is an intellectual sanctum sanctorum into which all entry is sinful, must rely upon some claim of special revelation, or some other nonrational restriction that has no rightful authority to limit inquiry in a university or research institution.

Principles of privacy, it is true, may render certain sorts of knowledge about individuals not suitable for public scrutiny. But there is a vast difference between the claim that some knowledge is not properly public and the claim that some knowledge is intrinsically unfit for human acquisition. Individuals are free, of course, to limit themselves if they honestly hold beliefs of the latter sort. The search here, however, is not for principles that some persons may cling to but for the principles research institutions ought to defend.

Note that this principle, (1), is widely attractive. Much of the anxiety that attends DNA research, I submit, flows from vague, unformulated doubts about whether this probe into "the code of life itself" might not be a form of human presumption, a playing of God. One is understandably awed by the cumulative powers of human intelligence; those powers can be (and often have been) misused. But fear of that misuse does not give rational warrant for closing the avenues of exploration. If one did believe that there are domains in which human knowing is taboo, molecular genetics might indeed be one of them. Inquiry into nuclear fusion or celestial exploration might then be equally taboo, as might be the study of theories of relativity, or the development of contraceptive technics. The penetration of every intellectual frontier threatens deeply held convictions. Every striking advance in human prowess frightens many, horrifies some and appears to a few as the profane invasion of the holy of holies. The difficulty lies not in discriminating between the real holy of holies and those only mistakenly supposed; it lies in the unwarranted asssumption that there are any spheres of knowledge to which ingress is forbidden. This first principle is wholly untenable; a fortiori it is not tenable as applied to the biochemistry of genetics.

(2) "Research should not be permitted when it aims at (or is likely to result in) the discovery of knowledge that is not wise to place in human hands."

Of this principle I distinguish three varieties, depending on the degree of probability with which great injury may be anticipated as a result of the possession of that knowledge. Of course, there will be argument about what constitutes great injury, about how such probabilities are to be calculated or estimated, and about what the probabilities are in a particular case. But supposing rough agreement is reached on these matters, the rightness (or wrongness) of the principle here formulated remains to be determined, and is of profound importance.

Principle (2a) [that prohibition of research is justified when there is any probability of very injurious consequences] may be rejected categorically; it verges on the absurd. On that principle one ought not rise from bed.

Principle (2b) [that prohibition of research is justified when there is moderate probability of very injurious consequences] must be more seriously considered—but it too deserves rejection in the end. It is true, of course, that the results of inquiry will often be such that there is some moderate likelihood that their use will prove very injurious, even disastrous. But the ubiquity of such possibilities renders (2b) [as it does (2a)] so sweeping as to entail the cessation of a great deal of the research—both in biologic and in physical sciences—best calculated to improve the human condition.

Nevertheless, serious thinkers have urged the adoption of some such principle. Two especially—one a historian, and the other a biophysicist—deserve response.

Shaw Livermore, professor of history at the University of Michigan, in concluding that his university should not proceed with the development of recombinant DNA technology, argues as follows[2]:

(i) Research on recombinant DNA promises the development of a special, elemental capability: that of overcoming the natural genetic barriers that separate the species, and (ultimately) of uniting genetic components of different species to produce new forms of life.

(ii) this capability would be so great, so overwhelming, as to exceed the capacity of society to direct and control it.

Therefore, (iii) success in this research "will bring with it a train of awesome and possibly disastrous consequences,"[2]

and (iv) decisions demanded by this technology may well have effects that are "unintended but irreversible."[2]

Livermore suggests, in effect, that scientists here are like the Sorcerer's Apprentice, conjuring into existence what they do not fully understand and none of them can control. Although appealing, the argument fails upon careful test. Consider its elements in reverse order.

(iv) That decisions regarding DNA will sometimes have unintended and irreversible effects is surely true, but not very weighty. That is precisely the case for every important human enterprise in research and development—it leaves the world in an irreversibly different condition from that in which it was before, and has consequences that could not have been foreseen, and therefore could not have been intended. Many of the discoveries that have proved the greatest boons to mankind have arisen from basic research in ways that were—when that research was first pursued—wholly unforeseen and unintended.

That some consequences (bad and good) of any major inquiry will be irreversible and unintended is evident, and cannot reasonably be taken as grounds for the prohibition of inquiry.

(iii) But the consequences of this inquiry may be awesome—possibly disastrous. Awesomeness, again, may be for good as well as evil. One should bear in mind, in weighing arguments like these, that recombinant DNA technology also opens possibilities for monumental improvements in the human condition. Both sides must be weighed. But it is the "possibly disastrous" results that are the nub of this complaint—a complaint that cuts either not at all or entirely too well. There are no grounds for supposing that the likelihood of disaster is greater in this arena than in other research arenas that one would not seriously think of foreclosing. There is "moderate probability," I suppose, that the results of research into nuclear fusion will one day be put to malevolent uses—but one would not on this ground seriously suggest a prohibition of inquiry into the ways in which the nuclei of atoms may combine. In any sphere knowledge may be put to devilish use; that is a poor reason for prohibiting its acquisition.

(ii) It is suggested that the acquisition of certain awesome capabilities be barred because the capacity to direct them, once acquired, is lacking. But do we lack that power? The supposition is very doubtful. Many reflective historians and philosophers would insist that we have the capacity for the direction and control of the products of research. Whether we will sharpen such capacities as finely as we ought remains to be seen. Recent self-imposed restraints, followed by extended public deliberation, precisely in this sphere of recombinant DNA, strongly suggest that the capacity to control does exist and is being applied. Some present uncertainty about the outcome of this application surely does not justify the cessation of the inquiry. And even if only the potential for wise control is now present, the realization of that potential can be stimulated and encouraged only with the advance of the inquiry in question. Professor Livermore, although reflectively, gives up hope for Dame Reason; I judge that one is ill advised to join him in despair.

(i) His anxieties—and indeed most arguments of this variety—stem largely from the "elemental" nature of the capabilities in view. But there is confusion hidden in the slippage between fears arising from the alleged probabilities of disaster (probabilities not ever established) and fears arising from the allegedly special, extraordinary properties of the knowledge to be discovered. The implicit suggestion that the knowledge sought is too godlike for human frailty gives seeming (but unjustifiable) plausibility to the claim that its acquisition will bring catastrophe. Once it is clearly seen that knowledge is not to be feared, that it may prove valuable everywhere, risky anywhere, and intrinsically improper nowhere, it will also be seen that the specialness of the discoveries in view, though in some ways real, ceases to serve as any ground for prohibition. Research in genetics, as in every science, moves ever onward; inquiring into the controlled manipulation of genetic macromolecules is a natural and inevitable phase of that advance. Fears that human beings are incapable of dealing with the products of their own intelligence are as much and as little justified on every other research continuum as on this one.

A differing effort to provide a tenable variant of this principle, (2b) is made by Sinsheimer. He writes:

[One] may extend inquiry into the ends of inquiry and question whether, in particular instances, we want to know the answer in every case. Given the nature of man and of human society, are the secondary consequences of such knowledge, on balance, likely to be beneficial? Here it may be that the highest wisdom is to recognize that we are not wise enough to know what we do not want to know, and thus to leave the ends of inquiry unrestrained. Indeed, I expect there are only a few instances where prudence would be in order. But the set may not be null.[1]

What does this say? Sinsheimer is guarded, tentative, unsure. From his questions and modalities emerge at last his suggestion of four actual spheres in which—because the secondary consequences of knowledge are not likely, on balance, to prove beneficial—he seriously believes that inquiry might appropriately be restricted.

(i) "Should we attempt to contact presumed 'extraterrestrial intelligences'?" Sinsheimer believes that "the impact upon the human spirit" if it should develop that there are vastly superior forms of life, and the impact of that knowledge upon science itself would be "devastating."[1]

(ii) "Research upon improved, easier, simpler, cheaper methods of isotope separation?" Sinsheimer doubts whether such research is in man's best interest, yielding "slightly cheaper power, far easier bombs."[1]

(iii) "Research upon a simple means for the predetermination of the sex of children?" Sinsheimer appears to believe that the resultant potential for "a major imbalance in the human sex ratio" shows advances here to be undesirable.[1]

(iv) "Indiscriminate research upon the aging process?" Sinsheimer appears to believe that the stated goal accompanying legislation to advance such research, "keeping our people as young as possible, as long as possible," is not, on balance, desirable.[1]

It is hard to know what to make of these suggestions. They are very cautiously put, half in interrogative form. But (whatever Sinsheimer believes or may find desirable), if such speculations are treated as arguments for the principle of restriction here involved, they fail utterly. Two observations will suffice.

First. The most that such apprehensions could establish—supposing that everyone shared them—is that it might be that certain inquiries will not prove beneficial on balance. Of course that may be. What follows? Precisely that argument has been presented (with greater force than in most of Professor Sinsheimer's instances) against every scientific advance: against Galileo, against Darwin, against Freud. Such obstinacy (it was urged that good men not even look through Galileo's "infernal glass") is now considered indefensible. It is not an iota more defensible now than it was then. It was entirely correct for the opponents of these seminal thinkers to insist that inquiry of the kinds that they opposed might not prove beneficial in the end. What does that tell about the principle invoked? If, now, the same principle is used not merely to discourage but to prohibit research—in recombinant DNA, for example—one will operate under strictures of essentially the same character as those that persuaded so many rational men to condemn the teaching of the Copernican hypothesis.

Second. The illustrations given by Professor Sinsheimer of the applicability of his principle, his pleas for "prudence," where ignorance seems to him more desirable than knowledge, are self-convicting. If principle (2b) when applied means—as it appears to for him—that researches into the aging process, into nuclear power, into extraterrestrial contact and so on are to be blocked or restricted because of what may transpire if they are successful, the upshot of the argument is revealed. He helps one to see the extreme consequences forced upon everyone, unacceptable to most, if the principle of restriction that he has put forward is taken seriously.

Finally respecting (2b), one variety of great injury that some foresee (unlike catastrophic decisions having unintended impact) deserves remark. It is the gradual deterioration of human culture resulting from ever more extended subjection to technical control. As technology comes to pervade culture (some contend), human values must retreat—even wither. So we can defend our most humane interests only by disarming the technologists. Well, the probability of this feared outcome is very difficult to estimate. Its likelihood, in my judgment, though not trivial, is not great. To prohibit research on such grounds would be intolerably repressive. On this interpretation of disaster, too, the principle would cut against technological advance in every sphere, not that of molecular genetics alone.

For principle (2c) [that research be prohibited when the probability of its very injurious consequences is high or very high] the case is different. Were we to believe that in a given case, the prohibition of that specific inquiry would be, I judge, at least arguable. In such circumstances—the only persuasive candidate I can think of is research into nuclear explosives—the alleged probability would have to be explored, documented, established as fully as resources would then permit. Even here potentiality for benefit would aslo need to be weighed. Recognizing that rational men may ultimately differ in the resolution of such cases,

one must allow that for some research ventures the probability of disastrous use of the products might be so high as to justify prohibition.

Again, two observations respecting (2c). First. Our rational commitment to freedom of inquiry is such that, in judging any claim of highly probable disaster, the burden of proof clearly rests upon those who would prohibit on that basis. They must present a convincing account of what concrete disasters are envisaged, what the methods are for determining the probability of such outcomes, and how those methods establish the high probability of the catastrophe pictured. The burden here is not light, nor ought it to be. Scientific inquiry should not be blocked simply upon the presentation by critics of a parade of imagined horribles of unspecified nature and doubtful likelihood.

Secondly, principle (2c) does not, in any case, apply to research with recombinant DNA. There is some probability (it may be supposed) that, after years of further development, the products of such research might be put to malevolent use—as instruments of war (although better, more convenient killers are already at hand) or in the realization of some (now farfetched but then realizable) brave new world. There is some probability of that, one must grant. But that probability, on the best evidence now available, is slight; at its gravest interpretation, which very few would accept, that probability is no more than moderate. A high probability it is not. Hence in this sphere principle (2c) does not apply.

I conclude that principle (2) is generally inapplicable in most of its forms, and that in none of its forms may it properly serve to prohibit any research in the biochemistry of genetics now contemplated.

(3) "Research should not be permitted when it aims specifically at the development or perfection of instruments for killing or injuring human beings."

This is a reasonable principle for both persons and institutions; it is now accepted and applied by some universities. There are times, circumstances and some institutions to which it might not properly apply.

Although this principle may serve as major premise in a practical syllogism forbidding some kinds of research in some contexts, it cannot serve in a syllogism forbidding recombinant DNA research in any context at present. Research now contemplated with recombinant DNA does not faintly resemble the "munitions" development that would be the target of such a principle. If such an aim were proposed, or even seriously entertained, this principle might, indeed, be called into play. Under present and foreseeable circumstances, however, principle (3) simply has no bearing on the problem at hand.

I conclude that no tenable principle for the prohibition of research based upon its product can now serve to restrict research into recombinant DNA.

Principles Based upon the Process of Research (#4-#6)

(4) "Research should not be permitted when it is not conducted openly, for all to examine the ongoing process and results."

This attractive principle is of a kind very different from the others so far reviewed. Rightly understood, it presents not a limitation upon research but the statement of an ideal—one that we all properly share and promote. The realization of this ideal cannot and should not be taken as an inviolable condition for the conduct of the inquiry. It simply is not that. National security, proprietary interests (of firms or individuals) justly acquired, or other special concerns may render full openness an impractical ideal in many circumstances, certainly not justifying the cessation of all research whose conduct falls short of that ideal.

Openness—both in the research process and for the results of research—is an ideal widely and genuinely honored. Some universities do not permit in their precincts (or are inhospitable toward) research so classified as to restrict access to its results. But complete openness of the research process is very deliberately not applied as a necessary condition by universities, governmental institutions or private enterprises. If it were to be so applied, a great deal of research in progress would have to be discontinued. Much research that is planned would not (under such restriction) go forward. One would not seriously wish to insist upon this discontinuation and blockage. I conclude that

the publicity principle is not even remotely acceptable as a basis for prohibition. Since it cannot serve for prohibition generally, it cannot serve so for research in recombinant DNA unless this inquiry can be shown to be specially prone to the evils of secrecy. That cannot be shown. There is no reason to believe that review of the research process in this field, and timely publication of its results, will fail to meet normal standards of the scientific community.

In fact, the circumstances surrounding DNA research lead to the very opposite conclusion. The nature, location and conditions of recombinant DNA research have been subject to a publicity surpassing that in any other comparable scientific sphere. Largely as a result of initiatives taken by the scientific community itself, public scrutiny in this area has been intense, and the researchers' standards of openness have been, and are sure to continue to be, much higher than normal. Therefore, even if the demand for openness in the process were an appropriate ground for restricting some inquiries in some contexts, it could not serve to restrict, in this context, inquiry using recombinant DNA.

(5) "Research should not be permitted when its continuation is unfair, either to the subjects of the experimentation or to those otherwise involved in the research."

This principle is sound; research whose process does substantial injustice ought not to be pursued, no matter its kind. Often disregarded in the past, this principle is now generally accepted, and is applied concretely to research activities in which unfairness can become a problem. To this end, all experiments proposing to put human subjects at risk—in any way, and to any degree, even the slightest—must be screened by a specially organized human-subjects review committee (HSRC), one kind of institutional review board. No such research may go forward without the explicit approval of an HSRC—and this restriction applies fully to any work with DNA that proposes to put human subjects at risk in any way.

Restrictions for the protection of human subjects being already in force, they need no special restatement for a specific sphere of inquiry. Experiments with recombinant DNA involving human beings have not yet been proposed. If they become a real possibility, and are proposed, the task of the HSRC screening that enterprise may be a delicate one. One will surely agree, in any case, that fairness (non-coercion, full information and so on) toward proposed subjects must be a condition for the continuation of that investigation.

Fairness to other researchers—respect for the present state of the work of others, full information to all investigators involved about what is in view and what is at risk—is also a demand reasonably made. But it, like openness, is a principle for the guidance of conduct, not the restriction of it. It cannot serve for the prohibition of research of a given kind.

Principle (5), I conclude, although important and sound, has no special application to research in recombinant DNA. So far as it does have institutional applicability, its application must be (and is) general, screening out research protocols in every sphere that fail to measure up to the requirements of justice. But measuring up to this standard is not a function of the subject matter of the research.

(6) "Research should not be permitted when the conduct of such research (as distinct from its product) presents risks (either of misfire or of accident) so great as clearly to outweigh the benefits reasonably anticipated." A misfire might be, for example, the creation, through DNA recombination, of an organism with unintended pathogenic capacity against which ordinary antibiotics proved ineffective. An accident might be, for example, the undetected escape, from a laboratory thought to be sealed, of a micro-organism giving rise to contagion.

This principle also is sound and applicable. Bringing it to bear upon DNA research, however, is complicated, and the outcome of that that application is uncertain. Just here lie the major technical problems that have been and remain the focus of much scientific debate. The problem of containing the recombined DNA, either by physical retention within the laboratory or by weakening the host organism so as to render it not viable outside the laboratory, has been the major topic in controversy over what is unreasonably risky and what is not. Only in the light of the present state of effectiveness of containment measures can

risks be rationally estimated. Hence the emergence of guidelines (laid down by the National Institutes of Health) for containment, and for permissible risks given known levels of effective containment. Hence, too, the need to reassess what is reasonably safe to do in the light of existing technical capacities to contain—especially since the capacity to contain biologically, by "disarming the bug," is being steadily improved. Recombined DNA molecules do create special dangers, which do, rightly, require special attention to the conditions and precautions under which specific research activities are carried on.

Still, the principle accepted here, that risks must be minimized, and never allowed to exceed the reasonably anticipated benefits, is one of general application. It applies to all research in medicine, in physics, in biology, in aeronautics, and so on. It has a bearing upon DNA research, to be sure—but only to the extent that the risks encountered in a specific experimental project within that domain appear to equal or to outweigh the anticipated benefits of that project.

Critical here are the risks to persons other than those involved in the research (6b): the people in the street who may be endangered by accident or misfire. Risks to experimental subjects (6a1) must be screened by human-subjects review committees [described above under (5)] designed precisely for that purpose. Risks to researchers themselves or to others formally involved in the research project (6a2) may be grouped for present purposes with risks to outsiders. It is for this combined group that the key question arises.

That key question, now heatedly argued, is this: Are the risks of recombined DNA, whether of misfire or of accident, of such enormity and such probability as to justify prohibition of further research in that sphere?

The first thing to notice about this question is that although here framed in the singular, it must in fact be asked about a host of very different research proposals. Estimating risk-benefit balance for some proposed investigation is often a vexing task. But it should be emphasized that the decisions called for in this family of cases are not, in principle, different from those we are commonly obliged to make when data are incomplete, the time-frame long, the object risky but promising. In this family of cases, as elsewhere, we will do the best we can.

Some contend that in this sphere of research, unlike others, the general sum of anticipated risks, taking into consideration both their degree of seriousness and their probability, outweighs the general sum of anticipated benefits, their value and likelihood similarly weighed. Therefore (they conclude) the proper estimate of risk-benefit balance calls for cessation now of all further research in this sphere.

This argument is unsound. Consider:

First, the key premise is false; it makes a stronger claim than the evidence supports. Granting that the present state of knowledge is short, all indications are that, if one weighed, as on a balance scale, the expected goods in view, multiplied by the likelihood of their probability, the result would be very different from that supposed by this argument. Everyone will allow that there are dangers, some not yet fully known, but the most careful and sophisticated discussions of these dangers, taking severity and probability into account, do not begin to show that they outweigh, or even approach, the sum of advantages likely to accrue from such research over the long term.[1]

The fact remains that some future proposals for investigation in molecular genetics, because of the special risks entailed in the process (and with full consideration of the nature and probability of the benefits in view) may, after thoughtful deliberation, then be rejected by the research institution. Clearly, such rejections, if they transpire, will require the continuing activity of an institutional review board, on the model of a human-subjects review committee, but with a differing focus. Rejection on the grounds of excessive risk is a step that must not be taken lightly, but it probably will be taken in some cases.

Since general prohibition is not in order, and approval for individual proposals must be given on a case-by-case basis, it is appropriate that such continuing review bodies set the conditions for the permissible pursuit of the risky inquiry proposed. Here lies the operative force of the general conviction that, whatever the level of risks found tolerable, there must be a commensurate level of precaution. Only through a process of ongoing review will it be possible to adjust restriction to enterprise rationally. Only through such deliberation can improvements in the effectiveness of containment (both physical and biologic) be weighed, as well as any special likelihood of misfire that the specific nature of the investigation at hand may present.

Finally, it is the singularity of this sphere of research, the uniqueness of its risks and promises, that is so specially provocative. That singularity must be taken account of, but should not be overplayed. Special attentions are rightly given, on a continuing basis, to proposals for experimentation with recombinant DNA, all agree. But it has been my aim to show that the form of the questions to be answered is not essentially different in this domain of scientific research from that in any other. There is a temptation to treat the recombination of DNA as fundamentally different just because of the character of the knowledge aimed at. But if I am right about the first set of principles entertained (#1–#3) pertaining to the product of research, this temptation should not be yielded to.

In summary, for the general prohibition of scientific research in any sphere, the only arguments that might suffice require premises vastly stronger than any now available or likely soon to be available. There is no valid practical syllogism, having true premises, whose conclusion is that research into recombinant DNA should be stopped. Of proposed arguments to this end it may be fairly said either that the major premise (the principle of prohibition) is false, or when true principles are provided, that the minor premise (specifying recombinant DNA research as defective in the ways indicated) is very far from established.

Note

1. A number of bodies, with members both in the sciences and in the humanities, have deliberated long and carefully upon the likely balance of risk and benefit, over long term and short, of recombi-

nant DNA research. Perhaps the two most thorough and probing studies are the Report of the Working Party on the Experimental Manipulation of the Genetic Composition of Micro-Organisms. Presented to Parliament by the Secretary of State for Education and Science, London, January, 1975 (this document is widely known as the Ashby Report, after the Chairman of the Working Party, Lord Eric Ashby), and the report of the University Committee to Recommend Policy for the Molecular Genetics and Oncology Program, presented to the vice-president for research at the University of Michigan, Ann Arbor, March, 1976 (attached to this document, widely known as the Report of Committee B, is a dissent and a reply to the dissent). Subsequently appeared a critique of the Report of Committee

B, a response to that critique by Committee B, and a separate endorsement of the Committee's original report, all presented to the Regents of the University of Michigan.

References

1. SINSHEIMER R: Inquiry into inquiry. Hastings Cent Rep 6(4):18,1976
2. LIVERMORE S: Statement of dissent, Report of the University Committee to Recommend Policy for the Molecular Genetics and Oncology Program Office of the Vice President for Research, University of Michigan, Ann Arbor, March, 1976. Appendix B1, pp 46–47.

Human Experimentation: New York Verdict Affirms Patient's Rights

Elinor Langer

New York, N.Y. Two years ago this month, New York City's yellow and not-so-yellow journalists had a feast with the disclosure that, as part of a research project, live cancer cells were being injected into hospitalized patients under circumstances in which the nature of their consent to the proceedings was exceedingly ambiguous (*Science*, 7 February 1964). A number of circumstances made the case particularly newsworthy. The patients in question were 22 seriously ailing and debilitated inhabitants of a relatively obscure Brooklyn institution, the Jewish Chronic Disease Hospital (JCDH). The research in question, studies in cancer immunology, was generally rated with the scientific community as among the most significant of all lines of research on malignant diseases. And both the researcher in question, Chester Southam, and his institution, Sloan-Kettering, held unassailable posi-

tions in the forefront of American medical science.

After considerable time the sensational charges and accusations of "Nazi tactics" disappeared from the headlines, although an article on the case, entitled "How doctors use patients as guinea pigs," appeared in a national women's magazine as recently as last fall. But in the labyrinths of New York State's administrative machinery, under the direction of a unit of the department of education known as the Division of Professional Conduct, the case was being subjected to intensive review. Last month the Regents of the University of the State of New York, acting under this responsibility for licensing the medical profession, issued their verdict.* Southam and Emanuel

*The Board of Regents consists of 15 individuals elected by joint resolution of the two houses of New York's legislature for terms of 15 years. The Regents have jurisdiction over all education in the state, public and private, and over all licensed professions excluding the law. The three Regents most intimately involved in this decision were the three

Mandel, medical director of the Chronic Disease Hospital, were found guilty of ''unprofessional conduct'' and of ''fraud and deceit in the practice of medicine.'' Their licenses were suspended for 1 year, although execution of the sentences has been stayed. The men will be on probation, but allowed to practice.

In the course of their review, the Regents and the medical grievance committee which advised them explored many questions of serious importance to the entire medical research community. On two key questions—when is consent ''informed,'' and how far may the physician exercise his physician's authority when he is acting in the role of experimenter—the Regents have developed definitions which, while not legal precedents (except perhaps in New York), represent a major attempt to put some precision into the vague ethical concepts now governing experimentation with human subjects.

Some of the arguments raised by the defense lawyers are also important, for they suggest that Southam and Mandel were stumbling through a signless desert and that, if they lost their way, they did no more than other researchers have done before them or than, in the absence of clearer standards, researchers will continue to do after them.

Finally, the fact of the proceedings is in itself significant, confirming what the large-scale publicity itself hinted—that the question of medical experimentation is already outside the house of science. The Regents' decision is an affirmation that there is a public interest to be protected in the field of medical research; it is an omen that the public may begin to set the rules. (The body of the Regents' decision is given on pages 630–32.)

The nondisputed facts in the case are these: Southam's work involved the injection of tissue-cultured cancer cells into human subjects

---

members of a special committee on discipline: Joseph W. McGovern, a lawyer; Joseph T. King, a lawyer; and Carl H. Pforzheimer, Jr., an investment banker. The remaining Regents, who concurred in the decision, are drawn from a variety of business and professional interests, including law, banking, education and philanthropy.

and measurement of the speed with which the injected substance was rejected by the body. Earlier phases of the work had established that healthy persons would reject the tissue culture in 4 to 6 weeks, and that individuals already ill with advanced cancer would reject them in a longer period, ranging from 6 weeks to several months. To test the hypothesis that the slower rate of rejection in the cancer patients was in fact attributable to their cancer and not to the general debility that accompanies any chronic illness, it was necessary to perform the experiment on patients severely ill with nonmalignant diseases. A chronic-disease hospital was a logical place to look for patients with the required characteristics. Southam approached Mandel, who agreed to the collaboration, and, in July 1963, 22 patients (including three cancer patients used as controls) were subjected to the experiment. The patients were asked by Mandel, Southam, and their assistants if they would consent to an injection which was described as a test to discover their resistance or immunity to disease. They were told that a lump would form, and that in a few weeks it would go away. They were not told in plain language that the procedure was a research project unrelated to medical treatment of their own condition. And they were not told that the substance to be injected consisted of live cancer cells. The record indicates that all the patients approached agreed to the injection and, further, that none suffered any ill effects other than the transient discomfort of the injection and the nodule it produced.

MOTIVATIONS

Both men had reasons for acting as they did. Their thinking is extensively set out in the records of the administrative hearings, and their views were restated in interviews with *Science* last week.

Southam's practices, developed in the earlier experimentation on cancer patients at Memorial and James Ewing hospitals in New York, rested on the conviction that the procedure involved no risk of transplanting cancer to the experimental subjects. ''I saw no reason why we should use [the word *cancer*] because it is not pertinent to the phenomenon which is going to follow," he told the hearing board. "We are not doing something which is going to induce cancer. We are not going to do something which is going to cause them any harm. . . . We are going to observe the growth and rejection of these transplanted cancer cells. The fact then that they are cancer cells does not mean that there is any risk of cancer to this patient." In addition, Southam believes that the word *cancer* "has a tremendous emotive value, disvalue to everybody. . . . What the ordinary patient, what the nonmedical person, and even many doctors . . . whose knowledge of the basic science behind transplantation is not great—to them the use of a cancer cell might imply a risk that it will grow and produce cancer, and the fear that this word strikes in people is very great." The suggestion was raised in the hearing that, having recognized the emotional impact of the word *cancer,* the doctors avoided it through fear that its use would discourage consent and thus hinder the research. But Southam sees his action as an act of professional judgment and solicitude, based on an unwillingness to scare or arouse the patients when such fright was not in fact relevant to the objective situation. And he believes that his formula gave the patients all the information they needed to make an intelligent decision about participation.

On the basic question of the type of explanation to be given to the patients, Mandel followed, and endorsed, the practice described to him by Southam. But many factors influenced Mandel's agreement to the project. A relative newcomer to the Chronic Disease Hospital, he was alarmed by what seemed to him disastrously insufficient medical attention to the long-term, chronically ill patients. "I could tell you stories which would curdle your blood," he told *Science* last week, and he did. The experiment involved a number of visits to the patients by the JCDH resident working with Southam to check on the development and regression of the nodules, and Mandel believed that the added attention would improve their care. He saw some hope of using the injections as a diagnostic device, to discover undetected cancer in patients hospitalized for other illnesses.

And he looked forward to the possibility of a more prolonged collaboration with the Sloan-Kettering, which would contribute to upgrading his own institution.

Within the hospital, Mandel's decision to permit the experiment to proceed became the focus of an intense disagreement which led to a battle with one of the hospital's directors over the confidentiality of patients' records and to the resignation of several staff physicians. The bad feeling between Mandel and the physicians, whether it preceded the Sloan-Kettering issue, as Mandel contends, or was the result of it, as the physicians imply, seriously impeded the efforts of the examining committees to evaluate one of the ugliest charges in the case—that the patients used were in such a debilitated physical and mental state that they were incapable of giving informed consent. Almost every patient became the subject of conflicting testimony from the opposing sides. In his report to the Regents, a physician member of the medical grievance committee which conducted the bulk of the hearings summarized descriptions of patients that had been supplied by the physicians who resigned. Patient No. 26 is fairly typical: "Suffering from advanced Paget's disease, with overgrowth of bone, pressing on the brain. This patient was suffering from severe deafness, blindness, mental condition." Another patient was described as suffering from "Parkinson's disease, lung abscess, was running and falling, speech was unintelligible." A chart stated that the patient "was misunderstood by the orderly, drools, and tries to avoid speech." Another patient, a 75-year-old man described as senile, was diagnosed as "impaired mentally, with easy crying and laughing, tendency to repeat the same sentence several times. Also it is difficult to obtain the patient's attention." In all these cases, Mandel and the resident, supported by Southam, testified basically that, if you knew the patients (as the resident did), it was possible to communicate adequately with them and that they had an alert appreciation of what was going on.

Although the Regents were unable to come to a definitive conclusion about the alertness of all the patients, they did find that at least "some . . . were incapable of understanding the nature of this experiment or of giving informed consent thereto.'' While agreeing with Southam's contention that he was not responsible for the internal practices of the Chronic Disease Hospital, the Regents argued that he had a clear responsiblity nonetheless: ''As a physician in charge of the experiment, it was his duty to pay enough attention to what was going on to make sure that he was dealing with persons capable of being volunteers and sufficiently informed to consent to the use of their bodies for the experiment and not merely with people who were too confused or too sick or too resigned to object to the injection.'' Southam believes, the Regents continued, that ''it is important to make it clear to the patients that what is being done is an experiment and is not for the treatment or diagnosis of their own condition, yet he was present, this was not adequately done, and he did not complain. A physician may not shirk his ethical responsibility or violate basic human rights so easily.'' As for Mandel, the Regents concluded that although he had, legitimately, delegated responsibility for the actual conduct of the experiment to a resident, he was nonetheless ''directly responsible for the determination of the procedure followed'' in the selection of patients and the explanations he permitted them to be offered. In addition to the substantive arguments, lawyers for Mandel and Southam raised two technical points of some interest. First, they claimed that, because ''no clear-cut medical or professional standards were in force or were violated'' by the two physicians, the attempt to find them guilty had an ex post facto quality. They also argued that the charges did not accurately fit the case. Testimony was introduced from well-known cancer and other professional researchers, including I. S. Ravdin, vice president for medical affairs of the University of Pennsylvania, and George E. Moore, director of Roswell Park Memorial Institute, to the effect that Southam's practices did not differ dramatically from those of other researchers. ''If the whole profession is doing it,'' one of the lawyers remarked in an interview, ''how can you call it 'unprofessional conduct'''? The lawyers also argued that the ''fraud and deceit'' charge was more appropriate to lowbrow scoundrels, such as physicians who cheat on insurance, supply illegal narcotics, or practice medicine without a license, than to their respectable and well-intentioned clients.

VOICE OF THE PUBLIC

To all arguments of humane motivations, extenuating circumstance, conflicting testimony, or legal ambiguities, the final answer of the Regents was very simple: It is no excuse. There was never any disagreement on the principle that patients should not be used in experiments unrelated to treatment unless they have given informed consent. But in the Regents' decision, two refinements of that principle are heavily stressed. The first is that it is the patient, and not the physician, who has the right to decide what factors are or are not relevant to his consent, regardless of the rationality of his assessment. ''Any fact which might influence the giving or withholding of consent is material,'' the Regents said. ''A patient has the right to know he is being asked to volunteer and to refuse to participate in an experiment for any reason, intelligent or otherwise, well-informed or prejudiced. A physician has no right to withhold from a prospective volunteer any fact which he knows may influence the decision. It is the volunteer's decision to make, and the physician may not take it away from him by the manner in which he asks the question or explains or fails to explain the circumstances. There is evidenced in the record . . . an attitude on the part of some physicians that they can go ahead and do anything which they conclude is good for the patient, or which is of benefit experimentally or educationally and is not harmful to the patient, and that the patient's consent is an empty formality. With this we cannot agree.''

The second principle stressed by the Regents is that the physician, when he is acting as experimenter, has no claim to the doctor-patient relationship that, in a therapeutic situation, would give him the generally acknowledged right to withhold information if he judged it in the best interest of the patient. In the absence of a doctor-patient relationship, the Regents said, ''there is no basis for the exercise of their usual professional judgment applicable to patient care." Southam, in an interview, disagreed. "An experimental relation has some elements of a therapeutic relationship," he said last week. "The patients still think of you as a doctor, and I react to them as a doctor, and want to avoid frightening them unnecessarily." Mandel takes a similar position. In a letter to the editor of a medical affairs newspaper he stated: "In accordance with the age-old motto—primum non nocere—it would seem that consideration of the patient's well-being may, at times, supersede the requirement for disclosure of facts if such facts lack pertinence and may cause psychologic harm." But on this point, the Regents are clear: "No person can be said to have volunteered for an experiment unless he had first understood what he was volunteering for. Any matter which might influence him in giving or withholding his consent is material. Deliberate nondisclosure of the material fact is no different from deliberate misrepresentation of such a fact."

In closing their case, and acknowledging that the penalties imposed were severe—they might have just authorized a censure and reprimand—the Regents were pointed and succinct: "We trust that this measure of discipline will serve as a stern warning that zeal for research must not be carried to the point where it violates the basic rights and immunities of a human person."

What the impact of the case will be is by no means clear. The Regents' decision outlines clear rules for a very narrow situation and attempts to set out some broad principles as well. But it is by no means binding, and it by no means covers the variety of situations with which researchers seeking to use human subjects are faced. The question is, What will cover these situations? Codes and declarations, of which there are already several, are too general to offer specific guidance. Researchers and patients alike are too vulnerable to await a slow case-by-case accretion of specific rulings. One alternative is the development within each hospital or research institution of "ethical review committees" that could define the consent-and-disclosure requirements for each proposed experiment and see that they were adhered to. In theory, this is already taking place. During the Southam-Mandel hearings, the state at-

tempted to prove that Southam, a recipient of an NIH grant, had violated regulations of the Public Health Service. In fact, the regulations in question govern only the normal volunteer program of the NIH Clinical Center in Bethesda. The PHS response to an inquiry from New York's Attorney General made clear that the rules were not generally applicable and stated that, "in supporting extramural clinical investigations, it is the position of the Public Health Service that proper ethical and moral standards are more effectively safeguarded by the processes of review and criticism by an investigator's peers than by regulation."

That is the theory, but the trouble is, it is not yet being done. And, given the tremendous growth and variety of medical research involving human beings, if it is not done by the scientific community, someone else will start to do it. The New York Regents may be only the beginning.

THE REGENTS' DECISION

We are of the opinion that there are certain basic ethical standards concerning consent to human experimentation which were involved in this experiment and which were violated by the respondents. When a patient engages a physician or enters a hospital he may reasonably be deemed to have consented to such treatment as his physician or the hospital staff, in the exercise of their professional judgment, deem proper. Consent to normal diagnostic tests might similarly be presumed. Even so, doctors and hospitals as a matter of routine obtain formal written consents before surgery, and in a number of other instances, and whether or not a specific consent is required for a specific act must be decided on the facts of the particular cases.

No one contends that these 22 patients, by merely being in the hospital, had volunteered their bodies for any purpose other than treatment of their condition. These injections were made as a part of a cancer research project. The incidental and remote possibility, urged by Dr. Mandel, that the research might have been beneficial to a patient is clearly insufficient to bring these injections within the area of procedures for which a consent could be implied. Actual consent was required.

What form such an actual consent must take is a matter of applying common sense to the particular facts of the case. No consent is valid unless it is made by a person with legal and mental capacity to make it, and is based on a disclosure of all material facts. Any fact which might influence the giving or withholding of consent is material. A patient has the right to know he is being asked to volunteer and to refuse to participate in an experiment for any reason, intelligent or otherwise, well-informed or prejudiced. A physician has no right to withhold from a prospective volunteer any fact which he knows may influence the decision. It is the volunteer's decision to make, and the physician may not take it away from him by the manner in which he asks the question or explains or fails to explain the circumstances. There is evidenced in the record in this proceeding an attitude on the part of some physicians that they can go ahead and do anything which they conclude is good for the patient, or which is of benefit experimentally or educationally and is not harmful to the patient, and that the patient's consent is an empty formality. With this we cannot agree.

In his testimony . . . Dr. Mandel took the position that he regards these experiments as beneficial to the patients both because the experiment might result in a diagnosis of an advanced cancer which had not been discovered by the hospital, and also because the participation in the experiment would result in extra medical attention to the patients involved and possibly other patients in the hospital.

The record indicates that the only additional medical care any of these patients received as a result of this experiment was that the injections were made and they were occasionally checked thereafter as to the progress of the growth and disappearance of the nodule. The inference that participation in the experiment benefited the patients because of such additional medical care is without foundation in the record. Since the purpose of the experiment was to obtain verification of Dr. Southam's hypothesis that diseased patients would reject the implant in the same manner as healthy patients and that their rejection would not be delayed as was that of patients suffering from an advanced cancer, it is somewhat inconsistent for Dr. Mandel to say before the experiment was completed that he authorized it as a diagnostic measure. In any event, it was clearly not treatment, not experimental therapy, and not a diagnostic test which would reasonably be given to these particular patients. Nevertheless, from the manner in which they were asked for their consent and from the statement made to them that this was a test to determine their immunity or resistance to disease, the patients could naturally assume that it was being given to help in the diagnosis or treatment of their condition. They were not clearly and unequivocally asked if they wanted to volunteer to participate in an extraneous research project.

There is one point which is undisputed, namely, that the patients were not told that the cells to be injected were live cancer cells. From the respondents' standpoint this was not considered to be an important fact. They regarded the experiment as medically harmless. There was not appreciable danger of any harmful effects to the patients as a result of the injection of these cancer cells. It is not uncommon for a doctor to refrain from telling his patient that he had cancer where the physician in his professional judgment concludes that such a disclosure would be harmful to the patient. The respondents testified that they felt that telling these patients that the material did consist of live cancer cells would upset them and was immaterial to their consent. They overlooked the key fact that so far as this particular experiment was concerned, there was not the usual doctor-patient relationship and, therefore, no basis for the exercise of their usual professional judgment applicable to patient care. No person can be said to have volunteered for an experiment unless he has first understood what he was volunteering for. Any matter which might influence him in giving or withholding his consent is material. Deliberate nondisclosure of the material fact is no different from deliberate misrepresentation of such a fact. The respondents maintain that they did not withhold the fact that these were cancer cells because they thought that some of the patients might have refused to consent to the injection of live cancer cells into their bodies. This was, however, a possibility and a decision that had to be made by the patients and not for them. Accordingly, the alleged oral consents that they obtained after deliberately withholding this information were not informed consents and were, for this reason, fraudulently obtained.

Although there is conflicting testimony and evidence in this point, it is our opinion that some of these patients were in such a physical and mental condition that they were incapable of understanding the nature of this experiment or of giving an informed consent thereto. . . . We note that in no case were any relatives of any of these patients told about the experiment nor were any of these patients asked if they wished to think the matter over or discuss it with their relatives. It is noteworthy that one of these same patients was operated on two days

after the injections and that prior to making the operation, which was a part of the patient's treatment, the hospital obtained two separate written consents each signed by both the patient and a relative. If there was any doubt at all concerning a patient's ability to fully comprehend and consent to this experiment, it was the duty of the physicians involved to resolve that doubt before proceeding further. . . . We do not say that it is necessary in all cases of human experimentation to obtain consents from relatives or to obtain written consents, but certainly upon the fact of this case and in view of the fact that the patients were debilitated, the performance of this experiment on the basis of alleged oral consents from these particular patients falls short of the ethical standards of the medical profession.

ALTRUISM, MARKETS, AND MEDICAL RESOURCES

Why Give to Strangers?

Richard M. Titmuss

In Alexander Solzhenitsyn's novel *Cancer Ward* Shulubin is talking to Kostoglotov:

> "We have to show the world a society in which all relationships, fundamental principles and laws flow directly from moral ethics, and from them *alone*. Ethical demands would determine all calculations: how to bring up children, what to prepare them for, to what purpose the work of grown-ups should be directed, and how their leisure should be occupied. As for scientific research, it should only be conducted where it doesn't damage ethical morality, in the first instance where it doesn't damage the researchers themselves."

Kostoglotov then raises questions. "There has to be an economy after all doesn't there? That comes before everything else." "Does it?" said Shulubin. "That depends. For example, Vladi-

Reprinted with permission from *The Lancet,* 123–125, January 16, 1971.

mir Solovyov argues rather convincingly that an economy could and should be built on an ethical basis."

"What's this? Ethics first and economics afterwards?" Kostoglotov looked bewildered.

The questions raised by Solzhenitsyn could as well be directed at social policy institutions. What, for example, are the connections between what we in Britain conventionally call the social services and the role of altruism in modern industrial societies? And have we a convenient model for studying such relationships? Blood as a living tissue and as a bond that links all men and women so closely that differences of colour, religious belief, and cultural heritage are insignificant beside it, may now constitute in Western societies one of the ultimate tests of where the "social" begins and the "economic" ends.

THE WORLD DEMAND FOR BLOOD

The transfer of blood and blood derivatives from one human being to another represents one of the greatest therapeutic instruments in the hands of modern medicine. But these developments have set in train social, economic, and ethical consequences which present society with issues of profound importance.

The demand for blood and blood products is increasing all over the world. In high-income countries, in particular, the rate of growth in demand has been rising so rapidly that shortages have begun to appear. In all Western countries, demand is growing faster than rates of growth in the population aged 18–65 from whom donors are drawn. And, despite a massive research effort in the United States to find alternatives, there is often no substitute for human blood.

Many factors are responsible for this increase in demand. Some surgical procedures call for massive transfusions of blood (as many as 60 donations may be needed for a single open-heart operation, and in one American heart-transplant case over 300 pints of blood were used); artificial kidneys require substantial volumes of blood; and developments in organ transplants could create immense additional demands. Furthermore, more routine surgery is now used more frequently and is made available to a larger proportion of the population than formerly. A more violent or accident-prone world insistently demands more blood for road casualties and for war injuries (in 1968 more than 300,000 pints of blood were shipped from the U.S.A. and elsewhere to treat victims of the Vietnam war).

There seems to be no predictable limit to the demand for blood supplies, especially when one remembers the as-yet unmet needs for surgical and medical treatment.

SUPPLY OF BLOOD

On the biological, technical, and administrative side, three factors limit the supply of blood.

Only about half of a population is medically eligible to donate blood. Furthermore, the amount any one person can give in a year is restricted—two donations in the British National Blood Transfusion Service (probably the lowest limit and the most rigorous standard in the world); five in the United States, a minimum often exceeded by paid donors, commercial blood-banks, and pharmaceutical companies using techniques such as plasmapheresis; in Japan, where 90% of blood is bought and sold, the standard is even lower. These differences can be analysed as a process of redistribution of life chances in terms of age, sex, social class, income, ethnic group, and so on.

Human blood deteriorates after three weeks in the refrigerator, and this perishability presents great technical and administrative problems to those running transfusion services. But it does mean that, by measuring wastage (i.e., the amount of blood that has to be thrown away) the efficiencies of different blood collection and distribution systems can be compared.

Blood can be more deadly than any drug. Quite apart from the problems of cross-matching, storage, labelling, and so on, there are serious risks of disease transmission and other hazards. In Western countries a major hazard is serum hepatitis transmitted from carrier donor to susceptible patient. Since carriers cannot yet be reliably detected, the patient becomes the laboratory for testing "the gift." Donors, therefore, have to be screened every time they come to give blood, and the donor's truthfulness in answering questions about health, medical history, and drug habits becomes vital. Upon the honesty of the donor depends the life of the recipient of his blood. In this context we need to ask what conditions and arrangements permit and encourage maximum truthfulness on the part of the donors. Can honesty be pursued regardless of the donor's motives for giving blood? What systems, structures, and social policies encourage honesty or discourage and destroy voluntary and truthful gift relationships?

TYPES OF DONOR

To give or not to give, to lend, repay, or even to buy and sell blood are choices which lead us, if we are to understand these transactions in the context of any society, to the fundamentals of social and economic life.

The forms and functions of giving embody moral, social, psychological, religious, legal, and aesthetic ideas. They may reflect, sustain, strengthen, or loosen the cultural bonds of the group, large or small. They may inspire the worst excesses of war and tribalism or the tolerances of community.

Customs and practices of non-economic giving—unilateral and multilateral social transfers—thus may tell us much, as Marcel Mauss so sensitively demonstrated in his book *The Gift,* about the texture of personal and group relationships in different cultures. In some societies, past and present, gifts to men aim to buy peace; to express affection, regard, or loyalty; to unify the group; to fulfil a contractual set of obligations and rights; to function as acts of penitence, shame, or degradation; and to symbolise many other human sentiments. When one reads the work of anthropologists and soiciologists such as Mauss and Lévi-Strauss, who have studied the social functions of giving, a number of themes relevant to any attempt to delineate a typology of blood-donors may be discerned.

From these readings and from statistics for different countries a spectrum of blood-donor types can be constructed. At one extreme is the paid donor who sells his blood for what the market will bear: some are semi-salaried, some are long-term prisoner volunteers, some are organised in blood trade-unions. As a market transaction, information that might have a bearing on the quality of the blood is withheld if possible from the buyer, since such information could affect the sale of the blood. Thus in the United States blood-group identification cards are loaned, at a price, to other sellers, and blood is illegally mislabelled and updated, and other devices are used which make it very difficult to screen out drug addicts, alcoholics and hepatitis carriers, and so on.

At the other extreme is the voluntary, unpaid donor. This type is the closest approximation in social reality to the abstract idea of a "free human gift." There are no tangible immediate rewards, monetary or non-monetary; there are no penalties; and donors know that their gifts are for unnamed strangers without distinction of age, sex, medical illness, income, class, religion, or ethnic group. No donor type

can be characterised by complete disinterested spontaneous altruism. There must be some sense of obligation, approval, and interest; some awareness of the need for the gift; some expectation that a return gift may be needed and received at some future date. But the unpaid donation of blood is an act of free-will: there is no formal contract, legal bond, power situation; no sense of shame or guilt; no money and no explicit guarantee of or wish for reward or return gift.

Almost all the 1 ½ million registered donors in Britain and donors in some systems in European countries fall into this category. An analysis of blood-donor motives suggests that the main reason people give blood is most commonly a general desire to help people; almost a third of the British donors studied said that their gift was in response to an appeal for blood; 7 % said it was to repay a transfusion given to someone they knew.

By contrast, in the United States less than 10 % of supplies come from the voluntary community donor. Proportionately more and more blood is being supplied by the poor, the unskilled, the unemployed, Negroes, and other low-income groups, and with the rise in plasmapheresis there is emerging a new class of exploited high blood yielders. Redistribution in terms of "the gift of blood and blood products" from the poor to the rich seems to be one of the dominant effects of the American blood-banking system.

WHICH SYSTEM?

When we compare the commercial blood-bank, such as that found in the United States, with the voluntary system functioning as an integral part of the National Helath Service in Britain we find that the commercial bloodbank fails on each of four counts—economic efficiency, administrative efficiency, price, and quality. Commercial blood-bank systems waste blood, and shortages, acute and chronic, characterise the demand-and-supply position. Administratively, there is more paperwork and greater computing and accounting overheads. The cost varies between £10 and £20 per unit in the United States, compared with £1 16s, (£2 if processing costs are included) in Britain. And, as judged by statistics for post-transfusion hepatitis, the risk of transfusing contaminated blood is greater if the blood is obtained from a commercial source.

Paradoxically—or so it may seem to some—the more commercialised blood-distribution becomes (and hence more wasteful, inefficient, and dangerous) the more will the gross national product be inflated. In part, and quite simply, this is the consequence of statistically "transferring" an unpaid service (voluntary donors, voluntary workers in the service, unpaid time), with much lower external costs, to a monetary and measurable paid activity involving costlier externalities. Similar effects on the gross national product would ensue if housewives were paid for housework or childless married couples were financially rewarded for adopting children or if hospital patients cooperating for teaching purposes charged medical students. The gross national product is also inflated when commercial markets accelerate "blood obsolescence"; the waste is counted because someone has paid for it.

What *The Economist* described in its 1969 survey of the American economy as the great "efficiency gap" between that country and Britain clearly does not apply to the distribution of human blood. The voluntary, socialised system in Britain is economically, professionally, administratively, and qualitatively more efficient than the mixed, commercialised, and individualistic American system.

Another myth, the Paretian myth of consumer sovereignty, has also to be shattered. In the commercial blood market the consumer is not king. He has less freedom of choice to live unharmed; little choice in determining price; is more subject to scarcity; is less free from bureaucratisation; has fewer opportunities to express altruism; and exercises fewer checks and controls in relation to consumption, quality, and external costs. Far from being sovereign, he is often exploited.

What also emerges from this case-study is the significance of the externalities (the values and disvalues external to but created by blood-distribution systems treated as entities) and the multiplier effects of such externalities on what we can only call "the quality of life." At one end of the spectrum of externalities is the individual affected by hepatitis; at the other end, the market behaviour of economically rich societies seeking to import blood from other societies who are thought to be too poor and economically decadent to pay their own blood-donors.

CONCLUSION

We started with blood as a model for examining how altruism and social policy might work together in a modern industrial society. We might equally have chosen eye banks, patients as teaching material, fostering, or even the whole concept of the community-based distribution of welfare to those in need. All these involve in some degree a gift relationship. The example chosen suggests, firstly, that gift exchange of a non-quantifiable nature has more important functions in a complex society than the writings of Lévi-Strauss and others might indicate. Secondly, the application of scientific and technological developments in such societies is further accelerating the spread of such complexity, and has increased rather than decreased the scientific as well as the social need for such relationships. Thirdly, for these and many other reasons, modern societies require more rather than less freedom of choice for the expression of altruism in the daily life of all social groups. This requirement can be argued for on social and ethical grounds, but, as we have seen for blood donors, it can also be argued for on scientific and economic criteria.

I believe that it is a responsibility of government, acting, for example, through social policy, to weaken market forces which put men in positions where they have little opportunity to make moral choices or to behave altruistically if they wish to do so. The voluntary blood-donor system is a practical example of a fellowship relationship operating on an institutional basis, in this instance the National Health Service. It shows how social policy decisions can foster such relationships between free and equal individuals. If we accept that man has a social and biological need to help then he should not be denied the chance to express this need by entering into a gift relationship.

Letter: Ethics and Economics in Blood Supply

A.J. Culyer

Sir,—Professor Titmuss, in his discussion of the role of giving in blood-supplies, is likely to mislead many of your readers (a) by suggesting a distinction between "economic" and "social" man and (b) by asserting that payment for blood causes higher social costs, acute and chronic shortages of blood, and a high risk of infection of recipients through viral hepatitis and other diseases, compared with donation. Although I do not "urge" and have not "urged" the introduction of payment to blood suppliers in Britain, as Titmuss asserts, the case for payment (if there is or ever will be one) does not stand or fall on these claims.

(*a*) Man is a social animal with economic problems that are a subset of "social problems." They are not mutually incompatible categories. As a science, economics is the study of the *means* of achieving ends and only the ends can ever justify any specific means. In this sense nobody will dispute that "ethics" comes before "economics." So far as I know nobody (except Titmuss) has ever suggested otherwise.

(*b*) The problem of post-transfusion hepatitis was barely discussed in my original study with M.H. Cooper of the role of "price," and I should like briefly to indicate some of the economic possibilities here. It is clearly not "price" *per se* that causes the disease but the social condition of those who are frequently drawn by "price" to supply blood. A variety of possibilities suggest themselves once this fallacy has been identified:

A. Assume there is no clinical test by which hepatitis carriers can be identified before donation. One could (1) collect all blood, including infected blood, and distribute as usual on the grounds that it is better to incur a risk (of less than unity) that recipients contract hepatitis than to suffer even greater shortage. This seems a wrong policy since better choices are available. It is a valid criticism of Americans that they have largely adopted this policy; (2) offer a sufficiently high price that an excess supply is produced from

Reprinted with permission from *The Lancet,* 1, 602-3, March 20, 1971.

amongst which those individuals with obviously undesired characteristics may be rejected—this is costly; (3) offer a "price" *in kind* of a sort to appeal to the appropriate social class (e.g., theatre tickets, free parking, Wine Society membership)—this is costly; (4) discriminate at the point of collection by offering "prices" only to certain prechosen categories of population (e.g., university students, teachers, residents of well-to-do districts)—this too will be costly.

B. Retain donation only and encourage donation by advertising, jogging consciences, public lectures on ethics, offsetting costs of attendance (e.g., provide baby-sitting services), etc. In short, vary the non-price determinants of supply. This will be costly.

C. It seems highly likely that in the near future a clinical test for detecting viral hepatitis will become generally available. It could be used to screen both donors and paid suppliers to remove the problem (almost) entirely. This would be costly.

These are some possibilities (by no means an exhaustive list) suggested by the economics of blood supply and demand whereby supplies could be increased if it were felt desirable to do so. It seems to me wrong to be complacent about the adequacy of current supplies in Britain. Apart from the postponement of operations, which occurs in all countries with an unknown relative frequency, one would wish to know how frequently patients are transfused with imperfectly matched blood; how often blood is used for purposes in which it is less useful than other purposes; how often a current or expected shortage affects *future* demand via the planned amounts of complementary inputs to be made available in the future; and other questions of a similar type. We are so ignorant about such things that complacency is irresponsible in implying that we ought not to bother to find out.

Regarding Titmuss's views on the wider role of altruism in the blood market, I have little to say. His assertions, however, strike me as lacking both the theory to predict and the facts to sustain the extraordinary view that *supplementing* (not replacing) donation with compensation in some form will have serious long-term disruptive effects on society. But even if that is on the cards, the choice is not for Titmuss, or me, or doctors, to make, but for the whole of society, since it affects the whole of society. In the limit, adherence to giving and giving alone would countenance the death of patients should suppliers turn out to be less philanthropic than he hopes, and I doubt if society would hesitate much between choosing between these conflicting ends. I doubt also whether the Americans would be much impressed by Titmuss's ideas as the solution to their problem. By contrast, the electicism of the economic approach may be useful to them.

Fundamentally, Titmuss does not understand economics. This leads him falsely to assert that the American system exploits the poor and redistributes real income to the relatively rich, whereas whatever the faults of the American system this is most unlikely to be one of them! It leads him to present totally misleading comparative cost statistics (ignoring costs not revealed in cash; the fact that cost is not independent of supply; the irrelevance of *unit* compared with *incremental* cost in policy decisions). It leads him falsely to be concerned about "inflating" G.N.P. (of all things). Finally, it leads him falsely to identify "Paretian" improvements in social welfare with "consumer sovereignty," whereas the latter is wholly inconsistent with the former.

All this is to sacrifice truth for the sake of special pleading. This dispassionate analyst must recognise that payment for blood, if suitably engineered, can be effective and may be desirable, but actual choice of donation-only/ payment-only/donation-with-payment ought to be dependent upon the relative social costs of different methods in getting a given increase in supply. At the moment we have neither this information nor enough knowledge about present or future demand and adequacy to decide. Without this knowledge (which *economics* suggests is needed) a-priori reasoning cannot dictate policy, Professor Titmuss notwithstanding.

From "Organ Transplants: Ethical and Legal Problems"

Paul A. Freund

Until we secure an adequate supply of organs—natural or artificial—to meet the needs, there will be problems of allocation of these resources: from whom they should come and to whom they should be transferred. By what critiera should these decisions be made? The question implicates moral, legal, and medical considerations, which differ in the cases of removal after death and removal during life.

The moral and legal problems attending the taking of an organ from a cadaver appear to be

Reprinted with permission of author and publisher from *Proceedings of the American Philosophical Society* 115:4, 276–81, August 1971.

well on the way to resolution. Although objection to the mutilation of a corpse has been traditional in Orthodox Judaism, as the life-saving potential of transplants has become clearer the resistance on religious grounds has weakened.[1] Legal obstacles have been more widespread. Under the principles of the common law a person could not in his lifetime determine by will or agreement how his bodily organs should be treated after death; and the authority of the next of kin was essentially limited to providing a decent burial. While more recent legal precedents could be construed to authorize the next of kin to donate organs, the authority was not beyond peradventure clear, and since the next of kin might be unknown, or unavailable, or hostile, the procedure for securing approval was at best unsatisfactory, especially in situations where the utmost promptness in removal was essential for the viability of the organ.[2]

The problem of obtaining the necessary consent has now been resolved from another direction. The Uniform Anatomical Gift Act, which has been adopted in forty-eight states, authorizes an individual to donate his body, or certain organs or tissues, for purpose of transplantation or other scientific use, by means of a relatively simple witnessed document, and there is a growing practice of using a card to signify his authorization. Many persons are now card-carrying potential donors of organs. Alternatively, the Act authorizes the next of kin (in order of priority, beginning with a surviving spouse) to grant authorization. The most serious problems that remain in the field of transplants from cadavers are thus the biological ones: the medical requirement that certain organs, notably the heart, be utilized in an oxygenated condition, precluding storage or even appreciable delay, and so necessitating early typing and matching of tissues.

Turning from the donation of organs after death to their donation for live transplants, we have to differentiate between paired and unpaired organs.

In the case of paired organs, like kidneys, the law is permissive, where the loss and the risk of further injury to the donor are moderate in relation to the anticipated benefit to the recipient. Indeed, a renal transplant has been authorized by a Massachusetts court even between minors who were twins, despite the rule that a child may not be made the subject of harm unless for his own benefit; the court reasoned, after interviewing the healthy twin, that he would suffer lasting psychic trauma if he were not allowed to contribute an organ to his brother so that they could continue to enjoy the blessings of life together.

From the ground of permitting the donation of a paired organ to save a life, should the law move to the position of requiring such contributions, through a process of random selection? In Kantian terms, would we will a universal rule imposing an obligation on others to save us, and in return accept an obligation to save others in the same way? Compulsory vaccination is of course a different matter, since an unvaccinated person may be a positive menace. The law has hesitated to equate a duty to come to the aid of another with a duty to refrain from doing harm. Why should this reluctance persist? Three possible reasons can be suggested. First, there is a practical calculus. Compulsory giving may range along a spectrum from taxation to enforced martyrdom. There is an intuitively felt difference between the taking of one's substance and of one's selfhood. In a situation of catastrophe one can imagine a conscription of blood, which is self-replenishing, more readily than a conscription of organs. The disproportion between risk to the donor and expected benefit to the donee would have to be greater and surer to warrant compulsion than to support a voluntary sacrifice; otherwise we might be in the position of the traveler in the desert, carrying a canister of water sufficient for one person, who is obliged to share it with another and thereby causes two deaths. Secondly, there would be practical problems of selection among all possible donors, since randomness is not a self-defining concept. And finally, enforced giving would diminish the moral quality of the act, though this consideration would be less relevant if scope were also left for voluntary donations. . . .

There is one further question that ought to be raised in connection with the selection of donors: should a person be encouraged or permitted to sell his organs for purposes of transplant? In the case of donations of blood, where the risk to the donor is negligible, the question is relatively unimportant. We would not object on moral grounds to paying someone to stand in line for us at a ticket counter, though we would have the most serious moral qualms about paying for someone to take our place in a conscript army.[3] To save oneself by putting another in mortal danger through trading on his poverty strikes one as an immoral bargain. Is the case different if the bargain is struck not by the more affluent beneficiary but more impersonally by the state or a philanthropic institution? The question is analogous to that raised by a so-called volunteer army, using the inducement of higher pay for service, and the answer is equally debatable. The Uniform

Anatomical Gift Act takes no position on the issue, leaving it to state law, although it can be said that the acceptability of compensation is strongest where the donation is to be made after death. In the case of an *inter vivos* transplant of serious nature, the allowance of a pecuniary motive is repugnant, as if society has a vested interest in maintaining an impoverished class of citizens to serve as risk-takers for others. If the need for organs is felt to be crucial, and if both payment and conscription are ruled out, a possibility remains of liberalizing the law concerning bodies at death, by enacting that postmortem removal of organs may be effected unless the decedent or next of kin have affirmatively interposed an objection.[4] This is a step whose consideration ought to await evidence on the adequacy of the Uniform Act.

It is time to turn from the selection of donors to that of donees. Few decisions can be as harrowing as the choice of who shall live and who shall die, as any judge or governor can attest; and yet in those cases the law is dealing with persons whose guilt, at least in a legal sense, has been found, and where there is no constraint on sparing the lives of all. In our problem we are dealing with the constraints of scarcity and the consequent necessity of preferences for secular salvation and doom of innocent persons.

In 1943, when penicillin was in short supply for our forces in North Africa, two groups of soldiers could have benefited from its use: those who had contracted venereal disease, and those who suffered from infected battle wounds. The consulting surgeon advised, on moral grounds, that the wounded be given priority, but the medical officer in charge ruled that preference be given to the other group. The latter, he reasoned, could be restored to active duty more quickly, and immediate manpower was needed; moreover, if untreated they could be a threat to others. For good or ill, life's values are seldom so one-dimensional as they are on the front lines in wartime. Nevertheless efforts have been made to assess the comparative worth of patients to society in the rationing of scarce medical resources, notably renal dialysis equipment. At the center in Seattle, after a medical and psychiatric screening to identify those patients who could benefit substantially from the treatment, they are evaluated by an anonymous but predominantly lay committee, operating under no more definite criteria than social worth, which in practice has been judged by such factors as the number and need of dependents and civic service performed, such as scout leadership, religious-social teaching, and Red Cross activities.[5] One less confident that one's middle-class values represent eternal verities or even the clear hope of the future might well find it impossible to serve on such a committee. More pointedly, where the facilities are operated by a public agency there is a real question whether some more articulated and warrantable standards must be formulated to satisfy the demands of the constitutional guarantees of due process of law and equal protection of the laws.[6] When mortals are called on to make ultimate choice for life or death among their innocent fellows, the only tolerable criterion may be equality of worth as a human being. Translated into practical terms this means a procedure for selection based on randomness within a group, or on objective factors like age or priority of application.

Scarcity of resources presents not only a problem of selection of donors and donees but of allocation of medical facilities and personnel between transplant and other undertakings. At a large teaching hospital in Boston the decision was made not to engage in heart transplant surgery at the present time. To have done so would have required a material inroad on the program of open-heart surgery, where the operative results have been favorable in eighty to ninety per cent of the cases. Meanwhile basic work on the biological aspects of transplantation continued. Not every institution that has undertaken heart transplants, it can be said, was ideally suited for the mission. Should the decision to engage or not to engage in this form of surgery be left to the individual institution, or should not an effort be made to ration this enterprise in order to achieve a minimum of dislocation and a maximum of scientific progress in the experimental stage of a promising therapeutic procedure?

The upshot of our whole discussion is that the choices enforced by a scarcity of resources, and the awesome moral questions raised by deliberate programs to increase the number of donors of viable organs, point to a search for a solution that would by-pass these issues, so uncomfortable for human decision. It may not be thought an evasion, one hopes, to suggest that what is urgently needed is a program for the development of artificial organs, like teeth and limbs, to supersede the transplant of natural organs. The physical obstacles are admittedly formidable: how, for example, to provide a lasting and safe power supply for an implanted mechanical heart, and how to overcome the problem of clotting presented by a large foreign surface at the site of the heart. Yet the eventuality of biologists and engineers supplanting moralists and lawyers in the collaborative quest for bodily renewal is a consummation devoutly to be wished.

Notes

1. D. Daube, "Limitations on Self-Sacrifice in Jewish Law and Tradition," *Theology* 72 (1969): pp. 291, 299; Carroll, "The Ethics of Transplantation," *Amer. Bar Assn. Jour.* **56** (1970): pp. 137,

138. (The Chief Rabbi of Israel hailed the first heart transplant in that country; the rabbinate, at the same time, asserted that post-mortem operations are prohibited by the Torah.)
2. ". . . in the light of current medical advances . . . existing 'anatomical' statutes, such as [the law providing for surrender of unclaimed bodies for the advance of medical science] are inadequate, and the need for appropriate statutory provision to implement the desires of the dying to aid the living is increasingly urgent." *Holland v. Metalious,* 105 N.H. 290, 293, 198 Atl. 2d 654, 656 (1964).
3. Nevertheless it is to be recalled that in our early history it was customary to condition the exemption of conscientious objectors from military service on their providing a substitute or the money necessary to engage one. See J. Cardozo, in *Hamilton v. Regents,* 293 U.S. 245, 266–277 (1934).
4. D. Sanders and J. Dukeminier, "Medical Advance and Legal Lag: Hemodialysis and Kidney Transplantation," *U.C.L.A. Law Rev.* **15** (1968): pp. 357, 410–413.
5. *Idem* at pp. 366–380.
6. See Note, "Patient Selection for Artificial and Transplant Organs," *Harv. Law Rev.* **82** (1969): pp. 1322, 1331–1337.

Who Shall Live
When Not All Can Live?

James F. Childress

Who shall live when not all can live? Although this question has been urgently forced upon us by the dramatic use of artificial internal organs and organ transplantations, it is hardly new. George Bernard Shaw dealt with it in "The Doctor's Dilemma":

SIR PATRICK: Well, Mr. Savior of Lives: which is it to be? that honest decent man Blenkinsop, or that rotten blackguard of an artist, eh?

Reprinted with permission from the author and *Soundings: An Interdisciplinary Journal,* vol. 53, No. 4, Winter 1970, pp. 339–355.

RIDGEON: It's not an easy case to judge, is it? Blenkinsop's an honest decent man; but is he any use? Dubedat's a rotten blackguard; but he's a genuine source of pretty and pleasant and good things.

SIR PATRICK: What will he be a source of for that poor innocent wife of his, when she finds him out?

RIDGEON: That's true. Her life will be a hell.

SIR PATRICK: And tell me this. Suppose you had this choice put before you: either to go through life and find all the pictures bad but all the men and women good, or go through life and find all the pictures good and all the men and women rotten. Which would you choose?[1]

A significant example of the distribution of scarce medical resources is seen in the use of penicillin shortly after its discovery. Military officers had to determine which soldiers would be treated—those with venereal disease or those wounded in combat.[2] In many respects such decisions have become routine in medical circles. Day after day physicians and others make judgments and decisions "about allocations of medical care to various segments of our population, to various types of hospitalized patients, and to specific individuals,"[3] for example, whether mental illness or cancer will receive the higher proportion of available funds. Nevertheless, the dramatic forms of "Scarce Life-Saving Medical Resources" (hereafter abbreviated as SLMR) such as hemodialysis and kidney and heart transplants have compelled us to examine the moral questions that have been concealed in many routine decisions. I do not attempt in this paper to show how a resolution of SLMR cases can help us in the more routine ones which do not involve a conflict of life with life. Rather I develop an argument for a particular method of determining who shall live when not all can live. No conclusions are implied about criteria and procedures for determining who shall receive medical resources that are not directly related to the preservation of life (e.g. corneal transplants) or about standards for allocating money and time for studying and treating certain diseases.

Just as current SLMR decisions are not totally discontinuous with other medical decisions, so we must ask whether some other cases might, at least by analogy, help us develop the needed criteria and procedures. Some have looked at the principles at work in our responses to abortion, euthanasia, and artificial insemination.[4] Usually they have concluded that these cases do not cast light on the selection of patients for artificial and transplanted organs. The reason is evident: in abortion, euthanasia, and artificial insemination, there is no conflict of life with life for limited but indispensable resources (with the possible exception of thera-

peutic abortion). In current SLMR decisions, such a conflict is inescapable, and it makes them so morally perplexing and fascinating. If analogous cases are to be found, I think that we shall locate them in moral conflict situations.

ANALOGOUS CONFLICT SITUATIONS

An especially interesting and pertinent one is *U.S. v. Holmes.*[5] In 1841 an American ship, the *William Brown,* which was near Newfoundland on a trip from Liverpool to Philadelphia, struck an iceberg. The crew and half the passengers were able to escape in the two available vessels. One of these, a longboat, carrying too many passengers and leaking seriously, began to founder in the turbulent sea after about twenty-four hours. In a desperate attempt to keep it from sinking, the crew threw overboard fourteen men. Two sisters of one of the men either jumped overboard to join their brother in death or instructed the crew to throw them over. The criteria for determining who should live were "not to part man and wife, and not to throw over any women." Several hours later the others were rescued. Returning to Philadelphia, most of the crew disappeared, but one, Holmes, who had acted upon orders from the mate, was indicted, tried, and convicted on the charge of "unlawful homicide."

We are interested in this case from a moral rather than a legal standpoint, and there are several possible responses to and judgments about it. Without attempting to be exhaustive I shall sketch a few of these. The judge contended that lots should have been cast, for in such conflict situations, there is no other procedure "so consonant both to humanity and to justice." Counsel for Holmes, on the other hand, maintained that the "sailors adopted the only principle of selection which was possible in an emergency like theirs,—a principle more humane than lots."

Another version of selection might extend and systematize the maxims of the sailors in the direction of "utility"; those are saved who will contribute to the greatest good for the greatest number. Yet another possible option is defended by Edmond Cahn in *The Moral Decision.*

He argues that in this case we encounter the ''morals of the last days.'' By this phrase he indicates that an apocalyptic crisis renders totally irrelevant the normal differences between individuals. He continues,

> In a strait of this extremity, all men are reduced—or raised, as one may choose to denominate it—to members of the genus, mere congeners and nothing else. Truly and literally, all were ''in the same boat,'' and thus none could be saved separately from the others. I am driven to conclude that otherwise—that is, if none sacrifice themselves of free will to spare the others—they must all wait and die together. For where all have become congeners, pure and simple, no one can save himself by killing another.[6]

Cahn's answer to the question ''who shall live when not all can live'' is ''none'' unless the voluntary sacrifice by some persons permits it.

Few would deny the importance of Cahn's approach although many, including this writer, would suggest that it is relevant mainly as an affirmation of an elevated and, indeed, heroic or saintly morality which one hopes would find expression in the voluntary actions of many persons trapped in ''borderline'' situations involving a conflict of life with life. It is a maximal demand which some moral principles impose on the individual in the recognition that self-preservation is not a good which is to be defended at all costs. The absence of this saintly or heroic morality should not mean, however, that everyone perishes. Without making survival an absolute value and without justifying all means to achieve it, we can maintain that simply letting everyone die is irresponsible. This charge can be supported from several different standpoints, including society at large as well as the individuals involved. Among a group of self-interested individuals, none of whom volunteers to relinquish his life, there may be better and worse ways of determining who shall survive. One task of social ethics, whether religious or philosophical, is to propose relatively just institutional arrangements within which self-interested and biased men can live. The question then becomes: which set of arrangements—which criteria and procedures of selection—is most satisfactory in view of the human condition (man's limited altruism and inclination to seek his own good) and the conflicting values that are to be realized?

There are several significant differences between the *Holmes* and SLMR cases, a major one being that the former involves *direct* killing of another person, while the latter involve only *permitting* a person to die when it is not possible to save all. Furthermore, in extreme situations such as *Holmes,* the restraints of civilization have been stripped away, and something approximating a state of nature prevails, in which life is ''solitary, poor, nasty, bruitish and short.'' The state of nature does not mean that moral standards are irrelevant and that might should prevail, but it does suggest that much of the matrix which normally supports morality has been removed. Also, the necessary but unfortunate decisions about who shall live and die are made by men who are existentially and personally involved in the outcome. Their survival too is at stake. Even though the institutional role of sailors seems to require greater sacrificial actions, there is obviously no assurance that they will adequately assess the number of sailors required to man the vessel or that they will impartially and objectively weigh the common good at stake. As the judge insisted in his defense of casting lots in the *Holmes* case: ''In no other than this [casting lots] or some like way are those having equal rights put upon an equal footing, and in no other way is it possible to guard against partiality and oppression, violence, and conflict.'' This difference should not be exaggerated since self-interest, professional pride, and the like obviously affect the outcome of many medical decisions. Nor do the remaining differences cancel *Holmes'* instructiveness.

CRITERIA OF SELECTION FOR SLMR

Which set of arrangements should be adopted for SLMR? Two questions are involved: Which standards and criteria should be used? and, Who should make the decision? The first question is basic, since the debate about implementation, e.g. whether by a lay committee or physician, makes little progress until the criteria are determined.

We need two sets of criteria which will be applied at two different stages in the selection of recipients of SLMR. First, medical criteria should be used to exclude those who are not "medically acceptable." Second, from this group of "medically acceptable" applicants, the final selection can be made. Occasionally in current American medical practice, the first stage is omitted, but such an omission is unwarranted. Ethical and social responsibility would seem to require distributing these SLMR only to those who have some reasonable prospect of responding to the treatment. Furthermore, in transplants such medical tests as tissue and blood typing are necessary, although they are hardly fully developed.

"Medical acceptability" is not as easily determined as many non-physicians assume since there is considerable debate in medical circles about the relevant factors (e.g., age and complicating diseases). Although ethicists can contribute little or nothing to this debate, two proposals may be in order. First, "medical acceptability" should be used only to determine the group from which the final selection will be made, and the attempt to establish fine degrees of prospective response to treatment should be avoided. Medical criteria, then, would exclude some applicants but would not serve as a basis of comparison between those who pass the first stage. For example, if two applicants for dialysis were medically acceptable, the physicians would *not* choose the one with the *better* medical prospects. Final selection would be made on other grounds. Second, psychological and environmental factors should be kept to an absolute minimum and should be considered only when they are without doubt critically related to medical acceptability (e.g., the inability to cope with the requirements of dialysis which might lead to suicide).*

The most significant moral questions emerge when we turn to the final selection.

*For a discussion of the higher suicide rate among dialysis patients than among the general population and an interpretation of some of the factors at work, see H.S. Abram, G.I., Moore, and F.B. Westervelt, "Suicidal Behavior in Chronic Dialysis Patients," *American Journal of Psychiatry* (in press). This study shows that even "if one does not include death through not following the regimen the incidence of suicide is still more than 100 times the normal population."

Once the pool of medically acceptable applicants has been defined and still the number is larger than the resources, what other criteria should be used? How should the final selection be made? First, I shall examine some of the difficulties that stem from efforts to make the final selection in terms of social value; these difficulties raise serious doubts about the feasibility and justifiability of the utilitarian approach. Then I shall consider the possible justification for random selection or chance.

Occasionally criteria of social worth focus on past contributions but most often they are primarily future-oriented. The patient's potential and probable contribution to the society is stressed, although this obviously cannot be abstracted from his present web of relationships (e.g., dependents) and occupational activities (e.g., nuclear physicist). Indeed, the magnitude of his contribution to society (as an abstraction) is measured in terms of these social roles, relations, and functions. Enough has already been said to suggest the tremendous range of factors that affect social value or worth.† Here we encounter the first major difficulty of this approach: How do we determine the relevant criteria of social value?

The difficulties of quantifying various social needs are only too obvious. How does one quantify and compare the needs of the spirit (e.g., education, art, religion), political life, economic activity, technological development? Joseph Fletcher suggests that "some day we may learn how to 'quantify' or 'mathematicate' or 'computerize' the value problem in selection, in the same careful and thorough way that diagnosis has been."[7] I am not convinced that we can ever quantify values, or that we should attempt to do so. But even if the various social and human needs, in principle, could be quantified, how do we determine how much weight we will give to each one? Which will have priority in case of conflict? Or even more basically, in the light of which values and principles do we recognize social "needs"?

One possible way of determining the values

† I am excluding from consideration the question of the ability to pay because most of the people involved have to secure funds from other sources, public or private, anyway.

which should be emphasized in selection has been proposed by Leo Shatin.[8] He insists that our medical decisions about allocating resources are already based on an unconscious scale of values (usually dominated by material worth). Since there is really no way of escaping this, we should be self-conscious and critical about it. How should we proceed? He recommends that we discover the values that most people in our society hold and then use them as criteria for distributing SLMR. These values can be discovered by attitude or opinion surveys. Presumably if fifty-one percent in this testing period put a greater premium on military needs than technological development, military men would have a greater claim on our SLMR than experimental researchers. But valuations of what is significant change, and the student revolutionary who was denied SLMR in 1970 might be celebrated in 1990 as the greatest American hero since George Washington.

Shatin presumably is seeking criteria that could be applied nationally, but at the present, regional and local as well as individual prejudices tincture the criteria of social value that are used in selection. Nowhere is this more evident than in the deliberations and decisions of the anonymous selection committee of the Seattle Artificial Kidney Center where such factors as church membership and Scout leadership have been deemed significant for determining who shall live.[9] As two critics conclude after examining these criteria and procedures, they rule out "creative nonconformists, who rub the bourgeoisie the wrong way but who historically have contributed so much to the making of America. The Pacific Northwest is no place for a Henry David Thoreau with bad kidneys."[10]

Closely connected to this first problem of determining social values is a second one. Not only is it difficult if not impossible to reach agreement on social values, but it is also rarely easy to predict what our needs will be in a few years and what the consequences of present actions will be. Furthermore it is difficult to predict which persons will fulfill their potential function in society. Admissions committees in colleges and universities experience the frustrations of predicting realization of potential. For

these reasons, as someone has indicated, God might be a utilitarian, but we cannot be. We simply lack the capacity to predict very accurately the consequences which we then must evaluate. Our incapacity is never more evident than when we think in societal terms.

Other difficulties make us even less confident that such an approach to SLMR is advisable. Many critics raise the spectre of abuse, but this should not be overemphasized. The fundamental difficulty appears on another level: the utilitarian approach would in effect reduce the person to his social role, relations, and functions. Ultimately it dulls and perhaps even eliminates the sense of the person's transcendence, his dignity as a person which cannot be reduced to his past or future contribution to society. It is not at all clear that we are willing to live with these implications of utilitarian selection. Wilhelm Kolff, who invented the artificial kidney, has asked: "Do we really subscribe to the principle that social standing should determine selection? Do we allow patients to be treated with dialysis only when they are married, go to church, have children, have a job, a good income and give to the Community Chest?"[*]

The German theologian Helmut Thielicke contends that any search for "objective criteria" for selection is already a capitulation to the utilitarian point of view which violates man's dignity.[11] The solution is not to let all die, but to recognize that SLMR cases are "borderline situations" which inevitably involve guilt. The agent, however, can have courage and freedom (which, for Thielicke, come from justification by faith) and can

---

[*] "Letters and Comments," *Annals of Internal Medicine*, 61 (Aug. 1964), 360. Dr. G. E. Schreiner contends that "if you really believe in the right of society to make decisions on medical availability on these criteria you should be logical and say that when a man stops going to church or is divorced or loses his job, he ought to be removed from the programme and somebody else who fulfills these criteria substituted. Obviously no one faces up to this logical consequence" (G.E.W. Wolstenholme and Maeve O'Connor, eds. *Ethics in Medical Progress: With Special Reference to Transplantation*, A Ciba Foundation Symposium [Boston, 1966], p. 127).

go ahead anyway and seek for criteria for deciding the question of life or death in the matter of the artificial kidney. Since these criteria are . . . questionable, necessarily alien to the meaning of human existence, the decision to which they lead can be little more than that arrived at by casting lots.[12]

The resulting criteria, he suggests, will probably be very similar to those already employed in American medical practice.

He is most concerned to preserve a certain *attitude* or *disposition* in SLMR—the sense of guilt which arises when man's dignity is violated. With this sense of guilt, the agent remains "sound and healthy where it really counts."[13] Thielicke uses man's dignity only as a judgmental, critical, and negative standard. It only tells us how all selection criteria and procedures (and even the refusal to act) implicate us in the ambiguity of the human condition and its metaphysical guilt. This approach is consistent with his view of the task of theological ethics: "to teach us how to understand and endure—not 'solve'—the borderline situation.[14] But ethics, I would contend, can help us discern the factors and norms in whose light relative, discriminate judgments can be made. Even if all actions in SLMR should involve guilt, some may preserve human dignity to a greater extent than others. Thielicke recognizes that a decision based on any criteria is "little more than that arrived at by casting lots." But perhaps selection by chance would come the closest to embodying the moral and nonmoral values that we are trying to maintain (including a sense of man's dignity).

THE VALUES OF RANDOM SELECTION

My proposal is that we use some form of randomness or chance (either natural, such as "first come, first served," or artificial, such as a lottery) to determine who shall be saved. Many reject randomness as a surrender to non-rationality when responsible and rational judgments can and must be made. Edmond Cahn criticizes "Holmes' judge" who recommended

the casting of lots because, as Cahn puts it, "the crisis involves stakes too high for gambling and responsibilities too deep for destiny."[15] Similarly, other critics see randomness as a surrender to "non-human" forces which necessarily vitiates human values. Sometimes these values are identified with the process of decision-making (e.g., it is important to have persons rather than impersonal forces determining who shall live). Sometimes they are identified with the outcome of the process (e.g., the features such as creativity and fullness of being which make human life what it is are to be considered and respected in the decision). Regarding the former, it must be admitted that the use of chance seems cold and impersonal. But presumably the defenders of utilitarian criteria in SLMR want to make their application as objective and impersonal as possible so that subjective bias does not determine who shall live.

Such criticisms, however, ignore the moral and nonmoral values which might be supported by selection by randomness or chance. A more important criticism is that the procedure that I develop draws the relevant moral context too narrowly. That context, so the argument might run, includes the society and its future and not merely the individual with his illness and claim upon SLMR. But my contention is that the values and principles at work in the narrower context may well take precedence over those operative in the broader context both because of their weight and significance and because of the weaknesses of selection in terms of social worth. As Paul Freund rightly insists, "The more nearly total is the estimate to be made of an individual, and the more nearly the consequence determines life and death, the more unfit the judgment becomes for human reckoning . . . . Randomness as a moral principle deserves serious study."[16] Serious study would, I think, point toward its implementation in certain conflict situations, primarily because it preserves a significant degree of *personal dignity* by providing *equality* of opportunity. Thus it cannot be dismissed as a "non-rational" and "non-human" procedure without an inquiry into the reasons, including human values, which might justify it. Paul Ramsey stresses this point about the *Holmes* case:

Instead of fixing our attention upon "gambling" as the solution—with all the frivolous and often corrupt associations the word raises in our minds—we should think rather of *equality* of opportunity as the ethical substance of the relations of those individuals to one another that might have been guarded and expressed by casting lots.[17]

The individual's personal and transcendent dignity, which on the utilitarian approach would be submerged in his social role and function, can be protected and witnessed to by a recognition of his equal right to be saved. Such a right is best preserved by procedures which establish equality of opportunity. Thus selection by chance more closely approximates the requirements established by human dignity than does utilitarian calculation. It is not infallibly just, but it is preferable to the alternatives of letting all die or saving only those who have the greatest social responsibilities and potential contribution.

This argument can be extended by examining values other than individual dignity and equality of opportunity. Another basic value in the medical sphere is the relationship of trust between physician and patient. Which selection criteria are most in accord with this relationship of trust? Which will maintain, extend, and deepen it? My contention is that selection by randomness or chance is preferable from this standpoint too.

Trust, which is inextricably bound to respect for human dignity, is an attitude of expectation about another. It is not simply the expectation that another will perform a particular act, but more specifically that another will act toward him in certain ways—which will respect him as a person. As Charles Fried writes:

Although trust has to do with reliance on a disposition of another person, it is reliance on a disposition of a special sort: the disposition to act morally, to deal fairly with others, to live up to one's undertakings, and so on. Thus to trust another is first of all to expect him to accept the principle of morality in his dealings with you, to respect your status as a person, your personality.[18]

This trust cannot be preserved in life-and-death situations when a person expects deci-

sions about him to be made in terms of his social worth, for such decisions violate his status as a person. An applicant rejected on grounds of inadequacy in social value or virtue would have reason for feeling that his "trust" had been betrayed. Indeed, the sense that one is being viewed not as an end in himself but as a means in medical progress or the achievement of a greater social good is incompatible with attitudes and relationships of trust. We recognize this in the billboard which was erected after the first heart transplants: "Drive Carefully. Christiaan Barnard Is Watching You." The relationship of trust between the physician and patient is not only an instrumental value in the sense of being an important factor in the patient's treatment. It is also to be endorsed because of its intrinsic worth as a relationship.

Thus the related values of individual dignity and trust are best maintained in selection by chance. But other factors also buttress the argument for this approach. Which criteria and procedures would men agree upon? We have to suppose a hypothetical situation in which several men are going to determine for themselves and their families the criteria and procedures by which they would want to be admitted to and excluded from SLMR if the need arose.* We need to assume two restrictions and then ask which set of criteria and procedures would be chosen as the most rational and, indeed, the fairest. The restrictions are these: (1) The men are *self-interested*. They are interested in their own welfare (and that of members of their families), and this, of course, includes survival. Basically, they are not motivated by altruism. (2) Furthermore, they are *ignorant* of their own talents, abilities, potential, and probable contribution to the social good. They do not know

*My argument is greatly dependent on John Rawls's version of justice as fairness, which is a reinterpretation of social contract theory. Rawls, however, would probably not apply his ideas to "borderline situations." See "Distributive Justice: Some Addenda," *Natural Law Forum*, 13 (1968), 53. For Rawls's general theory, see "Justice as Fairness," *Philosophy, Politics and Society* (Second Series), ed. by Peter Laslett and W.G. Runciman (Oxford, 1962), pp. 132–157 and his other essays on aspects of this topic.

how they would fare in a competitive situation, e.g., the competition for SLMR in terms of social contribution. Under these conditions which institution would be chosen—letting all die, utilitarian selection, or the use of chance? which would seem the most rational? the fairest? By which set of criteria would they want to be included in or excluded from the list of those who will be saved? The rational choice in this setting (assuming self-interest and ignorance of one's competitive success) would be random selection or chance since this alone provides equality of opportunity. A possible response is that one would prefer to take a "risk" and therefore choose the utilitarian approach. But I think not, especially since I added that the participants in this hypothetical situation are choosing for their children as well as for themselves; random selection or chance could be more easily justified to the children. It would make more sense for men who are self-interested but uncertain about their relative contribution to society to elect a set of criteria which would build in equality of oppurtunity. They would consider selection by chance as relatively just and fair.*

An important psychological point supplements earlier arguments for using chance or random selection. The psychological stress and strain among those who are rejected would be greater if the rejection is based on insufficient social worth than if it is based on chance. Obviously stress and strain cannot be eliminated in these borderline situations, but they would almost certainly be increased by the opprobrium of being judged relatively "unfit" by society's agents using society's values. Nicholas Rescher makes this point very effectively:

* Occasionally someone contends that random selection may reward vice. Leo Shatin (op. cit., p. 100) insists that random selection "would reward socially disvalued qualities by giving their bearers the same special medical care opportunities as those received by the bearers of socially valued qualities. Personally I do not favor such a method." Obviously society must engender certain qualities in its members, but not all of its institutions must be devoted to that purpose. Furthermore, there are strong reasons, I have contended, for exempting SLMR from that sort of function.

a recourse to chance would doubtless make matters easier for the rejected patient and those who have a specific interest in him. It would surely be quite hard for them to accept his exclusion by relatively mechanical application of objective criteria in whose implementation subjective judgment is involved. But the circumstances of life have conditioned us to accept the workings of chance and to tolerate the element of luck (good or bad): human life is an inherently contingent process. Nobody, after all, has an absolute right to ELT [Exotic Lifesaving Therapy]—but most of us would feel that we have "every bit as much right" to it as anyone else in significantly similar circumstances.†

Although it is seldom recognized as such, selection by chance is already in operation in practically every dialysis unit. I am not aware of any unit which removes some of its patients from kidney machines in order to make room for later applicants who are better qualified in terms of social worth. Furthermore, very few people would recommend it. Indeed, few would even consider removing a person from a kidney machine on the grounds that a person better qualified *medically* had just applied. In a discussion of the treatment of chronic renal failure by dialysis at the University of Virginia Hospital Renal Unit from November 15, 1965 to November 15, 1966, Dr. Harry Abram writes: "Thirteen patients sought treatment but were not considered because the program had reached its limit of nine patients."[19] Thus, in practice and theory, natural chance is accepted at least within certain limits.

My proposal is that we extend this principle (first come, first served) to determine who among the medically acceptable patients shall live or that we utilize artificial chance such as a lottery or randomness. "First come, first served" would be more feasible than a lottery

† Nicholas Rescher, "The Allocation of Exotic Medical Lifesaving Therapy," *Ethics,* 79 (April 1969), 184. He defends random selection's use only after utilitarian and other judgments have been made. If there are no "major disparaties" in terms of utility, etc., in the second stage of selection, then final selection could be made randomly. He fails to give attention to the moral values that random selection might preserve.

since the applicants make their claims over a period of time rather than as a group at one time. This procedure would be in accord with at least one principle in our present practices and with our sense of individual dignity, trust, and fairness. Its significance in relation to these values can be underlined by asking how the decision can be justified to the rejected applicant. Of course, one easy way of avoiding this task is to maintain the traditional cloak of secrecy, which works to a great extent because patients are often not aware that they are being considered for SLMR in addition to the usual treatment. But whether public justification is instituted or not is not the significant question; it is rather what reasons for rejection would be most acceptable to the unsuccessful applicant. My contention is that rejection can be accepted more readily if equality of opportunity, fairness, and trust are preserved, and that they are best preserved by selection by randomness or chance.

This proposal has yet another advantage since it would eliminate the need for a committee to examine applicants in terms of their social value. This onerous responsibility can be avoided.

Finally, there is a possible indirect consequence of widespread use of random selection which is interesting to ponder, although I do *not* adduce it as a good reason for adopting random selection. It can be argued, as Professor Mason Willrich of the University of Virginia Law School has suggested, that SLMR cases would practically disappear if these scarce resources were distributed randomly rather than on social worth grounds. Scarcity would no longer be a problem because the holders of economic and political power would make certain that they would not be excluded by a random selection procedure; hence they would help to redirect public priorities or establish private funding so that life-saving medical treatment would be widely and perhaps universally available.

In the framework that I have delineated, are the decrees of chance to be taken without exception? If we recognize exceptions, would we not open Pandora's box again just after we had succeeded in getting it closed? The direction of my argument has been against any exceptions, and I would defend this as the proper way to go. But

let me indicate one possible way of admitting exceptions while at the same time circumscribing them so narrowly that they would be very rare indeed.

An obvious advantage of the utilitarian approach is that occasionally circumstances arise which make it necessary to say that one man is practically indispensable for a society in view of a particular set of problems it faces (e.g., the President when the nation is waging a war for survival). Certainly the argument to this point has stressed that the burden of proof would fall on those who think that the social danger in this instance is so great that they simply cannot abide by the outcome of a lottery or a first come, first served policy. Also, the reason must be negative rather than positive; that is, we depart from chance in this instance not because we want to take advantage of this person's potential contribution to the improvement of our society, but because his immediate loss would possibly (even probably) be disastrous (again, the President in a grave national emergency). Finally, social value (in the negative sense) should be used as a standard of exception in dialysis, for example, only if it would provide a reason strong enough to warrant removing another person from a kidney machine if all machines were taken. Assuming this strong reluctance to remove anyone once the commitment has been made to him, we would be willing to put this patient ahead of another applicant for a vacant machine only if we would be willing (in circumstances in which all machines are being used) to vacate a machine by removing someone from it. These restrictions would make an exception almost impossible.

While I do not recommend this procedure of recognizing exceptions I think that one can defend it while accepting my general thesis about selection by randomness or chance. If it is used, a lay committee (perhaps advisory, perhaps even stronger) would be called upon to deal with the alleged exceptions since the doctors or others would in effect be appealing the outcome of chance (either natural or artificial). This lay committee would determine whether this patient was so indispensable at this time and place that he had to be saved even by sacrificing the values preserved by random selection. It would make it quite clear that exception is warranted, if at all, only as the "lesser of two evils." Such a defense would be recognized only rarely, if ever, primarily because chance and randomness preserve so many important moral and nonmoral values in SLMR cases.*

Notes

1. George Bernard Shaw, *The Doctor's Dilemma* (New York, 1941), pp. 132–133.

2. Henry K. Beecher, "Scarce Resources and Medical Advancement." *Daedalus* (Spring 1969), pp. 279–280.

3. Leo Shatin, "Medical Care and the Social Worth of a Man." *American Journal of Orthopsychiatry,* 36 (1967), 97.

4. Harry S. Abram and Walter Wadlington, "Selection of Patients for Artificial and Transplanted Organs," *Annals of Internal Medicine,* 69 (September 1968), 615–620.

5. *United States v. Holmes* 26 Fed. Cas. 360 (C.C.E.D. Pa. 1842). All references are to the text of the trial as reprinted in Philip E. Davis, ed., *Moral Duty and Legal Responsibility: A Philosophical-Legal Casebook* (New York, 1966), pp. 102–118.

6. *The Moral Decision* (Bloomington, Inc., 1955), p. 71.

7. Joseph Fletcher, "Donor Nephrectomies and Moral Responsibility," *Journal of the American Medical Women's Association,* 23 (Dec. 1968), p. 1090.

8. Leo Shatin, op. cit., pp. 96–101.

9. For a discussion of the Seattle selection committee, see Shana Alexander, "They Decide Who Lives, Who Dies," *Life,* 53 (Nov. 9, 1962), 102. For an examination of general selection practices in dialysis see "Scarce Medical Resources," *Columbia Law Review* 69:620 (1969) and Harry S. Abram and Walter Wadlington, op. cit.

10. David Sanders and Jesse Dukeminier, Jr., "Medical Advance and Legal Lag: Hemodialysis and Kidney Transplantation," *UCLA Law Review* 15:367 (1968) 378.

11. Helmut Thielicke, "The Doctor as Judge of Who Shall Live and Who Shall Die," *Who Shall Live?* ed. by Kenneth Vaux (Philadelphia, 1970), p. 172.

12. Ibid., pp. 173–174.

13. Ibid., p. 173.

14. Thielicke, *Theological Ethics,* Vol. I, *Foundations* (Philadelphia, 1966), p. 602.

15. Cahn, op. cit., p. 71.

16. Paul Freund, "Introduction," *Daedalus* (Spring 1969), xiii.

17. Paul Ramsey, *Nine Modern Moralists* (Englewood Cliffs, N.J., 1962), p. 245.

18. Charles Fried, "Privacy," In *Law, Reason, and Justice,* ed. by Graham Hughes (New York, 1969), p. 52.

19. Harry S. Abram, M.D., "The Psychiatrist, the Treatment of Chronic Renal Failure, and the Prolongation of Life: II" *American Journal of Psychiatry* 126:157–167 (1969), 158.

*I read a draft of this paper in a seminar on "Social Implications of Advances in Biomedical Science and Technology: Artificial and Transplanted Internal Organs," sponsored by the Center for the Study of Science, Technology, and Public Policy of the University of Virginia, Spring 1970. I am indebted to the participants in that seminar, and especially to its leaders, Mason Willrich, Professor of Law, and Dr. Harry Abram, Associate Professor of Psychiatry, for criticisms which helped me to sharpen these ideas. Good discussions of the legal questions raised by selection (e.g., equal protection of the law and due process) which I have not considered can be found in "Scarce Medical Resources," *Columbia Law Review,* 69:620 (1969); "Patient Selection for Artificial and Transplanted Organs," *Harvard Law Review,* 82: 1322 (1969); and Sanders and Dukeminier, op. cit.

Index